Cosmetic Surgery

BASIC AND CLINICAL DERMATOLOGY

Series Editors

ALAN R. SHALITA, M.D.

Distinguished Teaching Professor and Chairman
Department of Dermatology
State University of New York
Health Science Center at Brooklyn
Brooklyn, New York

DAVID A. NORRIS, M.D.

Director of Research
Professor of Dermatology
The University of Colorado
Health Sciences Center
Denver, Colorado

1. Cutaneous Investigation in Health and Disease: Noninvasive Methods and Instrumentation, *edited by Jean-Luc Lévêque*
2. Irritant Contact Dermatitis, *edited by Edward M. Jackson and Ronald Goldner*
3. Fundamentals of Dermatology: A Study Guide, *Franklin S. Glickman and Alan R. Shalita*
4. Aging Skin: Properties and Functional Changes, *edited by Jean-Luc Lévêque and Pierre G. Agache*
5. Retinoids: Progress in Research and Clinical Applications, *edited by Maria A. Livrea and Lester Packer*
6. Clinical Photomedicine, *edited by Henry W. Lim and Nicholas A. Soter*
7. Cutaneous Antifungal Agents: Selected Compounds in Clinical Practice and Development, *edited by John W. Rippon and Robert A. Fromtling*
8. Oxidative Stress in Dermatology, *edited by Jürgen Fuchs and Lester Packer*
9. Connective Tissue Diseases of the Skin, *edited by Charles M. Lapière and Thomas Krieg*
10. Epidermal Growth Factors and Cytokines, *edited by Thomas A. Luger and Thomas Schwarz*
11. Skin Changes and Diseases in Pregnancy, *edited by Marwali Harahap and Robert C. Wallach*
12. Fungal Disease: Biology, Immunology, and Diagnosis, *edited by Paul H. Jacobs and Lexie Nall*
13. Immunomodulatory and Cytotoxic Agents in Dermatology, *edited by Charles J. McDonald*
14. Cutaneous Infection and Therapy, *edited by Raza Aly, Karl R. Beutner, and Howard I. Maibach*
15. Tissue Augmentation in Clinical Practice: Procedures and Techniques, *edited by Arnold William Klein*
16. Psoriasis: Third Edition, Revised and Expanded, *edited by Henry H. Roenigk, Jr., and Howard I. Maibach*
17. Surgical Techniques for Cutaneous Scar Revision, *edited by Marwali Harahap*
18. Drug Therapy in Dermatology, *edited by Larry E. Millikan*
19. Scarless Wound Healing, *edited by Hari G. Garg and Michael T. Longaker*
20. Cosmetic Surgery: An Interdisciplinary Approach, *edited by Rhoda S. Narins*

ADDITIONAL VOLUMES IN PREPARATION

Cosmetic Surgery

An Interdisciplinary Approach

edited by

Rhoda S. Narins

Dermatology Surgery and Laser Center
New York and White Plains
and New York University Medical Center
New York, New York

MARCEL DEKKER, INC. NEW YORK • BASEL

ISBN: 0-8247-0302-2

This book is printed on acid-free paper.

Headquarters
Marcel Dekker, Inc.
270 Madison Avenue, New York, NY 10016
tel: 212-696-9000; fax: 212-685-4540

Eastern Hemisphere Distribution
Marcel Dekker AG
Hutgasse 4, Postfach 812, CH-4001 Basel, Switzerland
tel: 41-61-261-8482; fax: 41-61-261-8896

World Wide Web
http://www.dekker.com

The publisher offers discounts on this book when ordered in bulk quantities. For more information, write to Special Sales/Professional Marketing at the headquarters address above.

Current printing (last digit):
10 9 8 7 6 5 4 3 2 1

PRINTED IN THE UNITED STATES OF AMERICA

To my wonderful staff,
several of whom have been with me for many years.
They make work a pleasure and provide expertise
as well as a warm and caring experience for patients.

Series Introduction

During the past decade there has been a vast explosion in new information relating to the art and science of dermatology as well as fundamental cutaneous biology. Furthermore, this information is no longer of interest only to the small but growing specialty of dermatology. Scientists from a wide variety of disciplines have come to recognize both the importance of skin in fundamental biological processes and the broad implications of understanding the pathogenesis of skin disease. As a result there is now a multidisciplinary and world-wide interest in the progress of dermatology.

With these factors in mind, we have undertaken a new series of books specifically oriented to dermatology. The series will be purposely broad in focus and will range from pure basic science to practical, applied clinical dermatology. Thus, while there will be something for everyone, all editions in the series should ultimately prove to be valuable additions to the dermatologist's library.

Since the inception of this series of books on Basic and Clinical Dermatology, there has been an expanding interest in the field of dermatological surgery, in general, and cosmetic surgery in particular. The current volume: *Cosmetic Surgery: An Interdisciplinary Approach*, edited by Dr. Rhoda Narins, fulfills an obvious need for a broad-based interdisciplinary approach to a subject of great interest and timeliness. I sincerely believe that this volume will be a valuable edition to the libraries of all physicians interested in cosmetic surgery.

Alan R. Shalita, M.D.
Distinguished Teaching Professor & Chairman
Department of Dermatology
SUNY Downstate Medical Center

Preface

Very few substantial cosmetic surgery texts integrate the knowledge of dermatological, maxillofacial, and plastic surgery procedures. There is a growing demand for cosmetic enhancement with heightened media attention on the numerous treatments available. The level of expertise and the number of new treatments have risen dramatically. It is necessary to know and understand all the latest technology and innovative techniques available in order to choose the optimal proecdure for each patient. This book includes chapters by dermatological cosmetic surgeons as well as plastic and oral maxillofacial surgeons from an international faculty, providing a comprehensive perspective and combined expertise to offer each patient the best possible surgical treatment. I would like to gratefully acknowledge all the authors whose hard work has enabled this book to be realized.

This is a how-to manual that will take you step-by-step through surgical procedures and will thoroughly explain every aspect of the surgical techniques. Contributors have been encouraged to make each chapter readable as an independent entity. Pre-op information and instruction sheets, consent forms, and post-op instructions are included. Each chapter discusses the indications and contraindications for the procedure, techniques, and possible innovative results in the future, along with the limitations and potential complications.

This book is designed to be comprehensive in scope and to provide information for the novice as well as the experienced cosmetic surgeon. We hope it will appeal to cosmetic surgeons of many different specialties worldwide. The topics covered range from facelifts, filling substances, laser procedures, and liposuction to consultations and office and OR set-ups as well as handling the dissatisfied patient. The effectiveness of any practicing cosmetic surgeon ultimately depends on making the right choice of treatment. The extensive experience of the authors enables them to give invaluable practical tips about each procedure. After reading this book, the cosmetic surgeon will be able to plan the best combination of treatment and maintenance programs for each patient.

Rhoda S. Narins

Contents

Series Introduction Alan R. Shalita, M.D. *v*
Preface *vii*
Contributors *xiii*

1. Designing the Surgical Suite 1
C. William Hanke and Jenette A. Buening

2. Aesthetic Analysis of the Aging Face 17
Richard G. Glogau

3. Superficial Chemical Peels 27
Seth L. Matarasso and Karyn Grossman

4. Medium and Deep Chemical Peels 37
Gary D. Monheit

5. The Total Body Peel: Peeling the Skin of the Neck, Chest, Hands, and Other Areas 69
Kim K. Cook

6. Peel Complications and Management 79
Harold J. Brody

7. CO_2 Laser Resurfacing 99
Tina S. Alster

8. Erbium Skin Remodeling 123
Cynthia Weinstein

9. The Effective Use of Resurfacing Lasers 163
Stephen O. Kovacs, Arielle N. B. Kauvar, and Roy G. Geronemus

10. Dermabrasion 179
Stephen Mandy

11. Filling Substances: Collagen 193
Arnold William Klein

12. Structural Lipoaugmentation 221
Lisa M. Donofrio

13. Fat Transplantation and Autologous Collagen 241
Kevin S. Pinski

14. Human-Derived Filling Materials for Soft-Tissue Augmentation 267
Tina B. West

15. Gortex 289
Naomi Lawrence

16. New Filling Substances on the Horizon 313
Arnold William Klein

17. Botulinum A. Exotoxin 333
Alastair Carruthers and Jean Carruthers

18. Moles, Cysts, and Lipomas: Surgical Treatment of Cutaneous Cysts 355
Vicki J. Levine

19. Flaps and Grafts 379
David A. Davis and Christopher J. Arpey

20. Topical Anesthetics and Local and Regional Blocks 411
Tri H. Nguyen

21. The Pharmacology of Tumescent Liposuction 443
Jeffrey A. Klein

22. Laser Removal of Vascular Lesions, Scars, Warts, and Poikiloderma 455
Robin Ashinoff

23. Laser Treatment of Pigmented Lesions and Tattoos 489
David J. Goldberg

24. Treatment of Varicose and Telangiectatic Veins: Sclerotherapy, Ambulatory Phlebectomy, and Laser 513
Robert A. Weiss and Margaret A. Weiss

25. Tumescent Liposuction 545
Rhoda S. Narins

26. Liposuction Using General Anesthesia: A Plastic Surgeon's Viewpoint 573
Mehdi N. Adham, Bahman Teimourian, and Michael Chiaramonte

27. The Cook Weekend Alternative to the Facelift™ 641
William R. Cook, Jr.

28. Abdominal Contouring: Liposuction, Abdominal Rectus Plication, and Crescent Tuck Abdominoplasty to Contour the Abdomen 661
Edward B. Lack

29. Multivector Face/Neck/Browlift: An Anatomical and Biomechanical Approach 679
Elliot H. Rose

30. Blepharoplasty 719
Gregg M. Menaker, Ronald L. Moy, and Philina Lamb

31. Cosmetic Upper and Lower Eyelid Blepharoplasty: The Ophthalmologist's Perspective 749
Jean Carruthers and Alastair Carruthers

32. Brow Rejuvenation 771
Alan Matarasso, Ivo Pitanguy, Henrique N. Radwanski, and Giulio Gherardini

33. Combination Cosmetic Procedures 785
William P. Coleman, III

34. Hair Transplantation with Alopecia Reduction 795
Walter P. Unger and Paul C. Cotterill

35. Earlobe Repair, Scar Revision, Actinic Cheilitis, and Other Lip Lesions 847
Nancy Marchell and Yardy Tse

36. Ancillary Aesthetic Dermatologic Treatments and Procedures 871
Zoe Diana Draelos

37. Laser Hair Removal 881
Wendy W. Lou and Arielle N. B. Kauvar

38. Office Photography in Cosmetic Surgery 896
David J. Narins

39. Handling the Dissatisfied or Difficult Patient 911
Timothy Corcoran Flynn and Mark A. Chastain

40. Facial Implants 925
Tracy M. Pfeifer

41. Cosmetic Benefits of Oral and Maxillofacial Surgery 939
Arthur C. Elias

Index *961*

About the Editor *987*

Contributors

Mehdi N. Adham, M.D. University of Oklahoma Health Sciences Center, Oklahoma City, Oklahoma

Tina S. Alster, M.D. Washington Institute of Dermatologic Laser Surgery, and Department of Medicine, Georgetown University, Washington, D.C.

Christopher J. Arpey, M.D. Department of Dermatology, University of Iowa College of Medicine, Iowa City, Iowa

Robin Ashinoff, M.D. Department of Dermatology, New York University, New York, New York

Harold J. Brody, M.D. Department of Dermatology, Emory University School of Medicine, Atlanta, Georgia

Jenette A. Buening, M.D. Laser and Skin Surgery Center of Indiana, Carmel, Indiana

Alastair Carruthers, M.D. University of British Columbia, Vancouver, British Columbia, Canada

Jean Carruthers, M.D. University of British Columbia, Vancouver, British Columbia, Canada

Mark A. Chastain, M.D. Tulane University School of Medicine, New Orleans, Louisiana

Michael Chiaramonte, M.D. University of Maryland, Baltimore, Maryland

William P. Coleman, III, M.D. Department of Dermatology, Tulane University School of Medicine, New Orleans, Louisiana

Kim K. Cook, M.D. Coronado Skin Medical Center, Inc., Coronado, California

William R. Cook, Jr., M.D. Coronado Skin Medical Center, Inc., Coronado, California

Paul C. Cotterill, M.D. Private Practice, Toronto, Ontario, Canada

David A. Davis, M.D. Department of Dermatology, University of Iowa College of Medicine, Iowa City, Iowa

Lisa M. Donofrio, M.D. Department of Dermatology, Yale University School of Medicine, New Haven, Connecticut

Zoe Diana Draelos, M.D. Department of Dermatology, Wake Forest University School of Medicine, Winston-Salem, North Carolina

Arthur C. Elias, D.M.D. Private Practice, New York, New York

Timothy Corcoran Flynn, M.D. Tulane University School of Medicine, New Orleans, Louisiana

Roy G. Geronemus, M.D. Laser and Skin Surgery Center of New York, New York, New York

Giulio Gherardini, M.D., Ph.D. The National Centre for Cosmetic Surgery, Birmingham, United Kingdom

Richard G. Glogau, M.D. Department of Dermatology, University of California at San Francisco, San Francisco, California

David J. Goldberg, M.D. New Jersey Medical School, Newark, New Jersey

Karyn Grossman, M.D. Private Practice, Santa Monica, California

C. William Hanke, M.D. Laser and Skin Surgery Center of Indiana, Carmel, and Indiana University School of Medicine, Indianapolis, Indiana

Arielle N. B. Kauvar, M.D. Laser and Skin Surgery Center of New York, and New York University School of Medicine, New York, New York

Arnold William Klein, M.D. University of California at Los Angeles School of Medicine, Los Angeles, California

Jeffrey A. Klein, M.D. Department of Dermatology, University of California at Irvine, Irvine, California

Stephen O. Kovacs, M.D. Laser and Skin Surgery Center of New York, New York, New York

Edward B. Lack, M.D. The Center for Liposculpture and Cosmetic Surgery, Ltd., Des Plaines, Illinois

Philina Lamb, M.D. Division of Dermatology, VA–West Los Angeles Medical Center, University of California at Los Angeles, Los Angeles, California

Naomi Lawrence, M.D. Department of Dermatologic Surgery, Cooper Health System, Marlton, New Jersey

Vicki J. Levine, M.D. Department of Dermatology, New York University School of Medicine, New York, New York

Wendy W. Lou, M.D. Laser and Skin Surgery Center of New York, New York, New York

Stephen Mandy, M.D. Department of Dermatology, University of Miami, Miami, Florida

Nancy Marchell, M.D. Laguna Hills Dermatology, Inc., Laguna Hills, California

Alan Matarasso, M.D. Albert Einstein College of Medicine, New York, New York

Seth L. Matarasso, M.D. University of California School of Medicine, San Francisco, California

Gregg M. Menaker, M.D. Departmen of Dermatology, Harvard Medical School, Boston, Massachusetts

Gary D. Monheit, M.D. University of Alabama at Birmingham, Birmingham, Alabama

Ronald L. Moy, M.D. Division of Dermatology, VA–West Los Angeles Medical Center, University of California at Los Angeles, Los Angeles, California

David J. Narins, M.D. New York University School of Medicine, New York, New York

Rhoda S. Narins, M.D. Dermatology Surgery and Laser Center, New York and White Plains, and Department of Dermatology, New York University Medical Center, New York, New York

Tri H. Nguyen, M.D. Department of Dermatology, Mayo Clinic Foundation, Rochester, Minnesota

Tracy M. Pfeifer, M.D. Department of Plastic Surgery, Manhattan Eye, Ear and Throat Hospital, New York, New York

Kevin S. Pinski, M.D. Department of Dermatology, Northwestern University Medical School, Chicago, Illinois

Ivo Pitanguy, M.D. Pontifical Catholic University of Rio de Janeiro and Carlos Chagas Institute of Post-Graduate Medical Studies, Rio de Janeiro, Brazil

Henrique N. Radwanski, M.D. Pontifical Catholic University of Rio de Janeiro and Carlos Chagas Institute of Post-Graduate Medical Studies, Rio de Janeiro, Brazil

Elliot H. Rose, M.D. Division of Plastic Surgery, The Mount Sinai/NYU Medical Center, and The Aesthetic Surgery Center, New York, New York

Bahman Teimourian, M.D. Georgetown University Medical Center, Bethesda, Maryland

Edward O. Terino, M.D. Plastic Surgery Institute of Southern California, Thousand Oaks, California

Yardy Tse, M.D. Division of Dermatology, Department of Medicine, University of California at San Diego, San Diego, California

Walter P. Unger, M.D. University of Toronto, Toronto, Ontario, Canada

Cynthia Weinstein, M.D. Laser House, Laser Surgery Institute of Melbourne and Freemason's Hospital, East Melbourne, Victoria, Australia

Margaret A. Weiss, M.D. Johns Hopkins University School of Medicine, Baltimore, Maryland

Robert A. Weiss, M.D. Johns Hopkins University School of Medicine, Baltimore, Maryland

Tina B. West, M.D. Department of Dermatology, The Washington Hospital Center, Washington, D.C.

1

Designing the Surgical Suite

C. William Hanke
Laser and Skin Surgery Center of Indiana, Carmel, Indiana, and Indiana University School of Medicine, Indianapolis, Indiana

Jenette A. Buening
Laser and Skin Surgery Center of Indiana, Carmel, Indiana

FACILITY TYPE

The number of outpatient surgery procedures has surpassed the number of inpatient procedures, and currently makes up 60 to 80% of the surgery market. States have established regulations and accrediting organizations have developed standards in an attempt to assure quality care in the outpatient setting. The California Assembly passed AB 595, which requires regulatory oversight of outpatient surgery facilities that use general anesthesia or intravenous sedation. This California Statute mandates accreditation of office surgical facilities by the Accreditation Association for Ambulatory Health Care (AAAHC), the Joint Commission on Accreditation of Healthcare Organizations (JCAHO), Institute for Medical Quality (IMQ), or the American Accreditation Association for Ambulatory Surgical Facilities (AAAASC); state licensure of an outpatient surgical facility; and Medicare certification of an ambulatory surgery center. Other states have adopted similar policies or are considering them.

Consequently, three key questions must be answered to determine what type of facility to design and develop:

1. What types of surgical procedures do you perform?
2. What types of anesthesia do you require?
3. What regulations regarding office surgery have been implemented in your state?

Ambulatory Surgery Centers

Some physicians prefer to do procedures under local anesthesia in the office, and will use an ambulatory surgery center or hospital operating room when intravenous sedation or general anesthesia is necessary. Many free-standing or hospital-based ambulatory surgery centers will grant privileges to dermatologic surgeons who can document proper training and experience. A minority of dermatologic surgeons have developed their own ambulatory surgery centers as an extension of the office. The cost to develop an office ambulatory surgery center is much higher than that for an office alone. Therefore, a high volume of insurance-reimbursable ambulatory surgery center procedures is required to support the facility. In dermatologic surgery, this usually necessitates a large case load of flaps, grafts, and complex repairs.

Ambulatory surgery centers are highly regulated. Some states require a Certificate of Need (CON) before a new ambulatory surgery center can be built. Some states have a state licensure requirement for ambulatory surgery centers that is distinct from Medicare certification. Currently, AAAHC and other accrediting bodies have "deemed status" which allows them to survey for AAAHC accreditation and Medicare Healthcare Financing Administration (HCFA) certification during a single survey. However, the Medicare survey does not satisfy state licensure requirements and the state will schedule a separate survey for state licensure. As was stated earlier, ambulatory surgery centers are highly regulated.

A Medicare-certified, state-licensed ambulatory surgery center will have a number of very specific design requirements depending on the particular state. A typical list of requirements includes operating rooms as large as 400 sq ft, recovery room(s), soiled utility room, clean utility room, separate waiting room for the ambulatory surgery center, 8-ft wide corridor access to operating rooms, special air filtration requirements, emergency power, emergency cart, special fire protection, and special ceiling and wall coverings. One or more registered nurses are required for staffing. The exact requirements for a particular state can be obtained from the ambulatory care division of the state department of health.

Office Surgical Facilities

It is possible to develop a high-quality office surgical facility (OSF) without the expense of an ambulatory surgical center. Many physicians would use only local anesthesia or light oral or intramuscular sedation in a facility of this type. Other physicians would contract with a Certified Registered Nurse Anesthetist (CRNA) or anesthesiologist to deliver intravenous sedation or general anesthesia. An appropriately sized procedure room for an OSF would be 144 to 256 sq ft. If general anesthesia or intravenous sedation is used, a recovery area should be available. However, we have surveyed OSFs and ambulatory surgery centers where patients were recovered in the operating rooms after the procedure. Full emergency preparedness is necessary, and includes emergency cart and emergency power.

ACCREDITATION BY AAAHC

The AAAHC currently has 1000 ambulatory health care facilities under accreditation. The American Society for Dermatologic Surgery (ASDS) is one of 12 sponsoring healthcare organizations for AAAHC, and has two seats on the AAAHC Board of Directors (Table 1). The ASDS and the other sponsoring healthcare organizations have input into the AAAHC accreditation standards. The standards are under continuous review and revision by the AAAHC Board of Directors. The purpose of AAAHC is delineated in Table 2.

AAAHC accredits many different types of ambulatory healthcare organizations (Table 3). AAAHC Core Standards must be satisfied by all organizations, but Adjunct Standards are applied only when appropriate (Tables 4, 5).

TABLE 1 AAAHC Sponsoring Organizations and Initial Year of Sponsorship

Sponsoring organization	Year of sponsorship
American Academy of Cosmetic Surgery (AACS)	1989
American Academy of Dental Group Practice (AADGP)	1987
American Academy of Facial Plastic and Reconstructive Surgery (AAFPRS)	1983
American Association of Oral and Maxillofacial Surgeons (AAOMS)	1989
American College Health Association (ACHA)	1979
American College of Occupational and Environmental Medicine (ACOEM)	1987
American Society for Dermatologic Surgery (ASDS)	1993
Association of Freestanding Radiation Oncology Centers (AFROC)	1989
Federated Ambulatory Surgery Association (FASA)	1979
Medical Group Management Association (MGMA)	1979
National Association of Community Health Centers (NACHC)	1979
Outpatient Ophthalmic Surgery Society (OOSS)	1982

TABLE 2 Purpose of AAAHC

Conduct a survey and accreditation program that will promote and identify high-quality, cost-effective ambulatory health care programs and services

Establish standards for accreditation of ambulatory health care organizations and services

Recognize compliance with standards by issuance of certificates of accreditation

Conduct programs of education and research that will further the other purposes of the corporation; to publish the results thereof; and to accept grants, gifts, bequests, and devices in support of the purposes of the corporation

Provide programs that will facilitate communication, sharing of expertise, and consultation among ambulatory health care organizations and services

Assume such other responsibilities and conduct such other activities as are compatible with such survey, standard-setting, accreditation, and communication programs

TABLE 3 Types of Ambulatory Health Care Organizations Accredited by AAAHC

Ambulatory health care clinics
Ambulatory surgery centers
Birthing centers
College and university health services
Community health centers
Dental group practices
Diagnostic imaging centers
Endoscopy centers
Health maintenance organizations (HMOs)
Hospital-sponsored ambulatory care clinics and surgery centers
Occupational health services
Office surgery centers and practices
Oral and maxillofacial surgeons' offices
Radiation oncology centers
Single-specialty group practices
Surgical recovery centers
Urgent or immediate care centers

TABLE 4 AAAHC Core Standards

Rights of patients
Governance
Administration
Quality of care provided
Quality management and improvement
Clinical records
Professional improvement
Facilities and environment

TABLE 5 AAAHC Adjunct Standards

Anesthesia services
Surgical services
Overnight care and services
Dental services
Immediate/urgent care services
Pharmaceutical services
Pathology and medical laboratory services
Diagnostic imaging services
Radiation oncology treatment services
Occupational health services
Other professional and technical services
Teaching and publication activities
Research activities

It generally takes a healthcare organization 3 to 6 months to prepare for a AAAHC survey. Some organizations send staff members to AAAHC educational conferences in advance of the survey. The organization fills out a pre-survey questionnaire, which is reviewed by AAAHC staff.* The survey is then scheduled. For a single-physician office practice, the survey is usually performed by a single-physician surveyor over 1.5 days at a cost of approximately $2500.00. The size of the team and cost are greater for larger facilities.

More dermatologic surgery practices are seeking AAAHC accreditation surveys each year. The ASDS has sent a number of its members through AAAHC surveyor training but more volunteers are needed. It is not always possible to match each dermatologic surgery facility requesting a survey with an ASDS/AAAHC surveyor. Consequently, dermatologic surgeons are sometimes surveyed by a physician from another specialty. During the survey the surveyor will review multiple materials, which include:

Accreditation Association for Ambulatory Health Care, Inc., 3201 Old Glenview Rd., Suite 300, Wilmette, IL 60091. Phone: (847) 853-6060, FAX: (847) 853-9028.

1. Governing body and committee minutes
2. Personnel records for physicians, dentists, and other health care practitioners
3. Policies governing physician and staff credentialing
4. Personnel policies for physician and nonphysician staff members
5. Most recent audit, balance sheet, and related financial records
6. Continuing education schedules for physician and nonphysician staff members
7. The most recent statistical reports for pathology, laboratory, radiology, and other technical services
8. Policies and procedures for fire, bomb, and other emergency situations
9. Information reflecting patient satisfaction with services provided
10. Statement of patient rights and responsibilities
11. Any patient handouts and other marketing materials
12. Reports of surveys conducted by Medicare
13. Reports of surveys conducted by state or local fire marshals, state or local health departments, or other code enforcement agencies
14. Reports from companies providing maintenance and calibration of equipment used in providing patient care

The surveyor's purpose is to verify that the organization is doing what it says it is doing in the pre-survey questionnaire. After the survey, the surveyor's report is reviewed by the AAAHC Accreditation Committee. An accreditation decision can be 3-year accreditation, 1-year accreditation, nonaccreditation, or deferral pending another survey (Table 6).

ADMINISTRATION AND STAFFING

Mission Statement

An important element to identify the goals and objectives of an ambulatory surgery practice is a mission statement. The mission statement serves to proactively educate patients and employees. The statement should be shared with new employees during orientation. It has proven beneficial to include the statement as part of the personnel manual that is required reading for all employees. Goals are clearly defined to assure that expectations within the practice are met. The goals should define how the practice strives to maximize the quality of patient care.

TABLE 6 Advantages and Disadvantages of Accreditation

Advantages	Disadvantages
Enhanced quality of care	Increased operating expense
Reduced liability	Increased numbers of personnel
Increased reimbursement	Increased staff time to satisfy documentation
Prestige/marketing advantages	
Satisfies state regulations	

Order of Authority

It is important for all employees to be clear about their position within the organization. A visual outline containing the hierarchy of command should be available for all employees. In a practice where there are 6 to 10 staff members, an administrator oversees the day-to-day activities of the staff. The administrator serves as the liaison between the managers within the practice, and the physician. The managers supervise the employees in their respective job duties. The division of supervisory responsibility is diffused from the physician to the administrator, and from the administrator to the managers. Managers may include Office, Insurance, Nursing, Laboratory, and Clinical Research.

Personnel Manual

Employees have a right to know what is expected of them. It is wise for an organization to implement employee policies that clarify what is acceptable and what is not. In addition to learning what is expected through the code of ethics, employees should become aware of benefits, working hours, holiday schedules, paid time off, insurance plan, and employee rights. A personnel manual should be prepared to document office policy. Each employee should be given a copy of the personnel manual during orientation. It is best to have the employee sign an acknowledgment that they have read the manual. The signed acknowledgment should be kept in the employee's personnel file.

The personnel manual should include the mission statement of the organization; a brief overview of the manual; job classifications, including an explanation of the probationary period; details of the compensation policy, including salary program, paychecks, overtime, and time records; a summary of benefits including paid holidays, paid time off, insurance, retirement, the hierarchy of authority, employees with disabilities, and standards of conduct. The manual should also include a policy on Equal Employment Opportunity and sexual harassment and discrimination.

Job Descriptions

Job descriptions are essential in a well-organized, efficient surgical practice. Clearly defined job descriptions delineate the responsibilities of the employee. Although there may be some degree of cross-training between employees, it is essential that each employee maintain specific job duties. A job description should include an estimate of the time needed for each task, as well as a detailed description of the duties to be performed (see Appendix 1). The job description should also leave space for new responsibilities. This can be accomplished by adding the phrase "other duties assigned as needed" to each employee's job description. The employee should be presented with the job description during orientation. It is the responsibility of the employee's supervisor to clarify all duties and responsibilities. Job descriptions serve as an outline for employee evaluations, which may directly affect bonuses or probationary action.

Personnel Files

Personnel files are important for the development of employees and the practice. Personnel files should contain documentation of job experience, education, and licensure. Orientation paperwork containing social security number and tax forms should be included. Documentation of met OSHA requirements, including Hepatitis-B vaccination, annual TB test results, and annual bloodborne pathogen, hazardous communication, and fire safety training should be included in the file, as well as CPR certification cards. Employee performance evaluation forms should be kept in the file along with continuing education activities. All personnel files should be confidential. Personnel files may be separated into payroll/non-payroll files. The pay roll files should contain employee time cards (if needed), insurance application, salary documentation, and tax forms including social security number and current address. All other forms should be kept in the non-payroll personnel file. Files should be updated regularly, especially with regard to continuing education and safety training. Personnel files should be retained for 5 years after resignation or termination of an employee.

Salary and Benefits

The majority of high-performance employees prefer work environments that offer rewards. An appealing benefits package presented to new employees often serves as a source of enthusiasm. One of the first questions a prospective employee may ask is about salary. Competitive salaries are set by taking into account the responsibilities of the position, and then researching the salaries of similar positions in other practices. Salary ranges for a geographic area may be determined by contacting local medical societies, hospital human resource departments, and the chamber of commerce.

Employee Rights

Employees should understand their rights within the organization. Employee rights should include safety in the workplace, encouragement to sensibly discuss complaints with supervisors, air grievances, and maintain a voice in decisions that affect work policies and procedures. Employee rights should be included in the personnel manual, which is given to the employee during orientation.

Orientation

All new employees should receive appropriate orientation. On the first day of employment, the employee will be given a copy of the personnel manual and will be encouraged to discuss the manual with the supervisor. Orientation should also include the following: a tour of the facility with introductions to the staff, detailed explanation of the employee's job description, key agreement (if they are given keys), confidentiality agreement, equipment demonstration including a check-off form, patient and employee rights, and the completion of insurance and tax forms. In addition, OSHA training and fire safety/evacuation procedures should be explained by the Safety Coordinator. If applicable, Hepatitis-B vaccination forms should be completed and the series started immediately. The employee should also receive a TB skin test. All forms signed during orientation should be placed in the employee's personnel file. The orientation period should lay the groundwork for the establishment of successful relationships among the new employee, supervisors, and co-workers.

Professional Development

A highly efficient, motivated staff should strive for continuous improvement. Most employees appreciate the opportunity to increase knowledge and upgrade skills. An employer who takes an active role in professional development of employees will be rewarded. Professional development may include continuing education seminars or periodic reading materials. It may also include in-service sessions held at the office on a certain day of the month, or when the need arises. Employees should be encouraged to actively learn about the specialty in which they work. Compensation for attendance at national meetings or seminars should be offered in order to encourage employee growth.

Risk Management/Quality Improvement

A risk-management plan is designed and maintained to prevent potentially harmful situations from occurring and to protect the life and welfare of the organization's patients and employees. The plan should identify and address areas of potential liability, and promote activities to minimize legal and physical risk to patients and staff. A healthcare organization can implement a risk-management program by using the following guidelines

1. Establish a risk-management committee to superintend risk management of the practice. The chair of the committee should be the physician implementing the risk-management plan. This committee should meet quarterly.
2. Apply the risk-management program throughout the organization, including all departments and all service locations.
3. Establish a method by which a patient may be dismissed from care and treatment discontinued. This method should provide adequate explanation to the patient for the withdrawal.
4. Develop procedures for collection of unpaid accounts, allowing for the review of unpaid accounts before referral to a collection agency.
5. Establish procedure for the analysis of patient and staff incident reports. Incidents include serious accidents, trauma, adverse events, and fatalities.
6. The risk-management committee meets periodically to review litigation involving the organization and its staff. Minutes from these meetings are kept.
7. Establish procedure for the review of patient complaints. All complaints are discussed by the risk-management committee and corrective action is taken.
8. Maintain correspondence with the professional liability insurance carrier.
9. Develop methods of responding to inquiries from government agencies, attorneys, consumer advocate groups, reporters, and the media.
10. Establish methods for addressing the relationships with competing health care organizations in order to avoid antitrust and restraint of trade concerns.
11. Provide a policy to be implemented in the event that the physician becomes incapacitated during a surgical procedure or becomes an impaired health care provider.

12. Establish methods for complying with all applicable government regulations and contractual agreements.
13. Establish staff accessibility after usual office hours.
14. Implement procedure for the periodic review of clinical records and policies concerning clinical records.
15. Provide risk-management education to all employees with documentation.

A quality-improvement program should be implemented to guide the coordination, integration, and operation of a plan that ensures and promotes the optimum of quality patient care. The program should function to

1. Maintain and deliver quality health care through the identification, evaluation, and resolution of problems. Quality-improvement studies should be completed regularly.
2. Provide assistance and guidance to the administrative and clinical staff in the identification of problems or opportunities for improvement.
3. Promote efficient use of resources through regular monitoring of patient care and patient satisfaction.
4. Improve employee satisfaction by encouraging their participation in improving the delivery of care.
5. Review key indicators in comparison with other practices.
6. Quantify and ascertain outcomes via quarterly status reports to the governing body.

FACILITY DESIGN

Space Planning

Ambulatory surgery center and office surgical facility designs vary greatly depending on the procedures to be performed. Whatever style may be used within the suites, it is important to maintain compliance with the requirements of regulatory agencies and accreditation organizations. It is important to consult with agencies such as AAACHC, the state department of health, and the National Fire Protection Agency before constructing an ambulatory surgical center or office surgical facility.

Patient flow is the first factor to consider when designing the layout of the surgical facility. The recovery rooms, operating rooms, and nursing station should allow for the quick transfer of patients. The time required for the physician to travel between rooms should be minimized. The operating rooms should be in close proximity to the recovery rooms. The doorways of the operating rooms should be wide enough to accommodate emergency code equipment in the unlikely event of an emergency. In order to maximize efficiency for nursing staff, the location of instruments, surgical supplies, and sterilization equipment should be easily accessible. A clean utility room should be separate from a soiled utility room to eliminate the possibility of contamination.

The front office area should be separated from the surgical area. The patient's first interactions will take place at the front desk, so care should be taken to maximize organization of the area. The activity of the busy front office should not hinder the physician and nursing staff from remaining efficient in patient care.

The sizes of surgical suites may vary significantly to accommodate different procedures. Many prefer an operating room of 20 × 20 ft to maximize movement around the room. Recovery rooms containing large equipment should be 9 × 12 ft. An operating room 15 × 15 ft would easily accommodate large lasers or liposuction equipment. It is important to develop room plans and blueprints including all equipment to be certain that rooms will provide ample space for efficient patient care.

Space in the surgical suite should be allotted for recovery rooms, scrub areas near the operating rooms, patient dressing room, patient and employee restrooms, medical records storage, equipment and supply storage, and physician office(s). It is important to initiate early contact with regulatory agencies that will be reviewing the facility in order to eliminate the inconvenience and cost of retrofitting.

Walls and Ceilings

A variety of materials are available for wall coverings and ceilings. The materials for ceilings should provide a smooth surface for easy cleaning. Materials that are porous are not easily cleaned and should not be used.

Paint and wall coverings should be washable. Regulations concerning smoke and flame resistance should be followed to comply with building codes and the state department of health.

Flooring should be cleanable without risk of cracking. Seamless vinyl or similar material should be used to promote disinfection of the operating and procedure rooms. If ceramic tile is chosen for ease of cleaning, it must be inspected regularly for chips or cracks. If damage to the tile occurs, it is necessary to replace the damaged sections immediately in order to avoid the accumulation of dust and contaminants.

Lighting

Standard

Surgical lighting may vary greatly depending on the procedures to be performed. Lighting may be installed in the ceilings of the surgery suite for a moderate price. Many ceiling lamps offer multiple light sources and flexible arms to maximize lighting efficiency and eliminate shadows. Both high-intensity halogen and fluorescent lamps are available and have replaced many reflector lights. Many lamp units are lightweight and can emit up to 1000 foot candles at 18 inches. Small lamps may be attached to the physician's magnifier for use as a headlamp.

Emergency

It is important to have an auxiliary power supply available in the event of an emergency. Emergency power lighting can be maintained through battery backup systems. When a power outage occurs, the battery system will allow sufficient power to maintain lighting. In addition, battery powered flashlights and lamps should be located in convenient places throughout the office.

Emergency Power

Maintaining access to auxiliary power may ensure the safety of patients undergoing procedures in the operating room. In the event of a power outage, a backup power supply enables the physician to finish the procedure. There are several choices and varying price ranges for auxiliary power supplies.

Electrical generators that run on natural gas are powerful enough to supply an entire office with power. Although the generator may produce an unlimited supply of power, it may prove to be the most expensive option.

A second option for back-up power is an electric inverter. Activation of the inverter takes place in one-fortieth of a second. The inverter is ideal to maintain memory for computer systems. The space needed for the inverter is minimal and little maintenance is required. The inverter will provide battery backup power for essential pieces of surgical equipment.

Ventilation

Ventilation for operating rooms is important to keep airborne contaminants from causing infection. If the operating room is not set up with its own ventilation system, it may be necessary to install high efficient particular air (HEPA) filters or electrostatic filters. Filters will sufficiently decrease the number of airborne contaminants that enter the operating room. The filtration system should be monitored to ensure proper operation.

Maintenance and Repair

In order to ensure the proper performance and maintenance of equipment, biomedical engineering specialists should evaluate office and surgical equipment annually. Hospitals can usually provide these equipment checks through their clinical engineering departments. Equipment checks should be documented in writing.

Restrooms

A patient restroom should be available in close proximity to the operating rooms or procedure rooms. Wide corridors and doorways are beneficial for postsurgical patients that may require assistance. Hand rails installed on the wall of the restroom are useful for elderly and postsurgical patients. A restroom should be large enough to include lockers for patient belongings.

Storage

Storage space is a high priority in a surgical facility. Space should be allotted for storage of supplies inside and outside the operating and procedure rooms. Clean, sterile storage rooms should contain cabinet doors that close to inhibit dust. Cabinetry located above countertops and sinks maximizes work space as well as storage space. Closets with locks are necessary for pharmaceutical supplies.

Laboratory

If laboratory facilities are not located near the office, space can be allotted within the office. Durable countertops and sinks should be provided, with ample cabinet space for storage. If chemicals are to be used in the laboratory, it is necessary to provide for proper storage. A flammables cabinet may be needed in addition to chemical waste containers. It is important to consider how many people will work in the lab, and allow 150 sq ft per technician. A refrigerator in the lab may be used to store surgical and laboratory supplies, but not food.

Surgical Practices

Sterilization

Sterilization is a daily process in a busy surgical practice. Sterilization equipment should be easily accessible and reliable. The most effective sterilization of instruments is achieved with a steam autoclave. Because of high heat and pressure, steam sterilization is efficient for removing spores.

Before instruments are sterilized, they should be washed in warm water and a neutral pH detergent. Dried blood and debris can be dislodged from instruments with an ultrasonic cleaner. After the instruments are removed from the ultrasonic bath, they should be rinsed with an oil-in-water emulsion for lubrication. The emulsion will minimize rust and corrosion of stainless steel instruments.

Instruments may be placed in clear packs for sterilization. An indicator strip should be placed in the pack to monitor sterilization. Biological indicators should be used every 2 to 4 weeks to be sure that all spores are eliminated through sterilization.

Many options are available in addition to steam sterilization. Dry heat and chemical sterilization including ethylene oxide may be acceptable, although more staining and damage to instruments may occur.

Surgical Site Preparation

Care should be taken to ensure that surgical sites are appropriately prepared before the first incision. Proper surgical site preparation significantly decreases the rate of infection. Cutaneous surgical wounds are usually in the clean or clean-contaminated categories. Clean surgical wounds necessitate sterile technique throughout the procedure. Care is taken to avoid entry into the respiratory, genitourinary or alimentary tracts and oropharyngeal cavity. Clean-contaminated wounds may allow minor breaks in sterile technique. The wounds may enter the respiratory, genitourinary or alimentary tracts, or oropharyngeal cavity with little spillage. Major breaks in sterile technique define contaminated wounds, and old traumatic wounds, infected tissue, and devitalized tissue constitute dirty wounds.

Cutaneous surgery carries a very low risk of infection when appropriate preparation and scrub is performed before surgery.

Preparatory Solutions

Surgical preparatory solutions are used to disinfect the patient's skin and to remove as much surface bacteria as possible. A preparatory solution with prolonged antibacterial activity offers the greatest bacterial eradication both during and after surgery.

Several effective skin preparatory solutions are currently available. Isopropyl alcohol (70%) and ethyl alcohol (90%) are active against gram-positive and gram-negative bacteria. Alcohol is flammable and must be allowed to dry completely before electrosurgical equipment can be used. It is relatively inexpensive and easily accessible, and is a reliable bacteriocidal agent.

Chlorhexidine (Hibiclens, Hibitane, Hibistat) is a skin disinfectant that is effective against gram-positive and gram-negative bacteria. Chlorhexidine binds well to the skin and has a very long duration of activity. It is ideal for length surgical procedures and in patients who are allergic to iodine. Caution should be used around the ears, eyes, and tendons.

Iodine (Lugol's solution, iodine topical solution, iodine tincture) and iodophor (Betadine) are effective against gram-positive and gram-negative bacteria. To effectively disinfect, they must remain on the skin for 3 to 5 minutes. Iodine-containing agents should not be allowed to enter open wounds because they are toxic to cells. Iodine allergy is common.

Benzalkonium chloride (Zepharin) is a quarternary ammonium cationic detergent. It may be used to disinfect skin, although it is more easily contaminated than chlorhexidine or iodine. It rarely causes allergic contact dermatitis.

Considerations in choosing the proper antiseptic surgical scrub are the estimated length of surgical procedure, patient allergies, and surgical site. Several different scrub solutions should be available for all cases.

Surgical Scrub

Bacteria on the skin surface should be minimized for a patient undergoing surgery. Patients should be encouraged to shower on the evening before surgery. A dramatic reduction in bacteria occurs after showering.

The removal of patient hair on the scalp, beard, or groin may be necessary in order to sufficiently scrub the surgical site. Trimming the hair with scissors is preferred to shaving in order to minimize cuts and nicks. It is necessary to scrub the surgical site and surrounding areas with a preparatory solution to remove the maximum number of organisms.

The surgeon should include hand washing as a regular part of patient interaction. Hand washing between patients reduces the risk of contamination between patients. Scrubbing before surgery should include a solution such as chlorhexidine, parachlorometaxylenol, povidone-iodine, or benzalkonium chloride. Watches, jewelry, and nail polish should be removed before the surgical scrub. The surgeon should use the scrub solution on hands, wrists, and forearms up to the elbows. Special attention should be given to scrubbing under fingernails. Scrubbing should take 3 to 5 minutes.

Surgical Attire

Cotton surgical scrub suits should be worn under fluid-resistant gowns in the operating room. Gowns may be disposable or reusable. Street clothes should not be worn in the operating rooms because they are likely to harbor contaminants.

Eyewear such as goggles or glasses with side shields are required for the entire surgical staff during operating room procedures. The eyes must be protected from the splashing of blood, anesthetic, bodily fluids, or chemicals.

The surgical team must protect itself and the patients by using masks. The mask should cover the nose and mouth in order to decrease wound contamination during surgery. Masks should be disposable and fluid-resistant in order to protect the surgical team from splashing blood, anesthetic, bodily fluids, or chemicals. Masks should be used with laser surgery and electrodesiccation to protect from viral particles found in the smoke plume.

Gloves

Surgical gloves should be sterile latex, vinyl, hypoallergenic, powder-free, or powdered. The gloves protect the surgical team from being exposed to bloodborne pathogens such as Hepatitis B and the human immunodeficiency virus. The use of gloves decreases the number of bacteria transmitted from the surgical team to the patient. Gloves should be visually examined during surgical procedures to be sure that no punctures have occurred. If a glove becomes torn or perforated during surgery, it should immediately be removed and replaced.

Equipment

Tables

The operating table should be easily maneuvered and tilted to provide comfort for patients. The table should provide adequate head, neck, upper and lower back, and leg support without inconvenience to the surgical team.

An operating table with multiple adjustments allows for multiple uses. A table that fully reclines may be ideal for lengthy cases. A table that adjusts into an upright seated position is convenient for less lengthy procedures. A table should not be bulky or excessively wide. Floor pedals allow the surgeon to raise and lower the table during surgery. A surgical table should offer as much comfort to the surgeon as it does the patient.

Electrosurgical Equipment

Many choices for electrosurgical equipment are available. Depending on the requirements of the surgeon, the unit may be monopolar using a grounding plate or dispersive electrode. The electrode may be a forceps type or the standard pencil type. Touching the electrode to the blood vessel causes immediate coagulation. When using forceps the vessel is pinched and sealed off by touching the electrode to the forceps.

In bipolar electrocoagulation, less power is used which decreases damage to surrounding tissue. Bipolar electrocoagulation requires the use of special forceps to pinch the vessel and allows the current to pass from one tip of the forceps to the other.

Options for sterilization of the electrosurgical unit and electrodes should be considered when choosing a system. Disposable tips may be used, but electrodes are designed for multiple uses with the appropriate sterilization.

Mayo Stands and Back Tables

Mayo surgical stands and back tables are important for the accessibility of surgical instruments during a procedure. A tray containing instruments and gauze sponges can be sterilized and placed directly on the Mayo stand. The stand may contain two or four wheels for ease of movement in the operating room.

Back tables should be placed in close proximity to the operating table. A sterilized tray may be placed on the table allowing for accessibility to instruments and sterile surgical supplies. Back tables are found in many sizes, and should be chosen to fit the operating room. A table should be large enough for appropriate use during surgery, but should not be so large that it inhibits personnel moving around the room.

Waste Receptacles

Waste should be separated into contaminated and noncontaminated waste containers. Contaminated waste is most often placed in a visible red container or bag that is marked with a biohazard sticker. Contaminated waste includes gauze or surgical aids that have been in contact with patient blood, tissue, or bodily fluids. All noncontaminated waste, such as paper towels and instrument and supply wrappers, should be placed in a separate trash container identified by a black garbage bag or labeled as noncontaminated waste.

Kick buckets on wheels are useful within the operating room. They can easily be moved to the desired location. Kick buckets are not as large as traditional waste cans, and multiple bag changes may be necessary during the day. It will be necessary to have a large contaminated waste container for temporary storage of multiple waste bags.

Suction

Suction may be used in addition to electrosurgical units in cases where excessive bleeding occurs. Suction may allow the surgical team to efficiently pinpoint a bleeding vessel. Suction is most efficient when attached to a small vacuum pump. Suction units may add substantial noise to the operating room.

Crash Cart

A crash cart should be in close proximity to the operating rooms for immediate use in the event of an emergency. In the event of a medical emergency, employees certified in ACLS and CPR should be responsible for procedures involving restoring cardiac, circulatory, ventilatory, and metabolic function. The following equipment should be included on the crash cart: cardiac monitor with defibrillator, oxygen, Ambu bag, portable suction machine for aspiration, laryngoscope, oropharyngeal airways, tracheotomy kit, stethoscope and blood pressure cuff, intravenous (IV) access equipment, IV fluids, and emergency drugs. Emergency drugs include: 10% calcium chloride, bretylium tosylate, 2% lidocaine, epinephrine multidose, diphenhydramine, and naloxone.

The crash cart should be checked regularly to ensure proper operation of the defibrillator and monitor as well as to replace expired emergency drugs.

Monitors

Monitoring equipment should be used during office surgery, especially when IV sedation and general anesthesia are used. Strict monitoring of a surgical patient allows for rapid response in the event of a medical emergency. Equipment for patient monitoring should include a pulse oximeter, electrocardiograph, and blood pressure. Many monitoring units are included as part of resuscitation units. The monitoring equipment should be kept in close proximity to the crash cart to facilitate quick action if necessary.

RECOMMENDED READING

Accreditation Handbook for Ambulatory Health Care. Wilmette, IL: Accreditation Association for Ambulatory Health Care, Inc. 2000 edition.

Coleman WP, Hanke WE, Alt TH, Asken S, eds. Accreditation of the Office Surgical Facility in Cosmetic Surgery of the Skin. 2nd ed. St. Louis: Mosby Publishers, 1997, pp. 81–84.

APPENDIX 1: SAMPLE JOB DESCRIPTION

Position:	Office Manager
Qualifications:	High School Diploma/College Courses Typing skills (60 wpm) A minimum of five years experience in a business office managing customer service, clerical operations, and accounting. Proficient word processing skills, strong verbal and written communications are required as well as organization and efficiency.
Physical Requirements:	Good physical health required Visual and audio acuity Clear and distinct speech Neat, clean, particular appearance
Reports to:	Administrator
Supervises:	Office Staff

Position Primary Responsibilities:

1. Schedule appointments and input into computer database.
2. Handle all incoming calls and route as needed.
3. Handle all general correspondence for physician including dictation.
4. Supervise office staff.
5. Distribute mail.
6. Maintain inventory of office supplies.
7. Maintain responsibility for communication with physicians, officers, Board of Directors and staff.
8. Develop appropriate marketing for practice.

Position Secondary Responsibilities:

1. Patient check in/check out.
2. Run daily schedule, distribute to nursing/laboratory staff.
3. Medical Record management
4. Mailings/new patient packets

Terms of Employment: Permanent, full-time position

Approved by: ______________________________ Date ___________

Reviewed and agreed by: ______________________ Date ___________

2

Aesthetic Analysis of the Aging Face

Richard G. Glogau
University of California at San Francisco, San Francisco, California

Wrinkles should merely indicate where smiles have been. Mark Twain. (1987).

As a member of the so-called Baby-Boomer generation turns 50-years old every 8 seconds, aging appearance has taken center stage as a presenting complaint for many patients. The motivations behind their unhappiness with their appearance include the following:

- job pressures in a highly competitive and increasingly technical job market
- a high rate of divorce and successive remarriage
- incessant visual advertising media
- awareness of the wider availability of cosmetic services
- a sustained decade of economic growth, with higher discretionary income
- a wider social acceptance of cosmetic rejuvenation procedures
- a logarithmic explosion of medical and surgical techniques introduced to the standard armamentarium

Many techniques, such as liposuction surgery, were literally unheard of only two decades ago, and now liposuction is the most commonly performed cosmetic surgical procedure in the United States. Now lasers, which didn't exist two decades ago, have probably surpassed liposuction in sheer number of cases performed. Use of injectable soft-tissue fillers and the newest aesthetic agent, botulinum toxin, may even surpass the number of laser procedures performed in the next year or two.

ANATOMIC BASIS FOR AGING APPEARANCE

One can approach the analysis of the aging face using an anatomical model to provide a systematic framework to counsel patients and rationally select among a wide variety of therapeutic options. Too often, patients encounter physicians who have a therapeutic "hammer," and they all become "nails." Inappropriate application of a given therapeutic technique to a clinical situation in aging appearance because of inability or unwillingness to correctly recognize and categorize the anatomical basis for the cosmetic defect leads to mediocre results at best and disasters at worst.

The human face ages in response to the following factors, which appear in varying degrees in different individuals:

1. Chronic ultraviolet (UV) light damage to the skin,
2. Loss of subcutaneous fat,
3. Changes in the intrinsic muscles of facial expression,
4. Gravitational changes from loss of elasticity of the tissue, and
5. Remodeling of the underlying bony and cartilaginous structures.

Identifying the relative mix and proportion of these factors in the patient, selecting the proper procedure knowing the risk/benefit ratio, and communicating this information to the patient constitutes the essential ingredients of the cosmetic consultation. Clearly there is a great deal of confusion among cosmetic professionals because we still see patients with distinct cosmetic defects being mismatched with the wrong therapeutic procedure on a regular basis. Examples include the following:

- patients with severe sun damage as their main aesthetic problem having face-lifts without resurfacing
- patients with jowls and platysmal banding of the neck getting liposuction without redraping the submuscular aponeurotic system (SMAS)
- patients with not a gram of fat left in their face getting laser resurfacing and rhytidectomy, accentuating their presurgical gaunt appearance
- patients with deep glabellar furrows being treated with collagen or other fillers without botulinum toxin being used to address the intrinsic muscles of the glabellar complex

Mismatching the procedure to the patient is the result of failing to take into account the individual variables that go into the aging appearance of the face. Considered in turn, each lends itself to some aspect of therapy that may be used individually or combined to give the desired aesthetic effect.

PHOTOAGING

With the increase in leisure time, air travel, and outdoor activity, "Boomers" spent their formative years out in the sun without the benefit of currently available sunscreens. Years of "baby oil and iodine," more revealing clothing, and the desire of the physically fit to acquire the oxymoronic "healthy tan," have produced high rates of skin cancer and premature aging skin. Cumulative exposure to sun remains the largest factor in aging skin and is responsible for a large portion of the unwanted aesthetic effects. Clinical signs of photoaging of the skin include rhytids, lentigines, keratoses, telangiectasia, loss of translucency, loss of elasticity, and sallow color [1,2].

A simple systematic classification of patient photoaging types, Types I through IV (Table 1), has been developed by the author [3]. Younger patients, usually in their second or third decade, show only the earliest signs of photoaging, usually as a change in homogeneity of color, but generally have no rhytids at all, even when the face is animated by talking or expression. They are categorized as Type I, or "no wrinkles" (see Fig. 1). They generally wear no makeup foundation at all because they do not require it for either color or lines.

TABLE 1 Glogau Photoaging Classification

Type I: No wrinkles
early photoaging
mild pigmentary changes
no keratoses
minimal wrinkles
patient age, twenties or thirties
minimal or no makeup
Type II: Wrinkles in motion
early to moderate photoaging
early senile lentigines visible
keratoses palpable but not visible
parallel smile lines beginning to appear
patient age, late thirties or forties
usually wears some foundation
Type III: Wrinkles at rest
advanced photoaging
obvious dyschromia, telangiectasia
visible keratoses
wrinkles even when not moving
patient age, fifties or older
always wears heavy foundation
Type IV: Only wrinkles
severe photoaging
yellow-gray color of skin
prior skin malignancies
wrinkled throughout, no normal skin
patient age, sixth or seventh decade
cannot wear makeup—"cakes and cracks"

As the patient ages, the UV damage to the elastic fibers becomes chronic, and the inherent "snap back" quality of the skin becomes impaired. At first, wrinkles begin to appear only when the face is in motion, usually as expression lines parallel to the meilolabial fold, the corners of the mouth, and the lateral canthal areas and over the zygomatic arch and malar eminences. These patients frequently use makeup foundation to conceal the irregularity in color or the sallow tones that result from chronic sun exposure. These patients are commonly in their thirties or forties and look unlined when their face is at rest. However, as soon as they begin to talk, the lines appear. They are classified as Type II, or "wrinkles in motion" (see Fig. 2).

As the photoaging proceeds, the damage to the elastic fibers becomes more severe. Eventually the wrinkles produced by dynamic movement of the face persist even when the face is at rest. Generally by the fifth decade of life, there are visible parallel lines at the crow's feet, parallel to the corners of the mouth, radiating down from the lower eyelids onto the malar cheeks, and across the upper lip and lower lip. Makeup foundation still helps with the color problem in these patients, but tends

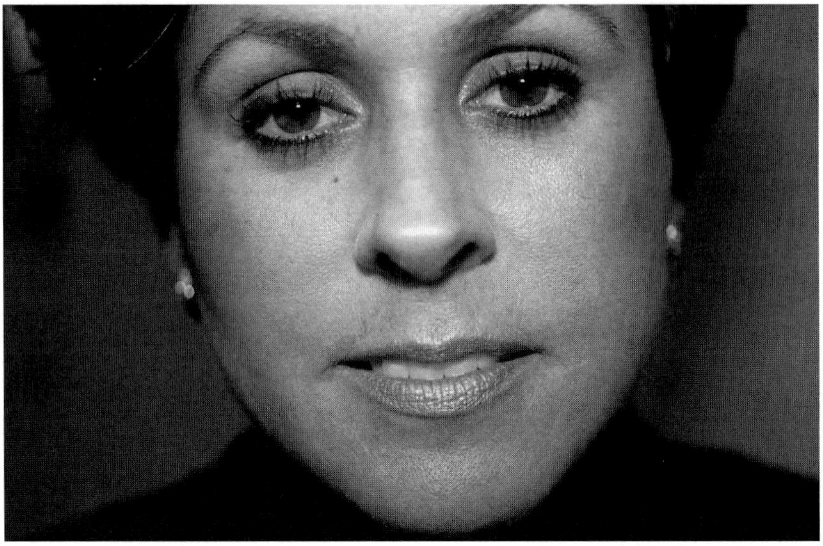

FIGURE 1 Type I: No wrinkles. Skin is uniform in color. There is an absence of lines even at the corners of the eyes and mouth.

to accentuate the appearance of the lines. These patients appear lined even when their face is at rest, and are classified as Type III, or "wrinkles at rest."

With continued photoaging, the wrinkles gradually spread to cover the majority of the facial skin while the dermis becomes totally engorged with thick debris or poorly staining ground substance, giving a thickened, coarse quality of the skin. Usually this occurs by the sixth or seventh decade of life, but earlier in the severest cases. Many of these patients have already had one or more skin cancers. Makeup is completely impractical because it gives the appearance of cracked mud when applied to such an uneven surface. These patients really have no unlined skin at all anywhere on their face, and are classified as Type IV, or "only wrinkles."

PIGMENTARY SYSTEM

Patients must also be categorized according to their Fitzpatrick Sun-Reactive Skin Type [4]. This classification (Table 2) is based on the skin's response to erythema producing doses of UV light. Patients differ in their sun reactivity and the scale gives a very good indication of potential dyschromia after epidermal/papillary dermal injury and the likelihood of developing postinflammatory hyperpigmentation during the short-term postsurgical period, as well as the potential for permanent hypopigmentation resulting from destruction of melanocytes. Evaluating the degree of photodamage present and the pigmentary UV response can be expressed as shorthand

→

FIGURE 2 Type II: Wrinkles in motion. (a) When the face is at rest, the patient appears similar to Type I. But when the face is animated by expression (b and c), there are many parallel lines that appear, first at the corners of the mouth, then parallel to the nasolabial folds, then at the corners of the eyes, and finally over the malar cheeks.

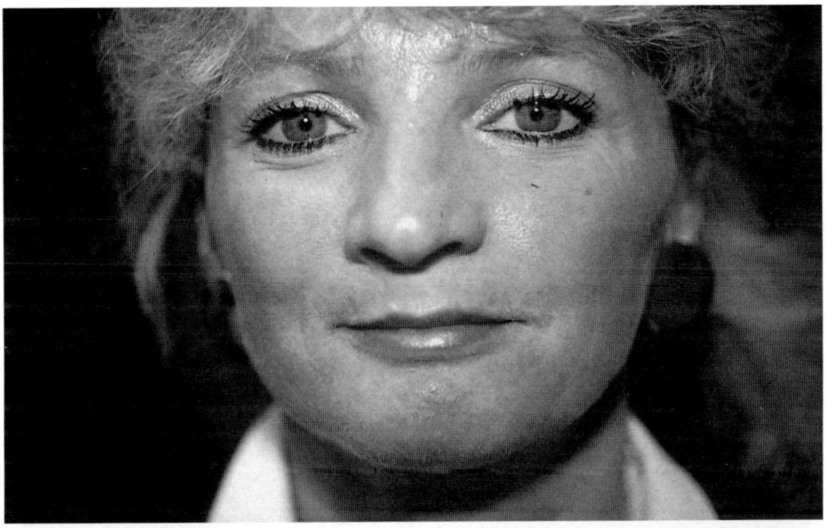

(a)

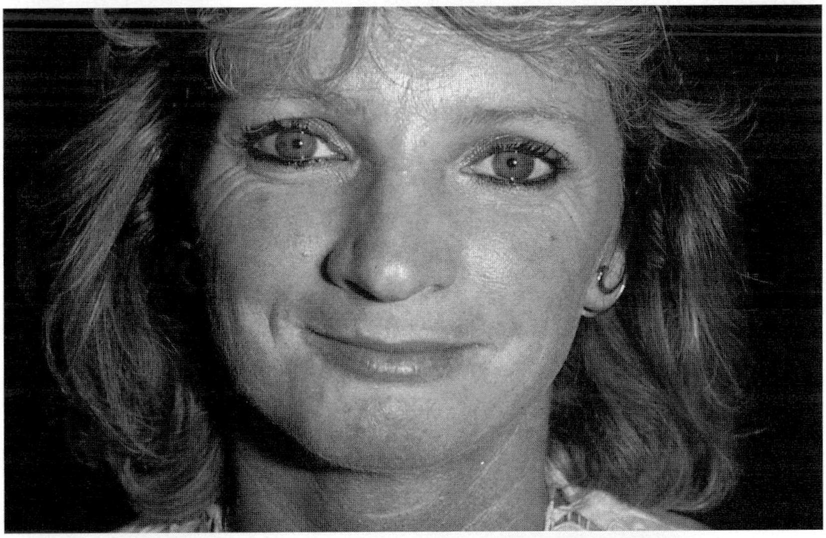

(b)

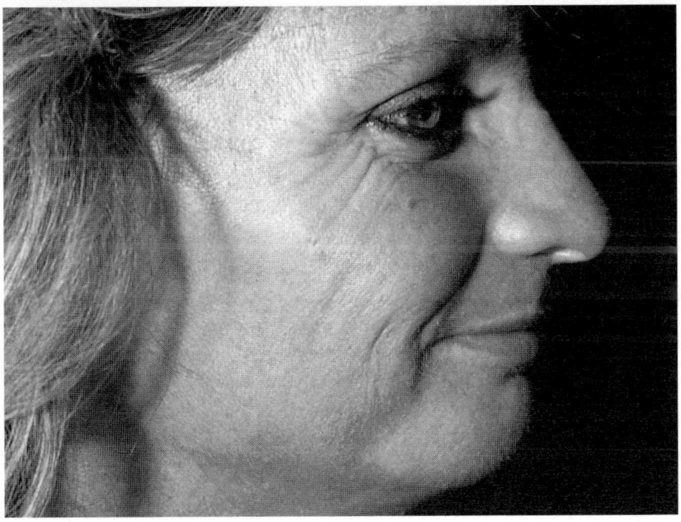

(c)

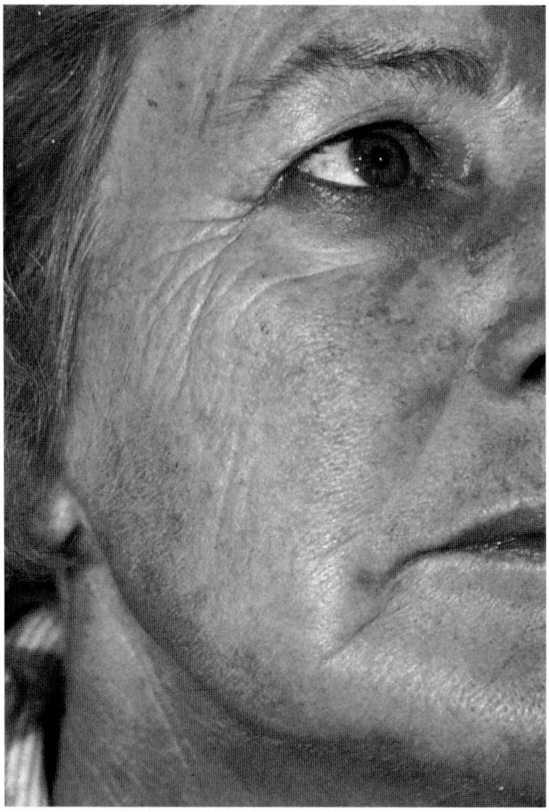

FIGURE 3 Type III: Wrinkles at rest. This patient clearly shows the parallel lines seen with animation in Type II except they are now present with the face at complete rest.

to classify the patient's degree of damage. A patient, who is a Fitzpatrick III, Glogau Photoaging III is a very different candidate for resurfacing than a Fitzpatrick I, Glogau Photoaging II. The risk benefit ratios are entirely different in these two patients. The presence of lines and wrinkles alone is not sufficient indication for resurfacing.

As a general rule, patients with Fitzpatrick Skin Types I to III will tolerate resurfacing without significant risk of color change. Although resurfacing may be undertaken in Fitzpatrick Skin Types IV to VI, the risk of pigmentary change is certainly high enough that the patient should be warned that there can be color change in the treated skin.

THE LOSS OF SUBCUTANEOUS FAT

An aspect of the aging face that is a major component of aesthetic disharmony is the redistribution and loss of subcutaneous fat. Although some compartments, such as the submental fat, may lend themselves to removal via liposuction, in general there is a growing appreciation that removal of fat should be performed with caution because of the flattening or hollowing of contours that may occur. Aging produces

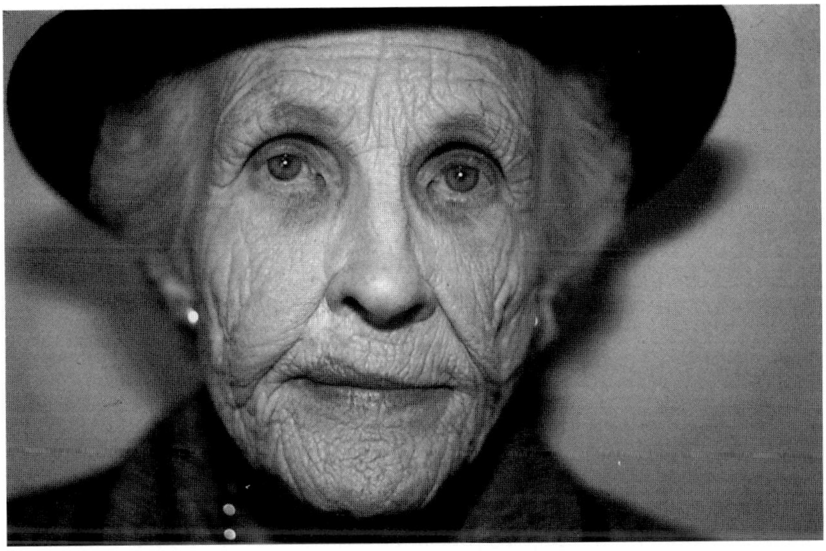

FIGURE 4 Type IV: Only wrinkles. The perioral skin in particular is likely to show the total replacement of normal skin with minute, rhomboid, and geometric rhytids, clearly seen in this patient. The entire face shows similar rhytids on close inspection.

a profound loss of subcutaneous fat in the perioral area, temporal fossae, premalar areas, chin, and forehead. The older face has a flattened quality to the cheekbones, a sunken appearance to the lips, a bulging of the inferior fat pads of the eye, and a general loss of the fullness and roundness of youth. Experienced plastic surgeons have recognized this and are moving away from excessive fat removal to fat repositioning or augmentation. S. Hoefflin has written, "[i]n the aging face it is not the tightness of the SMA (platysma aponeurosis) or skin that makes the difference, but the quantity and position of subcutaneous fat" [6].

The routine removal of the infraorbital fat as a part of blepharoplasty, which often accentuated the deep grooves between the lower eyelid and the cheek, has become outdated. Now surgeons prefer to use an arcus marginalis release and mobilize the fat medially and anteriorly to fill in that groove and return a more youthful appearance to the lower eyelids through restoration of fullness. Similarly, repositioning of the premalar fat has become an important part of routine face-lifting, or

TABLE 2 Fitzpatrick's Sun-Reactive Skin Types

Skin type	Skin color	Tanning response
Type I	White	always burn, never tan
Type II	White	usually burn, tan with difficulty
Type III	White	sometimes mild burn, tan average
Type IV	Brown	rarely burn, tan with ease
Type V	Dark brown	very rarely burn, tan very easily
Type VI	Black	no burn, tan very easily

reversing the aged appearance that comes from flattening of the cheekbone contours. The ultimate recognition of the importance of the subcutaneous volume of the face comes from the work of surgeons like Fournier, Coleman, and others who have developed techniques of fat transfer to restore the volume contours of the aged face. Microlipoinjection in small and larger volumes, placed subcutaneously and intramuscularly has been used with great success to reshape the aging face. Although, difficulties remain in the predictability and longevity of fat transfers, the aesthetic effects are often impressive in the naturalness of the resulting appearance. Restoration of loss of volume lies behind the appeal of injectable fillers such as collagen, hyaluronic acid get, and microdroplet silicone. Lip augmentation with injectables remains one of the most frequently sought after cosmetic procedures performed in aesthetic medicine today. The market is literally overflowing with introduction of new injectable agents and alloplastic implants of expanded polytetrafluorethylene (SoftForm, Gore-Tex).

Analysis of the aging face must include an assessment of the quality and position of the subcutaneous fat. Are the lips thin? Have they lost their shape? Are the cheekbones flattened? Is there wasting in the temporal fossae, above the eyebrows, or in the buccal pads? Resurfacing and/or face-lifting will not address these problems, and may make them stand out even more.

CHANGES IN FACIAL MUSCULATURE

Perhaps nothing else has driven home the impact of facial musculature on facial aging like the introduction of botulinum toxin for selective chemical denervation of selected muscles of the face. Paralysis or partial weakening of the glabellar corrugator/procerus complex, the forehead frontalis, and the lateral orbicularis muscles has simply revolutionized the management of the upper third of the aging face. Deep glabellar lines, which could only be briefly improved with injectable fillers, now melt away with the placement of botulinum toxin in the corrugator/procerus complex. Crow's feet lines, which routinely reappeared after deep resurfacing now, vanish in a few days. Even the troublesome horizontal lines and creases of the lower eyelid, which persisted after blepharoplasty and/or resurfacing, can now be treated with botulinum toxin. The toxin is both safe and temporary. It has now become a mainstream tool in cosmetic surgery.

The interesting thing about the use of botulinum toxin is that it allows us to see precisely what the components of the various anatomic compartments may be in the aging face. For example, the patient who has deep photoaging lines may not get complete resolution of the flabellar furrows with initial treatment with botulinum toxin. Having repeatedly folded the sun-damaged skin, a line may still be visible for several months after botulinum toxin has completely paralyzed the corrugators. These patients require either resurfacing or a dermal filler such as Zyderm collagen to address the remaining component of the glabellar line. Similarly, the occasional male patient will have such hypertrophy of the glabellar muscle complex that with botulinum-induced paralysis and atrophy of the muscles, the underlying contour of the bone becomes more prominent and the patient perceives a "bump" appearing on the brow. Volume in the face can be at least partly related to musculature as well as subcutaneous fat.

INHERENT LOSS OF ELASTICITY

As the facial soft tissue ages, the skin and underlying supporting structures, while sagging under the effects of gravity, lose their inherent resiliency or ability to resist stretching. The most striking example of this is the development of brow ptosis with age. The most common problem in patients' own analysis of the aging face is their inability to relate the hooding of the upper eyelid skin to malposition of the brows and forehead. How many patients ask for (and receive) upper-lid blepharoplasty when the source of their problem is ptosis of the upper brow and forehead? In a similar vein, inappropriate and overzealous use of botulinum toxin in the upper third of the face routinely produces brow ptosis, a feeling of "heaviness," and a slightly Neanderthal-like appearance because the older forehead does not have the inherent resiliency to maintain any brow position without the support of the underlying frontalis. In contrast, the surgeon who inappropriately elevates the brow to a position that would be mismatched to the patient's gender or age does the patient no aesthetic favor. Careful consideration of the quality of elasticity of the skin and soft tissue must be taken into account before attempting to address the position of the brow either surgically or with botulinum toxin.

In the lower third of the face, the face-lift is the *sine qua non* of the successful aesthetic outcome. Redraping, repositioning, and judicious removal of skin and soft tissue that has lost elasticity achieves a restoration of youthful appearance that cannot be achieved with resurfacing, fillers, fat transfer, or botulinum toxin. Although in truth many of these other techniques properly applied have made it possible for patients to delay and defray, virtually no one escapes the effects of gravity and the loss of intrinsic elasticity. The face-lift procedure is not in danger of extinction, although it now requires more selective application and execution that is mindful of the other components of aging previously discussed.

CHANGES IN UNDERLYING CARTILAGE AND BONE

The aging nose elongates and the tip droops. The aging mouth is affected by bony remodeling of the maxilla. The chin sharpens and protrudes. The ears appear to lengthen as the lobes droop. The tarsal plate softens and no longer holds the lower-lid margin in proper curve or position. Various surgical procedures address these problerms, such as tip rhinoplasty, tarsal lid tightening, and canthoplasty. Newer dental implant procedures and maxillofacial surgery can address intrinsic changes affecting the lower face.

But the practiced diagnostic eye of the cosmetic surgeon should not overlook the contribution of the underlying hard structures of the face—particularly when assessing presence (or more commonly absence) of facial symmetry. Patients often present with requests for treatment of facial problems without appreciating the contribution of underlying structures to their facial asymmetry. Although subtle, the asymmetry is not attributable to the soft tissue. No amount of collagen is going to correct an underlying difference in maxillary structure of the cheekbones, for example.

These pre-existing differences in facial asymmetry need to be identified so they can be pointed out to the patient and discussed. We have seen too many patients who are unhappy with their face-lift results and rail against the surgeon when it is their underlying facial structures that are the root cause of the difference in the appearance of their lifts. Recognizing pre-existing facial asymmetry attributable to underlying bony or cartilaginous structural differences is an important part of setting realistic patient expectations.

The most common example of pre-existing asymmetry is in cosmetic ear piercing. Patients recognize that their earlobes differ in size, volume, position, and orientation. They know how difficult it is to pierce ear lobes so that their jewelry will hang at the proper angle. The surgeon can often use this example to point out other asymmetries and put them in terms the patients can recognize.

COMBINATION THERAPIES

Optimal improvement in appearance can more often be obtained by combining procedures. At one end of the therapeutic spectrum, topical medical therapy using agents like tretinoin, alpha-hydroxy acids, hydroquinones, and 5-fluoruracil can inhibit or reverse UV-associated changes in aging skin. At the other end of the therapeutic spectrum, rhytidectomy, blepharoplasty, brow-lift, and suction-assisted lipectomy often provide dramatic results in facial rejuvenation. The choice of therapy rests on the ability of the surgeon to look at the face, analyze the anatomical components of the aging appearance, and then prioritize them, matching procedure risk/benefit ratio to each element. Is the predominant problem sun damage, sagging, or loss of volume? Often there are overriding constraints, e.g., the "down time," surgical risk, cost, and likelihood of benefit all weigh in the selection of the appropriate therapy. But underlying all of these choices must be a rational analysis of the various elements that go into making up the aging face.

REFERENCES

1. Balin A, Pratt L. Physiological consequences of human skin aging. Cutis 1989; 43:431–436.
2. Montagna W, Carlisle K, Kirchner S. Epidermal and Dermal Histological Markers of Photodamaged Human Facial Skin. Shelton, CT: Richardson-Vicks, 1988.
3. Glogau RG. Chemical peeling and aging skin. J Geriatr Dermatol 1994; 2(1):30–35.
4. Fitzpatrick T. The validity and practicality of sun-reactive skin types I through VI. Arch Dermatol 1998; 124:869–871.

3

Superficial Chemical Peels

Seth L. Matarasso
University of California School of Medicine, San Francisco, California

Karyn Grossman
Private Practice, Santa Monica, California

INTRODUCTION

Over the past several years, patients have become increasingly concerned with the appearance of their skin, and this has been further fueled in part by the media's interest in youth and facial rejuvenation. Patients want to both reverse the sun damage they have already sustained and to prevent future signs of aging. The vocabulary and the vast array of topical products aimed at rejuvenating the skin are routine and part of the modern vernacular. Contemporary patients and "baby boomers" are in search of procedures that will improve their appearance, but without causing substantial morbidity or down time. "Quick fixes" in facial appearance are not limited to women, because men too are also increasingly looking for rejuvenation without surgery and the stigma associated with cosmetic procedures. As such, superficial or light chemical peels that are primarily aimed at subtly and gradually refreshing the skin have gained in popularity. However, it is imperative for the physician to understand the indications, mechanism of action, potential complications, and the limitations of superficial chemical peels.

BACKGROUND

Chemical peels are defined as the application of a caustic agent to the skin resulting in partial-thickness injury and necrosis, with subsequent healing secondarily with reepithelialization by adnexae. This results in a skin surface that is more homogeneous and improved in both texture and appearance. Peels are loosely categorized based on the percutaneous penetration of the solution (Table 1). Although superficial chemical peels create a wound of approximately 0.06 mm in depth, corresponding to the epidermis and papillary dermis in whole or in part, there is a continuum between peel categories, and precise classification should be considered only as guidelines and not rigid indicators of biological effect. Indeed, many factors (Table 2) may affect the actual penetration of the peel, and agents normally considered "superficial"

TABLE 1 Classification of Peel Depths

Peel	Cutaneous depth	Layers affected
Light	0.06 mm	Stratum granulosum to superficial papillary dermis
Medium	0.5–0.60 mm	Papillary to upper reticular dermis
Deep	0.61–0.80 mm	Midreticular dermis

may actually penetrate deeper in the tissue, and hence create a deeper peel with the consequent risk profile.

The more common superficial resurfacing agents include alpha-hydroxy acids (specifically glycolic acid), beta-hydroxy acids, low-concentration trichloroacetic acid (TCA), Jessner's solution, and, recently, microdermabrasion (Table 3). Although many of these agents create a similar cutaneous injury and comparable results, they can be used to complement one another. Hence, the physician should become familiar with several of them. Ultimately, however, agent selection will be based on the patient's facial anatomy and deformity, as well as the physician's preference.

One of the more popular and diverse superficial peeling agents is glycolic acid. Because there are many different concentrations, formulations, and preparations, it is important to be aware of the specifications of the products being used. In general, the higher the concentration, the stronger the product; however, many commercially available products are buffered, which increases the pH and diminishes the effectiveness of the acid. At concentrations less than 15%, glycolic acid works by diminishing corneocyte cohesion, and at higher concentrations, there is epidermolysis. Epidermal penetration corresponds to the development of erythema, whereas dermal penetration can be seen as a whitish blanch. Recently, the addition of strontium nitrate to glycolic acid preparations has been suggested to decrease any mild irritation associated with these peels. Beta-hydroxy acids have recently become repopularized because of the potential for increased penetration into the pilosebaceous unit, and therefore can be particularly helpful for patients with acne and rosacea. They are available as prepackaged kits of 20% and 30% salicylic acid. TCA is a versatile agent and can be used in various concentrations. Superficial peels can be obtained with low TCA concentrations in the range of 10 to 30%. Precipitation of the epidermal protein imparts a faint and oftentimes incomplete white frost. The application

TABLE 2 Factors Determining Depth of Peel

Agent	Integrity of epidermal barrier	Skin type	Physician variation
Solution	Pretreatment	Atrophy/dermal thickness	Pressure
Concentration	Degreasing (soap, alcohol, acetone)	Epidermal lesions or cicatrix	Mode of application
Number of applications		Location (facial vs. nonfacial)	
Duration (glycolic acid)		Pilosebaceous unit density	

TABLE 3 Superficial Resurfacing Agents

Alpha-hydroxy acids	Jessner's (Combes') solution
Glycolic acid	Trichloroacetic acid 10–30%
Lactic acid	Azelaic acid
Malic acid	5-Fluorouracil
Tartaric acid	Carbon dioxide
Citric acid	Resorcinol
	Unna's paste
Beta-hydroxy acids	Retinoic acid
Salicylic acid	Microdermabrasion
Alpha/Beta-hydroxy acids	
Glycolic/salicylic acid	

of Jessner's solution (Table 4) breaks intercellular bridges and also serves as an effective superficial peeling agent.

CONSULTATION AND PRESURGICAL CONSIDERATIONS

Indications for superficial peels include mild photodamage inclusive of fine lines, lentigines, and acne. They are also appropriate in areas where wound healing may be unpredictable, such as nonfacial skin. Epidermal melasma may also be improved with repeated light peels, and the use of a Wood's lamp will help to localize the dyschromia before the peel. However, it is important for the patient to understand that, in order to maximize the benefits, they will need to undergo multiple peels as well as maintain an adequate intrapeel skin care regimen (Table 5).

During the initial consultation it is imperative to determine the patient's ultimate cosmetic goals. The patient is handed a mirror and instructed to verbalize his or her concerns. A chemical peel of any depth is aimed at resurfacing and retexturing the skin, and will not address the underlying structural anatomy. Thus, it is equally important that the physician also understand what the patient wishes modified, and then determine if, indeed, a chemical peel will address these issues. A patient complaining of blepharochalasia, brow ptosis, facial laxity, or fat atrophy may be best served by other procedures or a combination of another procedure with skin resurfacing. During this initial consultation it is also important to determine the patient's

TABLE 4 Jessner's Solution (Combes' Formula)

Resorcinol, 14 g
Salicylic acid, 14 g
Lactic acid (85%), 14 g
Ethanol 95% q.s.a.d., 100 mL

Table 5 Skin Care Regimen

Morning	Evening
Bland cleanser/bland cleanser with low percentage alpha- or beta-hydroxy acid	Bland cleanser/bland cleanser with low percentage alpha- or beta-hydroxy acid
Ascorbic acid or other antioxidant	Bleaching agent (4% hydroquinone, kojic acid)
Sunscreen SPF 15 or greater	Exfoliating agent (alpha- or beta-hydroxy acid or tretinoin cream)

lifestyle (with emphasis on sun exposure) and ability to tolerate multiple office visits, down time, and subtlety of the eventual results. Some patients would rather undergo many minor procedures with minimal recovery, whereas others would prefer one comprehensive procedure even with the attendant recovery period.

Once the physician and patient have determined that skin resurfacing is appropriate, then the type and depth of skin resurfacing will need to be agreed on. As chronological and photoaging begin, fine rhytides develop when the face is in motion, and, as the process continues, these wrinkles persist even when the face is at rest. Simultaneously, dyschromia, telangiectases, and epidermal lesions will appear. In general, the more profound the photodamage with attendant deep rhytides, the deeper the cutaneous injury will be needed to accomplish the desired results (Fig. 1). Con-

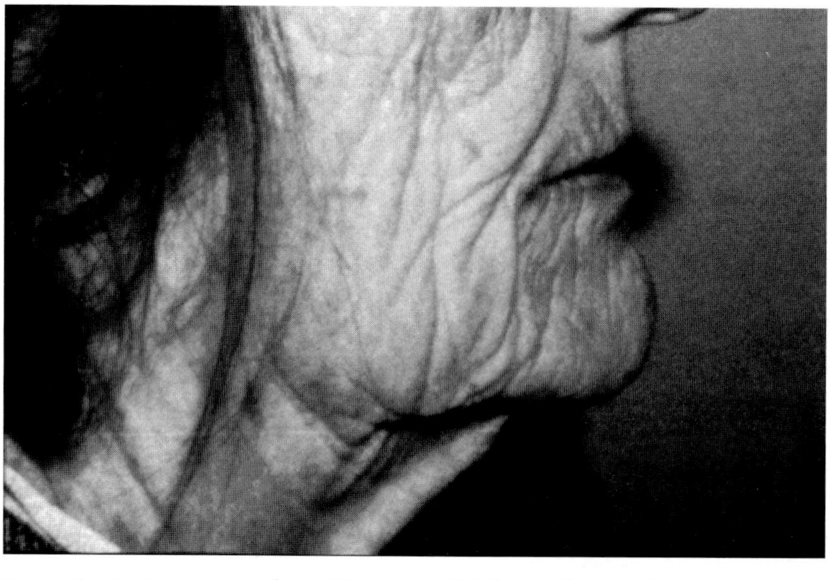

Figure 1 Patient was referred for superficial resurfacing; however, profound photodamage with deep rhytides and actinic damage would be more responsive to deeper resurfacing modalities and/or facial plasty surgery.

versely, a patient with mild photodamage, which consists of fine lines and minimal dyschromia, would perhaps be best suited to a series of light peels.

PRESURGICAL INSTRUCTIONS

Once realistic goals have been established and the patient has committed to a regiment of superficial chemical peels, she or he begins a rigorous home skin care regimen (Table 5) that ideally should begin 2 to 3 weeks before the first peel. This interval allows the physician to determine patient compliance and diligence with sun protection as well as any potential contact hypersensitivities. The regimen and their vehicles should be individualized, and can be altered contingent on the patient's skin type and degree of exfoliation. Ultimately the regimen will also cause a uniform epidermal desquamation which aids in an even intraoperative peel application. It is often helpful to provide the patient with detailed written instructions regarding the presurgical skin care regimen to maximize compliance.

TECHNIQUE

All of the equipment for superficial peels is readily available and can be assembled on a Mayo stand (Fig. 2). Having all of the agents in one location allows for maximum flexibility when the patient arrives and facilitates a possible change and a tailoring of the peel to accommodate the patient's precise needs.

On the day of the procedure the patient is instructed to arrive without make-up. The risks, benefits, and expectations are reviewed with the patient. The rare

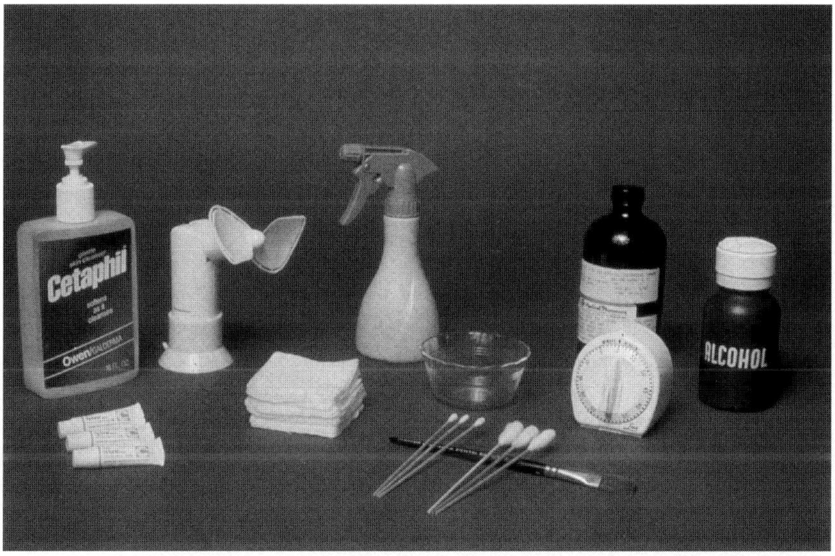

FIGURE 2 Equipment set-up: superficial peeling agent [glycolic acid (70%), salicylic acid (30%), Jessner's solution, trichloroacetic acid (20%)], degreasing agent (alcohol), applicator (cotton-tipped, single/proctology), gauze, paintbrush, neutralizing solution, emollient, and handheld fan.

complications of infection and postinflammatory pigmentary anomalies are again discussed, and the postsurgical instructions and sequence of events are also reviewed. Patients are also reminded that they may feel a mild burning sensation on peel application and, depending on the agent used, erythema and skin flaking can last from minutes to days.

The patient's skin is cleansed with soap and tepid water and blotted dry. The face is inspected for small lacerations and/or alterations in the epidermal barrier that would result in isolated areas of deeper peel penetration (Fig. 3). The patient's head should be elevated to a roughly 45° angle to aid in preventing the acid from accidentally spilling into the eye. A small handheld fan should also be available to reduce any mild burning sensation. The hair is pulled back with a headband or surgical cap. The patient typically remains in his or her own clothes, but a gown or drape can be placed around the neck to absorb any fluids that may spill onto the patient's garments. Petrolatum ointment can be placed on areas that should be avoided, such as open wounds or the lips.

The face can be degreased with alcohol, acetone, or astringent solutions that contain glycolic acid. This removes the residual make-up, debris, and sebum from the skin, allowing for uniform application and penetration of the acid. A more vigorous and complete debridement permits deeper penetration of the acid; however, care should be taken to avoid frank epidermal abrasion.

The acid can be applied in many fashions and with many different applicators. However, to avoid skip areas, the acid is applied in a methodical fashion, starting on the forehead and progressing in a clockwise pattern. In general, the more acid or pressure applied, the greater the penetration. Broad passes should essentially paint

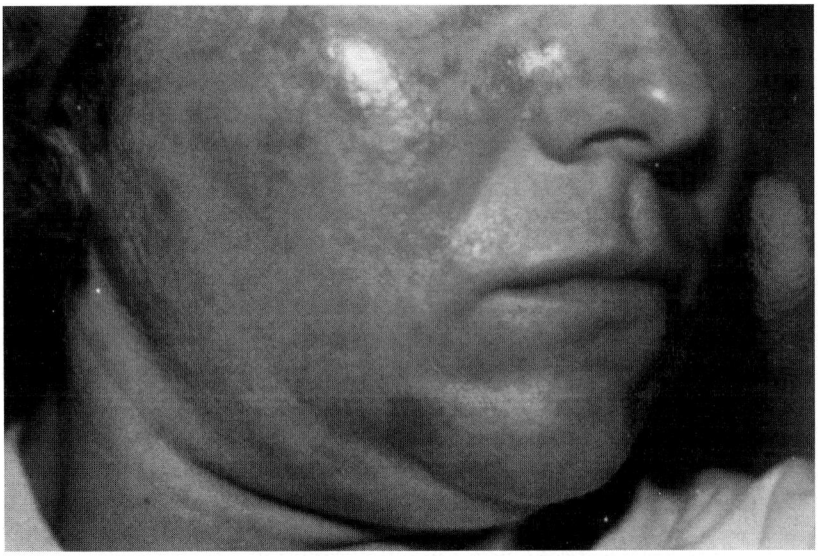

FIGURE 3 Area of deep glycolic acid penetration with resulting excoriation after intralesional administration of corticosteroid for an acne cyst.

TABLE 6 Glycolic Acid Protocols

Indication-Based Protocol	Concentration (%)	Time (min)
Acne	50–70	1–3
Melasma	50–70	2–4
Actinic keratoses	70	5–7
Fine wrinkles	70	4–8
Solar lentigines	70	4–8
Back or chest (any indication)	70	5–10
Concentration-Based Protocol	35	3
	35	4
	50	3
	50	4
	70	3
	70	4
Time-Based Protocol	70	2
	70	3
	70	4
	70	5
	70	6
	70	7

the entire facial surface, with feathering into the hairline and periocular area and, when indicated, onto the neck and chest. Once an even application has been achieved, repeat applications may be performed over the entire face or in select areas where there is significant damage, such as dyschromia or keratoses. After acid application, most light peels result in faint erythema and occasionally a transient mild frost. TCA, Jessner's solution, and beta-hydroxy acids remain intact after application. On drying, the salicylic acid found in beta-hydroxy peels and Jessner's solution leave a fine, white powder residue. This can serve as marker indicating completeness of the peel and can be left in place or removed with a dry gauze. Uniquely, glycolic acid peels are neutralized with either tepid water or sodium bicarbonate on completion. Glycolic acid removal is time- and/or concentration-dependent, and is predetermined by a set protocol (Table 6). After acid removal, as with other superficial peels such as TCA, a topical corticosteroid (Class VI) and emollient cream may be applied.

POSTSURGICAL CARE

After most superficial chemical peels, patients can resume their schedules without interruption. However, those with residual erythema or desquamation are instructed to gently cleanse the face and apply moisturizer followed by a sunscreen until all the flaking has subsided and, if so desired, they may apply make-up. If significant erythema is present, a mild topical corticosteroid can be continued twice daily for the first 3 to 5 days. Some patients who receive a deeper injury to their skin will

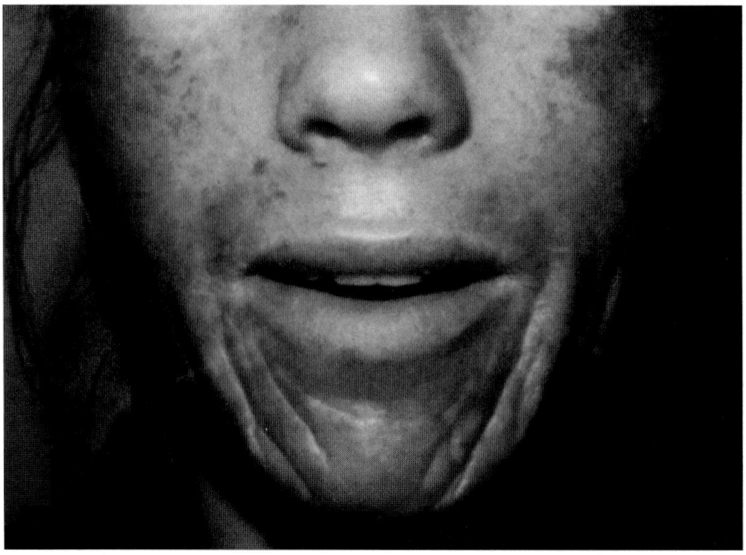

FIGURE 4 Patient requested "refreshing lunchtime peel." Three days after multiple coats of Jessner's solution by nonphysician practitioner, the patient was referred for treatment of "scarring." Skin tightness with inability to open mouth and hyperpigmentation resolved uneventfully after appropriate patient education and wound care.

have a taut feeling and then progressively develop fine wrinkles and some isolated areas of hyperpigmentation (Fig. 4). Over the next several days the skin will begin to peel, and the patient should be instructed not to prematurely remove any of the flaking skin. During this time, increased lubrication is warranted, and the patient is instructed to use a gentle cleanser and apply a mild corticosteroid to the area twice daily. On resolution of the normal sequelae of erythema and mild flaking, to maintain the results the patient is instructed to resume the presurgical skin care regimen and is encouraged to receive peels on a regular basis (4–12 weeks).

COMPLICATIONS

The complications resulting from superficial chemical peels are relatively infrequent. The mild discomfort and burning from these peels are normal sequelae, as are temporary erythema and scale. Persistent erythema, however, can be disquieting, and a source of an occult contact dermatitis should be excluded. Possibly because of overzealous lubrication or interruption of the normal cutaneous flora, on occasion patients may also experience a flare of acne. Postinflammatory hyperpigmentation rarely occurs, and fortunately, with judicious sun protection and topical bleaching agents, this condition will resolve uneventfully (Fig. 5). Perhaps of greatest concern with superficial resurfacing is the subtlety of improvement. Adequate and appropriate patient selection and patient education, however, should mitigate confusion and result in a satisfied patient.

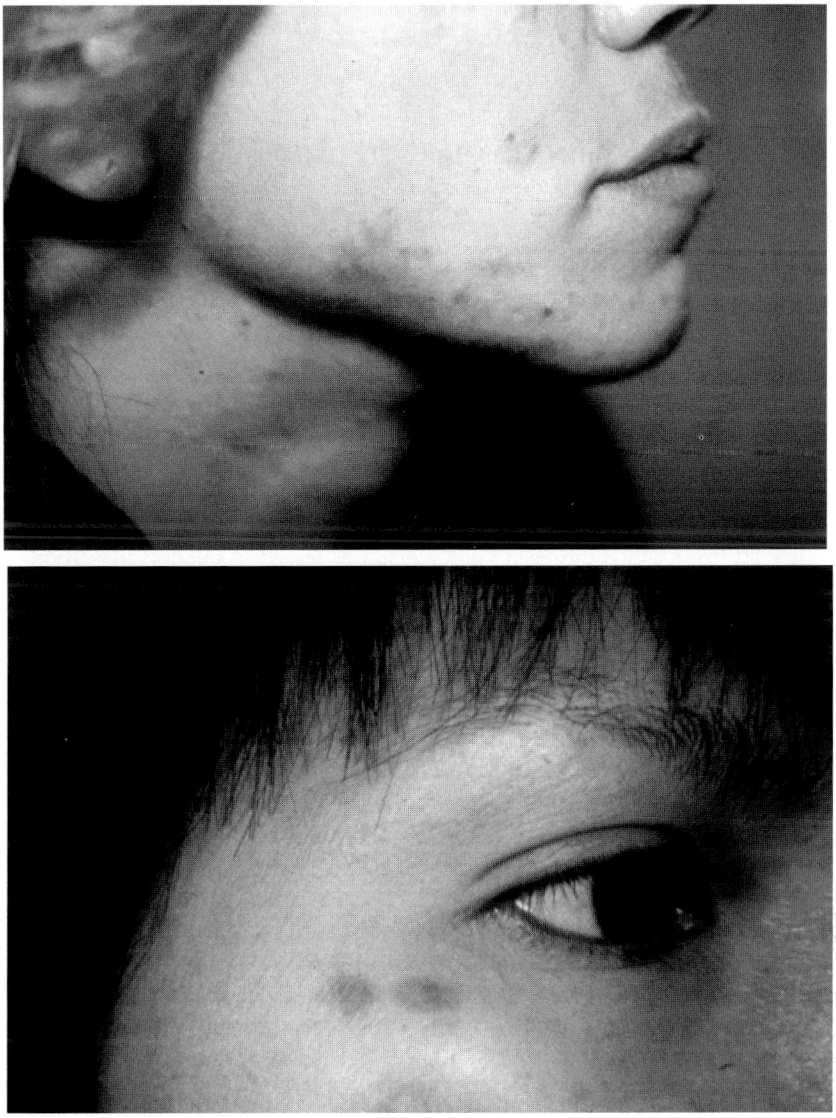

(a)

(b)

FIGURE 5 (a) Postinflammatory hyperpigmentation after 70% glycolic acid peel. (b) Accentuation of nevi after 70% glycolic acid peel.

REFERENCES

1. Becker FF, Langford FPJ, Rubin MG, et al. A histological comparison of 50% and 70% glycolic acid peels using solutions and various pHs. Dermatol Surg 22:463–468, 1996.
2. Berger R. Initial studies show salicylic acid promising as antiaging preparation. Cosmet Dermatol 10(1):31–32, 1997.
3. Brody HJ. Histology and classification. In: Brody HG, ed. Chemical Peeling and Resurfacing (2nd ed). St. Louis: Mosby Yearbook, 1997, pp. 1–6.
4. Brody HJ. Trichloroacetic acid application in chemical peeling: operative techniques. Plast Reconstr Surg 2:127–128, 1995.

5. Brody HJ. Variations and comparisons in medium-depth chemical peeling. J Dermatol Surg Oncol 15:953–963, 1989.
6. Clark CP III. Office-based skin care and superficial peels: the scientific rationale. Plast Reconstr Surg 104(3):854–864, 1999.
7. Coleman WP, Futrell JM. The glycolic acid/trichloroacetic acid peel. J Dermatol Surg Oncol 20:76–80, 1994.
8. Combes FC, Sperber PA, Reisch M. Dermal defects: treatment by a chemical agent. NY Physician Am Med 56:36, 1960.
9. Ditre CM, Griffin TD, Murphy GF, et al. The effects of alpha hydroxy acids on photoaged skin: a pilot clinical, histological and ultrastructural study. J Am Acad Dermatol 34:187–195, 1996.
10. Garcia A, Fulton JE. The combination of glycolic acid and hydroquinone or kojic acid for the treatment of melasma and related conditions. Dermatol Surg 22:443–444, 1996.
11. Grimes PE. The safety and efficacy of salicylic acid chemical peels in darker racial-ethnic groups. Dermatol Surg 25:18–22, 1999.
12. Hahn GS. Strontium is a potent and selective inhibitor of sensory irritation. Dermatol Surg 25:689–694, 1999.
13. Horvath PN. The light peel. Bull Assoc Milit Dermatol 18:2, 1970.
14. Lawrence NL, Cox SE, Brody HJ. A comparison of Jessner's solution and glycolic acid in the treatment of melasma in dark-skinned patients: a double-blind study. J Am Acad Dermatol 36(4):589–593.
15. Leyden JJ, Lavker RM, Grove G, et al. AHAs are more than moisturizers. J Geriatr Dermatol 3(suppl A):33A–37A, 1995.
16. Matarasso SL. Cutaneous resurfacing. Semin Cutan Med Surg 15:131–214, 1996.
17. Matarasso SL, Glogau RG, Markey AC. Wood's lamp for superficial chemical peels. J Am Acad Dermatol 30:988–992, 1994.
18. Matarasso SL, Glogau RG. Chemical face peels. Clin Dermatol 9:131–150, 1991.
19. Matarasso SL, Glogau RG. The role of chemical peeling in the treatment of photodamaged skin. J Dermatol Surg Oncol 17:622–623, 1991 (letter).
20. Moy LS, Howe K, Moy RL. Glycolic acid modulation of collagen production in human skin fibroblasts cultures in vitro. Dermatol Surg 22(5):439–441, 1996.
21. Moy LS, Murad H, Moy RL. Glycolic acid peels for the treatment of wrinkles and photoaging. J Dermatol Surg Oncol 19:243–246, 1993.
22. Newman N, Newman A, Moy LS, et al. Clinical improvement of photoaged skin with 50% glycolic acid: a double-blind vehicle-controlled study. Dermatol Surg 22:455–462, 1996.
23. Stagnone JJ. Superficial peeling. J. Dermatol Surg Oncol 15:924–930, 1989.
24. Swinehart JM. Salicylic ointment peeling of the hands and forearms. J Dermatol Surg Oncol 18:495–498, 1992.
25. Van Scott EJ, Yu RJ. Hyperkeratinization, corneocyte cohesion and alpha hydroxy acids. J Am Acad Dermatol 11:867–879, 1984.
26. Van Scott EJ. Alpha hydroxy acids: procedures for use in clinical practice. Cutis 43: 222–228, 1989.

4

Medium and Deep Chemical Peels

Gary D. Monheit
University of Alabama at Birmingham, Birmingham, Alabama

The explosion of interest in chemical peeling and laser resurfacing on the part of cosmetic surgeons has paralleled the general public's interest in acquiring a youthful appearance by rehabilitating the photoaged skin. The public's interest has been further heightened by advertising for cosmetic agents and over-the-counter chemicals and treatment programs that have entered the general market of products meant to rejuvenate skin and erase the marks of sun damage and age. Most of these over-the-counter do-it-yourself home programs have been tried by patients, and by the time they consult their dermatologist, plastic surgeon, or cosmetic surgeon, they are ready for a more definitive procedure performed with either chemical peeling or laser resurfacing. It is the obligation of the physician to analyze the patient's skin type and the degree of photoaging skin, and accordingly prescribe the correct facial rejuvenation procedure. This should be the procedure or combination of procedures that will give the greatest benefit for the least risk factors and morbidity. The cosmetic surgeon should have available for the consumer the options of medical or cosmoceutical topical therapy, dermabrasion, chemical peeling, and lasers available for selective skin destruction and resurfacing. Each of these techniques maintains a place in the armamenteria of the cosmetic surgeon to provide the appropriate treatment for each individual patient and his specific problem.

The approach to photoaging skin has expanded beyond a one-stage procedure to now include preparatory medical therapy and posttreatment cosmoceutical topical therapy to maintain results and prevent further photodamage. Thus, the cosmetic surgeon's office has become not only the site for a surgical treatment session, but also an educational setting for skin protection and care, and a marketplace for the patient to obtain the necessary topicals for skin protection. It is up to the physician to fully understand the nature of skin and sun damage, protective techniques available, and active agents that work as cosmoceutical preparations. Having available multiple procedures to solve these problems will make patients better candidates for the right procedure to restore and rehabilitate their skin.

Chemical peeling involves the application of a chemical exfoliant to wound the epidermis and dermis for the removal of superficial lesions and improve the texture of skin. Various acidic and basic chemical agents are used to produce the varying effects of light to medium to deep chemical peels through differences in their ability to destroy skin. The level of penetration, destruction and inflammation determines the level of peeling. The stimulation of epidermal growth through the removal of the stratum corneum without necrosis consists of light superficial peel. Through exfoliation, it thickens the epidermis with qualitative regenerative changes. Destruction of the epidermis defines a full superficial chemical peel inducing the regeneration of the epidermis. Further destruction of the epidermis and induction of inflammation within the papillary dermis constitutes a medium-depth peel. Then, further inflammatory response in the deep reticular dermis induces new collagen production and ground substances which constitutes a deep chemical peel [1]. These have now been well classified and usage has been categorized for various degenerative conditions associated with photoaging skin based on levels of penetration. The physician thus has tools capable of solving problems that may be mild, moderate, or severe, with very superficial, superficial, medium-depth, and deep peeling chemicals. The physician must choose the right agent for each patient and condition.

INDICATIONS AND PATIENT SELECTION

Analysis of the patient with photoaging skin must take into account skin color and skin type as well as degree of photoaging. Various classification systems have been available, and a presentation of a combination of three systems that may simplify and help the physician define the right program or therapeutic procedure for the patient follows. The Fitzpatrick skin-type system classifies degrees of pigmentation and ability to tan [2]. Graded I through VI, it prognosticates sun sensitivity, susceptibility to photodamage, and ability to facultative melanogenesis (the skin's intrinsic ability to tan). In addition, this system classifies skin as to its risk factors for complications during chemical peeling. Fitzpatrick divides skin types I through VI, taking into account both color and reaction to the sun. Skin types I and II are pale white and freckled with a high degree of potential to burn with sun exposure. Types III and IV can burn but usually are an olive to brown coloration. Types V and VI comprise dark brown to black skin that rarely ever burns and usually does not need sunscreen protection (Table 1). The patient with type I or II skin with significant photodamage needs regular sunscreen protection before and after the procedure. However, this patient has little risk for hypopigmentation or reactive hyperpigmentation after a chemical peeling procedure. The patient with type III through VI skin has greater risk for pigmentary dyschromia—hyper or hypopigmentation—after a chemical peel and may need pre- and posttreatment with both sunscreen and bleach-

TABLE 1 Fitzpatrick's Classification of Skin Types

Skin type	Color	Reaction to sun
I	Very white or freckled	Always burns
II	White	Usually burns
III	White to olive	Sometimes burns
IV	Brown	Rarely burns
V	Dark brown	Very rarely burns
VI	Black	Never burns

ing to prevent these complications [3]. Pigmentary risks are generally not a great problem with very superficial and superficial pigment chemical peeling, but may become a significant problem with medium and deep chemical peeling. It can also be a significant risk when regional areas such as lips and eyelids are peeled with a pulsed laser, creating a significant color change in these cosmetic units from the rest of the face. The porcelain-white shiny skin seen after taped deep chemical peels in regional areas has been classified as the "alabaster look." This is an objectionable side effect of deep taped phenol peeling and should be avoided because patients demand a natural look. The physician must inform the patient of this and other potential problems, especially if the skin is type III through VI. He must justify whether the benefits of the procedure outweigh these risks and, in addition, plan for the appropriate techniques to prevent these unwanted changes in color.

The Glogau system classifies severity of photodamage, taking into account the degree of epidermal and dermal degenerative effects [4]. The categorization is I through IV, ranging from mild, moderate, advanced, and severe photodamaged skin. These categories are devised to project which patients need therapeutic intervention. Category I or minimal-degree photodamage can be treated with light chemical peeling and medial treatment. Category II and III would entail medium-depth chemical peeling whereas category IV would need deep peeling or resurfacing as well as cosmetic surgical intervention for gravitational changes (Table 2). Monheit and Fulton have devised a system of quantifying photodamage by developing numerical scores that fit into corresponding rejuvenation programs [5]. In analyzing photodamage, the major categories include dermal with textural changes and epidermal with skin lesions. Dermal changes include wrinkles, cross-hatched lines, sallow color, leathery appearance, crinkly thin parchment skin, and the pebblish white nodules of milia. Each of these is quantitated, giving the patient a point score of 1 through 4. In addition, the number and extent of lesions are categorized from freckles, lentigenes, telangiectasias, actinic and seborrheic keratoses, skin cancers, and senile comedones. These also are added in a classification system of 1 through 4 and the final

TABLE 2 Photoaging Group—Glogau's Classification

Group I Mild (typically age 28–35 yrs)
Little wrinkling or scarring
No keratoses
Requires little or no make-up
Moderate (age 35–50 yrs)
Early wrinkling, mild scarring
Sallow color with early actinic keratoses
Little make-up
Advanced (age 50–65 yrs)
Persistent wrinkling or moderate acne scarring
Discoloration with telangiectasias and actinic keratoses
Wears make-up always
Severe (age 60–75 yrs)
Wrinkling: photoaging, gravitational and dynamic
Actinic keratoses with or without skin cancer or severe acne scars
Wears make-up with poor coverage

score results are tabulated. A total score of 1 through 4 would indicate very mild damage, and the patient would adequately respond to a five-step skin care program including sunscreen protection, retinoic acid, glycolic acid peels, and selective lesion removal. A score of 5 through 9 would include all of the aforementioned plus repetitive superficial peeling agents program such as glycolic acid, Jessner's solution, or lactic acid peels. A score of 10 to 14 would need a medium-depth chemical peeling, and a score of 15 or above would include deep chemical peeling or laser resurfacing. The patient thus understands during the consultation the degree of photodamage and the necessity for an individual skin rejuvenative program (Fig. 1).

The peeling agent is a chemical eshcarotic that damages the skin in a therapeutic manner. It is important that the physician understand the patient's skin and its ability to withstand this damage. The epidermis and stratum corneum have a barrier function against noxious chemicals, and some skin types withstand the damage to a greater degree than others while particular skin disorders have a greater tendency to produce side effects and complications from chemical peels because of poor barrier function or exaggerated inflammatory reactions. Patients with skin disorders such as atopic dermatitis, seborrheic dermatitis, psoriasis, and contact dermatitis may find their disease exacerbated in the postoperative period or may even develop problems with postoperative healing such as prolonged wound healing, posterythema syndrome, or contact sensitivity. Rosacea is a disorder of vasomotor instability in the skin and may develop an exaggerated inflammatory response to the peeling agents. Other important factors include a history of radiation therapy to the proposed facial skin, because chronic radiation dermatitis decreases the body's ability to heal properly. A general rule of thumb is to examine the facial hair in the area treated by radiation, and if it is intact there are enough pilosebaceous units to heal the skin properly after medium or even deep chemical peeling. This, however, is not absolute and one should find in the patient's history the dates of radiation treatment and how many rads were used for each individual treatment. Some of my patients with the greatest amount of radiation dermatitis, however, had treatments that were given for acne in the mid 1950s and over the years the skin developed the resultant degenerative changes [6]. On the other hand, patients with extensive photodamage may require stronger peeling agents and repeated applications of medium-depth peeling solutions to obtain therapeutic results. It is for this reason a careful evaluation of skin types and problems must be assessed.

Herpes simplex can be a postoperative problem with significant morbidity. Patients susceptible should be pretreated with antiherpetic agents such as acyclovir or valcyclovir to prevent herpetic activation. These patients can be identified in the preoperative consultation and placed on appropriate therapy at the time of the chemical peel. All antiherpetic agents act by inhibiting viral replication in the intact epidermal cell. The significance of this in peeling is that the skin must be re-epithelialized before the agent has its full effect. Thus, the antiviral agent must be continued in deep chemical peeling for the entire 2 weeks, or in medium-depth peeling for at least 10 days [7].

The chief indications for medium and deep chemical peeling are associated with the reversal of actinic changes such as photodamage, rhytides, actinic growths, pigmentary dyschromias, and acne scars [8]. The physician can thus use his classification systems to quantitate and qualitate the level of photodamage and prescribe the appropriate chemical peeling combination.

TEXTURE CHANGES	POINTS				SCORE
Wrinkles (% of potential lines)	1 <25%	2 <50%	3 <75%	4 <100%	
Cross-latched line (% of potential lines)	1 <10%	2 <20%	3 <40%	4 <60%	
Sallow color	1 Dull	2 Yellow	3 Brown	4 Black	
Leathery appearance	1	2	3	4	
Crinkly (thin & parchment)	1	2	3	4	
Pebbly (deep whitish nodules) (% of face)	2 <25%	4 <50%	6 <75%	8 <100%	

LESIONS	POINTS				SCORE
Freckles-mottled skin (# present)	1 <10	2 <25	3 <50	4 >100	
Lentigenes (dark & irregular) & SKs (Size)	2 <5mm	4 <10mm	6 <15mm	8 >20mm	
Telangiectasia-erythema flush (# present)	1 <5	2 <10	3 <15	4 >15	
AK's and SK's (# present)	2 <5	4 <10	6 <15	8 >15	
Skin Cancers (# present-now or by history)	2 1ca	4 2ca	6 3ca	8 >4ca	
Senile Comedones (in cheek bone area)	1 <5	2 <10	3 <20	4 >20	

Total Score________________

CORRESPONDING REJUVENATION PROGRAM

SCORE	NEEDS
1-4	Skin care program with tretinoin, glycolic acid peels
5-9	Same plus Jessner peels; pigmented lesion laser and/or vascular laser
10-14	Same plus medium peels - Jessner/TCA peel; skin fillers and/or Botox
15 or more	Above plus laser resurfacing

Staff Signature Date   Patient Signature Date

FIGURE 1 Index of phototyping.

MEDIUM-DEPTH CHEMICAL PEELING

Medium-depth chemical peeling is defined as controlled damage from a chemical agent to the epidermis and papillary dermis resulting in specific regenerative changes that can be performed in a single setting. Agents currently used include combination products—Jessner's solution, 70% glycolic acid, and solid carbon dioxide with 35% trichloroacetic acid. The benchmark for this level peel was 50% trichloroacetic acid. It has traditionally achieved acceptable results in ameliorating fine wrinkles, actinic changes, and preneoplasia. However, since TCA itself is an agent more likely to be fraught with complications, especially scarring, in strengths of 50% or higher, it has fallen out of favor as a single agent chemical peel [9]. It is for this reason that the combination products along with a 35% TCA formula have been found equally effective in producing this level of control damage without the risk of side effects.

Brody first developed the use of solid CO_2 applied with acetone to the skin as a freezing technique prior to the application of 35% trichloroacetic acid. The preliminary freezing appears to break the epidermal barrier for a more even and complete penetration of the 35% trichloroacetic acid [10].

Monheit then demonstrated the use of Jessner's solution prior to the application of 35% trichloracetic acid. The Jessner's solution was found effective in destroying the epidermal barrier by breaking up individual epidermal cells. This also allows a deeper penetration of the 35% TCA and a more even application of the peeling solution [11]. Similarly, Coleman has demonstrated the use of 70% glycolic acid prior to the application of 35% trichloroacetic acid. Its effect has been very similar to that of Jessner's solution (Table 3) [12].

All three combinations have proven to be as effective as the use of 50% trichloroacetic acid with a greater safety margin. The application of acid and resultant frosting are better controlled with the combination so that the "hot spots" with higher concentrations of TCA can be controlled, creating an even peel with less incidence of dyschromias and scarring. The combination peel produces an even, uniform peel. The Monheit version of the Jessner's solution—35% TCA peel is a relatively simple and safe combination. The technique is used for mild to moderate photoaging including pigmentary changes, lentigines, epidermal growths, dyschromias, and rhytids. It is a single procedure with a healing time of 7 to 10 days. It is also useful as an alternative to chemical exfoliation with topical 5-fluorouracil chemotherapy in the removal of diffuse actinic keratoses. Topical chemotherapy is applied for 3 weeks creating erythema, scabs, and crusts for up to 6 weeks [13]. The

TABLE 3 Agents for Medium-Depth Chemical Peel

Agent	Comment
50% TCA	Not recommended because of risk of scarring
Combination 35% TCA–solid CO_2 (Brody)	The most potent combination
Combination 35% TCA–Jessner's (Monheit)	The most popular combination
Combination 35% TCA–70% Glycolic (Coleman)	An effective combination
89% Phenol	Rarely used

combination peel will produce similar therapeutic benefits within 10 days of healing. It thus reduces the morbidity significantly and gives the cosmetic benefits of improved photoaging skin.

The procedure is usually performed with mild preoperative sedation and nonsteroidal anti-inflammatory agents. The patient is told that the peeling agent will sting and burn temporarily, and aspirin is given before the peel and continued through the first 24 hours if the patient can tolerate the medication. Its inflammatory effect is especially helpful in reducing swelling and relieving pain. If given before surgery, it may be all the patient requires during the postoperative phase. For full-face peels, however, it is useful to give preoperative sedation (5 to 10 mg diazepam orally) and mild analgesia, 25 to 50 mg meperidine (Demerol; Winthrop, NY), and 25 mg hydroxyzine hydrochloride intramuscularly (Vistaril; Lorec, NY). The discomfort from this peel is not long lasting, so short-acting sedatives and analgesics are all that are necessary [14].

Vigorous cleaning and degreasing is necessary for even penetration of the solution. The face is scrubbed gently with Ingasam (Septisol; Vestal Laboratories, St. Louis, MO) 4 × 4 inch gauze pads and water, then rinsed and dried. Next, an acetone preparation is applied to remove residual oils and debris. The skin is essentially debrided of stratum corneum and excessive scale. A thorough degreasing is necessary for an even penetrant peel. The physician should feel the dry, clean skin to check the thoroughness of degreasing. If oil is felt, degreasing should be repeated. A splotchy peel is usually the result of uneven penetration of peel solution attributable to residual oil or stratum corneum and inadequate degreasing.

After thorough cleaning, the Jessner's solution is applied with either cotton-top applicators or 2 × 2 inch gauze (Table 4). The Jessner's solution is applied evenly with usually one or two coats to achieve a light but even frosting. The frosting achieved with Jessner's solution is much lighter than that produced by TCA and the patient is usually uncomfortable, feeling only hat. A mild erythema appears with a faint tinge of splotchy frosting over the face. Even strokes are used to apply the solution to the unit area covering the forehead to the cheeks to the nose and chin. The eyelids are treated last creating the same erythema with blotchy frosting (Fig. 2).

The TCA is painted evenly with one to four cotton-tipped applicators that can be applied over different areas with light or heavier doses of the acid. Four cotton-tipped applicators are applied in broad strokes over the forehead and also on the medial cheeks. Two mildly soaked cotton-tipped applicators can be used across the lips and chin, and one damp cotton-tipped applicator on the eyelids. Thus, the dosage of application is technique-dependent on the amount used and the number of cotton-

TABLE 4 The Jessner's Solution Formula

Resorcinol	14 g
Salicylic Acid	14 g
Lactic Acid	14 mL
Ethanol (qs)	100 mL

(a)
(b)
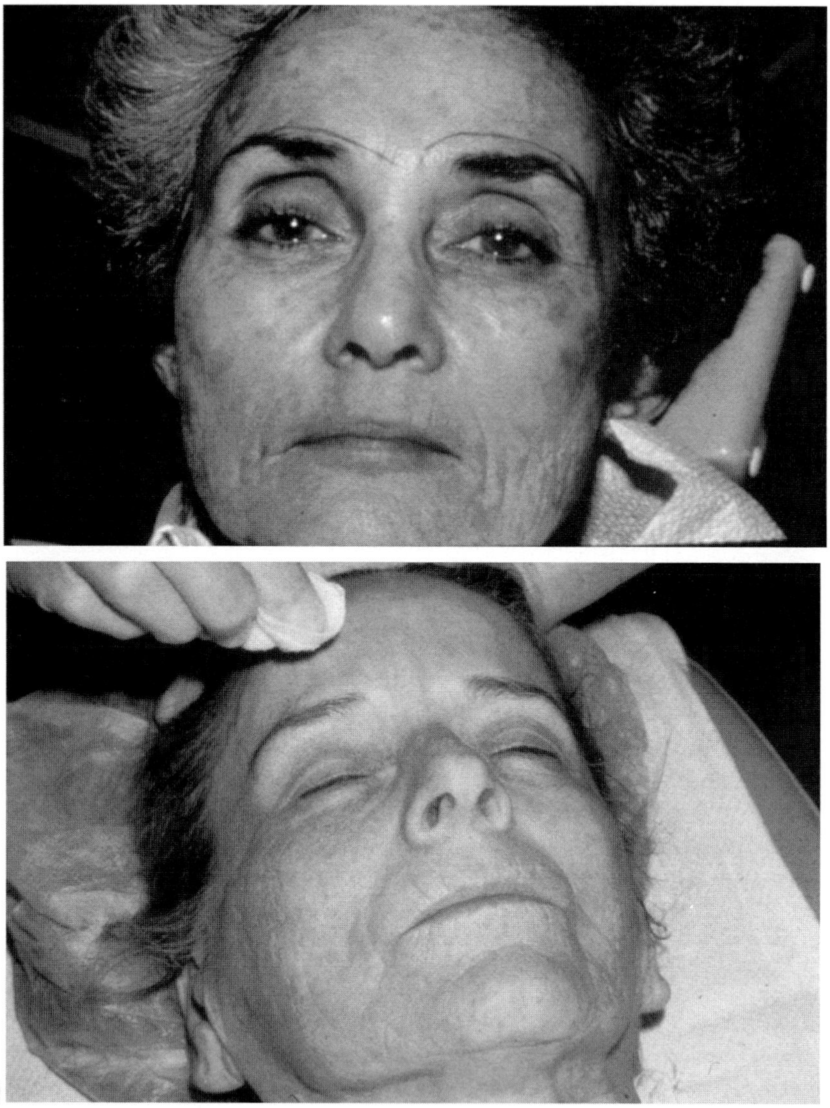

FIGURE 2 Chemical peeling for photoaging skin. (a) Presurgical appearance of Glogau II photoaging facial skin, (b) Jessner's solution applied with 2 × 2 gauze pads, (c) appearance of skin after Jessner's solution, (d) full application of 35% TCA with frosting, (e) appearance 4 days after surgery, and (f) appearance 6 months after surgery.

tipped applicators applied. The cotton-tipped applicator is useful in quantitating the amount of peel solution to be applied.

The white frost from the TCA application appears complete on the treated area within 30 seconds to 2 minutes. Even application should eliminate the need to go over areas a second or third time, but if frosting is incomplete or uneven the solution should be reapplied. TCA takes longer to frost than Baker's formula or straight phenol, but shorter than the superficial peeling agents. The surgeon should wait at

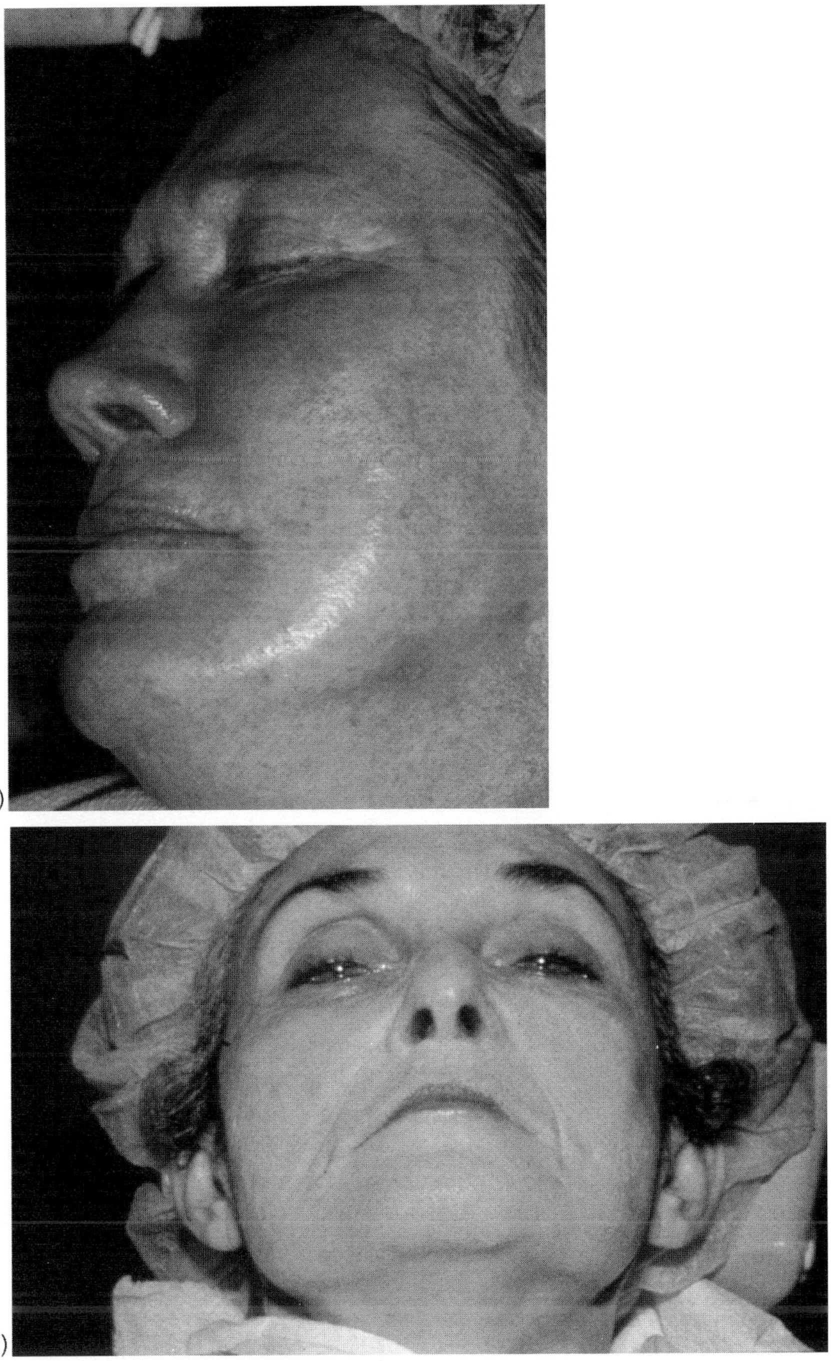

(c)

(d)

FIGURE 2 **Continued**

(e)
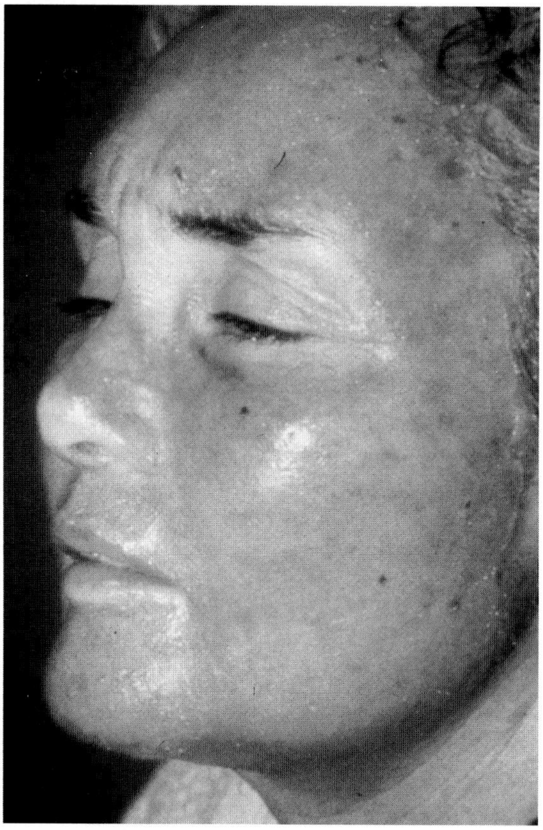

FIGURE 2 Continued

least 3 to 4 minutes after the application of TCA to ensure the frosting has reached its peak. He can then document the completedness of a frosted cosmetic unit and touch up the area as needed. Areas of poor frosting should be retreated carefully with a thin application of TCA. The physician should achieve a level II to level III frosting. Level I frosting is erythema with a stringy or blotchy frosting and is seen with light chemical peels. Level II frosting is defined as white-coated frosting with erythema showing through. A level III frosting, which is associated with penetration through the papillary dermis, is a solid white enamel frosting with little or no background of erythema [15]. A deeper level III frosting should be restricted only to areas of heavy actinic damage and thicker skin. Most medium-depth chemical peels use a level II frosting, and this is especially true when used on eyelids and areas of sensitive skin. Those areas with a greater tendency to scar formation, such as the zygomatic arch, the bony prominences of the jawline, and chin, should only receive up to a level II frosting. Overcoating trichloroacetic acid will increase its penetration so that a second or third application will drive the acid further into the dermis, creating a deeper peel. One must be careful in overcoating only areas in which the take-up was not adequate or the skin is much thicker (Fig. 3).

Anatomic areas of the face are peeled sequentially from forehead to temple to cheeks, and finally to the lips and eyelids. The white frosting indicates keratocoag-

(f) 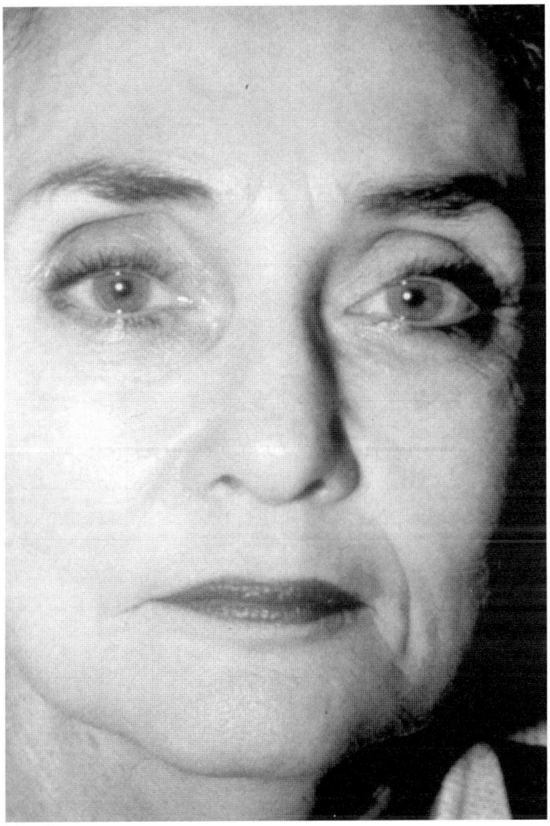

FIGURE 2 Continued

ulation or protein denaturation of keratin, and at that point the reaction is complete. Careful feathering of the solution into the hairline and around the rim of the jaw and brow conceals the line demarcation between peeled and nonpeeled areas. The perioral areas has rhytids that require a complete and even application of solution over the lip skin to the vermilion. This is accomplished best with the help of an assistant who stretches and fixates the upper and lower lips to which the peel solution is applied.

Certain areas and skin lesions require special attention. Thicker keratoses do not frost evenly and thus do not pick up peel solution. Additional applications rubbed vigorously into the lesion may be needed for peel solution penetration. Wrinkled skin should be stretched to allow an even coating of solution into the folds and troughs. Oral rhytides require peel solution to be applied with the wood portion of a cotton-tipped applicator and extended into the vermilion of the lip. Deeper furrows such as expression lines will not be eradicated by peel solution and thus should be treated like the remaining skin.

Eyelid skin must be treated delicately and carefully. A semidry applicator should be used to carry the solution within 2 to 3 mm of the lid margin. The patient should be positioned with the head elevated at 30 degrees and the eyelids closed.

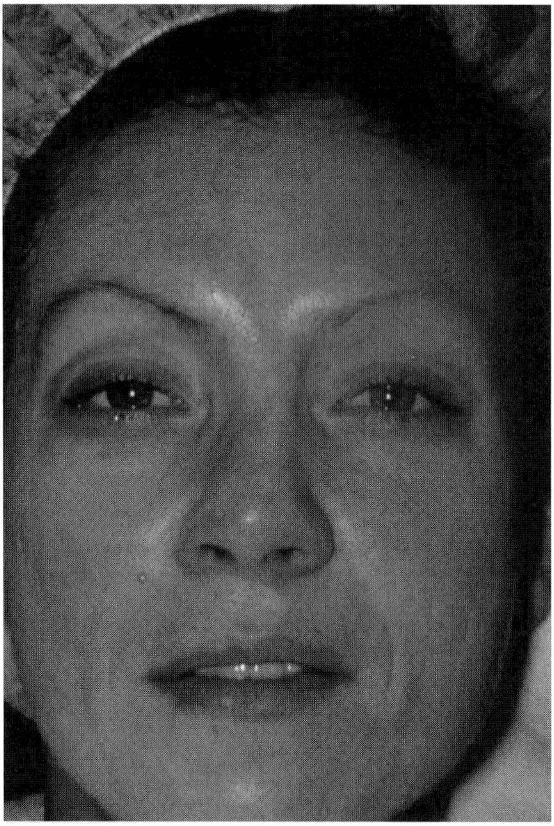

(a)

FIGURE 3 Skin appearance with levels of frosting. (a) Level I: Erythema with streaky frosting. (b) Level II: Even white frosting with erythema showing through. (c) Level III: Solid white enamel frosting.

Excess peel solution on the cotton tip should be drained gently on the bottom before application. The applicator is then rolled gently on the lids and periorbital skin. Never leave excess peel solution on the lids because the solution can roll into the eyes. Dry the tears with a cotton-tipped applicator during peeling because they may pull peel solution to the puncta and eye by capillary attraction (Fig. 4). The solution should be diluted immediately with cool saline compresses at the conclusion of the peel. The Jessner's–TCA peel procedure is as follows:

1. The skin is cleaned thoroughly with Septisol to remove oils.
2. Acetone or acetone alcohol is used to further debride oil and scale from the surface of the skin.
3. Jessner's solution is applied.
4. 35% TCA is applied until a light frost appears.
5. Cool saline compresses are applied to dilute the solution.
6. The peel will heal with 0.25% acetic acid soaks and a mild emollient cream.

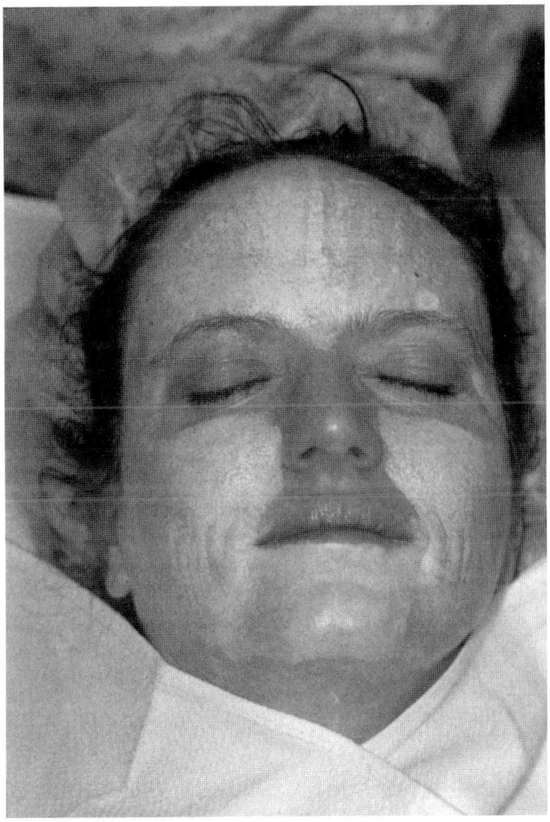

(b)

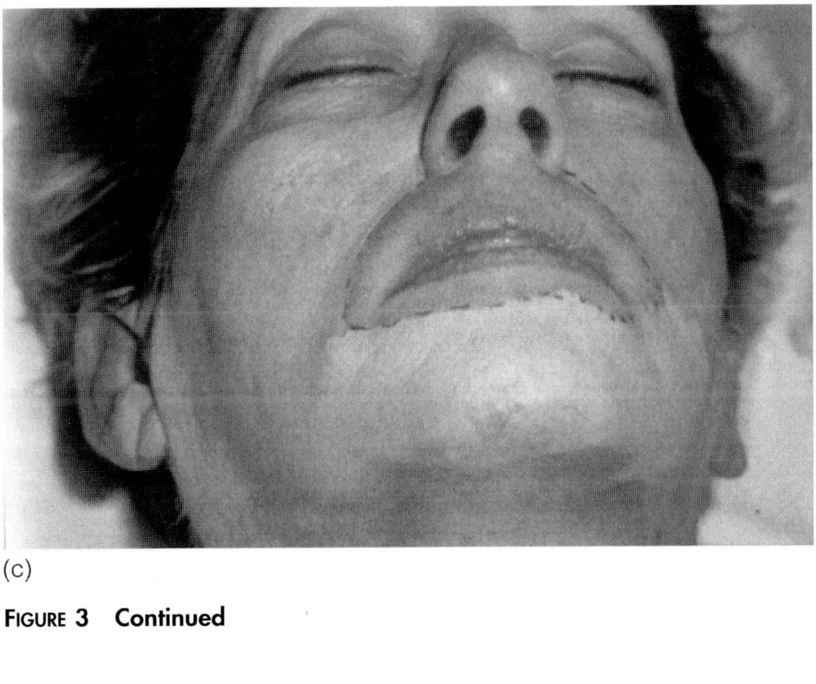

(c)

FIGURE 3 Continued

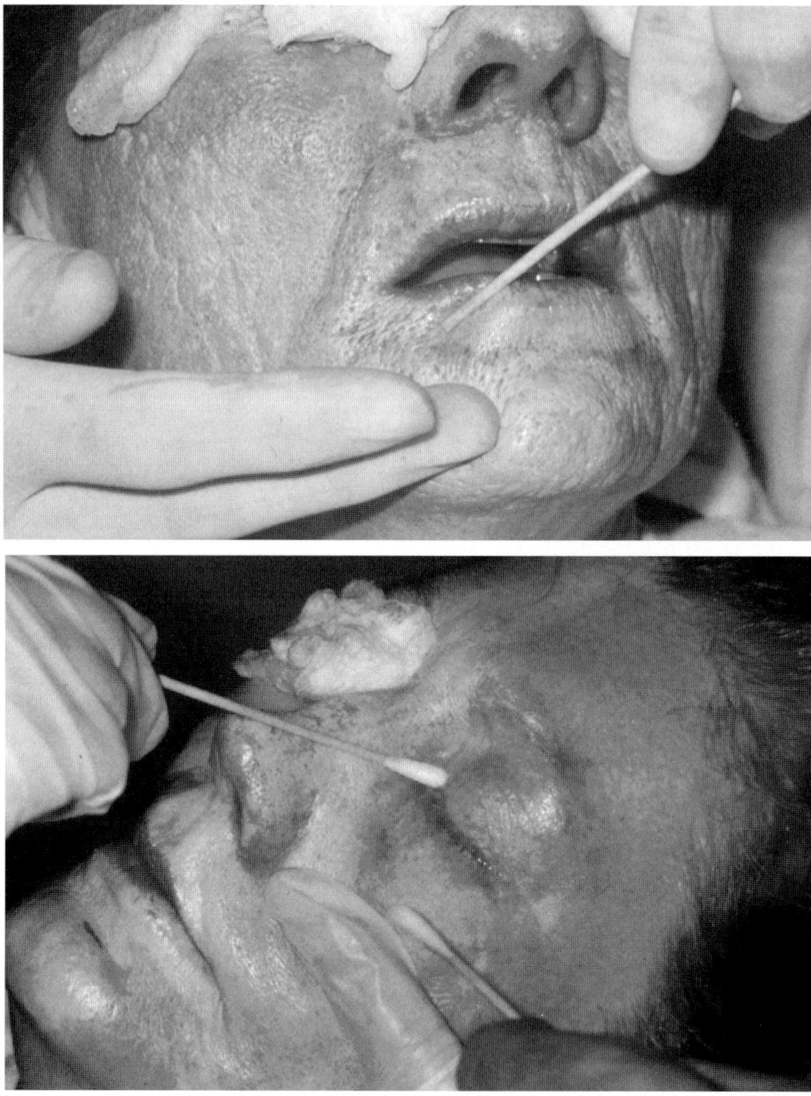

(a)

(b)

FIGURE 4 (a) Oral rhytids are treated with wood portion of cotton tip for deeper penetration. (b) Eyelids are painted cautiously with damp cotton-tip applicators; dry cotton tips are used to blot the tears.

There is an immediate burning sensation as the peel solution is applied, but this subsides as frosting is completed. Cool saline compresses offer symptomatic relief for a peeled area as the solution is applied to other areas. The peel reaction is not neutralized by saline solution as the reaction is completed when frosting occurs [16]. The compresses are placed over the face for 5 to 6 minutes after the peel until the patient is comfortable. The burning subsides fully by the time the patient is ready to be discharged. At that time, most of the frosting has faded and a brawny desquamation is beginning.

Postoperatively, edema, erythema, and desquamation are expected. With periorbital peels and even forehead peels, eyelid edema can occur and may be enough to close the lids. For the first 24 hours, the patient is instructed to soak four times a day with a 0.25% acetic acid compress made of 1 tablespoon white vinegar in 1 pint of warm water. A bland emollient is applied to the desqumating areas after soaks. After 24 hours, the patient can shower and clean gently with a mild nondetergent cleanser. The erythema intensifies as desquamation becomes complete within 4 to 5 days. Thus, healing is completed within 1 week to 10 days. At the end of 1 week, the bright red color has faded to pink and has the appearance of a sunburn. This can be covered by cosmetics and will fade fully within 2 to 3 weeks.

The medium-depth peel is dependent on three components for therapeutic effect: (1) degreasing, (2) Jessner's solution, and (3) 35% TCA. The amount of each agent applied creates the intensity and thus the effectiveness of this peel. The variables can be adjusted according to the patient's skin type and the areas of the face being treated. It is thus the workhorse of peeling and resurfacing in my practice as it can be individuated for most patients I see.

The medium-depth chemical peel thus has five major indications: (1) destruction of epidermal lesions–actinic keratoses, (2) resurfacing the level II or III moderate photoaging skin, (3) pigmentary dyschromias, (4) mild acne scars, and (5) blending photoaging skin with laser resurfacing and deep chemical peeling.

1. *Actinic keratoses*. This procedure is well suited for the patient with epidermal lesions, such as actinic keratoses, that have required repeated removal with either cryosurgery or chemoexfoliation (5-fluoruracil). The entire face can be treated as a unit or subfacial cosmetic unit such as forehead, temples, and cheeks, and can be treated independently. Active lesions can be removed, along with incipient growths as yet undetected, as the epidermis is sloughed. Advantages for the patient with photodamaged skin include a limited recovery period of 7 to 10 days, with little postoperative erythema after healing. There is little risk of pigmentary changes such as hypopigmentation or hyperpigmentation; therefore, the patient can return to work after the skin has healed (Fig. 5).

2. *Moderate photoaging skin*. Glogau level II or III damage responds well to this peeling combination by removing epidermal lesions and dermal changes, thereby freshening photoaging which is characterized as sallow, atrophic skin with fine rhytides. This peel is favored over deeper resurfacing procedures such as laser and deep peel because it will heal in 10 days with minimal risk of textural or color complications. However, it is only designed for medium-depth damage (Fig. 6).

3. *Pigmentary dyschromias*. Although color change can be treated with repetitive chemical peeling, the medium-depth peel will be a single treatment preceded and followed by the use of bleaching agents and retinoic acid [17]. In most cases, the pigmentary problems are resolved with this single peel as an adjunct to the skin care program (Fig. 7).

4. *Blending other resurfacing procedures*. In a patient in whom there is advanced photoaging changes, such as crow's feet and rhytides in the periorbital and/or perioral area with medium-depth changes on the remaining face, a medium-depth peel can be used to integrate these procedures. Laser resurfacing or deep chemical peeling can be performed over the periorbital and perioral areas that have more advanced photoaging changes, while the medium-depth chemical peel is used for the rest of the face. This will blend the facial skin as a unit so that the therapeutic

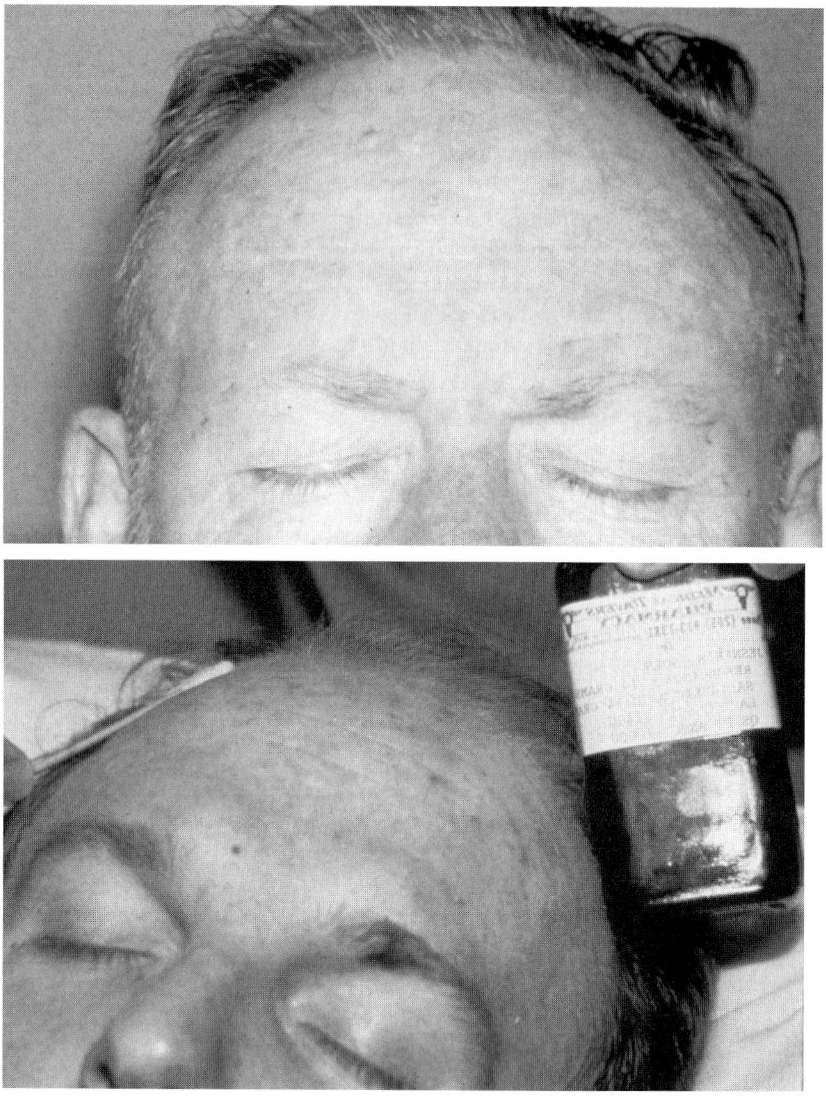

(a) (b)

FIGURE 5 Treatment of actinic keratoses with Jessner's 35% TCA peel. (a) Presurgical appearance, (b) application of Jessner's Solution, (c) Jessner's solution with 35% TCA, (d) after surgery—4 days with desquamation and brisk erythema, and (e) 3 months after surgery.

textural and color changes will not be restricted to one area. The patients requiring laser resurfacing in a localized cosmetic unit will have the remaining areas of their face blended with this medium-depth chemical peel. Patients having laser resurfacing or deep peeling to the perioral or periorbital areas alone develop a pseudohypopigmentation that is a noticeable deformity. The patient requiring laser resurfacing at a localized cosmetic unit will have the remaining areas of their face blended with this medium-depth peel. The alternative—a full-face deep peel or laser resurfacing—has

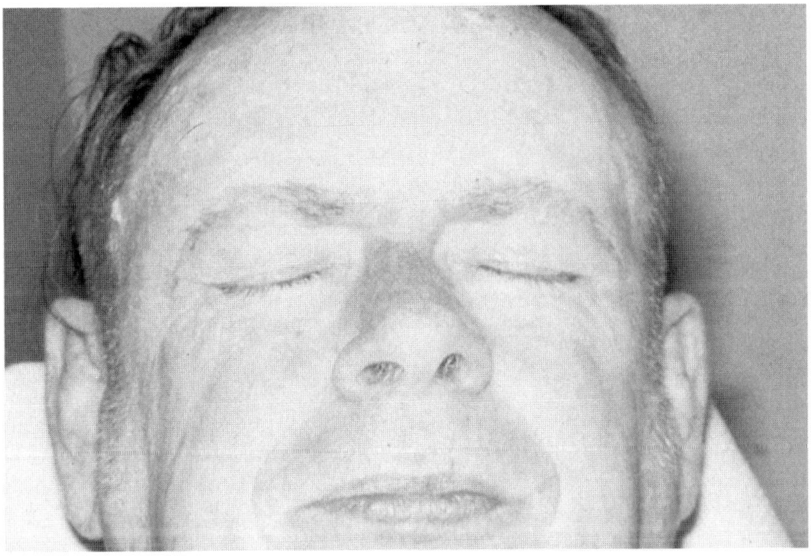

(c)

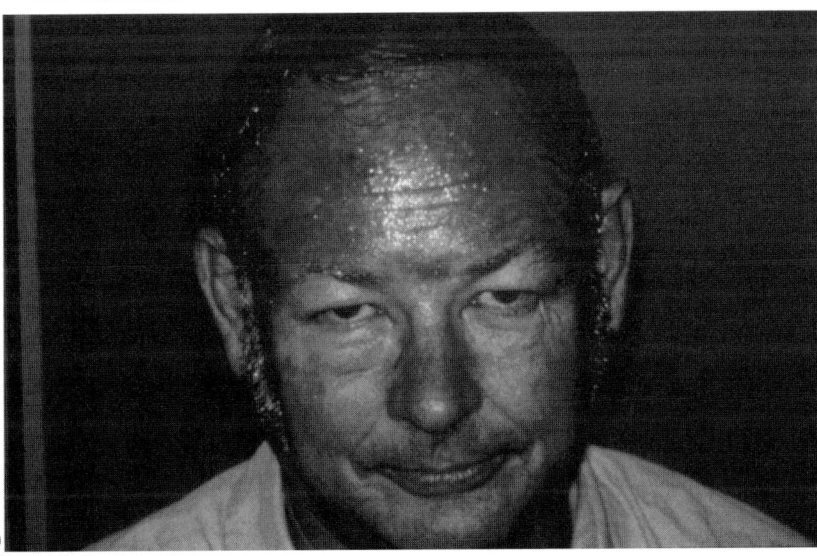

(d)

FIGURE 5 Continued

an increased morbidity, longer healing, and risk of scarring over areas such as the lateral jaw line, malar eminences, and forehead. If deep resurfacing is only needed over localized areas such as perioral or periorbital face, a blending medium-depth peel reduces morbidity and healing time (Fig. 8) [18].

DEEP CHEMICAL PEELING

Glogau level III and IV photodamage requires deep chemical peeling. This entails the use of either trichloroacetic acid above 50% or the Gordon-Baker phenol peel. Laser resurfacing can also be used to reliably reach this level of damage. TCA above

(e) 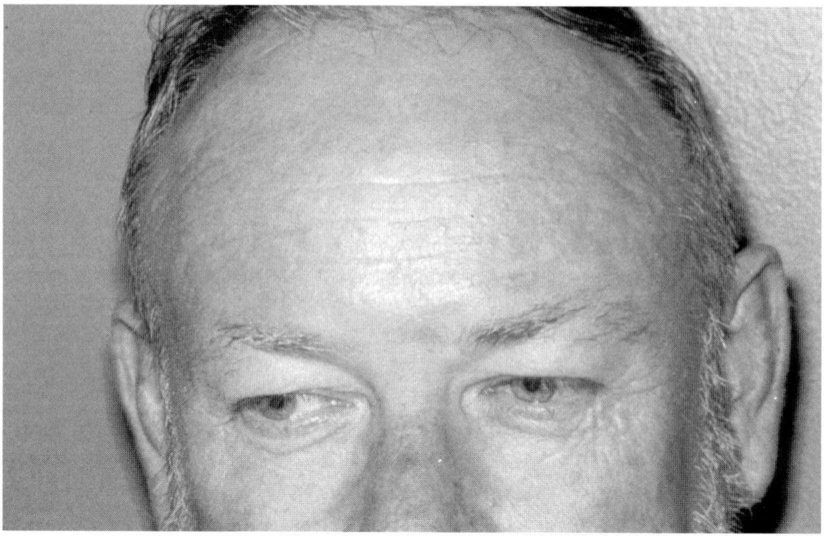

FIGURE 5 Continued

45% has been found to be unreliable and dangerous with a high incidence of scarring and postoperative complications. For this reason, it is not included as a preferred treatment method for deep chemical peeling. The Baker-Gordon phenol peel has been used successfully for over 40 years for deep chemical peeling and produces reliable results (Fig. 9) (Table 5). It is a labor-intensive procedure that must be taken seriously as all major surgical procedures are.

The patient requires preoperative sedation with an intravenous line and preoperative IV hydration. Usually a liter of fluid is given preoperatively, and in addition a liter of fluid is given during the procedure. This is helpful in decreasing the phenol concentration from the serum. For this reason, one must be concerned with phenol absorption through the skin and the resultant serum concentration of phenol through cutaneous absorption. Methods to limit this include

1. IV hydration prior to the procedure and during the peel to flush the phenolic products through the serum.
2. Extending the time of application for a full-face peel over 1.5 hours. Baker's solution is applied to each cosmetic unit with a 15-minute wait in between each unit. That is, the forehead, cheeks, chin, lips, and eyelids are each given a 15-minute period of time for a total of 1 to 1.5 hours for the procedure.
3. All patients are monitored, and if there is any electrocardiographic abnormality, i.e., PVC or PAC, the procedure is stopped and the patient is watched carefully for other signs of toxicity.
4. Many physicians believe that O_2 given during the procedure can be helpful in preventing arrhythmic complications.
5. Any patient with a history of cardioarrhythmia, hepatic or renal compromise, or who is on medications that give a propensity for arrhythmias should not undergo the Baker-Gordon phenol peel [19].

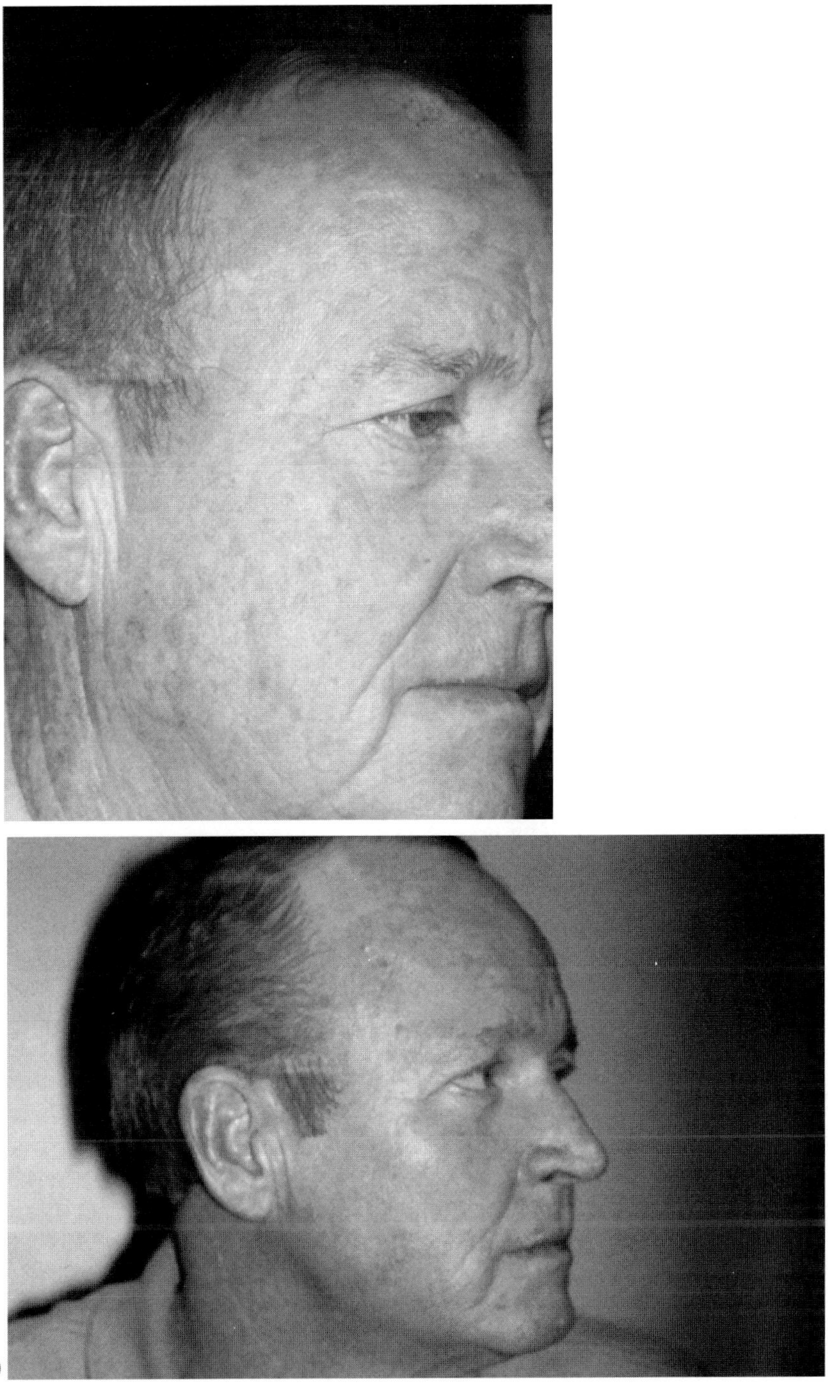

(a)

(b)

FIGURE 6 Treatment of moderate photoaging skin. (a) Presurgical appearance. (b) Appearance 6 months after surgery.

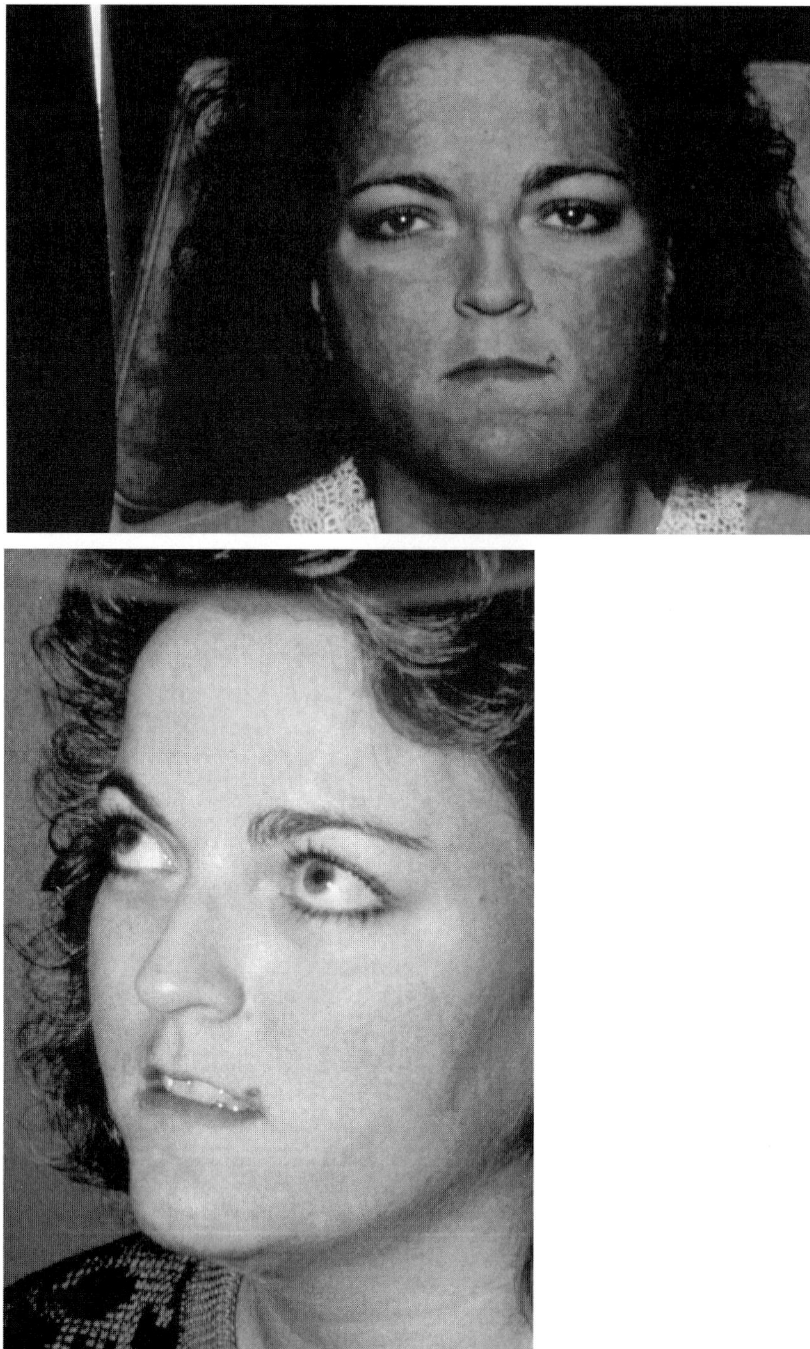

(a)

(b)

FIGURE 7 Treatment of pigmentary dyschromias with medium-depth chemical peel and cosmoceutical treatment with tretinoin and hydroquinone 4%. (a) Appearance before surgery. (b) Appearance 6 months after surgery.

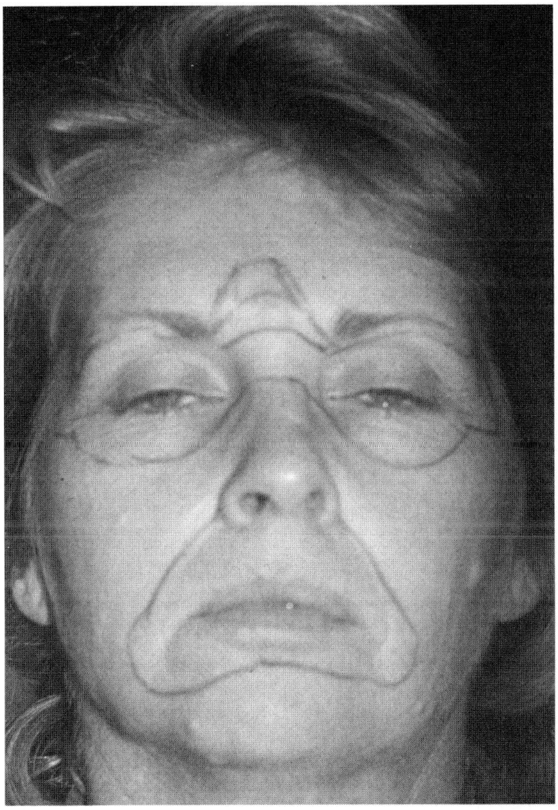

(a)

FIGURE 8 Combination deep chemical peel—perioral area with medium-depth peel over remaining face. (a) Before surgery, (b) peel solution applied, and (c) after surgery.

The patient undergoing deep chemical peeling must recognize the significant risk factors, the increased morbidity, and possible complications involved in this procedure so that the benefits can be weighed positively against these particular factors. In the hands of those that perform this technique regularly, it is a reliable and safe method of rejuvenating advanced to severe photoaged skin including deeper perioral rhytids, periorbital rhytids and crow's feet, forehead lines and wrinkles, as well as the other textural and lesional changes associated with the more severe photoaging process.

There are two methods for deep chemical peeling: Baker's formula phenol unoccluded and Baker's formula phenol occluded with tape (Fig. 10). Occlusion is accomplished with the application of waterproof zinc oxide tape such as 0.5 in Curity tape. The tape is placed directly after the phenol is applied to each individual cosmetic unit. Tape occlusion increases the penetration of the Baker's phenol solution and is particularly helpful for deeply lined "weather-beaten" faces. A taped Baker's formula phenol peel creates the deepest damage in midreticular dermis and this form of chemical peeling should only be performed by the most knowledgeable and experienced cosmetic surgeons who understand the risks of overpenetration and deep

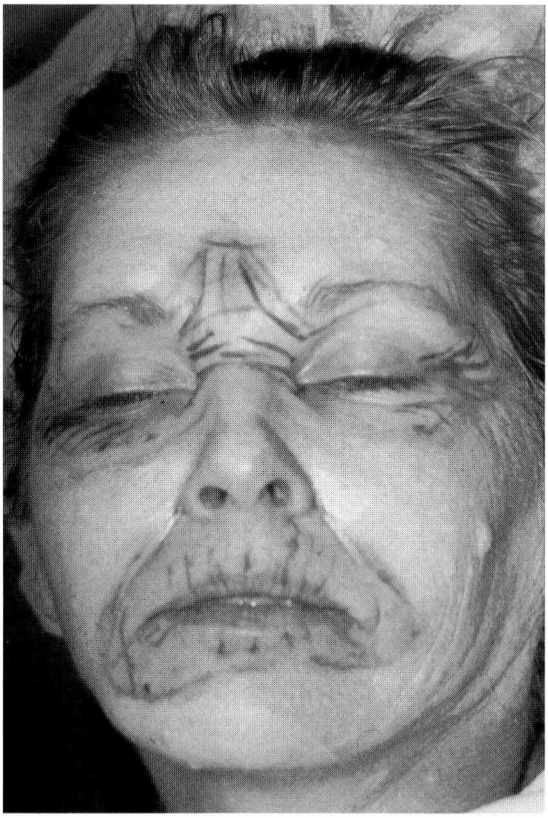

(b)

FIGURE 8 Continued

damage to the reticular dermis [20]. The unoccluded technique as modified by McCollough involves more skin cleansing and application of more peel solution. On the whole, this technique does not produce as deep a peel as the occluded method [21].

When the Baker's peel was first popularized in the 1970s, taping and dry healing would produce both color and textural changes on most patients. This included hypopigmentation with alabaster skin texture. Most patients were told that they would need make-up to disguise the color and textural changes. This is currently unacceptable because natural appearance of skin texture has become more important.

The Baker-Gordon formula for this peel was first described in 1961, and since then has been used successfully for over 25 years. The Baker-Gordon formula of phenol (Table 3) penetrates further into the dermis than full-strength undiluted phenol, because full-strength phenol allegedly causes an immediate coagulation of epidermal keratin proteins and self-blocks further penetration. Dilution to approximately 50 to 55% in the Baker-Gordon formula causes keratolysis and keratocoagulation resulting in greater penetration. The liquid soap, Septisol, is a surfactant that reduces skin tension, thereby allowing a more even penetration. Croton oil is a vesicant and epidermolytic agent that enhances phenol absorption. The freshly prepared formula

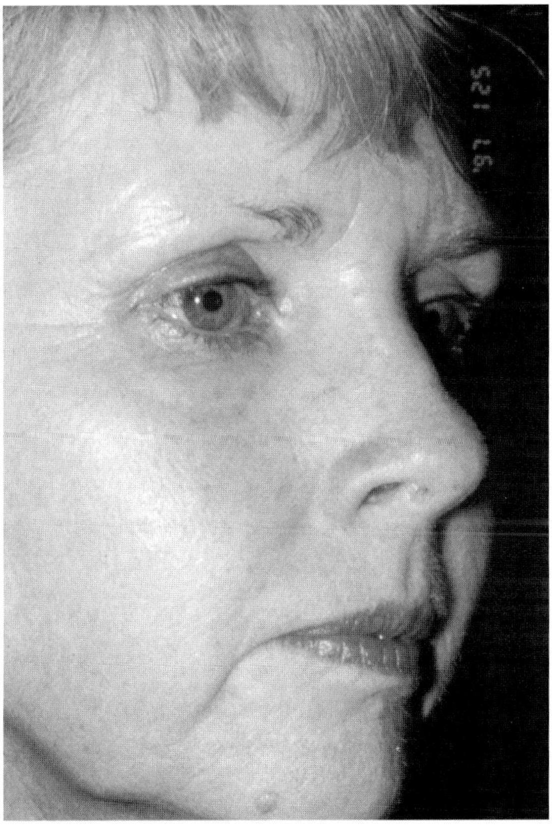

(c)

FIGURE 8 Continued

is not miscible, but rather is a suspension and must be stirred in a clear glass medicine cup immediately before application to the patient. Although the mixture can be stored in an amber glass bottle for short periods, this is usually unnecessary and it should be reformulated on a regular basis.

TECHNIQUES

Before the administration of anesthesia, the patient's face is marked in seated position noting landmarks such as the mandibular angle, the chin, the preauricular sulcus, the orbital rim, and the forehead. The markings delineate the borders of the peel throughout the limits of the face and slightly over the mandibular rim to blend any color change. This peel does require sedation. An intravenous combination such as fentanyl citrate (Sublimaze) and midazolam (Versed) can be administered intravenously by an anesthetist while the patient is monitored and given intravenous sedation. It is helpful to use local nerve blocks along the supraorbital and infraorbital nerve, and along the mental nerve with Marcaine, which should provide some local anesthesia for up to 4 hours. This is helpful with postoperative pain.

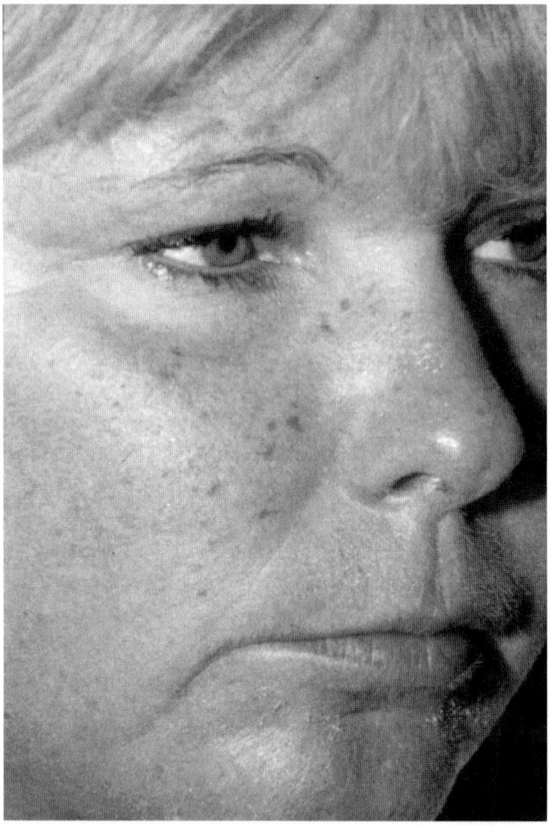

(a)

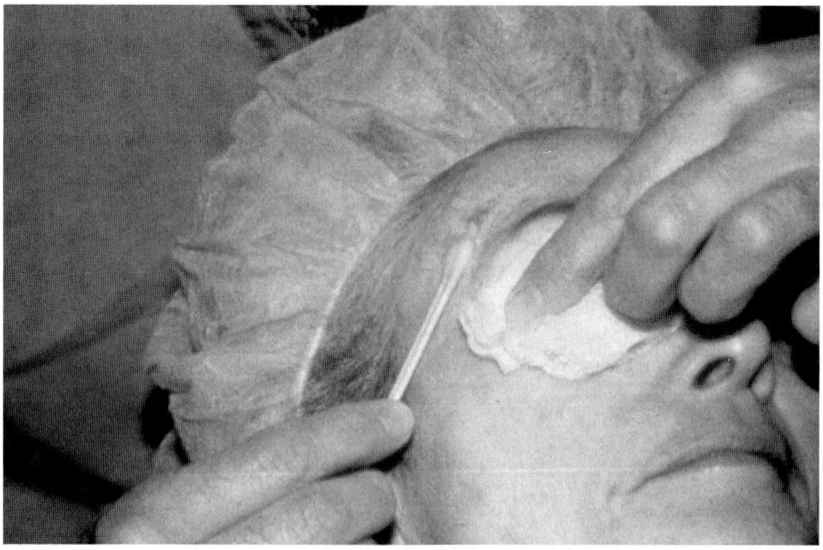

(b)

FIGURE 9 Baker-Gordon Phenol Peel performed for rhytids—unoccluded technique. (a) Before surgery, (b) application of Baker's solution, (c) frosting appearance (which fades rapidly), (d) appearance 3 days after surgery, and (e) appearance 6 months after surgery.

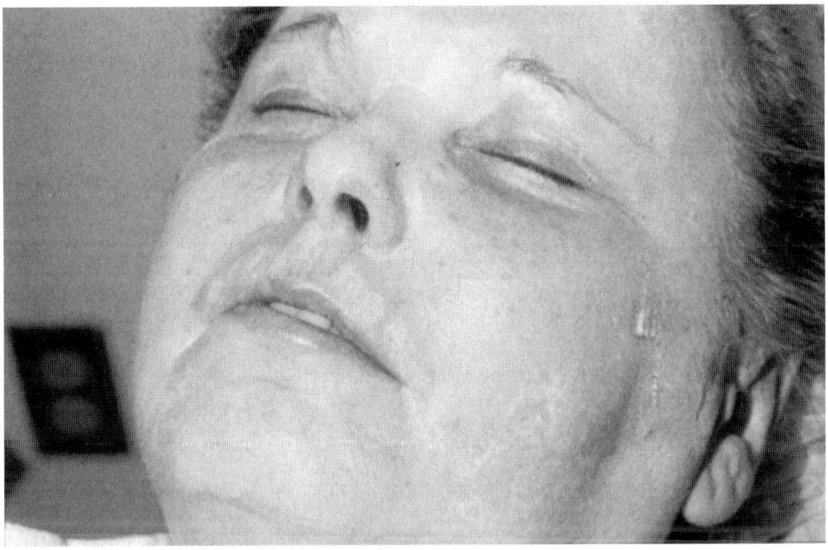

(c)

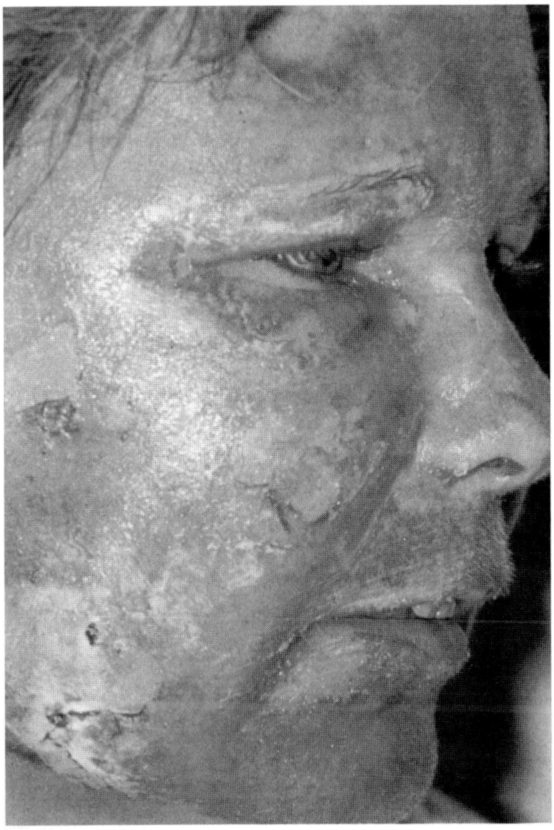

(d)

FIGURE 9 Continued

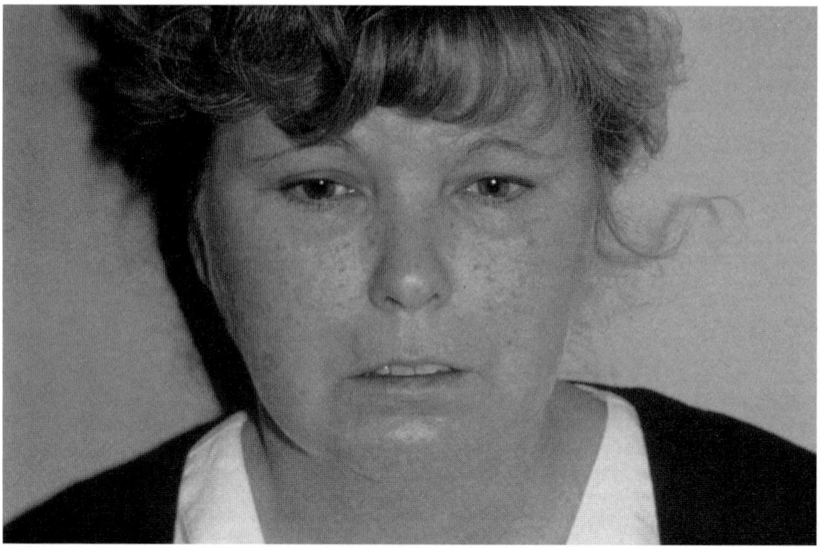

(e)

FIGURE 9 Continued

The patients should arrive n.p.o., and have shaved and cleansed their face the morning of surgery. The face then is cleansed and degreased with a keratolytic agent such as hexochlorophine with alcohol (Septisol) over the entire face with emphasis placed on oily areas such as the nose, the hairline, and midfacial cheeks. A thorough and evenly distributed cleansing or degreasing of the face will assure a more uniform peel without skipped areas.

The phenol chemical agent is then applied sequentially to the six aesthetic units: forehead, perioral, right, and left cheeks, nose, and periorbital areas. Each cosmetic area takes 15 minutes for application, allowing 60 to 90 minutes for the entire procedure. Cotton-tipped applicators are used with a similar technique as discussed on the medium-depth Jessner–35% TCA peel. However, less agent is used because frosting occurs very rapidly. The last area for the peel is the periorbital skin on which the chemical is applied with damp cotton-tipped applicators, taking care to keep the drops away from the eye and tears off the skin. Tearing may allow the peel solution to reach the eye by capillary attraction. It is important to remember that water dilution of this chemical may increase the absorption; therefore, if the chemical does get into the eye, these should be flushed with mineral oil rather than water. An immediate

TABLE 5 Formula for the Baker-Gordon Phenol Peel

3 mL USP liquid phenol 88%
2 mL tap water
8 drops liquid soap (Septisol)
3 drops croton oil

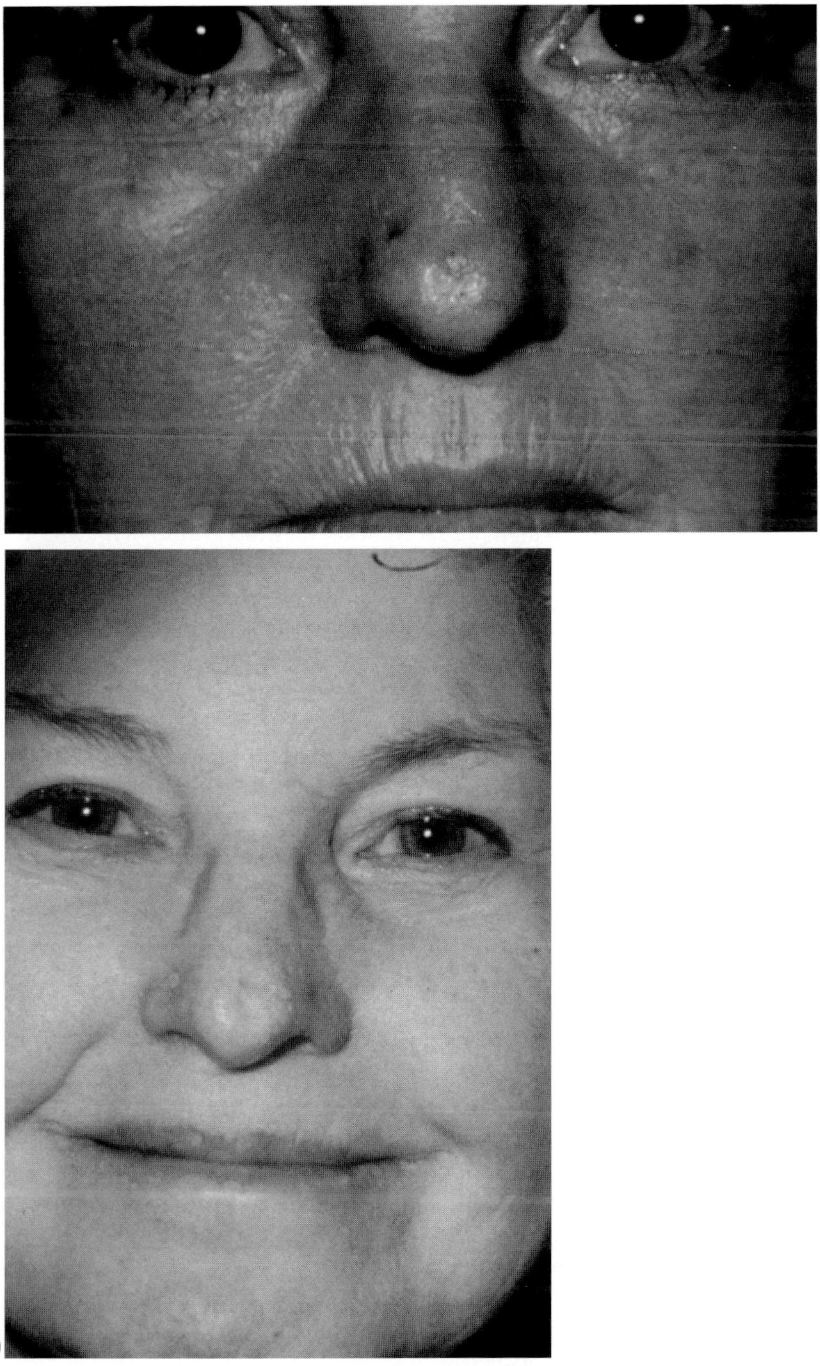

(a) (b)

FIGURE 10 Baker's Phenol Peel for photoaging skin, Glogau III. (a) Appearance before surgery. (b) Appearance 6 months after surgery.

burning sensation is present for 15 to 20 seconds, and then subsides. The pain returns in 20 minutes and persists for 6 to 8 hours.

After the full application of peel solution, the white frosting gradually develops a brawny brown color and the tape can be applied for an occluded peel. Ice packs can be applied at the conclusion of the peel for comfort, and if this is an untaped peel, petrolatum is used. A biosynthetic dressing such as Vigilon or Flexzan can be used for the first 24 hours. The patient is usually seen in 24 hours to either remove the tape or the biosynthetic dressing and to monitor the healing. It is at this time the patient is again reinstructed in the method of compresses and occlusive ointments or dressings. It is important to keep the skin crust-free.

The four stages of wound healing are apparent after a deep chemical peel. They include: (1) inflammation, (2) coagulation, (3) re-epithelialization, and (4) fibroplasia [23]. At the conclusion of the chemical peel, the inflammatory phase has already begun with a brawny, dusky erythema that will progress over the first 12 hours. This is an accentuation of the pigmented lesions on the skin as the coagulation phase separates the epidermis, producing serum exudation, crusting, and pyoderma. It is during this phase that it is important to use debridant soaks and compresses as well as occlusive salves. These will remove the sloughed, necrotic epidermis and prevent the serum exudate from hardening as crust and scab. I prefer the use of 0.25% acetic acid soaks found in the vinegar/water preparation (1 teaspoon white vinegar, 1 pint warm water) because it is antibacterial, especially against pseudomonas and gram negatives. In addition, the mildly acidic nature of the solution is physiological for the healing granulation tissue, and mildly debridant, as it will dissolve and cleanse the necrotic material and serum. I prefer to use bland emollients and salves such as Vaseline petrolatum, Eucerin, or Aquaphor, as the skin can be monitored carefully day by day for potential complications.

Re-epithelialization begins on day 3 and continues until day 10 to 14. Occlusive salves promote faster re-epithelialization and less tendency for delayed healing, which may occur with dry crusting. The final stage of wound healing, fibroplasia, will continue well beyond the initial closure of the peeled wound and continues with neoangiogenesis and new collagen formation for 3 or 4 months. Prolonged erythema may last 2 to 4 months in unusual cases of sensitive skin or with contact dermatitis. New collagen formation can continue to improve texture and rhytides for a period up to 4 months during this last phase of fibroplasia.

COMPLICATIONS

Many of the complications seen in peeling can be recognized early on during healing stages. The cosmetic surgeon should be well acquainted with the normal appearance of a healing wound and its time frame for both medium and deep peeling. Prolongation of the granulation tissue phase beyond a week to 10 days may indicate delayed wound healing. This could be the result of viral, bacterial, or fungal infections, contact dermatitis interfering with wound healing, or other systemic factors. A red flag should alert the physician to carefully investigate and institute prompt treatment to forstall potential irreparable damage that may result in scarring [24].

Complications can be caused either intraoperatively or postoperatively. The two inherent errors that lead to intraoperative complications are incorrect peel pharmacology and accidental solution misplacement. It is the physician's responsibility to know the solution and its concentration is correct. Trichloroacetic acid concentrations should be measured weight by volume as this is the standard for measuring depth of peel. Glycolic acid and lactic acid solutions as well as Jessner's solution must be checked for expiration date as the potency decreases with time. Alcohol or water absorption may inappropriately increase the potency, so one must assure the shelf life is appropriate. The peel solution should be applied with cotton-tipped applicators, and in medium and deep peels it is best to pour the peel solution in a secondary container rather than apply the solution spun around the neck of the bottle. Intact crystals may give the solution a higher concentration as it is taken directly from its container. One should be careful to apply the solution to its appropriate location and not to pass the wet cotton-tipped applicator directly over the central face where a drop may inadvertently get on sensitive areas such as the eyes. Saline and bicarbonate of soda should be available to dilute TCA or neutralize glycolic acid if placed in the wrong area. Likewise, mineral oil should be present for Baker's phenol peels. Post-operative complications can result from local infection or contact dermatitis. The best deterrent for local infection is the continuous use of soaks to debride crusting and necrotic material. Streptococcus and staphylococcus infection can occur under biosynthetic membranes or thick occlusive ointments. The use of 0.25% acetic acid soaks seems to deter this as well as the judicious removal of the ointment with each soak. *Staphylococcus*, *e. coli*, or even *pseudomonas* may result from improper care during healing and should be treated promptly with the appropriate oral antibiotic.

Frequent postoperative visits are necessary to recognize the early onset of a bacterial infection. It may present itself as delayed wound healing, ulcerations, build-up of necrotic material with excessive scabbing, crusting, purulent drainage, and odor. Early recognition and institution of appropriate antibiotics will prevent the spread of infection, heal the skin, and prevent scarring.

Herpes simplex infection is the result of reactivation of the herpes simplex virus (HSV) on the face and most commonly on the perioral area. A history of previous HSV infection should necessitate the use of prophylactic oral antiviral medications. Patients with a positive history can be treated with 400 mg of acyclovir three times a day beginning on the day of the peel and continuing for 7 to 14 days, depending on whether it is a medium-depth or deep chemical peel. I prefer to treat all patients with antiviral agents irregardless of a positive history as many patients do not remember prior herpes simplex infection that may have occurred years ago. The mechanism of action of all antiviral agents is to inhibit viral replication in the intact epidermal cell. This would mean that the drug would not have an inhibitory effect until the skin is re-epithelialized, which is 7 to 10 days in medium and deep peels. In the past, these agents were discontinued at 5 days, and in treated patients, clinical infection became apparent in 7 to 10 days [24]. Active herpetic infections can be easily treated with antiviral agents and, caught early, they usually do not result in scars.

Delayed wound healing and persistent erythema are signs that the peel is not healing normally. The cosmetic surgeon must know the normal timetable for each of the healing events so that he may recognize when healing is delayed or the erythema is not fading adequately. Delayed wound healing may respond to physician debridement if an infection is present, to corticosteroids if caused by contact allergic or contact irritant dermatitis, along with the change of the offending contact agent, or to protection with a biosynthetic membrane such as Flexzan or Vigilon. When this diagnosis is made, these patients must be followed daily with dressing changes and a close watch on the healing skin.

Persistent erythema is a syndrome where the skin remains erythematous beyond what is normal for the individual peel. A superficial peel loses its erythema in 3 to 5 days, a medium-depth peel within 15 to 30 days, and a deep chemical peel within 60 to 90 days. Erythema and/or pruritus beyond this period of time is considered abnormal and fits this syndrome. It may be contact dermatitis, contact sensitization, re-exacerbation of prior skin disease, or a genetic susceptibility to erythema. It is also a red flag that indicates a sign of potential scarring. Erythema is the result of the angiogenic factors stimulating vasodilation which indicates that the phase of fibroplasia is being stimulated for a prolonged period of time. For this reason, it can be accompanied by skin thickening and scarring. It should be treated promptly and appropriately with topical steroids, systemic steroids, intralesional steroids if thickening is occurring, and skin protection which would eliminate the factors of irritancy and allergy. If thickening or scarring becomes evident, other measures that can be helpful include the daily use of silicone sheeting and the dye pulsed vascular laser to treat the vascular factors. With prompt intervention, scarring in many cases can be averted.

CONCLUSION

The physician has the responsibility of choosing the correct modality to treat skin conditions such as photoaging skin, scars, dyschromias, and the removal of skin growths. There are many agents available including the three levels of chemical peels reviewed. It is the responsibility of the physician to have thorough knowledge of all of these tools to give each patient the treatment his condition warrants.

REFERENCES

1. Stegman SJ. A comparative histologic study of the effects of three peeling agents and dermabrasion on normal and sun-damaged skin. Aesthetic Plast Surg 1982; 6:123–125.
2. Fitzpatrick TB. The validity and practicality of sun-reactive skin types I through VI. Archiv Dermatol 1988; 124:869–871.
3. Monheit GD. Chemical peeling for pigmentary dyschromias. Cosmet Dermatol 1995; 8(5):10–15.
4. Glogau RG. Chemical peeling and aging skin. J Geratr Dermatol 1994; 2(1):30–35.
5. Monheit GD. Presentations at the American Academy of Dermatology in New Orleans. March 25, 1999.
6. Wolfe SA. Chemical face peeling following therapeutic irradiation. Plastic Reconstr Surg 1982; 69:859.
7. Monheit GD. Facial resurfacing may trigger the herpes simplex virus. Cosmet Dermatol 1995; 8(7):9–16.
8. Glogau RG. Chemical peeling and aging skin. J Geratr Dermatol 1994; 2(1):30–35.
9. Brody HJ. Trichloroacetic acid application in chemical peeling, operative techniques. Plast Reconstr Surg 1994; 2(2):127–128.
10. Brody HJ. Variations and comparisons in medium depth chemical peeling. J Dermatol Surg Oncol 1989; 15:953–963.
11. Monheit GD. The Jessner's + TCA peel: a medium depth chemical peel. J Dermatol Surg Oncol 1989; 15:945–950.
12. Lawrence N, Brody H, Alt T. Chemical peeling. Resurfacing Techniques, p. 95.

13. Katz B. The 5-FU TCA peel. J Derm Surg
14. Monheit GD. The Jessner's-trichloroacetic acid peel. Dermatol Clin 1995; 13(2):277–283.
15. Rubin M. Manual of chemical peels. Philadelphia: Lippincott, 1995:120–121.
16. Monheit GD. The Jessner's-TCA peel. Facial Plast Surg Clin N Am 1994; 2(1):21–22.
17. Monheit GD. Skin preparation: an essential step before chemical peeling or laser resurfacing. Cosmet Dermatol 1996; 9(9):13–14.
18. Monheit GD, Zeitouni NC. Skin resurfacing for photoaging: laser resurfacing versus chemical peeling. Cosmet Dermatol 1997; 10(4):11–22.
19. Baker TJ, Gordon HL. Chemical face peeling. Surgical Rejuvenation of the Face. Mosby, 1986.
20. Alt T. Occluded Baker/Gordon chemical peel. Review and update. J. Dermatol Surg Oncol 1989; 15:998.
21. McCollough EG, Langsdon PR. Chemical peeling with phenol. In: Roenigk H, Roenigk R, eds. Dermatologic Surgery: Principles and Practice. New York: Marcel Dekker, 1989.
22. Falanga V. Occlusive wound dressings. Arch Dermatol 1988; 124:877.
23. Goslen JB. Wound healing after cosmetic surgery. In: Coleman WP, Hanke CW, Alt TH, et al., eds. Cosmetic Surgery of the Skin. Philadelphia: BC Decker, 1991:47–63.
24. Monheit GD. Facial resurfacing may trigger the herpes simplex virus. Cosmet Dermatol 1995; 8(7):9–16.

5

The Total Body Peel: Peeling the Skin of the Neck, Chest, Hands, and Other Areas

Kim K. Cook
Coronado Skin Medical Center, Inc., Coronado, California

INTRODUCTION

Patients seeking cosmetic surgery often show many epidermal and dermal lesions. Irregular pigmentation, lentigines, keratoses, wrinkling, roughness, striae distensae, and other problems may be present, caused by sun damage and aging skin. Facial skin resurfacing with a laser or chemical peel can greatly improve the patient's appearance. This treatment in properly selected patients not only minimizes wrinkles, roughness, and pigmented lesions, but also gives the skin a more vigorous and youthful quality by the formation of new collagen and reorganization of elastic fibers in the skin [1,2].

Resurfacing procedures have traditionally been limited to the face for technical reasons. However, when the face alone is resurfaced, the result in some patients may be a sharp line of demarcation between the treated skin of the face and the untreated skin of the neck and chest. This results in an unnatural looking appearance and can leave the patient with a less than optimal cosmetic result.

For this reason, I have developed a method of more "controlled" chemical peeling that has proven to be safe and effective in peeling nonfacial skin. I call this technique the Cook Total Body Peel. (The term "Total Body Peel" does not mean that I peel the entire body of every patient, but that the technique can be used on any part of the body.) This controlled chemical peel technique uses a combination of glycolic acid gel and trichloroacetic acid (TCA). Neutralization with copious quantities of sodium bicarbonate solution permits precise timing and limits the extent and depth of the peel [3].

The Cook Total Body Peel reduces or eliminates the sharp transition in appearance that can occur between treated and untreated areas. It permits a blending of the facial skin with the neck, chest, hands, and other areas. It can be performed on almost all areas of the body and most skin types. It is particularly helpful on patients with freckled or actinically damaged necks, chests, and hands.

The result is a peel ranging in depth from light to medium. The depth is controlled by the physician and is almost entirely technique-dependent. I have used this method for the past 7 years on more than 2800 patients, with consistently good results on the neck, chest, hands, arms, legs, back, and even the face.

HISTORY

Historically, the standard techniques for skin peeling have not proven to be satisfactory for nonfacial skin. Superficial chemical peels are too light to produce the desired results on the nonfacial skin [4,5]. Uncontrolled medium or deep peels of the nonfacial skin can give unpredictable results and may penetrate beyond the desired depth [1].

PRESURGICAL CONSIDERATIONS

When I perform a facial peel on a patient, I generally also perform a Cook Total Body Peel on the neck, chest, and hands, as well as other body areas as indicated. Each patient must be carefully examined to determine their cosmetic concerns and the peeling agent or laser technique that would best suit their lifestyle. I may use a combination of laser and chemical peels on various parts of the face for a more customized peel. I am careful to respect cosmetic units on the face and body, so that each area will blend smoothly with adjacent areas.

Factors I consider in evaluating a patient include:

- Fitzpatrick skin type [6]
- Degree of actinic or age damage [7]
- Prior cosmetic surgery or scarring
- General medical and physical condition of the patient
- Any history of hypertrophic scarring, keloids, allergies, or acne
- Current medications, including isotretinoin (Accutane)
- The degree of sun exposure the patient currently experiences and will experience in the future
- The degree and extent of poikiloderma on the neck, and whether it extends onto the facial areas
- Whether the patient has realistic expectations

In evaluating prior cosmetic surgery, it is important to obtain the history of any allergies, including "sensitive skin," so that the postsurgical regimen can be adjusted appropriately. If the patient has a history of acne, the postsurgical use of emollients should be less extensive and for a shorter period of time.

PRESURGICAL TREATMENT AND INSTRUCTIONS

Before any skin resurfacing procedure, the patient is placed on prophylactic antibiotics and antiviral medication after review of the patient's allergic status. If patients can tolerate tretinoin (Retin-A), they will benefit from its presurgical application to the face. However, I prefer that patients not use high concentrations of alpha-hydroxy acids or tretinoin on the nonfacial skin for approximately 1 week before the body peel procedure, as it may increase the speed of penetration of the peeling substance.

MATERIALS

The materials needed for this technique are acetone, 70% glycolic acid gel (not glycolic acid liquid), 40% trichloroacetic acid (TCA), and 10% sodium bicarbonate solution.

ANESTHESIA

No pretreatment with intramuscular or local anesthetic is needed for the Cook Total Body Peel. No sedation is required.

PROCEDURE

Application of the Peeling Agents

The skin is cleansed with acetone. Then a 70% glycolic acid gel is applied with a folded 4 × 4 gauze, followed immediately by 40% TCA. The glycolic acid gel is not removed before applying the TCA. Several additional coats of TCA may be applied directly over the glycolic acid gel with a folded 4 × 4 gauze as needed, until the desired depth is obtained. It is important to use glycolic acid gel for this technique, rather than liquid, because the gel acts as a partial barrier to the TCA penetration. Liquid glycolic acid does not act as a barrier and can result in too deep a peel on the body skin.

The skin should be observed carefully during treatment, so that the physician can determine the proper endpoint and immediately neutralize with 10% sodium bicarbonate solution.

Endpoint

The endpoint of each area is determined visually. It will vary from one patient to another and from one body area to another, according to the patient's skin type, actinic damage, and "age damage."

When undergoing a chemical peel, the skin goes through a series of color changes. Careful attention to the color change is key to obtaining the best cosmetic result. First, the skin becomes pink or erythematous, then small white speckles develop. The speckles increase in number and size until the skin reaches a "frosted" appearance, with the underlying pink still showing through.

A typical endpoint for the Cook Total Body Peel would be characterized by erythema with small scattered white speckles, or an expression by the patient of a slight burning sensation. In patients with darker skin types and/or less sun damage, the peeling process may be stopped earlier. In patients with severely weathered or sun-damaged skin, the peeling may be allowed to proceed to a more speckled or lightly frosted endpoint. The nonfacial skin below the level of the upper neck is rarely peeled to the point of blanching.

The artistry of the Cook Total Body Peel lies in the blending and consistency in depth of the peel from one body area to another. For example, the upper neck should be peeled "deeper" than the more distal areas of the neck and chest for smoother blending between deeper peeled areas of the face and peeled areas of the body. Careful attention to the color change (endpoint) is key to the cosmetic result.

Some skin areas may require more time or more TCA to "speckle" to the same degree as neighboring skin. The physician can allow more time before neutralizing or apply an additional coat of TCA.

The desired result is a lighter peel than a typical 40% TCA peel. This is in contrast to medium-depth peels using TCA plus glycolic acid liquid, which produce a "heavier" peel [8].

Neutralization

When the desired point is reached, I immediately neutralize the peeling agents with copious amounts of 10% sodium bicarbonate solution. The sodium bicarbonate solution is applied at least five times, with care taken to remove all glycolic acid gel from the skin.

POSTSURGICAL CONSIDERATIONS

After a skin resurfacing treatment, patients are placed on emollients. They are instructed to bathe twice a day and then reapply emollient. I prefer that they not exercise extensively until re-epithelialization has occurred. Sun exposure should be strictly avoided for approximately 1 month or more after treatment. If possible, I like to have all patients use retinoic acid (Retin-A) and hydroquinone on the treated areas after the skin has finished peeling.

The treated skin will peel in the form of flaking and scaling for 2 to 4 weeks postsurgically, depending on the area treated. This peeling is not usually a major cosmetic concern because the body areas can be covered with clothing.

A small percentage of patients choose to repeat the body peel more than once, and their skin improves after each peel. The Cook Total Body Peel can be repeated as often as every month, as soon as the flaking is complete.

COMPLICATIONS

The Cook Total Body Peel shows a markedly decreased incidence of postinflammatory pigmentation compared with treatment by TCA alone. If postinflammatory pigmentation occurs, it resolves quickly with local hydroquinone treatment. Pretreatment with prophylactic antibiotics and antiviral medications should prevent infection. I have not seen any scarring or other major complications as a result of the Cook Total Body Peel.

SUMMARY

When a laser or chemical peel of the face is combined with a Cook Total Body Peel of the neck, there is excellent blending of the face and neck skin. The Cook Total Body Peel can be applied to the neck and chest (Fig. 1), arms (Fig. 2), hands (Fig. 3), legs, back, abdomen, and even the face. Wrinkling is reduced, pigmented lentigines are greatly reduced, and the skin texture is smoother. The skin appears more even in color and texture. Striae distensae become less obvious, with atrophic hyperpigmented striae showing a decrease in width and depth that continues to improve with successive treatments. Complications are minimal and patient satisfaction is high.

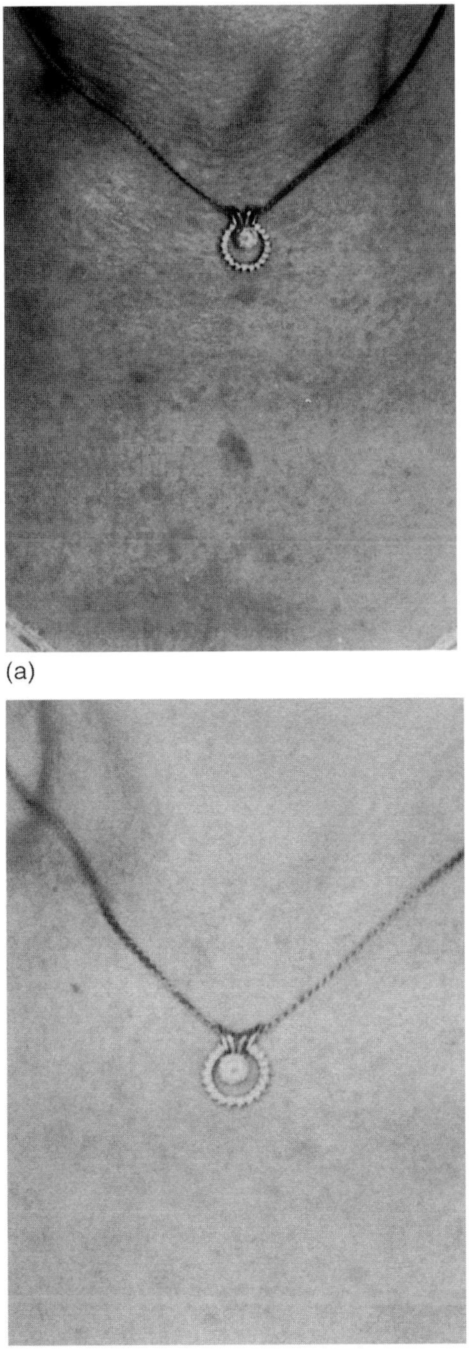

(a)

(b)

FIGURE 1 Patient before (a) and after (b) Cook Total Body Peel of neck and chest. One peel. Note improved texture of neck and chest skin.

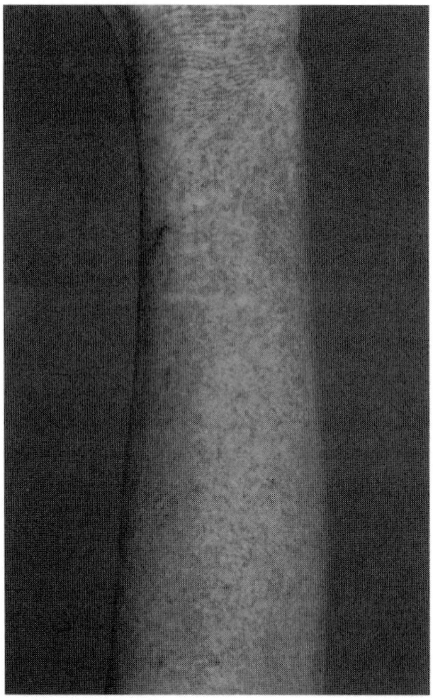

(a)

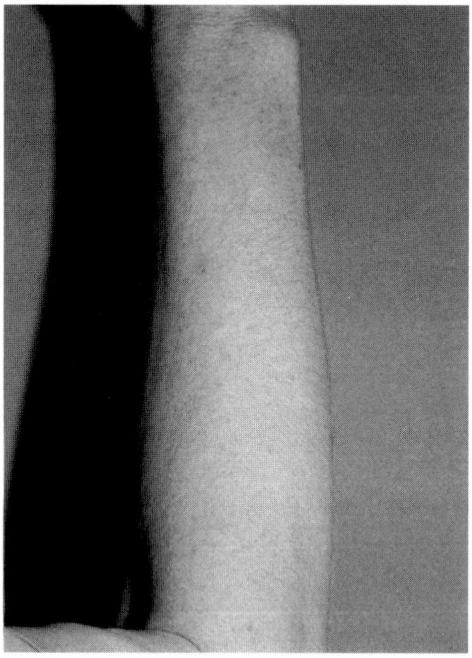

(b)

FIGURE 2 Patient before (a) and after (b) Cook Total Body Peel of the arms. One peel.

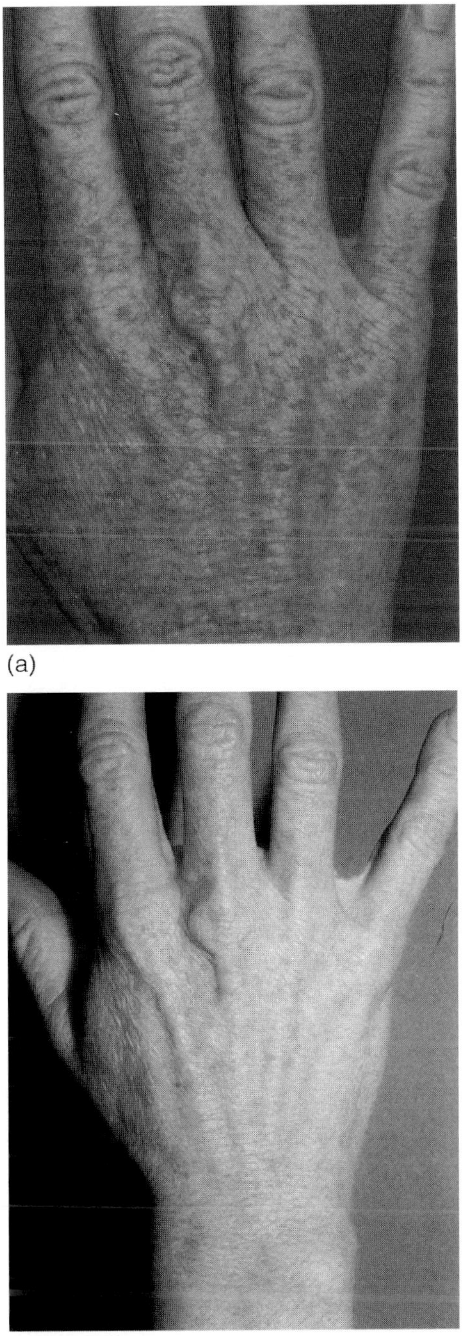

(a)

(b)

FIGURE 3 Patient before (a) and after (b) Cook Total Body Peel of the hands. One peel. Note lightening of the freckling on the hand and fingers.

REFERENCES

1. Brody H. Chemical Peeling. St. Louis: Mosby-Year Book, Inc., 1997.
2. Rubin MG. Manual of Chemical Peels: Superficial and Medium Depth. Philadelphia: Lippincott-Raven, 1995.
3. Cook WR Jr, Cook KK. Manual of Tumescent Liposculpture and Laser Cosmetic Surgery. Philadelphia: Lippincott Williams & Wilkins, 1999.
4. Moy LS, Murad H, Moy RL. Glycolic acid peels for the treatment of wrinkles and photoaging. J Dermatol Surg Oncol 1993; 19:243–246.
5. Newman N, Newman A, Moy L, et al. Clinical improvement of photoaged skin with 50% glycolic acid. Dermatol Surg 1996; 22:455–460.
6. Fitzpatrick TB. The validity and practicality of sun-reactive skin types I through VI. Arch Dermatol 1988; 124:869–871.
7. Glogau RG. Chemical peeling and aging skin. J Geriatr Dermatol 1994; 2:30–35.
8. Coleman WP 3rd, Futrell JM. The glycolic acid trichloroacetic acid peel. J Dermatol Surg Oncol 1994; 20:76–80.

APPENDIX 1a: CONSENT FORM FOR TCA AND BODY PEEL

1. I clearly understand and accept:

    a) The potential benefits of the proposed procedure;
    b) The possible alternate medical procedure;
    c) The probability of success;
    d) The reasonable anticipated consequences if the procedure is not performed;
    e) The possibility that additional services/fees may be required, including, but not limited to, anesthesia, laboratory, medications, and/or surgical facility or hospital use.

2. The goal of these procedures, as in any cosmetic surgery, is improvement, not perfection. Satisfaction is based on realistic expectations. No one should expect that the procedure will remove every abnormal pigment spot or every wrinkle, or result in perfectly smooth skin.

3. Although the procedures are intended to improve my appearance, in rare cases it may leave it unchanged or in some cases worsened.

4. The final result may not be apparent for 3 or more months postoperatively.

5. In rare instances, to achieve the best possible result, additional procedures may be necessary. There will be a charge for any additional operation performed.

6. Strict adherence to the postoperative regimen discussed by Dr. Cook (i.e. medications, creams, postoperative care instructions, avoidance of sun exposure, avoidance of skin irritation, and all other regimens discussed) is necessary in order to achieve the best possible results.

7. The surgical fee is paid for the peel procedure itself and subsequent postoperative visits.

8. There is no guarantee that the expected or anticipated results will be achieved.

9. I give my permission for the administration of anesthesia, as deemed appropriate by the physician.

Although complications following surgery are infrequent, I understand that the following may occur:

1. *Wound Healing*. These procedures may result in swelling, weeping, crusting, or flaking of the treated areas, which may require 1-3 weeks to heal. Once the surface has healed, it may be pink and sensitive to the skin for an additional 1-3 months or rarely longer.
2. *Infection*. Infection is rare, but should it occur, treatment with antibiotics and/or surgical drainage may be required.
3. *Changes in Pigment (Skin Color) and Texture*. During the healing process, there is a possibility of the treatment area becoming either lighter or darker in color or different in texture than the surrounding skin. This is usually temporary, but it may persist.
4. *Scarring*. Scarring is a rare occurrence, but it is a possibility when the skin's surface is disrupted. To minimize the chances of scarring, I understand that it is important that I follow all postoperative instructions carefully.
5. *Persistence of Lesion*. Some growths, birthmarks, wrinkles, scars, warts, keratoses, blood vessels, and tattoos may respond only partially or not at all to these procedures. If this situation arises, there may be other treatment alternatives available.
6. *Allergies*. Allergic or toxic responses to anesthetic are extremely rare, but possible.
7. *General Risks*. In addition to these possible complications, I am aware of the general risks inherent in all surgical procedures and anesthetic administration.

Patient signature: ______________________ Date: ______________________

APPENDIX 1b: AFTER-CARE INSTRUCTIONS FOR TCA AND BODY PEELS

1. Wash treated areas gently with your fingertips (no washcloth) twice a day with soap and water, and pat dry with a soft clean towel. Do not rub. You will not be able to wash off all your moisturizer, so do not try. Wash very gently.
2. Keep a thin coat of emollient on the treated parts of your face and body. Do not apply anything that we have not recommended.
3. Take Duricef, or other antibiotic prescribed, twice a day starting the day of surgery.
4. (For facial peels.) Take Valtrex twice a day starting the day of surgery.
5. During the healing process, your skin will peel. You may get a few sore spots or thick scabs or red spots (places that peeled a little deeper). Use cortisone cream on these areas twice a day. Do not pick at loose skin, as this can cause scarring.
6. After the skin has finished peeling, you may use moisturizing lotion.
7. Starting 1 week after your peel, apply hydroquinone and Retin-A every other night. Ask Dr. Cook when to start using this treatment. Do not put these substances on areas that have not completely peeled.
8. After you finish peeling, apply sunscreen every day. Ask Dr. Cook when to start doing this. Do not put sunscreen on areas that have not completely peeled.
9. You must avoid the sun for a period of 4 weeks after your peel. Be sure to wear sunscreen and protective clothing whenever you are outside and when driving.
10. If you have any questions, please call the office.

6

Peel Complications and Management

Harold J. Brody
Emory University School of Medicine, Atlanta, Georgia

The application of wounding agents to the skin to produce a controlled wound is the principal concept in chemical peeling. Despite attempts to standardize peeling to understand defect depth in addition to specific wounding agent depth, side effects may still occur. The total number of different types of complications that may occur increase with wound depth (Table 1). Superficial peels usually produce transient pigmentary reactions only, but scarring can occur if dermal invasion occurs inadvertently. Medium-depth peels can cause pigmentary changes and scarring. Deep peels are associated with the preceding and other, more serious, reactions (Table 2) [1].

Proper informed consent is suggested before all dermal peels. The form should mention the possibility of pigmentary alteration, scarring, and infection at minimum. Excellent instruction to patients before and after surgery leaves little room for misunderstanding. Photographs of the patient before and after peeling are deterrents to patient dissatisfaction or litigation because the patient may not be aware of previous skin defects or may forget the previous appearance of the skin.

A favorable test-spot result in patients at higher risk for pigmentation or scarring may allay the fears of the patient and the physician, but it does not guarantee the behavior of the rest of the facial skin to the procedure [2]. However, an unfavorable test result may help inform the high-risk patient or eliminate him or her from further consideration. A pertinent history should be taken to ascertain relative contraindications to chemical peeling. These are not absolute contraindications. Caution should be exercised with patients who cannot avoid sunlight; patients who cannot use cosmetic coverup; patients with inability to re-epithelialize because of isotretinoin or irradiation; patients with simultaneous or recent undermining cosmetic surgery; smokers; medications or disease that may predispose to infection or delayed healing; a strong history of recurrent herpetic infection; a history of hypertrophic scarring; and unrealistic expectations (Table 3). These factors in the history, in addition to the pigmentation of the patient's skin color, must be evaluated and the proper peel depth ascertained.

TABLE 1 Complications of All Types of Chemical Peeling

Pigmentary change
Scarring
Infection
Prolonged Erythema or Pruritus
Contact Dermatitis
Textural changes
Milia
Acne
Cold Sensitivity
Poor physician/patient relationship

COMPLICATIONS ARISING FROM ALL TYPES OF CHEMICAL PEELS

Pigmentary Changes

If a single cosmetic unit is to be peeled, applying solutions approximately 5 mm beyond the natural boundaries will make demarcation lines less noticeable. For example, when peeling periorally, peel beyond the nasolabial fold. Applying a more superficial agent on the remainder of the face is helpful. The contrast between phenol-peeled or laser-resurfaced and unpeeled areas may be quite noticeable in very sun-damaged Fitzpatrick type I skin. Feathering the edges of a peel with a superficial agent like 25% TCA onto the neck under the angle of the jaw is very helpful.

Although hyperpigmentation can occur after any depth of chemical peel, lighter complexions have lower risk. Fitzpatrick type V skin is the most unpredictable. Hyperpigmentation is more likely to occur after superficial or medium-depth peels and hypopigmentation after peels involving phenol or after laser resurfacing. If patients use birth control pills, exogenous estrogens, photosensitizing drugs, or if they become pregnant within 6 months after peeling, hyperpigmentation is more likely despite strict sun avoidance [3]. If this occurs, the areas may be repeeled 3 to 6 months later [4], possibly but not necessarily with a less potent wounding agent. Nevi have been reported to hyperpigment after deep peeling (Fig. 1) [5].

Hypopigmentation after Baker's phenol application is a function of patient selection and mode of application with subsequent wound care. The inherent color of the un–sun-damaged skin of the patient, the axillary skin, for example, may forecast the color after phenol peeling. Fitzpatrick type I photodamaged skin (the

TABLE 2 Complications Arising Exclusively from Deep Phenol Peeling

Atrophy
Cardiac arrhythmias
Laryngeal edema
Exacerbation of concurrent disease

TABLE 3 Relative Contraindications

Sun exposure
Cosmetic usage
Isotretinoin or radiographic history
Time of prior cosmetic surgery
Smokers
Health and medications
History of Herpes simplex
Hypertrophic scar formers
Unrealistic expectations

redheaded patient) is most likely to be the porcelain or alabaster white color after peeling. Hypopigmentation after phenol is proportional to the amount of phenol applied, and a small pigment loss is an expected result and not a complication (Table 5).

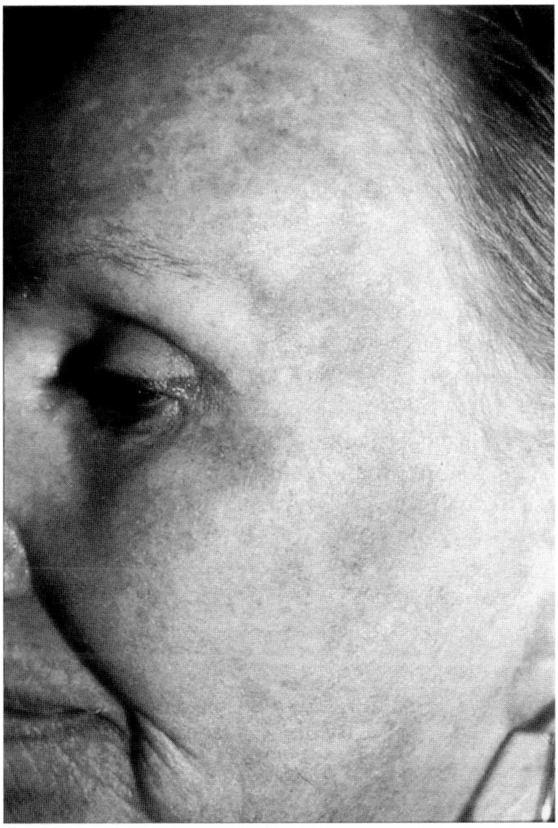

FIGURE 1 Hyperpigmentation from probable sun exposure 6 weeks after medium-depth peeling in Fitzpatrick type III skin.

TABLE 4 Bleaching Formula for Darker Skin Types: "Bleach-eze"

Hydroquinone, 6–10%*
Ascorbic acid, 0.05%*
Retinoic acid, 0.1%*
Propylene glycol, 4%
In Hytone cream 2.5%, (Dermik), 30 g, Mix
Dissolve the crystals* in propylene glycol and mix with the cream. Apply twice a day.

*The initial concentration of hydroquinone is 6%. This may be increased if pigmentation returns after peeling. Ascorbic acid prevents the hydroquinone from oxidizing. Hytone™ (hydrocortisone) cream (Dermik) is paraben-free. Creams with high concentrations of hydroquinone should be discontinued as soon as the appropriate amount of pigment loss is achieved to avoid paradoxical hyperpigmentation. This cream may be locally compounded or ordered for individual patients by prescription in concentrations up to 15% from Medical Center Pharmacy, 4600 N. Habana Ave., Tampa, FL 33614. Phone: 1-800-226-7094; FAX: 813-876-9095. Its potency decreases if not used in 2 months.

After severe rhytides of photoaging IV have been treated with the laser or Baker's phenol, residual hypopigmentation may be slight, but unbothersome, with both modalities. The rate of hypopigmentation with laser resurfacing may be as high as 16%.

Stark porcelain white (alabaster) skin with clinical depigmentation, commonly seen around the mouth in the 1970s when only partial-face perioral peels were performed, may be more likely to result from larger amounts of Baker's phenol and greater occlusion. It is rarely seen today. In addition, the use of the original thymol iodine powder mask may have also contributed to these appearances. Depigmentation is more likely to occur with a very heavy application of phenol to only mildly sun-damaged skin as opposed to heavily sun-damaged skin. This improper patient selection was a major factor to producing depigmentation. Phenol produces hypopigmentation and not depigmentation by impairing melanin synthesis from melanocytes [6]. Treatment of hyperpigmentation can be instituted by twice-daily application of 4% hydroquinone gel, with or without tretinoin, after peeling in addition to sunscreen. There is no dispute that the postpeel use of hydroquinone and its potentiation by tretinoin have decreased postoperative hyperpigmentation. Optionally, corticosteroid cream no stronger than 0.1% triamcinolone may be added. A modification of the traditional depigmentation formula is especially helpful after peeling for Fitzpatrick types IV to VI skin (Table 4). There is a small subset of patients that may produce a better response when bleaching or prophylaxing against hyperpigmentation with

TABLE 5 Factors in Pigment Loss in Phenol Peeling

Quantity of phenol applied
Improper or inappropriate taping
Thymol iodine powder
Lighter skin types
Partial peels with demarcation lines on the face

the addition of glycolic acid lotion to their regimen [7]. The compound should be used daily or every other day as tolerated after re-epithelialization until the erythema is faint. There is no definitive evidence that pretreatment of the skin with hydroquinone affects the subsequent appearance of pigmentation after re-epithelialization.

Scarring

Medium-depth and deep peels have the risk of scarring, but as of yet the contributing factors are unresolved. Heredity, darker skin types, smoking, inadequate topical hydration, constrictive taping, previous cosmetic undermining surgery, excessive facial chewing, and infection during healing may be contributory. Most scars in chemical peeling are hypertrophic scars and not true keloids [8]. "Thin skin" has also been cited as a causal factor, but even thick-skinned individuals have "thin skin" at the temples or at the nasal bridges that may not scar [9,10]. Any previous chemical, laser, or abrasive resurfacing, as well as isotretinoin use, may be risk factors of uncertain degree for scarring. Medium-depth and deep dermal repeeling before the erythema has clinically resolved is also a hazard. Scarring is least likely to occur after superficial peeling because the dermis is rarely penetrated.

In the three combination medium-depth peels of solid CO_2, Jessner's solution, or glycolic acid followed by 35% TCA, the risk of scarring is less than 1% [3,11]. Care should be exercised when using 50% TCA because high-strength TCA is more caustic than full-strength phenol and may be more likely to produce scarring [12–15]. No contractile scarring has been reported with any of the three published medium-depth combination peels. Additives to TCA in attempts to slow absorption and frosting may force TCA into the deep dermis, possibly producing contractile scarring (Fig. 2).

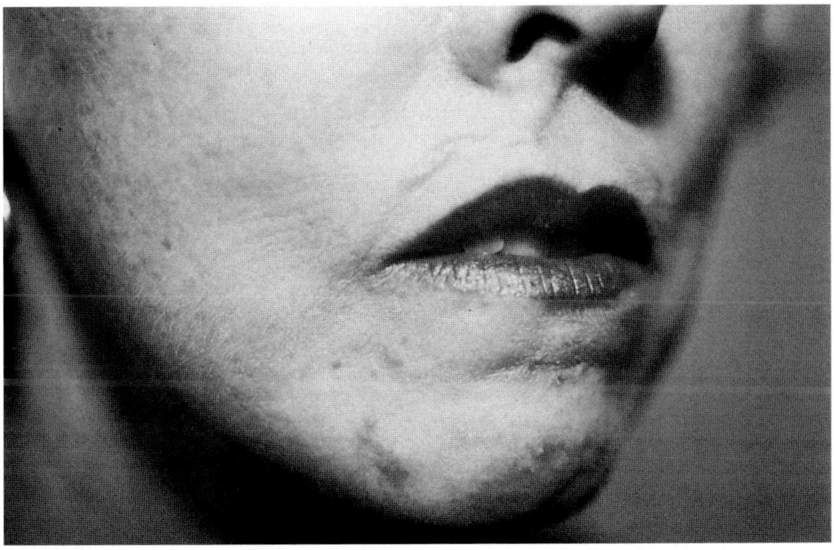

FIGURE 2 Perioral scarring after dermal peeling can be minimized with intralesional steroids.

The incidence of scarring with the traditional Baker's phenol formula in a series of over 1000 patients peeled by Drs. Baker and Gordon is less than 1%. These are patients who were peeled without preliminary overtreatment with tretinoin or other topicals. The rate of scarring may increase with deviations from the original description of various peels, the use of preliminary skin treatments to increase absorption, or improper patient selection. Comparison with CO_2 laser resurfacing reveals comparable safety if proper peeling methodology is followed.

Nonfacial skin has a greater incidence of scarring. Superficial peeling can be performed in these areas with a very low risk. Full-thickness skin sloughs are associated with simultaneous peeling and rhytidectomy, probably as a result of undermining and compromised vascular and lymphatic circulation [5]. A time interval of 1 to 3 months should separate deep or medium-depth peeling and rhytidectomy or brow lift. Deep-plane face lifting may carry less risk, but TCA application technique and cosmetic surgery varies considerably among surgeons [16–18].

Lower eyelid ectropion after chemical face peeling can develop if deep peeling is performed in conjunction with a blepharoplasty [19,20]. The lower eyelids should be peeled with caution in individuals with subclinical or partial ectropion and minimal loss of apposition of the lid to the sclera. Less risk is apparent with transconjunctival blepharoplasty and peeling. The role of isotretinoin in scarring after chemical peeling is uncertain [21–24]. The technique and depth of dermabrasion as well as laser resurfacing is very operator sensitive, and therefore exact guidelines for peeling are difficult to establish. The generalization of a 6-month interval in dermabrasion, for example, may or may not be appropriate depending on physician technique and total drug dosage. The incidence of scarring with chemical peeling in relationship to isotretinoin is a real but rare risk. The use of the drug during the 6 months before or after a peel may be a factor in scar formation, perhaps because tissues have not returned to normal metabolism from insult with either the drug or the peel. Certainly the dose and duration of the drug and the depth of the peel are factors to consider when judging time intervals.

The phenomenon of delayed healing (Table 6) has been noted after both medium depth TCA and deep phenol peeling as well as laser resurfacing [25,26]. These patients give no indication during the peel process that they will have aberrant re-epithelialization. The immediate frost in a case with TCA peeling does not reflect the forthcoming complication. Multiple or single friable stellate-bordered nonindurated slightly tender erosions with serous granulation tissue are present by the expected final days of the healing process. They are noticed by day 8 in medium-depth peeling and day 10 to 14 in deep peeling or laser resurfacing. Because these areas resemble bacterial infection, the lesions should be cultured and treated systemically

TABLE 6 Delayed Healing

Friable, stellate, nonindurated painful unhealed erosions with serous granulation tissue
Persists 10 days after peeling
Unpredictable
May heal with hypopigmented flat scarring
Effective treatment with artificial wound dressings

for bacteria and yeast with oral antibiotics and antifungals to confirm the diagnosis. Antibiotics are not effective (Fig. 3).

Treatment of delayed healing with artificial wound dressing (Vigilon-Hermal Labs, Delmar, NY) is very effective in reducing wound healing time. After 2 to 3 days, Duoderm (ConvaTec, Bristol Meyers Squibb, Princeton, NJ) or Opsite (Smith and Nephew Research, UK) may be substituted as less-wet occlusive dressings are needed. These are changed daily until healing [26]. Because keloids have increased water content [27] and pathologic states such as eczema have increased transepidermal water loss [28,29], this implies that the use of an artificial dressing will restore normal epidermal barrier function and facilitate epithelial cell migration and healing. Injection of the edge of the wound with very dilute intralesional triamcinolone (2 mg/ml in 1% xylocaine) will also reduce inflammation and speed epithelial migration with wound healing. They characteristically may heal with scars that resemble the smooth hypopigmented scars resembling cryosurgery.

Treatment options of scars during or after their formation are listed in Table 7. If erythema without induration is present, a nonfluorinated but potent steroid cream (hydrocortisone valerate; (Westcort-Westwood-Squibb Co., Buffalo, NY), aclometasone dipropionate (Aclovate-Schering Co., Kenilworth, NJ), or desonide (Desowen-

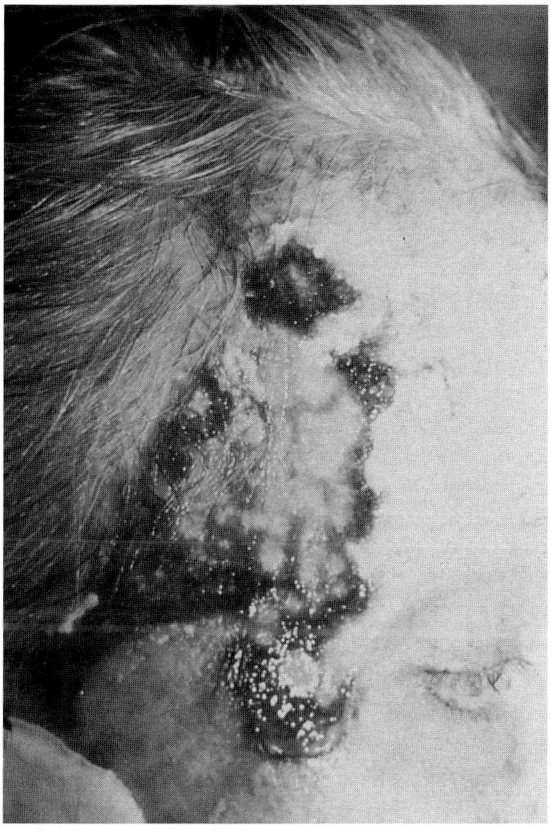

FIGURE 3 Erosions of delayed healing 8 weeks after resurfacing.

TABLE 7 Treatment of Hypertrophic Scars

Topical nonfluorinated steroids
Topical fluorinated steroids
Steroid-impregnated tape
Intralesional steroids
Silicone gel sheeting
Flashlamp-pumped pulsed dye laser at 585 nm
Surgical excision
Observation with or without the above intervention

Galderma Labs, Ft. Worth, TX) may be used to avoid skin atrophy. More aggressive topical and intralesional intervention is indicated if induration is present. The use of a class I topical steroid (clobetasol [Temovate-Glaxo], halobetasol propionate [Ultravate-Westwood-Squibb]), diflorasone diacetate (Psorcon [Dermik]), or a fluocinonide-impregnated tape (Cordan; Oclassen Pharm., San Rafael, CA) may too quickly reduce erythema but produce atrophy or striae. The tape should be used only at night, and signs of overusage necessitate close follow-up. Some physicians advocate aggressive treatment of any slightly indurated persistent erythematous linear or curved lesions with topical or intralesional fluorinated corticosteroids [30]. Diluting the injection strength down to as low as 2 mg/ml for early questionable indurated erythema, 4 mg/ml for indurated erythema, and as high as 20 to 40 mg/ml of triamcinolone for actual hypertropic scarring and injecting every 2 to 4 weeks is justified based on the aggressiveness and the time of intervention of the erythematous scarring process. Time alone or compression and massage may resolve mild, small scars. Combined scar revision with intralesional steroids may be necessary in severe cases.

A semiocclusive scar cover made of silicone gel, a cross-linked polydimethylsiloxane polymer, applied to the area for a minimum of 12 hours daily is helpful [8,31–33]. The gel can be alternated with steroid-impregnated tape and may be initiated at night at the first sign of deep erythema without induration.

Erythematous and hypertrophic scars can also be improved with the flashlamp-pumped pulsed dye laser (FLPDL) at 585 nm with or without intralesional triamcinolone [34–36]. Patients who receive combination treatment achieve greater resolution. Facial scars and scars less than 1-year old respond more readily to 2 to 4 sequential monthly treatments.

Risk factors for scarring after resurfacing occur as a result of a combination of risk factors based on hereditary predisposition; the time interval between multiple peels or courses of isotretinoin; the concentration and application of specific wounding agent and peel depth; the location with varying appendages for healing, dermal actinic quality, and possible motion of the skin being peeled (e.g., the perioral area); the quality of wound care after peeling with the presence of infection [3,37]; and too short an interval between peeling and undermining from cosmetic surgery. Poor nutritional status in vegetarians may affect epithelialization and collagen reorganization after TCA or phenol peels [38]. Excessive dissolution of epidermal integrity from atopic dermatitis, overuse of abrasive scrubs or facials, or unwarranted pretreatment may cause undue absorption of wounding agents.

Infection

The best deterrent to infection (Table 8) after peeling is to minimize crusting by treating the skin with wet to dry soaks. Occlusive ointments may rarely promote folliculitis that may become secondarily infected with Streptococcus, Staphylococcus, or Pseudomonas. All suspected infections should be cultured for identification and sensitivity and the patient given appropriate antibiotics. Acne flare-ups after peeling respond best to an infectious approach with a culture and appropriate antibiotics. Five percent acetic acid or white vinegar diluted 1:1 with tap water is a safe, effective, and inexpensive topical soaking agent for twice daily use [39]. Toxic shock syndrome, induced by an exotoxin elaborated by Staphylococcus aureus, has been reported after Baker's phenol face peels [40,41].

Herpes simplex infection may be reactivated by peeling of any depth (Fig. 4) [42]. Unusual and unexpected postpeel pain may reflect the onset of viral infection. Patients with a positive history of herpes can be treated prophylactically during healing with 400 mg of acyclovir (Zovirax; Glaxo Wellcome, West Caldwell, NJ) three times daily if undergoing a deep peel beginning on the day of the peel. Valacyclovir HCl (Valtrex; Glaxo Wellcome, West Caldwell, NJ) 500 mg two times daily or famciclovir (Famvir; SmithKline Beecham, Philadelphia, PA) 500 mg three times daily are effective alternative antivirals. Scarring from recurrent herpes with medium-depth or superficial peeling is rare, and prophylaxis to every patient with a rare history of "fever blisters" who is undergoing these peels is probably not necessary. Active herpes during the postpeel period should be treated with appropriate increased therapeutic doses of antivirals. Because the barrier layer is removed in laser and abrasive resurfacing, prophylaxis is more likely indicated in this setting.

A patient that is exposed to herpes simplex for the first time during the healing period may become infected with primary inoculation herpes and experience severe pain with lymphadenopathy and fever. These patients are candidates for treatment with intravenous antivirals.

Epstein-Barr virus keratitis after a Baker's peel, perhaps from the Croton oil, manifested as blurred vision with fever and joint pain 4 days after peeling [43]. Candidiasis (yeast) has been reported more frequently after dermabrasion and CO_2 laser resurfacing [44]. The partially protective presence of a nonviable epidermis remaining intact after peeling and lack of occlusive dressing in peels make yeast less likely.

Prolonged Erythema or Pruritus

Erythema after peeling usually disappears in 30 to 90 days, depending on the wounding agent. Fourteen to 30 days after superficial peeling, 30 to 60 days after medium-depth peeling, and 90 days after deep peeling are reasonable resolution times, but different patients may manifest longer intervals especially if they are using tretinoin before and after peels [3]. Isotretinoin administration before peeling, genetic or atopic factors of the patient, rosacea, or minimal amounts of alcoholic beverages [5] may also affect redness. It is never permanent, but intermittent flushing may occur for as long as 4 years afterward. Generally, the erythema after laser resurfacing is more prolonged than after chemical resurfacing.

Topical hydrocortisone 2.5% lotion or other nonfluorinated steroid cream may be helpful. Oral antihistamines, short-term systemic steroids, silicone gel sheeting,

TABLE 8 Infectious Complications

Bacterial pyoderma
Toxic shock syndrome
Herpes simplex virus
Epstein-Barr virus keratitis
Candidiasis

and the application of a green foundation under base makeup can also be useful. Pruritus is a common occurrence after re-epithelialization and typically persists for about 1 month. In addition to the above drugs, aspirin and propranolol in low doses will relieve some symptoms [6]. Pruritus occurring during the healing period can signal a contact dermatitis to the ointment used in wound care, especially when accompanied by slow healing, increased erythema, or follicular pustules on the neck or outside of the peel region.

Textural Changes

Enlarged pores may result after peeling because of removal of the stratum corneum, but the appearance is temporary [3]. Pore size is not consistently changed by chemical peeling of any depth. A diffuse, grainy, porous, peau d'orange texture can follow any form of chemical, abrasive, or laser resurfacing [10]. This may be produced after 50% TCA as well as phenol, and may be more noticeable in sebaceous patients. Temperature and wind sensitivity may occur.

If an agent is too weak to peel evenly below the defect, lacks the surfactant to provide an even depth of wounding, or has too high a surface tension, an irregular

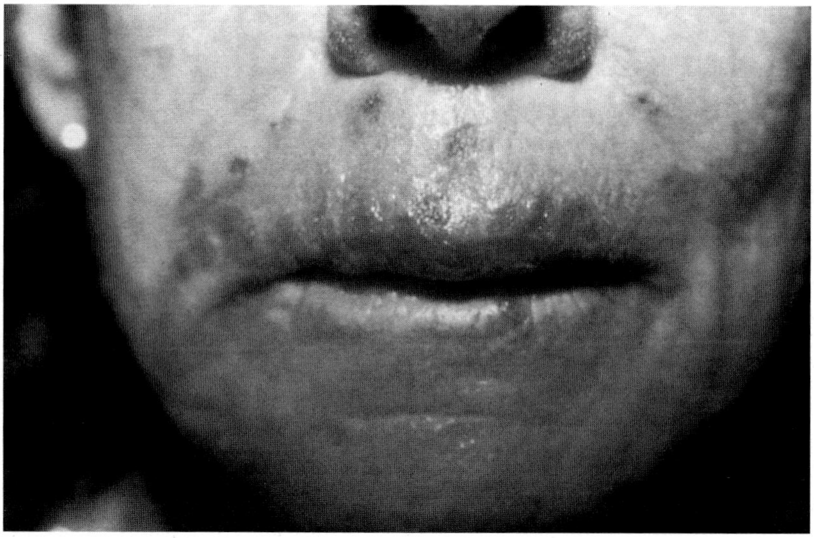

FIGURE 4 Herpes simplex infection after a perioral deep chemical peel.

texture change may be produced. Telangiectasia is not predictably altered by chemical peeling alone.

Milia

Milia, sometimes called inclusion cysts, appear as part of the healing process and are more common after dermabrasion than after chemical peeling. They typically do not appear until 2 to 3 weeks after re-epithelialization and may be aggravated by thick ointments that occlude the upper pilosebaceous units [4]. In dermabrasion, saline scrubs immediately postsurgery may minimize milia [3]. After peeling, the use of gentle epidermabrasion (Buf-Puf; 3M, St. Paul, MN) after re-epithelialization or topical tretinoin both before and after peeling may decrease their occurrence. Treatment with electrodessication or extraction by using a number 11 scalpel blade is effective.

Acne

The entire spectrum of pustular to cystic acne may appear during the healing process or immediately after re-epithelialization from depth of peel. A previous history of the disorder may not be present and the lesions may produce scarring (Fig. 5). Recent

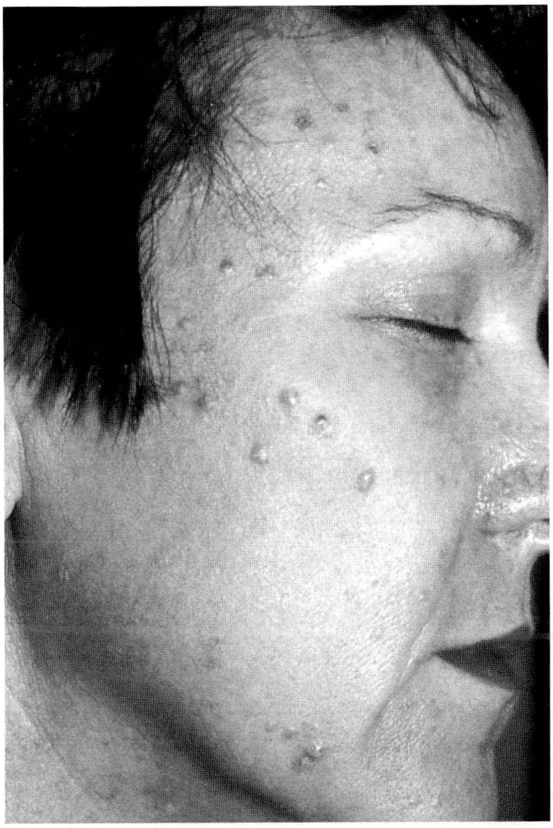

FIGURE 5 Acne papules and pustules appearing 5 days after peeling with 35% TCA.

institution of tretinoin or overgreasing with moisturizers or ointments during postoperative re-epithelialization may be causes. Culture and sensitivity should be obtained to eliminate bacteria and yeast infection. The patient should be placed on treatment with topical and oral antibiotics for 5 days. If the cultures are negative, aggressive acne treatment in the form of tetracycline and topical antibiotics should be instituted. Intralesional triamcinolone acetonide 1 mg/ml and a rapidly tapering dose of prednisone for 1 week may be considered if cystic lesions are present to prevent scarring. Low-dose isotretinoin may be required. It is unlikely that any inhibition of the sebaceous apparatus would affect the wound healing mechanisms when using a low dose for a short period of time in this setting, but the patient should be apprised of the potential risk.

Superficial peeling agents, glycolic acid, or 15% TCA, for example, are used for adjunctive acne vulgaris or acne rosacea therapy. When flaring of acne occurs during this treatment, it is especially disconcerting. This situation should not require aggressive treatment.

Cold Sensitivity or Cold Urticaria

When using solid CO_2 (dry ice) to freeze the skin either alone or in combination with TCA in medium-depth peeling, transient swelling or urticaria can be produced in distant areas [3]. Because CO_2 has minimum temperature of only $-78.5°C$ and is rarely concentrated in any one area for more than 20 seconds, it is limited in its ability to produce cold reactions. The application of a 10-second liquid nitrogen spray to the entire face for acne scar treatment has resulted in full-thickness necrosis and scarring because of the presence of occult cryofibrinogenemia and would be a risk in this type of cryosurgical peeling [45].

Poor Physician/Patient Relationship

Loss of confidence in the physician in the face of minor, manageable complications can result in a loss of follow-up and the possibility of litigation. The physician-patient relationship is critical and must withstand any complication of the greatest gravity. Good preoperative counseling with thorough comprehension of the patient's desires by the physician and of the procedural risks by the patient are imperative. Informed consent should be obtained. Patients with some psychiatric illnesses or untreated endogenous depression and patients who have unrealistic expectations should not be peeled or should have their primary disorders treated before peeling. Being housebound for a week or more can be traumatic for some patients.

COMPLICATIONS ARISING EXCLUSIVELY FROM DEEP PHENOL PEELS

Atrophy

Atrophy, or clinical loss of the normal skin markings in the absence of scarring, may occur after multiple deep peels with phenol but has not been observed after superficial or medium-depth peeling involving multiple applications of TCA. Atrophy may result also from applying a deep wounding agent on very thin, relatively un–sun-damaged skin. For example, using periorbital Baker's solution on a relatively un–

sun-damaged 27-year-old produces almost transparent skin so that the muscle is seen when light is transmitted through the epidermis [3], especially as chronologic aging proceeds. This skin is not histologically atrophic [6,46].

Cardiac Arrhythmias

Phenol is the only chemical peeling agent that can produce cardiotoxic complications with improper adherence to guidelines. There has never been a death from properly applied phenol peeling. TCA applied to the skin is neutralized by serum in the superficial dermal plexus and is nontoxic to internal body organs [47]. Hepatorenal or central nervous system problems have not been reported in the literature with properly performed chemical peels and occur only as results of industrial accidents. It is not necessary to use more than 2 to 3 ml of phenol for each procedure [48]. The extent of cutaneous absorption depends more on the total area of skin exposed than on the concentration of phenol. Deaths attributed to phenol toxicity may have other causes. Predisposed individuals may have idiosyncratic cardiac death from an adrenalin release because of facial pain transmitted from the trigeminal nerve to the cardiac vagal nerve or from the cerebral cortex directly to the cardiac sinoatrial node [49]. This adrenal release could trigger a hypodynamic cardiac status or ventricular ectopic impulses. There is a wide variability in susceptibility to the cardiac effects of the agent.

Cardiac arrhythmias have been associated with phenol application in full face peeling. In patients peeled rapidly in 30 minutes' time, tachycardia was noted first, followed by premature ventricular contractions, bigeminy, paroxysmal atrial tachycardia, and ventricular tachycardia [50]. Atrial fibrillation has also been reported but was self-reversing after phenol serum clearance [51]. Diuresis with intravenous fluids promotes metabolism and excretion of phenol and reduces arrhythmias. Pausing 10 to 15 minutes between applications to cosmetic units in full face peeling and allowing 90 to 120 minutes for the procedure is safe technique for phenol application. If minor supraventricular arrhythmias occur despite proper technique and pausing between cosmetic units, the application should be discontinued until normal sinus rhythm has returned for 15 minutes. The procedure may be resumed and the peel intervals extended for an additional 15 minutes [52,53]. Holter monitor electrocardiographic (ECG) studies on 10 patients performed 24 hours before, during, and after Baker's phenol peels [54] showed that there were many spontaneously occurring ventricular ectopic beats unrelated to the actual application of the chemical peel formula. There was no correlation between a screening ECG and the Holter monitor tracings. In most patients there were more abnormalities in the preoperative data than in the intraoperative and postoperative data. Most ectopic beats occurred in the period after the completion of formula application, which suggests that the beats were random or spontaneous in nature or attributable to stress, anxiety, or unrecognized causes. Spontaneously occurring arrhythmias in normal individuals are not uncommon. Monitoring during application to more than one cosmetic unit and immediately thereafter allows the detection of possible cardiac complications, irrespective of cause.

The application of phenol to one cosmetic unit or less is equivalent to or less than the application of phenol into a nail matrix for chemical nail matrixectomy. Cardiac precautions and monitoring are not necessary for this, and oral hydration with 8 to 16 oz of water can be given to the patient if they have not been drinking many fluids on the day of the peel.

Laryngeal Edema

Laryngeal edema associated with stridor, hoarseness, and tachypnea developed within 24 hours of phenol peeling in 3 of 245 women (approximately 1.2%) [55]. All 3 women were heavy smokers, and their symptoms resolved within 48 hours with warm mist inhalation therapy. Perhaps the cause was a hypersensitivity reaction to phenol or ether fumes in a larynx already chronically irritated by cigarette smoke.

Exacerabation of Concurrent Disease

A local pemphigus-like blister developed on the cheek of a 66-year-old woman 4 weeks after the second of two local phenol peels on the face within a 3-month interval [56]. Immunofluorescent-positive acantholytic lesions developed slowly months later on the body in the absence of oral lesions. The physical trauma of the peel may have Koebnerized the disease although she had no preexisting history. The isomorphic response of Koebner refers to the development of lesions in previously normal skin that has been traumatized. Patients with psoriasis, a much more common disease with an isomorphic response, have not experienced such problems during chemical peeling.

INHERENT ERRORS DURING THE PEEL PROCEDURE

Inherent errors during the peel procedure may occur and can lead to complications (Table 9). With resorcinol combinations, TCA, or phenol formulas, errors in compounding or evaporation of the alcohol or water vehicle base can occur and inadvertently produce a stronger solution. Lactic acid and ethanol can both absorb water from moist air over time if unsealed. Resorcinol and salicylic acid may sit on the pharmacy shelf for 10 to 15 years. Phenol solutions should be prepared fresh for each peel. TCA solutions that are uncontaminated by cotton-tipped applicators are stable under natural office conditions for at least 6 months. It is best to pour all wounding agents into a 1 oz. glass cup to avoid touching applicators to the neck of a bottle that may contain evaporated crystals from solution.

To avoid spilling wounding agents, never hold an open container of the peeling agent and never move the applicator or brush directly over the eye area. A syringe of saline or an eyewash bottle for dilution should be available for the eye if wounding agent is accidentally introduced. Thirty-five percent TCA is not caustic enough to cause major corneal abrasions [57]. If phenol is spilled on the skin the most easily practiced decontamination procedure is to flood the area with propylene glycol or glycerol, the former being readily available. Olive oil, castor oil, and cottonseed oil may also reduce penetration [9,10,58]. Mineral oil in a dropper bottle should be available if phenol is inadvertently placed into the eye.

TABLE 9 Inherent Errors Producing Complications

Incorrect wounding agent compounding or pharmacology
Accidental solution spilling

We live in a litigious society. The risk-to-benefit ratio should be evaluated by both the dermatologic surgeon and the patient. As long as this ratio can be balanced in the proper perspective, complications can be reduced to a minimum.

REFERENCES

1. Matarasso SL, Glogau RG. Chemical face peels. Dermatol Clin 1991; 9:131–150.
2. Swinehart JM. Test spots in dermabrasion and chemical peeling. J Dermatol Surg Oncol 1990; 16:557–563.
3. Brody HJ. Complications of chemical peeling. J Dermatol Surg Oncol 1989; 15:1010–1019.
4. Collins PS. The chemical peel. Clin Dermatol 1987; 5:57–74.
5. Spira M, Gerow FJ, Hardy SB. Complications of chemical face peeling. Plast Reconstr Surg 1974; 54:397–403.
6. Kligman AM, Baker TJ, Gordon HL. Long-term histologic follow-up of phenol face peels. Plast Reconstr Surg 1985; 75:652–659.
7. Rubin M. Symposium on AHAs, Orlando, FL, Dec 1994.
8. Nemeth AJ. Keloids and Hypertrophic Scars. J Dermatol Surg Oncol 1993; 19:738–746.
9. Stegman SJ, Tromovitch TA. Chemical peeling. In: Cosmetic Dermatologic Surgery. St Louis; Mosby-Year Book, 1984:27–46.
10. Stegman SJ, Tromovitch TA, Glogau RG. Chemical peeling. In: Cosmetic Dermatologic Surgery. St Louis; Mosby-Year Book, 1990:35–58.
11. Brody HJ, Hailey CW. Medium-depth chemical peeling of the skin: a variation of superficial chemosurgery. J Dermatol Surg Oncol 1986; 12:1268–1275.
12. Sperber PA. Chemoexfoliation for aging skin and acne scarring. Arch Otolaryngol 1965; 81:278–283.
13. Ayres S III. Superficial chemosurgery. Arch Dermatol 1964; 89:395–403.
14. Ayres S. Dermal changes following application of chemical cauterants to aging skin. Arch Dermatol 1960; 82:578.
15. Monheit G. The Jessner's-Trichloroacetic Acid Peel. Dermatol Clin 1995; 13(2):277–283.
16. Dingman DL, Hartog J, Siemionow M. Simultaneous deep-plane face lift and trichloroacetic acid peel. Plast Reconstr Surg 1994; 98:86–93.
17. Baker TJ. Discussion on simultaneous deep-plane face lift and trichloreoacetic acid peel. Plast Reconstr Surg 1994; 93:94–95.
18. Baker TJ, Gordon HL, Stuzin JM. Reply to Letter to the Editor (on simultaneous deep-plane face lift and trichloroacetic acid peel.) Plast Reconstru Surg 1995; 95:602.
19. Litton C, Trinidad G. Chemosurgery of the eyelids. In: Aston ST, et al. (eds). Third International Symposium of Plastic and Reconstructive Surgery. Baltimore: Williams & Wilkins, 1982:341–345.
20. Wojno T, Tenzel R. Lower eyelid ectropion following chemical face peeling. Ophthalmic Surg 1984; 15:596–597.
21. Rubenstein R, Roenigk HH, Stegman SJ, et al. Atypical keloids after dermabrasion of patients taking isotretinoin. J Am Acad Dermatol 1986; 15:280–285.
22. Roenigk HH, Pinski JB, Robinson KJ, et al. Acne, retinoids, and dermabrasion. J Dermatol Surg Oncol 1985; 11:396–398.
23. Dzubow LM, Miller WH. The effect of 13-cis-retinoic acid on wound healing in dogs. J Dermatol Surg Oncol 1987; 13:265–268.
24. Moy RL, Moy LS, Bennett RG, et al. Systemic isotretinoin: effects on dermal wound healing in a rabbit ear model in vivo. J Dermatol Surg Oncol 1990; 16:1142–1146.
25. Szachowicz EH, Wright WK. Delayed healing after full-face chemical peels. Facial Plast Surg 1989; 6:1:8–13.

26. Glogau RG. Delayed healing. Chemical Peel Symposium, American Academy of Dermatology, 1992.
27. Murray JC, Pollack SV, Pinnell SR. Keloids: a review. J Am Acad Dermatol 1981; 4: 461–470.
28. Aalto-Korte K. Improvement to skin barrier function during treatment of atopic dermatitis. J Am Acad Dermatol 1995; 33:969–972.
29. Ghadially R, Halkier-Sorensen L, Elias PM. Effects of petrolatum on stratum corneum structure and function. J Am Acad Dermatol 1992; 26:387–396.
30. Asken S. Unoccluded Baker/Gordon phenol peels: review and update. J Dermatol Surg Oncol 1989; 15:998–1008.
31. Mercer NSG. Silicone gel in the treatment of keloid scars. Br J Plast Surg 1989; 42: 83–87.
32. Gold MH. A controlled clinical trial of topical silicone gel sheeting in the treatment of hypertrophic scars and keloids. J Am Acad Dermatol 1994; 30:506–507.
33. Katz BE. Silicone gel sheeting in scar therapy. Cutis 1995; 56:65–67.
34. Goldman MP, Fitzpatrick RE. Laser treatment of scars. Dermatol Surg 1995; 21:685–687.
35. Alster RS. Improvement of erythematous and hypertrophic scars by the 585-nm flash-lamp-pumped pulsed dye laser. Ann Plast Surg 1993; 31:1–5.
36. Alster TS, Kurban AK, Grove GL, Grove MJ, Tan OT. Alteration of argon laser–induced scars by the pulsed dye laser. Lasers Surg Med 1993; 13:368–373.
37. Brody HJ. Update on chemical peeling. Adv Dermatol 1992; 7:275–289.
38. Perez IR. Vegetarians may heal more slowly after chemical face peels. American Academy of Cosmetic Surgery, Los Angeles, CA, Feb 1995.
39. Milner SM. Acetic acid to treat Pseudomonas aeruginosa in superficial wounds and burns (Letter). Lancet 1992; 340:61.
40. Dmytryshyn JR. Chemical face peel complicated by toxic shock syndrome. Arch Otolaryngol 1983; 109:170.
41. LoVerme WE, et al. Toxic shock syndrome after chemical face peel. Plast Reconstr Surg 1987; 80:115–118.
42. Rapaport MJ, Kamer F. Exacerbation of facial herpes simplex after phenolic face peels. J Dermatol Surg Oncol 1984; 10:57–58.
43. Pflugfelder SC, Huang A, Crouse C. Epstein-Barr virus keratitis after a chemical face peel. Am J Ophthalmol 1990; 110:571–573.
44. Fitzpatrick RE, Goldman MP, Satur NM, Tope WD. Pulsed carbon dioxide laser resurfacing of photoaged facial skin. Arch Dermatol 1996; 132:395–402.
45. Stewart RH, Graham GF. A complication of cryosurgery in a patient with cryofibrinogenemia. J Dermatol Surg Oncol 1978; 4:743–744.
46. Brown AM, Kaplan LM, Brown ME. Phenol induced histological skin changes: hazards, techniques, and uses. Br J Plast Surg 1960; 13:158–169.
47. Ayres S. Superficial chemosurgery in treating aging skin. Arch Dermatol 1962; 85:125–133.
48. Litton C. Chemical face lifting. Plast Reconstr Surg 1962; 29:371–380.
49. Stagnone JJ, Stagnone GJ. A second look at chemabrasion. J Dermatol Surg Oncol 1982; 8:701–705.
50. Truppman F, Ellenbery J. The major electrocardiographic changes during chemical face peeling. Plast Reconstr Surg 1979; 63:44.
51. Gross D. Cardiac arrhythmia during phenol face peeling. Plast Reconstr Surg 1984; 73: 590–594.
52. Beeson WH. The importance of cardiac monitoring in superficial and deep chemical peeling. J Dermatol Surg Oncol 1987; 13:949–950.

53. McCollough EG, Langston PR. Dermabrasion and Chemical Peel, A Guide for Facial Plastic Surgery. New York: Thieme Medical Publishers Inc, 1988:53–112.
54. Price NM. EKG changes in relationship to the chemical peel. J Dermatol Oncol 1990; 16:37–42.
55. Klein DR, Little JH. Laryngeal edema as a complication of chemical peel. Plast Reconstr Surg 1983; 71:419–420.
56. Detwiler SP, Saperstein HW. Physically induced pemphigus after cosmetic procedures. Int J Dermatol 1993; 32:100–103.
57. Morrow DM. Chemical peeling of eyelids and periorbital area. J Dermatol Surg Oncol 1992; 18:102–110.
58. Gleason MD, Gosselin RF, Hodge HC, et al. Clinical Toxicology of Commercial Products. Baltimore: Williams & Wilkins, 1969:189–192.

APPENDIX 1: CHEMICAL PEELS AND DERMABRASIONS—WHAT THEY CAN AND CANNOT DO

Dermatologic surgeons have been using peeling agents for the last 50 years. Light peels to correct mild defects, medium depth peels to correct moderate defects, and deep peels to correct severe defects can be used over the entire face and neck area uniformly, or in combining light, medium depth and deep peels on the same face to correct different skin problems. Today with rejuvenation of the skin and reversal of the aging process paramount in the minds of many, chemical peeling has emerged as an exciting supplement to a total skin care program.

Most chemical peels today are supplemented by the peeling effects of creams, such as retinoic acid (Retin-A) on a daily basis, which gives a constant turnover of the top layers of the skin further improving its integrity. Peels can also be used to eradicate superficial sun damage and prevent the reoccurrence of precancers of the skin.

WHAT CHEMICAL PEELS CAN DO

I. Correction of sun damage (Actinic Degeneration)
II. Flattening mild scarring
III. Removing rhytids (Wrinkles)
IV. Improving irregular hyperpigmentation

The mild and moderate peels are called freshening peels because they improve the quality of the skin without altering its normal architecture. The ability of the skin to tan again and return to the same color after peeling or sunlight exposure is unchanged.

With deeper peels, usually involving phenol, the color of the skin is lighter after peeling and may not ever tan again; instead it may freckle.

WHAT CHEMICAL PEELS CANNOT DO

I. Chemical peels cannot change pore size - if anything they might increase pore size temporarily.
II. Chemical peels cannot improve lax skin; removal of fine wrinkling and cross-hatching may not make any difference if there is profound lax skin that needs a face lift.
III. Chemical peels cannot improve deep scarring. Dermabrasion, punch grafting, punch elevation, or excision of scarring is much more effective.
IV. Chemical peeling cannot always totally remove hyperpigmentation in dark skinned Caucasians, Asians, or blacks and may not be indicated.
V. Chemical peeling cannot remove broken blood vessels on the face.

APPENDIX 2: CHEMICAL PEEL CONSENT

I, ____, consent to the treatment known as a chemical peel. The treatment has been explained to me, and I have had an opportunity to ask questions. The procedure will cause swelling of my face which may be uncomfortable. The skin will turn red, blister and crust, and look like a very bad sunburn before it heals. The peeling usually lasts about 1-2 weeks, although it may last longer. I understand that there is a risk of developing a temporary or permanent pigment color change in the skin. There is a small incidence of the reactivation of "cold sores" (herpes infection) in patients with a prior history of herpes. Acne may be aggravated or appear temporarily after a peel. There is also a rare incidence of allergy to the creams used after the peel. There is a rare incidence of scarring. The actual degree of improvement cannot be predicted or guaranteed. I also consent to the taking of medical photographs

______________________________________ ____________________

Patient's Signature Date

______________________________________ ____________________

Witness Date

APPENDIX 3: POST–SKIN PEEL

You have been peeled with chemicals that may cause water blisters that may break, crust, turn brown, and peel off over a period of a week.

Washing with a mild soap (Dove) and povidone-iodine skin cleanser (Betadine) twice daily in the shower or over the sink is necessary to prevent any infection. Use your fingertips and not a Buf-Puf since the skin is very sensitive at this time. A tube of petrolatum-containing ointment (Aquaphor, Vaseline) or Preparation H should be used during this week all over the face after washing. A tube is more sterile than a jar. Do not pick at the peeled skin.

Three (3) aspirin or ibuprofin are to be taken 3-4 times daily to reduce swelling. Sleep on several pillows the first night.

Total sunblock and a hat should be used after the first week, but remember, your skin will be more sensitive than usual.

If <u>pain</u> begins, which may signal a fever blister, call us immediately.

APPENDIX 4: POST–SKIN PEEL INSTRUCTIONS—SUPERFICIAL

You have been peeled with chemicals that contain superficial agents that may contain alpha hydroxy acids or other mild acids. Typically the skin turns dark the following day and peels without blistering over the next 3-5 days. Flaking may persist longer than this. Stop your skin cream regimen, wash and shampoo normally, and apply only sunscreen moisturizer or bland moisturizer if the sunscreen stings. You may return to your regimen after the skin has peeled and is pink, usually by 5-7 days. Do not pick at the peeling skin or scarring could result. Allow the skin to come off naturally with cream application. Sometimes the first peel produces very little reaction. Successive superficial peels may result in more redness and reactivity, but this can usually be adjusted by you and your doctor. You may apply makeup over this peel at any time, but coverage of the peeling skin may not be complete.

Severe swelling or crusting of an area does not usually occur but may happen if you are sensitive to one of the ingredients. Any swelling that occurs is not permanent and will recede in several days. If you develop a fever blister during the recovery period after your peel, you should begin acyclovir (Zovirax) or your antiviral pills immediately as prescribed. Please contact our office if severe swelling, local crusting, or fever blisters develop.

7

CO_2 Laser Resurfacing

Tina S. Alster

Washington Institute of Dermatologic Laser Surgery, and Georgetown University, Washington, D.C.

INTRODUCTION

Despite the advent of new laser surgery technologies, the carbon dioxide (CO_2) laser remains unparalleled in its versatility for cosmetic cutaneous resurfacing. Currently available CO_2 lasers ablate tissue by emitting brief pulses of high energy which greatly minimizes cutaneous thermal damage—an effect of older continuous wave (CW) laser systems that commonly led to unwanted tissue fibrosis and scarring.

HISTORY

The development of today's superior resurfacing lasers is attributable to the successful application of the principles of selective photothermolysis, wherein employment of the correct wavelength and pulse duration of laser light could effect selective destruction of a particular cutaneous target without unwanted thermal injury to normal surrounding skin. This theory, first proposed in the early 1980s [1], revolutionized the role of lasers for cutaneous resurfacing, leading to their transformation into precise tissue ablation tools. Numerous CO_2 laser systems are now available for vaporizing rhytides, atrophic scars, and a variety of epidermal and dermal lesions [2–16].

At a wavelength of 10,600 nm, the CO_2 laser is ideal for cutaneous resurfacing because of the strong absorption of its infrared wavelength by water-containing tissue (water constitutes 70% of skin tissue volume). However, early CO_2 lasers emitted light in a continuous wave (CW) mode that far exceeded the 0.001 second thermal relaxation time of the 20 to 30 μm of laser-absorbing skin, resulting in unintended tissue fibrosis and scarring [17–21]. When pulsed and scanned CO_2 lasers were subsequently developed in the early 1990s, thin layers of skin (20–30 μm per pass) could be removed through the delivery of very high peak fluences in less than 0.001 seconds [22–24]. Thus, successful vaporization of tissue could be achieved while leaving an acceptably narrow zone of residual thermal damage (25–70 μm in comparison with 200–600 μm produced by the CW systems) [20–25]. In addition, the thermal effect of the pulsed and scanned CO_2 lasers in the dermis could effect excellent hemostasis and visible collagen shrinkage during tissue irradiation [26–28].

Thus, the goal of CO_2 laser resurfacing is the clean, char-free, layer-by-layer ablation of skin, resulting in the absolute or relative effacement of lesions while avoiding the creation of excessive dermal injury that could result in scarring or other untoward complications. Obliteration of the epidermis and partial ablation or coagulative necrosis of the upper dermis is achieved. Re-epithelialization occurs from the migration of normal, well-organized cells from follicular adnexae which effectively replace atypical, disorganized photodamaged skin cells. In addition, normal compact collagen and elastic fibers replace the amorphous elastotic dermal elements that are removed with laser vaporization. Collagen shrinkage (up to 25%) is seen intraoperatively and during the collagen remodeling phase of wound healing, presumably because of either the production of a new collagen matrix that recapitulates the contracted postoperative "scaffolding" or the production of immunofactors by fibroblasts that migrate into the laser-induced wounds [29,30].

PATIENT SELECTION

The ideal patient for CO_2 laser resurfacing has a fair skin type (phototype I or II), laser-amenable epidermal or dermal lesions, and realistic expectations (Table 1) (Fig. 1) [31–34]. Although individuals with darker complexions (phototypes III–VI) can also be treated, they are more prone to develop undesirable postoperative pigmentary changes, and thus must be approached more cautiously (Fig. 2).

The type of lesion(s) present is a major criterion in determining whether the CO_2 laser resurfacing procedure is appropriate. Patients with photodamaged skin, evidenced by non-movement-associated rhytides and dyspigmentation, as well as

TABLE 1 Patient Selection

Ideal Treatment Candidate
Pale skin tone (skin phototype I or II)
Non-movement-associated rhytides
Actinic cheilitis
Atrophic facial scars
Epidermal lesions
Mild dermatochalasis
Less-than-Ideal Treatment Candidate
Dark skin tone (phototype III–VI)
Dynamic (movement-associated) rhytides
Pitted scars
Diffuse dyspigmentation
Extensive dermal lesions
Contraindications
Prior lower blepharoplasty +/− ectropion
Fibrosis due to prior treatment
Collagen vascular disease, immunologic dysfunction, Koebnerizing skin condition
Concurrent skin infection
Medical problems or medication that could interfere with surgery and/or anesthesia
Unrealistic expectations
Noncompliance

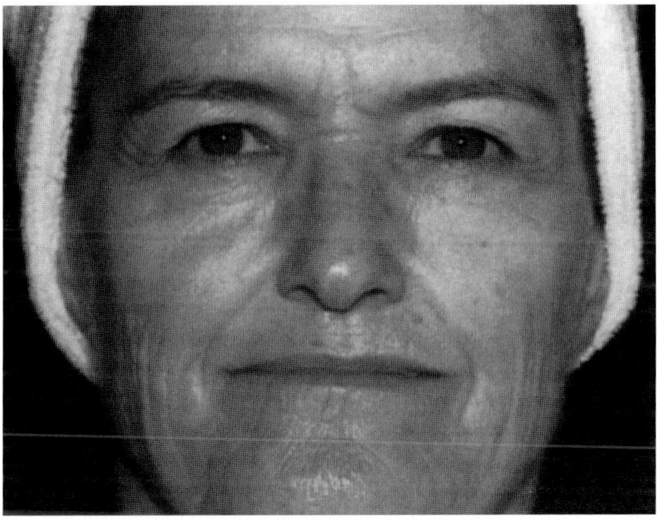

FIGURE 1 Ideal laser surgery candidate has skin phototype I to II, predominantly non-movement-associated rhytides (perioral, cheeks, periorbital, chin), and no prior history of treatment.

atrophic scars can achieve excellent results with CO_2 laser vaporization [2–8,12–14]. Dynamic (movement-associated) rhytides in the glabellar and brow regions are not as amenable to laser resurfacing and have a high recurrence rate [31,35]. Mild dermatochalasis can be ameliorated because of the collagen-tightening effect of CO_2 laser vaporization [36]. Epidermal and dermal lesions responsive to laser resurfacing include seborrheic and actinic keratoses, molluscum contagiosum, syringomas, epi-

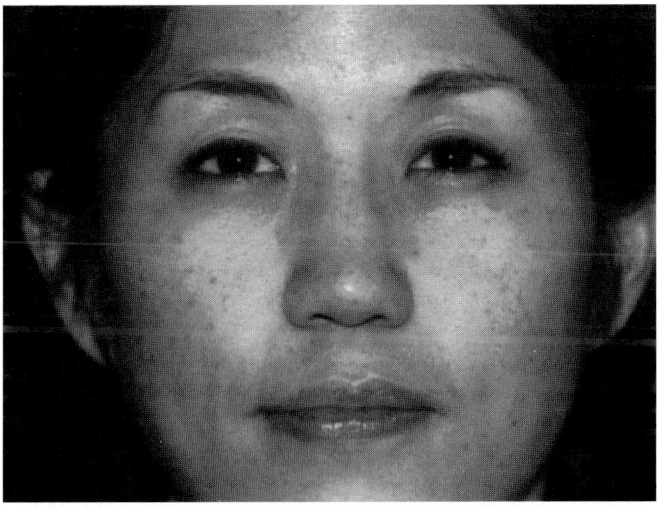

FIGURE 2 Less-than-ideal treatment candidate has skin phototype III (or darker) and melasma.

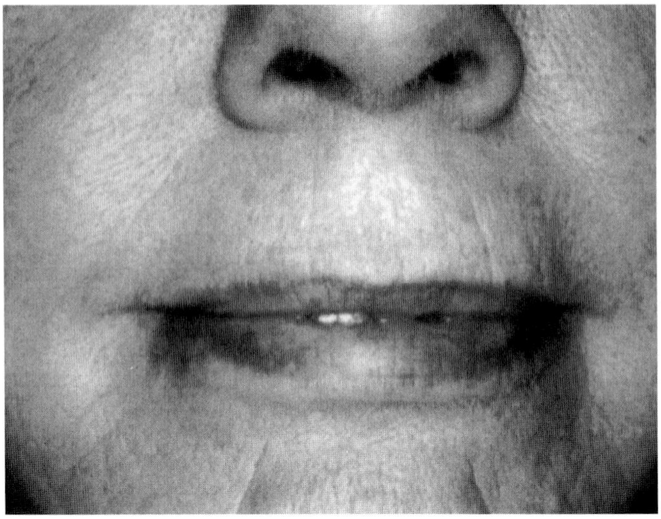

FIGURE 3 Active herpes labialis is an absolute contraindication to cutaneous laser resurfacing. Once infection has cleared, the patient may be resurfaced with concomitant use of prophylactic antiherpetic therapy.

dermal nevi, diffuse lentigines, verrucae, actinic cheilitis, xanthelasma, sebaceous hyperplasia, trichoepitheliomas, and rhinophyma [9–11].

The patient's ability to tolerate the extended period of convalescence after the laser procedure must also be considered. Re-epithelialization typically requires 7 to 10 days and erythema can persist for several months postoperatively. Thus, individuals whose practical obligations prevent them from being able to take the time necessary for healing or those who are temperamentally unsuited to remaining housebound for an extended period are not suitable candidates for CO_2 laser resurfacing. In addition, some patients may have psychological difficulty dealing with the immediate negative effects of laser resurfacing on their physical appearance, and should therefore be given other treatment options (eg, botulinum or collagen injections) that would not require a significant or prolonged healing course.

Absolute contraindications to laser resurfacing include isotretinoin use within 6–12 months of surgery, active cutaneous infection, presence of ectropion (for infraorbital resurfacing), poor patient compliance, and unrealistic patient expectations [31–34] (Fig. 3). Relative contraindications include perpetual sun exposure; collagen, vascular, or immunologic disease; previous lower blepharoplasty (for infraorbital resurfacing); and history of radiation therapy or extensive tissue fibrosis in the involved area (eg, from previous dermabrasion, deep chemical peels) (Fig. 4).

PATIENT EDUCATION

Once the patient has been determined to be a good treatment candidate for laser resurfacing, extensive patient education begins. The relative benefits and risks of the procedure should be thoroughly detailed. Patients should be given a realistic view of the anticipated postoperative course and eventual clinical results without absolute

1. Are the patient's lesion(s) amenable to laser resurfacing? While a variety of epidermal and dermal lesions as well as rhytides and scars respond favorably to laser vaporization, unusual pigmented lesions or other suspicious growths should be biopsied for histologic examination prior to laser irradiation.
2. Has the patient ever had the lesions treated? Laser resurfacing may unmask hypopigmentation or fibrosis produced by prior dermabrasion, cryosurgery, or phenol peels. In addition, the presence of fibrosis may limit the vaporization potential of the CO_2 laser, thereby decreasing clinical efficacy. Patients who have had prior lower blepharoplasties (using an external approach) are at greater risk of ectropion formation after infraorbital resurfacing due to the collagen tightening effect of the CO_2 laser on residual dermal tissue.
3. What is the patient's skin type? Paler skin tones have a lower incidence of undesirable postoperative hyperpigmentation compared to darker skin tones after CO_2 laser resurfacing.
4. Does the patient have a history of herpes labialis? Reactivation and/or dissemination of prior herpes simplex infection can occur with laser resurfacing. The de-epithelialized skin is also particularly susceptible to primary inoculation by herpes simplex virus.
5. Does the patient have an autoimmune disease or other immunologic deficiency? Because the postoperative course associated with CO_2 laser resurfacing is prolonged, intact immunologic function and collagen repair mechanisms are necessary to optimize the tissue healing response. In addition to possible delayed wound healing, patients with scleroderma, lupus erythematosus, and vitiligo may also exhibit worsening of their conditions after CO_2 laser resurfacing. The procedure may exacerbate underlying immunodeficiencies in patients with HIV disease and make them more susceptible to secondary infection.
6. Are there other dermatologic conditions present which could potentially spread after treatment? Psoriasis, eczema, verrucae, and molluscum are but a few conditions that could conceivably koebnerize after CO_2 laser vaporization. Thus, the skin should be carefully inspected to rule out the presence of these and other inflammatory or infectious cutaneous lesions so that the final clinical result is optimized.
7. Is the patient taking any medications that are contraindicated? Concomitant isotretinoin use could potentially lead to an increased risk of postoperative hypertrophic scar formation due to its detrimental effect on wound healing and collagenesis. Because the alteration in healing is idiosyncratic, a safe interval between the use of oral retinoids and laser resurfacing is difficult to calculate; however, most practitioners delay the treatment for at least 6 to 12 months after cessation of the drug.
8. Does the patient have a tendency to form hypertrophic scars or keloids? Patients with a propensity to scar will be at greater risk of scar formation after laser resurfacing, independent of the laser's selectivity and the operator's skill level. If unsure of a patient's scarring tendency, a test area can be lased before making a determination as to whether laser treatment in that particular individual is a viable treatment option.
9. Is the patient prone to acne breakouts? Complete control of acne eruptions should be obtained prior to laser resurfacing with appropriate topical or systemic antibiotics. The presence of inflamed papules, pustules or cysts could lead to excessive intraoperative bleeding and limit operator visibility or could impair postoperative wound healing and thus affect the ultimate clinical results.
10. Are there medical conditions present or medications being taken that would preclude the use of intravenous anesthesia? Patients with a history of heart disease, asthma, or emphysema should either receive medical clearance from their primary care physicians to undergo the resurfacing procedure and/or have a recent (within the preceding 6 months) chest x-ray and electrocardiogram that can be examined. In addition, a review of the patient's current medications and known allergies should be made to exclude possible adverse drug reactions.
11. Does the patient have realistic expectations of the procedure and will he/she be compliant with postoperative instructions? Patients who believe that every rhytide or scar will be removed with the laser resurfacing procedure are not good treatment candidates. In addition, those who can not physically or emotionally handle the prolonged postoperative course should also be dissuaded from pursuing laser treatment.

FIGURE 4 Questionnaire for patient selection.

guarantees of outcomes. Patients should not only be prepared for the initial 1 to 2 weeks of postoperative erythema, pain, and edema, but also to the fact that return of the skin to its normal coloration will take several weeks to several months. Because pigmentary alteration of skin after laser resurfacing is common, patients need to understand that sun exposure is contraindicated until wound healing is complete (eg, when all erythema has subsided).

In addition to helping to establish a sense of rapport between physician and patient, good preoperative teaching can also positively affect the postoperative course by ensuring patient compliance and preventing adverse psychological sequelae. Ideally, such information should be presented repetitively and in a variety of formats: verbally with the physician and with various staff members, through observation of pertinent patient photographs and videotape demonstrations, and in written form (see Appendix 1).

Informed consent (see Appendix 2) and representative preoperative photographs of the involved areas should be obtained. Postoperative instructions should also be provided (see Appendix 3). A preoperative checklist ensures that all of the necessary information has been received and considered (see Appendix 4).

PREOPERATIVE SKIN PREPARATION

Preoperative regimens differ widely, and there remains a lack of consensus on whether the patient's skin should be pretreated for several weeks before surgery with topical tretinoin, alpha-hydroxy acids, and/or bleaching agents such as hydroquinone in order to enhance healing or to reduce the incidence of postoperative hyperpigmentation [37–39]. Although topical tretinoin in particular may be expected to accelerate postoperative re-epithelialization, its benefit in laser resurfacing remains problematic because laser-induced cutaneous wounds differ substantially from those produced by dermabrasion or deep chemical peels. The use of hydroquinone or other bleaching agents would be expected to reduce the incidence of postoperative hyperpigmentation by their cytoxic effects on melanocytes and/or inhibition of tyrosinase (with decreased melanosome formation); however, a recent study has shown no significant effect of the pretreatment use of hydroquinone, or retinoic or glycolic acid on posttreatment hyperpigmentation [40]. Topical antioxidants such as vitamin C serve to block ultraviolet light–induced tissue damage and may stimulate fibroblasts as well as photoprotect the skin during the wound-healing process. In addition, ascorbic acid has been shown to reduce the duration of postoperative erythema, presumably because of its anti-inflammatory effect [41].

As previously discussed, antiviral prophylaxis is recommended in all patients undergoing resurfacing, regardless of personal herpetic history [31–34]. Antiherpetic medications such as acyclovir, famciclovir, and valacyclovir are typically initiated 24 hours before the procedure and continued for 10 days at which time re-epithelialization is complete.

Prophylactic antibiotics with gram-positive coverage are often used because of the thermal injury produced and presumed predisposition of the wound bed to infection. New research, however, indicates that the use of antibiotics may instead lead to suprainfection with more pathogenic organisms such as pseudomonas and serratia species [42]. Therefore, as has been shown by wound healing research of burns, antibiotics may best be reserved for clinical and/or laboratory findings indicative of infection.

INTRAOPERATIVE CONSIDERATIONS

On the day of surgery, patients should be instructed to avoid make-up application, to tie back hair, and to wear comfortable clothing (eg, button or zip-front rather than pullover top). Once in the operating suite, the periphery of the patient's face and neck should be draped with dampened cloths and the skin prepared with a nonflammable solution (eg, Septisol or Betadine). Treatment boundaries should be marked with patient in an upright position using a felt-tip pen (Fig. 5). Metal eye shields should then be inserted after instillation of tetracaine drops and an ophthalmic lubricant (Fig. 6). When treating isolated facial regions such as the perioral or periorbital areas, local anesthesia, sensory nerve blocks (Fig. 7), and/or tumescent anesthesia can be used. For full-face procedures, intravenous sedation with a mixture of anesthetic agents (eg, propofol, midazolam, fentanyl, ketamine) are typically used. These anesthetics provide short-acting sedation, analgesia, and amnesia, thereby making the procedure more comfortable for the patient. Appropriate monitoring equipment, including blood pressure monitor, pulse oximeter, and electrocardiogram, as well as emergency resuscitation equipment (oxygen delivery system, intubation supplies, defibrillator) should be present (Table 2).

LASER PROTOCOL

Multiple different CO_2 lasers are available for cutaneous resurfacing: pulsed, scanned, and superpulsed. High-energy pulsed systems include the Coherent Ultrapulse, Paragon ClearPulse, and Tissue Technologies TruPulse. Scanned systems include the Sharplan/ESC FeatherTouch and SilkTouch lasers which effectively serve

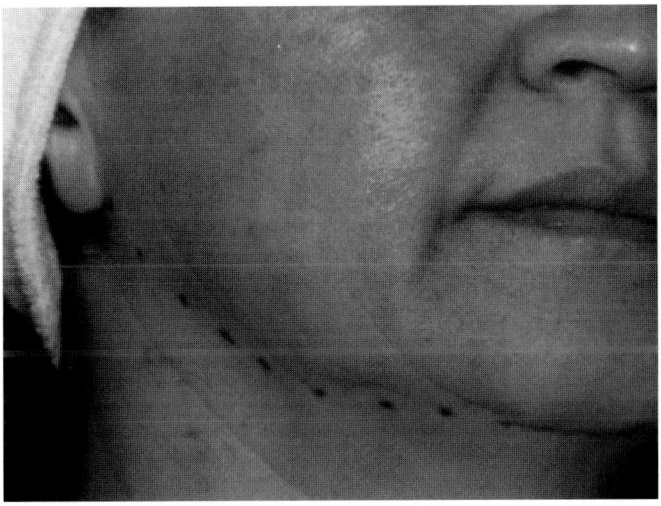

FIGURE 5 Treatment boundaries are ink-marked with patient in an upright position prior to surgery.

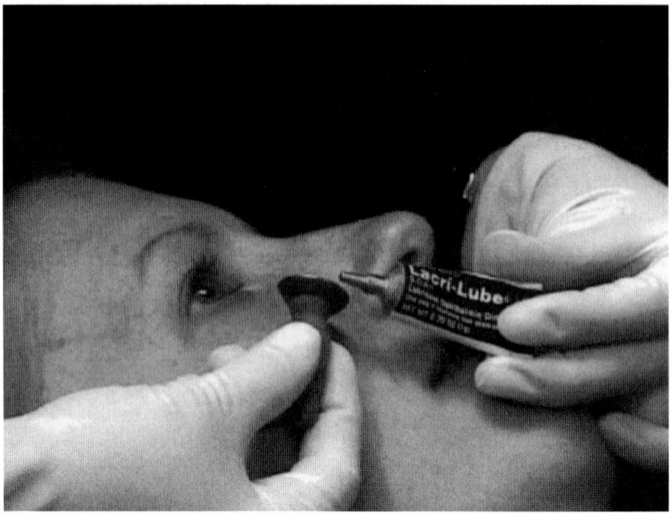

FIGURE 6 Sand-blasted metal eye shields are carefully inserted after instillation of tetracaine eye drops and ophthalamic lubricant.

as pulsed systems with tissue-dwell times shorter than 1-ms. Superpulsed lasers include the Luxar NovaPulse and Nidek UniPulse.

The UltraPulse laser produces individual 600 μs to 1 ms pulses with peak energies of 500 mJ, resulting in production of fluences exceeding the 2 to 5 J/cm^2 ablation threshold of skin. A computer pattern generator (CPG) handpiece, which places 2.25 mm spots in present patterns at maximum energies of 300 mJ and 60 watts power can be used with this laser. Most surgeons select square or rhomboid

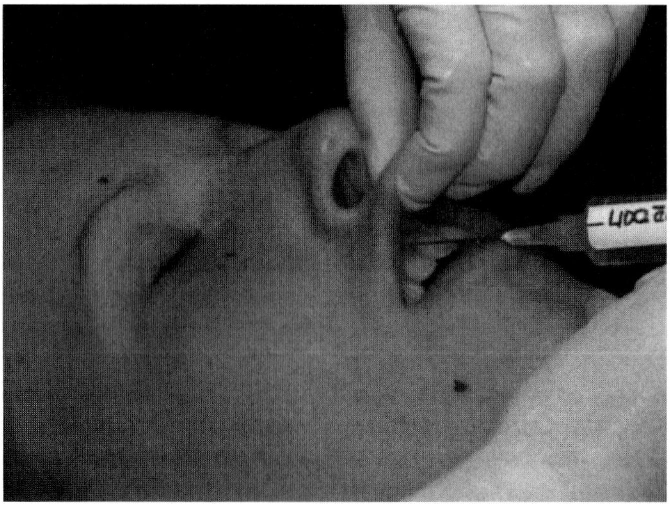

FIGURE 7 Cutaneous sensory nerve blocks are delivered intraorally using lidocaine with 1:200,000 units epinephrine. (Nerve exit sites are marked with ink pen).

TABLE 2 Intraoperative Checklist

Laser Tray
Gauze (4 × 4 in)
Lacrilube ophthalmic ointment
Tetracaine eye drops
Normal saline
Laser Safety Equipment
Smoke evacuator
Metal eyeshields/contacts (patient)
Laser goggles (surgical room personnel)
Fire extinguisher
Anesthetics
Lidocaine with epinephrine
Fentanyl
Ketamine
Propofol
Versed
Monitoring Equipment
Blood pressure monitor
EKG
Pulse oximeter
Resuscitation Equipment
Oxygen and delivery system
Emergency medications
Intubation equipment
Defibrillator

patterns at varying sizes (up to 9 mm^2). Pattern densities can be adjusted so that spots are placed adjacent to each other, either overlapping by 10 to 60% (higher density) or nonoverlapping (lower density). The 3 mm collimated handpiece is usually applied at 350 to 500 mJ/pulse and 3 to 7 watts to treat difficult-to-reach areas such as the medial canthal regions, which require more manual dexterity and precise laser spot placement, or at the completion of a resurfacing procedure to "sculpt" raised edges of scars or ragged treatment edges (eg, mandibular ridge, frontal scalp line, preauricular area).

The SilkTouch and FeatherTouch laser systems incorporate the use of a flash-scanner (a microprocessor-controlled optomechanical device consisting of rotating mirrors that produces a spiral scan) that can be attached to many CO_2 laser systems. These lasers can deliver 0.2 mm spots in a spiral pattern so rapidly that the dwell time on any individual area is less than the 1 ms thermal relaxation time of skin. The resurfacing parameters of the SilkTouch/FeatherTouch systems include spot sizes of 4 to 6 mm and 5 to 20 watt powers. Delicate or thin tissue areas such as the periorbital regions require the use of lower power levels and fewer laser passes. Thicker perioral and cheek skin or more severely scarred or fibrotic areas are usually treated with a greater number of passes at higher energies.

The TruPulse laser is a 6 watt CO_2 system delivering individual 60 to 100 μs pulses at fluences exceeding 5 J/cm^2. Successive passes using 3 mm square spots are applied over the treatment region. Once the desired level of tissue ablation has been achieved, a "shrink spatula" can be used on thicker skin areas such as the cheeks and upper lip in order to obtain a tightening effect.

The superpulsed NovaPulse laser features a CO_2 system with pulse durations of 160 to 900 μs and peak powers of 5 to 8 watts. The preset programs used for light (A5) and heavy ablation (A14) are delivered through a 3 mm scanned handpiece at 4 to 7 watts, producing fluences of 60 to 80 mJ/mm^2. A larger scanner can also be attached to the system, thereby resulting in faster treatment times. While tissue vaporization is effected, greater residual thermal damage is seen with this system compared with the aforementioned pulsed lasers.

In addition to the clean layer-by-layer ablation of skin that can be achieved with these lasers, an immediate skin tightening effect has been observed. Tissue shrinkage has traditionally been explained by tissue dehydration and contracted dermal collagen; however, recent studies have indicated that new fibroblasts migrating into CO_2 laser–induced wounds express an increased number of immunofactors, including smooth muscle action, which may account for the creation of a smaller, contracted scaffold for further collagen deposition [29,30].

TREATMENT TECHNIQUE

Two or three passes using laser parameters yielding fluences exceeding the 2 to 5 J/cm^2 skin ablation threshold are performed with a scanning handpiece. The partially-desiccated tissue should be completely removed between each successive laser pass in order to limit residual thermal damage and subsequent risk of scarring (Fig. 8). Individual scar edges or residual rhytides can be further sculpted using a smaller scanner or spot size. A treatment log serves to document the laser parameters used and the tissue responses observed (see Appendix 5).

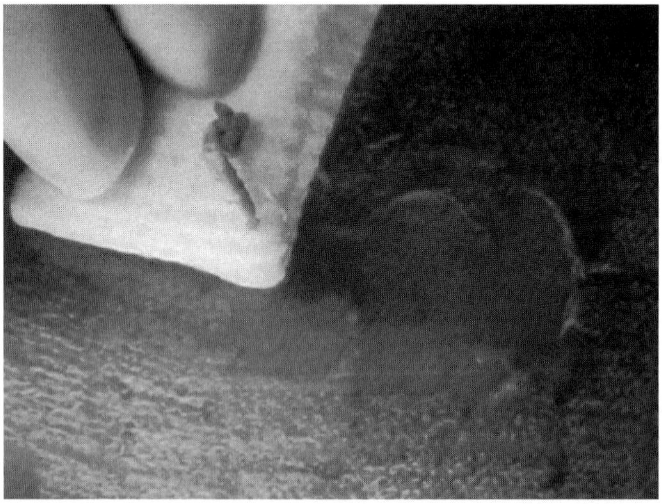

FIGURE 8 Partially-desiccated tissue is completely removed with saline-soaked gauze after each laser pass. Note clean, nonbleeding skin after residual debris from first laser pass has been removed.

TABLE 3 Postoperative Wound Care Options

Open	Closed
Ice packs, cool compresses, or cooling mask	Ice packs or cooling mask
Topical ointments:	Semiocclusive dressings:
Aquaphor	*Flexzan*
BiO_2 balm	*N-Terface*
Catrix-10	*Second Skin*
Elta	*Silon-SR*
Petrolatum	*Vigilon*
Recovery I balm	

POSTOPERATIVE MANAGEMENT

Postoperative healing is prolonged and requires close follow-up. During the re-epithelialization process, which takes place over the first 7 to 10 days, the lased skin must be kept moist using either an open or closed wound dressing (Table 3) [33,34,43–45]. The moist environment promotes healing by preventing dry crust or scab formation which could impede epidermal cell migration. Controversy continues over the best postoperative regimen to use in order to achieve expeditious and maximal wound healing. The closed technique, which involves the use of semiocclusive dressings (eg, Flexzan, Second Skin, Vigilon), offers more patient comfort and a "hands-free" approach to wound care; however it may also be responsible for wound maceration and higher rates of infection with opportunistic bacteria and fungi (Fig. 9) [46]. Open wound care techniques with such healing ointments as Aquaphor, BiO_2

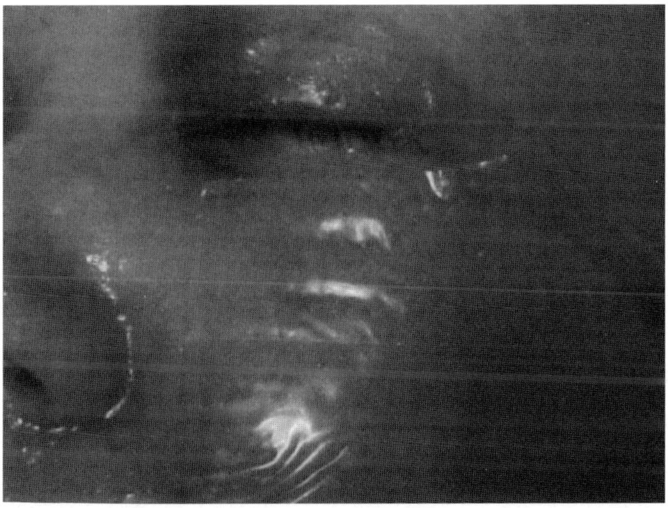

FIGURE 9 "Closed" postoperative technique involves the use of a semiocclusive dressing over the laser-irradiated skin, providing enhanced patient comfort, but limited visualization of the wound bed.

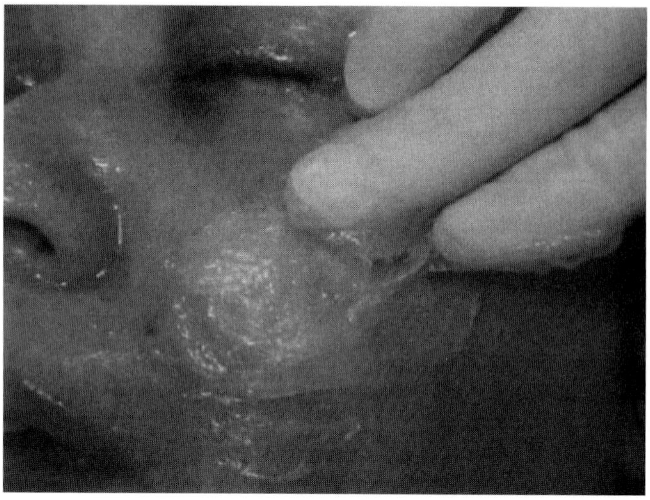

FIGURE 10 **An "open" wound healing technique involves the application of a viscous ointment that is cumbersome to the patient; however, the wound may be evaluated more readily.**

balm, Catrix-10, Elta, Recovery I balm, or plain petrolatum requires more patient involvement with postoperative care, but has shown lower infection rates and permits improved visualization of the wound bed in order to detect and treat problems early in their course (Fig. 10) [47]. Taking into account the advantages and disadvantages of each technique, some surgeons now advocate the use of a closed dressing system for a few days followed by an open technique until full re-epithelialization has occurred.

In all patients undergoing perioral or full-face laser resurfacing, prophylactic antivirals (acyclovir, famciclovir, or valacyclovir) are prescribed until re-epithelialization is completed (7–10 days). The use of prophylactic antibiotics is more controversial because of the potential for the development of drug-resistant strains of bacteria [48]. If used, the antibiotic should have good coverage against gram-positive organisms because they are most frequently responsible for cutaneous infection. Postoperative oral corticosteroids may also be prescribed on a short-term basis to reduce inflammation (edema).

RECOGNIZING AND TREATING SIDE EFFECTS AND COMPLICATIONS

Although the rate of complications after CO_2 laser resurfacing is low and most procedures yield highly favorable results (Figs. 11, 12), serious sequelae can occur even in the hands of experienced surgeons [47,49,50]. Early recognition of and intervention for side effects can limit their ultimate impact.

Mild side effects and complications observed after treatment include prolonged erythema, acne exacerbation, milia formation, and irritant or allergic contact dermatitis. More serious complications include localized bacterial or fungal infections, regional herpes simplex reactivation, and pigmentary alteration (hyper- and hypo-

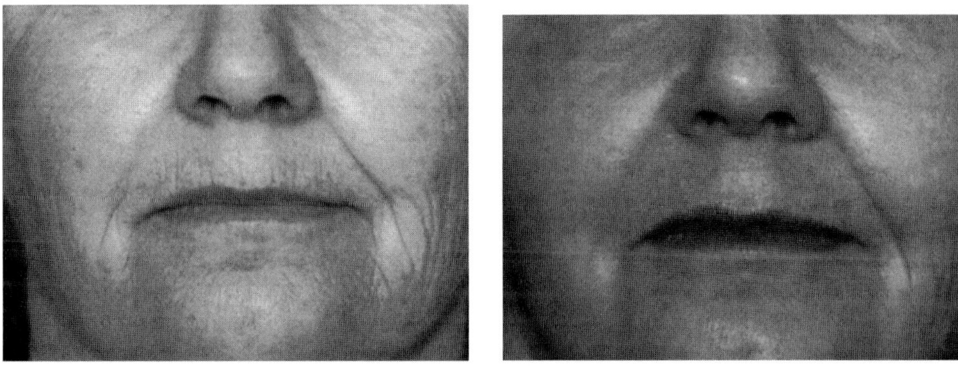

(a) (b)

FIGURE 11 63-year-old woman with photodamaged skin manifested by facial dyspigmentation and non-movement-associated rhytides before surgery (a) and 6 months after full face CO_2 laser resurfacing (b).

pigmentation). The most severe complications (and, fortunately, the most rare) are hypertrophic scarring, ectropion formation, and disseminated infection (Table 4).

Milia formation and acne exacerbation are fairly common occurrences after laser resurfacing because of the need for highly occlusive dressings and ointments in the immediate postoperative period (Fig. 13). After re-epithelialization is complete, topical retinoic, glycolic, and/or azelaic acid may reduce the incidence and severity of milia and acneiform lesions.

Allergic contact or irritant dermatitis may also occur more frequently in patients after laser treatment because of the decreased barrier function of the de-epithelialized tissue. As many as 65% of patients experience a reaction to topical preparations during or immediately after the re-epithelialization process. The most common irritants include antibiotic ointments (eg, neomycin, polysporin, or bacitracin), corticosteroid cream bases, fragrances, and chemical sunscreens.

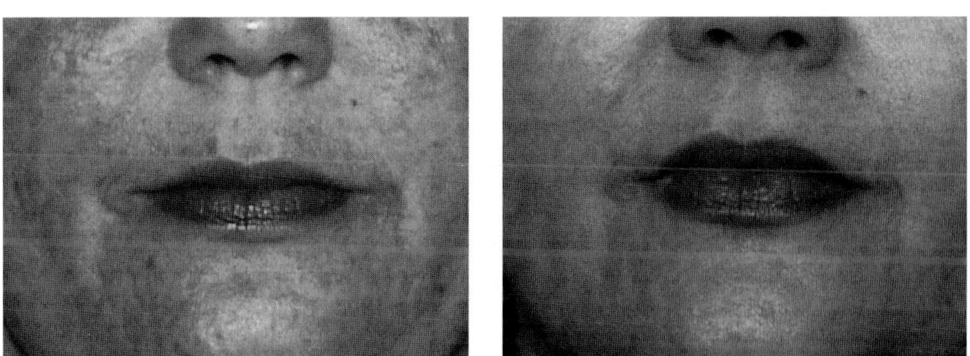

(a) (b)

FIGURE 12 45-year-old woman with atrophic acne scars before surgery (a) and 12 months later showing continued and prolonged improvement (b).

TABLE 4 Side Effects and Complications

Side effect/complication	Management
Erythema	Avoid irritants, use topical ascorbic acid, apply cosmetic camouflage
Allergic/irritant dermatitis	Discontinue irritating substances, use cool compresses/ oral antihistamine/petrolatum-based emollient/topical steroid ointment
Acne exacerbation/milia	Discontinue heavy ointments/occlusive dressings, use oral antibiotics (acne), manual extraction of milia
Hyperpigmentation	Topical retinoic, glycolic, or azelaic acids, hydroquinone, sunscreen, glycolic acid peels
Hypopigmentation	Glycolic or retinoic acid, camouflage makeup, progressive UVL exposure
HSV reactivation	Culture wound, maximize antiviral coverage (zoster dose), aggressive wound care
Bacterial/fungal infection	Culture wound, appropriate oral antibiotic coverage, aggressive wound care
Hypertrophic scarring	Topical/intralesional corticosteroids, silicone gel, pressure dressings, pulsed dye laser rx
Ectropion	Massage, topical corticosteroids, surgical repair

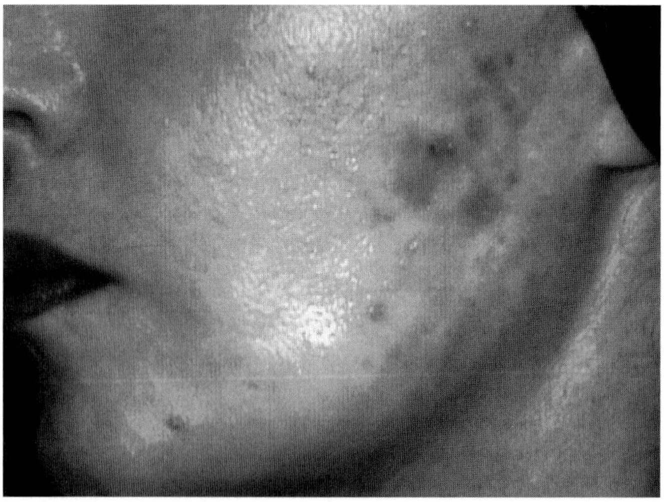

FIGURE 13 Acne exacerbation, milia, and dermatitis seen 1 to 2 months after laser resurfacing. Elimination or reduction of occlusive ointment use with or without topical corticosteroid application helps to alleviate the problem.

Pigmentary alterations are more problematic for patients postoperatively. Hyperpigmentation occurs in upwards of one third of those who undergo resurfacing, with nearly universal incidence in patients with dark skin phototypes (III or greater) (Fig. 14). It is typically observed within the first or second months after surgery and, although it usually resolves spontaneously, its resolution can be hastened with the topical use of glycolic, azelaic, or retinoic acid creams, light glycolic acid peels, and/or topical hydroquinone, along with regular sunscreen use. Avoidance of products that cause irritation is imperative, as postinflammatory hyperpigmentation can worsen. Hypopigmentation is less frequently seen, but unlike hyperpigmentation, its appearance is delayed (6–12 months) and relatively permanent [51]. The severity of the pigment loss may be reduced by the treatment of surrounding dyspigmented skin with peeling or lightening agents.

Viral, bacterial, and fungal infections usually occur within 7 to 10 days postoperatively during the re-epithelialization process (Fig. 15). Even with appropriate antiviral prophylaxis, herpes outbreaks have been shown to occur in 2 to 7% of all laser resurfacing patients [52]. The most common bacterial infections are those caused by *Staphylococcus aureus*; however, *Pseudomonas* and *Candida* infections have also occurred because of the necessity of maintaining a moist wound environment in the postoperative period. Because severe cutaneous infections can disrupt and prolong the healing process, prompt and aggressive treatment is necessary to prevent the development of scarring or the systemic spread of the infection. Wound cultures should, thus, be obtained and the patient placed on appropriate antibiotic coverage with optimal wound care.

Hypertrophic scarring, ectropion formation, and systemic infection are the most severe complications of cutaneous laser resurfacing and, fortunately, are also the most rare, occurring in fewer than 1% of cases [47,49,50]. Hypertrophic scarring usually becomes apparent within the first or second months postoperatively. Areas

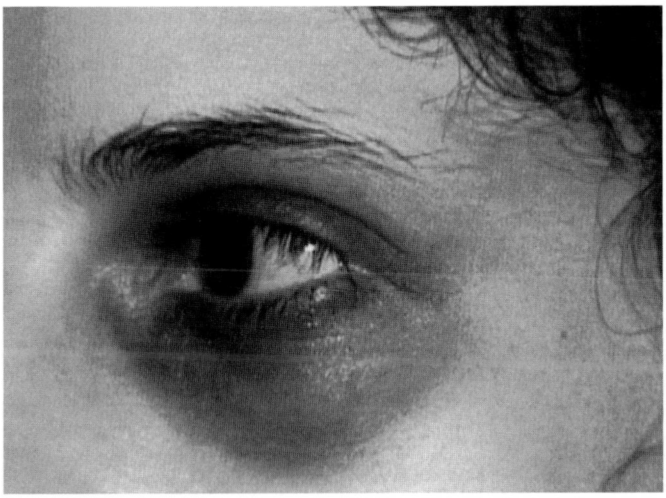

FIGURE 14 Hyperpigmentation seen 1 month after periorbital laser resurfacing. Spontaneous resolution occurs; however, topical retinoic, glycolic, azelaic acid and/or hydroquinone application can hasten the process.

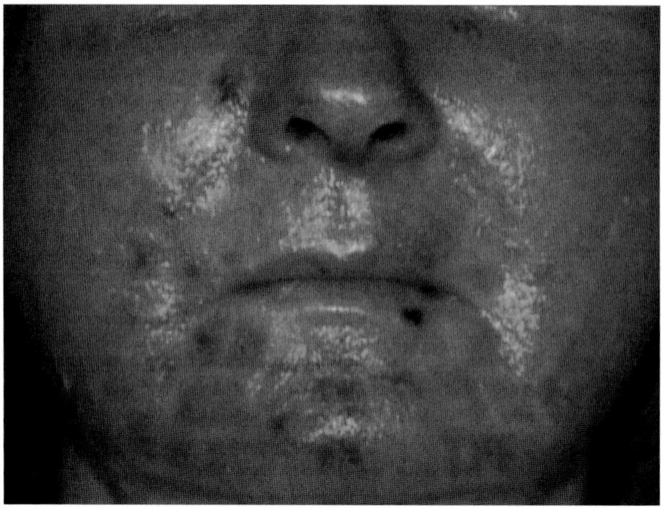

FIGURE 15 Bacterial infection seen 5 days after full face CO_2 laser resurfacing despite use of antibiotic prophylaxis. Early intervention with appropriate broad spectrum antibiotics (after obtaining wound cultures) and aggressive topical wound management prevents continued infectious spread and possible scarring.

most prone to scar formation include the perioral, chin, mandibular, and neck regions, but the aggressiveness of treatment (eg, energy density used, number of passes performed, overlapping placement of spots/scans) can also impact scar development. In addition to conventional intralesional steroid use, topical silicone gel, and pressure dressings, 585 nm pulsed dye laser irradiation can improve the clinical and histopathologic appearance of hypertrophic scars and also reduce associated pruritus and dysesthesia [53]. Although the rate of ectropion formation is also low, it occurs most often in those patients who have previously undergone an external lower blepharoplasty and/or in those who have had overly aggressive infraorbital laser resurfacing. Topical corticosteroids and massage can improve ectropion to a certain extent; however, surgical intervention is often necessary for its full correction.

SUMMARY

CO_2 laser vaporization remains the "gold standard" for cutaneous resurfacing. The latest CO_2 laser technology has revolutionized the approach to facial rejuvenation of rhytides and scar treatment. Complications, however, can still occur despite the use of precise laser parameters and improved visualization of treatment endpoints. The common notion that the laser resurfacing procedure is "easy in, easy out" is not only untrue, but has led to unrealistic patient expectations. Thus, in addition to providing the patients with basic laser education, it is important to determine the patient's suitability for treatment based on the medical and dermatologic history, previous and concurrent treatments, and actual lesions at presentation. The relative benefits and risks of the laser procedure should be discussed as well as the specifics of the postresurfacing healing period. The importance of close postoperative follow-up cannot be overemphasized. In summary, proper patient selection, laser technique, and postoperative management with early recognition and treatment of side effects and complications are all essential in reducing the risk of long-term sequelae and ensuring successful clinical results.

REFERENCES

1. Anderson RR, Parrish JA. Selective photothermolysis: precise microsurgery by selective absorption of pulsed radiation. *Science* 1983; 220:524–527.
2. Alster TS, West TB. Resurfacing of atrophic scars with a high-energy, pulsed carbon dioxide laser. *Dermatol Surg* 1995; 22:151–155.
3. Waldorf HA, Kauvar ANB, Geronemus RG. Skin resurfacing of fine to deep rhytides using a char-free carbon dioxide laser in 47 patients. *Dermatol Surg* 1995; 21:940–946.
4. Lask G, Keller G, Lowe NJ, Gomley D. Laser skin resurfacing with the Silktouch flashscanner for facial rhytides. *Dermatol Surg* 1995; 21:1021–1024.
5. David LM, Sarne A, Unger WP. Rapid laser scanning for facial resurfacing. *Dermatol Surg* 1995; 21:1031–1033.
6. Alster TS, Garg S. Treatment of facial rhytides with a high-energy pulsed carbon dioxide laser. *Plast Reconstr Surg* 1996; 98:791–794.
7. Fitzpatrick RE, Goldman MP, Satur NM, Tope WD. Pulsed carbon dioxide laser resurfacing of photoaged facial skin. *Arch Dermatol* 1996; 132:395–402.
8. Alster TS. Comparison of two high-energy, pulsed carbon dioxide lasers in the treatment of periorbital rhytides. *Dermatol Surg* 1996; 22:541–544.
9. Alster TS, West TB. Ultrapulse CO_2 laser ablation of xanthelasma. *J Am Acad Dermatol* 1996; 34:848–849.
10. Rosenbach A, Alster TS. Multiple trichoepitheliomas successfully treated with a high-energy, pulsed carbon dioxide laser. *Dermatol Surg* 1997; 23:708–710.
11. Hruza GJ. Laser treatment of warts and other epidermal and dermal lesions. *Dermatol Clin* 1997; 15:487–506.
12. Apfelberg DB. Ultrapulse carbon dioxide laser with CPG scanner for full-face resurfacing of rhytids, photoaging, and acne scars. *Plast Reconstr Surg* 1997; 99:1817–1825.
13. Bernstein LJ, Kauvar ANB, Grossman MC, Geronemus RG. Scar resurfacing with high-energy, short-pulsed and flashscanning carbon dioxide lasers. *Dermatol Surg* 1998; 24: 101–107.
14. Walia S, Alster TS. Prolonged clinical and histologic effects from CO_2 laser resurfacing of atrophic acne scars. *Dermatol Surg* 1999; 25:926–930.
15. West TB, Alster TS. Improvement of infraorbital hyperpigmentation following carbon dioxide laser resurfacing. *Dermatol Surg* 1998; 24:65–66.
16. Gross EA, Rogers GS. A side-by-side comparison of carbon dioxide resurfacing lasers for the treatment of rhytides. *J Am Acad Dermatol* 1998; 39:547–553.
17. Walsh JT Jr, Deutsch TF. Pulsed CO_2 laser tissue ablation: measurement of the ablation rate. *Lasers Surg Med* 1988; 8:264–275.
18. Walsh JT Jr, Flotte TJ, Anderson RR, Deutsch TF. Pulsed CO_2 laser tissue ablation: effect of tissue type and pulse duration on thermal damage. *Lasers Surg Med* 1988; 8: 108–118.
19. Lanzafame RJ, Naim JO, Rogers DW, et al. Comparisons of continuous-wave, chop-wave, and super-pulse laser wounds. *Lasers Surg Med* 1988; 8:119–124.
20. Zweig AD, Meierhofer B, Muller OM, et al. Lateral thermal damage along pulsed laser incisions. *Lasers Surg Med* 1990; 10:262–274.
21. Fitzpatrick RE, Ruiz-Esparza J, Goldman MP. The depth of thermal necrosis using the CO_2 laser: a comparison of the superpulsed mode and conventional mode. *J. Dermatol Surg Oncol* 1991; 17:340–344.

22. Alster TS, Kauvar ANB, Geronemus RG. Histology of high-energy, pulsed CO_2 laser resurfacing. *Seminar Cutan Med Surg* 1996; 15:189–193.
23. Stuzin JM, Baker TJ, Baker TM, Kligman AM. Histologic effects of the high-energy pulsed CO_2 laser on photoaged facial skin. *Plast Reconstr Surg* 1997; 99:2036–2050.
24. Alster TS, Nanni CA, Williams CM. Comparison of four carbon dioxide resurfacing lasers: a clinical and histopathologic evaluation. *Dermatol Surg* 1999; 25:153–159.
25. Kauvar ANB, Waldorf HA, Geronemus RG. A histopathological comparison of "char-free" carbon dioxide lasers. *Dermatol Surg* 1996; 22:343–348.
26. Ross E, Naseef G, Skrobal M, et al. In vivo dermal collagen shrinkage and remodeling following CO_2 laser resurfacing. *Lasers Surg Med* 1996; 18:38.
27. Fulton JE, Barnes T. Collagen shrinkage (selective dermaplasty) with the high-energy pulsed carbon dioxide laser. *Dermatol Surg* 1998; 24:3–41.
28. Kirsch KM, Zelickson BD, Zachary CB, Tope WD. Ultrastructure of collagen thermally denatured by microsecond domain pulsed carbon dioxide laser. *Arch Dermatol* 1998; 134:1255–1259.
29. Smith KJ, Skelton HG, Graham JS, et al. Increased smooth muscle actin, factor XIIIa, and vimentin-positive cells in the papillary dermis of carbon dioxide laser-debrided porcine skin. *Dermatol Surg* 1997; 23:891–895.
30. Alster TS. Commentary on increased smooth muscle actin, factor XIIIa, and vimentin-positive cells in the papillary dermis of carbon dioxide laser-debrided porcine skin. *Dermatol Surg* 1998; 24:155.
31. Alster TS. Manual of Cutaneous Laser Techniques. 2nd ed. Philadelphia: Lippincott, Williams & Wilkins, Inc., 2000.
32. Alster TS. Preoperative preparation for CO_2 laser resurfacing. In: Coleman WP, Lawrence N, eds. *Skin Resurfacing*. Baltimore: Williams and Wilkins, 1998:171–179.
33. Alster TS. Cutaneous resurfacing with CO_2 and erbium: YAG lasers: preoperative, intraoperative, and postoperative considerations. *Plast Reconstr Surg* 1999; 103:619–632.
34. Horton S, Alster TS. Preoperative and postoperative considerations for carbon dioxide laser resurfacing. *Cutis* 1999; 64:399–406.
35. West TB, Alster TS. Effect of botulinum toxin type A on movement-associated rhytides following CO_2 laser resurfacing. *Dermatol Surg* 1999; 25:259–261
36. Alster TS, Rosenbach A, Huband L. Improvement of dermatochalasis with carbon dioxide laser resurfacing. *Dermatol Surg* 1999; 25.
37. Alster TS. Combined laser resurfacing and tretinoin treatment of facial rhytides. *Cosmetic Dermatol* 1997; 10:39–42.
38. Duke D, Grevelink JM. Care before and after laser skin resurfacing: a survey and review of the literature. *Dermatol Surg* 1998; 24:201–206.
39. Apfelberg DB. Summary of the 1997 ASAPS/ASPRS laser task force survey on laser resurfacing and laser blepharoplasty. *Plast Reconstr Surg* 1998; 101:511–518.
40. West TB, Alster TS. Effect of pretreatment on the incidence of hyperpigmentation following cutaneous CO_2 laser resurfacing. *Dermatol Surg* 1999; 25:15–17.
41. Alster TS, West TB. Effect of topical vitamin C on postoperative carbon dioxide resurfacing erythema. *Dermatol Surg* 1998; 24:331–334.
42. Walia SS, Alster TS. Cutaneous CO_2 laser resurfacing infection rate with and without prophylactic antibiotics. *Dermatol Surg* 1999; 25:857–861.
43. Weinstein C, Ramirez OM, Pozner JN. Postoperative care following CO_2 laser resurfacing: avoiding pitfalls. *Plast Reconstr Surg* 1997; 100:1855–1865.
44. Ruiz-Esparza J, Gomez JMB, de la Torre OL. Wound care after laser skin resurfacing. *Dermatol Surg* 1998; 24:79–81.
45. Newman JP, Koch RJ, Goode RL. Closed dressings after laser skin resurfacing. *Arch Otolaryngol Head Neck Surg* 1998; 124:751–757.

46. Sriprachya-Anunt S, Fitzpatrick RE, Goldman MP, Smith SR. Infections complicating pulsed carbon dioxide laser resurfacing for photoaged facial skin. *Dermatol Surg* 1997; 23:527–536.
47. Nanni CA, Alster TS. Complications of carbon dioxide laser resurfacing: an evaluation of 500 patients. *Dermatol Surg* 1998; 24:315–320.
48. Haas AF. Practical thoughts on antibiotic prophylaxis (letter). *Arch Dermatol* 1998; 143: 1–2.
49. Bernstein LJ, Kauvar ANB, Grossman MC, Geronemus RG. The short- and long-term side effects of carbon dioxide laser resurfacing. *Dermatol Surg* 1997; 23:519–525.
50. Fulton JE. Complications of laser resurfacing: methods of prevention and management. *Dermatol Surg* 1997; 24:91–99.
51. Laws RA, Finley EM, McCollough ML, Grabski WJ. Alabaster skin after carbon dioxide laser resurfacing with histologic correlation. *Dermatol Surg* 1998; 24:633–636.
52. Alster TS, Nanni CA. Famciclovir prophylaxis of herpes simplex virus reactivation after laser resurfacing. *Dermatol Surg* 1999; 25:242–246.
53. Alster TS, Nanni CA. Pulsed dye laser treatment of hypertrophic burn scars. *Plast Reconstr Surg* 1998; 102:2190–2195.

APPENDIX 1: LASER RESURFACING INFORMATION SHEET

The pulsed or scanned carbon dioxide (CO_2) laser is capable of removing superficial portions of the skin in a layer-by-layer manner. The skin literally evapoates because of the high water content of the epidermis and upper dermis (superficial skin layers). Thus, this laser is best used to treat fine lines, wrinkles, indented acne or surgical scars, and other benign skin growths (keratoses, warts).

The laser procedure is quick and bloodless and can be performed using local or light intravenous sedation ("twilight" anesthesia). Immediately after the procedure and for the first few postoperative days, the treated skin appears bright red and swollen. Ice packs and healing ointments or dressings are used for the first several days. You will be required to return to the office for regular skin examinations and cleaning during the first week or until full re-epithelialization has occurred (usually by the 10th day after surgery). Thus, the initial healing process takes place during the first 1 to 2 weeks after the procedure, after which time the skin will appear pink and more smooth. Return of your skin to its normal color requires several weeks to months. It is expected that you will be able to return to work or your usual daily activities within 10 to 14 days after surgery wearing makeup to camouflage the residual skin redness.

The risk of complications using this advanced laser technology is relatively small, but skin sensitivity, prolonged redness, skin lightening or darkening, infection, development of cold sores, scarring, or acne may occur. We will take all necessary precautions to prevent the development of any untoward side effects and to diagnosis and treat any suspected complication early in its course.

APPENDIX 2: CONSENT FORM

My doctor has explained to me that I am a good candidate for laser skin resurfacing treatment. While laser surgery has been shown to be highly effective, I understand that no guarantees can be made that I will benefit from treatment. I further understand that possible side effects and complications of this laser treatment include:

1. PAIN. The sharp, burning sensation of each laser pulse may produce a moderate to severe amount of discomfort. Anesthetic injections or intravenous sedation will be used to block the pain during the procedure. Oral pain mediation will be prescribed for the postoperative period.

2. SWELLING and OOZING. The eyes and neck are areas most likely to swell. A clear fluid (serum) will also be present in the treated areas and may create a crust or scab if the skin is not kept moist. Swelling, crusting, and oozing usually subsides within 5 to 7 days with the use of the postoperative skin care regimen prescribed.

3. PROLONGED REDNESS. The treated skin will initially appear bright red in color. After the first week or two, the redness can be camouflaged with opaque makeup. The redness gradually fades to normal skin color over several months.

4. SKIN DARKENING (*Hyperpigmentation*). Darkening of the skin may be seen 1 month or more after treatment and will fade over the next several months. This occurs more commonly in patients with olive or dark skin tones and can worsen if the laser-treated skin is exposed to the sun or is irritated.

5. SKIN LIGHTENING (*Hypopigmentation*). Lightening of the skin can occur as a delayed response to laser treatment or may simply be "uncovered" as a result of prior surgical treatments (for example, dermabrasion). The light spots may darken with time, but could be permanent.

6. ACNE OR MILIA FORMATION. Flare-up of acne or formation of milia (tiny white bumps) can occur in the postoperative period even in individuals who do not have a prior history of acne. It is usually associated with over-use of healing ointments, but may be a normal healing response.

7. ALLERGIC OR IRRITANT REACTION. It is possible that an adverse reaction to an anesthetic, topical cream/ointment, or oral medication can occur.

8. INFECTION. A skin infection can result in the laser wound in the postoperative period despite the use of good skin care and antibiotics.

9. SCARRING. While the risk of scar formation is minimal, it can conceivably occur whenever there is disruption of the skin's surface. Strict adherence to all advised postoperative instructions will reduce the possibility of injury and subsequent scarring.

10. ECTROPION. A downward pull of the eyelids can result after treatment of the skin under the eyes.

By signing below, I acknowledge that I have read and understood the information presented above. I feel that I have been adequately informed of other treatment options, the risks of the proposed surgery, and have had my questions answered to my complete satisfaction.

Patient's or Guardian's Signature Date Witness' Signature Date

APPENDIX 3: POSTOPERATIVE INSTRUCTION SHEET

Day 1	Your skin will appear more red than it did immediately after surgery and you may be swollen (especially around your eyes). It is critical to keep the areas *cold* and *moist* using an ice pack or cooling gel mask on top of your wound dressing (if using a "closed" technique) or application of ointment (if using an "open" technique) in order to provide comfort and reduce swelling. Take your pain and sleeping medications as needed and your antibiotics as prescribed.
Day 2	It is normal to have even *more* swelling and pain as well as oozing (clear "straw" or "amber" color) from the treated areas. Continue to ice and apply cold moist compresses and healing ointments ("open" technique) Take your antibiotics as prescribed and the pain and sleeping medications as needed.
Days 3-4	Redness and swelling may be even more prominent. Continue wound care and medications as previously outlined. You may be seen in the office for an evaluation of your skin and further wound care management (dressing change if using "closed" technique or gentle cleansing/steaming if using "open" technique).
Days 5-7	Healing will continue with decreased swelling, oozing, and discomfort. The skin will remain red and it may itch. This is *normal*, but if you are unable to keep from scratching your skin, please let the doctor know so that an appropriate treatment can be prescribed. You will be finishing several of your medications at this time.
Days 7-10	Continue to moisturize your skin. It is typical for makeup to be applied at this juncture (when oozing has ceased).

APPENDIX 4: PREOPERATIVE CHECKLIST

Skin type: ____
Age: ____
Diagnosis: ___Rhytides (periorbital, perioral, glabellar, forehead, cheeks, ears, other____)
___Atrophic scars (acne, traumatic, surgical)
___Epidermal/dermal lesions (keratoses, verrucae, other_____________)
___Rhinophyma
___Other (dermatochalasis, dyspigmentation, jowling)

Prior Treatments *(list with dates)*: ____

History of: ___oral/genital HSV
___collagen vascular disease
___valvular heart disease
___other____________________________
___isotretinoin use (dates used_______)
___immunodeficiency (HIV)
___immunologic disorder (vitiligo, anemia)

Current Skin Care: ____
Current Medications: ____
Allergies: _______________________________________

If >50 years or if H/O cardiac/lung disease: ___EKG _____Chest x-ray

Information sheet given to patient and reviewed: _______ *(date)*
Informed consent reviewed and signed: _________ *(date)*
Preoperative HSV/antibiotic prophylaxis: _______________________ *(list med/dose/time taken)*
Preoperative photos obtained: ________ *(date)*
Postoperative wound care reviewed and written instructions provided: ________ *(date)*
Surgery scheduled: __________ *(date/time/location)*
Confirmation phone #: __________________
Emergency phone #: __________________

APPENDIX 5: LASER RESURFACING TREATMENT LOG

Date of Operation: _______________
Patient Name: ___________________
Age: ________
Diagnosis: ___________________
Previous Treatments: ____

LASER USED	FLUENCE/ POWER	SPOT/SCAN SIZE/PATTERN	LOCATION/ AREA TREATED	TOTAL RX TIME
POSTOP SKIN APPEARANCE	**OINTMENTS/ DRESSINGS**	**ANESTHESIA USED**	**ANESTHESIA TIME**	**REMARKS**

8

Erbium Skin Remodeling

Cynthia Weinstein
Laser Surgery Institute of Melbourne and Freemason's Hospital, East Melbourne, Victoria, Australia

INTRODUCTION

Skin resurfacing for facial rejuvenation is not a new procedure, but has become increasingly popular over the last decade with the introduction of pulsed carbon dioxide (CO_2) lasers. Many of the results produced by CO_2 lasers were indeed spectacular, and improvement lasted for many years because of the new collagen formation that was produced [1]. However, the morbidity and complications associated with CO_2 laser resurfacing have encouraged the search for alternative methods of skin resurfacing [2–5].

In the short term, the prolonged and often intense erythema associated with CO_2 laser resurfacing posed a major problem after surgery for most individuals, especially men, as well as for those undergoing regional resurfacing. Postsurgical hyperpigmentation is a major problem for those of darker skin types. In the long term, hypopigmentation has become a major problem following CO_2 laser resurfacing, which in some individuals can be cosmetically unsightly.

Many of the complications resulting from CO_2 laser resurfacing occurred because of the nonspecific thermal effects generated by the laser when treating dermal problems, eg, wrinkles. As collagen is exquisitely heat sensitive, extensive destruction of dermal tissue may result in scarring and hypopigmentation [6]. CO_2 lasers were initially introduced for the treatment of epidermal lesions because the epidermis consists of 90% water [7]. However, the dermis consists mainly of structural proteins with little water (approximately 30%). After the first laser pass into the dermis, most of the water is vaporized and the blood vessels coagulated. Further passes lead to nonspecific thermal effects.

The Erbium:YAG laser, with wavelength 2940 nm, is more avidly absorbed by water than CO_2 lasers (Fig. 1). It will ablate more superficially than CO_2 and will produce less thermal conduction. The threshold ablation for Erbium:YAG is 1.5 J/cm^2, compared with 4 to 5 J/cm^2 for CO_2 laser, while the thermal relaxation time for Erbium:YAG is 50 microseconds, compared with 1 millisecond with CO_2 laser (Table 1). Consequently, more precision in skin ablation is possible. Dermal ablation is also possible, because the Erbium:YAG does not coagulate vessels and so produces

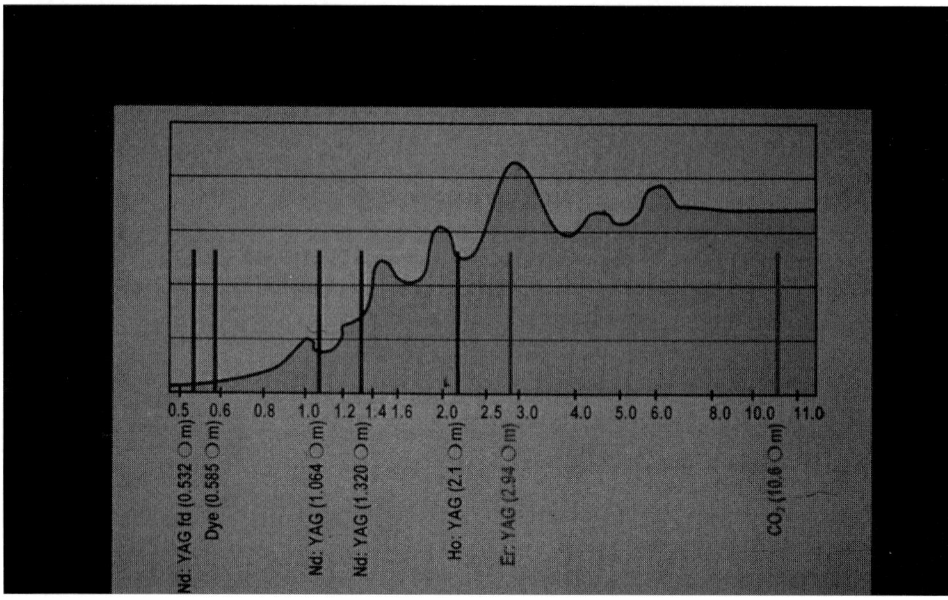

FIGURE 1 Comparison of water absorption between Erbium:YAG laser (A = 2940 mm) and CO_2 (A = 10,600).

a transudate that "wets" the dermis, thus allowing precise removal of dermal collagen without significant thermal injury [8–12].

In my experience of more than 700 patients over a 20 month period, the Erbium:YAG has proven extremely successful in rejuvenating sun-damaged skin, wrinkles, acne scars, and other skin lesions. Furthermore, the morbidity associated with Erbium:YAG skin resurfacing appears to be considerably less than with the CO_2 laser.

HISTORY

Many methods of skin resurfacing exist, each with advantages and disadvantages. Chemical peeling in its various forms has been practiced for centuries by both medical practitioners and lay peelers. Precision in depth control has always been a limitation of this procedure, although superficial chemical peeling will continue to enjoy

TABLE 1 Physical Properties of CO_2 and Erbium Lasers

	Erbium:YAG	CO_2
Wavelength	2940 nm	10,600 nm
Threshold ablation	1.5 J/cm^2	4–5 J/cm^2
Thermal relaxation time	50 u sec	1000 u sec
Zone thermal injury	5–20 um	20–100 um
Relative water absorption	10	1

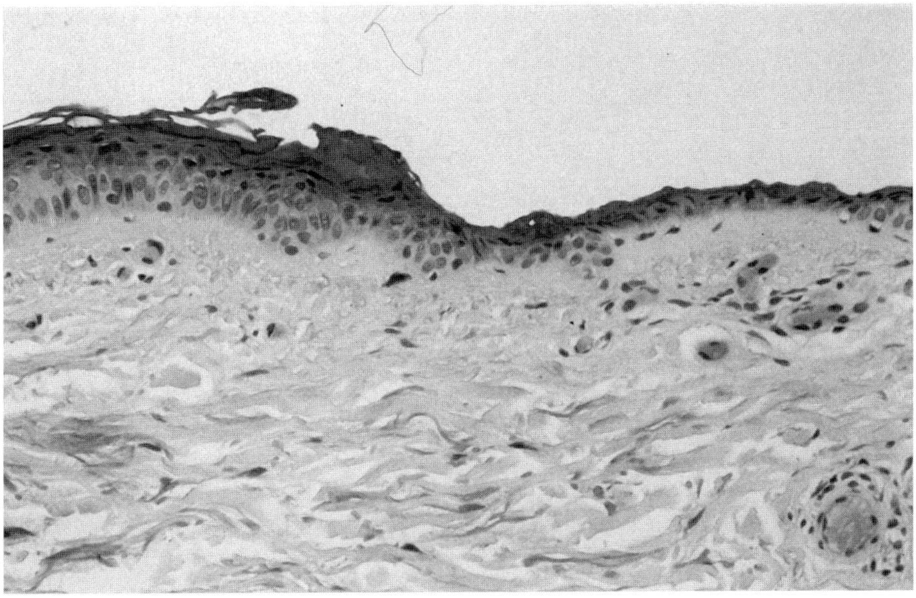

FIGURE 2 Histology of Erbium resurfacing at 5 J/cm^2 showing precise epidermal ablation with no significant zone of thermal necrosis.

popularity in the foreseeable future [13,14]. Dermabrasion, which has proven extremely effective for the treatment of wrinkles and acne scars, has become largely superseded by laser resurfacing techniques [15].

CO_2 lasers have been used in dermatology since the 1970s for the treatment of epidermal lesions. It was not until the development of the high-energy pulsed and rapid scanning CO_2 lasers in the 1990s that their use for resurfacing skin became feasible [7,16,17]. Yet despite these technological advances, CO_2 lasers were not ideally suited for resurfacing dermal abnormalities, including wrinkles and acne scars, because of their unwanted thermal effects [6,18].

The Erbium:YAG laser, with its high absorption coefficient in water, is "ideally" suited for superficial ablation of skin (Fig. 1). The early studies by Kaufmann, Hibst, and others in the late 1980s, show that the Erbium:YAG was successful in precisely ablating skin and soft tissues, with sparing of adjacent structures (Figs. 2, 3) [8–10]. The earlier Erbium:YAG lasers were single-spot, short-pulse duration (350 microsecond) systems which, although effective, were slow and cumbersome to use. Reproducibility was difficult because of the variable overlap of pulses that resulted from changes in hand speed. Excessive overlap of pulses may lead to deeper ablation than intended, along with some thermal effects. The introduction of rapid computerized scanners has allowed Erbium:YAG resurfacing to be performed efficiently, accurately, and with a great degree of reproducibility [11].

INDICATIONS AND PRESURGICAL CONSIDERATIONS

Following are some of the many indications for Erbium:YAG resurfacing (Table 2).

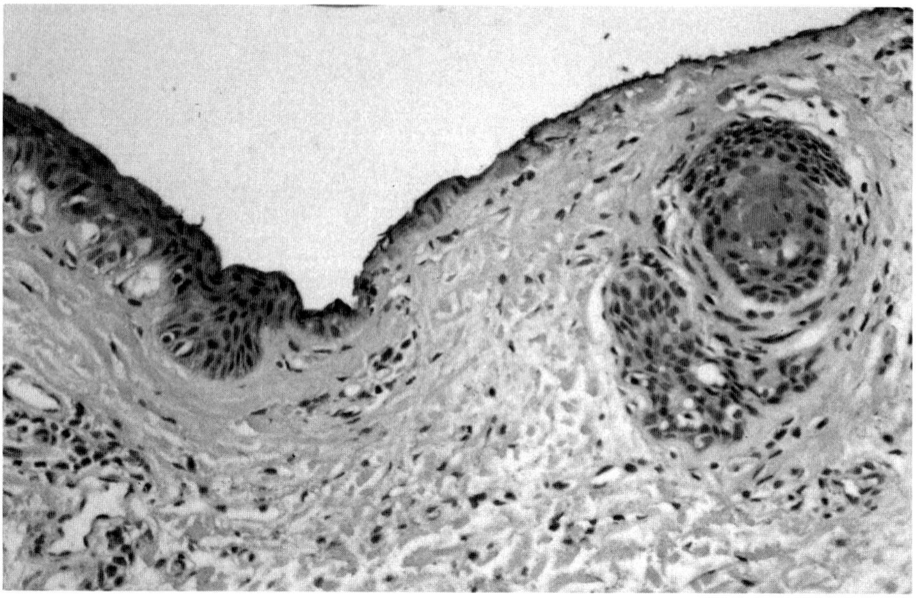

FIGURE 3 Histology of Erbium resurfacing at 20 J/cm^2 showing dermal ablation with a narrow band of thermal necrosis (<20 microns). Note excellent preservation of hair follicle.

TABLE 2 Indications for Erbium:YAG Resurfacing

Wrinkles
static
superficial (Erbium alone)
deep (simultaneous combined Erbium and CO_2)
Acne
atrophic
pitted
combined with fat grafting, punch excision, grafts
Pigmentation
epidermal (lentigenes, chloasma)
dermal (lentigenes, chloasma)
Exophytic skin lesions
epidermal (solar keratoses, seborrhoeic keratoses)
dermal (syringomas, xanthelasmas, compound naevi)
Birth marks
cafe au lait, Becker's naevi
Neck
pigmentation
Hands
solar keratoses
lentigenes

Wrinkles

Wrinkles attributable to solar damage are ideally suited to Erbium:YAG resurfacing (Figs. 4–6). Those that are present without animation respond best, whereas dynamic lines, eg, glabella and crow's feet, require adjunctive treatment either with Botox or surgical muscle modification. Superficial and moderately deep wrinkles will respond to Erbium:YAG alone. Deep wrinkles will also respond, but bleeding makes this procedure cumbersome and messy. For deep wrinkles, especially in the perioral region, I have found it best to use the simultaneous combined Erbium:YAG/CO_2 (Derma K) laser. This allows deeper penetration per pulse and more coagulation of blood vessels, which reduces (but does not eliminate) bleeding, making the procedure easier and cleaner.

Full-Face Versus Regional Erbium Resurfacing

Because there is minimal thermal injury produced by the Erbium:YAG laser, regional resurfacing produces satisfactory cosmetic results without cosmetically unacceptable color and texture changes between lasered and nonlasered areas. Postsurgical erythema is usually considerably milder than with CO_2 laser and is of shorter duration, lasting an average of 6 weeks. Regional laser resurfacing is particularly indicated for perioral rhytids and for fine periocular wrinkles.

Erbium:YAG Resurfacing Combined With Other Procedures

Erbium resurfacing can be readily combined with Botox injections for movement lines, especially in the glabella and crow's feet region (Figs. 7, 8). Erbium resurfacing may also be combined with other surgical procedures, eg, blepharoplasty, face-lifting, and endoscopic brow-lifting.

Skin Types

Although all skin types are suitable for Erbium skin resurfacing (Fig. 9), darker skins, ie, types 4, 5, and 6, have a tendency to hyperpigment after erbium laser resurfacing, and bleaching preparations must be used in the postsurgical period.

Consultation

Consultation and communication are of paramount importance when assessing patients for Erbium laser resurfacing or any other cosmetic procedures. Understanding patient expectations in terms of results and healing times will help to minimize patient complaints.

Many patients have unrealistic expectations, especially about the postsurgical course, based on advertising and media hype. A useful checklist during the consultation includes:

1. *What does the patient feel is his or her main problem?* If the patient is worried about wrinkles around the mouth or cheeks, Erbium resurfacing will definitely be helpful. Wrinkles around the eyes pose a more difficult problem. Wrinkles that are present without animation will respond well to laser resurfacing. Many patients demonstrate periocular wrinkles only when they smile. Those patients should be advised to consider Botox injections first and resurfacing if Botox is insufficient. Similarly, wrinkles on the forehead, both glabella, and horizontal, may respond better to either Botox alone or a combination of Botox and laser resurfacing. Wrinkles on

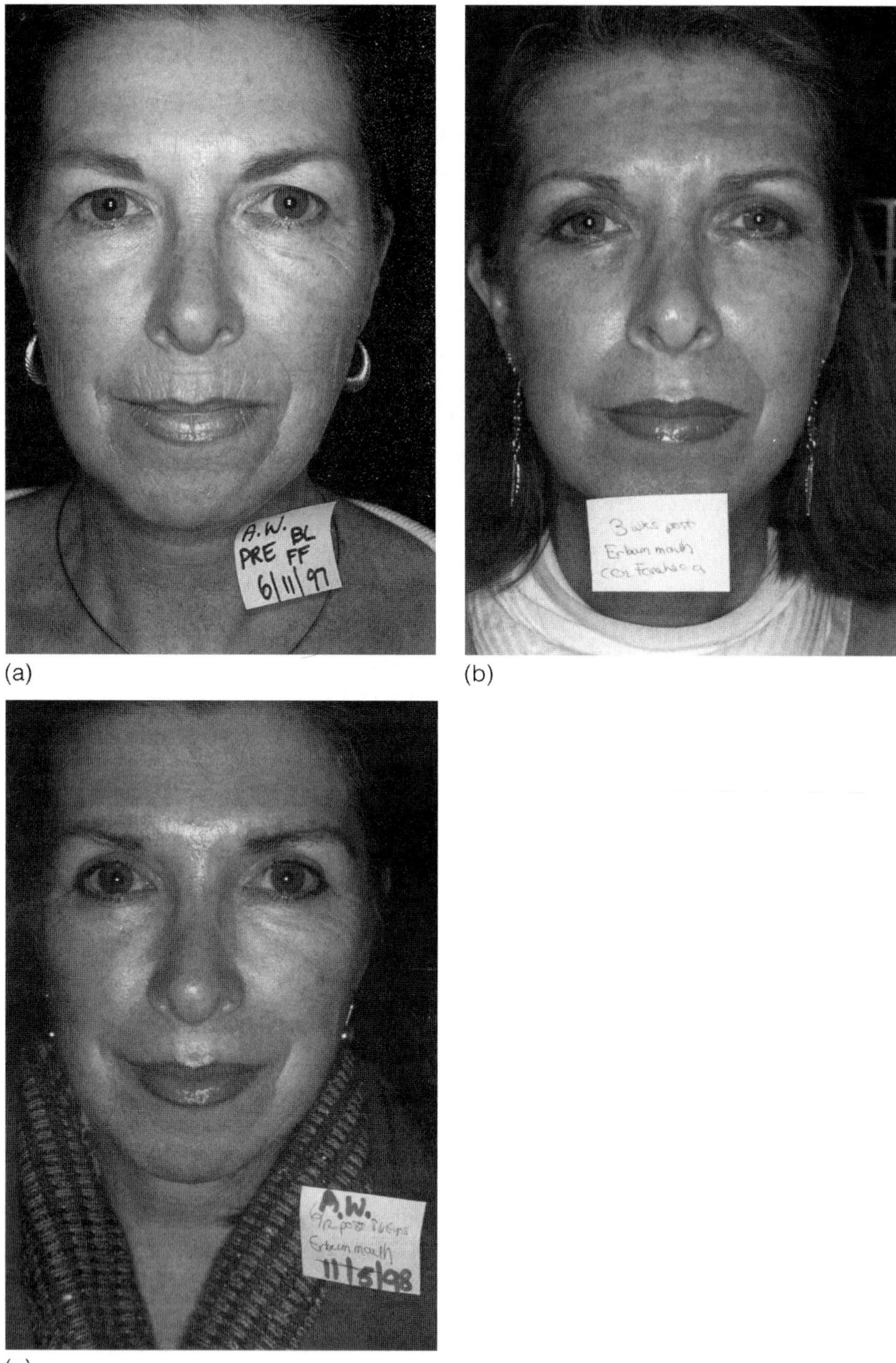

FIGURE 4 (a) Fifty-two–year-old female before Erbium resurfacing in perioral region as well as CO_2 resurfacing periocular and forehead skin, 35% TCA peel cheeks, and laser blepharoplasty. (b) Same patient 3 weeks after surgery. Note homogenous appearance of perioral area compared with CO_2 area on forehead. (c) Same patient 6 months after surgery. Note complete disappearance of perioral wrinkles after Erbium resurfacing. Total fluence of Erbium was 60 J/cm^2.

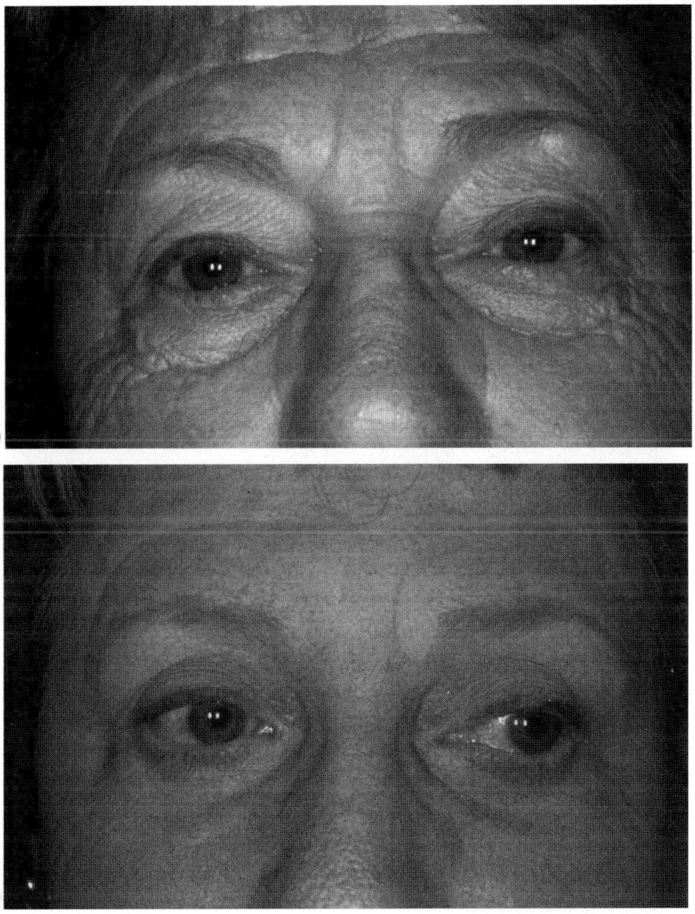

(a)

(b)

FIGURE 5 Sixty-nine–year-old female before laser blepharoplasty combined with Erbium resurfacing of periocular skin. (b) Same patient 6 months after surgery. Total fluence of Erbium used was 30 J/cm^2.

the neck do not respond well to Erbium laser resurfacing, and other procedures, eg, neck-lifting or ultrasonic liposuction of the neck, should be considered as an alternative. Perhaps in the future, nonablative lasers will be helpful for this region. Loose skin attributable to gravity changes, eg, jowls, will not show any lasting benefit from Erbium resurfacing, and surgical face-lifting is more appropriate.

2. *How much time does the patient have to recover from surgery?* Recovery time after laser resurfacing is a most important issue. In order to produce lasting improvement in wrinkles, Erbium resurfacing must be carried down to the level of the papillary dermis. Re-epithelialization will take 7 to 10 days, so time away from work is needed. If the patient needs to return to work in 2 to 3 days, only superficial, ie, intraepidermal resurfacing, is possible, which may freshen the skin but will not produce lasting improvement in wrinkles. The use of a nonablative laser may be more appropriate in such an individual.

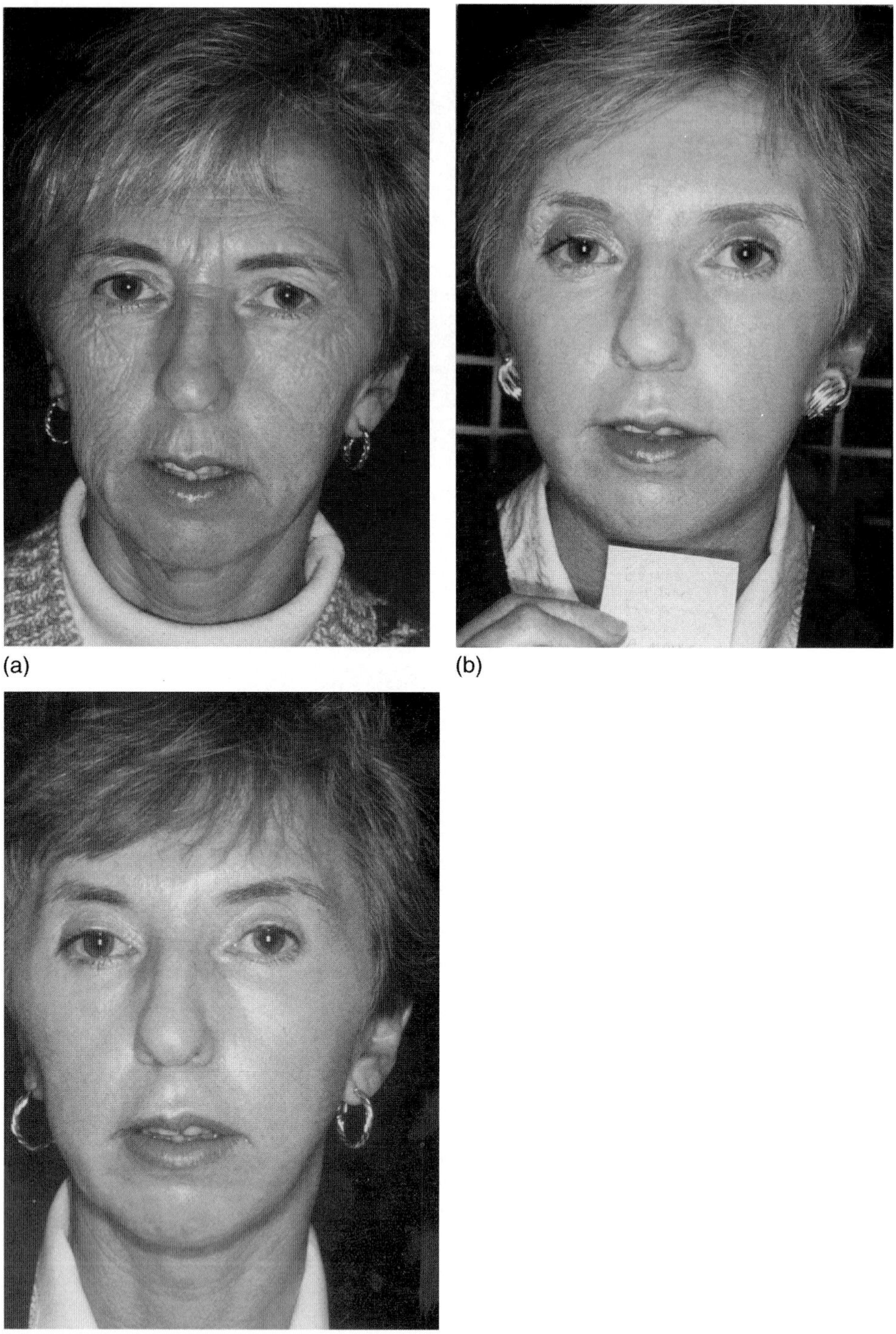

(a) (b) (c)

FIGURE 6 (a) Fifty-three–year-old female with severe wrinkles before resurfacing with combined Erbium and CO_2 laser. However, the periocular region was treated with Erbium at total fluence of 42 J/cm^2. She also underwent laser blepharoplasty and endoscopic browlift. (b) Same patient 6 weeks after surgery. (c) Same patient 6 months after surgery.

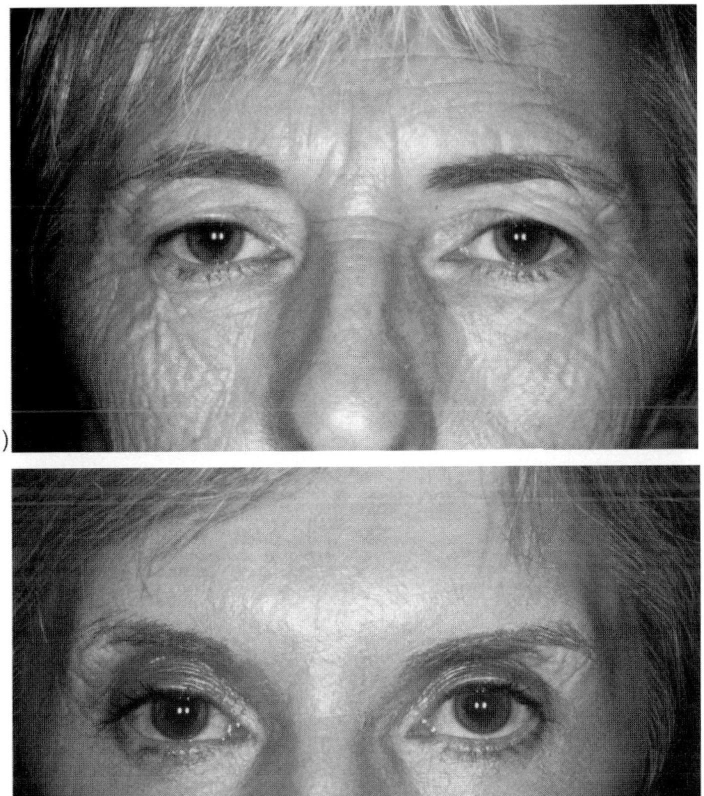

(d) (e) (f)

FIGURE 6 Continued (d) Same patient before surgery. Close-up view of the periocular region. (e) Same patient 6 weeks after surgery. Close-up view of periocular region. (f) Same patient 6 months after surgery. Close-up view of periocular region.

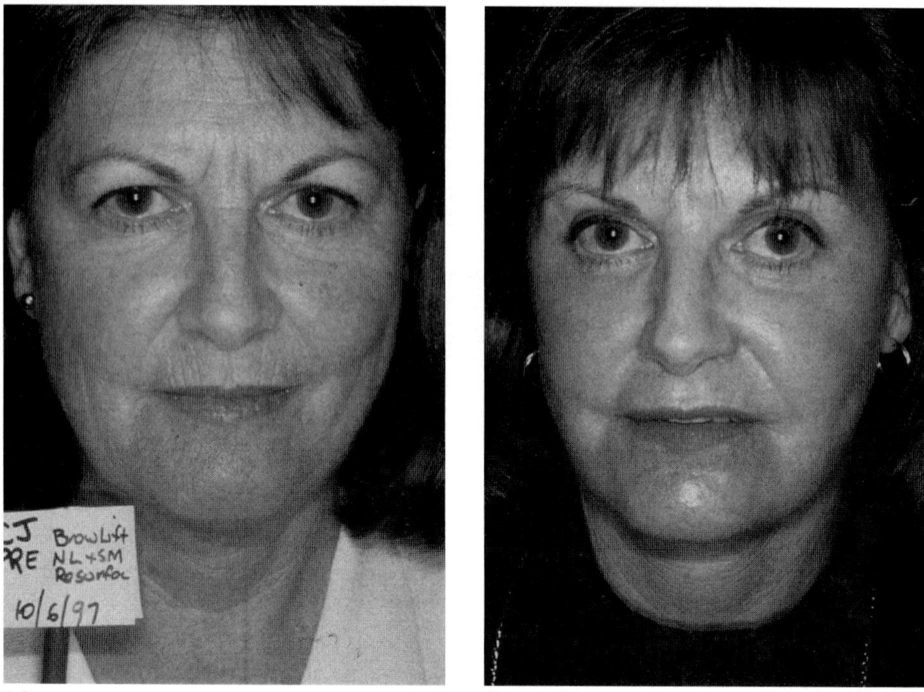

(a) (b)

FIGURE 7 (a) Fifty-five–year-old female before endoscopic brow-lift and face- and neck-lift combined with Erbium skin resurfacing. (b) Same patient 6 weeks after surgery.

3. *Is the patient a smoker or does he or she spend considerable time outdoors?* Although in my experience smokers heal no more slowly than nonsmokers and do not appear to have any more complications, recurrence of wrinkles will certainly occur more rapidly if they continue to smoke. Similarly, if the patient spends much time in outdoor pursuits, recurrence of wrinkles will occur more quickly unless meticulous sun protection is practiced.

4. *Does the patient normally wear makeup?* After Erbium laser resurfacing, there may be a slight change in skin color and texture that may not be apparent for some 6 months after the procedure. Although it is less marked with the Erbium laser compared with the CO_2 laser, it may be troublesome for the patient who does not like to wear makeup. It can be particularly annoying after regional resurfacing. Patients must be carefully counseled about these possible skin changes that may require makeup for concealment.

5. *Are the patient's expectations realistic?* Many patients believe that laser resurfacing will fix all the effects of aging. They mistakenly believe that laser resurfacing will remove eyelid bags, jowls, and loose necks. Although it is possible to explain the different effects, patients have little imagination and rarely fully understand what laser resurfacing can really achieve. For this reason, I have found computerized imaging an invaluable tool to point out what laser resurfacing can and cannot achieve. Also, computerized imaging can clearly show the sometimes unde-

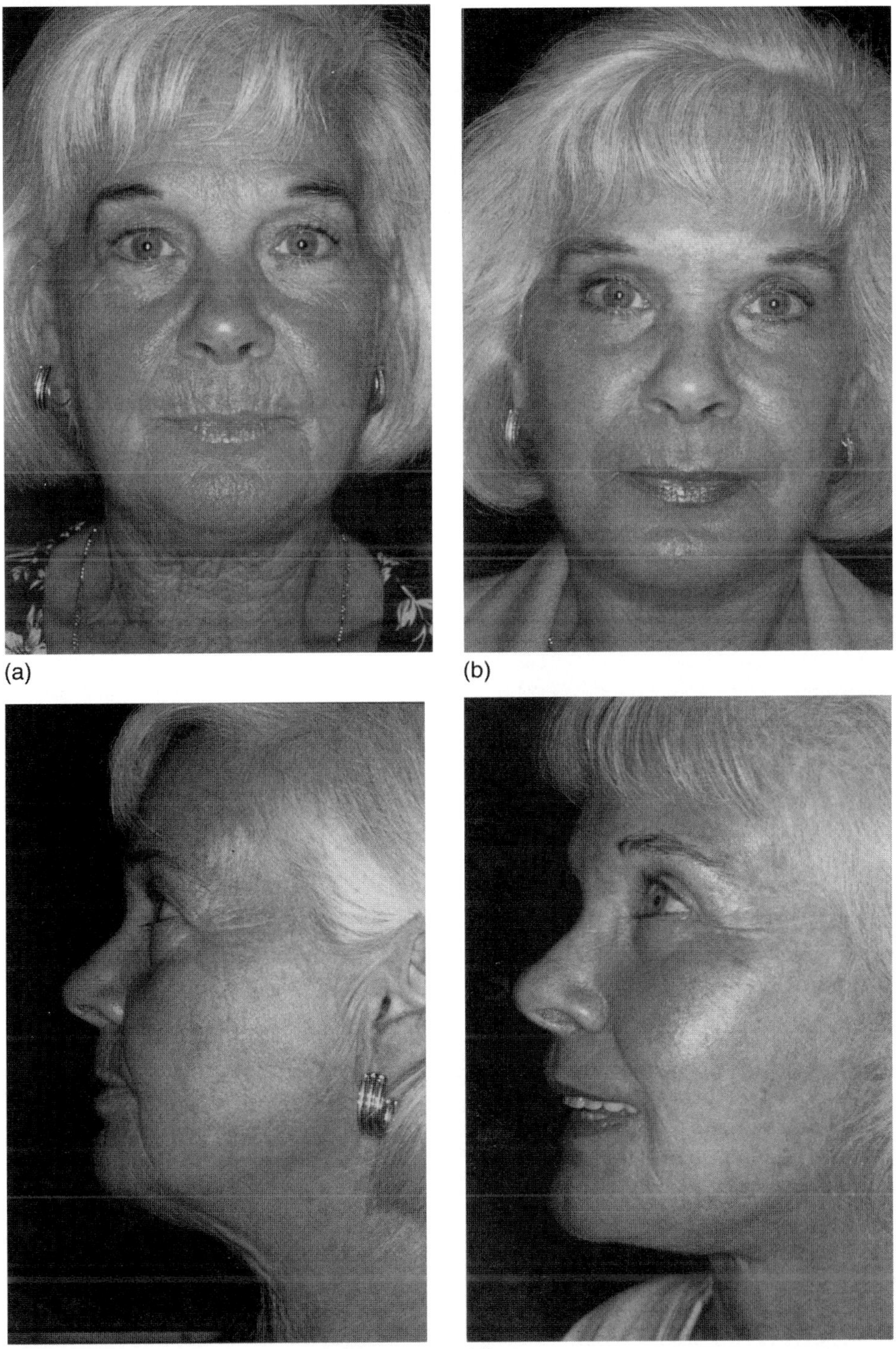

FIGURE 8 (a) Sixty-three–year-old female with loose neck and facial wrinkles before laser blepharoplasty and face- and neck-lift combined with Erbium skin resurfacing. (b) Same patient 6 weeks after surgery. (c) Same patient before surgery. Side view. (d) Same patient 6 weeks after surgery. Side view.

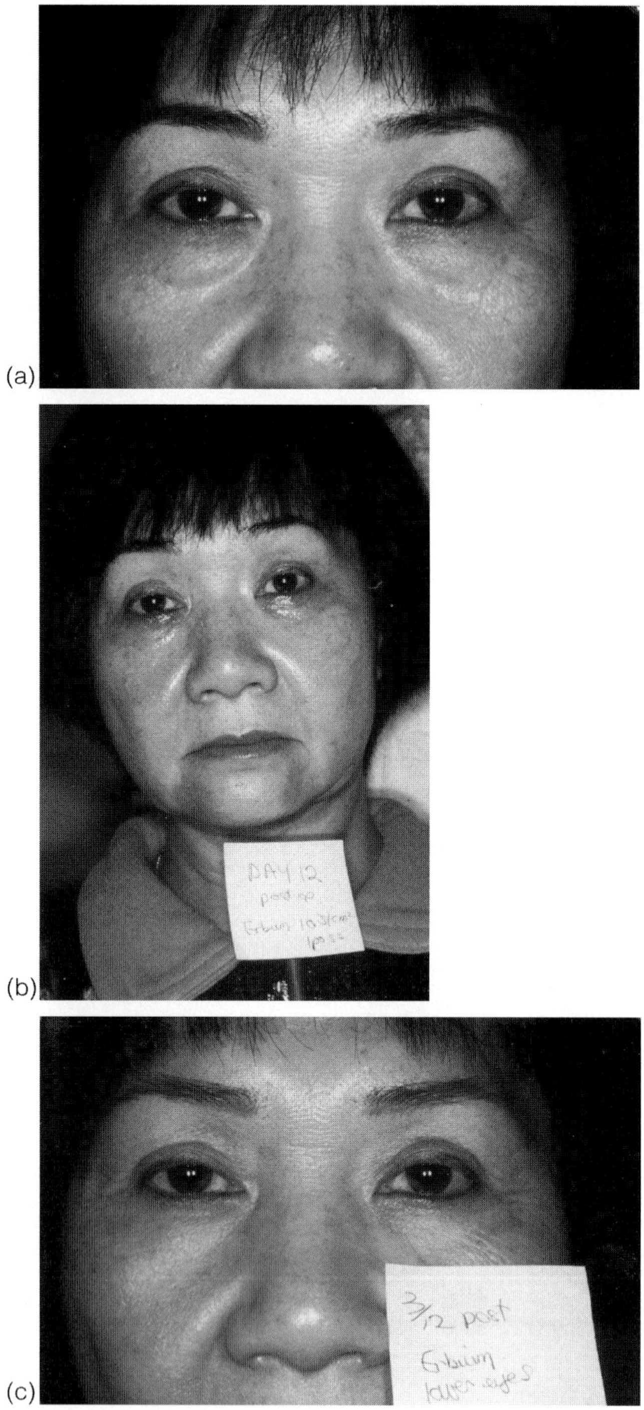

FIGURE 9 (a) Forty-seven–year-old Asian female before transconjunctival lower-lid laser blepharoplasty combined with Erbium skin resurfacing of periocular skin. (b) Same patient 12 days after surgery. (c) Same patient 3 months after surgery.

sirable results from regional resurfacing, especially color and texture differences in the resurfaced areas relative to the untreated adjacent skin.

6. *Does the patient have a history of herpes infection?* As widespread herpes infection can occur after laser resurfacing, the prophylactic use of an antiviral drug, eg, Famvir or Valtrax, is mandatory in those with a previous history of cold sores.

7. *Is the patient taking any medication that may interfere with healing?* As Erbium resurfacing relies on re-epithelialization for healing to occur, drugs, eg, isotretinoin, that interfere with healing need to be assessed. In my experience, even if the patient ceased oral isotretinoin 2 years before resurfacing, delayed healing and atypical scarring may result. However, if the skin has become oilier and a few acne lesions are present, I would feel more reassured about performing laser resurfacing on such an individual. High doses of vitamin A, either in tablet form or diet, can pose similar problems. Patients taking the oral contraceptive pill may be at higher risk of developing post-treatment hyperpigmentation, and should be warned of this possibility or asked to cease this medication, at least temporarily.

Acne Scarring

Acne scarring (Figs. 10–12) is a good indication for Erbium laser resurfacing. However, because acne scarring is usually deeper than wrinkles, a patient can realistically

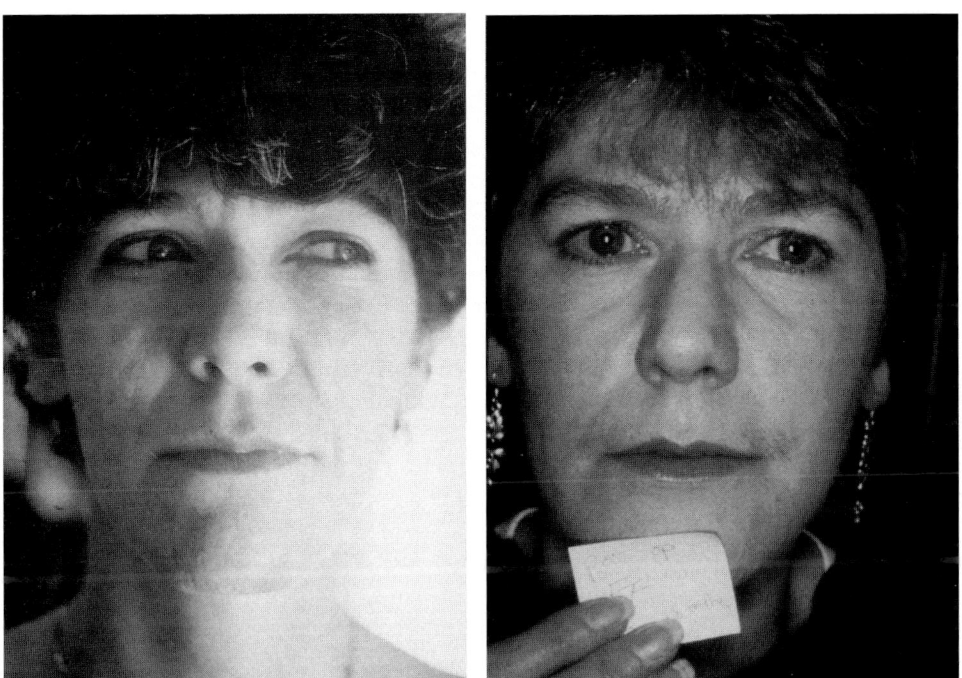

(a) (b)

FIGURE 10 Forty-five–year-old female with acne scarring before fat grafting combined with Erbium skin resurfacing. (b) Same patient 18 months after surgery.

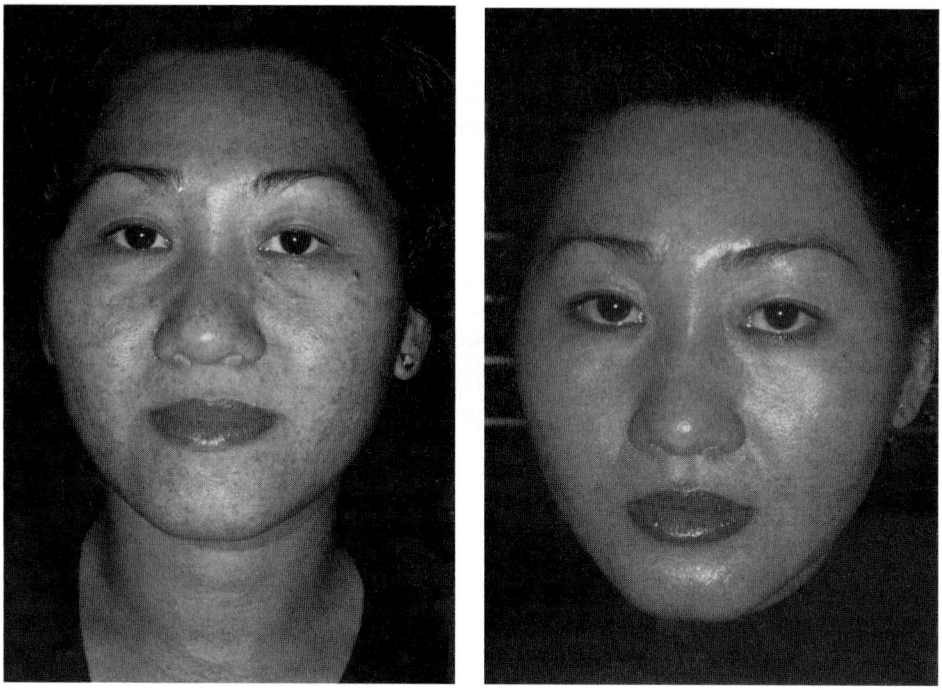

(a) (b)

FIGURE 11 (a) Forty-three–year-old Asian female with pitted acne scars before Erbium skin resurfacing alone. (b) Same patient 4 weeks after surgery. Note mild erythema, but no hyperpigmentation.

achieve only 50 to 70% correction. Apart from general presurgical considerations as for wrinkles, there are issues specifically relevant to acne scarring.

1. *What type of acne scarring is present?* Erbium laser resurfacing is particularly beneficial for atrophic and pitted acne scars, while valley-type scars respond poorly and require filling agents. In most individuals there is a combination of scar types, so a combined approach will produce optimal results. Erbium laser resurfacing may be combined with the use of filling agents, eg, fat grafting, as well as punch excision and punch grafting of deeper pitted acne scars.

2. *Is active acne present as well as scarring?* Although active acne is not a contraindication to Erbium laser resurfacing, ideally laser resurfacing is best delayed until the acne is quiescent. On the other hand, it is better to have some active acne rather than treat the patient with isotretinoin. Although many experts advocate waiting 6 months after isotretinoin therapy before undertaking any resurfacing procedure, it is my experience that delayed healing and atypical scarring may result even if the patient has ceased isotretinoin therapy 2 years previously. It is often better to control acne with antibiotics before resurfacing and commence oral isotretinoin 6 months after skin resurfacing.

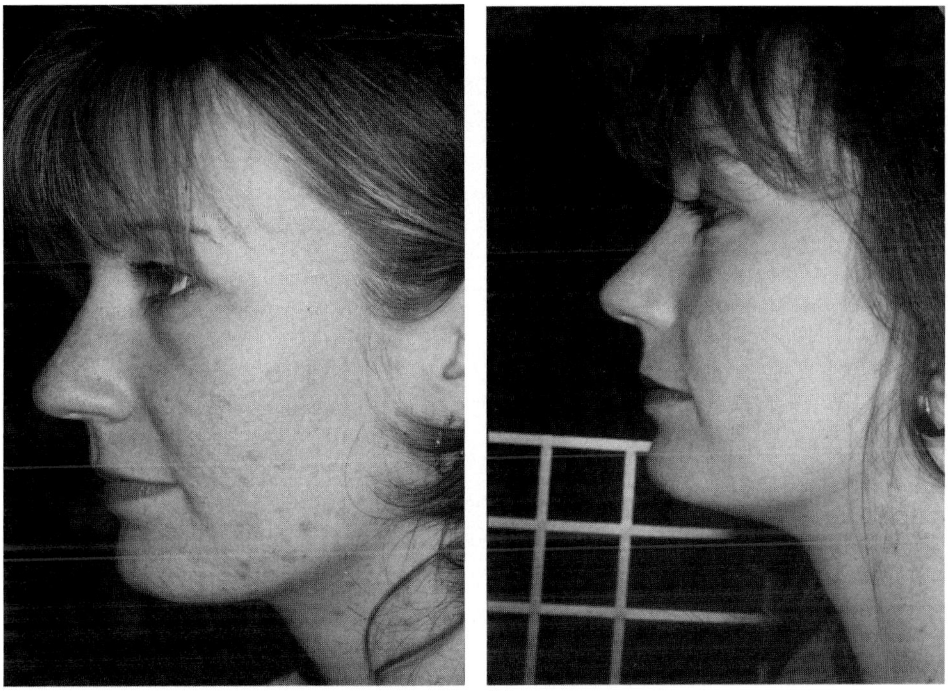

(a) (b)

FIGURE 12 (a) Twenty-six–year-old female with active acne and old acne scars before Erbium skin resurfacing alone. (b) Same patient 6 months after surgery.

3. *How much improvement does the patient expect?* Because improvement in acne scarring after laser resurfacing is modest at best, it is important that the patient understands this to avoid disappointment. Computer imaging is invaluable to show the anticipated improvement.

Pigmentation

Pigmentation attributable to solar damage responds extremely well to Erbium laser treatment (Figs. 13–15). In Caucasians, this is usually manifest as epidermal lentigenes, whereas in Asian patients and those with darker skins the lentigenes may be either epidermal or dermal. Clinically, epidermal lentigenes are well defined and brownish in color, whereas dermal lentigenes are more poorly defined and are greyish black in appearance. A Wood's lamp may also help to distinguish between epidermal and dermal pigment.

Chloasmal pigmentation will also respond well to Erbium laser treatment, but will tend to recur after surgery and will require the use of a bleaching preparation on a continuing basis. Chloasmal pigment, like lentigenes, may be epidermal or dermal or both. Patients must be warned that despite the Erbium laser treatment, they will need to strictly apply an ultraviolet A blocking sunscreen and a bleaching preparation for the rest of their lives.

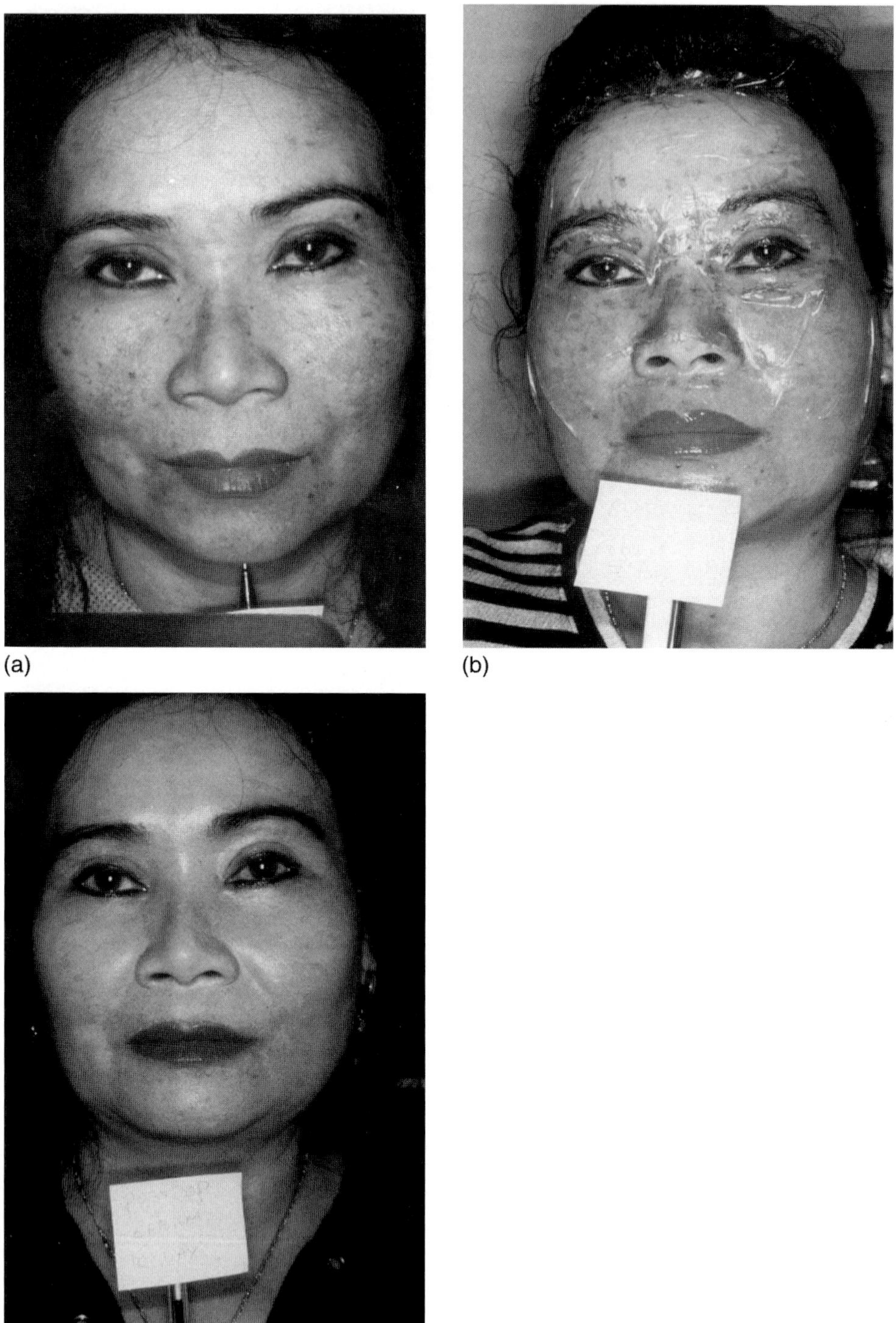

FIGURE 13 (a) Forty-nine–year-old Asian female with superficial epidermal lentigenes before Erbium skin resurfacing. (b) Same patient 5 days after surgery with "Opsite" semiocclusive dressing. (c) Same patient 10 days after surgery. Note minimal erythema.

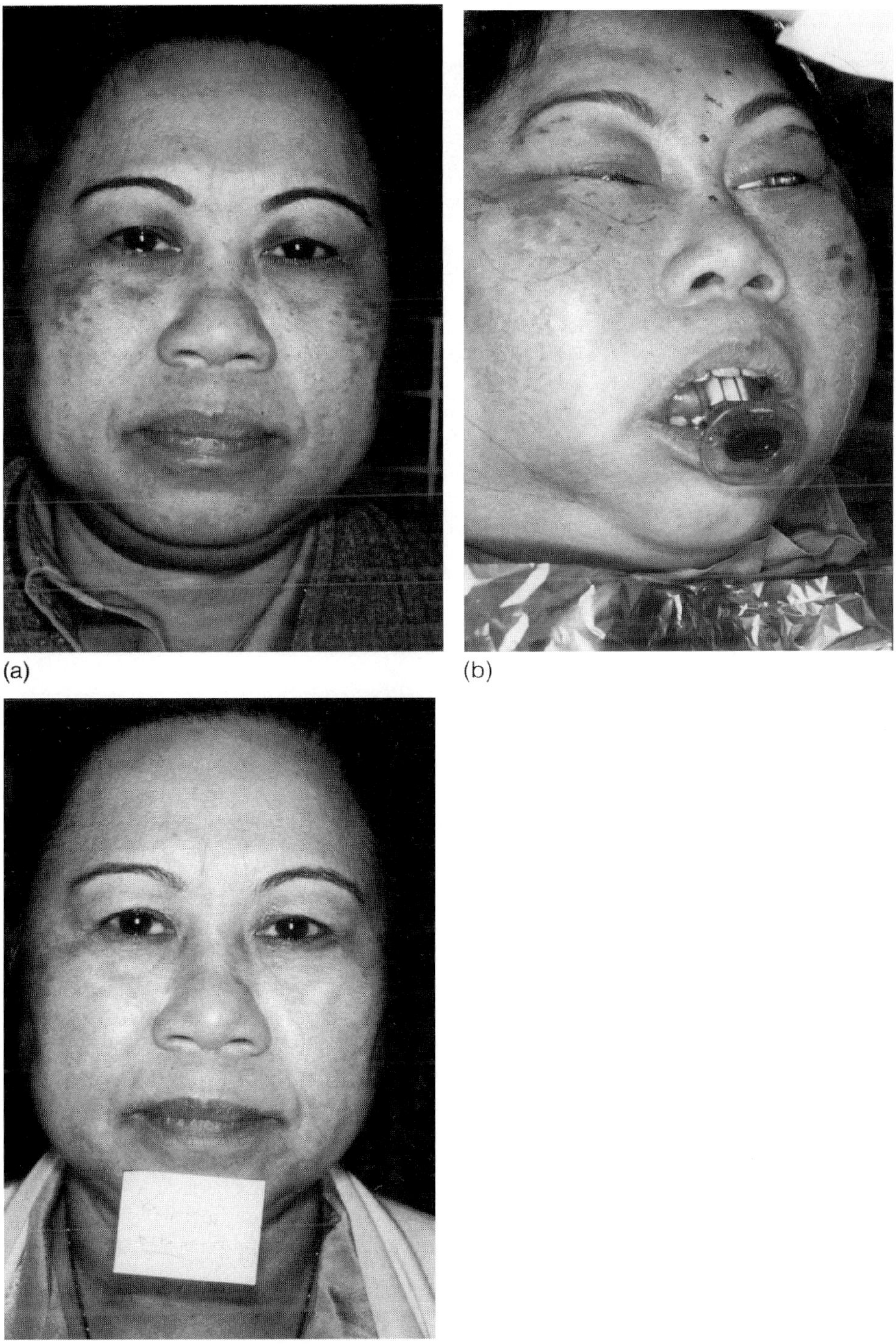

FIGURE 14 **Fifty-four–year-old female with deep dermal lentigenes before Erbium skin resurfacing. Total of 60 J/cm^2 of Erbium was used to eradicate the deeper lentigenes. (b) Same patient, intrasurgical view. Note splotchy bleeding over deep dermal pigment indicative of penetration into upper reticular dermis. (c) Same patient 6 months after surgery. Deep dermal pigment has completely cleared.**

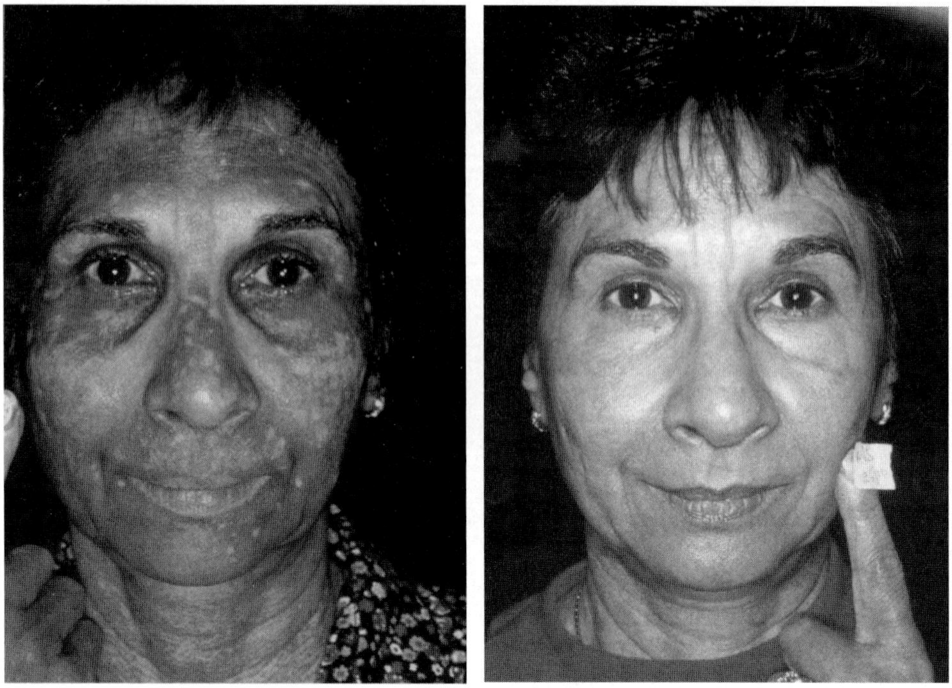

(a) (b)

FIGURE 15 Fifty-six–year-old female with dermal chloasma before full-face Erbium resurfacing. (b) Same patient 1 year after surgery with continuing use of bleaching preparation containing hydroquinone with retinoic acid.

Exophytic Skin Lesions

Epidermal exophytic lesions, eg, solar keratoses, and seborrhoeic keratoses respond well to erbium treatment, whereas dermal lesions, eg, syringomas, xanthelasmas, and compound naevi, show an initial improvement but inevitably recur.

Birth Marks

Epidermal naevi usually respond well to Erbium laser treatment, although some may recur. Melanocytic naevi, cafe au lait marks, and Becker's naevi often show good results, although some do recur.

Neck Lesions

The neck is a particularly difficult region to treat because scarring and hypopigmentation readily occur. Wrinkles on the neck are unsuitable for treatment with the Erbium laser, and either a neck-lift or ultrasonic liposuction will produce better results. Pigmentation on the neck can be removed, although long-term hypopigmentation is a real risk.

Hands

Wrinkles on the hand (Fig. 16) are not suitable for Erbium laser treatment because scarring occurs readily. However, solar keratoses and pigmented lentigenes respond well.

PRESURGICAL INSTRUCTIONS AND TREATMENT

If the patient wishes to undergo treatment with the Erbium laser, they are scheduled for a presurgical visit with a nurse counselor 10 days before the procedure. This allows adequate time for the patient to discuss the treatment and postsurgical care before the day of surgery. The consent forms (see Appendix 1) are explained and signed on this day and photographs are taken. The patient is given a prescription for oral Famvir 250 mg daily to commence 24 hours before the procedure. Valtrax may be used as an alternative. I no longer use acyclovir, as it is less effective because of its poor absorption and low bioavailability. The patient is also given a separate prescription for postsurgical medications which include oral broad spectrum antibiotics, oral steroids, and pain killers.

Presurgical Skin Care

Although there are a multitude of presurgical skin care regimes advocated, a great deal of controversy exists as to their efficacy and necessity [3,19,20]. I have found

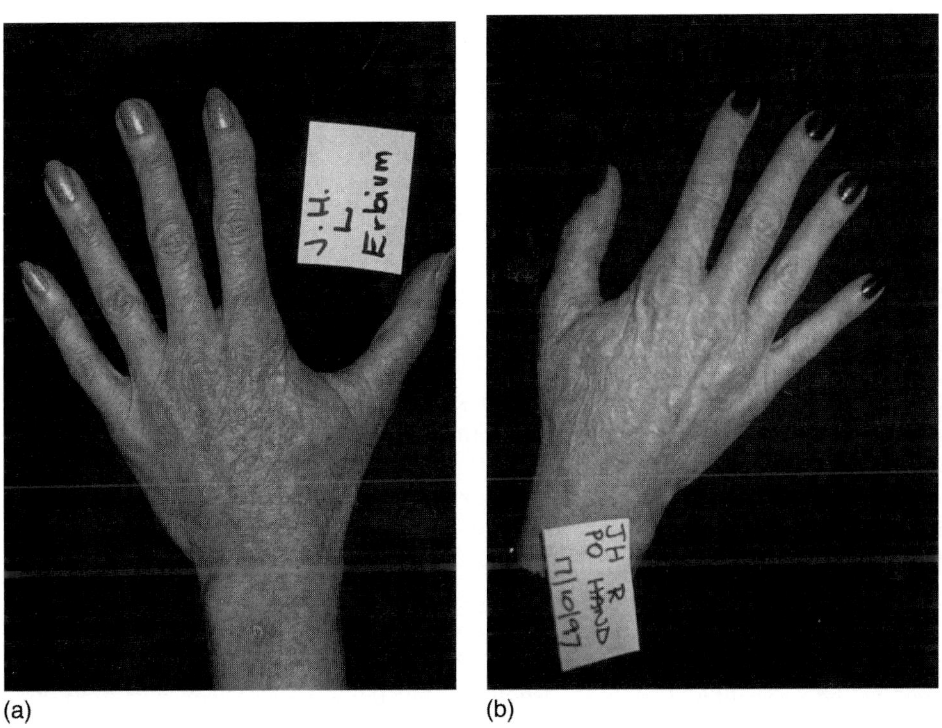

(a) (b)

FIGURE 16 (a) Presurgical view of patient with solar keratoses of the hand before Erbium treatment. (b) Same patient 6 months after surgery.

that none of the presurgical skin care programs are advantageous in prevention of hyperpigmentation or speeding up re-epithelialization. In fact, the presurgical use of topical retinoic acid caused more telengiectasia which led to troublesome bleeding during Erbium resurfacing.

The rationale for the use of presurgical bleaching creams is spurious because topical hydroquinone influences melanin production in the melanocytes that are present in the basal layer of the epidermis which will be destroyed during the resurfacing procedure. The melanocytes that are responsible for postresurfacing hyperpigmentation are presurgically present in the bases of the appendages where they are out of reach from topical bleaching creams. Postsurgically, these melanocytes migrate to the surface and produce and release melanin, leading to postresurfacing hyperpigmentation which normally commences 3 to 4 weeks postsurgically. It is far more important to commence bleaching preparations as soon as re-epithelialization is complete after surgery.

Some investigators favor the use of topical Vitamin C presurgically; however, in my experience it has not been beneficial. I favor the use of a vascular laser or Photoderm before Erbium resurfacing if the patient has telangiectasia so that troublesome bleeding will be minimized.

Paperwork

In our modern litigation environment, documentation of patient information is essential because most patients tend to forget at least 50% of the information given to them. Consent forms should be easy for the patient to understand in order to comply with the standards of informed consent (see Appendix 1). Signing consent forms on the day of the operation is not recommended because it may be construed that the patient was too nervous to understand all the implications within the consent form. Although I favor signing consent forms 10 days before the procedure, others may choose a time closer to the surgery date. Postsurgical instructions should be clear and easy for the patient to comprehend in order to avoid errors (see Appendix 2).

Equipment

Erbium Laser Machine

Although there are a number of Erbium laser machines (Fig. 17) available on the market, there are a few features that I would recommend in order to perform successful Erbium laser resurfacing which include the following:

1. The Erbium laser should be capable of generating fluences of at least 15 J/cm^2 in order to produce successful remodeling of the papillary dermis in a time-efficient manner.

2. A computerized scanner capable of producing 30 to 50% pattern overlap is particularly helpful. Many investigators use no scanners and obtain satisfactory results. However, it is possible to inadvertently produce too little or too deep penetration without a scanning system. Scanners with pattern overlap of less than 30% tend to produce a nonhomogeneous appearance resembling a cookie cutter.

3. The computerized scanner should be able to produce a large scan size so that large areas, eg, cheeks, can be resurfaced efficiently.

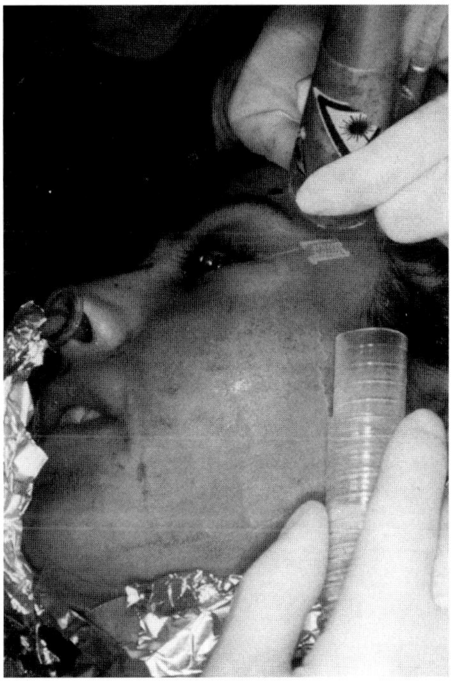

FIGURE 17 An Erbium machine with a computerized scanner makes resurfacing more efficient and reproducible.

4. Combined Erbium/CO_2 laser machine, eg, Derma K, is a luxury rather than a basic necessity. Patients who have deeper wrinkles can be resurfaced more efficiently and with less troublesome bleeding using the simultaneously combined Erbium and CO_2 machine. These laser machines work on the basis that a preselected amount of low fluence CO_2 is introduced for a preselected time during the rest phase of the Erbium cycle. Depending on the parameters chosen, variable amounts of coagulative changes are produced within the dermis while still allowing the Erbium pulse to provide ablation of the skin. The major advantage of the simultaneously combined Erbium and CO_2 machine is the reduction of bleeding which makes the procedure easier and less messy to perform, particularly when treating deeper wrinkles. The postsurgical morbidity of the simultaneously combined Erbium/CO_2 is less than for CO_2 laser alone because the zone of thermal coagulative necrosis remains constant and small (30-50 microns) with each laser pass.

Smoke Evacuation Systems

When performing Erbium resurfacing ablation of live tissue occurs, causing a great deal of debris to be released into the plume. A powerful evacuation system is needed to evacuate the debris and prevent spread of live viruses into the surgery room. I have used the Buffalo Whisper and the Stackhouse systems, both of which are suitable for Erbium resurfacing. However, great expense is incurred with replacement of filters and prefilters, which only last for a few cases.

Ear Muffs for Noise Protection

Erbium ablation produces a great deal of noise because of the tissue explosion. Industrial ear muffs are recommended for all surgery room personnel.

Face Masks

Erbium ablation produces a significant amount of debris and plume, which may be inhaled. Although laser face masks are somewhat protective, I have found the use of a facial welding shield to be a great advantage.

Eye Protection

Surgery room personnel and patients require eye protection. Surgery room personnel should wear plastic glasses with lateral shields. I usually wear magnifying plastic glasses so that the end points may be more clearly visualized. The patient's eyes should be protected with sand-blasted metal eye shields, wet gauze, or plastic glasses.

Drapes

Regular cloth or paper drapes are unsuitable for Erbium resurfacing, as they may ignite and cause a fire in the surgery room. Either wet drapes or dull crumpled silver foil should be used.

Surgery Room

Although regional Erbium resurfacing can be performed with local anesthesia alone, widespread areas and full-face resurfacing usually require intravenous sedation. It is now becoming regulation in many countries that procedures requiring intravenous sedation must be performed in a registered Day Surgery Center or hospital. Dermatologists who perform a significant number of laser resurfacing cases should seriously consider registering their surgery facility or obtain surgical privileges at a registered facility.

DAY OF SURGERY

On the day of surgery, patients should arrive early after fasting for 6 hours (if intravenous sedation is planned). Patients should not wear makeup, and should wear clothing that is loose so it can easily be pulled over the head after the procedure without disturbing their dressings. After the preliminary observations are taken, the wrinkle lines, acne scars, and cosmetic units are marked because local anesthesia may distort these during the procedure.

If intravenous sedation is planned, a friend or relative should pick up the patient after the procedure and be given a written postsurgical instruction sheet.

ANESTHESIA

The anesthesia required for Erbium resurfacing will depend on the area treated, depth, and fluence needed to treat the problem. The following anesthetic regimes have, in my experience, been found to be most useful.

EMLA Cream

Topical EMLA cream has limited use in Erbium skin resurfacing. Its main use is for very superficial intraepidermal resurfacing at low laser fluences, ie, less than 10 j/cm^2. Once the dermo-epidermal barrier is passed, EMLA cream is rarely sufficient for adequate analgesia.

Local Anesthetic Infiltration

Local anesthetic alone is suitable for localized areas of Erbium resurfacing, eg, the periocular region. Furthermore, the epinephrine used in conjunction with the local anaesthetic agent minimizes bleeding during Erbium resurfacing. Although xylocaine has traditionally been used, I favor the use of the newer, long-acting local anesthetic drug ropivocaine (Narapin). Ropivocaine, unlike Marcaine, has a rapid onset of action, negligible cardiotoxicity, and lasts 6 to 8 hours, thereby providing longer postsurgical analgesia.

Nerve Blocks

Nerve blocks are suitable for resurfacing the forehead (supraorbital nerve block) and the perioral area (infraorbital and mental nerve blocks). These may be used alone or in conjunction with intravenous sedation. I favor the use of ropivocaine with 1/150,000 epinephrine to provide a longer duration of action.

Tumescent Infiltration

Infiltration of a large quantity of dilute lignocaine 0.1% with 1/1,000,000 epinephrine is useful when resurfacing the cheeks because nerve blocks do not satisfactorily block the lateral cheeks. This technique also reduces bleeding from the Erbium laser. One major disadvantage of tumescent infiltration is the distortion of the abnormalities to be treated.

Intravenous Sedation

When full face Erbium resurfacing is undertaken, intravenous sedation is preferable. A combination of propafol, midazolam, and fentanyl are administered.

General Anesthesia

The main role of general anesthesia in Erbium skin resurfacing is when resurfacing is combined with other surgical procedures, eg, face-lifting.

TECHNIQUE

When performing Erbium resurfacing, I generally prefer to use the scanning system (Table 3) whereas the single spot is reserved for small exophytic lesions, eg, seborrhoeic keratoses, compound naevi, the shoulders of acne scars, and perioral wrinkles. The major advantages of scanning systems are their speed and evenness of depth penetration. With nonscanning systems it is possible to produce too little overlap of laser spots, leading to a cookie-cutter effect or too-deep penetration, which leads to

TABLE 3 Technique for Erbium Resurfacing

Scan pattern
square, rectangle
Scan pattern density
30–50% overlap → maximum homogeneity
Number passes
at least two → maximum homogeneity
Orientation
change orientation after each pass
Feathering
at edge cosmetic unit, avoid obvious demarcation
Single spot
small lesions, shoulder acne scars, perioral wrinkles

scarring. After each laser pass, the ablated tissue is automatically removed so wiping is unnecessary. This differs from CO_2 laser resurfacing.

Scan Pattern

Although various scan patterns and sizes are available, I always use the square or rectangular pattern because they fit easily next to one another. Pattern overlap also varies from 0 to 50%. To ensure the most homogeneous clinical result, 30 to 50% pattern overlap is selected. The size of the scan varies from 3 to 13 mm and the size is selected according to the region being treated.

After each laser pass, the orientation of the pattern should be changed to ensure a more homogeneous result and avoid printing the pattern on the skin. In all cases, it is best to perform more than one pass so a more even clinical result is obtained.

Laser Parameters

Laser parameters will vary according to the region and the pathology being treated (Table 4). To treat dermal pathology, ie, wrinkles and acne scars, fluences greater than 10 j/cm^2 must be used. Because the eyelid has thinner skin than the rest of the face, lower fluences are selected for this region.

When treating wrinkles, the whole cosmetic unit must be treated evenly because the solar elastosis is present as a fairly uniform band in the upper dermis. Extra passes may be occasionally needed to lower the shoulders of the perioral wrinkles. Acne scars are more focal in nature, and so require more passes than the surrounding skin.

Visual End Points

With the use of scanning systems, it is relatively easy to visualize how deep within the dermis the laser has reached (Table 5, Figs. 18, 19). These end points may be somewhat modified when local anesthetic infiltration with epinephrine is used. To better appreciate these changes, magnification (2–3×) helps greatly.

TABLE 4 Laser Parameters

Wrinkles	
Eyelid skin	10–14 J/cm^2, two passes
Crow's feet	14 J/cm^2, three passes
Forehead	14–20 J/cm^2, two to three passes
Cheeks	14–20 J/cm^2, two to three passes
Perioral	14–20 J/cm^2, three to four passes simultaneously combined Erbium and CO_2 laser 18 J/cm^2 Erbium + 1.4 J/cm^2 CO_2, two passes
Acne Scars	
Cosmetic unit	14–20 J/cm^2, two passes
Acne scar shoulders	single spot, 8 J/cm^2, 5 Hz
Pigmentation	
Superficial	10–14 J/cm^2, two passes
Deep	14–20 J/cm^2, two to four passes
Extrafacial	
Neck, hands	<15 J/cm^2

Epidermis

The epidermis is clearly seen as yellowish brown keratinizing tissue.

Upper Papillary Dermis

Once the epidermal-dermal junction is passed, the yellowish brown opaque tissue gives way to a more shiny pinkish spongy dermis. Follicular openings are small and regular.

TABLE 5 Visual End Points (with Magnification)

Epidermis
brownish keratinizing tissue
Papillary dermis
pink spongy fine network
small follicular openings
fine regular collagen bundles
pinpoint bleeding
transudate
Reticular dermis
coarse haphazard collagen bundles
wider follicular openings, "stand out" from surrounding skin
splotchy bleeding

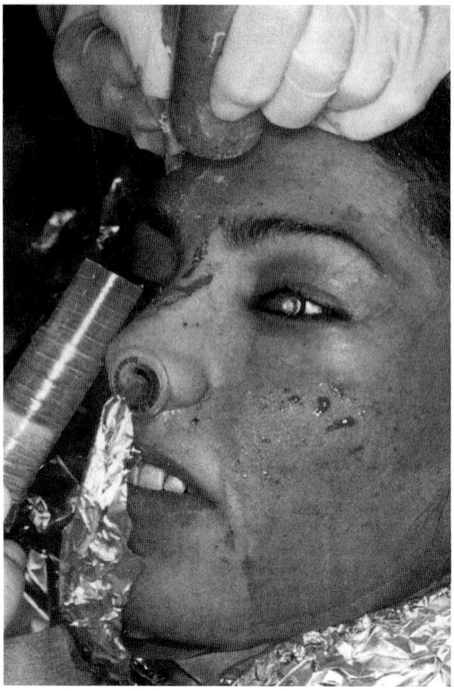

FIGURE 18 Visual end points of Erbium resurfacing. Pinpoint bleeding is seen readily when resurfacing in midpapillary dermis.

Midpapillary Dermis

Because small capillary blood vessels are present in the midpapillary dermis, pinpoint bleeding will be seen. If telangiectasia is present, there will be a larger number of vessels that bleed, whereas if epinephrine is used, bleeding may be considerably reduced.

A clear transudate will develop because of the "shock" waves being transmitted by the Erbium laser to these dermal vessels. It is this transudate that produces water within the dermis, allowing the Erbium laser to ablate dermal tissue. In the midpapillary dermis, the follicular openings become wider and begin to "stand out" from the surrounding skin.

Papillary-Reticular Dermal Junction

As the reticular dermis is approached, larger blood vessels are encountered and splotchy bleeding will occur. Transudate becomes heavier, and the follicular openings become wider. Collagen bundles become coarser and more haphazard in orientation. In some instances, bleeding obscures these changes. If the patient has a large number of telangiectasia, it is often advantageous to pretreat them with a vascular laser or Photoderm intensive light source. This will greatly reduce troublesome bleeding. If deeper resurfacing is required, the use of the simultaneously combined Erbium and CO_2 laser (Derma K) will coagulate some vessels and reduce bleeding. Once the reticular dermis is reached, resurfacing should cease to avoid deeper laser penetration with the risk of scarring.

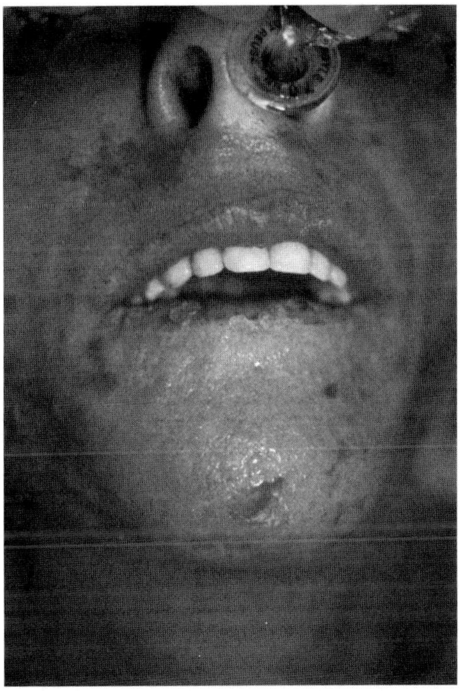

FIGURE 19 Deeper resurfacing into the upper reticular dermis will produce splotchy bleeding and a more profuse transudate. Follicular openings become wider.

Feathering at the Edge of a Cosmetic Unit

To avoid demarcation lines at the end of the Erbium-treated area, feathering is useful. This may be easily achieved by tilting the scanner to 45° and pulling the scanner away from the skin. By doing so, the pattern is spread out and the effective fluence reduced. I have found this a very useful technique to avoid a demarcation line at the jawline.

WRINKLES

Eyelid

To treat wrinkles around the upper and lower eyelid, the entire area is treated evenly and right up to the lash line. I use Erbium square scan pattern with 50% pattern overlap, keeping the eyelashes out of the firing line with a cotton-tipped applicator. Ten to 14 J/cm^2 are selected, depending on the age of the patient and perceived skin thickness. Two passes are made on the thinner eyelid skin, while three passes may be made in the thicker crow's feet region. Ideally, crow's feet resurfacing should be combined with Botox injections.

Forehead

The skin of the forehead is much thicker, so higher fluences may be used. The whole region is treated evenly using a large square pattern, 50% pattern overlap, and 15 to

20 J/cm^2. Generally, two to three passes are made. Erbium laser resurfacing is ideally combined with endoscopic forehead-lifting.

Cheeks

Cheek skin is similar to the forehead region. Similar parameters are used. Two passes are usually made over the entire cosmetic unit, while a third pass may be made selectively over deeper wrinkled areas. If the patient is undergoing face-lifting simultaneously, the lateral cheek must be resurfaced very conservatively using a total fluence of less than 15 J/cm^2.

Mouth

The perioral area is in many ways the most difficult area to successfully treat without causing scarring. I generally treat the whole cosmetic unit by first using a square pattern, 50% pattern overlap, at fluences of 15 to 20 J/cm^2. Two passes are made routinely. A single 3 mm spot is then used at 8 J/cm^2, 5 Hz, to lower the shoulders of the wrinkles. A further one to two passes are made using the single spot to localized areas only. Care should be taken to not violate the vermilion border. If wrinkles are present on the mucosa, they should be treated with the single spot while leaving the vermilion border itself intact.

Extrafacial Regions

Resurfacing off the face is at best unpredictable because scarring and hypopigmentation may result. Wrinkles on the neck rarely respond predictably, so only superficial resurfacing is recommended, ie, total fluence less than 15 J/cm^2.

ACNE SCARRING

Because acne scarring can be deep, resurfacing alone will produce at best only modest results. I often combine Erbium resurfacing with fat grafting and punch excision of deeper scars. These procedures may be performed simultaneously during the same operation. If fat grafting is used, it is performed before the resurfacing, whereas punch excisions are performed at the end of the procedure.

Initially the entire cosmetic unit is treated evenly by using two passes of the scanning Erbium laser. A large square pattern, 50% pattern overlap is chosen, and fluences of 15 to 20 J/cm^2. Two passes are made, taking care to change the pattern orientation after each pass.

The acne scars are then treated with further passes by using either a smaller pattern or a single 3 mm spot with the aim of lowering the shoulders of the acne scars. However, once the reticular dermis is entered, with splotchy bleeding and wide follicular openings, resurfacing should cease.

PIGMENTATION

Epidermal and dermal pigmentation may be successfully treated with the Erbium laser. Clinically, it is possible to determine whether the pigment is epidermal or dermal although it does not matter for the purposes of Erbium resurfacing because one can readily observe the pigment being removed as if by an eraser.

If the abnormal pigment is widespread, the scanning system is used with a 50% pattern overlap. Ten to 14 J/cm^2 are selected. Two passes will usually readily eliminate epidermal pigment and produce a homogeneous appearance. If the pigment is dermal, three to four passes will be necessary. I usually make two passes over the entire area, and then with a smaller scan pattern will make selective further passes to the areas of deeper pigment. If the pigmentation is lentigo like, it is easier to use a single spot at fluences of 5 to 8 J/cm^2 and lower repetition rates of 5 Hz until the pigment disappears. When using single spot, care is necessary to avoid going beyond the end point.

EXOPHYTIC SKIN LESIONS

Solar, seborrhoeic keratoses, compound naevi, and other exophytic skin lesions are treated by using a single spot at 8 J/cm^2, 5 Hz, until the exophytic component has been removed.

COMBINED ERBIUM AND CO_2 LASER RESURFACING

When treating deep wrinkles, especially in the perioral area and cheeks, deeper Erbium resurfacing often leads to bleeding, making the procedure difficult and messy. To overcome this problem, combining Erbium with CO_2 laser will help to minimize bleeding while the Erbium component continues to ablate tissue. The use of the simultaneously combined Erbium and CO_2 laser (Derma K) is ideal for treating deep wrinkles and acne scars. In most cases, I favor using the minimum fluence of CO_2 that will coagulate superficial vessels without causing excessive thermal injury to dermal collagen. In most cases, I use the simultaneously combined laser at Erbium 18 J/cm^2 with CO_2 1.4 J/cm^2 (2 watts CO_2 at 50% duty cycle). Two passes are sufficient to treat most deeper rhytids.

IMMEDIATE POSTSURGICAL CARE

Early postsurgical care is made up of topical and oral treatment (Table 6).

TABLE 6 Postsurgical Operative Care

Wound care
semipermeable dressings
24–48 hours (absorbent, eg, Second skin, Vigilon)
Oral medications
antiviral drugs (Famvir, Valtrax)
antibiotics (broad spectrum)
oral steroids
Topical preparations
ultraviolet A blocking sunscreen, titanium dioxide
moisturizer, bland, oil free
cleanser bland, oil free
bleaching preparation, pigment gel forte, hydroquinone and retinoic acid
Vitamin C?

Topical Therapy

There has always been much debate about the relative merits of a closed technique with semipermeable dressings versus an open technique after laser resurfacing. If superficial intraepidermal resurfacing is performed, no dressings are needed. The use of bland moisturizers and sunscreens are used immediately after surgery.

Once the epidermis is removed, I favor the use of semipermeable dressings because many studies have shown that semiocclusion speeds up re-epithelialization and decreases postsurgical pain [21–23]. Although there are many biosynthetic dressings available, I have found the following regiment to be helpful.

1. *First 24 to 48 hours.* Bionet 2nd skin (Little Rock, AR) or Vigilon are used because these dressings are highly absorbent and there is a considerable transudate after Erbium resurfacing. The semipermeable dressings, eg, Flexzan, that are normally recommended for CO_2 laser resurfacing are less suitable because of their relatively poor absorbing capacity. Dressings are held in place by a stockingette and left for 24 or 48 hours. Many patients request a dressing change after 24 hours because it feels wet and uncomfortable. If an open technique is used, the transudate will form a dry crust that may be painful and is fairly unsightly to the patient and their relatives. Vaseline and other creams generally "slip off" the face and are not very effective.

2. *48 hours to 7 days.* Once the transudate has been fully absorbed, a thin clear adherent dressing, eg, Opsite or Tegaderm, is used because it is more comfortable and aesthetic. It will normally "stick" until re-epithelialization is complete, after which time it can be readily removed.

If an open technique is adopted at this stage, a bland moisturizer, eg, Vaseline or Aquafore, should be used. In my experience, Vaseline often causes acne and many other moisturizers cause irritant reactions. It is important to avoid topical antibiotic preparations because contact dermatitis often develops and can be difficult to diagnose.

Oral Therapy

Oral Antiviral Medications

To prevent widespread herpes infection, it is imperative to use an antiviral agent beginning 24 hours before the procedure and continuing until re-epithelialization is complete, which may be 7 to 10 days. Even if the patient has no previous history of herpes infection, it is still wise to use an antiviral drug. The newer antiviral drugs, eg, Famvir and Valtrax, are more bioavailable and so should be selected over the older drugs, eg, acyclovir. In most patients, a dose of Famvir 250 mg daily is sufficient, although if active herpes is present 500 dg daily is used. In elderly patients, there is a significant risk of herpes zoster so a higher dose, ie, 750 mg Famvir daily, is suggested.

Oral Antibiotics

Infection following Erbium facial resurfacing is rare because of the excellent blood supply to the face and the lack of necrotic tissue. Despite this, broad spectrum oral antibiotics are used prophylactically, eg, cephalosporin and Zithromax.

Oral Steroids

Although there is much debate about the use of oral steroids, they are of advantage when extensive areas are resurfaced to minimize swelling. I favor the use of oral steroids for 48 hours in a dose of 50 mg prednisolone daily.

Oral Painkillers

With the use of semiocclusive dressings, painkillers are usually unnecessary. Tylenol should be adequate for Erbium resurfacing.

LATE POSTSURGICAL CARE

Once the skin has fully re-epithelialized, it is still prone to acne, irritant dermatitis, and pigmentation. To minimize these potential problems, the following regime is recommended.

Moisturizer

The skin is slightly flaky after Erbium skin resurfacing, so a moisturizer is needed. It is best to use an oil-free (silicone-based), bland moisturizer. It is best to avoid moisturizers that contain alpha hydroxy acids, perfume, and chemical sunscreens because they may irritate the skin. Greasy preparations, eg, Vaseline, tend to cause acne in many individuals. I have used the Skin tech moisturizer successfully in most patients after Erbium resurfacing.

Cleanser

Cleansers also have the ability to irritate the skin and so should be relatively bland, eg, Cetaphil lotion.

Sunscreen

Postsurgical pigmentation can occur after Erbium resurfacing, especially in patients with skin types 4 to 6. This may occur in the absence of sun exposure, but is exacerbated by ultraviolet light. It is ultraviolet A rather than ultraviolet B light that is mostly responsible for postsurgical pigmentation. Using sunscreens that specifically block out ultraviolet A light are therefore most important. It is best to use sunscreens that contain predominantly titanium dioxide because they block out ultraviolet A light most effectively and do not cause irritant or allergic contact dermatitis. Minimizing the use of chemical-based sunscreens will help to minimize irritant and allergic reactions. If pigment is added to titanium dioxide, a broader spectrum of ultraviolet light protection is obtained while the cosmetic appearance of the sunscreen is improved.

Bleaching Preparations

Because postsurgical pigmentation is common in patients with skin types 4 to 6, prophylactic use of bleaching preparations postsurgically in patients with these skin types if advisable. Although skin types 1 to 3 may pigment occasionally, routine prophylactic use of bleaching preparations in this group is not usually necessary. If pigmentation does occur, then a bleaching preparation is introduced, eg, Pigment gel forte (Physician's Choice).

Bleaching creams are used on skin types 4 to 6 as soon as re-epithelialization is complete. The preparation is initially used on alternate nights until tolerance develops after which time it is used nightly for 4 to 6 weeks.

For skin type 4, I have found that Pigment gel forte (Physician's Choice) and Skin lightening gel (Mene & Moy) both work well. Hydroquinone alone appears to be less effective. Skin types 5 and 6 do not regularly respond to these preparations and require hydroquinone with retinoic acid to prevent hyperpigmentation. If tolerated, Kligman formula (5% hydroquinone, 0.1% retinoic acid, 1% hydrocortisone) is ideal. If it is too irritating, then half-strength Kligman formula is used.

Other Topical Creams

Although there are many other preparations recommended for use after Erbium laser resurfacing, I have not found them to be particularly useful. These include topical vitamin C and steroids, among others. As a general rule, it is best to keep the postsurgical skin care routine as simple as possible. Complicated skincare programs are confusing for patients and have the potential for causing unwanted side effects, especially acne and contact irritant and allergic reactions.

COMPLICATIONS AND THEIR TREATMENT

One of the major reasons for the introduction of Erbium skin resurfacing was to find a more precise tool of skin remodeling that produced less morbidity and complications than existing, more established techniques, namely CO_2 laser resurfacing (Table 7).

As with all new techniques, there is a significant learning curve to produce optimal results and minimize side effects. With increased experience in Erbium resurfacing, complications have become relatively uncommon. A complication does not equal disaster, and in most cases may be satisfactorily treated. Dermatologists are ideally suited to detect and manage complications if and when they occur, so frequent follow-up is recommended, especially in the first 6 to 8 weeks after laser resurfacing.

Erythema

Erythema is an inevitable sequela to most resurfacing procedures. The degree and duration of erythema after Erbium laser resurfacing is less than CO_2 laser for the same depth of resurfacing. Erythema will be greater with increasing depth of penetration. In most cases, erythema is mild and has largely resolved by 6 to 8 weeks after surgery. With the simultaneously combined Erbium and CO_2 laser treatment at the parameters used, the erythema is more intense than Erbium alone but less intense than CO_2 alone. Erythema will be more pronounced and longer lasting if bleaching preparations containing glycolic or retinoic acid are used after surgery. Erythema may be somewhat modified with the use of topical steroid creams, although in some cases, these creams produce acne. I have not found topical vitamin C cream to be particularly beneficial in reducing erythema secondary to Erbium treatment, although some investigators have found it useful after CO_2 laser resurfacing [24]. Certainly,

TABLE 7 Complications

Hyperpigmentation
skin types 4–6, temporary, responsive to bleaching preparations
Hypopigmentation
loss sun damage
dermal fibrosis
skin types 1-4
mild, less severe than CO_2
Scarring
excessive depth resurfacing
extrafacial regions
infection
patient factors
early treatment with intralesional steroids and 5FU
Infection
bacterial
viral
fungal
Contact dermatitis
topical antitiotics
topical irritants, perfumed creams, glycolic acid, chemical sunscreens
Ectropion
rare
Synechiae
lower eyelid skin

the use of a yellow-based tinted sunscreen was most helpful in concealing the erythema.

Pigmentation

Postsurgical pigmentation will universally occur in patients with skin types 4 to 6 unless bleaching preparations are introduced early in the postsurgical period, ie, as soon as re-epithelialization is complete. In fair-skinned patients, pigmentation may still occur because of inadvertent sun exposure. If this occurs, a bleaching preparation, eg, Pigment gel forte (Physician's Choice) may be introduced. In my experience, postinflammatory pigmentation will almost always resolve.

Hypopigmentation

Hypopigmentation may occur with any resurfacing procedure and is usually evident after 6 months. It occurs because of two major factors:

1. Removal of sun damage. Newly resurfaced skin shows a loss of pigment dyschromia, which is a feature of solar damage, and leads to a contrast between resurfaced skin and surrounding sun damaged skin.

2. Dermal fibrosis. After any resurfacing procedure, sun-damaged dermal collagen fibers are replaced by new collagen formation. As maturation occurs, collagen bundles become tightly organized, leading to loss of light reflectance and a relative opacification of the dermis. As the epidermis in light-skinned patients is relatively transparent, the opaque dermal tissue becomes apparent. The deeper the resurfacing procedure, the more intense the dermal fibrosis and the more apparent is the hypopigmentation. Vascular fibrosis also occurs as part of this process, contributing further to skin pallor.

When comparing equivalent depths of Erbium and CO_2 laser resurfacing procedures, Erbium produces less severe hypopigmentation. This is probably because of the lack of unnecessary thermal injury to collagen fibers, resulting in less intense fibrosis. Some degree of new collagen formation, or fibrosis, is necessary for the removal of wrinkles, but the greater precision of the Erbium laser allows for sufficient, but not excessive, fibrosis.

Once hypopigmentation develops, it is irreversible. Topical retinoic acid may be helpful in promoting new vessel formation, thereby giving the skin a more rosy appearance. Significant hypopigmentation rarely occurs in the darker-skinned patients because of the denser melanin production within the epidermis, which obscures the changes within the dermis. It may, however, occur in these patients secondary to scarring.

Scarring

Scarring may occur with any resurfacing procedure because of several factors, which include the following:

1. *Excessive depth of penetration.* Resurfacing too deeply, in particular destroying appendages, will result in delayed re-epithelialization and scarring. This may occur with Erbium lasers if the surgeon is not familiar with the end points or is using a nonscanning system with stacking of laser pulses. Scanning Erbium lasers should help to minimize this problem.
2. *Infection.* Although infection is relatively uncommon in the well-vascularized face, poor wound care can lead to bacterial infection and scarring. Herpes infection can also lead to scarring. Candidal infection does not usually scar.
3. *Oral retinoid or high-dose vitamin A therapy.* Patients who have recently taken oral retinoids may experience abnormal healing and scarring, so patients should wait at least 6 months or longer after completion of oral retinoid therapy before undergoing laser resurfacing. Some experts have noted that vegetarians may also exhibit impaired healing and scarring, although the reasons are unclear [25–28].
4. *Appendageal abnormalities.* Patients who have scarred or abnormal appendages, eg, electrolysis therapy, may have delayed re-epithelialization and scarring.
5. *Patient factors.* Some patients scar more easily than others, eg, Asians, the exact reasons for which are unknown.

In the resurfaced skin, scarring appears as an area of induration and intense erythema, usually beginning at about 6 weeks after surgery. Early and aggressive treatment will usually resolve the problem. If untreated, however, true hypertrophic scarring will tend to follow (Fig. 20).

In some cases, strong fluorinated topical steroids, with or without occlusion, will clear the indurated areas. However, in most cases, early use of intralesional

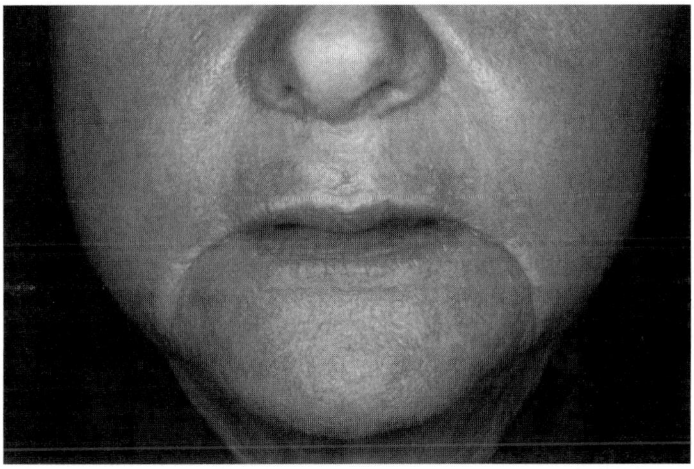

FIGURE 20 Patient at 6 weeks after surgery with induration indicative of early hypertrophic scarring. Early injection of triamcinolone and/or 5FU will prevent true hypertrophic scarring.

triamcinolone 10 mg/mL is much more effective. Weekly injections may be needed until the induration resolves. If scarring does not respond to intralesional steroids, intralesional 5FU will help in most patients. Repeated injections may be necessary. Occasionally, the use of a vascular laser or Photoderm may be helpful.

Infection

Bacterial Infection

If bacterial infection does occur, a swab should be taken of the skin and an appropriate antibiotic started. Even more important is attention to wound care. The area should be left open until infection has cleared.

Herpes Infection

With adequate herpes prophylaxis, significant herpes infection should not occur. If it does, a higher dose of the oral antiviral drug is recommended. The area should be left open and treated with acetic acid soaks.

Fungal Infection

Candidal infection may occur if the skin is kept too moist, either with overly occlusive ointments or inadequate change of moist dressings. The mainstay of treatment is to dry out the area with acetic acid soaks along with cessation of the occlusive ointment. Although local measures alone suffice in most cases, patients with severe infection may require oral antifungal agents, eg, ketoconazole.

Contact Dermatitis

Contact dermatitis may occur secondary to the use of any active ingredient, especially while the skin is re-epithelializing. It is particularly likely if a topical antibiotic ointment is used. As the epidermis has been removed, the usual features of contact dermatitis are not present but the patient will usually complain of swelling and itching. The offending agent should be ceased and oral steroids introduced for 48 hours. Contact dermatitis may also occur after complete re-epithelialization, especially to chemical sunscreens, perfumed creams, and any other active ingredient. A high index of suspicion is needed to detect this readily treatable problem.

Ectropion

Scleral show and temporary ectropion commonly occur after CO_2 laser resurfacing, requiring the frequent use of canthopexy procedures. Scleral show is uncommon after Erbium resurfacing unless the patient has pre-existing lower eyelid laxity or has previously undergone a transcutaneous lower eyelid blepharoplasty.

Synechiae

Synechiae under the lower eyelid are relatively common after Erbium laser resurfacing because of the wet surfaces of the skin "sticking" to one another. To minimize this problem, taping over the dressing may be helpful. If it does occur, resurfacing gently over the synechia with a single spot at low Erbium fluence (7 J/cm^2) will usually release it.

CONCLUSION

Erbium laser resurfacing is a very precise tool for skin resurfacing, offering a lower morbidity and complication rate compared with CO_2 laser resurfacing. It is suitable for all skin types and can be satisfactorily performed in localized areas. Erbium laser resurfacing does have shortcomings, especially for treating deeper wrinkles, because of bleeding. To overcome these problems, the introduction of simultaneously combined Erbium and CO_2 lasers combines the advantages of the two different technologies while minimizing their disadvantages. The simultaneously combined Erbium and CO_2 laser is particularly useful for treating lighter-skinned female patients with deep wrinkles or acne scars.

REFERENCES

1. Fitzpatrick RE, Goldman MP, Satur NM, Tope WD. Pulsed carbon dioxide laser resurfacing of photoaged facial skin. Arch Dermatol 1996; 132:395–402.
2. Weinstein C, Pozner JN, Ramirez OM. Complications of carbon dioxide laser resurfacing and their prevention. Aesth Surg J 1997; July/August.
3. Weinstein C, Raminez OM, Pozner JN. Post operative care following carbon dioxide laser resurfacing. Avoiding Pitfalls. J Deramtol Surg 1998; 24:51–56.
4. Nanni CA, Alster TS. Complications of carbon dioxide laser resurfacing. Dermatol Surg 1998; 24:315–320.
5. Bernstein LJ, Kauver AN, Grossman MC, Geronemus RG. The short and long term side effects of carbon dioxide laser resurfacing. Dermatol Surg 1997; 23:519–525.
6. Gardner ES, Reinisch L, Stricklin GP, et al. In vitro changes in non-facial human skin following CO_2 laser resurfacing. A comparison study. Lasers Surg Med 1996; 19:379–387.
7. Wheeland RG. Clinical uses of lasers in dermatology. Lasers Surg Med 1995; 16(1):2–23.

8. Hohenleutner V, Hohenleutner S, Baumer W, et al. Fast and effective skin ablation with an Er:YAG laser: determination of ablation rates and thermal damage zones. Lasers Surg Med 1997; 20:242–247.
9. Kaufmann R, Hartmann A, Hibst R. Cutting and skin ablative properties of pulsed mid-infrared laser surgery. J Dermatol Surg Oncol 1994; 20:112–8.
10. Kaufmann R, Hibst R. Pulsed Erbium:YAG laser ablation in cutaneous surgery. Lasers Surg Med 1996; 19:324–330.
11. Weinstein C. Computerised scanning Erbium:YAG laser for skin resurfacing. J Dermatol Surg 1998; 24:83–89.
12. Weinstein C. Erbium laser resurfacing current concepts. Plast Reconstr Surg. In Press.
13. Lawrence N, Brody HJ, Alt TH. Chemical peeling. In: Coleman WP, ed. Cosmetic Surgery of the Skin. St. Louis: Mosby, 1997:85–111.
14. Baker TJ. Chemical face peeling and rhytidectomy. Plast Reconstr Surg 1962; 29–199.
15. Alt TH, Goodman GJ, Coleman WP, et al. In: Coleman WP, ed. Dermabrasion Cosmetic Surgery. St. Louis: Mosby, 1997; 112–152.
16. Weinstein C. Ultrapulse carbon dioxide laser rejuvenation of facial wrinkles and scars. Am J Cosm Surg 1997; 14:3–11.
17. Weinstein C, Alster TS. Skin resurfacing with high energy pulsed carbon dioxide laser. In: Alster TS, Apfelberg DG, eds. Cosmetic Laser Surgery. Wiley & Sons, 1996; 9–27.
18. Ross VE, Domankevitz Y, Skrobal M, et al. Effects of CO_2 laser pulse duration ablation and residual thermal damage; implications for skin resurfacing. Laser Surg Med 1996; 19:123–129.
19. Mandy SH. Tretinoin in the preoperative and postoperative management of dermabrasion. J Am Acad Derm 1986; 15:87–88.
20. Hevia O, Nemeth AJ, Taylor R. Tretinoin accelerates healing after trichloracetic acid chemical peel. Arch Dermatol 1991; 127:678–683.
21. Eaglestein WH, Mertz PM. "Inert" vehicles do affect wound healing. J Invest Dermatol 1980; 74–90.
22. Eaglestein WH, Davis SC, Mehle AL, et al. Optimal use of an occlusive dressing to enhance healing. Effect of delayed application and early removal on wound healing. Arch Dermatol 1988; 124:392.
23. Wheeland RG. New surgical dressings aid post operative healing. Dermatol Perspect 1991; 7:1–5.
24. Alster TS, West TB. Effects of topical Vitamin C on post operative carbon dioxide laser resurfacing erythema. J Dermatol Surg 1998; 24:3, 331–336.
25. Moy RL, Moy LS, Bennett RG, et al. Systemic isotretinoin. Effects on dermal wound healing in rabbit ear model in vivo. J Dermatol Surg Oncol 1990; 16:1142–1146.
26. Rubinstein R, Roenigk H, Stegman SJ, et al. Atypical keloids after dermabrasion of patients taking isotretinoin. J Am Acad Dermatol 1986; 15:280–285.
27. Williams ML, Elias PM. Nature of skin fragility in patients receiving retinoids for systemic effect. Arch Dermatol 1981; 117:611–619.
28. Ehrlich HP, Hunt TK. Effects of cortisone and Vitamin A on wound healing. Ann Surg 1968; 167:324.

APPENDIX 1: CONSENT FORM FOR SKIN RESURFACING

CONSENT FORM FOR REMOVAL OF WRINKLES, ACNE SCARS

AND BROWN SPOTS BY LASER RESURFACING

I ....

OF ....

Hereby voluntarily consent to undergo laser resurfacing of my skin.

I understand that Cosmetic Procedures are to improve my appearance and cannot always achieve a perfect result.

I also agree to carefully carry out all given instructions to ensure satisfactory healing.

This procedure has been explained to me and I understand the possible complications which may occur. All my questions have been answered to my satisfaction.

I understand the possible complications of the procedure which may occur.

These possible complications include:

1. **Scarring**
2. **Increased skin pigmentation**
3. **Decreased skin pigmentation**
4. **Infection**
5. **Cold Sores**
6. **Demarcation lines**
7. **Patchiness in the skin**
8. **Incomplete removal of damaged skin and/or wrinkles and acne scars**
9. **Depression in the skin**
10. **Swelling**
11. **Prolonged redness of skin**
12. **Flareup of acne**

If medical complications do occur, I agree that I am obliged to immediately inform Dr Weinstein's surgery.

I have read this Consent Form before signing and have had it fully explained to me.

PATIENT'S SIGNATURE:____

WITNESS:____

DATE:____

APPENDIX 2: POSTSURGICAL INSTRUCTIONS FOR SKIN RESURFACING

SKIN RESURFACING PRE-OPERATIVE INSTRUCTIONS

1. You may use your normal skin care products prior to skin resurfacing.

2. 24 hours prior to your procedure you must take Famvir (1 tablet) and continue taking Famvir tablets for 10-14 days. This will help prevent cold sores erupting during the healing phase.

SKIN RESURFACING POST-OPERATIVE INSTRUCTIONS

1. You will go home with a special dressing and bandage. **This must be left in place.** The dressing allows your skin to heal more quickly and prevents pain.
2. You will need to apply Vaseline (on a cotton bud) around the lips and under the eyes to prevent the skin becoming dry and crusty. **Keep it slightly moist.**

3. Take all your medications:
    a) Famvir – 1 tablet daily for 10-14 days.
    b) Keflex – 2 capsules twice daily for 10-14 days.
    c) Prednisolone – 4 tablets in the morning for 3 days. **STOP** after 3 days.
    d) Pain killers – Panadeine Forte as necessary.
    e) Sleeping tablets (Temazepam) 1-2 tablets at night
    It is important to take sleeping tablets as it is difficult to sleep on 3-4 pillows especially with dressings. Also, Prednisolone tends to make you stay awake.
4. Sleep on 3-4 pillows to minimise eyelid swelling. Continue doing this for 5 days if possible.

5. Use ice packs on your eyes – 20 minutes on and 5 minutes off for first 24 hours (while awake only).

THE NEXT DAY:

1. Return to our Clinic the day after your procedure to have your dressing changed. It is advisable to take some painkiller before you come. Please have a shower and wash your hair before you come in – if comfortable but do not remove the dressing on your face.
2. Take your medications (Keflex, Famvir, Prednisolone).

FOLLOWING DAYS:

1. You will need to come for dressing changes **ONLY** if dressing becomes loose.
2. Continue to apply Vaseline to any exposed areas of the skin (e.g. mouth & eyelid areas)
3. Continue taking medications (Keflex, Famvir).
4. It is normal to feel quite anxious and maybe even depressed. As your skin heals, your anxiety will disappear. If you feel anxious, please telephone our office – we can prescribe a sedative.

ON DAY 7:

1. Return to our Clinic – dressing will be removed. **Please wash your hair** before your visit.
2. When dressing is removed, your skin will be pink to red and slightly scabby – this will resolve over approximately the next 7 days.
3. You will need to apply the following preparations:
   a) **Moisturiser** – oil free, fragrance free as often as you like. If this is not sufficiently moist use Aqueous cream sparingly – if you use too much Aqueous cream you may get pimples and white heads.
   b) **Cleanser** - use Cetaphil lotion gently twice daily (this may be bought at a Chemist).
   c) Use **Ego Sunsense or Skin Tech** ($39) sunscreen daily. This will help protect you from ultraviolet A light. It will also help to cover the redness of your skin.
   d) To help reduce skin redness, Dr Weinstein may prescribe hydrocortisone 1% cream. Use this sparingly twice daily.

DAYS 10-14:

Continue to use moisturiser, cleanser and sunscreen.

1. You will need to use a **bleaching cream** e.g. – Pigment Gel Forte ($65) for 6-8 weeks. Start by applying this every second night. As you develop tolerance to this cream, you can use it each night. This bleaching cream may cause redness and peeling. If too much peeling occurs, reduce using it to every third night.

<u>YOU MUST NOT USE THE BLEACHING CREAM ON ANY BROKEN SKIN</u>

2 WEEKS – 3 MONTHS:

1. You will notice that the new skin will become less red and less flaky – this indicates that the new skin is maturing.
2. Your new skin will be sensitive to sunlight for 3 months, so **make certain you wear sunscreen** (e.g. – tinted sunscreen).
3. Your skin will be more prone to pimples due to the stimulation of oily glands. Therefore **use oil free skin creams and sunscreens only.** It is helpful to use glycolic acid or equivalent to minimise pimples.
4. Your skin will be more fragile for 3 months or so. You should:
   a) sleep on a soft pillow (e.g. satin)
   b) wash your face gently with cotton wool – do **NOT** use a face washer
   c) be careful at the hairdresser so that any chemical does not contact the skin.
   d) use **<u>bland</u>** skin care products e.g. creams that do not have any perfumes or alphahydroxy acids.

AFTER 3 MONTHS:

Your skin will gradually toughen so that you can resume use of your normal cosmetics.

9

The Effective Use of Resurfacing Lasers

Stephen O. Kovacs and Roy G. Geronemus
Laser and Skin Surgery Center of New York, New York, New York

Arielle N. B. Kauvar
Laser and Skin Surgery Center of New York, and New York University School of Medicine, New York, New York

INTRODUCTION

Until recently, chemical peeling and mechanical dermabrasion have been the standard modalities of treating photoaged skin [1]. With these techniques, the epidermis and variable portions of the dermis are destroyed. Improvements in skin texture and contour and a more youthful appearance are achieved by re-epithelialization and collagen remodeling, which occur after these procedures. Superficial chemical peeling with alpha-hydroxy acids, 10 to 30% trichloroacetic acid, Jessner's solution, or salicylic acid produces epidermal wounding to a depth of approximately 0.060 mm, resulting in mild desquamation and minimal dermal change [2]. Rhytides are not significantly altered by this process [3,4]. Medium-depth peels, such as those achieved with pyruvic acid or higher concentration trichloroacetic acid alone or in combination with Jessner's solution, produce more extensive wounding and dermal inflammation. Improvement of some fine lines and hyperpigmentation is the result. With deeper peeling agents, such as the Baker's phenol solution, injury to the epidermis, papillary dermis, and superficial reticular dermis to approximate depths of 0.45 to 0.6 mm is observed. This peeling agent improves textural irregularities and fine lines. Histological studies have shown that CO_2 resurfacing lasers ablate the epidermis and coagulate the superficial dermis in just one or two passes, depending on the laster parameters and system being used.

Extensive clinical experience suggests that laser resurfacing has the advantage of improved reproducibility and control compared with chemical peeling and dermabrasion. Chemical absorption may vary by anatomical location, from patient to patient, and with physician technique, whereas laser pulses vaporize predictable depths of tissue [5]. Medium-depth chemical peels can improve fine lines and textural irregularities but generally do not improve distinct rhytides. Baker-Gordon phenol peels improve deep rhytides but produce deeper injury and slower healing than CO_2 laser resurfacing. The injury to the reticular dermis results in prolonged and painful healing, as well as a higher risk of scarring, textural change, and permanent hypopigmentation. Clinical experience has shown that CO_2 laser resurfacing can produce improvement comparable to deep peeling without damaging the reticular dermis. Moreover, periorbital and perioral rhytides are more effectively treated with the laser than with other modalities. It also appears that CO_2 laser resurfacing can achieve comparable results in other areas of the face relative to dermabrasion with a lower risk of complications [6]. Although appropriate training is required, it is believed that compared with dermabrasion laser resurfacing is slightly less dependent on the skill of the surgeon, and the incidence of permanent pigmentary alteration, textural change, and scarring appear to be lower [7,8].

INTERACTION OF LASERS WITH THE SKIN

Modifications of the conventional CO_2 lasers (continuous wave) and the development of the erbium:YAG lasers have allowed for improved therapeutic results for precise tissue ablation. The original CO_2 lasers were developed as continuous wave light sources with a steady low level power output over time with light emitted at 10,600 nm. The duration of exposure of the CO_2 laser light was controlled by the physician with shuttering of brief pulses in the tenths or hundredths of seconds. The continuous wave CO_2 lasers were effective for tissue ablation and when used in the focused mode for tissue excision; however, their inability to limit the degree of thermal injury minimized their efficacy in the treatment of many cosmetic conditions [9–12]. With the continuous wave CO_2 lasers, the power emitted from the laser remains low and uniform throughout the laser emission despite the fact that the pulse is electronically shuttered.

In the early 1990s, efforts to modify CO_2 lasers resulted in new systems capable of minimizing thermal injury. The first of the modified CO_2 lasers was the Coherent Ultrapulse laser, which created a single pulse of very high peak power and a short exposure time, between 600 and 950 microseconds. An energy fluence of 5 J/cm^2 or greater and an exposure time less than the thermal relaxation time for tissue heated by the laser (less than 1 msec) has allowed for adherence to the principle of selective photothermolysis which provides a theoretical basis for the limitation of thermal energy to the tissue target and surrounding skin [13–16]. The theory states that selective heating of a target structure in tissue can be achieved by preferential laser light absorption and heat production in the target by a single pulse duration shorter than or equal to the thermal relaxation time, measured as the time required to cool the target by 63%. Thus the area that is thermally affected by the laser is more confined. Shortly after Coherent's development of their Ultrapulse system, an alternative method for tissue ablation within the confines of selective photothermolysis was developed. This method involved the use of a computer-driven optico-mechanical scanner for continuous wave CO_2 lasers, allowing the focus beam of continuous wave CO_2 laser light to be delivered in a spiral pattern over tissue with a "dwell" time of less than 1 msec. This technique uses a small spot size of 0.2 mm, and the computer-driven rapid movement of the laser emission around the preset pattern allows for precise tissue ablation with minimal collateral thermal injury. The individual patterns comprise a series of 2.25 mm collimated beams, which are overlapped by varying degrees (10–60%) to determine the total energy delivered to the tissue and the depth of ablation. In the past several years, additional CO_2 laser systems have been developed using variations of the Ultrapulse and scanning systems.

Subsequent to the use of the CO_2 lasers, the erbium:YAG laser has also been developed for laser resurfacing. This laser emits radiation at a wavelength of 2940 nm, matching the peak absorption spectrum of water. Because of the tenfold higher degree of absorption by water, the optical penetration depth of the erbium:YAG laser is 1 micron compared with 30 microns for the CO_2 laser. Although there are many different erbium:YAG lasers available, the maximum pulse energy developed to date is 2 J with a 200 microsecond train of 1 microsecond pulses at a maximum frequency of 10 Hz. Because there is a high degree of absorption by water with the erbium:YAG laser there is a very rapid rise in tissue temperature, creating an explosive ablation of the tissue with minimal thermal necrosis. The erbium:YAG laser requires two to three passes to reach the dermo-epidermal junction, whereas the high energy, shorter pulsed CO_2 laser requires one pass. With the lesser degree of thermal injury per pass, the rate of re-epithelialization and the duration of postsurgical erythema are greatly reduced compared with the CO_2 laser. Because the thermally coagulated layer of tissue produced by the erbium:YAG laser is less than the 50 mm zone necessary to coagulate small blood vessels, pinpoint bleeding may occur with dermal ablation.

The histological effects of the CO_2 lasers vary among the specific type of laser used. After attempting to equate the parameters of different laser systems, the Silktouch and SurgiPulse lasers ablate the entire epidermis, producing a measurable zone of coagulation necrosis in the superficial papillary dermis [17]. The Ultrapulse laser, however, can leave behind residual epidermis. The depth of ablation measures from 20 to 50 mm, with increasing zones of thermal damage from the first three successive laser passes, and usually does not exceed 150 mm on the third pass. In contrast, zones of thermal damage greater than 500 mm are produced with one pass of a continuous wave CO_2 laser [18,19]. With the erbium:YAG lasers, thinner layer tissue ablation with narrower zones of residual thermal damage are obtained because of the higher water absorption coefficient at a wavelength of 2940 nm.

Less tissue is ablated with the CO_2 lasers with subsequent passes, as each pass decreases the water content of tissue, the target chromophore. The depths of residual thermal necrosis increase with the first one to four laser passes up to approximately 150 mm, and then become constant for each CO_2 laser system. Pulse stacking, the successive application of multiple laser passes without allowing for cooling between passes, increases residual thermal damage and cell death by up to 100%.

One day after laser treatment there is extensive epidermal necrosis and coagulation necrosis of the superficial papillary dermis and a mixed upper dermal infiltrate [20,21]. Increasing doses of laser energies produce greater depths of thermal wounding. By day 3 after laser treatment, partial or complete re-epithelialization can be observed, and by day 90 half of patients have a normal rete ridge pattern and most have a subepidermal repair zone consisting of compact collagen bundles in parallel alignment to the skin surface with solar elastosis evident in the dermis beneath this repair zone.

Clinical improvement seen after laser resurfacing procedures results in part from the re-epithelialization and new collagen formation that follows the removal of the epidermis and portions of the dermis. Clinically evident skin contracture is produced with the application of each laser pulse or scan after epidermal vaporization. This tissue shrinkage is likely to be a manifestation of heat-induced shortening of collagen fibrils, which occurs at temperatures of 55 to 60°C via conformational changes and shrinkage of as much as two thirds of collagen fibril length. This heat-induced collagen shrinkage may contribute to the skin tightening effect that has been observed with CO_2 laser resurfacing but not with dermabrasion or chemical peeling, which leads to re-epithelialization and new collagen formation only after removal of the epidermis and portions of the dermis [22]

LASER SAFETY

Laser safety considerations are a critical part of the skin resurfacing procedure. Laser safety includes protecting the patient, the physician and staff, and the surgical room environment.

One of the greatest concerns in protecting the patient lies in protection of the patient's eyes during the procedure. Many laser resurfacing procedures involve the periorbital skin, which includes the eyelids. The CO_2 laser has the potential to injure the sclera of the eye, and appropriate precautions must be taken. When the periorbital area is treated by this technique, metal eye shields are required with or without the use of a topical anesthetic such as tetracaine hydrochloride ophthalmic 0.5%. Plastic shields are not efficacious. Hair is potentially flammable when it comes into contact with the CO_2 laser. Eyelashes, eyebrows, facial hair, and the close proximities of scalp hair should be protected with viscous ointments such as surgilube. Wet drapes over scalp hair also decrease potential problems. Moreover, the patient should be instructed not to use potentially flammable make-up or hair sprays before the procedure.

Protective eyewear must be worn by the physician and staff in the room where the treatment procedure is performed. High filtration masks, which filter particles less than 0.1 mm in diameter, are also recommended because the plume is more carcinogenic than cigarette smoke [23]. The use of a high filtration suction machine is important to minimize the inhalation of the laser plume, in which viral DNA particles such as those of human papilloma virus and human immunodeficiency virus have been shown to survive. The suction apparatus should be held within 1 cm from the actual site where the laser is ablating tissue. Reflective surfaces within the surgical field should be avoided; surgical instruments can be ebonized to avoid reflectance.

There is a potential for fire, and appropriate precautions must be taken to avoid any potential hazard. Any dry drapes, sponges, or gowns should be removed from the surgical field. There are flame retardant drapes that can be purchased; however, avoiding drapes altogether is the simples manner in which to address this problem. A fire extinguisher should be located in the surgical room. The use of oxygen should be eliminated or minimized if possible. If oxygen is required, it should be administered in a closed system such as by endotracheal intubation or laryngeal mask. Inadvertent firing of the laser can be avoided by placing the laser in stand-by mode while the procedure is not being performed. In order to avoid inadvertent entry, appropriate signs should be posted on the doors of the room specifying requirements for entry.

INDICATIONS AND RISKS FOR RESURFACING

Numerous conditions can be improved with the CO_2 laser. The more common conditions include rhytides, acne scars, traumatic scars, verruca, rhinophyma, syringomas, epidermal nevi, xanthelasma, and in-situ squamous cell carcinoma such as actinic cheilitis and erythroplasia of Queyrat [24]. With rhytides and scars, tissue re-epithelialization, new collagen formation, and collagen tightening play active roles in improving the cosmetic appearance of the skin. Tissue ablation is the primary treatment purpose with verruca, rhinophyma, syringomas, epidermal nevi, xanthelasma, and squamous cell carcinoma in situ. It is important for the potential patient to understand that swelling, slight burning, and pruritus are common whereas pain is not [25].

There are myriad risks that accompany the use of the CO_2 laser as a surgical tool, and adequate explanation of possible problems should be discussed before the treatment is begun [26]. Scarring, permanent and transient pigment changes, infection, and therapeutic laser limitations are the most common risks associated with CO_2 laser resurfacing [27]. Scarring occurs in a small minority of patients (<2%), usually on the cheeks and involving less than 10% of the total facial surface area [28].

The erbium:YAG laser is less effective at removing rhytides than is the CO_2 laser. However, it effectively improves fine rhytides on the lower eyelids and removes, at adequate fluences, hyperpigmented macules associated with sum damage. Moreover, it can be used to treat localized scars with the intention of blending the rim of the scar with the surrounding skin in order to minimize the "shadow effect." A younger patient with sun damage who wants a fresher appearance is an ideal candidate. The erbium:YAG laser can also be used with the CO_2 laser treatment of acne scars, whereby the former is used to initially treat the deeper scars and the latter is used for whole face resurfacing. The potential side effects are the same as those listed for the CO_2 laser but occur much less frequently.

Adequate assessment of skin type is necessary to predict possible pigment changes after laser treatment. The ideal candidate is a skin type I or II individual. Those patients with skin types III and above have increased risk of permanent hyper- or hypopigmentation, with skin type IV and V individuals at very high risk. Transient hyperpigmentation can be seen in patients who do not use sunscreen with an SPF greater than 45, wear a hat, or avoid the sunlight especially during the first 1 to 3 months after treatment when the erythema slowly resolves. Patients with significant sun damage that manifests itself in a permanent, slightly darker skin type on the face relative to non–sun-damaged areas like the buttocks will have hypopigmentation of the treated area, which can occur 9 to 12 months after the procedure. The postsurgical skin color is that of nonphotodamaged skin; however, the appearance relative to the presurgical state is hypopigmented. This can pose a problem if the neck is not treated and a contrast in skin pigment exists. Use of the erbium:YAG laser decreases but does not eliminate the chances of developing postsurgical hypopigmentation.

Infections occurring after skin resurfacing procedures can easily be avoided with the use of antibiotics and antiviral agents and with the avoidance of long-term (>1 day) occlusive dressings which often form a nidus for infections. Gram negative bacteria have been shown to colonize patients with significantly increased frequency with long-term occlusion. Oral antibiotics and antiviral agents should be administered for 10 days starting the day before the procedure. Intrasurgical intravenous antibiotics may also provide benefit. Women with a previous significant history of vaginal yeast infections can benefit from diflucan in a single dose on the oday of surgery in order to prevent candidal infection after surgery [29]. Preparing the skin with antibacterial washes immediately before the procedure is unnecessary because the laser sterilizes tissue as it evaporates [30,31].

Of utmost importance before treatment is an honest appraisal of the extent of improvement of the condition for which the patient is undergoing the laser procedure. False, high expectations can cause significant emotional problems, sometimes with legal consequences. Moreover, a thorough description of the extent to which the patient will be incapacitated after laser surgery is a necessity. Although the CO_2 laser is capable of creating some tightening of redundant skin through new collagen formation, the effects of redraping through a facialplasty or facelift are generally not seen. These lasers are effective for individual lines and mild to moderate skin laxity. A notable exception are lines subject to muscular movement such as nasolabial fold lines, lines, crow's feet, and forehead creases. Although dynamic lines, which are created through muscular movement, can be softened, this effect is often temporary relative to the long-lasting effect of fine rhytides.

With specific regard to scars, it is imperative to explain to the patient that scars are not eradicated, but improved. Deep, narrow acne scars are not ameliorated with resurfacing, whereas those that are wider based and atrophic can improve 20 to 50% by blending the border of the scar with the surrounding skin, thus creating a flatter surface which decreases the change of abnormal light reflection and shadows enhancing the delineation of the scar [32].

Patients undergoing a facelift should not have full-face resurfacing at the same time of the surgical procedure because impaired blood supply to the skin flap could impede healing and cause scarring [33]. Resurfacing an area in which herpes zoster occurred may cause increased, prolonged neuralgia and swelling.

PRESURGICAL EVALUATION OF THE PATIENT

A thorough history is necessary to minimize possible risks. A history outlining past incidence and frequency of herpes simplex virus infections, accutane treatment, keloid formation, radiation treatment, allergies to medications and soy products, previous chemical peels, and previous cosmetic procedures is of utmost importance. Moreover, cosmetic resurfacing patients often come into the office with preconceived ideas concerning their wish to have selective areas of the face treated rather than the entire face. The advantages of total face resurfacing include elimination of pigment and textural discrepancies and more effective skin tightening.

Because the prevalence of herpes simplex is high in our society, as shown by the vast majority of the population having positive titers to herpes simplex virus type 1, adequate understanding of the patient's frequency, extent, and location of outbreaks is necessary to guide pre- and postsurgical medications. All patients undergoing the procedure require adequate prophylaxis, and those with a strong history may require a longer treatment period with zoster dosages.

Accutane decreases the size of sebaceous glands in the hair follicles of the face, thus minimizing the effect of these physiologic units in aiding in the repair of de-epithelialized skin. The patient's last dose of accutane should be no sooner than 1 year before resurfacing, and it is recommended that the patient not start the medication until 1 year after the procedure. Noncompliance with this rule can lead to atypical scarring. Topical tretinion, however, minimizes postsurgical milia formation, enhances wound healing, and is used regularly for 2 weeks or more before the procedure [34].

A history of keloid formation, especially multiple keloids, can indicate an increased risk of scarring during the healing phase after laser treatment. A thorough history including questions referring to keloids or hypertrophic scarring after ear piercing or trauma to any part of the body is warranted. If a patient does have a positive personal history, especially one where he or she consistently develops keloids, resurfacing is contraindicated.

A previous history of radiation treatment, such as for acne, is not common, but it is surprising how many individuals, especially in the older population interested in facial resurfacing for rhytides, describe such experiences. Because of the decreased number of effective sebaceous glands, past radiation treatment may indicate slower healing and an extensive number of past radiation sessions is a contraindication for resurfacing.

A history of previous chemical peels as well as previous facial cosmetic procedures is important. A history of multiple light peels or a couple of deeper peels (eg, trichloroacetic acid) warrants close observation of the candidate to determine whether hypopigmentation has already resulted and whether resurfacing will cause more pigment anomalies. Phenol peels increase the risk of further hypopigmentation and resurfacing does not guarantee equilibration of previously hypopigmented skin with those areas that have never been treated.

Darker skin phototypes (IV–VI) require special consideration. Prolonged hyperpigmentation may be seen with the CO_2 laser and to a lesser degree with the erbium:YAG. Moreover, delayed hypo- or depigmentation may be seen 6 to 12 months after resurfacing with the CO_2 laser and to a lesser degree with the erbium–YAG laser.

Because each patient receives antibiotics intrasurgically and antibiotics and antiviral agents perisurgically, a thorough history of allergies is important. Relative contraindications to the use of resurfacing lasers include collagen vascular disease; infectious diseases such as AIDS/HIV, hepatitis C, and active herpes simplex; psoriasis; vitiligo; diabetes; labile hypertension; and significant cardiovascular or pulmonary disease [34].

Each patient is informed to avoid all nonsteroidal products, vitamin E, and alcohol 1 week before the procedure. Smoking should also be avoided in this period.

RESURFACING TECHNIQUES

Anesthesia

Topical anesthesia with EMLA cream or with 30% lidocaine may be helpful for superficial laser procedures with the erbium–YAG laser; however, this method does not provide total desensitization. Infiltration of the treated area or regional nerve blocks using local anesthetics usually provides adequate anesthesia for finite lesions or small areas. The treatment of large surface areas such as the entire face is facilitated with the use of intravenous anesthetics or general anesthesia. A combination of intravenous propofol and fentanyl works well when appropriately administered for excellent anesthesia, analgesia, and amnestic response. If general anesthesia is used with supplemental oxygen or nitrous oxide, then a closed system of gas administration as previously described is necessary. Wet drapes and flame-retardant materials are required to protect the tubes carrying the flammable substances.

Technique

Once the appropriate safety precautions have been taken, treatment may begin. The choice of laser and the laser parameters will vary with different clinical situations. It is important to realize that all resurfacing lasers do not provide the same degree of tissue ablation per pass across the skin's surface. CO_2 laser systems will be preferable when one is dealing with deeper lines and greater skin laxity, whereas the erbium:YAG laser may provide some benefit in treating superficial rhytides such as fine lines in the periorbital area. The patient's postsurgical considerations might also impact on the choice of laser because healing is faster and there is less postsurgical erythema with the erbium:YAG laser.

After the cosmetic unit(s) to be treated are demarcated with a pen, an initial pass is performed across the skin surface. This vaporized tissue should then be gently débrided with a wet surgical sponge. This will allow for the immediate visualization of the treated site. Additional passes with the laser may be required depending on the clinical circumstances, choice of laser, and specific parameters. For example, in the treatment of mild rhytides, one may require one to two passes with the Silktouch system, two to four passes with the Coherent system, or three to six passes with the erbium:YAG laser. After general débridement, the treated areas should be patted dry to allow for absorption of the laser light with the next pass. If the surgical field remains wet, the superficial water will absorb the laser light, limiting penetration into the skin. Immediately after CO_2 laser treatment for facial rhytides, it has been shown that use of the erbium:YAG over the same treated area quickens healing and minimizes the length of time redness is present.

The clinical endpoint will vary with each patient's response to the resurfacing laser used. Ideally one would like to see the removal of the lesion or cosmetic deformity at the completion of the procedure; however, this is not always possible. It is believed that a pink color of the skin after the procedure indicates ablation to the depth of the papillary dermis, a chamois-like color suggests a depth to the superficial reticular dermis, and a yellow color places one in the deep reticular dermis. This yellow color should be the absolute clinical endpoint to avoid scarring. It is important to note that it is not always necessary or desirable to remove the entire clinical lesion or deformity with the procedure. Neocollagenesis sometimes leads to continued or delayed clinical improvement for several to many months after the procedure. Thus, retreatment should not be an option for at least 6 months after surgery.

Treatment of the eyelids and periorbital skin should proceed with caution through the use of lower energy fluences and/or fewer passes with the laser. Treatment of the neck has not been established as safe or effective in the removal of rhytides or excessive jowls with the CO_2 laser. Some physicians have used the erbium:YAG laser safely and effectively on the neck; however, it is not anticipated that significant tightening of neck laxity would occur with this technique. Treatment below the head and neck may require fewer passes with lower energy fluences because healing may be slower in these anatomical areas. In the treatment of hypertrophic scars, complete flattening can be obtained during the procedure. Laser resurfacing can be used as an adjunct in the treatment of keloids, but it is not effective as the sole treatment modality. As previously discussed, atrophic scars can be treated with repetitive passes of the laser in an attempt to blend the circumference of the scar with surrounding, normal skin, but pitted acne scars do not improve with this technique.

In patients undergoing larger areas of resurfacing, the cosmetic unit (eg, of the periorbital or perioral regions) must be preserved. This concept implies that the whole unit be treated instead of parts of one unit.

POSTSURGICAL CARE AND TROUBLESHOOTING

The post surgical management of the resurfacing patient is a critical component to the success of this procedure. A moist wound healing open technique is of utmost importance in order to avoid eschar formation which would ultimately delay healing. Although the open technique generally requires much more patient involvement in the wound care process, this technique has a lower incidence of postsurgical infection and allows for a closer observation of the postsurgical wound. Regular steaming of the face to remove serious crust is necessary with the open technique. Conversely, there are other physicians who support the use of the closed technique with the use of occlusive dressings, and these investigators tend to report less postsurgical serous crusting but higher rates of wound infections.

Immediately after treatment, the skin appears pink to yellow without significant bleeding (see Fig. 1). Several hours after the procedure, there is an exudative response that requires postsurgical attention. Hydrophilic ointments such as Aquaphor healing ointment can minimize crusting of the exudate and provide symptomatic relief from the mild burning that occurs. Soaking with wet compresses will also minimize crust formation. With this open technique, there are variations in postsurgical care. The length of time that one would require this postsurgical regimen is dependent on the depth of procedure performed by the physician. Re-epithelialization generally occurs within 3 to 7 days after the procedure and, as healing progresses, the need for postsurgical care decreases. For example, one may consider having a patient use wet compresses every hour followed by the use of the healing ointment during the first 2 days after the procedure, and then decrease the frequency of soaking as the re-epithelialization process develops. After re-epithelialization, the skin requires moisturizers for approximately 1 to 3 more weeks; however, a lighter compound is necessary in order to avoid an acneiform eruption, especially in those patients who are at increased risk for this complication.

Antibiotics are prescribed to prevent bacterial colonization. The ideal medication should have staphylococcus and streptococcus coverage, and it should be started the day before the procedure and continued for 10 full days. Acyclovir, administered at the same time as the antibiotics, should be given to all patients regardless of history of herpes simplex. The patient should be advised to avoid contact with anyone infected with the herpes simplex virus. The standard doses are 400 mg of Acyclovir three times a day or 500 mg Valtrex twice a day. If a patient has a history of frequent bouts of herpes simplex, herpes zoster dosages (eg, 800 mg five times a day) can be prescribed.

During the re-epithelialization process, patients often complain of dryness and pruritus, which are easily treated with a mild topical corticosteroid and moisturizers. Sun avoidance and protection is particularly important for several months, especially during the red phase of healing, to help minimize hyperpigmentation. This is most critical for patients with darker skin phototypes. Recent data has shown that pro-

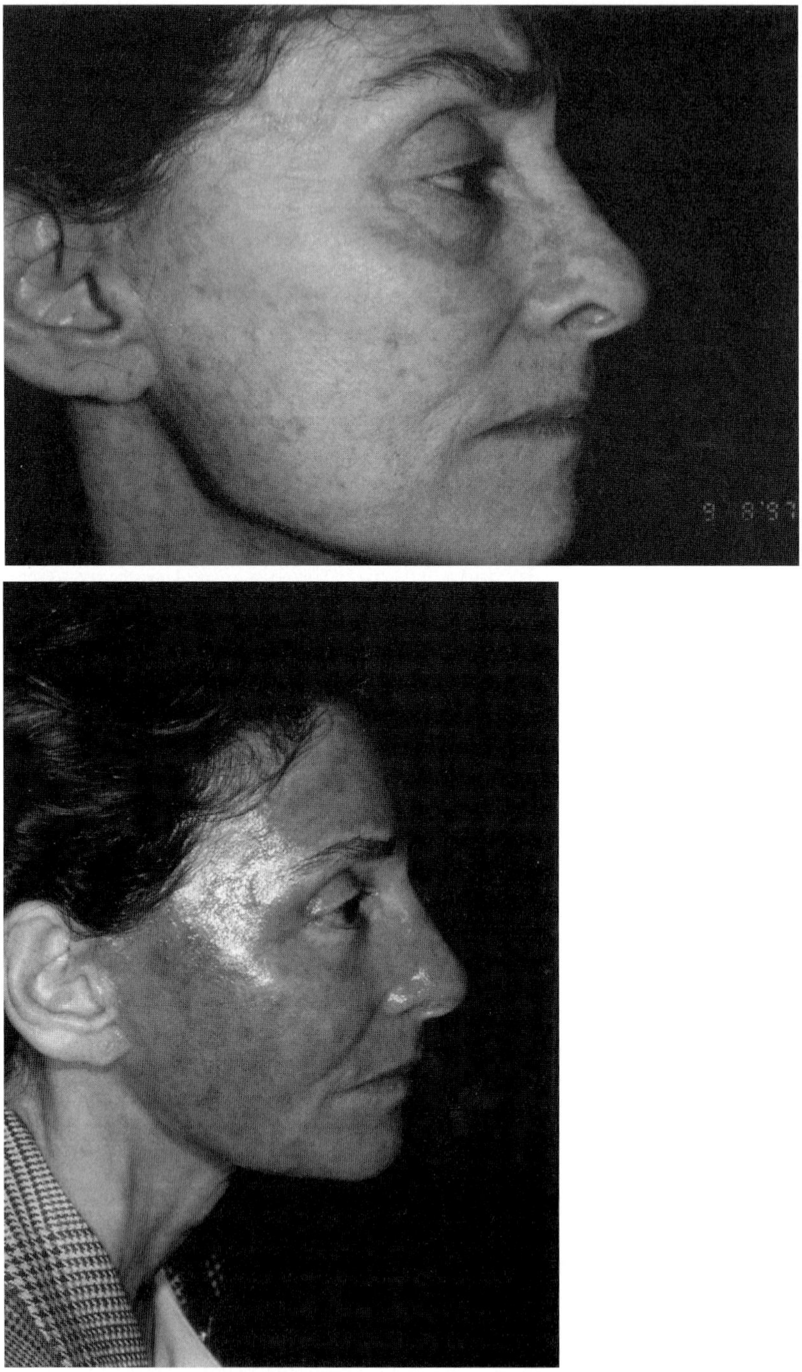

(a)

(b)

FIGURE 1 (a) Fifty-five-year-old female with facial rhytides, laxity, and actinic damage. (b) Five days after resurfacing with the CO_2 laser. (c) One month after laser resurfacing.

APPENDIX 1: LASER SKIN RESURFACING TREATMENT CONSENT FORM

□ Roy G. Geronemus, M.D., □ Arielle N.B. Kauvar, M.D., □ Melanie C. Grossman, M.D., □ Leonard J. Bernstein, M.D., □ Wendy Lou, M.D., has explained to me that I am a good candidate for laser resurfacing treatment and that although laser surgery has been shown to be highly effective, no guarantees can be made that I will benefit from treatment. I understand that the most common side effects and complications of this laser treatment are:

1. **PAIN** - The sharp, burning sensation of each laser may produce a moderate to severe amount of discomfort. Anesthetic injections or intravenous sedation will be used to block the pain during the procedure. Oral pain medications will be prescribed for the post-operative period.

2. **SWELLING AND OOZING** - Areas most likely to swell are around the eyes and neck. A clear fluid (serum) will also be present in the lasered areas and may create a crust (or scab) if the areas are not kept moist. The swelling, crusting and oozing stage subsides within 5 to 7 days with regular application of ice and prescribed healing ointments.

3. **PROLONGED SKIN REDNESS** - The laser-treated areas will initially appear bright red in color. After the first week, the redness can be camouflaged with opaque makeup. The redness fades to pink over the next several weeks and then to normal skin color in an average of 3 months.

4. **SKIN DARKENING (HYPERPIGMENTATION)** - This can occur in the treated areas and will eventually fade within 2 to 6 months. This reaction is more common in patients with olive or dark skin tones and can worsen if the laser-treated area is exposed to the sun.

5. **SKIN LIGHTENING (HYPOPIGMENTATION)** - This can occur in an area of skin which has already received prior treatment or can be a delayed response to the laser surgery. The light spots can darken or re-pigment in several months, but could be permanent. This is a very rare complication.

6. **SCARRING** - The risk of this complication is minimal, but can potentially occur whenever there is disruption of the skin's surface. Strict adherence to all advised post-operative instructions will reduce the possibility of this occurrence.

7. **INFECTION** - A skin infection in the post-operative period can result. This risk is minimized by the use of antibiotics and good skin care.

8. **ALLERGIC REACTION** - It is possible that an allergic reaction to an anesthetic, topical cream or oral medication can occur.

9. **ECTROPION** - In rare instances, a downward pull of the eyelids can result after periorbital laser resurfacing.

10. **ACNE OR MILIA FORMATION** - Flare-up of acne or formation of milia can occur in the post-operative period.

11. **PARTIAL OR NO IMPROVEMENT** - Although laser surgery is highly effective, there is no guarantee that you will achieve the desired degree of improvement.

12. **ACCUTANE** - I acknowledge that I have not used Accutane for the past year and agree not to use this drug for at least one year after my surgery.

By providing my signature below, I acknowledge that I have read and understood all of the information written above as well as that contained within the information sheet. I feel that I have been adequately informed of my alternative treatment options, the risks of the proposed laser surgery, and the risks of not treating my condition. I hereby freely consent to the laser surgery to be performed by □ Roy G. Geronemus, M.D., □ Arielle N.B. Kauvar, M.D., □ Melanie C. Grossman, M.D., □ Leonard J. Bernstein, M.D., □ Wendy Lou, M.D. and authorize the taking of clinical photographs which will be used solely for my medical records unless my physician deems their anonymous use (in lectures or scientific publications) could benefit medical research and education. They will not be used for advertising without my written permission.

____________________________________ ____________________________________

Patient's or Guardian's Signature Date Witness' Signature Date

\\Jennifer\d\Forms (from 6)\Consent Skin Resurfacing.wpd\July 14, 1999

10

Dermabrasion

Stephen Mandy
University of Miami, Miami, Florida

Dermabrasion is a mechanical, "cold steel" method of removing the epidermis and creating a papillary to upper reticular dermal wound. The subsequent manufacture of new collagen and a resurfaced epidermis germinated from deeper, less sun-damaged cells, yields excellent cosmetic improvement in actinically damaged, aged, or scarred skin. The pre and postoperative management that optimizes wound healing is well established and predictable, and morbidity and complications are encountered infrequently.

HISTORY

At the turn of the century, Kronmayer [1] first described modern dermabrasion technique, which was later modified in the 1940s and 1950s by Kurtin [2] and Burke [3]. Their wire brush techniques have changed little to this day. The basics of a rapidly rotating wire brush applied to the skin results in a controlled physical injury to the epidermis and papillary dermis which heals without scarring. Injury below the upper reticular dermis may result in scar formation. All areas of the skin may be dermabraded, but it is the face that is ideally suited to this procedure, as it is richly endowed with pilosebaceous follicles, which are the primordial germ cell of the healing process. Nelson [4,5] has shown that this injury results in significant increases in type I procollagen, type III procollagen, and transforming growth factor beta 1 in the papillary dermis. His results suggest that increased fibroblast activity and consequent collagen I and III synthesis underlie the clinical improvement and collagen reformation seen with dermabrasion.

PATIENT SELECTION AND INDICATIONS

Dermabrasive resurfacing is an effective treatment for acne scars, facial wrinkles, premalignant solar keratoses, rhinophyma, traumatic and surgical scars, and tattoos. Although perfection is impossible, dramatic improvement can be achieved with facial scarring caused by acne (Fig. 1). Realistic expectations must be conveyed to the patients before surgery, and patients who have extensive scarring must be warned of the possibility of further scarring, or hypo or hyperpigmentation postoperatively. For

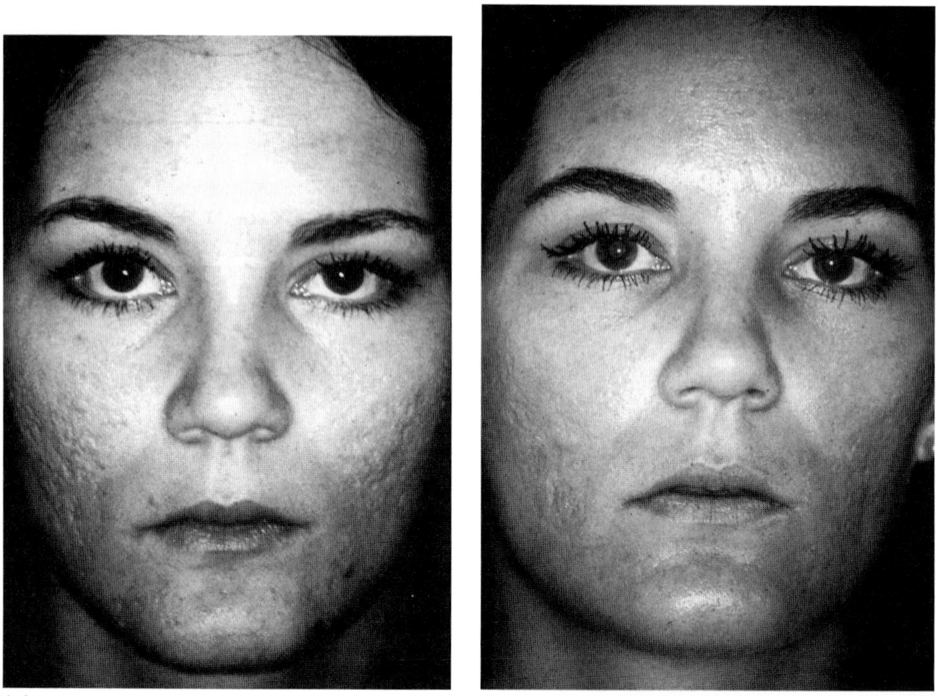

(a) (b)

FIGURE 1 Severe acne scarring (a) before dermabrasion and (b) after dermabrasion.

patients with deep ice-pick–type scarring, punch excisions followed by suture closure, or punch grafting, 4 to 6 weeks before dermabrasion will be the most likely to yield good results. Most dyspigmentation resulting from dermabrasion is temporary and the pigment will return to normal over the course of 6 or more months. However, the deeper the dermabrasion the greater the risk of permanent pigmentary alteration. This is especially true in patients of darker pigmentation.

Many patients requesting dermabrasion have been previously treated with 13 cis-retinoic acid systemically. This potent antiacne agent causes sebaceous gland atrophy, a cause for concern in the healing process. Initial reports suggested that dermabrasion patients were unaffected by previous treatment with Accutane [6], then later reports suggested that patients who were dermabraded after Accutane exhibited atypical scarring [7]. Subsequently, other surgeons have compiled numerous patients that have been treated with Accutane and dermabraded without difficulty. This controversy is clearly unsettling and has significant medical and legal implications. Although laboratory studies have failed to substantiate any abnormalities in fibroblast activity or collagen synthesis in Accutane-treated skin [8–10], there is still no definitive answer to the question of Accutane treatment and postdermabrasion scarring. Until such time as this issue is answered, it is prudent for physicians to suggest that Accutane patients be fully informed of the potential risks and wait a period of at least 6 months before undergoing dermabrasion.

Another preoperative consideration is the human immunodeficiency virus (HIV). Dermabrasion results in the aerosolization of blood and tissue products and, potentially, live infective viral particles. Wentzell [11] indicated that aerosolized particles produced during dermabrasion were of sufficient size to allow access to, and retention by, mucosal and pulmonary surfaces. Furthermore, his studies suggested that commonly used personal protection devices such as operatory masks, goggles, and scatter shields, do not prevent the inhalation of these particles. Additionally, the settling velocity of such small particles extends the exposure for many hours after the procedure has been performed, thereby endangering personnel not directly involved in the procedure. HIV may be difficult to detect if a patient is in the latent period between infection and positive antibody titers. Legal implications also exist if one refuses a patient who has a positive titer. Risks clearly exist to the physician, his assistants, and other personnel, as well as to the HIV-infected patient. Clearly, a thorough history, HIV titers, and all protective equipment must be used when doing dermabrasions, and there must be the realization that with all of these measures, there still remains a degree of risk. Similar precautions regarding hepatitis are also prudent.

Actinically damaged skin, and simply aging skin, is a growing indication for dermabrasion. Dermabrasion has been shown to be as effective as topically applied 5 Fluorouracil in the management of precancerous skin lesions [12]. In a study of half-face dermabrasion of actinically damaged skin, Burke [13] showed that precancerous lesions were substantially reduced and their future development was retarded over a 5-year period. This work has been corroborated by Coleman [14], et al., more recently. Aside from the benefit of the prophylactic effect on the development of new keratoses and the resolution of old ones, dramatic improvement in facial wrinkling is seen in dermabrasion patients (Figs. 2, 3). Because of the superficial nature of the pathology in actinically damaged and aged skin, the dermabrasion is subsequently more superficial and, therefore, there is less risk of scarring or pigmentary problems. The collagen restructuring is sufficient in this procedure to often yield dramatic results in terms of cosmesis.

Yarborough [15] showed that dermabrasion performed on traumatic or surgical scars approximately 6 weeks after injury often results in the complete disappearance or dramatic resolution of the scar (Fig. 4). Surgical scars respond so well to dermabrasion that patients who are receiving excisional surgery are told preoperatively that dermabrasion in 6 weeks may be a viable option as a "touch-up." Although this is often unnecessary, this does allow its anticipation by the patient should it be necessary. Varicella scars are also especially responsive to dermabrasion if treated 6 to 8 weeks after healing.

Although lasers very often can remove tattoos with minimal scarring and significant improvement, dermabrasion remains a viable inexpensive modality for this purpose. Superficial dermabrasion followed by the application of 1% gentian violet and a Vaseline gauze dressing changed daily for 10 days will result in at least 50% resolution of most tattoos without scarring. The gentian violet delays healing, causing the pigment to leach out onto the dressing and creating continued inflammation which causes phagocytosis of additional pigment. Limiting the dermabrasion to only the upper papillary dermis will avoid scarring. It should not be attempted to remove all the pigment by abrasion as this usually will result in too great a depth of injury. As a rule, professional tattoos are more responsive than amateur or traumatic tattoos, but all can be dramatically improved. Tattoos offer a very good training ground for the novice in dermabrasion (Fig. 6).

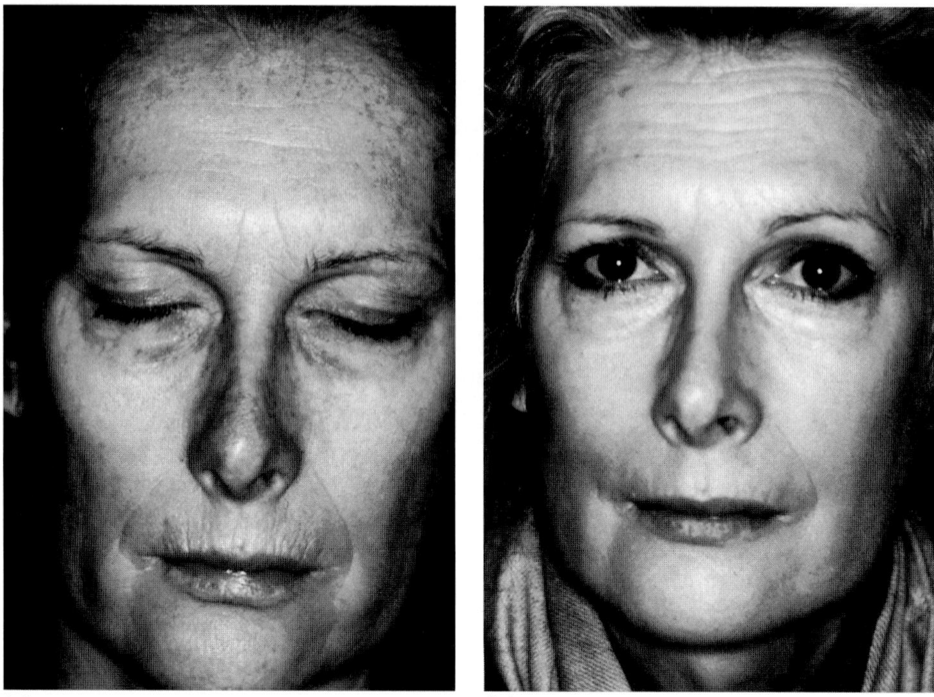

(a) (b)

FIGURE 2 **(a) Predermabrasion for actinic keratoses and wrinkles; (b) postdermabrasion.**

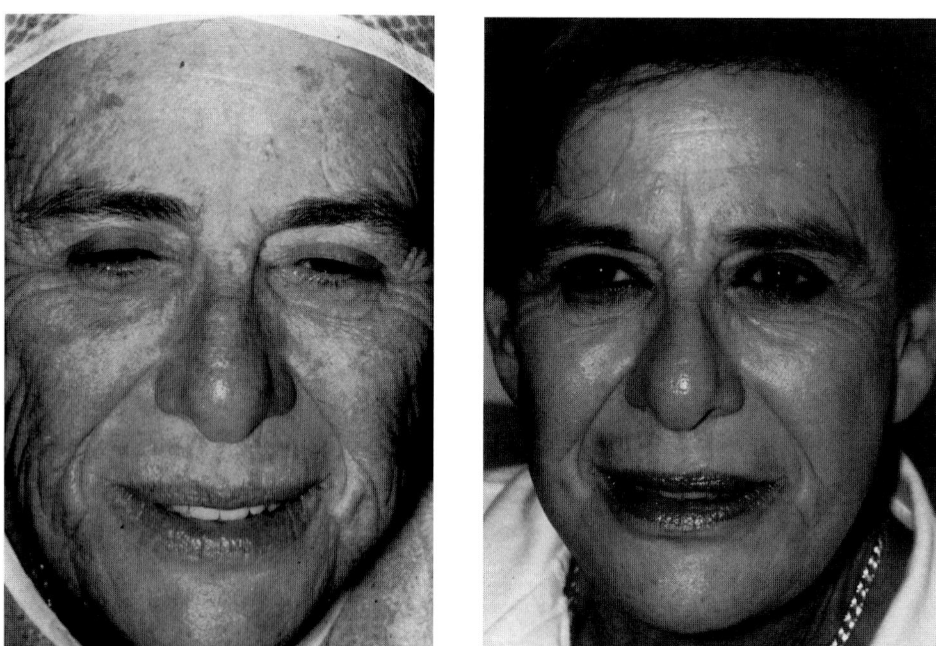

(a) (b)

FIGURE 3 **(a) Predermabrasion for actinic keratoses and wrinkles; (b) postdermabrasion.**

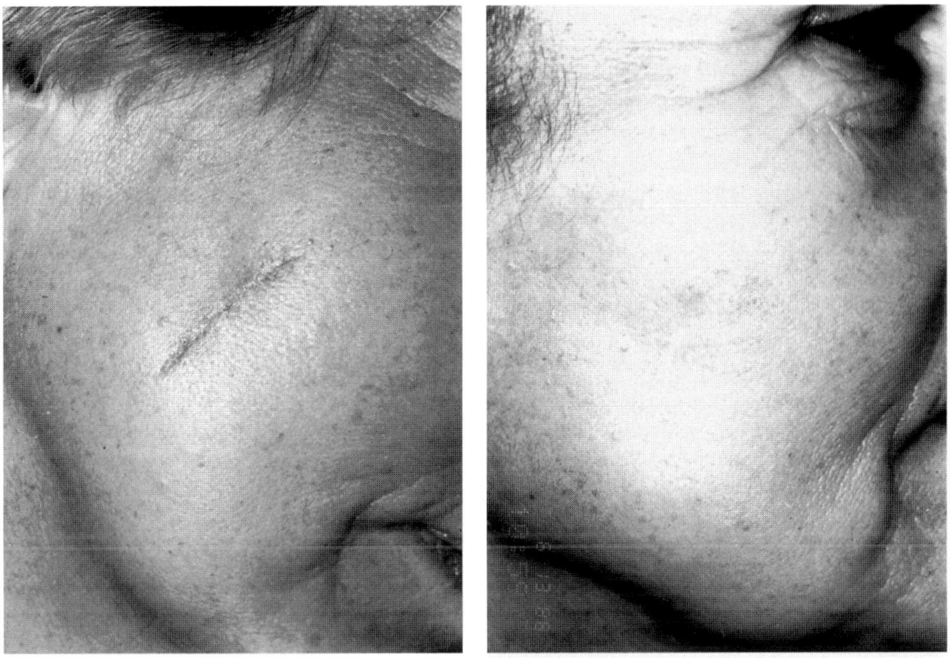

(a) (b)

FIGURE 4 (a) Predermabrasion of 6-week-old surgical scar and (b) postdermabrasion of scar.

Other indications for dermabrasion include benign tumors, such as adenoma, sebaceum, and syringomas (Fig. 5). These may be successfully dermabraded with marked cosmetic improvement, especially when combined with electrodesiccation of individual lesions. The patient should be forewarned that gradual recurrence is the usual event. Rhinophyma can be dramatically improved with dermabrasion when combined with electrofulguration (Fig. 7). Although a wide variety of abrading instruments are available, ranging from sand paper to salabrasion and air driven glass or aluminum particles, the wire brush and diamond fraise remain the mainstay of dermabrasive technique. Outstanding reviews by Yarborough [16] and Alt [17] of techniques using the wire brush and diamond fraise require little elaboration. It must be emphasized that dermabrasion is a hands-on technique that requires adequate preceptorship training under the auspices of someone experienced in this art. Most authors agree that a wire brush requires considerably more skill and runs higher potential risk for injury as it able to cut much deeper and more quickly than is the diamond fraise. Histologically, no difference can be found between diamond fraise and wire brush dermabrasion in terms of collagen synthesis [5], although it is this author's experience that with the exception of the extra-coarse diamond fraise, superior results for acne scarring appear to be achieved with the wire brush.

A continuing controversy in dermabrasive surgery is the use of preabrasive chilling of the skin. Materials that freeze the skin below −30°C and especially below −60°C have the risk of causing substantial tissue necrosis and subsequent scarring [18–20]. It is helpful to freeze the skin in dermabrasion in order to have a rigid

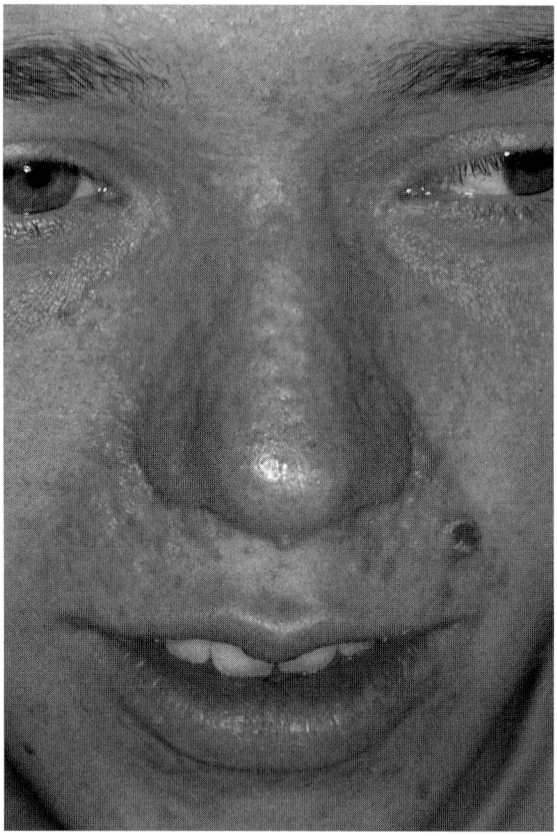

(a)

FIGURE 5 (a) Predermabrasion for multiple trichoepitheliomas and (b) postdermabrasion.

surface that will abrade evenly and to preserve anatomic markings which otherwise may be distorted when the tissue is thawed and stretched. As thermal injury may be a complicating factor resulting in scarring, caution would suggest that cryesthetic agents should be used that do not freeze the skin below −30°C. It is also increasingly difficult because of the regulation of fluorocarbons to obtain cryesthetic freezing agents. Increasingly, many dermabrasion surgeons are using tumescent anesthesia as a means of stabilizing the skin as well as inducing anesthesia.

TECHNIQUE

Outpatient dermabrasion has become much more feasible with the advent of sophisticated preoperative analgesia. Diazepam orally administered 45 minutes to an hour preoperatively in conjunction with 0.4 mg of atropine intramuscularly, which is an amnestic and antivagal agent, tends to make the patient more comfortable and less anxious. Before administering regional block anesthesia with a lidocaine-bupivacaine mixture, intravenously administered Fentanyl (Janssen Pharmaceutical) or intramuscular meperidine and Medazolam (Roche Dermatologics) gives the patient a great

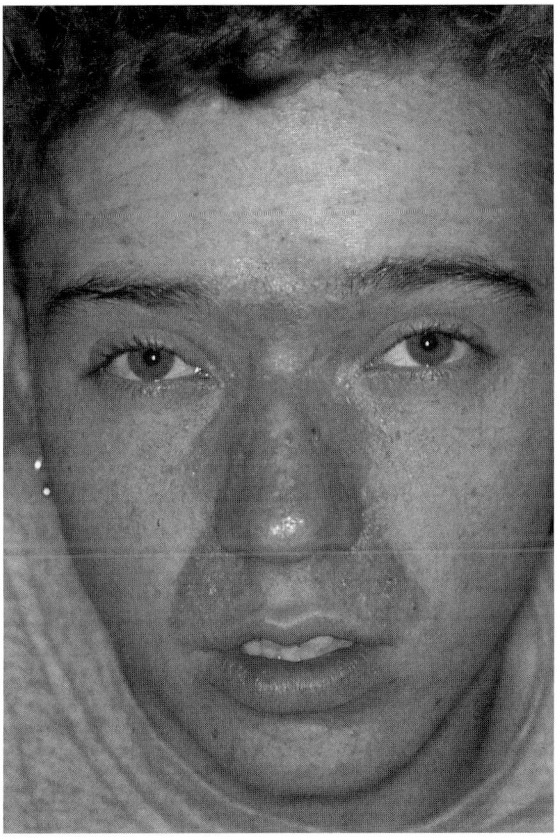

(b)

FIGURE 5 Continued

sense of euphoria while relieving the discomfort associated with the injection of the regional anesthesia. The regional anesthetic mixture is injected into the supraorbital, infraorbital, and mental foramina. This will usually result in anesthesia to approximately 60 to 70% of the entire face. When this is used in conjunction with the refrigerant spray or regional tumescent anesthesia, most patients can tolerate dermabrasion without pain. The dermabrasion is then conducted, dermabrading approximately a 1 in^2 area at a time, which is frozen before the sanding procedure. The dermabrasion instrument must be held firmly in the hand and pulled only in the direction of the handle and perpendicular to the plane of rotation. Back and forth or circular movements may result in gouging of the skin or "skipping." The wire brush or coarse diamond fraise require almost no pressure, and produce multiple microlacerations, which are a sign of the adequacy of the depth of the procedure. Progress through the skin is judged by several landmarks. The removal of skin pigmentation signifies the passage through the basal layer of the epidermis. As one advances into the papillary dermis, small capillary loops of the papillary plexus are identified as the tissue thaws and punctate bleeding results. As one advances further into the papillary dermis, small parallel strands of collagen become apparent. It is the fraying

(a)

(b)

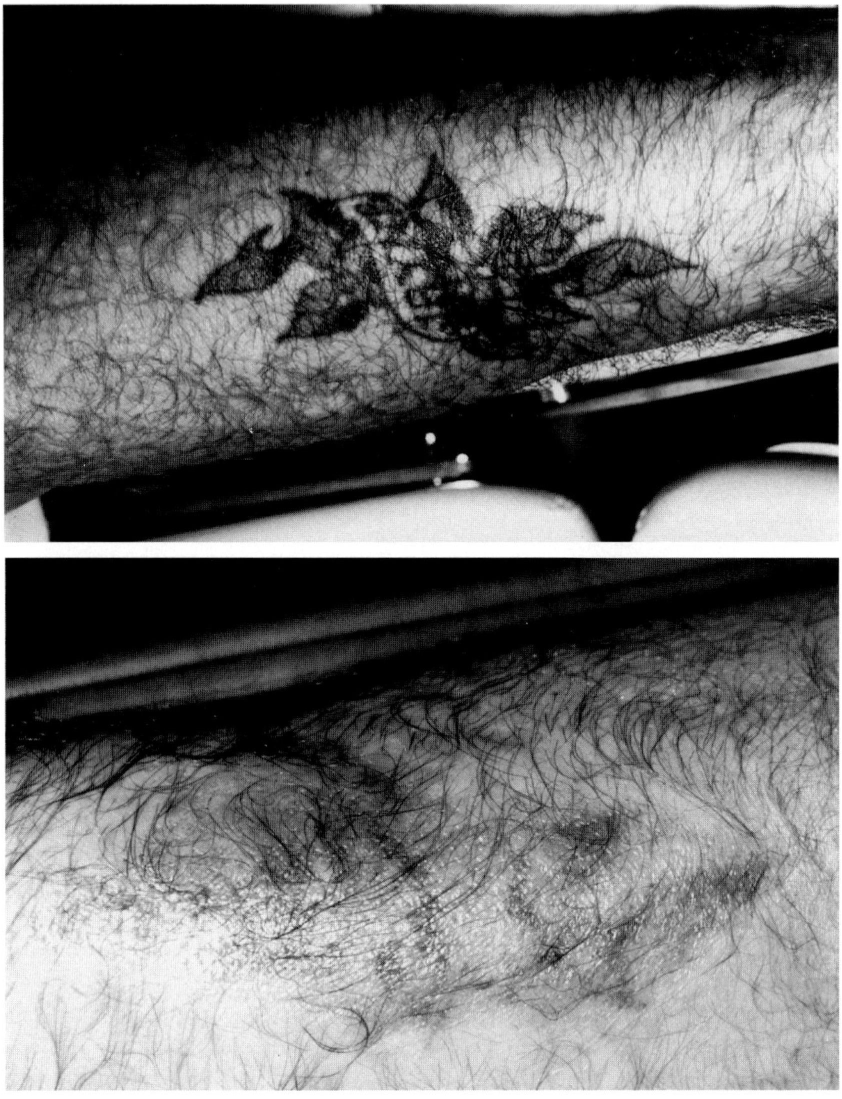

FIGURE 6 Commercial tattoo, (a) predermabrasion and (b) postdermabrasion.

of these collagen strands that signifies the dermabrasion is carried to the correct level. Going further may result in scarring. It is essential that one must fix, by traction, the skin surrounding the lip or eyelids as they may be ensnared by the dermabrader causing significant lacerations. Maintaining the dermabrader parallel to the surface is essential, especially in areas of complex curvature such as the chin, malar eminences, and jaw line. Although "spot" dermabrasion can be performed for isolated indications such as scars, when possible, dermabrasion should be carried out within facial units to avoid demarcation by pigmentary change. Dermabrasion to just below the jaw line, out to the preauricular area, and up to the suborbital areas insure

(a)

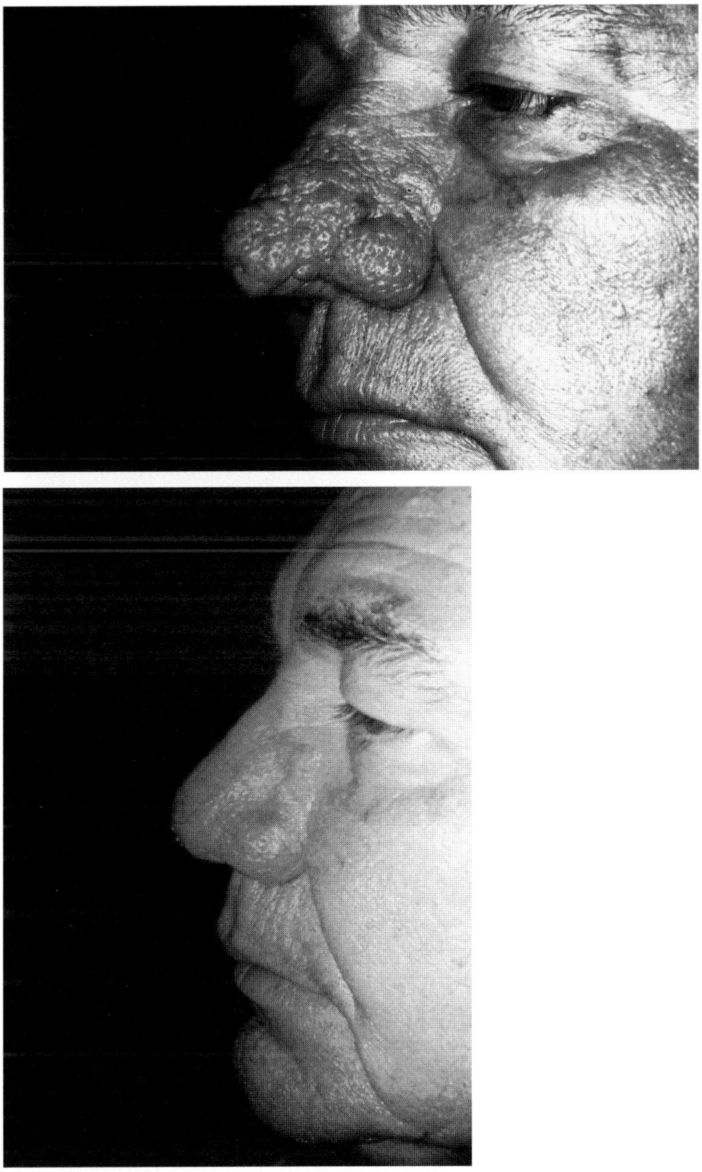

(b)

FIGURE 7 **Rhinophyme, (a) predermabrasion and (b) postdermabrasion.**

that uniform texture and appearance can be achieved. Blending of pigmentation by the application of 35% trichloracetic acid to unabraded skin such as the eyebrows and first few centimeters of the hairline and eyelids, ensures gradual blending of pigmentation. A frequent "combination" procedure of a perioral dermabrasion with a full face 35% TCA peel is often performed for patients with prominent perioral rhagades and mild to moderate actinic damage.

PRE- AND POSTOPERATIVE MANAGEMENT

The nightly preoperative application of tretinoin 0.5% for several weeks before partial thickness dermabrasive wounds has been shown clinically and in the laboratory to accelerate postoperative healing [21,22]. The use of occlusive dressings in the postoperative management of dermabrasive wounds has been well understood since the work of Rovee and Maibach [23] which reveal that wounds healed 40% faster when occluded rather than air dried. Modern biosynthetic dressings alleviate postoperative pain almost immediately upon their application and act to keep wounds moist, thereby allowing free epithelial migration across the surface [24]. They also cause wound fluids, which contain growth factors that stimulate wound healing, to remain in constant contact with the wound surface. There is evidence to suggest that the presence of occlusive dressings modulate collagen synthesis and produce a cosmetically more satisfying result [25]. When preoperative tretinoin and postoperative biosynthetic dressings have been used, most patients re-epithelialize within 5 to 7 days. There are a wide variety of biosynthetic dressings currently available, and the frequency with which they must be changed depends on the individual dressing. Changing the dressing daily does allow the physician or his assistant to monitor the patient's progress and be certain that complications have not appeared. Most biosynthetic dressings need to be covered with gauze and then held in place by a flexible surgical netting. This is especially true in the first 48 to 72 hours as drainage is considerable during that time.

Currently, most patients are started on acyclovir or other related antiviral agent before dermabrasion and continued until epithelialization is complete. Full therapeutic doses of these agents are used as opposed to recommended "prophylactic" doses. Postoperatively patients are placed on prednisone 40 mg a day, beginning the day of surgery, for 4 days. This reduces postoperative edema and patient discomfort and does not appear to interfere with wound healing.

After the skin has re-epithelialized, patients are usually restarted on topical tretinoin by the seventh to tenth postoperative day. Tretinoin helps to prevent the development of postoperative milia, a common complication, and dyspigmentation, which may occur following dermabrasion. In addition, recent studies by Griffiths [26] have shown that tretinoin also increases type I collagen production which should further enhance the long-term postoperative outcome. If patients have a history of previous pigmentary problems such as melasma, they are started on topical hydroquinone at the same time they begin tretinoin. If by the tenth to fourteenth day the patient shows signs of disproportionate erythema, a topical 1% hydrocortisone is begun. Patients are cautioned before surgery that it will take at least one month for their skin to become normal in its appearance. However, most patients are able to return to work within seven to ten days of surgery if a light coverup make up is applied. Compulsive daily application of sunscreens is essential for at least several months after dermabrasion.

COMPLICATIONS

Milia are the most common complication of dermabrasion, usually appearing in 3 to 4 weeks and rarely occurring if the patient is treated postoperatively with tretinoin. Postoperative erythema may be expected after dermabrasion for several weeks but rarely persists beyond 2 to 4 weeks. If it is intense, and persistent, it should be promptly treated with topical steroids as it may signify the beginning of hypertrophic scarring. Hyperpigmentation may occur beginning several weeks postoperatively and will usually resolve with the prompt institution of topical hydroquinone. Although infrequent, postoperative infection can occur as the result of dermabrasion. The most common organisms are Staphylococcus aureus, herpes simplex, and candida. Staph infections are usually manifest in 48 to 72 hours after dermabrasion and signified by facial swelling, honey crusting, and systemic symptoms such as fever. Herpes simplex infection may occur if the patient has not been pretreated with acyclovir and is recognized by severe pain, usually 48 to 72 hours after surgery. Candida infections usually result in delayed healing and are recognized somewhat later at 5 to 7 days with exudation and facial swelling. Cultures and treatment with the appropriate antibiotics, acyclovir, or anticandida agent usually result in resolution of the infection without sequella.

COMPARISON WITH OTHER MODALITIES

All resurfacing techniques result in a upper to mid-dermal wound. Dermabrasion relies on mechanical "cold steel" injury, acid peels result in a "caustic" injury, and lasers result in a thermal injury. Recent studies in the porcine model comparing carbon dioxide laser, trichloracetic acid, and dermabrasion by Fitzpatrick [27], and Campbell [28], have shown that histological and ultrastructural changes seen following these procedures are comparable. A study by Giese [29], revealed that when dermabrasion was compared with chemosurgical peels, significant alterations were seen in the elastic fibers in histological and mechanical properties. At 6 months after phenol treatment, the skin was both stiffer and weaker when compared with dermabraded skin. Holmkvist [30] reported that half-face perioral dermabrasion contrasted with half-face CO_2 laser resurfacing yielded identical clinical results but that dermabrasion healed in approximately half the time with significantly less postoperative erythema and morbidity. Most surgeons practicing resurfacing agree that extended postoperative erythema and delayed hypopigmentation are more common with phenol or laser than with dermabrasion. A review by Baker [31] points out that dermabrasion equipment is inexpensive, portable, widely available, requires no specialized accessory equipment and poses no fire hazard in the operating room.

CONCLUSION

In this era of computer-generated pulsed lasers and a potpourri of acid peels, there are those who might choose to recognize dermabrasion as an archeologic curiosity. However, dermabrasion is a well understood procedure with established pre and postoperative management and highly predictable and reproducible results. Healing is prompt with a minimum of morbidity and rare complications. The equipment is simple and the cost is reasonable. Dermabrasion offers a practical means of addressing a significant number of indications with the expectation of a positive outcome.

REFERENCES

1. Kurtin A. Corrective surgical planing of skin. Arch Derm Syphilol 1953; 68–389.
2. Kronmayer E. Die heilung der akne durch ein neves narben lases operations ver faren: das stranzen. Ilustr Monatssehr Aerztl Poly Tech 1905; 27:101.

3. Burke J. Wire Brush Surgery. Springfield: Charles C Thomas, 1956.
4. Nelson BR, et al. Clinical improvement following dermabrasion of photoaged skin correlates with synthesis of collagen I. Arch Derm 1994; 130:1136–1142.
5. Nelson BR, et al. A comparison of wire brush and diamond fraise superficial dermabrasion for photoaged skin. A clinical immunohistologic and biochemical study. JAAD 1996; 34:235–243.
6. Roenigk HH Jr, et al. Acne retinoids and dermabrasion. J Dermol Surg Oncol 1985; 11: 396–938.
7. Rubenstein R, Roenigk HH, Jr. Atypical keloids after dermabrasion of patients taking isotretinoin. J Am Acad Dermatol 1986; 15(LpLl):280–285.
8. Moy R, Moy L, Zitelli J, Mandy S. Effects of Systemic 13 Cis-Retinoic Acid on Wound Healing in Vivo-Exhibit. ADD, 1987.
9. Moy R, Zitelli J, Uitto J. Effect of 13 cis-retinoic on dermal wound healing, abstract. JID 1987; 88:508.
10. Dzubow CM, Miller WH Jr. The effect of 13 cis-retinoic acid on wound healing in dogs. J Derm Surg Oncol 13:265, 1987.
11. Wentzell J, Michael, et al. Physical properties of aerosols produced by dermabrasion. Arch Derm 1989; 125:1637–1643.
12. Field L. Dermabrasion versus 5 fluorouracil in the management of actinic keratoses. Controversies in Dermatology. In: Epstein I, ed. Philadelphia: WB Saunders Co., 1984: 62–102.
13. Burke J, Marascalco J, Clark W. Half-face planing of precancerous skin after five years. Arch Derm 1963; 88:140.
14. Coleman WP, Yarborough JM, Mandy SH. Dermabrasion for prophylaxis and treatment of actinic keratoses. J Derm Surg Oncol 1996; 22:17–21.
15. Yarborough JM. Dermabrasive Surgery State of the Art. In: Millikan, ed. Clinics in Dermatology, Advances in Surgery. Philadelphia: Lippincott, 1987; 5:75.
16. Yarborough JM. Dermabrasion by wire brush. J Derm Surg Oncol 1987; 13–610.
17. Alt T. Facial dermabrasion: advantages of the diamond fraise technique. J Derm Surg Oncol 1987; 13:618.
18. Hanke CW, O'Brien JJ, Solow EB. Laboratory evaluation of skin refrigerants used in dermabrasion. J Derm Surg Oncol. 11:45–49, 1985.
19. Dzubow LM. Survey of refrigerant and surgical techniques used for facial dermabrasion. J AA Derm 1985; 13:287–292.
20. Hanke CW, Roenigk HH, Pinske JB. Complications of dermabrasion resulting from excessively cold skin refrigeration. J Derm Surg Oncol 1985; 11:896.
21. Mandy SH. Tretinoin in the pre and postoperative management of dermabrasion. JAAD 1986; 115:878.
22. Hang VC, Lee JV, Zitelli JA, Hebda PA. Topical tretinoin and epithelial wound healing. Arch Derm 1989; 125:65–69.
23. Maibach H, Rovee D. Epidermal Wound Healing. Chicago: Yearbook Medical Publishers, 1972.
24. Mandy SH. A new primary wound dressing made of polyethylene oxide gel. J Derm Surg Oncol 1983; 9:153.
25. Alvarez OM, Mertz PM, Eaglestein WH. The effect of occlusive dressings on collagen synthesis in the superficial wounds. J Surg Res 1983; 35:142.
26. Griffths CE, et al. Restoration of collagen formation in photodamaged human skin by tretinoin. N Engl J Med 1993; 329(8):530–535.
27. Fitzpatrick RE, et al. Pulsed carbon dioxide laser trichloracetic acid, Baker-Gordon phenol, and dermabrasion: a comparative clinical and histologic study of cutaneous resurfacing in a porcine model. Arch Derm 1996; 132:469–471.

28. Campbell JP, et al. The ultrastructural comparison of mechanical dermabrasion and carbon dioxide laser resurfacing in the Minipig model. Arch Otolaryngeal Head Neck Surg 1998; 124:758–760.
29. Giese SY, McKinney P, Roth SI, Zukowski M. The effect of chemosurgical peels and dermabrasion on dermal elastic tissue. Plas Reconstr Surg 1997; 100:489–498.
30. Holmkvist KA. Treatment of perioral rhytides: a comparison of dermabrasion and superpulsed carbon dioxide laser treatment. Presented to The American Society for Dermatologic Surgery, May 1998.
31. Baker TM. Dermabrasion as a complement to aesthetic surgery. Clin Plast Surg 1998; 25:81–88.

11

Filling Substances: Collagen

Arnold William Klein
University of California at Los Angeles School of Medicine,
Los Angeles, California

INTRODUCTION

Over the years, many implantable substances and devices have been promulgated to cosmetically improve soft-tissue defects and deficiencies. The history of modern soft-tissue augmentation dates to the late 1800s when injectable fat was first used for tissue augmentation. Some of these agents, such as adulterated silicones and impure paraffins, frequently resulted in cosmetic disasters [1,2]. The injection of other substances, such as pure injectable-grade liquid silicone, although extremely useful in skilled hands, has been declared illegal by the Food and Drug Administration (FDA) and, thus, is not a consideration for the practitioner.

For a substance or device to be amenable for soft-tissue augmentation by the general medical community, it must meet certain criteria. It must have both a high *use* potential, producing pleasing cosmetic results with a minimum of undesirable reactions, and a low *abuse* potential, in that widespread and possibly incorrect or indiscriminate use would not result in significant morbidity [3]. It must be nonteratogenic, noncarcinogenic, and nonmigratory. In addition, the material must provide predictable, persistent correction through reproducible implantation techniques. Finally, if not autologous, the substance, agent, or device must be FDA approved. FDA approval of an agent or device assures purity and accessibility, as well as providing information regarding use.

Currently, in the United States, although many materials and substances are available, the most commonly used injectable filling agents are autologous fat and Zyderm®/Zyplast® collagen (Collagen Aesthetics, Palo Alto, CA). At the present time, the single most popular substance used for soft-tissue augmentation is injectable bovine collagen. Injectable bovine collagen, Zyderm I Collagen Implant (ZC-I), has been in use in the United States since 1977 [4]. It, together with Zyderm II (ZC-II) and Zyplast (ZP) Collagen Implants, have come to be regarded as the "gold standards" of injectable or implantable fillers. They are the standards against which all the newer materials are measured.

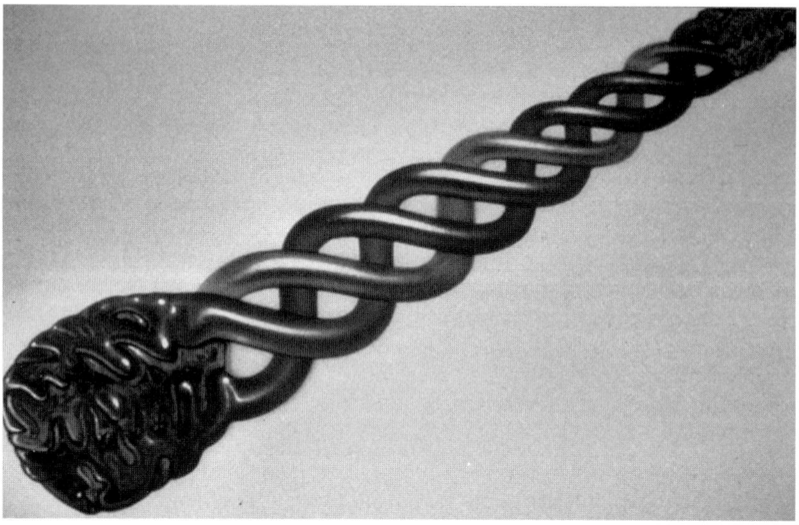

FIGURE 1 Bovine collagen molecule showing the helical structure with the telopeptides at each end. (Photograph courtesy of Collagen Aesthetics.)

STRUCTURE OF HUMAN COLLAGEN

The normal human dermis is composed of collagen proteins, which are the most abundant proteins in the human body. Collagen proteins are trimers involving three individual polypeptide chains known as alpha-chains (Fig. 1). Each alpha chain is composed of about 1000 amino acids, with glycine occupying every third position. About 96% of the collagen molecule is helical, and these helices are attached to nonhelical telopeptides at the amino and carboxy ends. The different types of collagens are each different combinations of alpha-chains. Normal human dermal collagen is roughly 80% type I collagen and 20% type III collagen. In the human body, similar to other secretory proteins, collagen is synthesized in the rough endoplasmic reticulum, modified in the Golgi apparatus, and transported to the cell surface where it is secreted as procollagen. The nonhelical telopeptide bonds are broken by specific peptidases extracellularly. The collagen molecules then cross-link to form collagen fibrils, which then associate to form collagen fibers. Collagen is broken down by specific extracellular collagenases [5,6].

HISTORY OF THE DEVELOPMENT OF ZYDERM/ZYPLAST COLLAGEN

In 1958 at the Harvard Medical School, Gross and Kirk showed that under physiological conditions a solid gel could be produced by gently warming a solution of collagen to body temperature [7]. In the 1960s, it was found that selective removal of the nonhelical amino and carboxy terminal telopeptides significantly reduced the antigenicity of collagen molecules (Fig. 2) [8,9]. A team of investigators at Stanford University in the early 1970s, Perkins, Daniels, Luck, and Knapp, began work on the development of a clinically useful collagen implant material [10]. This work led to Knapp, Luck, and Daniels reporting, in 1977, the successful injection of Pepsin-

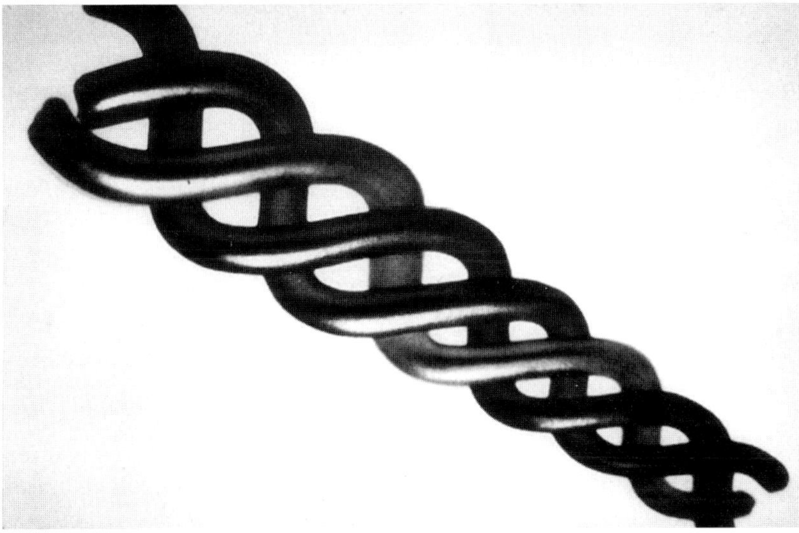

FIGURE 2 Bovine collagen with the telopeptides removed with preservation of the helical structure. (Photograph courtesy of Collagen Aesthetics.)

solubilized, telopeptide-poor, purified human, rabbit, and rat collagen into the subcutaneous tissue of rats. They studied the evolution of the implants over 152 days. They reported that the collagen implants remained as a stable graft and were progressively infiltrated by a matrix of viable host connective tissue [11]. These same investigators later conducted an initial trial of human and bovine collagen in 28 patients. Collagen was injected into the dermal and subcutaneous planes to correct depressed acne scars, subcutaneous atrophy, wrinkling, viral pock marks, and other contour defects with 50 to 85% improvement, which was maintained from 3 to 18 months [4].

Proceeding from these results, Zyderm collagen was developed by the Collagen Corporation and was initially tested by 14 investigators from 1977 to 1978. Subsequently, in 1979, the product became widely available to interested physicians in the United States under a Phase III protocol. This was called the Zyderm Clinical Verification Program and included 728 physician participants. In 1980, Stegman and Tromovitch, who were among the initial 14 investigators in the California Cooperative Study Group, reported on the use of Zyderm collagen in the correction of depressed acne and other types of scars [12]. Subsequently, a participant in the full Clinical Verification Program reported on their experience in 5109 patients who underwent testing and subsequent treatment with injectable Zyderm collagen. What became apparent from this study was the superb application this product had for correcting age-related rhytides. Among these 5109 patients, 3.0% developed positive test responses and 1.3% developed transient localized adverse reactions [13].

In July of 1981, after 6.5 years of development, clinical trials, and testing, Zyderm Collagen Implant received FDA approval. This was the first time an injectable xenogenic agent was FDA approved for soft-tissue augmentation. This approval reawakened interest in the entire field of filling agents and, since then, an estimated 1,900,000 individuals worldwide have received injectable collagen implants.

After the approval of the first injectable form, Zyderm I Collagen Implant (ZC-I), the FDA approved two other formulations, Zyderm II Collagen Implant (ZC-II) and Zyplast Collagen Implant (ZP) (Fig. 3). Additionally, a special packaging of Zyderm I Collagen that contains a 32-gauge needle has been made available (Z-FGN). The barrel of the syringe for this product–Zyderm I with Fine Gauge Needle–is specifically suited for use with the supplied 32-gauge, metal-hub needle (Fig. 4).

COMPOSITION OF ZYDERM/ZYPLAST COLLAGEN

Zyderm Collagen Implants (ZC-I, ZC-II, and ZP) are all sterile, purified fibrillar suspensions of bovine dermal collagen. Processing of the material involves purification, pepsin digestion, and sterilization. Pepsin digestion removes the more antigenic end portions of the bovine collagen molecule (the telopeptides) without disturbing the natural helical structure. This is critical so that the resulting agent is more immunologically compatible with the human host. Furthermore, the preservation of the helical structure is thought to contribute to substantivity of the product on implantation. Zyderm Collagen Implants are all 95 to 98% Type I collagen, with the remainder being type III [14]. The products are suspended in phosphate-buffered physiological saline containing 0.3% lidocaine. It should be indicated that these substances are all taken from the skin of a closed American herd, negating the possibility of contamination with the bovine spongiform encephalopathy virus or prion [15].

ZC-I, the original material, and ZC-II differ only in concentration. ZC-I is 3.5% by weight bovine collagen, whereas ZC-II (introduced in 1983) is 6.5% by weight bovine collagen. ZP, approved in 1985, is the third form of implantable collagen. In ZP, bovine dermal collagen is lightly cross-linked by the addition of 0.0075% glu-

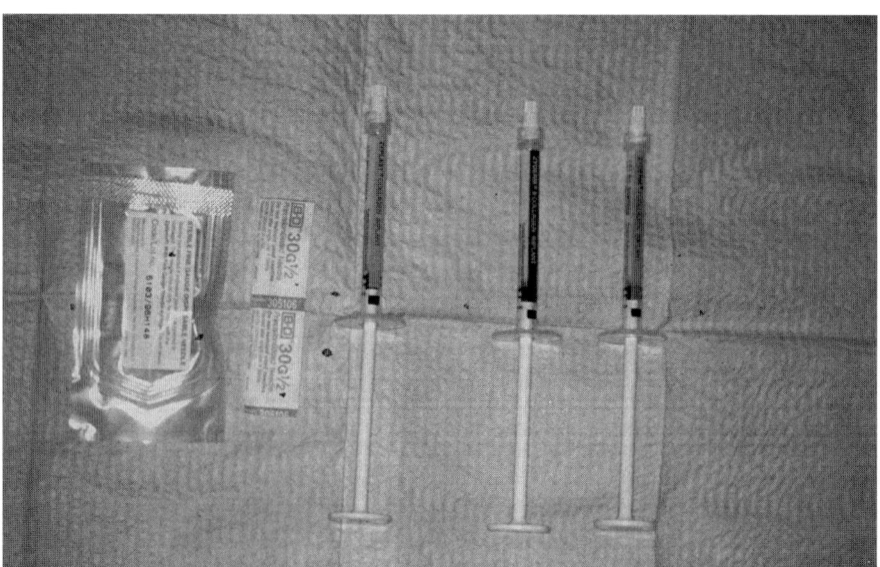

FIGURE 3 Zyderm I, Zyderm II, and Zyplast.

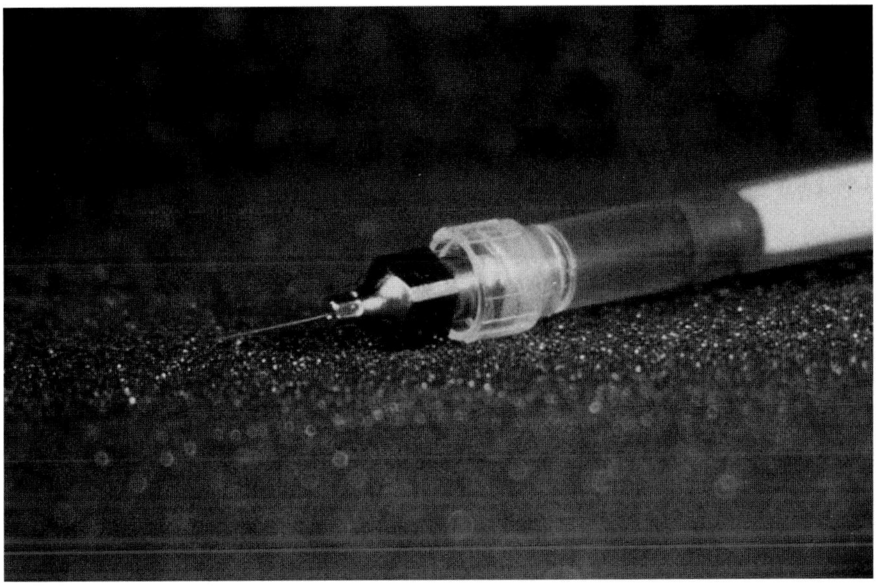

FIGURE 4 **32-gauge metal-hub needle.**

taraldehyde. Glutaraldehyde cross-links by producing covalent bridges between 10% of available lysine residues of the bovine collagen molecule. These bridges are intramolecular and intermolecular, as well as between fibrils, resulting in a more robust implant that is essentially an injectable latticework of bovine collagen [15]. As a result of this cross-linkage, ZP is more resistant to proteolytic degradation and less immunogenic [16–18]. Furthermore, the more substantive nature of ZP makes it applicable for deeper contour defects unresponsive to ZC-I or ZC-II [18,19].

All the products are provided in preloaded syringes that are stored at low temperature (4 °C) so the dispersed fibrils remain fluid and small. This allows passage of the products through small gauge needles. Once implanted, the human body temperature [5] causes the products to undergo consolidation into a solid gel as intermolecular cross-linking occurs in the injected suspension with the generation of a high proportion of larger fibrils. Obviously, Zyplast that is already chemically cross-linked probably could not be expected to undergo in vitro cross-linking to the extent of the other products.

In addition to the various forms of Zyderm Collagen, a special packaging of ZC-I collagen is available that contains a special syringe specially suited for use with a 32-gauge needle. This product, Zyderm I with fine Gauge needle (Z-FGN), contains a syringe barrel specifically designed for use with the supplied 32-gauge, metal-hub needle. Nevertheless, because 32-gauge metal-hub needles are easily affixed to the other ZC-I syringes, some individuals have not found this packaging particularly necessary.

PATIENT SCREENING AND SKIN TESTING

Proper patient screening and especially skin testing are of the utmost importance in the application of bovine collagen therapy. Individuals who have lidocaine sensitivity, a history of an anaphylactoid event, or previous sensitivity to bovine collagen are excluded from testing and treatment. Physicians must counsel patients as to the risks and benefits of injectable collagen therapy. Each physician must inform prospective patients about skin testing, the treatment procedure, and treatment expectations. The safety and contraindications of the various injectable collagen formulations have been described elsewhere [14,16–20].

Potential allergenicity to injectable collagen is reliably determined by skin testing. The skin test syringe contains 0.3 ml ZC-I and is used to screen allergy to all ZC-I and ZP therapy. Using only one third of the test syringe's contents, the dose is administered in a tuberculin manner in the volar forearm. The site is evaluated at 48 to 72 hours and again at four weeks. A positive skin test is defined as swelling, induration, tenderness, or erythema that persists or occurs 6 hours or longer after test implantation. This is a definite contraindication to treatment, and patients exhibiting any of these responses are excluded from therapy. A positive skin test response will be seen in 3.0 to 3.5% of individuals. Seventy percent of these reactions will become manifest in 48 to 72 hours, indicating a pre-existing allergy to bovine collagen [17,21–23]. Thus it is imperative to observe the test site at 48 to 72 hours as well as at the standard 4-week interval. Most authorities now recommend a second test as an additional precaution [3,24–26]. This can be placed in the contralateral forearm or the periphery of the face. It is administered either 2 weeks after the initial test, with treatment commencing at 4 weeks after initial testing, or 4 weeks after the initial test, with treatment commencing 6 weeks after the first test. The volume used for the second test is the same as that used for the first test and, again, skin test syringes are used. Because the majority of treatment-associated hypersensitivity reactions occur shortly after the first treatment, double testing greatly reduces the frequency of this most undesirable sequela by changing the first treatment exposure to a second test exposure. Additionally, treatment-associated hypersensitivity reactions that occur after two negative skin tests generally tend to be milder, indicating that, possibly, the physician has selected out the most severely allergic individuals.

Single retesting of individuals who have not been treated for more than 1 year or who were successfully tested or treated elsewhere is strongly recommended. After retesting, a minimum of 2 weeks is recommended for test site evaluation before commencing treatment.

IMPLANTATION TECHNIQUES

Injection technique is the single most important factor in the successful application of bovine collagen implants, and proper lighting, patient positioning, and magnification are the cornerstones of good injection technique. The patient must be in the seated position because many contour defects all but disappear when supine. Additionally, tangential halogen lighting is beneficial because it often reveals even the most subtle contour defects. Also, magnification greatly increases the precision of injection. The treating physician must remember that the ability to properly implant collagen is an evolutionary process that will improve with experience.

Zyderm Collagen is implanted in the superficial dermis by making serial punctures of the skin with syringes prefilled with the material. With ZC-I, a 30- or 32-gauge needle is used. Many experienced practitioners prefer the 32-gauge metal-hub needle because it produces less trauma to the skin and ultimately a better cosmetic result. For extraordinarily fine defects, a 33-gauge needle may be used. With ZC-II, a 30-gauge needle is necessary because its viscous nature prevents its use with a 32-gauge needle. When implanting ZC-I and ZC-II, a serial puncture technique is used with the syringe held all but parallel to the skin surface. Barely penetrating the skin with the needle tip, one must "flow" the material in the superficial dermis, observing a flat yellow blanching of the skin. While injecting, each subsequent injection volume should be placed at the advancing edge of the previously injected quantity, generating a continuous "flow" of material that smoothly fills in defects.

ZC-I is the most versatile of all forms of injectable collagen. It is also the most technique-sensitive and the most forgiving. Because it is not cross-linked, it has good flow characteristics. When placed correctly, it will smoothly fill superficial defects. This is best performed with a 30- or 32-gauge metal-hub needle, regardless of the syringe type chosen (0.5 ml, 1.0 ml, 2.0 ml, or Z-FGN). The physician prepares to inject the treatment site by holding it taut between the thumb and forefinger of the noninjecting hand. Next, the needle tip is guided horizontally with the bevel down along the skin surface until it barely penetrates the skin. The hub of the needle is then rocked gently over the thumb of the opposing hand, tenting up the skin with the needle tip, and a flow of material is created in the upper dermis as a smooth, yellowish mass that is both wide, flat and not three-dimensional in appearance. With ZC-I, upper dermal flow is created by applying each subsequent injection at the leading edge of the previously injected volume. This continuous, wide, and flat flow of ZC-I in the upper dermis smoothly augments the applicable soft-tissue defect, thereby providing the most cosmetically pleasing results. Although persistent beading and overcorrection can be problematic with superficial placement of ZC-II, they are rarely associated with ZC-I therapy.

Because ZC-I and ZC-II contain bovine collagen in the form of microfibrils, they both have excellent flow characteristics. However, ZC-II requires greater mechanical force to inject and one must always remember that it undergoes less condensation on implantation, leaving approximately 60% of the injected material at the implantation site, as opposed to ZC-I where 30% is deposited. "As superficial as possible" placement of ZC-I and ZC-II is no longer used, nor is excessive overcorrection because persistent whiteness at the injection site and elevation can be observed with overcorrection [27,28]. Initially, deliberate overcorrection was desired with ZC-I and ZC-II based on the theory that, after condensation and resorption of the saline and lidocaine, only a small proportion of the implant remained. Nevertheless, as one becomes more proficient with ZC-I and ZC-II implantation technique, significant overcorrection should be avoided because it will often create a persistent elevation above the site's normal contours. However, a slight degree of overcorrection (10–20%) should still be sought when injecting ZC-I and ZC-II.

ZC-II is useful for deep acne scars and deep glabellar furrows. Additionally, when certain defects that normally respond to ZC-I are unresponsive, ZC-II can be successfully used. Because of its more viscous nature, it can only be injected with a 30-gauge needle. Otherwise, techniques for injection with ZC-II are almost identical to those outlined above for ZC-I. Although I rarely use ZC-II, I am sure that some individuals find ZC-II a very useful adjunct to soft-tissue augmentation.

ZP was developed to correct deeper defects, which are often unresponsive to ZC-I. Because cross-linking forms a rigid lattice network, ZP does not flow well when placed superficially. Furthermore, superficial placement may cause persistent beading and long-lasting overcorrection. If ZP is placed too deeply, however, large amounts of material will be required for correction and improvement will be short lived. Thus, correct placement with ZP is as essential as it is with ZC-I (Fig. 5).

ZP is the most robust form of injectable bovine collagen presently approved for use in the United States. Two attributes—the rigid cross-linked structure and the absence of microfibrils—greatly affect the rheological character of this product and account for the decreased ability to smoothly flow this material. The resistance one often feels while implanting ZP may be explained by these characteristics, as well as possibly the density of the mid-dermal implantation site. In the use of ZP, a 30-gauge needle is used to create a mid-dermal flow of material, again using a serial puncture technique. ZP should neither be placed too superficially nor in the subdermal space. In the former situation it will result in persistent overcorrection with beading, and in the latter it will not provide lasting correction. With ZP the syringe is held at a 10 to 20° angle during the injection process and the material placed slightly deeper than ZC-I or ZC-II. While implanting ZP, the resistance of the dermal matrix is felt against the injecting hand and the plane of the injected site should elevate as the material is being placed. Deliberate overcorrection should be avoided because the material undergoes little syneresis or condensation on implantation. It should be noted that some individuals prefer a 90° angle for ZP implantation. If a 90° angle is chosen, only the needle tip should penetrate the skin with numerous serial punctures. Figures 6 through 11 are "before and after" photographs of patients injected with collagen. Although Collagen Aesthetics has offered the Adjustable Depth Gauge (ADG) to improve the accuracy of Zyplast implantation, I have not found it to increase one's technical accuracy. Additionally, the practice of molding or massaging ZP after implantation for an improved cosmetic result remains unsubstantiated and could result in the rapid loss of correction as the material is forced into the subdermal space.

Finally, the simultaneous use of two products can often provide an optimal result both in regard to cosmetic result and persistence of improvement. For example,

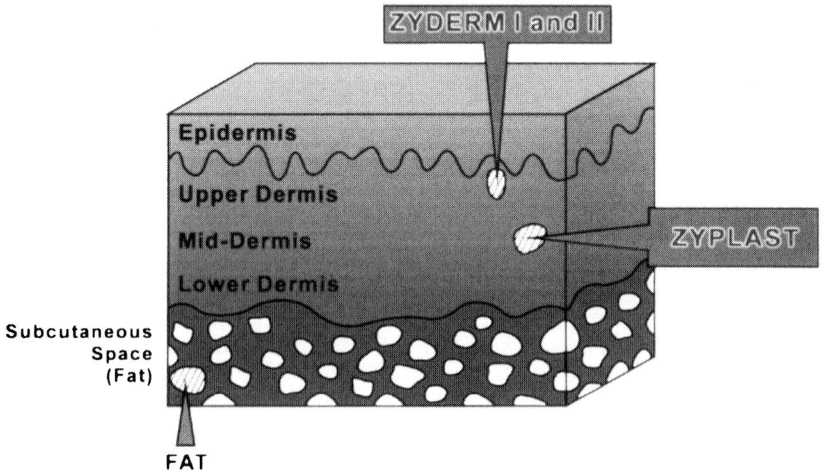

FIGURE 5 Applicable levels of injection in the dermis for Zyderm and Zyplast. (Photograph courtesy of Collagen Aesthetics.)

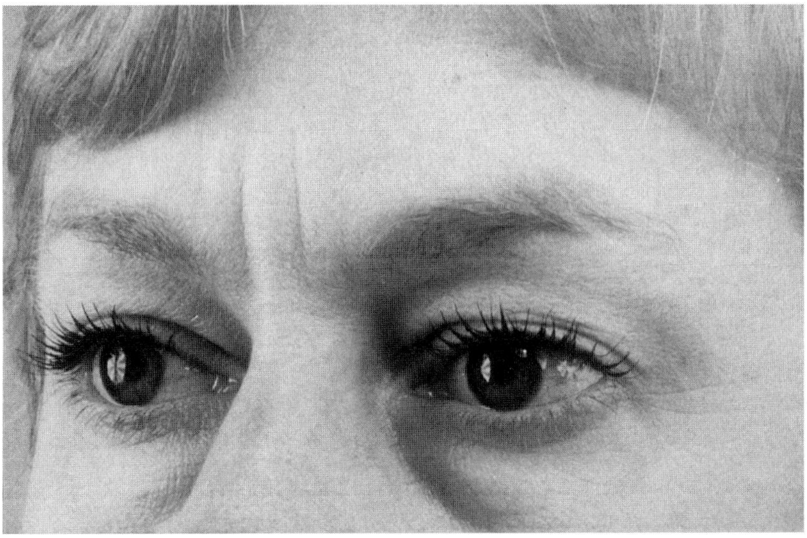

FIGURE 6 Before collagen implantation in the glabellar lines. (Photograph courtesy of Collagen Aesthetics.)

increased longevity of correction and improved aesthetic results can often be achieved by the "layering" technique wherein ZC-I or ZC-II is immediately implanted over Zyplast injection sites. Although Botox (Allergan Corp., Irvine, CA) has become extremely popular for the reduction of wrinkles and lines in the upper third of the face, its application in the lower two thirds is more problematic and collagen implantation is still the treatment of choice. Collagen can also be used in

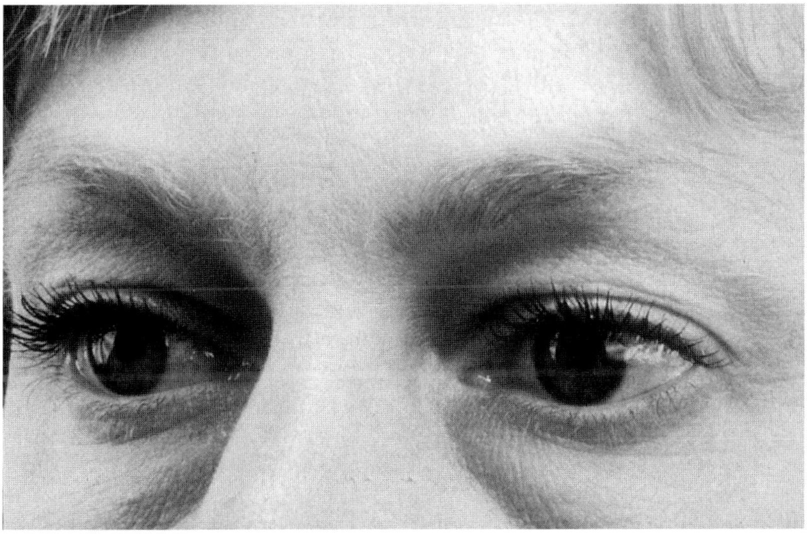

FIGURE 7 After collagen implantation in the glabellar lines. (Photograph courtesy of Collagen Aesthetics.)

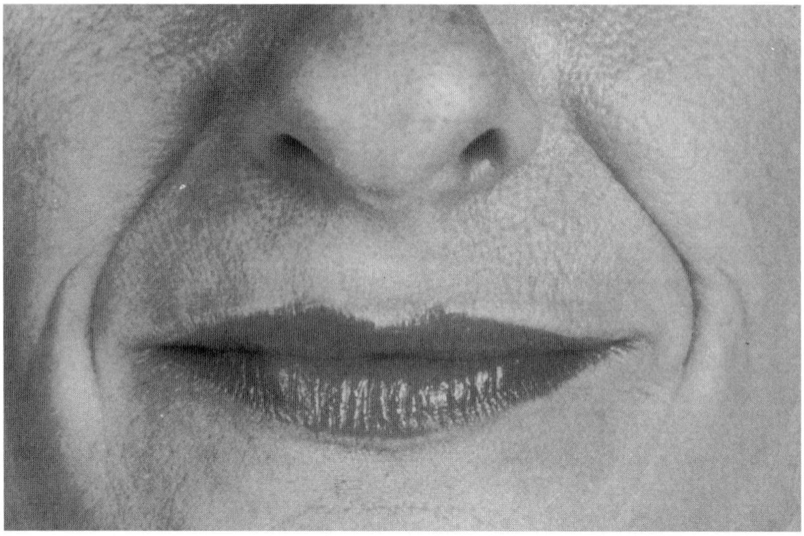

FIGURE 8 Before collagen implantation in the nasolabial folds. (Photograph courtesy of Collagen Aesthetics.)

concert with Botox in the upper face to achieve optimal results, eg, deep glabellar furrows, lower forehead lines, and so on.

MAINTENANCE OF CORRECTION

Although it was once stated that two to three treatment sessions were usually necessary to achieve optimal correction, full correction can be achieved at one visit if enough material is used. For all causal factors, 30% of individuals report 18-month longevity of correction, whereas 70% require touch-up treatments at intervals of 3 to 12 months. Correction with all forms of bovine collagen is temporary and requires periodic maintenance at 4 to 12 month intervals [29]. Glabellar frown lines and acne scars appear to retain correction the longest. Specifically, in regard to rhytides, correction appears to persist for periods of 6 to 24 months.

This variation in longevity could possibly be explained by continued mechanical stress at the treatment site, lesion location, and, possibly, the patient's individual response to Zyderm Collagen Implants [22,30,31]. Animal studies using ZC-I and ZP have suggested recipient collagen production after implantation [32,33]. This gradual colonization has been most marked with the use of ZP. Additionally, minimal inflammatory reactions and a high degree of biocompatibility have been noted. In humans, histological studies with both ZC-I and ZP have also shown excellent biocompatibility with minimal inflammation at sites of implantation. In humans, although histological studies of ZP, as opposed to ZC-I/ZC-II, have revealed some deposition of host collagen, there is no convincing evidence that this deposition contributes to longevity of correction [34,35]. Indeed, correction with all forms of bovine collagen appears to be lost because the material is displaced in the human from the site of implantation in the dermis into the subcutaneous space [36]. As previously stated, injectable collagen technique is an evolutionary process for the

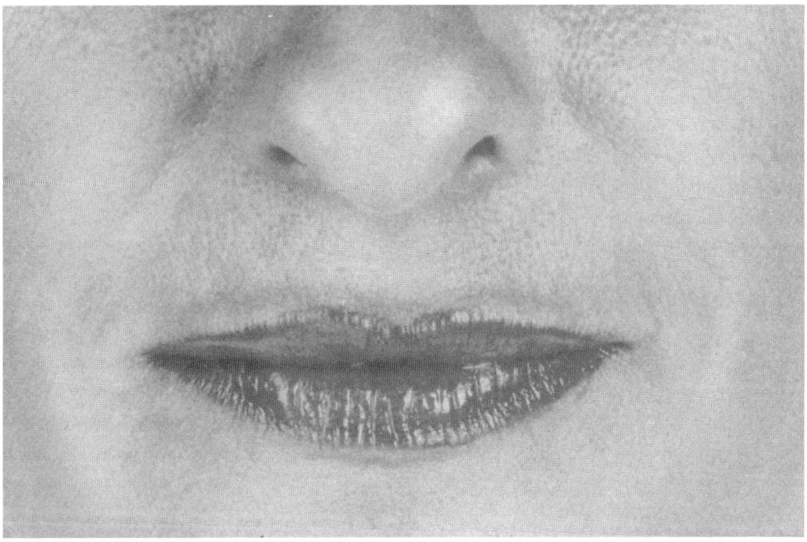

FIGURE 9 **After collagen implantation in the nasolabial folds. (Photograph courtesy of Collagen Aesthetics.)**

treating physician. In my experience with 70,000 patients, correction now requires fewer visits and less material.

INDICATIONS FOR COLLAGEN THERAPY

Among the indications for ZC-I/ZC-II are horizontal forehead lines, glabellar lines, crow's feet, nasolabial lines, fine lip lines, marionette lines, shallow acne scars, and excisional scars [30–33]. Soft, distensible superficial defects and lines are most amenable to ZC-I and ZC-II. Deep nasolabial folds, marionette grooves, deep acne scars, and the like respond best to ZP with or without ZC-I/ZC-II overlay. ZP is also best suited to resurface the vermilion border between the lip and skin for lip enhancement. Additionally, true "mucosal" injection of ZC-I, ZC-II, and ZP is often used in the lip enhancement process although the mucosal location is not an FDA-approved site for collagen implantation. ZP is not recommended for use in the glabellar frown lines (see adverse treatment responses) [28]. As one gains more experience, the practitioner will realize that although ZC-I is the most forgiving, it is also the most technique sensitive and versatile. Furthermore, as one's implantation techniques evolve, ZC-I, rather than ZC-II will be the preferred filler for shallow defects because as one becomes more proficient at superficial placement, ZC-II can often be associated with persistent whiteness at the injection site. Many experienced practitioners limit the use of ZC-II to deep acne scars and deep glabellar furrows that are unresponsive to ZC-I and the latter only in patients who are not accepting of the off-label adjunctive use of Botox.

ADVERSE TREATMENT RESPONSES

Adverse treatment responses to injectable collagen can be divided into nonhypersensitive and hypersensitive. Nonhypersensitive reactions include bruising, reactivation

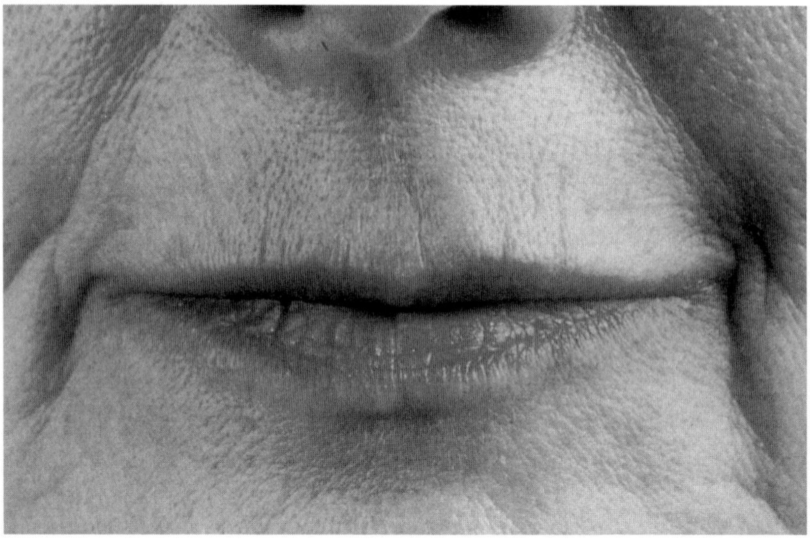

FIGURE 10 Before collagen implantation in the nasolabial folds and drool grooves. (Photograph courtesy of Collagen Aesthetics.)

of herpetic eruptions, as well as bacterial infection. Additionally, local necrosis caused by vascular interruption at the treatment site has been noted with ZP and rarely with ZC-I/ZC-II [32]. Because 56% of these locally necrotic events occur in the glabellar area, physicians are cautioned against using ZP at this site. If, on injection, a physician notes severe blanching of the area and pain, injection should be stopped immediately because local necrosis has possibly occurred. The value of

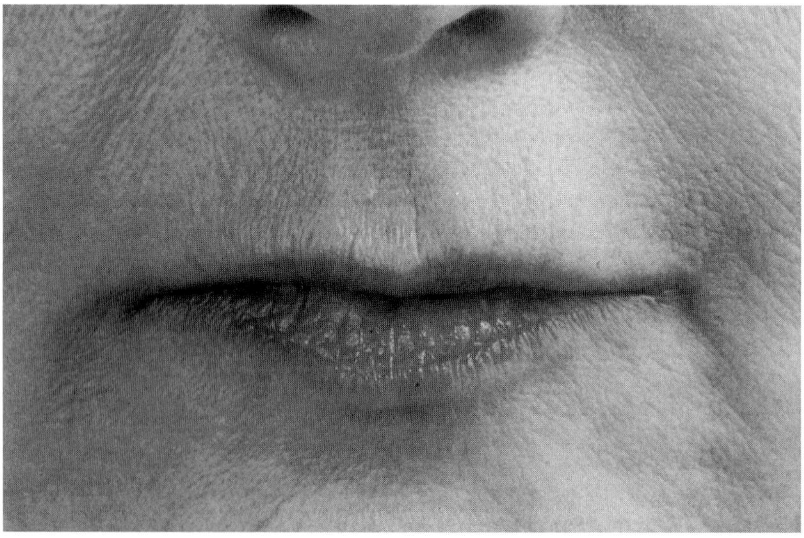

FIGURE 11 After collagen implantation in the nasolabial folds and drool grooves. (Photograph courtesy of Collagen Aesthetics.)

massage, warm compresses, or nitroglycerin gel in this situation is, as yet, unsubstantiated.

Two reports of partial vision loss after Zyderm Collagen therapy have been noted [37,38]. These are probably the result of an occlusive event involving the retinal artery. These serious consequences of a cosmetic procedure underscore the need to remember that the dermal site is the proper location for collagen implantation.

Treatment-associated hypersensitivity reactions to bovine collagen implants are, for the most part, cosmetic and consist of redness and swelling at the treatment site. It is rare, but mild systemic symptoms can accompany these reactions. Hypersensitive reactions are almost uniformly associated with anti-Zyderm antibodies [39–42]. These antibodies do not cross-react with human collagen [43,44]. "Cyst–Abscess" formation is a rare but severe hypersensitivity response occurring at a rate of four in 10,000 treated individuals [45]. Clinically, individuals develop painful, swollen cysts at the sites of treatment. These reactions are usually associated with ZP and rarely ZC-I/ZC-II. Eighty-six percent of these individuals have associated anti-bovine antibodies. Incision and drainage, as well as intralesional steroids, have been advocated to manage this most undesirable sequela. This is a long-lasting, severe hypersensitive response that can persist for more than 2 years. It should be noted that analysis of extruded material from these abscesses has revealed bovine collagen implant.

As to the possibility of bovine collagen inducing connective tissue disease in the human host, retrospective studies as well as an expert panel convened by the FDA have found no supporting evidence [44].

LIP AUGMENTATION: THEORY AND TECHNIQUE

The application of bovine collagen in the circumoral area is the largest single indication for which these products are used. Thus, an in-depth discussion of the use of bovine collagen as a tool for cosmetic enhancement in this area is warranted. The aging process of the mouth is often associated with the development of circumoral radial grooves as well as a loss of the three-dimensional aspects of the lips themselves. Therefore, even a small volumetric increase in the size of the lips in selected individuals can produce a most pleasing cosmetic result. Lip augmentation addresses both the age-related contour loss found in the lips and, by enhancing their size, the radial grooves. Furthermore, lips themselves are the cornerstone of the aesthetic appeal of the female, as well as male, face. Lip enhancement encompasses both the correctional age-related changes but also cosmetic psychosocial improvement. As previously indicated, it should be remembered that, although injection into the glabrous skin surrounding the lips is an FDA-approved indication, mucosal injection is an off-label use. One must be sure to counsel the patient regarding the cost as well as the frequent maintenance that is initially required. It has been my experience that frequency of injection will decrease over time, possibly as a result of subtle fibroplasia. Although various investigators have advocated the use of nerve blocks in association with this augmentation, others have unexpectedly found implantation more difficult and the result aesthetically less pleasing when nerve blocks are performed.

A review of the procedure of lip augmentation by six investigators revealed that the best results were achieved by first injecting ZP in the potential space between the lip mucosa and skin (along the vermilion border) in the upper and lower lip. This was then followed by ZC-I or ZP directly into the mucosa itself. It should be remembered that the major vascular supply to the lips runs in the mucosa and blind injections of ZP into this area will occasionally result in vascular events, especially after the lips are repeatedly treated. The ideal technique for lip enhancement is variable and is certainly not uniform between physicians or even from patient to patient. The following is an outline of a basic technique that the practitioner can individualize. Before the process is begun both the patient and the physician must be aware that this is a less-than-painless procedure. First the ZP must be placed in the potential space of the lip. The patient gently squeezes the nurse's hand and initial injection is begun at the right corner of the lower lip. While injecting, the lip is held taut with the thumb of the opposing hand slightly stretching the lip posteriorly from the corner of the mouth. Anterior to the opposing thumb, the potential space at the right corner is entered with ZP using a 30-gauge needle at about a 75° angle from the lip surface with the syringe held parallel to the lower lip. Once the treating physician feels the needle tip drop into the potential space, the injection angle is changed to about 45° from the lip and the flow of material begun across the lower lip in the potential space (Fig. 12).

If a spot is reached where the material will not easily advance, go to this spot and inject onward from this location (Fig. 13). A smooth, yellowish flow of ZP is desired in the potential space, not whitish lumps.

The vermilion potential space of the lower lip should be injected right corner to center and left corner to center (Fig. 14). It is very important to place sufficient ZP in the lateral sites of the lower lip because this will "lift" the mouth. In the upper lip, the potential space can be entered as in the lower lip, although some individuals prefer to enter the space centrally and inject center to left corner and then center to

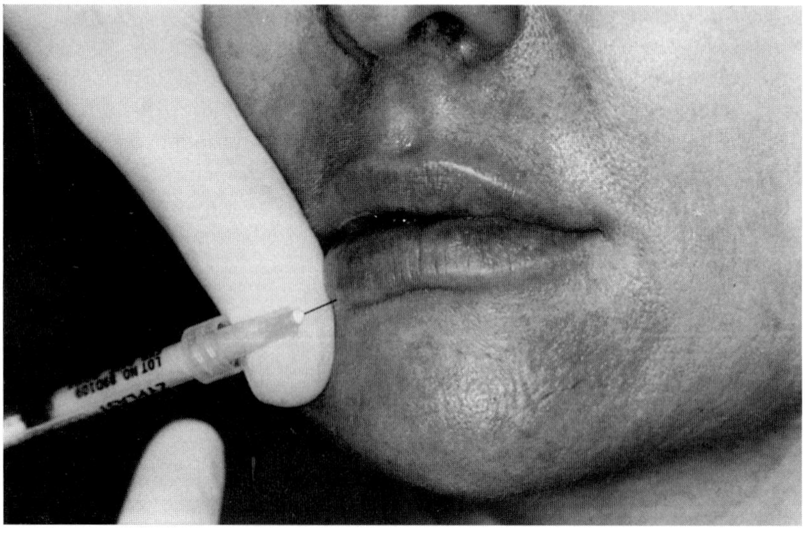

FIGURE 12 Entering the lip from the outside corner and flowing material across the lip.

right corner. This latter approach will preserve the patient's natural cupid's bow (Fig. 14). Once outlined, the lip can be further enhanced by placing ZP, ZC-I or ZC-II in the mucosa. All are flowed at this site in a manner similar to that used at other locations. Remember, mucosal injection is an off-label use. As stated previously, it has been my experience that, after repeated injections, the augmentation process in the lip begins to "hold" and touch-ups are only necessary two or three times a year.

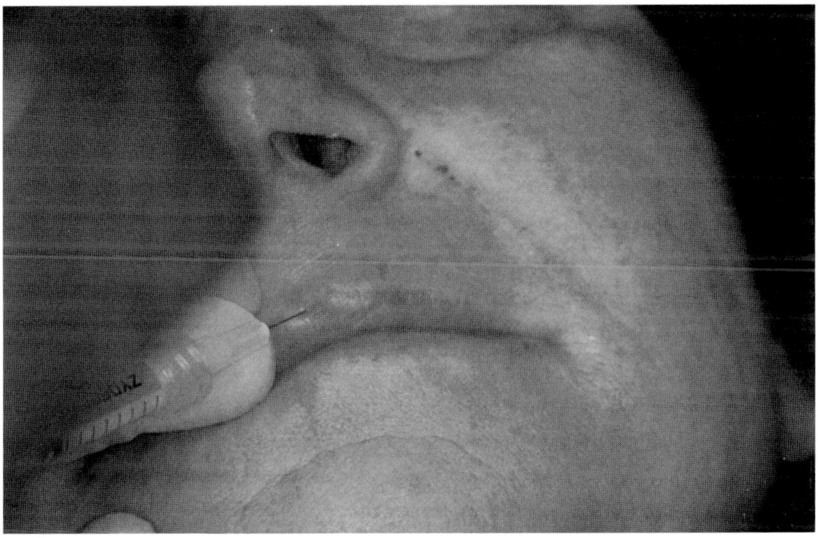

FIGURE 13 Continuation of injection by entering at the advancing edge of the previous injection.

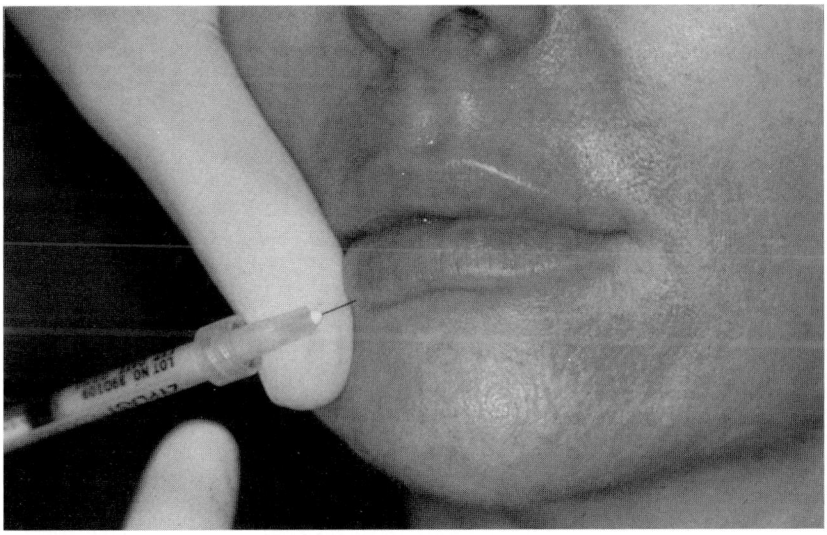

FIGURE 14 Injecting the lower lip from corner to center.

INJECTABLE COLLAGEN (ALTERNATIVE FORMS)

Koken Atelocollagen and Resoplast are nonfibrillar forms of implantable bovine collagen not approved for use in the United States. Although other investigators have found them quite beneficial, there remains no US experience. Recently, a sheet-like porcine collagen, Permacol, has been introduced abroad, but there is presently no injectable form of this agent available.

SUMMARY

Injectable collagens (ZC-I, ZC-II, and ZP) are tools that provide a physician with a manner in which to approach mild contour defects, the same defects that signify the aging process or the end result of scarring events. They are a temporary, biocompatible solution to many but certainly not all soft-tissue deficiencies. The adverse reaction profile is of an acceptably low level and indeed only of local significance. Nevertheless, for both the physician and patient to benefit from these agents, effective reproducible implantation technique(s) must be developed by the treating physician. As the physician's experience with these agents increases, so will his ability to produce aesthetically pleasing results.

REFERENCES

1. Urback F, Wilne SS, Johnson WC, Davies RE. Generalized paraffinoma (sclerosing lipogranuloma). Archiv Dermatol 103:277–285, 1971.
2. Klein JA, Cole G, Burr RJ, Bartlow G, Fulwider C. Paraffinomas of the scalp. Archiv Dermatol 121:382–385, 1985.
3. Klein AW, Rish DC. Injectable collagen: an adjunct to facial plastic surgery. Facial Plast Surg 4:87, 1987.
4. Knapp TR, Kaplan EN, Daniels JR. Injectable collagen for soft tissue augmentation. Plast Reconstr Surg 60:389, 1977.
5. Matton G, Answeeuw A, De Keyser F. The history of biomaterials and the biology of collagen. Aesth Plast Surg 9:133–140, 1985.
6. Hollister DW, Byers PH, Holbrook KA. Genetic disorders of collagen metabolism. In: Harris, Hirschorn, eds. Advances in Human Genetics 12. New York and London: Plenum Press, 1982, pp. 1–86.
7. Gross J, Kirk D. The heat precipitation of collagen from neutral salt solutions: some rate-regulating factors. J Biol Chem 233:355–360, 1958.
8. Davidson PF, et al. The serologic specificity of tropocollagen telopeptides. J Exp Med 126:331–349, 1967.
9. Schmitt FO, et al. The antigenicity of tropocollagen. Proc Natl Acad Sci USA 51:493–497, 1964.
10. Stegman SJ, Tromovich TA. Injectable collagen. In: Stegman SJ, Tromovich TA, eds. Cosmetic Dermatologic Surgery. Chicago and London: Yearbook Medical Publishers, 1984; pp. 131–149.
11. Knapp TR, Luck E, Daniels JR. Behavior of solubilized collagen as a bioimplant. J Surg Res 23:96–105, 1977.
12. Stegman SJ, Tromovitch TA. Implantation of collagen for depressed scars. J Derm Surg Onc 6:450–453, 1980.
13. Watson W, Kay RL, Klein AW, et al. Injectable collagen: a clinical overview. Cutis 31: 543–546, 1983.

14. Wallace DG, McPherson JJ, Ellingsworth LE, et al. Injectable collagen for tissue augmentation. In: Nimni ME, ed. Collagen, Vol. III, Biotechnology. (Boca Raton: CRC Press, Inc., 1988, pp. 117–144.
15. Bulletin Collagen Corporation. Bovine Spongiform Encephalopathy. Palo Alto, CA, April 14, 1996.
16. McPherson JM, Ledger PW, Sawamura S, et al. The preparation and physiochemical characterization of an injectable form of reconstituted, glutaraldehyde crosslinked, bovine corium collagen. J Biomed Meter Res 20:79, 1986.
17. DeLustro F, Smith ST, Sundsmo J, et al. Reaction to injectable collagen in human subjects. J Dermatol Surg Oncol 14(Suppl):49, 1988.
18. Elson ML. Clinical assessment of Zyplast implant: a year of experience for soft tissue contour correction. J Am Acad Dermatol 116:707, 1988.
19. Klein AW. Indications and implantation techniques for the various formulations of injectable collagen. J Dermatol Surg Oncol 14(Suppl 1):49, 1988.
20. Elson ML. Corrections of dermal contour defects with the injectable collagens: choosing and using these materials. Semin Dermatol 6:77, 1987.
21. Castrow FF II, Krull EA. Injectable collagen implant–update. J Am Acad Dermatol 9: 889, 1983.
22. Cooperman LS, Mackinnon V, Bechler G, Pharriss BB. Injectable collagen: a six-year clinical investigation. Aesth Plast Surg 9:145, 1985.
23. Kamer FM, Churukian XM. The clinical use of injectable collagen: a three-year retrospective study. Arch Otolaryngol 110:93, 1984.
24. Klein AW. In favor of double testing. J Dermatol Surg Oncol 15:263, 1989.
25. Elson ML. The role of skin testing in the use of collagen injectable materials. J Dermatol Surg Oncol 15:301, 1989.
26. Klein AW, Rish DC. Injectable collagen update. J Dermatol Surg Oncol 10:519, 1984.
27. Klein AW. Implantation techniques for injectable collagen: two-and-one half years of personal clinical experience. J Am Acad Dermatol 9:224, 1983.
28. Bailin PL, Bailin MD. Collagen implantation: clinical applications and lesion selection. J Dermatol Surg Oncol 14(Suppl 1):49, 1988.
29. Klein AW. Indications and implantation techniques for the various formulations of injectable collagen. J Dermatol Surg Oncol 14(Suppl):27–30, 1988.
30. Robinson JK, Hanke CW. Injectable collagen implant: histopathologic identification and longevity of correction. J Dermatol Surg Oncol 11:124, 1985.
31. Bailin MD, Bailin PM. Case studies: correction of surgical scars, acne scars, and rhytides with Zyderm and Zyplast Implants. J Dermatol Surg Oncol 14(Suppl 1):31, 1988.
32. Armstrong R, et al. Injectable collagen for soft tissue augmentation. In: Boretos JW, Eden M, eds. Contemporary Clinical Applications, New Technology and Legal Aspects. Parkridge, NJ: Noyes Publications, 1984, pp. 528–536.
33. McPherson JM, et al. An examination of the biologic response to injectable, glutaraldehyde cross-linked collagen implants. J Biomed Mater Res 20:93, 1986.
34. Kligman AM, Armstrong RC. Histologic response to intradermal Zyderm and Zyplast (glutaraldehyde cross-linked) collagen in humans. J Dermatol Surg Oncol 12:351, 1986.
35. Kligman AM. Histologic responses to collagen implants in human volunteers; Comparison of Zyderm Collagen with Zyplast implant. J Dermatol Surg Oncol 14(Suppl 1):35, 1988.
36. Stegman SJ, Chus S, Bensch K, Armstrong R. A light and electron microscopic evaluation of Zyderm Collagen and Zyplast Implants in aging human facial skin: a pilot study. Arch Dermatol 123:1644, 1987.
37. DeLustro F, Smith ST, Sundsmo J, et al. Reaction to injectable collagen: results in animal models and clinical use. Plast Reconstruct Surg 79:581, 1987.

38. McGraw R, et al. Sudden blindness secondary to injection of common drugs in the head and neck, pt 1: clinical experiences. Otolaryngology 86:147, 1978.
39. McCoy JP, et al. Characterization of the humoral immune response to bovine collagen implants. Arch Dermatol 121:990, 1985.
40. Cooperman LS, Michaeli D. The immunogenicity of injectable collagen, pt 2: a retrospective review of seventy-two tested and treated patients. J Dermatol Surg Oncol 10: 647, 1984.
41. Ellingsworth LR, et al. The human immune response to reconstituted bovine collagen. J Immunol 136:877, 1986.
42. DeLustro F, et al. Immune response to allogeneic and xenogeneic implants of collagen and collagen derivatives. Clin Orthop 260:263–279, 1990.
43. Siegle RJ, McCoy JP, Schade W, et al. Intradermal implantation of bovine collagen: humoral responses associated with clinical reaction. Arch Dermatol 120:183, 1984.
44. Klein AW. Bonfire of the Wrinkles. J Dermatol Surg Oncol 17:543–544, 1991.
45. Hane CW, Hingley HR, Jolivette DM, Swanson NA, Stegman SJ. Abscess formation and local necrosis after treatment with Zyderm or Zyplast collagen implant. J Amer Acad Dermatol 25:319–326, 1991.

APPENDIX 1: ZYDERM® COLLAGEN AND ZYPLAST® COLLAGEN EXPLAINED

Before you begin your Collagen treatments, please review this important information.

The way your skin looks is directly related to the way your skin is supported.

Aging, disease, injury – these are some of the factors that can weaken the collagen fibers that give your skin its underlying strength.

Until the 1970s, it wasn't possible for doctors to replace damaged collagen. Now, both Zyderm® Collagen and Zyplast® Collagen Implants are available. Made of highly purified bovine collagen, these materials can be injected into your skin to supplement your body's own collagen and actually fill certain lines and facial furrows.

This booklet will not take the place of a consultation with your doctor, but it will answer some of the questions often asked about treatment with injectable collagen. And it will help you and your doctor decide whether **Zyderm** or **Zyplast** Collagen treatments can help to smooth your skin.

What is collagen?

Collagen is a natural protein that provides structural support. It is found throughout the body – in skin, muscle, tendon, and bone. Fibers of collagen are woven together like threads in fabric to form a framework into which new cells can grow. In the skin, collagen provides texture, resiliency, and shape.

The collagen in human skin is very similar to the collagen found in certain animals. As a result, animal collagen has had many medical applications; for example, animal collagen has been used in sutures for over a century. Heart valves used during surgery are also made of collagen. Injectable **Zyderm** and **Zyplast** Collagen Implants are made of collagen from cow skin that has been highly purified.

How was injectable collagen developed?

In the early 1970s, a group of biochemists and physicians at Stanford University were researching alternatives to skin grafts. In the course of this work they developed the concept of purifying animal collagen so thoroughly that it could be used to replace lost skin tissue. Further research by Collagen Corporation led to the development of **Zyderm** and **Zyplast** Collagen Implants.

How long has injectable collagen been used?

Injectable collagen was first used to treat patients in 1976. Since then, over 500,000 people have been treated with either **Zyderm** or **Zyplast** Collagen Implants. The procedure is administered routinely by over 3,500 physicians nationally, and in more than 20 other countries.

How do Zyderm Collagen and Zyplast Collagen work?

Both **Zyderm** and **Zyplast** Collagen Implants lend additional support to the collagen network within the skin. When a physician injects small amounts of either material directly into areas where the body's own collagen has been weakened, depressions can be raised to the level of the surrounding skin. Thus, lines and scars can be minimized, texture is improved, and the skin has a softer and more even tone.

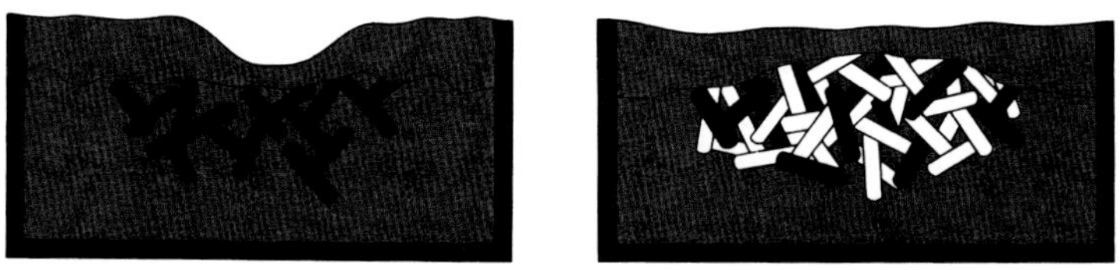

■ The body's collagen □ Injectable collagen

How does Zyderm Collagen differ from Zyplast Collagen?

Zyderm Collagen was formulated especially for people with small or superficial contour problems. It can be particularly effective in smoothing delicate frown and smile lines, as well as the fine creases that develop at the corners of the eyes and above and below the lips. It can also help correct certain kinds of shallow scars.

Zyplast Collagen was designed to treat depressions requiring a stronger material. It is used for more pronounced contour problems (such as deeper scars, lines, and furrows) and for areas upon which more force is being exerted (such as the corners of the mouth).

Zyderm and **Zyplast** Collagen Implants may be used alone or in conjunction with one another. Your physician will determine the potential benefits of each and an appropriate course of treatment.

Which skin depressions cannot be helped by either material?

Depressions with sharp edges and narrow "ice pick" acne scars do not usually respond to these materials.

Should injectable collagen take the place of surgical procedures such as face-lifts and dermabrasion?

No. Injectable collagen treatments are not meant for people who have excess facial skin or for those who want a major resurfacing of the skin. However, doctors often use **Zyderm** or **Zyplast** Collagen Implants in conjunction with surgery to fill in depressions not amenable to surgery. By using injectable collagen following a face-lift or dermabrasion, surgical results can be enhanced.

How do collagen creams differ from injectable collagen?

Regardless of the ingredients, moisturizers work only on the skin's surface as a temporary cap to help retain water. **Zyderm** and **Zyplast** Collagen Implants, however, are medical products that are injected below the skin's surface where contour problems begin and where collagen replacement can help.

Can anyone be treated with Zyderm Collagen or Zyplast Collagen Implants?

No. Your doctor will inquire about your medical history and administer a skin test to determine if you are an appropriate candidate for treatment. If you have a history of allergy to other bovine (cow) collagen products, severe allergies (indicated by a history of anaphylaxis [shock], or a history of presence of multiple severe allergies), if you are *currently* on corticosteroid or immunosuppressive therapy, e.g., prednisone, or are undergoing or planning to undergo desensitization injections to meat products, you cannot receive injectable collagen. Also, people who are sensitive to lidocaine cannot receive collagen implants, as a small amount of this anesthetic is contained in **Zyderm** and **Zyplast** Collagen Implants, and in the Collagen Test Implant. Furthermore, people who have had a previous allergic reaction to either **Zyderm** or **Zyplast** Collagen may not be re-treated. Neither **Zyderm** nor **Zyplast** Collagen Implant should be used for breast augmentation, and neither material should be injected into bone, tendon, ligament or muscle.

If you have a personal history of autoimmune disease which includes (but is not limited to) rheumatoid arthritis, psoriatic arthritis, scleroderma (including CREST syndrome), systemic or discoid lupus erythematosus, or polymyositis, a dietary allergy to beef, or if you have *recently* been on corticosteroid or immunosuppressive therapy, your physician may want to administer additional skin tests before deciding if you should be treated.

If you have any questions about these medical conditions, be sure to discuss them with your doctor. You will also be skin tested prior to treatment. Anyone who exhibits a sensitivity to the material, as demonstrated by the skin test, cannot proceed with treatment.

What is involved in injectable collagen treatment?

There are three steps: a skin test, the treatment series, and periodic touch-ups.

How does the skin test work?

To determine if you are eligible for treatment with either **Zyderm** or **Zyplast** Collagen Implant, your doctor will inject a small amount of collagen into your forearm, just below the skin's surface. Both you and your doctor should watch the test site closely for four weeks for any signs of sensitivity to the material such as redness, swelling, or itching. Pay special attention to your test site during the first three days since the majority of test reactions occur during this period. At the first sign of any of these problems, contact your doctor.

Only about three out of every 100 tested patients show a sensitivity to the test and cannot be treated with injectable collagen; 97 percent of all tested patients can be treated.

When does treatment start?

Treatment can begin after the four-week test observation period if you are not sensitive to the skin test. Treatment involves a series of office visits – usually two weeks apart. Most patients see considerable improvement in one to three treatment sessions depending on the size, shape, and texture of the area undergoing treatment.

Do the injections hurt?

You may find that the injections are somewhat uncomfortable, particularly around the nose or lips. However, both **Zyderm** and **Zyplast** Collagen Implants contain a small amount of lidocaine that helps numb the area temporarily, and most people report that the injections are relatively painless.

How will my skin look and feel *immediately* after treatment?

Most patients feel comfortable in resuming their normal activities following treatment. Temporary puffiness of the treated areas, however, should be expected, especially with **Zyderm** Collagen Implant.

With both **Zyderm** and **Zyplast** Collagen Implants, you may also notice temporary blushing, slight bruising, and tenderness around the treatment sites. Like the puffiness, these are normal occurrences and all should subside within a few days. Although the material is generally not visibly distinguishable from the surrounding skin, some patients have reported that they were initially able to feel the outline of the injected collagen.

However, as the new collagen is incorporated into your own skin, the treatment site takes on the natural look and feel of healthy skin. Any redness and/or visible swelling that persists for more than a few days may indicate a reaction to the material.
Be sure to report this or any other questionable symptoms to your doctor.

How common are treatment reactions?

With more than 500,000 people treated to date, only a small number of patients (approximately 1-2 percent) have developed an allergic reaction after one or more treatment injections. These reactions may consist of prolonged redness, swelling, itching and/or firmness at some or all injection sites. Most have lasted between three and four months, but in some cases have exceeded one year.

In less than 1% of treated patients, formation of a scab and sloughing (shedding) of the tissue at the treatment site have been noted, which can result in a shallow scar. On rare occasions, abscess formation has occurred at implantation sites. These reactions develop weeks to months following injections, and may result in induration and/or scar formation.

Also, in fewer than 2 per 1000 treated patients, the following have been reported: systemic complaints such as flu-like symptoms (nausea, fever, dizziness, headache, malaise, joint aches), rash, blurred vision, tingling, numbness or difficulty in breathing.

Of the patients who have developed an allergic reaction after treatment, one-half had an unreported or unrecognized response to the skin test. **With proper monitoring of the skin test, many of these reactions could have been prevented.** The remaining one-half of this group developed allergic reactions despite a response-free skin test.

An additional one percent of individuals experience symptoms similar to those of an allergic reaction that may, however, occur periodically. Recent research has shown that some of these patients are allergic to bovine collagen.

If you observe any symptoms such as redness and/or swelling, please inform your physician. He or she will determine if you should discontinue treatment; no further injectable collagen can be administered to anyone who has experienced an allergic reaction to the material.

Are there any other types of reactions I should be aware of?

Yes. There is a possibility that you could experience a reaction related to the injection process itself. However, this does not mean it is necessary to discontinue treatment. For instance, mild bruising or a slight blush could occur at the injection site. If you have previously had facial herpes simplex at the site of injection, there is a chance that the injection process itself could provoke another herpes simplex eruption. If you are using aspirin or non-steroidal anti-inflammatory drugs that reduce coagulation, you may experience increased bruising or bleeding at injection sites. In addition, any injection carries a small risk of infection.

Some physicians have reported the occurrence of connective tissue diseases such as rheumatoid arthritis, systemic lupus erythematosus, dermatomyositis (DM), and polymyositis (PM) subsequent to collagen injections, in patients with no previous history of these disorders. Statistical analysis comparing the number of collagen treated patients who were diagnosed with two rare connective tissue diseases (PM)/(DM) with the expected number of these diseases, suggests that the rate of occurrence of these two rare diseases appears to be higher than expected in the collagen treated population. However, a causal (cause and effect) relationship between collagen injection and the onset of autoimmune disease or systemic connective tissue disease has not been established.

Also, an increased incidence of cell-mediated and humoral immunity to various collagens have been found in systemic connective tissue diseases such as rheumatoid arthritis, juvenile rheumatoid arthritis, and progressive systemic sclerosis (scleroderma). Patients with these diseases may thus have an increased susceptibility to an allergic response and/or accelerated clearance of their implants when injected with bovine dermal collagen preparations. If you have any of these diseases, you should discuss this specifically with your doctor.

It is possible that, during the process of administering injectable collagen, the needle could be accidentally placed into or through a blood vessel. This has been reported to have occurred in less than 1% of patients treated. However, if it should happen, it could result in temporary discoloration of the treated area and/or formation of a scab, and sloughing (shedding) of this tissue at the treatment site can result in a shallow scar. Also, as with other substances that are injected (particularly local anesthetics and steroids injected into the head and neck area or the extremities), there is a remote possibility of accidental injection of the material into a blood vessel. This could result in blockage of the blood flow and loss of circulation to nearby sites, which in one case resulted in permanent loss of vision in one eye.

There have been infrequent reports of the injected collagen being visible in the skin, in the form of a small raised or white area at the treatment site, which may persist from a few weeks to several months. Also, some areas (such as compressed scars) resist precise placement of the material, resulting in a slight elevation beside the defect.

An understanding of the safety of injectable collagen is based on clinical data from 1978 to the present. Ongoing research will continue to provide more information.

Does the correction last forever?

No. Touch-up injections are usually needed to maintain maximum correction. Because both **Zyderm** and **Zyplast** Collagen Implants are similar to your own skin, they will be altered by the same ongoing mechanical forces such as smiling or other muscle activity and biochemical processes – such as aging and active acne – that caused the original skin depressions. It has been reported that the body may deposit its own collagen at the site of collagen implantation. You should therefore be aware that part or all of the correction may last for 2 years or longer.

How often will I need a "touch-up" injection?

Most patients who choose to receive touch-ups for lines or furrows do so within 3 to 12 months of the original treatment series. For scars, and perhaps those depressions treated with **Zyplast** Collagen, the time between touch-ups may be longer. But keep in mind that the amount of collagen used to restore full correction will be considerably less than that used in the initial treatment series.

Without touch-up injections, how will my skin look?

Correction may subside gradually until your skin looks like it did before treatment.

Touch-up injections will help you maintain your correction and can provide a long-term solution to skin contour problems.

For further information write:
Customer Relations
Collagen Corporation
1850 Embarcadero Road
Palo Alto, CA 94303

or call:
Toll-free (800) 227-4004
In Alaska call collect (415) 856-0200
In Canada call 1-(800) 227-4004

APPENDIX 2: RECORD OF CONSULTATION

I have read the brochure titled "Zyderm® Collagen and Zyplast® Collagen Explained" in its entirety and have discussed the risks and benefits of injectable collagen treatment with my physician or his/her representative. I understand the information provided.

____

(patient's signature)

____

(date)

I have discussed the risks and benefits of injectable collagen treatment with this patient, have answered his/her questions, and find him/her an appropriate candidate for test and treatment with injectable collagen.

____

(signature of physician or physician's representative)

____

(date)

[NOTE: Sign, remove, and file in patient record]

12

Structural Lipoaugmentation

Lisa M. Donofrio
Yale University School of Medicine, New Haven, Connecticut

INTRODUCTION

Structural lipoaugmentation is a specific technique for the harvesting of viable fat cells and their transplantation into recipient tissues. The cardinal principles involve the use of lipocytes to correct the loss of support of deep structures that commonly occurs with aging. Typically this involves atraumatic harvesting of autologous fat, and takes into account proper placement to ensure longevity of the fat graft and restore structural integrity to the recipient tissues. The history of lipoaugmentation is a long and tortuous one with many variations in techniques and results. The concept of restoring integral structure to the senescent face was first introduced by Fournier [1], but the majority of contributions have been made by Sidney Coleman and his Lipostructure® technique [2]. Structural lipoaugmentation is the compilation of many years of clinical observations and scientific correlations. It is a new standard in autologous fat transfer.

To fully understand the goal of structural augmentation, one must understand the atrophic changes that occur in the aging face. In youth, the soft tissues of the face are full and contiguous. There is a thick subcutaneous layer of fat and an even, ample distribution of the deeper fat pads. The jawline is full and round, the temples flat, and the periorbital area devoid of bony landmarks. In particular, the cheek is arced from the tarsus to the anterior jawline because of the abundance of malar and buccal fat. With aging, the subcutaneous fat diminishes diffusely, which leads to a demarcation of deeper landmarks [3,4]. The temporal, buccal, and malar fat pads diminish or change position and shape [5–7]. Loss of dentition causes bony erosion of the alveolar ridges and diminution of the height of the maxilla and mandible [8,9]. With advanced age, there is facial muscle atrophy and loss of muscle function of the orbicularis and masseter muscles [10]. Together these changes lead to an internal shrinkage of the foundation of the face and a relative excess of skin. Traditional facelift procedures ignore this dictum and stretch an already thin cutis over a bony framework, which produces a "skeletonized" face. More progressive facelift and blepharoplasty techniques acknowledge the importance of the facial fat compartments and reposition remaining fat over bony prominences [11–15]. Although the results are fuller and softer than with standard superficial musculo-aponeurotic system (SMAS) and skin envelope tightening procedures, they still carry with them the morbidity and scars common to all rhytidectomies and are again ignoring the true pathology of the aging face (Fig. 1).

The rationale for using autologous fat as a filler is plentiful: it is a readily available, nonallergenic substance that has the ability to "age" with the patient. Synthetic implants, although addressing the need for structural augmentation, may exacerbate the compartmentalization of the aging face, thereby causing sharp angles and valleys (Fig. 2). Autologous fat, when placed correctly, has the ability to diffusely fill and contour without lines of demarcation. It allows the dermatologic surgeon to be a sculptor, all at once changing and rejuvenating the aging face.

INDICATIONS FOR STRUCTURAL AUGMENTATION

In addition to restoring fullness to the aging face, structural augmentation may be used to correct liposuction defects, replenish fat loss secondary to facial hemiatropy syndromes and morphea, and for cosmetic enhancement in young patients desiring fuller lips or more prominent chins. It is an excellent way to correct the soft-tissue atrophy that occurs in acne scarring and can compliment resurfacing procedures used in that deformity. Traumatic atrophic scars and sunken skin grafts can also often benefit from this type of structural enhancement; however, "bound down" scars, ice pick scars, and poorly vascularized areas in general respond poorly.

PATIENT SELECTION

All patients can benefit from this procedure for the reasons previously mentioned; however, there are patients in whom the results are consistently dramatic. In general, nonsmokers who have maintained a stable, close-to-ideal body weight throughout life with early atrophic changes prove to be the best candidates. The senescent face displays topography of hills and valleys. It appears that the aging process causes specific areas of deep facial fat to selectively atrophy. This shrinkage commonly occurs in the buccal area, premalar area, lateral jawline, and supraorbital, temporal, premaxillary, and central chin areas. In contrast, persistence of fat is universally seen in the medial jawline (jowl area), lower medial cheek, medial upper eyelid, and suborbital area (Fig. 3). It is then understood why overweight patients display an even greater disparity between these areas and may need substantial augmentation of the "valleys" to bring them level with the "hills." In addition, the overweight patient may find the atrophy in the buccal area a desirable respite from a long-standing round-cheeked appearance and could in fact benefit from a facelift and suction procedure. Because the goal of structural fat transplantation is to effect a permanent change in the facial contour, the procedure is dependent on the ability of the transplanted fat to survive in the donor tissue. In the cases of advance aging, the atrophy may be so severe that it becomes difficult to find tissue with enough integrity to anchor the fat graft. This, in addition to the decreased cutaneous blood flow seen in advanced aging (and smoking), make this patient population less-than-ideal candidates [16].

PREOPERATIVE INSTRUCTIONS

Patients who smoke should refrain from smoking for 2 days prior to and 1 week after the procedure. Nonsteroidal, anti-inflammatory agents and Vitamin E supple-

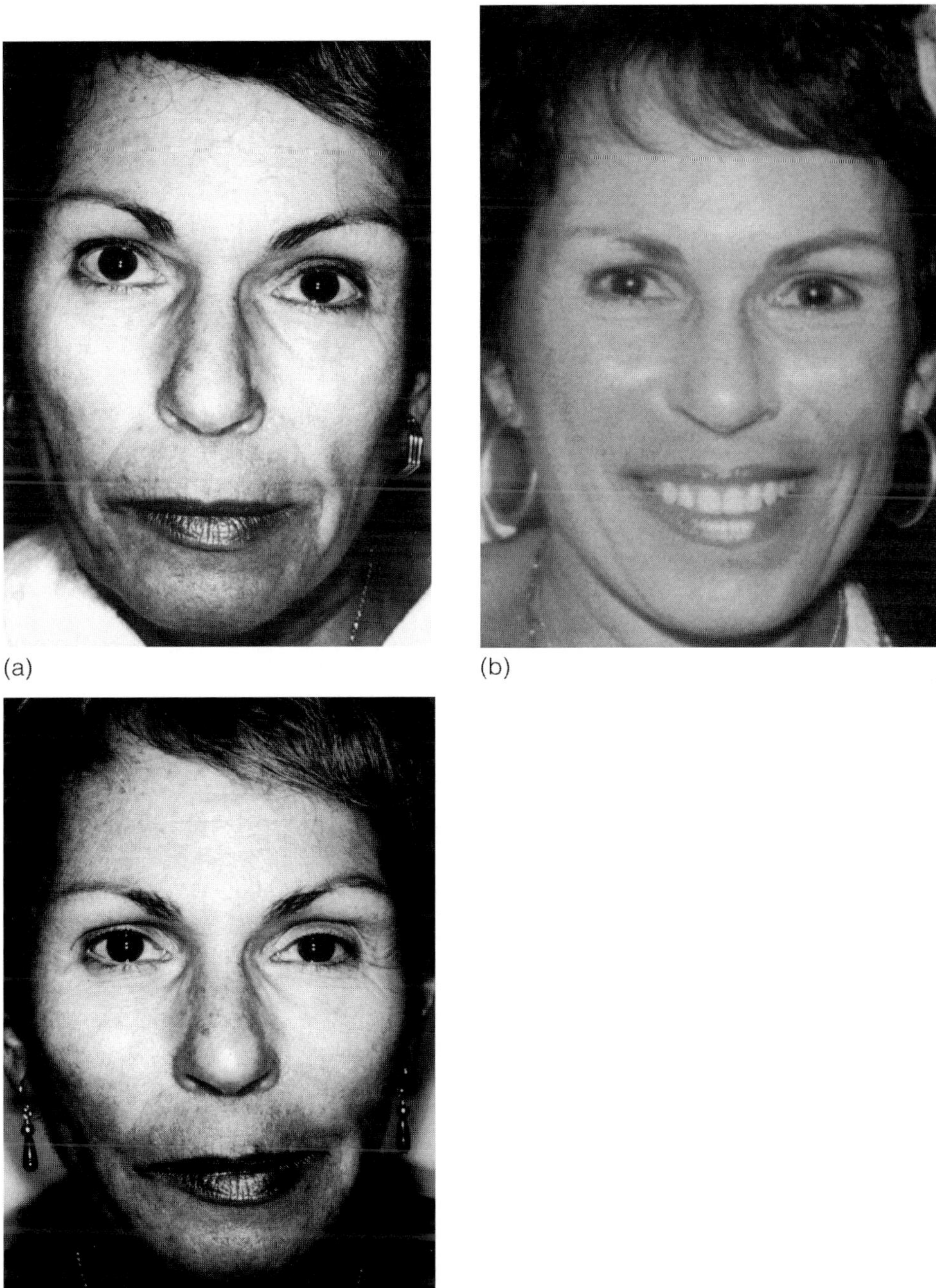

(a) (b) (c)

FIGURE 1 (a) 57-year-old female with significant atrophic changes leading to sunken appearance and relative skin excess. (b) Same patient age 44. (c) After five sessions of structural lipoaugmentation. Face lift procedure in this patient would have accentuated her bony framework. Replacing fullness makes her look more like she used to.

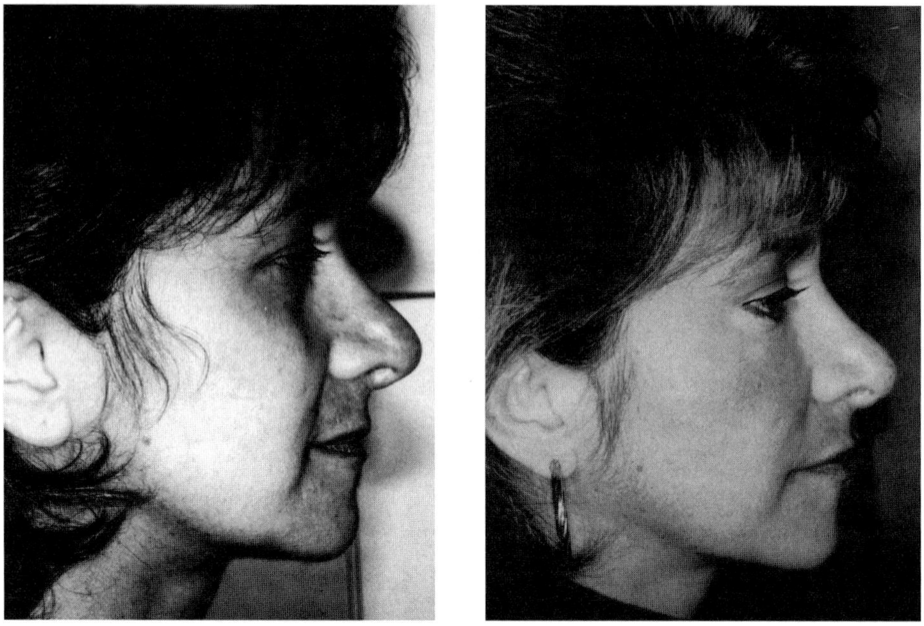

(a) (b)

FIGURE 2 (a) 44-year-old female with orbital hollow and accentuated angularity of cheek secondary to malar implants. (b) Same patient after structural lipoaugmentation. Note fullness in periorbital area and restoration of youthful arc of cheek.

ments are to be avoided starting 1 week before the surgery and continuing for 3 days after. Beginning the day before the procedure, azithromycin 500 mg is taken as a single dose and continued at a dose of 250 mg a day for the next 4 days. Patients with a history of oral herpes simplex virus who will be undergoing an aggressive perioral transfer should be prophylaxed with valcyclovir 500 mg twice a day starting the day before the procedure and continuing for 6 days afterward. Patients with a history of easy bruisability may warrant a coagulation profile and prechilling of the face with ice before the transfer. Anxious patients should be offered diazepam 5 to 10 mg orally one half hour before the procedure.

EXTRACTION TECHNIQUE

Selection of the donor site is from an area where the patient can benefit aesthetically, and should include, if possible, fat from the lateral thigh and/or buttocks. Studies have shown the lipogenic activity to be the greatest from these regions, and fat extracted from these areas appears to contain less fibrous cellular debris than abdominal fat [17–19]. However, in some patients, either the lack of peripheral fat stores or their lean body habitus make this site selection nearly impossible. In male patients, the flank area, although excessively fibrous, often proves to be the only accessible fat.

Fat is extracted with as little manual and chemical insult as possible. A dilute tumescent anesthetic solution in Ringers lactate is preferred over normal saline (Table

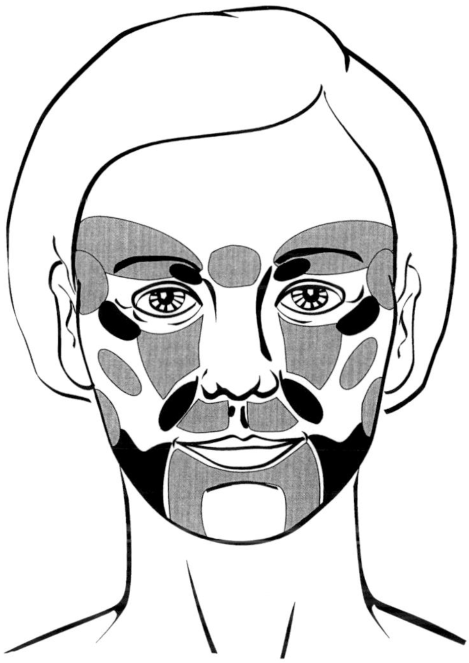

FIGURE 3 Solid markings represent areas prone to fat atrophy and collapse with aging. Shaded markings represent areas of persistent or hypertrophic aging changes.

1). Under sterile conditions, the donor area is tumesced until turgid. After waiting 20 minutes for the epinephrine to take effect, the extraction may proceed. Entry sites are placed in easily accessible areas and made with either an 18 g Nocor or a 1.5 mm punch. A 3 mm open cobra tipped cannula with a Luer Lok adjustment is attached to a 10 ml syringe (Fig. 4). The open tip and large diameter ensure that the lipocytes can fit through the opening in intact cylinders of fatty tissue. Fat obtained in this manner has shown an increased long-term survival after transplantation [20,21]. Care is taken to exert only minimal negative pressures when extracting by manually pulling the plunger back only 1 ml at a time. Locking mechanisms can generate large negative pressures and should not be used. It has been noted that adipocytes extracted at −1 atm of pressure (the pressure traditionally generated from a liposuction machine) are abnormally distended and possibly more prone to lysis [22]. Total volumes extracted will depend on availability of fat and estimated trans-

TABLE 1 Modified Klein Solution for Tumescent Anesthesia

1 L Lactated Ringer's solution
500 mg lidocaine
1 mg epinephrine
12.5 mg sodium bicarbonate

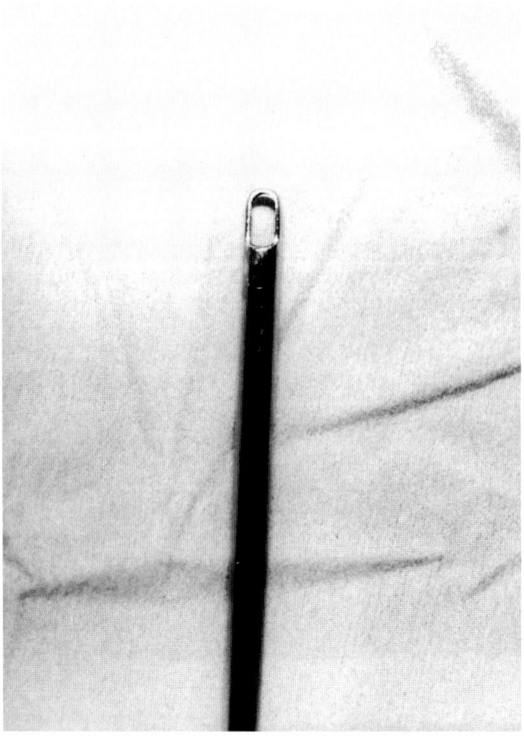

FIGURE 4 Luer Lok extraction cannula with open tip. (Byron, Tucson, AZ.)

plant volumes. In general, if fat is to be frozen and stored for sequential transplantation, a total of 100 to 150 ml of fat should be removed.

RECIPIENT SITE PREPARATION

It is often helpful to have the patient bring in photographs of themselves when they were young. By critically studying the changes that have occurred with aging, the surgeon can often see the obvious areas of atrophy. If the patient presents with exaggerated nasolabial folds and a "droopy" lower face it is instructive to manually suspend the cheek, thereby simulating the result of enhancement in this area (Fig. 5). The areas to be augmented are then shaded in with a washable marker and the face prepped with an antibacterial preparation or wash. Every surgeon will find his or her best method of encrypting the patient's face before augmentation.

RECIPIENT SITE ANESTHESIA

The infraorbital and mental nerves are blocked via the intraoral route. Topical anesthetic is applied with a cotton swab to the upper and lower anterior labial vestibule, and when adequate topical anesthesia is achieved, 1 to 2 ml of lidocaine 1% with epinephrine is infiltrated, keeping in the mid pupillary line. This effectively provides

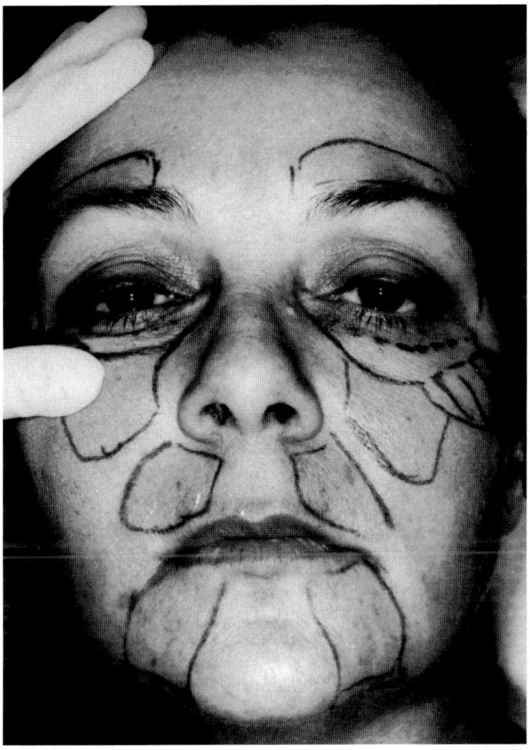

FIGURE 5 Amelioration of the nasolabial fold by suspension of the cheek manually is a good indicator that cheek atrophy has occurred.

anesthesia for the mid portion of the face. Supraorbital and supratrochlear blocks may also be performed for the forehead, or the area can be infiltrated locally. Areas that fall outside designated block sites have to be locally anesthetized. Incision sites are planned with easy access in mind and are best made with an 18 gauge Nocor needle. Additional local anesthesia at sites of planned incisions keeps bleeding to a minimum. These heal undetectably in a few days and are easily covered with make-up in the early postsurgical period.

PREPARATION OF THE FAT

The adipose tissue collected in the 10 ml syringes is kept under sterile conditions and is briefly centrifuged in sterilized central sleeves at 3300 rpm for 20 to 30 seconds (Fig. 6). This allows adequate time for separation into three distinct layers: the bottom layer of blood and tumescent fluid, middle layer of concentrated fatty tissue, and top layer of triglycerides from ruptured adipocytes (Fig. 7). Centrifugation for longer than 30 seconds is unnecessary and may in fact destroy the adipose cells [23]. The lowermost fluid layer is decanted off and a female-female adapter is placed on the Luer Lok apparatus. The compact adipose portion is then transferred to 1 ml syringes for augmentation (Fig. 8). Care is taken to stop short of the triglyceride

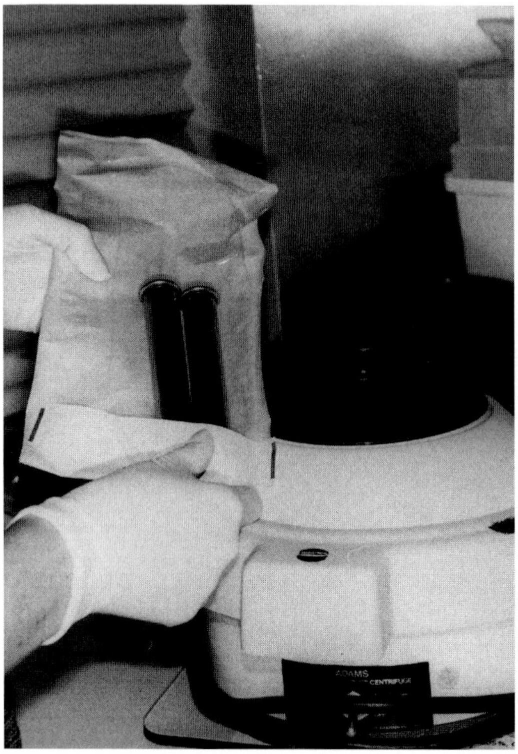

FIGURE 6 Centrifuge with sterilized stainless steel sleeves.

layer. The procedure is performed using only 1 ml syringes, thereby guaranteeing greater control over injected volumes and low injection pressures.

TRANSPLANTATION TECHNIQUE

At designated entry sites, small incisions are made with an 18 gauge Nocor needle (Fig. 9). Sterile technique is always observed and the tip of the infiltrator kept from contamination at all times. All transplantation is with a blunt infiltrator with an internal diameter of at least 18 gauges (Fig. 10). The blunt tip ensures that the recipient tissue is pushed aside rather than cored out. It also lessens the chance of vessel trauma, intravascular injection, and perforation. In all areas, the infiltrator advances through the recipient tissues at the lowest point structurally. In the malar, orbital, and jawline this means depositing the fat as close to bone as possible. Subsequent passes are made in higher planes until a final pass is placed in the dermis. The fat is deposited in 0.1 ml aliquots in the withdrawal phase of the movement only. If any significant resistance is encountered the infiltrator is withdrawn and cleared. Care is taken to only place the fat in virgin tunnels. It is very important to the longevity of the adipose graft for each 0.1 ml aliquot to be within 1.5 mm of direct contact with vascularized recipient tissue [24–27]. This is best achieved by depositing the fat in controlled linear streaks, avoiding globbing and lumping of fat.

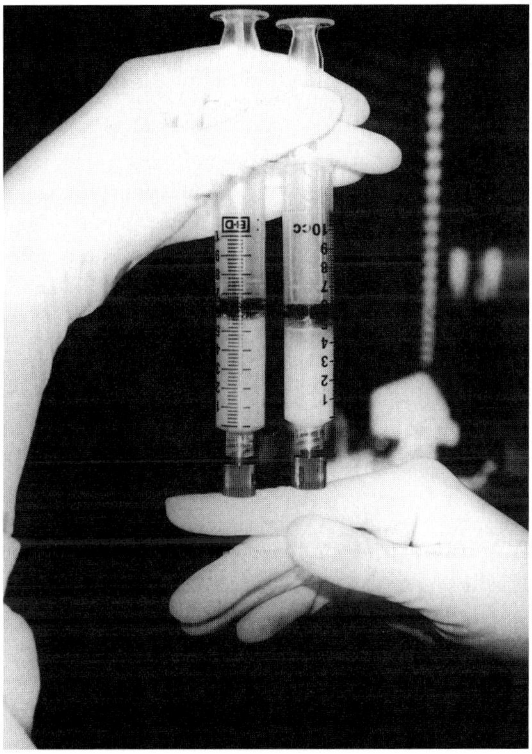

FIGURE 7 After decantation of infranate. Both syringes originally contained 6 ml of fat. Specimen on right has been centrifuged for 20 seconds at 3000 rpm. Notice compaction of intact cells and separation of triglyceride supranate.

To avoid infection, the lip should be treated last and the infiltrator changed should any frank contamination occur.

PERIORAL INFILTRATION

The nasolabial and melolabial creases define the perioral region. Atrophy of the lips and chin recede these areas, leading to prominence of the delineating folds. Incisions are best placed just lateral to the chin, at the base of the nasolabial folds, and in the oral commisure. From the mental incision, fat is woven in a superiolateral direction starting closest to bone and working up through to dermis. From this incision the lateral corners of the mouth can be accessed and lifted. By placing parcels of fat perpendicular to the marionette lines, the structural integrity of this area is regained and the fat is anchored and unable to migrate with mouth movements. This also provides access for central chin and jawline augmentation. In most patients, the lateral chin can hold no more than 2 to 3 ml of fat before passes have to be reintroduced into existing tunnels. Senile atrophy of the chin is addressed by "hugging" the anterior mandible, medial to the retaining ligaments, and depositing the fat next to the bone on its anterior and inferior surfaces. The upper lip is best accessed from the nasolabial fold incision, fanning the fat out in the premaxillary area. Fat can also

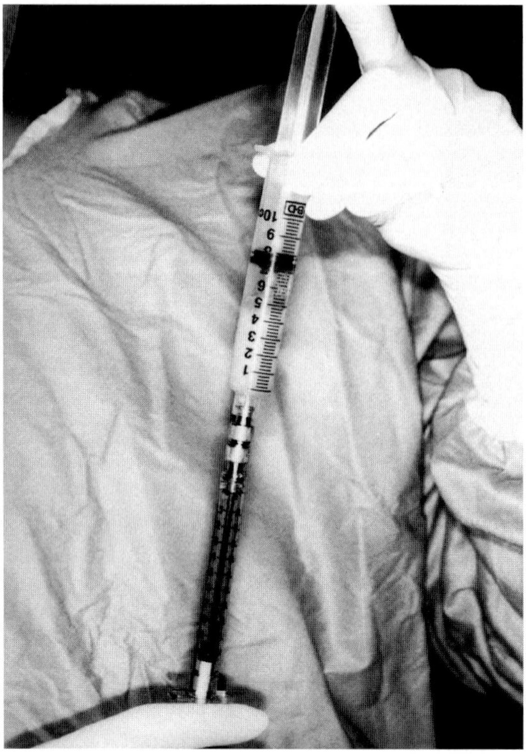

FIGURE 8 Female-female adapter is used to transfer fat to 1 ml syringes.

be placed adjacent to the fold, again in a weaving motion starting deep and ending at the surface. The nasolabial fold and premaxillary space can usually hold 2 to 3 ml of fat when placed in this manner. The mucosal lip should be the last area treated to avoid inadvertent contamination with oral bacteria. To efface the mucosa and get more vertical lip show, the incision should be just inferior to the vermilion at the upper oral commisure. The fat is placed deep to the undersurface of the mucosa starting high in the interior of the lip. Fat is deposited in an inferioanterior direction until the desired effacement is achieved. Because of the profound edema encountered postoperatively in this area, no more than 1 ml should be placed in each side. To accentuate the white roll and smooth out vertical lip rhytides, a Tuohy anesthesia needle, bevel facing posteriorly, can be threaded through the vermilion border and 0.1 to 0.3 ml of fat deposited on withdrawal. The lower lip is treated in a similar fashion according to the desires of the patient.

MANDIBULAR INFILTRATION

The angle of the mandible weakens with aging. It is often desirable to strengthen the line of the jaw when rejuvenating the rest of the face (Fig. 11). Preoperatively the areas of atrophy should be marked. They usually occur immediately posterior to the jowl area. One to 2 ml of fat can be placed starting close to the inferior surface of the bone and working up through to the surface. This is again performed by

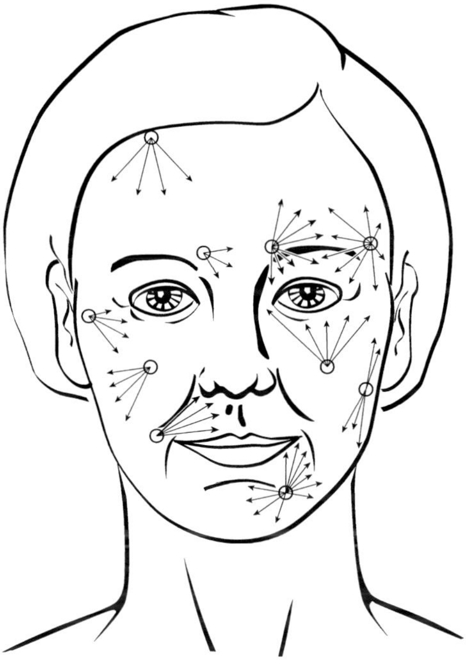

FIGURE 9 Suggested incision sites and direction of infiltration.

placing fat in 0.1 ml aliquots, trying for only virgin tunnels on each pass. Fat is placed deep moving up closer to the dermis with successive passes.

CHEEK INFILTRATION

There are two areas on the cheek that benefit from structural enhancement: the malar fat pad, which encompasses the "apple" of the cheek to the malar eminence, and the area of the buccal fat pad. The malar fat pad is perhaps the most significant area to change shape during aging. The lateral malar area is often persistent or even hypertrophic. Placing fat around this tenacious deposit can camouflage it and restore the full arc to the midface (Fig. 11). Fat in this area can be placed deep onto the body of the zygoma medially and advanced laterally and superiorly to suspend the midface. The cheek in its entirety can hold 3 to 5 ml of fat when placed correctly. In the buccal area, fat can only be placed subcutaneously and commonly fills in with 2 to 3 ml total volume.

PERIORBITAL INFILTRATION

The suborbital space should be filled at the same time as the cheek to give continuity to these areas. Fat is first placed in "beads" along the anterior portion of the bony suborbit advancing superiorly from an incision in the midcheek. The nondominant hand is used to palpate the placement along the wall of the orbital rim from medial to lateral. This area will need 1 to 2 ml of fat to substantially elevate the rim. By advancing the orbital rim anteriorly, one can change the relationship between the

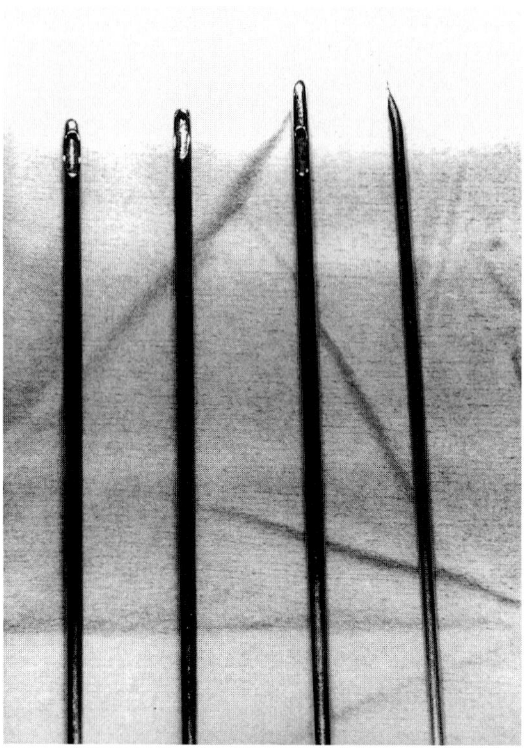

FIGURE 10 Blunt infiltrators. From left to right: Coleman I, Coleman II (Byron, Tucson, AZ), Modified Capistrano (Wells Johnson, Tucson, AZ) 18 g Tuohy epidural needle.

cheek and the suborbital area (Fig. 12). The tear trough, if shadowed, can also be augmented from this angle. Switching to a lateral approach, fat is then placed directly under the thin skin of the eyelid. Extreme care must be taken to ensure that tiny, even strands of fat are deposited in this area. A blunt cannula with a spatulate tip is helpful in obtaining the correct level of placement. Never should more than 1 ml of fat be infiltrated in this area unless the physician is extremely comfortable with the technique. From the lateral incision, the lateral orbital rim may be treated to attenuate "crow's feet." This can then be advanced to the inferior temple. Fat here is again placed bluntly in a deep bony plane to completely fill in the area of temporal atrophy. Another incision in the temple can then be placed for access to the supraorbital rim. Fat in this area is placed as close to the superior orbital bone as possible, using it as an anchoring plane. In this manner, fat is woven into the areas inferior and superior to the brow. Many patients display prominent atrophy in the medial superior sulcus, and this can be filled with a more medial direct approach. Filling the lid and brow in this way will redrape the eyelid and smooth out the redundant folds (Fig. 13).

FOREHEAD INFILTRATION

Because of the instability of fat placed against the areolar plane, fat in the forehead should be placed in a subcutaneous plane only. By diffusely filling the forehead with

for permanent augmentation [34,41–44]. In addition, fat cell viability has been shown after thawing frozen samples [41] (R. Alexander, personal communication, 1998). Fat should be stored in the original 10 ml syringes after centrifugation and decanting of the infranate. The triglyceride layer should remain as the supranate. It probably has cryoprotective effects that allow the fat to freeze evenly and slowly. Specimens must be meticulously labeled with patient's full name and social security number and date of procedure. They should then be placed in labeled freezer bags and stored at −30°C. The specimen freezer should have a digital readout and be equipped with an alarm that sounds when the temperature rises. The alarm can be hooked up with the office central alarm system, and if there is a temperature increase during off hours the physician can be called at home. Some may find it necessary to include in the informed consent absolution from any equipment failure or power outage. Generator backup is warranted in busy practices. On the day of "touch-up" procedures, the patients are asked to identify their name and social security number; this information is checked against the specimen label and initialed by the nurse and patient. The label taken off the syringe is then placed in the chart as part of the medical documentation of the procedure. The fat is defrosted by placing the syringes into a sterile glove and having the patients hold them close to their body. After about 10 minutes, the adipocytes are then transferred to 1 ml syringes, stopping short of the defrosted triglyceride layer, and the same guidelines on placement as previously mentioned adhered to. The surgeon and patient may choose to limit the touch-up to certain areas or lesser volumes. Because storage has contaminated the outside of the syringe, extreme care must be taken to keep the infiltrator tip sterile and uncontaminated. The operator should never touch the tip or shaft of the blunt infiltrator. It is usually not necessary for intramuscular cortisone administration after a minor touch-up, nor is it necessary for prophylactic antibiotics except in the cases where gross contamination has occurred. Most patients can benefit from regularly scheduled touch-up procedures at 4 to 8 week intervals over the course of a year. Frozen fat has been stored for up to 2 years with successful uncomplicated transplantation [43]; however, the optimal time to store fat is unknown.

CONCLUSIONS

Atrophic changes in facial structure lead to an excess of the skin envelope. Pulling the skin tightly over the bony skeleton does not reproduce the fullness associated with the youthful face.

Structural autologous lipoaugmentation is a safe and effective technique to achieve dramatic filling of the aging face (Fig. 14). Longevity of transfer has been well documented and seems to be largely technique dependent. Atraumatic collection principles, low injection pressures, and carefully placed small aliquots of fat are necessary for viability of the transplanted tissue. Frozen fat is a convenient way to perform additional touch-up procedures and may in fact prove to be superior in the long run.

REFERENCES

1. Fournier PF. Facial recountouring with fat grafting. Dermatol Clin 8(3):523–537, 1990.
2. Coleman SR. Facial recontouring with liposculpture. Clin Plast Surg 24(2):347–367, 1997.

3. Gonzalez-Ulloa M, Flores E. Senility of the face—basic study to understand its causes and effects. Plast Reconstr Surg 36(2):239–246, 1965.
4. de la Plaza R, de la Cruz L. Can some facial rejuvenation techniques cause iatrogenia? Aesthet Plast Surg 18(2):205–209, 1994.
5. Yousif NJ. Changes of the midface with age. Clin Plast Surg 22(2):213–226, 1995.
6. Yousif NJ, Gosain A, Sanger JR, Larson DL, Matloub HS. The nasolabial fold a photogrammetic analysis. Plast Reconstr Surg 93(1):70–77, 1994.
7. Gosain A, Amarante MTJ, Hyde JS, Yousif NJ. A dynamic analysis of changes in the nasolabial fold using magnetic resonance imaging: implications for facial rejuvenation and facial animation surgery. Plast Reconstr Surg 94(4):622–636, 1996.
8. Bartlett SP, Grossman R, Whitaker LA. Age-related changes of the craniofacial skeleton: an anthropometric and histologic analysis. Plast Reconstr Surg 90(4):592–600, 1992.
9. Adams D. Age change in oral structures. Dental Update 18(1):14–17, 1991.
10. Rastatter MP, McGuire RA, Bushong L, Loposky M. Speech motor equivalence in aging subjects. Percept Mot Skills 64(2):635–638, 1987.
11. Owsley JQ, Fiala TG. Update: lifting the malar fat pad for correction of prominent nasolabial folds. Plast Reconstr Surg 100(3):715–722, 1997.
12. Owsley JQ. Lifting the malar fat pad for correction of prominent nasolabial folds. Plast Reconstr Surg 91(3):463–476, 1993.
13. Owsley JQ. Elevation of the malar fat pad superficial to the orbicularis oculi muscle for correction of prominent nasolabial folds. Clin Plast Surg 22(2):279–293, 1995.
14. Hamra ST. Composite rhytidectomy and the nasolabial fold. Clin Plast Surg 22(2):313–323, 1995.
15. Lewis J. Augmentation blepharoplasty. Ann Plast Surg 21(5):434–438, 1988.
16. Smith JB, DeBenedette V. The extensive effects of smoking on the skin. Cosm Dermatol 9(11):24–26, 1996.
17. Hudson DA, Lambert EV, Bloch CE. Site selection for autotransplantation: some observations. Aesthet Plast Surg 14(3):195–197, 1990.
18. Lilleth H, Boberg J. The lipoprotein-lipase activity of adipose tissue from different sites in obese women and relationship to cell size. Int J Obes 2(1):47–52, 1978.
19. Arner P, Engfeldt P, Lithell H. Site differences in the basal metabolism of subcutaneous fat in obese women. J Clin Endocrinol Metab 53(5):948–952, 1981.
20. Moore JH, Kolaczynski JW, Morales LM, Considine RV, Pietrzkowski Z, Noto PF, Caro JF. Viability of fat obtained by syringe suction lipectomy: effects of local anesthesia with lidocaine. Aesthet Plast Surg 19(4):335–339, 1995.
21. Fagrell D, Enestrom S, Berggren A, Kniola B. Fat cylinder transplantation: an experimental comparative study of three different kinds of fat transplants. Plast Reconstr Surg 98(1):90–98, 1996.
22. Niechajev I, Sevcuk O. Long term results of fat transplantation: clinical and histologic studies. Plast Reconstr Surg 94(3):496–506, 1994.
23. Chajchir A, Benzaquen I, Moretti E. Comparative experimental study of autologous adipose tissue processed by different techniques. Aesthet Plast Surg 17(2):113–115, 1993.
24. Peer LA. The neglected free fat graft. Plast Reconstr Surg 18(4):233–250, 1956.
25. Carpeneda CA, Ribero MT. Study of the histologic alterations and viability of the adipose graft in humans. Aesthet Plast Surg 17(1):43–47, 1993.
26. Carpeneda CA, Ribero MT. Percentage of graft viability versus injected volume in adipose autotransplants. Aesthet Plast Surg 18(1):17–19, 1994.
27. Nguyen A, Pasyk KA, Bouvier TN, Hassett CA, Argenta LC. Comparative study of survival of autologous adipose tissue taken and transplanted by different techniques. Plast Reconstr Surg 85(3):378–386, 1990.

28. Coiffman F. Lipoinjection complications. In: Hinderer, ed. Plastic Surgery. Vol. 2. Amsterdam: Excerpta Medica, 1992, pp. 759–760.
29. Teimourian B. Blindness following fat injections (letter). Plast Reconstr Surg 82(2):361, 1988.
30. Dreizen NG, Framm L. Sudden unilateral visual loss after fat injection into the glabellar area. Am J Ophthalmol 107(1):85–87, 1989.
31. Egido JA, Arroyo R, Marcos A, Jimenez-Alfaro I. Middle cerebral artery embolism and unilateral visual loss after autologous fat injection into the glabellar area. Stroke 24(4): 615–616, 1993.
32. Coleman SR. Long term survival of fat transplants: controlled demonstrations. Aesthet Plast Surg 19:421–425, 1995.
33. Niechajev I, Sevcuk O. Long term results of fat transplantation: clinical and histologic studies. Plast Reconstr Surg 94(3):496–506, 1994.
34. Fulton J, Suarez M, Silverton K, Barnes T. Small volume fat transfer. J Dermatol Surg Oncol 24(8):857–865, 1998.
35. Matsudo PK, Toledo LS. Experience of injected fat grafting. Aesthet Plast Surg 12(1): 35–38, 1988.
36. Carraway JH, Mellow CG. Syringe aspiration and fat concentration: a simple technique for autologous fat injection. Ann Plast Surg 24(3):293–296, 1990.
37. Coleman WP III, Lawrence N, Sherman RN, Reed RJ, Pinski KS. Autologous collagen? Lipocytic dermal augmentation, a histopathologic study. J Dermatol Surg Oncol 19(11): 1032–1040, 1993.
38. Nguyen A, Pasyk KA, Bouvier TN, Hassett CA, Argenta LC. Comparative study of survival of autologous adipose tissue taken and transplanted by different techniques. Plast Reconstr Surg 85(3):378–386, 1990.
39. Chajchir A, Benzaquen I. Fat grafting injection for soft-tissue augmentation. Plast Reconstr Surg 84(6):921–934, 1989.
40. Billings E, May JW. Historical review and present status of free fat graft autotransplantation in plastic and reconstructive surgery. Plast Reconstr Surg 83(2):368–381, 1989.
41. Schuller-Petrovic S. Improving the aesthetic aspect of soft tissue defects on the face using autologous fat transplantation. Facial Plast Surg 13(2):19–24, 1997.
42. Wexler P. Presented at The World Congress on Liposuction Surgery, Pasadena, CA, October 9–11, 1998.
43. Sattler G, Sommer B. Liporecycling: immediate and delayed. Am J Cosmet Surg 14(3): 311–316, 1997.
44. Jackson RF. Frozen fat—does it work? Am J Cosmet Surg 14(3):339–343, 1997.

APPENDIX 1: INFORMED CONSENT AND PERMISSION FOR FAT TRANSFER (LIPOAUGMENTATION)

I, ______________________________ hereby authorize Dr. Lisa Donofrio and assistants to perform the following operation (s) / procedure (s) on me:
Fat removal from my ______________________ and / or transfer to my ______________________.

The nature and purpose of the operation (s) / procedure (s) as well as the therapeutic alternatives have been explained to me. No results have been guaranteed to me, and I understand that the filling achieved is occasionally temporary lasting 3-6 months. Dr. Donofrio or her agents have fully explained to me what will happen during the surgery and have answered all my questions. Specifically, the risks and / or complications of fat transfer surgery may include:

1) Persistence and / or recurrence of wrinkles or defects that are being augmented (filled).
2) Scar formation including both a depressed or raised (hypertrophic/keloidal) scar.
3) Bleeding, bruising and swelling.
4) Infection.
5) Discoloration including lighting or darkening of the skin.
6) Lumpiness or asymmetry in donor area as well as recipient site of transfer.
7) Allergic reaction to anesthetic solution

Side effects that have occurred as case reports in the scientific literature and would be extremely unlikely with Dr. Donofrio's technique include:

8) Nerve damage causing difficulty speaking or seeing.
9) Facial or eyelid droop.
10) Blindness.
11) Persistent numbness.
12) Parotid gland injury.

Dr. Donofrio has explained that the procedure works best and the results are the most satisfactory if I receive 6-12 treatments over the course of a year. I understand that each treatment will incur a separate additional charge.

______________________ ______________________
(Witness) (Patient signature)

______________________ ______________________
(Signature of person authorized to consent for patient) (Date) (Time)

13

Fat Transplantation and Autologous Collagen

Kevin S. Pinski
Northwestern University Medical School, Chicago, Illinois

INTRODUCTION

Aging of the face is influenced by loss of skin elasticity and by atrophy of subcutaneous fat. This results in loss of volume and fullness, which does not allow the skin to comfortably drape over the decreased facial framework, thus creating the illusion of facial sagging and wrinkling. Therefore, the answer to facial rejuvenation is not only skin resurfacing and/or tightening but also volume filling of the atrophied areas. In many cases, microlipoinjection may be the most sensible procedure to reverse some of the signs of aging.

Soft-tissue augmentation with adipose tissue has been used for many years. The more traditional approach has involved the placement of adipose tissue into the subcutis to correct cosmetic defects. More recently, constituents of this tissue have been used as a dermal filler substance termed "autologous collagen" or lipocytic dermal augmentation.

HISTORY

Fat transplantation surgery began almost a century ago when, in 1893, Neuber [1] reported on his technique of free-fat transplantation. He used 1 cm pieces of free fat from the upper arm to reconstruct depressed facial defects. In 1911, Bruning [2] reported the technique of fat injection. He placed small pieces of fat into a syringe and, by injecting this adipose tissue corrected postrhinoplasty deformities.

Free-fat transplants were largely neglected in the midtwentieth century because most surgeons preferred to use pedicle flaps. These preserved the blood supply to the fat, thereby making the outcome more predictable. In addition, artificial injectable substances such as paraffin and silicone became available and were used to fill defects in the skin. In 1950, Peer [3] reported a series of experiments with autologous human fat transplants in which over 50% of the fat remained as a viable transplant 1 year after grafting.

The current phase of fat transplantation began in 1976 when Fischer and Fischer [4] performed fat extraction with the cellusuctiotome. Two years later, Illouz

[5,6] introduced simplified instrumentation for the technique known today as liposuction. This new procedure provided the dermatologic surgeon with an abundant supply of viable adipose tissue that could be used to augment soft-tissue deformities.

Coincident with the appearance of liposuction surgery, there was a resurgence of interest in fat grafting as a natural mode of soft-tissue augmentation. Pierre Fournier pioneered a syringe-extraction fat-grafting technique called "microlipoinjection" [7]. Illouz reported a similar approach [8]. Microlipoinjection is currently performed as an outpatient surgical procedure for soft-tissue augmentation of the aging face and for minor contour defects.

Fournier soon began to experiment with other methods of soft-tissue transplantation [9]. He hypothesized that the extracted adipose tissue consisted of intracellular fat, adipocyte cell walls, and intercellular fibrous septae. He added distilled water to the extracted fatty tissue and then froze the mixture. Thawing caused the adipocytes to rupture and led to the production of an oily and solid fraction. The oily fraction contained intracellular triglycerides whereas the solid fraction consisted of cell walls and connective tissue. Decanting the oily fraction left supposedly collagen-rich autologous tissue suitable for soft-tissue injection. He referred to this tissue as "autologous collagen" [9]. He advocated freezing the unused portion for subsequent augmentation.

Recent histological and laboratory analyses have documented a small amount of actual collagen (<3%) in this collected tissue. Injections of this material into the dermis were shown to stimulate collagen production, thereby increasing dermal thickness [10]. In some ways, this is similar to the effects of microdroplet silicone and Fibrel [12,13]. However, because the tissue transplanted is autologous, there is no chance of an immune response to foreign tissue.

I have used Fournier's method since 1991, with some modification. Clinical results have been excellent with good patient acceptance. The longevity of the augmentation for wrinkles appears to be comparable to Zyplast, especially if a second "touch-up" procedure is repeated 1 to 2 months after the original injection [11].

PRESURGICAL CONSIDERATIONS/CONSULTATION

Aging of the face is most notable by fat wasting and deepening of wrinkles, all of which can be augmented with fat transplantation. Other areas such as acne scars, buccal fat wasting, facial asymmetries, and senile earlobes can also be improved with microlipoinjections. In addition, senile lipoatrophy of the hands and atrophy secondary to linear morphea or lupus panniculitis can be treated in a similar fashion.

Before beginning the procedure, the surgeon and the patient must sit together to discuss their goals and concerns. It is important for the surgeon to take a few moments to thoroughly examine the face for general proportions, asymmetries, and predicted volumes necessary to accomplish the desired results. The patient should be given a hand mirror to follow along.

It is imperative that the surgeon determine whether the cosmetic defect is of a superficial dermal or deeper subcutaneous nature. Subcutaneous defects are best augmented with fat transplants, whereas these are inappropriate for dermal defects. Superficial dermal defects, however, can be treated with lipocytic dermal augmentation (autologous collagen). Combined superficial and deep defects are best corrected with a layered approach (Fig. 1).

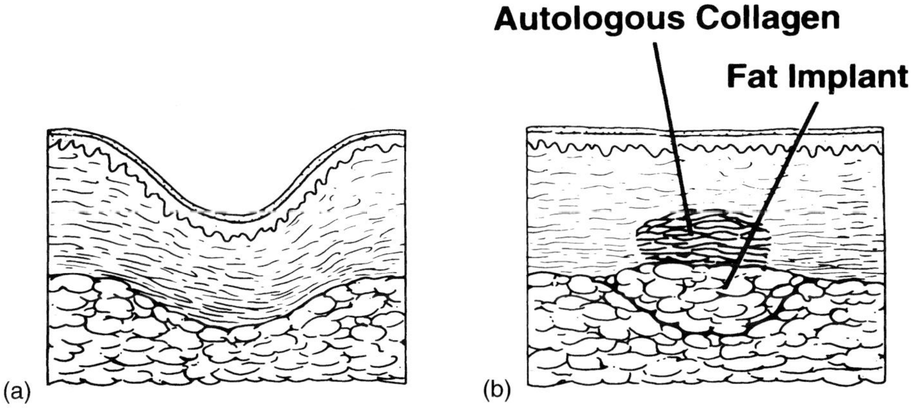

FIGURE 1 Proper placement of filler substances to correct a combined dermal and subcutaneous defect.

Presurgically it is also necessary to examine the patient's potential donor sites. Occasionally, it may be difficult to obtain a sufficient amount of fat from a very slender patient to perform even one procedure. In this situation, it may be prudent to suggest an alternative approach.

As previously mentioned, the nature of the cosmetic defect is an important consideration in regards to fat-graft longevity. Graft longevity varies with the nature of the cosmetic defect being treated and with the location of the recipient site [14]. The less mobile the recipient site, the greater the degree of graft longevity.

During the presurgical consultation, the patient should be informed that touch-up procedures will be required. It has been observed that long-term results are markedly improved when these transplants are repeated two to three times every 3 to 6 months after the initial procedure. Clinically, each subsequent transplant has a cumulative effect with higher percentages of fat surviving after each successive procedure. This has also been reported by other investigators [15] and documented by magnetic resonance imaging [16].

One final consideration is whether or not one should use freshly collected fat for each procedure. From a longevity standpoint, one should certainly use fresh material each time. In order for the fat transplant to survive as a true graft, it should be as unadulterated as possible. However, from a convenience standpoint, it is much easier to freeze any fatty tissue left after the initial procedure for subsequent touch-ups. It has been recently shown that frozen adipocytes are still viable on thawing [17,18]. Thus, frozen tissue should be adequate for microlipoinjections. It has been effectively and safely used after 1 to 2 years of storage [17].

PRESURGICAL INSTRUCTIONS/TREATMENT

Before the procedure, the consent form, presurgical instructions, as well as all post-surgical instructions should be thoroughly reviewed with the patient (see Appendixes 1 and 2). All aspirin and vitamin E should be discontinued at least 5 days before the procedure. Presurgical photographs should be taken for before and after comparison.

EQUIPMENT

A simple setup is used, which includes 500 ml of tumescent solution (Table 1). This is infiltrated by a Medex pressure cuff (Bernsco Surgical Supply, Inc.) by pushing the anesthetic solution through IV tubing to a connected Klein infiltrating cannula. The remainder of the tray consists of 3 ml and 60 ml syringes, a Johnnie-Lok device (The Tulip Co.), a 1 ml syringe, a 30-gauge needle, a 16-gauge needle, a #11 blade, a surgical marking pen, sterile gauze, a 15 cm 2.7 blunt-tipped uniport Toomey cannula (Byron Supply Co.), a fat-transfer adaptor (Byron Supply Co.), a Coleman 16-gauge injection cannula (Byron Supply Co.), a sterile basin or tray, and 100 ml of sterile saline solution (Figs. 2,3).

If lipocytic dermal augmentation is also planned, one will need an autologous collagen emulsifier (Bernsco Surgical Supply, Inc.), $\frac{1}{2}$ inch 25-gauge Lancet point needles (Bernsco Surgical Supply, Inc.), and a centrifuge (Fig. 4).

TECHNIQUE

Lipoextraction

Microlipoinjection involves extracting and reimplanting adipose tissue by a closed technique. Generally, the quantity of fat needed for correcting facial defects is small, approximately 10 to 20 ml. It is imperative that the surgeon respect the extracted tissue and minimize the hydraulic and chemical trauma.

The majority of fat transplantation procedures are performed under local anesthesia. If necessary, nerve blocks and/or Valium 5 mg PO can be administered. Great care must be taken to avoid causing pain as well as diminishing postsurgical swelling and ecchymosis. If these occur, the patient may be discouraged from following up with subsequent procedures, thereby diminishing one's chance for good long-term results.

Before beginning, the donor area is marked in a standing position as if to perform a standard liposuction, with attention paid to irregularities and asymmetrics. I prefer to use the upper outer quadrant of the buttocks whenever possible. The fat is easy to obtain here and if a resultant collection deformity occurs it is usually very unobtrusive. It is important to plan to remove adequate tissue for storage for subsequent touch-ups. Typically less than 100 ml is sufficient.

Using the tumescent anesthesia, an intradermal wheal is raised at the incision site of the chosen donor area. A 2 to 3 mm incision is made in the skin with a #11 blade. Tumescent anesthesia is then instilled using a 15 cm Klein infiltrating needle.

TABLE 1 Tumescent Anesthesia

500 ml	Normal saline
25 ml	1% lidocaine
0.5 ml	Epinephrine 1:1000
6.25 ml	8.4% sodium bicarbonate

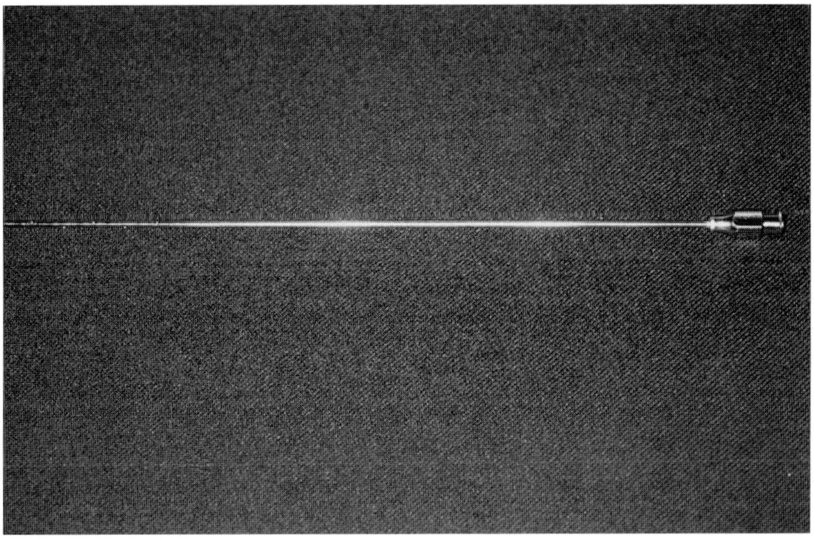

FIGURE 2 Klein infiltrating cannula.

The donor area should be tumesced in a very slow and nonpainful fashion, proceeding from the subcutaneous-fascial plane and progressing superficially.

Before collection, the surgeon must wait a minimum of 15 minutes for the maximum effect of the tumescent anesthesia. During this time, one should consider anesthetic options for the recipient areas. If EMLA or a regional nerve block are to be used, they can be safely administered at this time.

Lipoextraction begins by suctioning with a blunt-tipped 15 cm, 2.7 mm uniport cannula attached to a 60 ml syringe (Fig. 5). This is preferred over a 14-gauge needle,

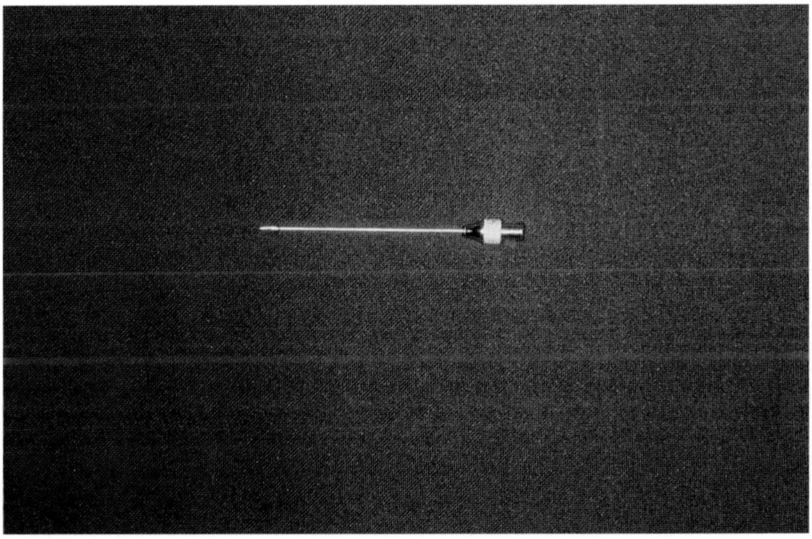

FIGURE 3 A Coleman 16-gauge injection cannula.

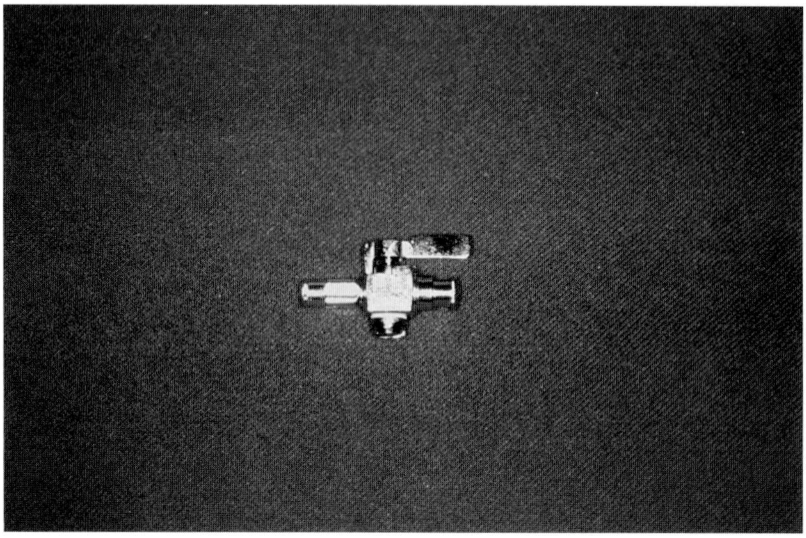

FIGURE 4 Dual luerlock device for processing autologous collagen (Bernsco Surgical Supply, Inc.).

multiple port cannulas, or Cobra tip cannulas, which tend to retrieve more fibrous tissue and are more traumatic to the fat [19]. It is important to respect this part of the procedure because a rough and hasty lipoextraction will result in destruction of fat cells, which will have little chance of survival. Keep in mind that this is collection of viable adipocytes for transfer and not destructive removal of fat by liposuction.

The syringe is primed for collection by submerging the distal end of the attached cannula into the basin filled with saline. All air should be expelled from the

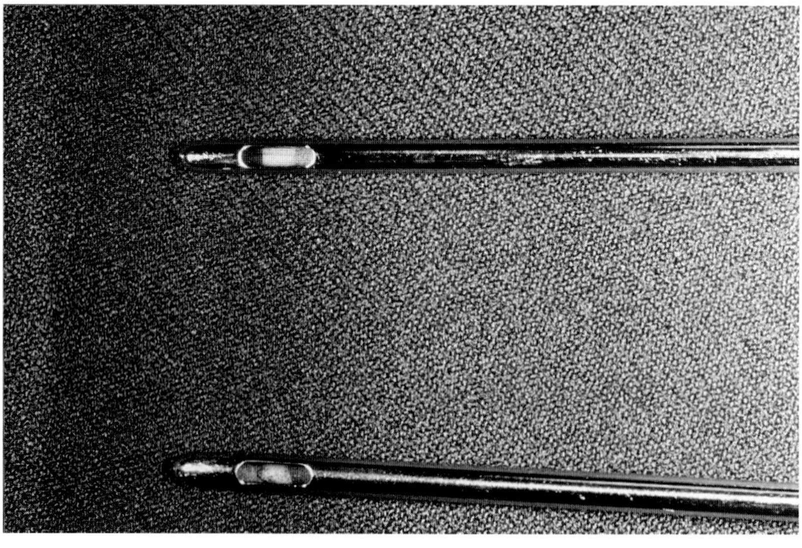

FIGURE 5 Close-up of the apertures of the extracting cannulas.

syringe and approximately 5 to 10 ml of saline should be aspirated. The cannula is then inserted into the fat through the incision site and the plunger of the syringe is pulled out to create negative pressure. This relative vacuum is sufficient to extract the fat as the cannula is maneuvered back and forth within the adipose layer (Fig. 6).

The cannula and syringe are moved back and forth five or six times in the same tunnel, after which the procedure is repeated in a radial fashion until sufficient fat has been aspirated. During the extraction the plunger is kept in the same position. A Johnnie-Lok device aids in maintaining the negative pressure of the syringe (Fig. 7). During the entire procedure, the skin is constantly palpated by the surgeon's free hand.

Treatment of the Collected Fat

When the extraction is complete, the filled syringe is capped, placed vertically (plunger up) and allowed to decant. It should be allowed to stand for 10 to 15 minutes. This will cause the tumescent fluid to accumulate near the tip of the syringe (Fig. 8). By removing the syringe cap this fluid is discarded, leaving only "pure fat" which is then transferred into 3 ml syringes (Fig. 9).

Some surgeons wash the fat with either saline or lactated Ringer's solution at this point. This is an unnecessary step if the tumescent technique is used at the donor site. In fact, excessive washing or manipulation of the fat cells may be detrimental to their survival.

Other methods of processing collected fat seem to decrease longevity of transplanted tissue. Profusing the cells with insulin increases resorption. Centrifrigation of collected fat also seems to destroy the adipocytes [20].

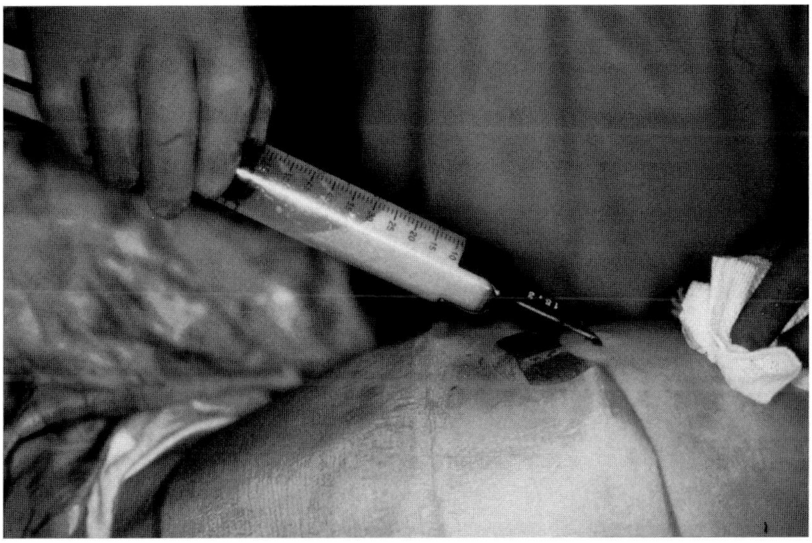

FIGURE 6 A sufficient vacuum is created with the syringe to atraumatically aspirate bloodless fat.

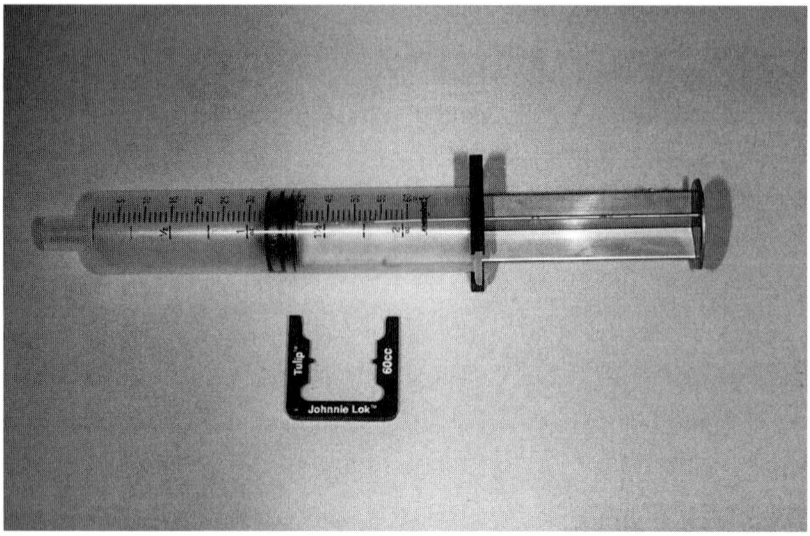

FIGURE 7 A Johnnie-Lok device aids in maintaining the plunger of the syringe withdrawn (The Tulip Company).

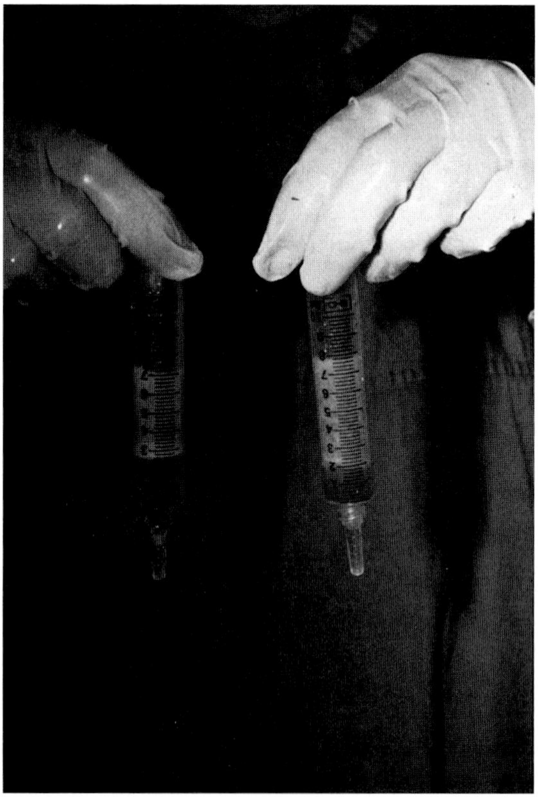

FIGURE 8 The aspirated fat will separate from anesthetic fluid and blood by gravitational pooling.

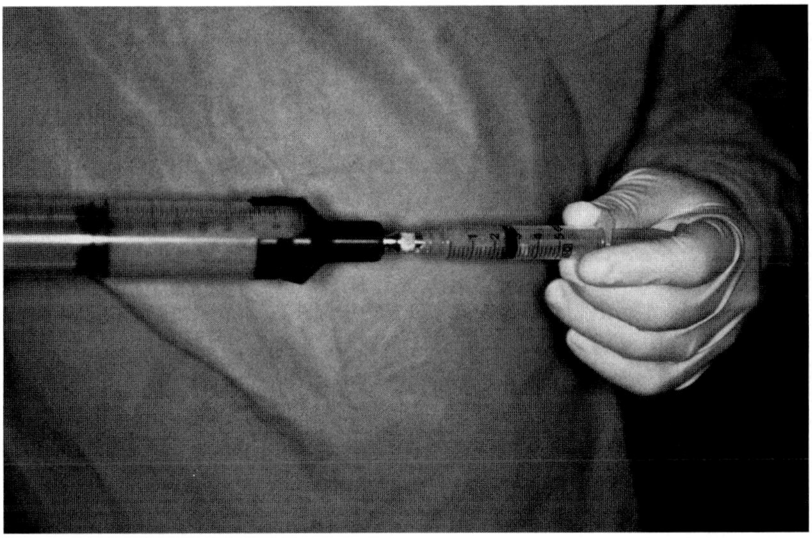

FIGURE 9 A fat-transfer adaptor maintains a closed system while transferring adipose tissue from Toomey tip syringes to luerlock syringes (Byron Supply Co.).

If a dermal filler is also required, some of the extracted fat should be prepared as autologous collagen. As previously mentioned, injections of adipocytes into the dermis have been shown to promote collagen formation. The dermis is not where fat cells belong and they don't appear to survive there. Thus, we are not concerned about preserving their integrity as in true fat transplantation.

Sterile distilled water is added to 2.5 to 3 ml of collected adipose tissue. The syringe is then attached to an empty 3-ml syringe by a dual luerlock device (Bernsco Surgical Supply, Inc.) and the material passed back and forth to thoroughly mix it (Fig. 10). This device has a stopcock, which when maneuvered will progressively decrease the aperture between the two syringes. The material should be pushed back and forth approximately five to six times while gradually diminishing the aperture. This pulverizes the tissue and creates an emulsion.

The syringes containing this mixture can be frozen in a commercial freezer for subsequent touch-ups. However, if immediate dermal augmentation is desired, syringes can be flash frozen by dipping them in liquid nitrogen. After thawing, two 3 ml syringes are centrifuged at low rpms for approximately 60 seconds. The resultant infranate is then expelled. One of the syringes is attached to an empty 3 ml syringe by the dual luerlock device and the material is again pushed back and forth to create the emulsified mixture. This should be performed again immediately before injection because the fat tends to harden and may be difficult to pass through a small gauge needle if left standing for 5 minutes or more.

Reimplantation

Lipoinjection is typically performed with a 3 ml syringe and a 16-gauge Coleman injection cannula. Fat injected through a lumen smaller than 18-gauge is damaged, as measured by nuclear, cellular, and globular morphology. This has been confirmed

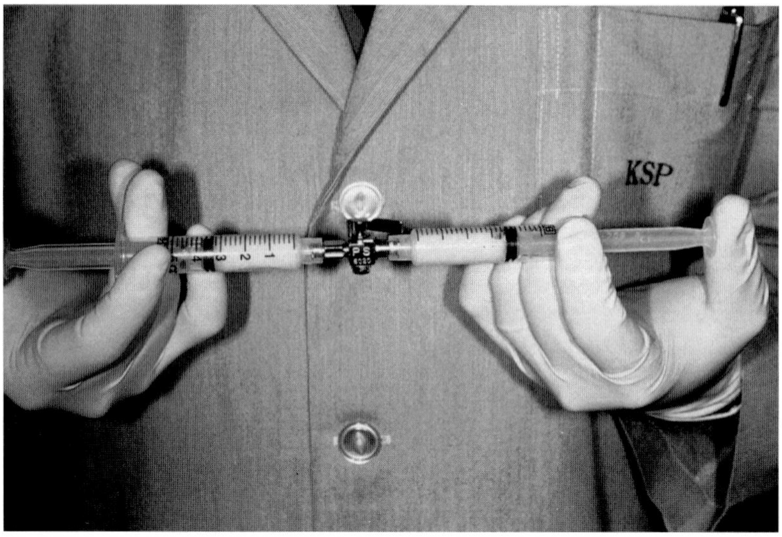

FIGURE 10 Processing adipocytes for autologous collagen implantation.

by checking the biochemical integrity of the adipocyte as measured by glucose metabolism, fatty acid synthesis, and insulin stimulation [21]. A 16-gauge cannula seems to be the optimal size for transferring fat, for both ease of injection and minimizing trauma to the transplanted adipocytes. In addition, it does not scar the skin and its blunt tip reduces the risk of vascular laceration.

A small intradermal wheal is raised at each injection site with 1% Xylocaine. A 16-gauge needle is used to pierce a hole in the skin to make the entry site for the transplant cannula. The cannula is then guided into the anesthetized recipient sites, parallel to the surface of the skin, sliding just along the dermal subcutaneous junction until it reaches its most distal point. As the cannula is slowly withdrawn, the fat is injected in a retrograde fashion in microdroplet amounts. Multiple passes are made at various levels extending from the superficial subcutaneous layer down to the subcutaneous fascial plane in a fan-shaped pattern.

The injection of fat in different areas and levels ensures sufficient peripheral circulation around each graft to allow its incorporation in the surrounding tissue. A column of injected fat seems to survive better than a large bolus. Therefore, the endpoint of microlipoinjection should be correction of the cosmetic defect. Overcorrection is not necessary and should be avoided. Control of fat deposition is maintained by applying manual pressure bilaterally along the edges of the defect. Once the injection is complete, the fat should be gently molded into a desired position.

If required, superficial defects can then be corrected with autologous collagen. A thawed 3 ml syringe of this emulsified mixture is attached to a 25-gauge Lancet point needle (Bernsco Surgical Supply, Inc.). Dermal wheals are raised by serial injections of the material into the lower dermis. Overcorrection is recommended because up to 50% of the augmentation may vanish within a few days after injection. Blanching is another endpoint to look for. Once adequate dermal augmentation has been achieved, the surgeon should then gently massage the area to smooth out individual lumps so the enitre defect is uniformly filled.

POSTSURGICAL CARE

Immediate

Postsurgical instructions for fat transplantation are relatively straightforward (Fig. 3). It should be stressed that ice packs for the first 8 hours will greatly minimize any edema or discomfort. Most importantly, the transplanted material is still potentially moldable for the first 6 to 8 hours. Therefore, the patient should avoid manipulating these areas after surgery.

Long Term

It is imperative that the patient understands that subsequent touch-up procedures will be required. Optimal long-term results are observed when these are repeated two to three times every 3 to 6 months. In addition, the longevity of the correction varies from person to person and with different cosmetic defects being treated.

INDICATIONS

Glabellar Furrows

Typically, less than 2 ml of fat are required. These furrows should be injected with the needle directed away from the eye to avoid intrusion of fat into the periorbital area. Marks left by a 16-gauge needle, if any, are not noticeable in the medial aspects of the eyebrows.

Nasolabial Furrows, Melolabial Furrows, and Oral Comissures

All these areas can be approached through the same entry point lateral to the commissures of the mouth (Fig. 11). Usually these can be adequately augmented with 3 to 4 ml per side. Patients should be cautioned about excessive facial expressions and exertion for the first 24 hours after surgery.

Lips

The same lateral entry points may be used. This will provide the lips with a fuller appearance (Fig. 12). Perpendicular rhytides or "smoker's lines" will not be eradicated. The majority of the fat transplant should be placed in the middle one third of the lower and upper lips.

Lip enhancement can most successfully be accomplished by visualizing three multilayered planes of augmentation. Approximately 0.5 to 1 ml are placed in each plane per lip. The first plane is very superficial and just underneath the vermillion border to create the natural curl of the lip. The second plane is up and over the top of the orbicularis muscle to the level of the mucocutaneous junction. The optional third site for lip augmentation is the intramuscular plane.

Cheeks

Whenever fat is injected into the face it should be directed away from orifices if possible. Hollow cheeks can be augmented with lipoinjection (Fig. 11). Atrophic and scars are amenable as well, but the scars should have associated atrophy of the

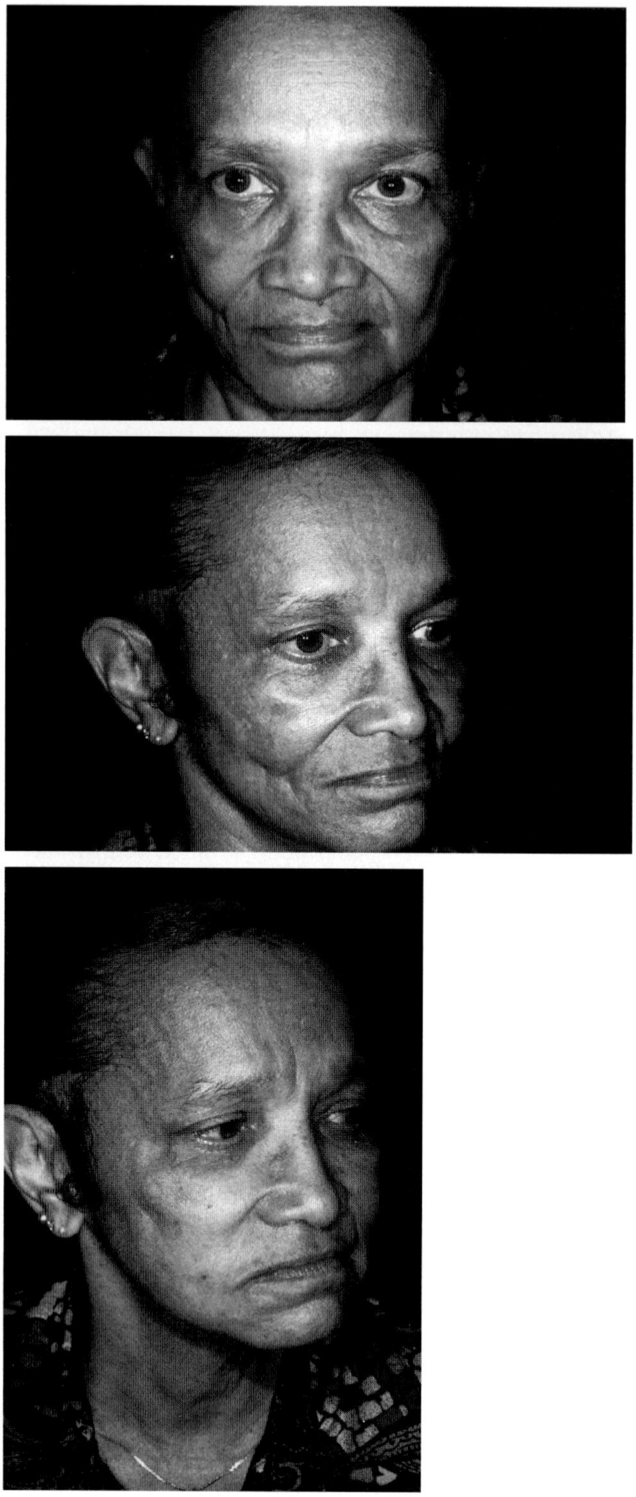

(a)

(b)

(c)

FIGURE 11 (a,b) Senile lipoatrophy of the cheeks before fat injections. (c) Three months after fat injections to cheeks and nasolabial furrows.

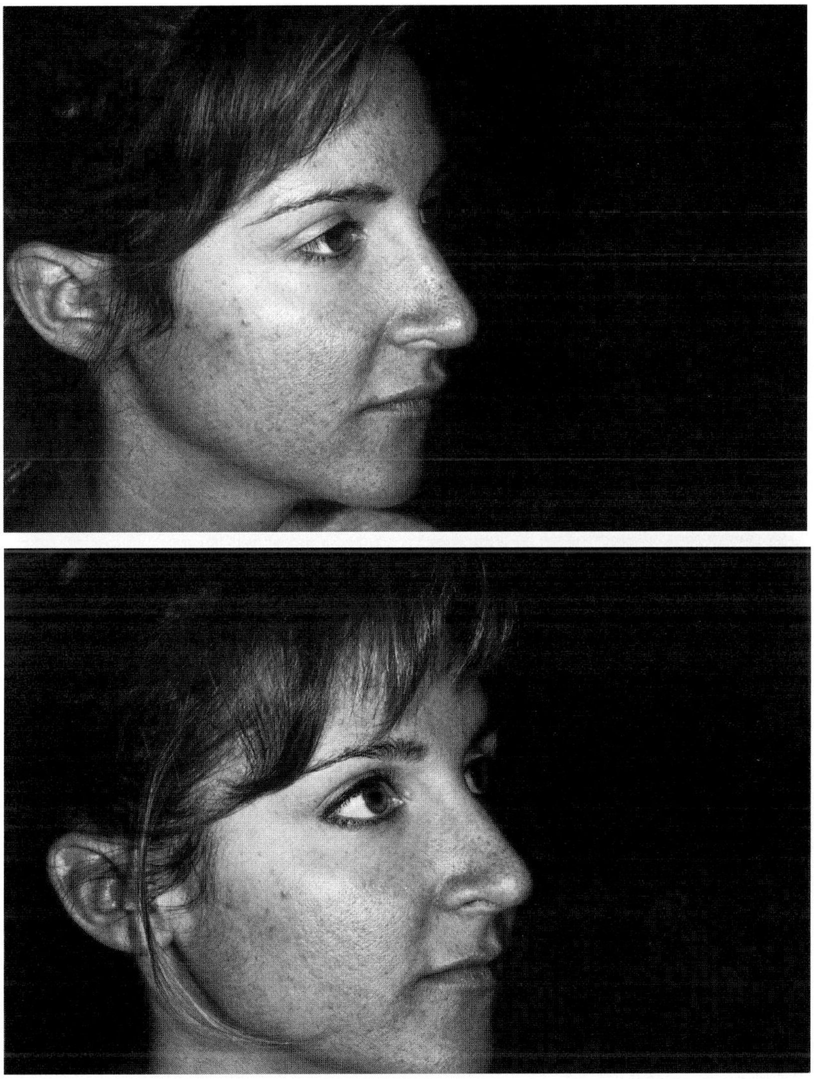

(a)

(b)

FIGURE 12 (a) Atrophic upper lip before fat injections. (b) One month after 3 ml of fat injected to the upper lip.

subcutis (Fig. 13). If the scars are purely dermal defects, autologous collagen is more appropriate for correction.

Cheeks may be augmented by entering over the malar eminence or below the lateral alar rim (at the top of the nasolabial fold).

Morphea and Lupus Profundus

Both of these conditions respond quite well to lipoinjections (Fig. 14). The disease process, however, should be inactive before beginning cosmetic correction. A biopsy may aid in documenting this.

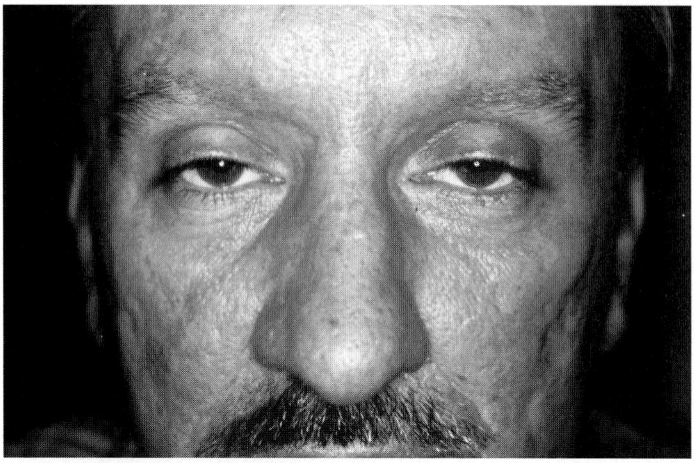

(a)

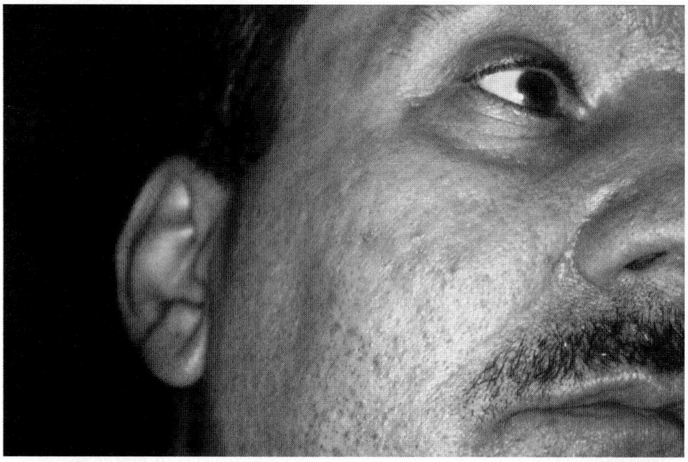

(b)

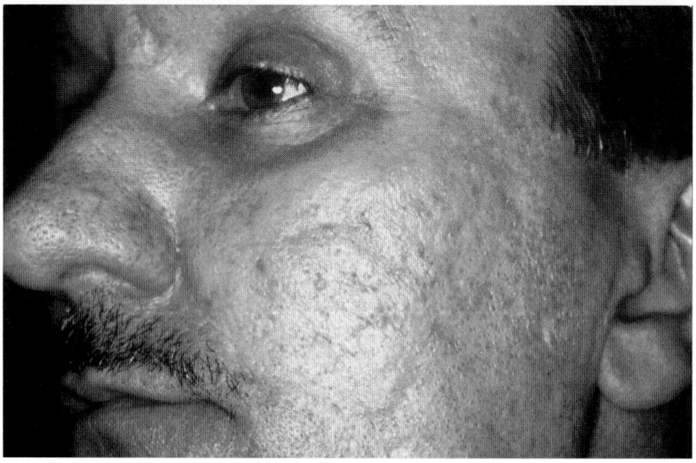

(c)

FIGURE 13 (a) Acne scars of cheeks with associated lipoatrophy. (b,c) One year after fat injections.

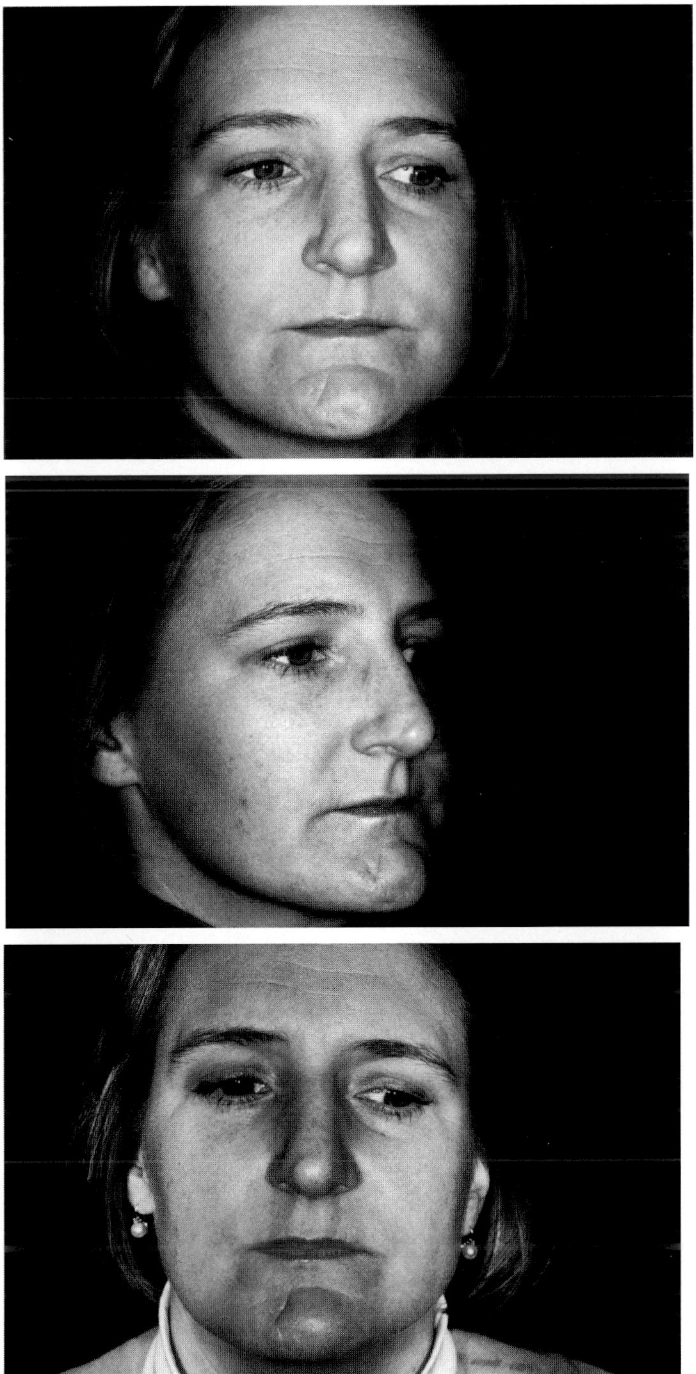

(a)

(b)

(c)

FIGURE 14 (a,b) Localized morphea of the right chin; note a central biopsy scar. (c,d) 3 months after 4 ml of fat injected.

(d)
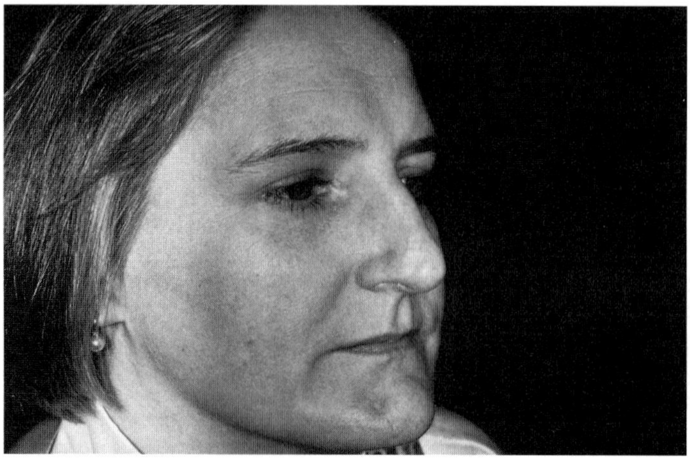

FIGURE 14 Continued

Facial Hemiatrophy

Congenital defects such as facial hemiatrophy can be successfully treated as well (Fig. 15). As more fat is injected into one area, be careful to place it at different levels.

Hands

Fat transplantation plays an integral role in hand rejuvenation. Transplanted fat provides thickness to an atrophic subcutaneous compartment, decreasing the prominence of blood vessels and tendons and giving the hands an overall younger appearance. The cannula is inserted at the dorsal wrist crease and threaded along the tendon sheath distally to each metacarpophalangeal joint. Approximately 5 to 10 ml are required for each hand. Be sure to massage the fat distally to avoid plump hands with skinny fingers (Fig. 16).

Dermal Defects

Dermal defects are better treated with autologous collagen as previously described (Fig. 17). This is typically best accomplished by using a serial puncture technique. It is important to overcorrect and produce blanching of the recipient sites.

COMPLICATIONS

To date this has been a relatively safe and effective procedure. Temporary swelling and minor bruising at the recipient site and mild tenderness at the donor site may occur. Rarely a hematoma or temporary lumpiness may develop. There has been one report of unilateral blindness after transplantation of autologous fat to the glabella [22]. Care must be exercised when injecting any particulate substance near the eye. Because of the large size of these particles, however, intravascular penetration of fat is a rare occurrence.

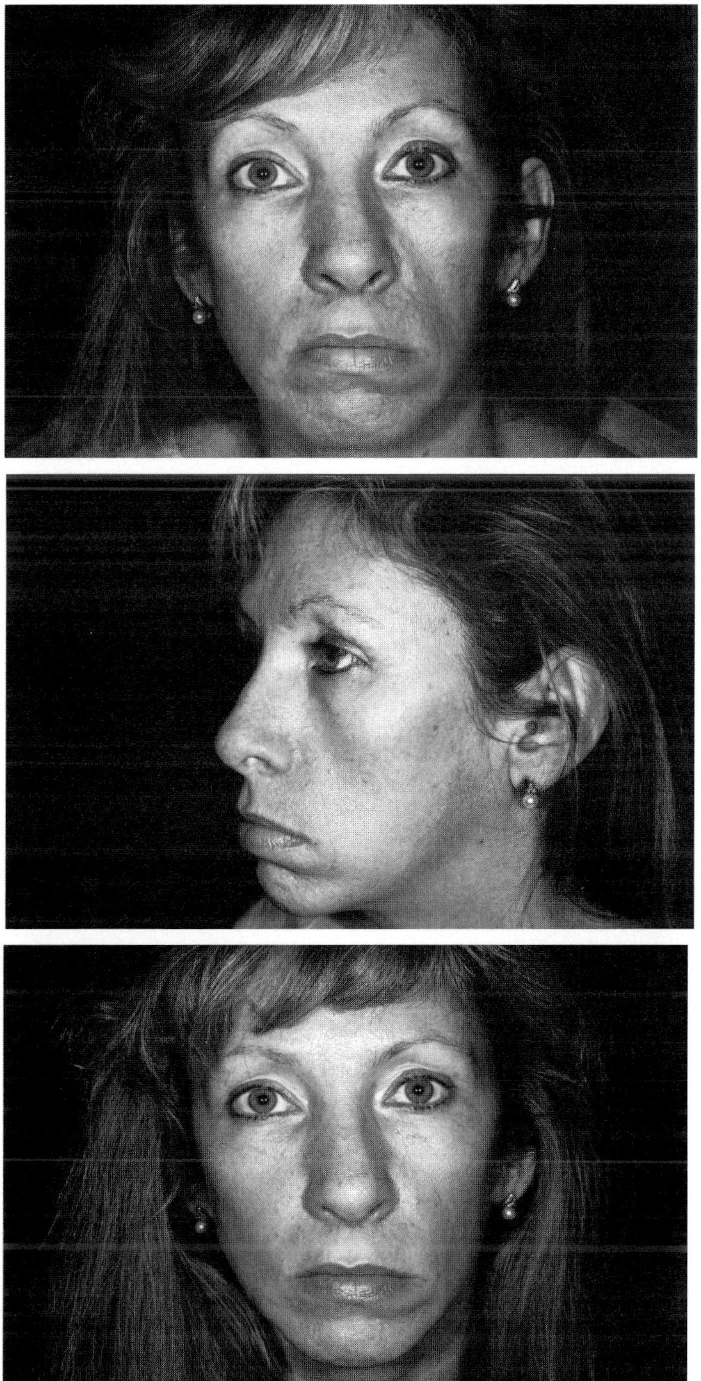

(a)

(b)

(c)

FIGURE 15 (a,b) Facial hemiatrophy before fat injections. (c,d) Three months after 4 ml of fat injected.

(d) 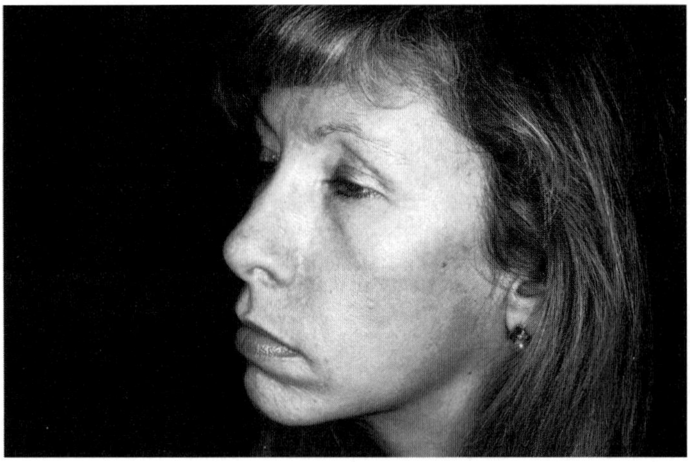

FIGURE 15 Continued

With injections of fat-derived autologous collagen patients typically develop immediate erythema and edema, which may last for 2 to 3 days. This can be minimized with the use of intramuscular corticosteroids. Postsurgical applications of ice are also recommended. Most patients can return to an active lifestyle within 2 days after treatment.

SUMMARY

My current procedure for fat transplantation has been progressively evolving since 1989. When I first began, adipose tissue was collected by a suction apparatus and a sterile-filter trap (Robbins Instrument Co.). Large volumes were injected into each recipient site because of high reabsorption rates. Most cases involved 30 to 50% overcorrection in an effort to compensate. However, this led to significant inflammation and swelling, which forced patients to heal for a period of days to weeks.

In the mid 1990s, being somewhat disenchanted with long-term results, I started to transplant smaller volumes of adipose tissue. I was also influenced by others who reported better graft viability with smaller injected volumes [23,24]. This, combined with less traumatic collecting, has led to more acceptable long-term results. The ideal fat graft appears to be tubular, less than 3 mm in diameter, and placed at various levels to insure adequate vascularity.

The other major change through the decade is the freezing of adipose tissue for subsequent touch-up procedures. I believe that using freshly extracted tissue each time would be ideal. However, as a matter of convenience, freezing excess tissue is more practical. In addition, a recent report has shown viability of adipocytes after freezing and thawing [18].

Touch-up procedures are repeated two to three times every 3 to 6 months. This is scientifically justified by work reported by Horl et al. with magnetic resonance imaging of fat transplants [16]. They identified 49% volume loss at 3 months and 55% loss at 6 months with negligible decrease in volume between 9 and 12 months.

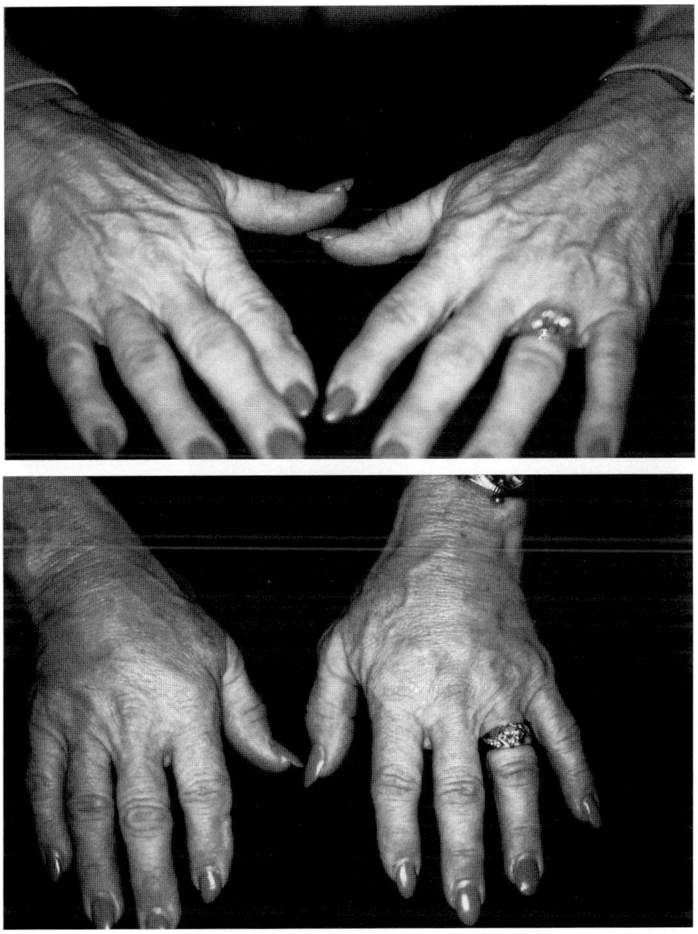

(a)

(b)

FIGURE 16 (a) Senile lipoatrophy of the hands. (b) Six months after injection of 8 ml of adipose tissue to each hand.

Finally, in regards to dermal filler substances, autologous collagen or lipocytic dermal augmentation shows promise. Although technically more difficult and time consuming to use than Zyplast, this technique is much more cost effective, especially for larger defects. When more than 1 ml of filler substance is required, the choice of Zyplast or other synthetically produced fillers becomes quite expensive. Adipose tissue is available in large quantities without appreciable additional effort. A 5 ml augmentation is not much more time consuming than a 1 ml correction. In addition, excess material can be stored for future touch-up procedures.

Because the transplanted tissue is autologous, there is no chance of an immune response to foreign tissue as with synthetic fillers. The notion of a potential autoimmune reaction after lipocytic dermal augmentation should be considered, but this is not consistent with modern immunology theory, nor has it been observed in autologous transplantation of other human tissues.

(a)
(b)
(c)
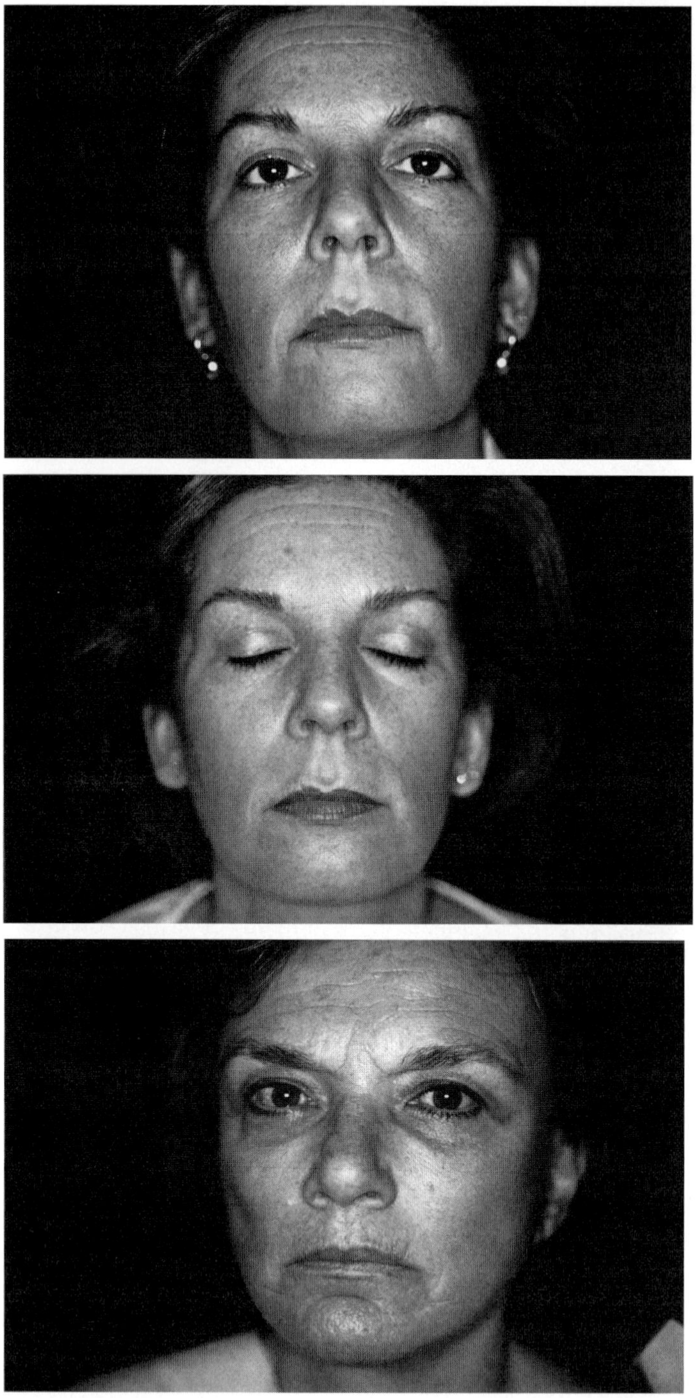

FIGURE 17 (a) Before and (b) 3 months after augmentation of glabellar furrows, melolabial furrows, and lips with autologous collagen; (c) before and (d) 3 months after augmentation of glabellar furrows, upper lip, and chin rhytides.

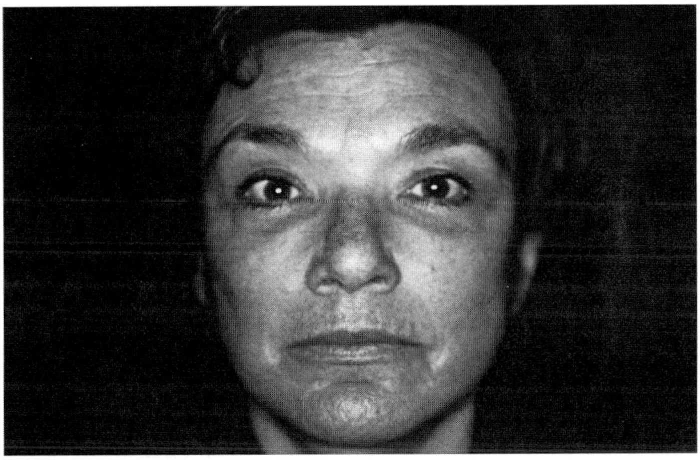

(d)

FIGURE 17 Continued

For soft-tissue defects with dermal and subcutaneous components, adipose tissue is ideal. Some of the extracted fat can be injected without mechanical processing into the subcutaneous defect. The dermal component can then be augmented with processed fat or autologous collagen. In conclusion, we can now effectively replace all the lost tissue of a given cosmetic defect with the patient's own adipose tissue.

REFERENCES

1. Neuber F. Fat grafting. Cuir Kongr Verh Otsum Ges Chir 20:66, 1893.
2. Brockaert TJ. Contribution a l'etude des greffes adipeueses. Bull Acad R Med Belg 28: 440, 1919.
3. Peer LA. Loss of weight and volume in human fat grafts. Plast Reconstr Surg 5:217, 1950.
4. Fischer A, Fischer GM. Revised technique for cellulite fat. Reduction in riding breeches deformity. Bull Int Acad Cosm Surg 2:40, 1977.
5. Illouz Y-G. Communications at the Societe Francaise de Chirurgie Esthetique. June 1978–1979.
6. Illouz Y-G. L'Avnir de la reutilisation de la graisse apres liposuction. Rev Chir Esthet Lang Franc 10, 1985.
7. Fournier PF. Facial recontouring with fat grafting. Dermatol Clin 8:523–537, 1990.
8. Illouz Y-G. The fat cell "graft," a new technique to fill depressions. Plast Reconstr Surg 78:122–123, 1986.
9. Fournier PF. Collagen Autologue: Liposculpture ma Technique. Paris: Arnette, 1989, pp. 277–279.
10. Coleman WP, Lawrence N, Sherman RN, Reed RJ, Pinski KS. Autologous collagen? Lipocytic dermal augmentation: a histopathologic study. J Dermatol Surg Oncol 19: 1032–1040, 1993.
11. Pinski KS, Coleman WP. Microlipoinjection and autologous collagen. Dermatol Clin 13: 339–351, 1995.
12. Orentriech D, Orentriech N. Injectable fluid silicone. In: Roenigk RK, Roenigk HH Jr, eds. Dermatologic Surgery. New York: Marcel Dekker, 1988.

13. Millikan LE. Long term safety and efficacy with Fibrel in the treatment of cutaneous scars—results of a multicenter study. J Dermatol Surg Oncol 15:837–842, 1989.
14. Pinski KS, Roenigk HH. Autologous fat transplantation. A long-term follow-up. J Dermatol Surg Oncol 18:179–184, 1992.
15. Brandow K, Newman J. Facial multilayered micro lipo-augmentation. Internat J Aesth and Restor Surg 4:95–110, 1996.
16. Horl HW, Feller AM, Biemer E. Technique for liposuction fat reimplantation and long-term volume evaluation by magnetic resonance imaging. Ann Plast Surg 26:248–257, 1991.
17. Sattler G, Sommer B. Am J Cosm Surg 14:311–316, 1997.
18. Jones JK. Am Acad Cosm Surg Mtg, Rancho Mirage, CA, 1997.
19. Newman J, Levin J. Facial lipo-transplant surgery. Am J Cosm Surg 4:131–140, 1987.
20. Chajchir A, Benzaquen I, Moretti E. Comparative experimental study of autologous adipose tissue processed by different techniques. Aesth Plast Surg 17:113–115, 1993.
21. Campbell G-Lem, Laudenslager N, Newman J. The effect of mechanical stress on adipocyte morphology and metabolism. Am J Cosm Surg 4:85–87, 1987.
22. Temourian B. Blindness following fat injections, correspondence and brief communications. Plast Reconstr Surg 80:361, 1988.
23. Lewis CM. The current status of fat grafting. Aesth Plast Surg 17:109–112, 1993.
24. Carpaneda C, Ribeiro MT. Study of the histological alterations and viability of the adipose graft in humans. Aesth Plast Surg 17:43–47, 1993.

APPENDIX 1

FAT TRANSPLANT/AUTOLOGOUS COLLAGEN

Dr. Pinski has carefully explained to me the nature, goals, limitations and possible complications of this procedure. He has also discussed alternative forms of treatment. I have had the opportunity to ask questions about the procedure, its limitations and possible complications.

By placing my initials next to the following items, I clearly understand and accept the following:

______ The goal of any cosmetic procedure is improvement, not perfection.

______ Because in most cases this is a nonpermanent filler substance, touch-up procedures are to be expected. There will be a charge for any touch-up procedure performed.

______ There is no charge for routine follow-up care after the surgery. There is no guarantee that the expected or anticipated results will be achieved.

______ I agree to allow Dr. Pinski to photograph me before, during, and after the operation. The photographs shall be his property and may be used for teaching, publication, or scientific research purposes. The patient's identity will not be revealed.

______ Although complications are infrequent, they may occur. These can include but are not limited to: swelling, bruising, bleeding, infection, skin irregularities, bumpiness, and numbness.

______ Allergic or toxic responses to anesthetic are extremely rare, but possible.

______ Dimpling of the donor area is unlikely but can occur.

______ In addition to these possible complications, I am aware of the general risks inherent in all surgical procedures and anesthetic administration.

APPENDIX 2

INSTRUCTIONS FOLLOWING FACIAL SURGERY/FAT TRANSPLANTATION

Swelling and discoloration may be present after facial surgery. The amount is usually minimal, but varies from person to person. The following may help minimize your swelling and discoloration after surgery.

1. ACTIVITY:

   a) Elevate your head at all times and sleep on two pillows the night of surgery. You may want to sleep in a recliner or lounge chair.

   b) Apply cold compresses to your face and eyes: 15 minutes on alternating with 15 minutes off for the first 8 hours. Bags of frozen peas or soft ice packs are excellent compresses — buy four bags so you can keep two in the freezer while you are using the other two. You may want to put the compresses in plastic wrappers to keep the bandages dry.

c) After 24 hours you may walk at a normal pace but do not resume exercise for at least 3 days after surgery — check with Dr. Pinski about this. If at any point in your recovery you experience swelling, resume the application of cold compresses.

2. DIET: Please eat soft foods and do not chew hard foods for 24 hours.
3. BATHING: Please keep any bandages dry. You may shower or bathe in lukewarm water only after the bandages are removed.
4. MEDICATIONS: Take any medications as prescribed. Elevate your head and use cold compresses for relief of mild discomfort.
5. ALCOHOL: No alcoholic beverages are allowed for 1 week after the surgery, or as long as you are taking medications.
6. COVERING DISCOLORATION: Cover creams may be used to camouflage discoloration. Do not put cover creams on sutures or incisions until they are healed (when no crusting or moisture are present). The nurse will instruct you on cover creams.
7. SUN: Avoid sunburning your face and incisions. Please wear a hat and protect yourself from the sun.

14

Human-Derived Filling Materials for Soft-Tissue Augmentation

Tina B. West
The Washington Hospital Center, Washington, D.C.

INTRODUCTION

Soft-tissue augmentation represents an essential treatment option for rejuvenation of the aging face. In addition, filling agents play an important role in the treatment of atrophic scars. Unfortunately, however, there have been various problems associated with the use of exogenous agents for the purpose of soft-tissue augmentation. Although xenogenic (bovine) collagen has emerged as the gold standard of this treatment modality because of its safety and reproducibility of results, it lasts only 3 to 6 months in vivo and therefore requires frequent reimplantation [1]. In addition, approximately 3 to 5% of the population is allergic to bovine collagen [1–4].

The ideal substance for soft-tissue augmentation would be biocompatible, nonimmunogenic, easily obtainable, low cost, nonresorbable, and easily stored. Autologous tissue preparations are theoretically the ideal material for replacing or repairing damaged or defective tissue. Inflammation accompanying tissue reactions results in elevated levels of active proteases, which may accelerate the degradation of biological replacement materials [5]. Autologous material should theoretically be devoid of the potential for allergic phenomena and tissue rejection. In fact, such complications have not been observed after autotransplantation of human tissues [6]. Homologous or allograft tissue would be less desirable because of concerns of viral transmission and potential immunological reactions. Heterologous material carries an even greater risk of immunogenicity and associated tissue reactions.

HISTORY

Bovine collagen implants consist of sterile, purified, reconstituted fibrillar bovine collagen (type I and type III) that are injected into the dermis for soft-tissue augmentation. After its injection, bovine collagen is detected as a foreign substance and is subsequently degraded by human collagenases and inflammatory cells over several months. In vivo investigations have shown that bovine collagen cannot be detected in the dermis 3 months after injection; however, up to 30% of patients report correction lasting up to 18 months [7–9]. It has been hypothesized that prolonged clinical improvement observed after injection of bovine collagen is caused by stimulation of fibroblasts that synthesize new collagen around the implant [7,8]. However, there is no convincing evidence in humans that host collagen production contributes to the longevity of clinical correction [9]. Displacement into the subcutaneous space from the overlying dermis also contributes to loss of correction [10]. Bovine collagen must therefore be administered frequently to maintain clinical results.

Because it is xenogenic, the largest drawback to the use of bovine collagen is the potential for hypersensitivity. Although the rate of allergic reactions is low (3–5%), it remains a concern [1–4]. Erythema and induration correlate with the presence of circulating antibodies to bovine collagen. Granulomatous responses in the absence of positive skin tests have been shown to occur in 0.5% of patients in a large retrospective study [2–4]. Lastly, serum sickness-like reactions have been documented [11,12]. Unfortunately, other implantation techniques, including plasma gel matrix (Fibrel) and silicone, have also been wrought with technical, systemic, and/or regulatory (eg, FDA) difficulties. Because of hypersensitivity and inflammatory reactions in particular, the development of autologous or allogeneic material for soft-tissue augmentation represents a significant advance (Table 1).

PRESURGICAL CONSIDERATIONS/CONSULTATION

The most important aspect of the patient consultation (Table 4) involves the determination of whether the patient and the desired treatment areas are amenable to correction with injectable or implantable filling materials. The assessment of treatment results is subjective. The efficacy of treatment depends on the selection of a filler material suited to a specific lesion and the use of proper injection technique (Tables 2, 3). Pre- and post-treatment photographs are particularly useful in documenting the efficacy of soft-tissue augmentation. During the consultation, specific information pertaining to the injection of human-derived fillers should be reviewed. Patients should receive an information form at the time of the pretreatment visit to advise them of the specifics of the treatment session, short and long-term postprocedural expectations, and medications to avoid. Exclusion criteria should be outlined.

Are the Lesions Amenable to Treatment With Injectable/Implantable Fillers?

As with all elective procedures for cosmetic enhancement, it is important to establish which lesions are of concern to the patient. Once is is determined that the lesions are suitable for treatment, it is important to thoroughly discuss with the patient risks and benefits of all other appropriate treatment options. In addition, the patient must be made fully aware of the expected treatment outcome and must express realistic expectations.

Does the Patient Have a History of Facial Herpes Simplex?

Trauma of any type, including that associated with multiple injections, may reactivate herpes simplex virus (HSV) infections. Prophylactic antiviral agents are prescribed for patients with a positive history of HSV involving the treatment area.

TABLE 1 Human-Derived Filling Substances

	Category	Treatment method	Pt. preparation	Anesthesia	Onset of correction	Duration of correction	Complications
Isolagen	Autologous	Injection × 3 sessions	Biopsy; skin test	+/−	Delayed	Up to 2 or more years	Burning/stinging
Autologen	Autologous	Injection × 3 sessions	Skin resection	+/−	Immediate	75% at one year	Placement-dependent
Dermalogen	Allogeneic	Injection × 3 sessions	Skin test	+/−	Immediate	Up to 50% at one year	Placement-dependent; burning/stinging
Alloderm	Allogeneic	Implantation	Incisions at implantation site	+	Immediate	Prolonged	Infection

TABLE 2 Patient Selection: Indications for Human-Derived Fillers

	Isolagen	Dermalogen/Autologen	Alloderm
Patient Factors			
Allergy to bovine collagen	X	X	X
Desires "natural" treatment	X	X	X
Desires long lasting correction	X	X	X
<60 years old	X		
Lesion Factors			
Fine lines—perioral/periorbital	+/−	+/−	
Prominent nasolabial folds	X	X	X
Glabellar furrows	X	X	
Atrophic scars (acne, varicella)	X	X	X
Lip atrophy	X	X	X
Oral commissures/marionette lines	X	X	X

Are There Any Other Medical Conditions or Medications That Could Affect Treatment?

Patients with autoimmune conditions, including scleroderma, lupus, or vitiligo, are probably not treatment candidates. Further studies are indicated to determine the safety of injecting autologous or allogeneic material in this population. In addition, the treatments are not recommended for immunocompromised hosts. Pregnancy, history of anaphylaxis, and keloid scar formation are also contraindications to treatment. The use of isotretinoin within the preceding 6 months is a contraindication for treat-

TABLE 3 Injection Technique

	Angle to skin surface (Degrees)	Implantation site (serial injections)	Degree of overcorrection	Technique
Isolagen	10–20	Upper dermis	300%	Bleb formation
Autologen	30–45	Mid dermis	10–20%	Min. blanching; inject on entry/exit
Dermalogen	30–45	Mid dermis	10–20%	Min. blanching; inject on entry/exit

TABLE 4 Preoperative Patient Consultation

Identify appropriate regions/patients for treatment
Prominent nasolabial folds/oral commissures/marionette lines
Rhytides
Atrophic scars
Atrophic lips
Postsurgical irregularities
Discuss risks/benefits
Allergic reactions (bovine vs. human collagen)
Discomfort on injection/implantation
Erythema
Swelling
Scar/abscess
Contraindications
Connective tissue disease
Immunologic disease
Active oral HSV
Nondistensible or rigid scars
Rhytides that do not improve with manual skin distention
Unrealistic expectations
Limitations
Variable response of movement-associated rhytides (glabellar, forehead)
Tissue source
Duration of correction
Onset of correction
Expense

Abbreviation: HSV, herpes simplex virus.

ment because of the potential for hypertrophic scarring after manipulation of the skin [13]. Oral vitamin E or corticosteroids should be discontinued before treatment because of adverse effects on wound healing [14]. In addition, patients should be advised that aspirin, products containing aspirin, other NSAIDs, and anticoagulants increase the likelihood of postprocedural bruising.

PATIENT INFORMATION AND CONSENT

Patients should be educated thoroughly regarding the expected outcome and possible risks of treatment. Alternative treatment options for the specific types of lesions being treated should be reviewed. All consent forms for human-derived fillers should discuss the fact that 3% of the population is allergic to bovine collagen [1–4]. In addition, although double skin testing before facial injection of bovine collagen usually determines whether one is allergic, an allergic reaction may rarely occur at the treatment site despite negative (nonallergic) test results [9]. Specific consent forms for each of the human-derived filling materials discussed may be obtained from the manufacturer.

The consent form should include a detailed description of the procedure to be followed by both patient and physician. The patient should be advised that there is no guarantee of results. Possible side effects should be outlined clearly. If appropriate, the option of tissue storage and its annual fee should be provided. In the event that the patient wishes to discontinue storage of autologous tissue at any point in time, permission must be obtained to dispose of stored skin or cells or make use of it for education, research, or commercial purposes as determined by the company in possession of the material. If desired, permission should also be obtained for pre- and post-treatment photographs.

AUTOLOGOUS HUMAN COLLAGEN

Autologous materials are commonly, and successfully, used to replace or augment body tissues. The availability and use of autologous dermal fillers to smooth wrinkle lines and scars have been limited to intact dermal grafts and injectable fat. Both of these procedures require extraction and manipulation of the patient's tissues [5]. Resorption rates of up to 20% have been reported for autologous dermal grafts and up to approximately 60% for autologous fat grafts [15,16]. Fat grafts and injectable processed fat have provided variable long-term correction [17,18].

Isolagen

Isolagen is a new process that has been approved by the FDA to provide living autologous cells for injection. The use of autologous human fibroblast injections is based on the hypothesis that injection of collagen-producing cells leads to prolonged correction of dermal defects. After injection, increased local production of collagen as well as decreased degradation by human collagenases should occur. A further theoretical advantage of the Isolagen process includes cryopreservation of extracted cells, providing a permanent, renewable, living tissue source for future injections. As the patient continues to age, access to younger, previously extracted cells is maintained [19]. Therefore, an older patient may be injected with "younger" cells, which are thought to produce collagen more effectively than cells of the patient's chronological age. The same concept implies that patients greater than 60 years of age are not ideal candidates based on the decreased ability of their cells to produce vigorous fibroblasts [14,19].

Before treatment with Isolagen, it is important to advise patients that onset of correction may be delayed until up to 3 months after the injection series [19,20]. Patients should also be advised to discontinue the use of oral vitamin E and corticosteroids based on their potential interference with normal wound-healing mechanisms [14].

Technique

The physical characteristics of each material reviewed dictate the preferred level of placement and injection method (Table 3).

As the initial step in the Isolagen process, a 3 mm punch excision specimen is obtained from the ultraviolet-protected skin of the postauricular scalp. It is important to avoid the thin skin immediately posterior to the ear because it contains insufficient dermis to provide an adequate supply of cells. The specimen is packaged in media provided by Isolagen laboratories and is chilled and shipped overnight to the Isolagen facility. Type I collagen and fibroblasts are collected from the biopsy specimen after 4 to 6 weeks in tissue culture, at which time a 0.1 ml intradermal test dose is

inconspicuous site such as the suprapubic region or buttocks to provide tissue specifically for Autologen preparation [23]. In general, the first 3 in^2 of skin yield 1 ml of injectable collagen and each additional 1.5 in^2 yield an additional 1 ml [24]. Therefore, one standard rhytidectomy yielding 6 to 8 in^2 of skin yields approximately 3 ml of Autologen. Exact tissue yield varies among individual patients as well as anatomic areas of varying dermal thickness. The dermis is pulverized in sterile buffer to form a dispersion of intact collagen fibers. The dispersed collagen fibers are washed in sterile phosphate buffer and concentrated by centrifugation. The resulting material is packaged into sterile, 1 ml Luer-Lock syringes and hand labeled with the donor-recipient's unique identification codes. Tissue processing requires 3 to 4 weeks. The final product is then suitable for storage in an office refrigerator for up to 6 months.

Autologen provides advantages similar to those of autologous human collagen and fibroblasts (Isolagen) in terms of its negligible potential for allergic or other tissue reactions because donor tissue originates from the patient (autologous). The relative permanence of Autologen compared with bovine collagen is postulated to be attributable to maintenance of the physical and chemical structure of collagen fibers. Transmission electron micrographs of collagen fibers in Autologen show intact fibers with intermolecular cross-links of each fiber present as in vivo. Similar micrographs of bovine collagen show minimal banding [5,25]. The intact dermal collagen fibers retaining their native cross-links should theoretically enhance collagenesis. In addition, the intact collagen fibers should exhibit greater resistance to protease degradation than reconstituted bovine collagen in which antigenic telopeptides have been removed [5]. The most obvious disadvantage of Autologen is the requirement of a large amount of skin from the donor-recipient for processing and, subsequently, the limited supply.

Autologous injectable collagen has been used to treat rhytids, depressed scars, and nasolabial folds, as well as lip augmentation (Fig. 3) [5,23,25]. Because the material is autologous and a sufficient number of patients have been treated with no incidence of allergic reactions, the FDA has deemed that skin testing is not necessary.

Technique

Autologen is injected through a 30-gauge needle into the mid-dermal plane. Preinjection with lidocaine locally or as nerve blocks is frequently necessary because there is no anesthetic in the preparation. A serial injection technique is recommended to achieve approximately 10 to 20% overcorrection. The material should be injected both on entering and exiting the mid-dermis, so that it flows into the tissue with a streamlike effect rather than as a series of discrete "beads." Most patients require three treatment sessions initially consisting of 1 to 1.5 ml followed by 1 ml at each subsequent session. The injections are delivered approximately 2 weeks apart.

Results

In a study evaluating 25 patients who received one to three injections (0.5–1 ml) for the treatment of rhytids in various facial locations, follow-up evaluations ranged from 1 month to more than 1 year [5]. A single injection provided 50 to 75% correction for up to 3 months and 50% correction for up to 6 months. Two injections provided 75% correction for up to 6 months. Three or more injections provided greater than 75% correction beyond 12 months. Excellent correction after four Au-

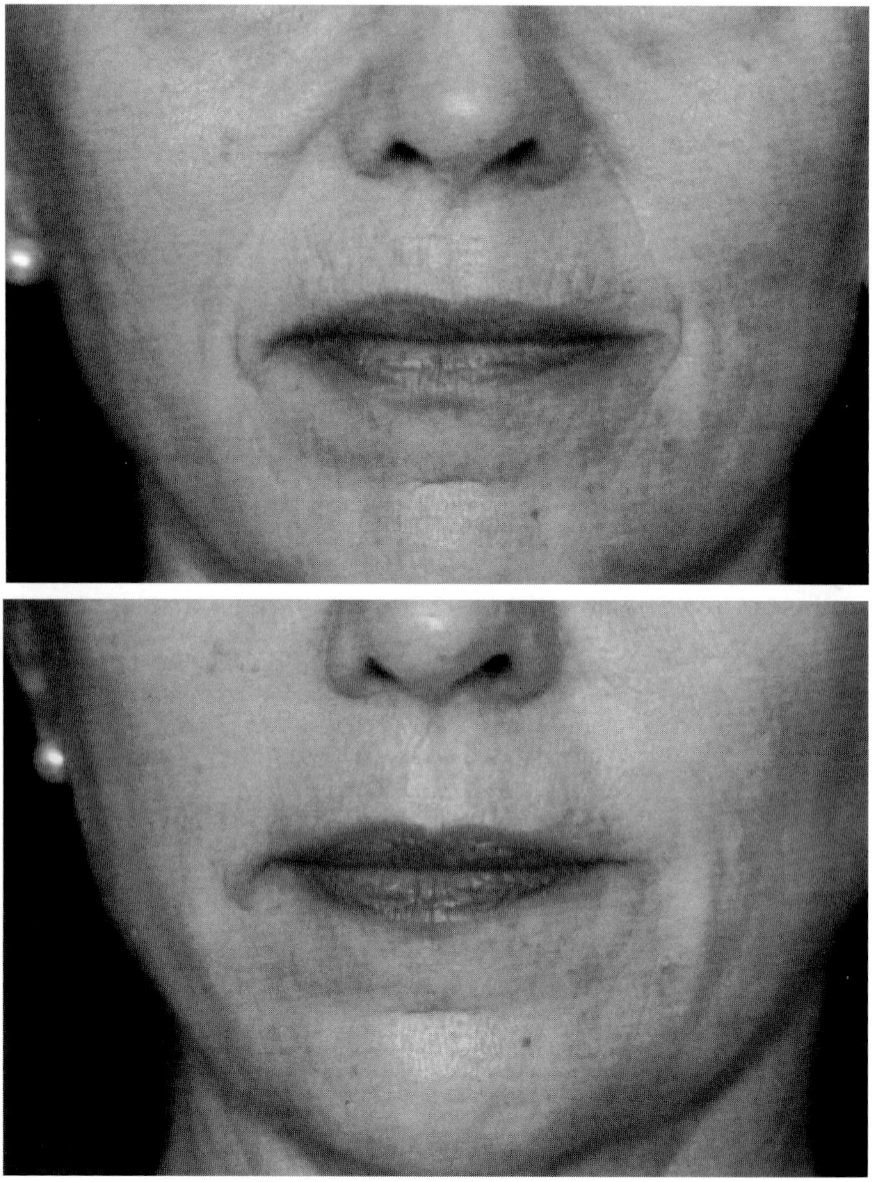

(a)

(b)

FIGURE 3 45-year-old woman with prominent nasolabial folds and upper lip rhytides (a) before and (b) 3 months after the third autologous collagen injection (Autologen).

tologen injections over a 6 month period (totaling 1.5 ml) was documented in the treatment of a deep glabellar furrow [23]. Ninety percent correction was maintained 12 months after the final treatment. Postinjection sequelae are minimal and primarily include transient redness at the injection site [5]. Although no significant adverse reactions have occurred, mild erythema may be present for up to 48 hours after injection [24]. Histological study of Autologen at 1 month in one human volunteer showed no inflammation or irritation [5].

Allogeneic Human Collagen

Dermalogen

Allografts represent tissue that is transplanted from one person to another. Allogeneic human dermis obtained from AATB-approved tissue banks has recently been approved for soft-tissue augmentation. Dermalogen human tissue implant consists of collagen, elastin, and glycosaminoglycans. Similar to Autologen, one major difference from the digested and fragmented fibrils of bovine collagen is the intact nature of the collagen fibrils in Dermalogen (Fig. 4). The tissue is processed to ensure safety, including two viral and prion inactivation steps and standardized sterilization procedures.

The most common indications for Dermalogen implantation include prominent nasolabial folds, perioral rhytides, vermilion ridge atrophy, glabellar frown lines, pronounced oral commissures, and depressed scars (Fig. 5). Neovascularization and host collagen deposition are induced. Neither Dermalogen or Autologen are best suited for correcting fine rhytides around the eyes and lips because skin in these areas is thin and these viscous materials are visible as tiny bumps that may last for weeks [26]. During initial clinical trials, the use of local anesthetics or nerve blocks was occasionally required because of pain on injection. More recently, the suspension has been buffered to approach neutral pH to reduce discomfort.

Bovine collagen produces clinical results largely because of an inflammatory response or scar formation. Dermalogen provides soft-tissue augmentation by virtue of the physical characteristics of the material itself [26]. Two to three treatment sessions (1 ml each) are therefore required over a 6 to 12 month period to provide prolonged clinical correction [22,26].

Technique

The injection techniques for Dermalogen and Autologen are essentially the same (Table 3). The key to successful injection of Dermalogen and Autologen is placement in the mid to deep dermis. The material is implanted in a series of injections through a 30-gauge needle at an approximately 30 to 45° angle from the skin surface with the bevel pointing downward. Slight blanching should be achieved. If resistance of collagen bundles in the dermis is not apparent, the material should not be injected. Subcutaneously placed material dissipates quickly and correction is lost within days. In contrast, if Dermalogen is placed too superficially, milia-like elevations may remain in the skin for months. As with Zyplast collagen, the defect should be slightly (10–20%) overcorrected. The area may be then massaged with the fingers to mold the material into the desired shape. An average of three injection sessions separated by approximately 2 weeks is generally required to achieve full correction. Progressive improvement is noted after each Dermalogen injection session [26].

Results

As part of a multicenter trial, Alster and West evaluated 28 patients in a blinded, randomized study to determine the comparative responses of nasolabial fold or oral

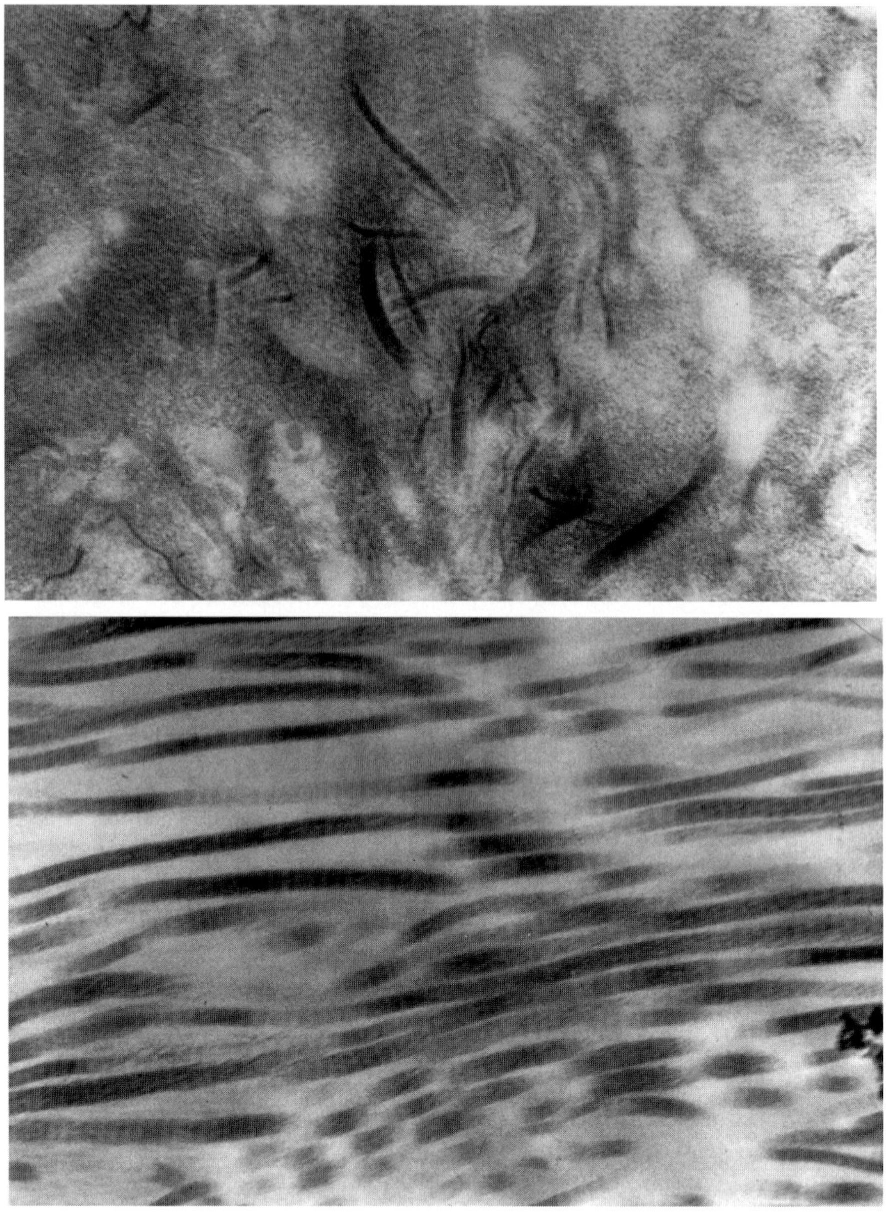

(a)

(b)

FIGURE 4 (a) Fragmented collagen fibers of reconstituted bovine collagen (Zyplast). (b) Intact human collagen fibers with normal banding pattern (Dermalogen). (Courtesy of Collagenesis, Inc., Beverly, MA.)

commissure deformities to Dermalogen versus bovine collagen injections [22]. Dermal implantations of 1.0 ml of Dermalogen or bovine collagen (Zyderm I or Zyplast) were delivered to the involved regions on a biweekly basis for a maximum total of 3.0 ml to achieve full correction. Patients were followed every 3 months for 1 year. Six months after the final injection, sustained clinical improvement was observed in

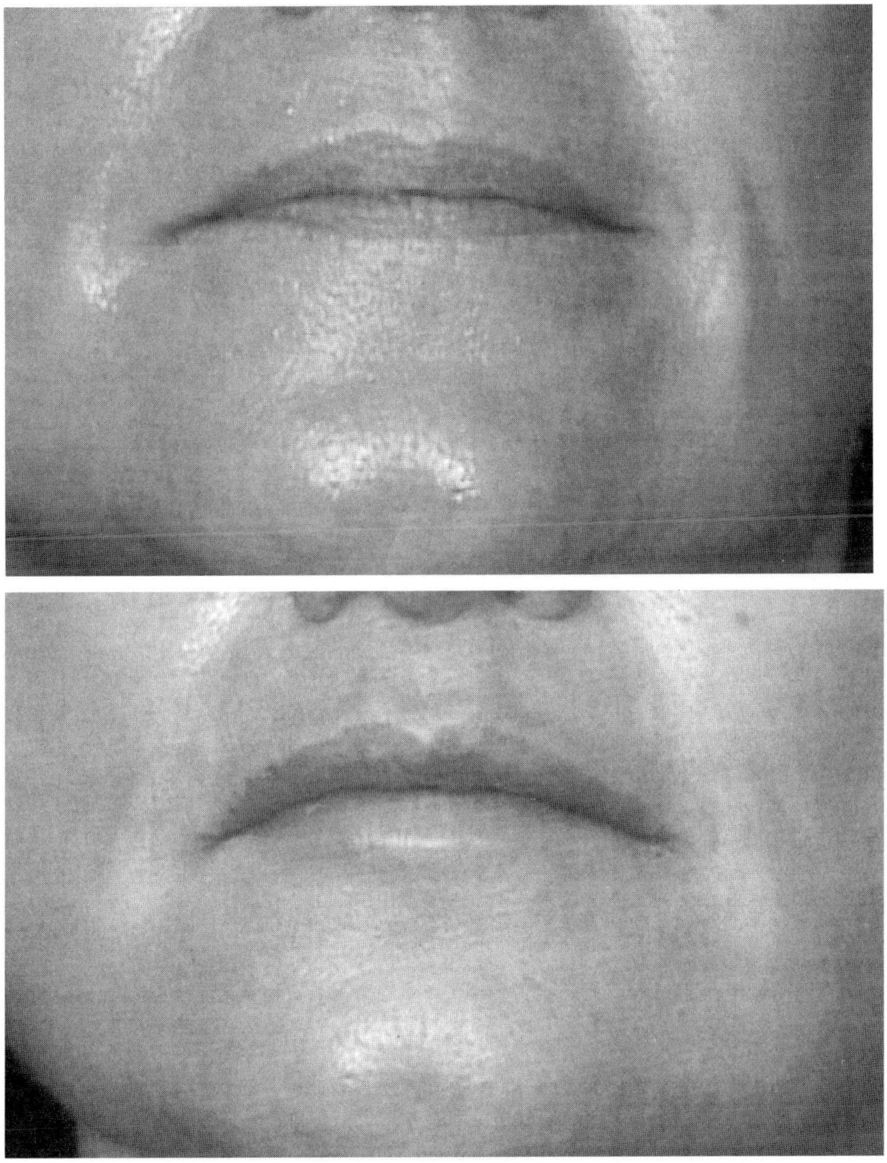

(a) (b)

FIGURE 5 43-year-old woman (a) before and (b), (c) immediately after lip augmentation with human dermal matrix (Dermalogen).

patients who received Dermalogen. The 12 month follow-up results of the multicenter study will be helpful in assessing the duration of correction of Dermalogen compared with bovine collagen. Results from the study center cited above indicate that Dermalogen persists at least as long as bovine collagen.

Clinical side effects of Dermalogen included stinging and burning at the injection sites, frequently necessitating facial nerve blocks. In addition, prolonged erythema and occasional acneiform eruptions were observed in 10% of patients. Other

(c) 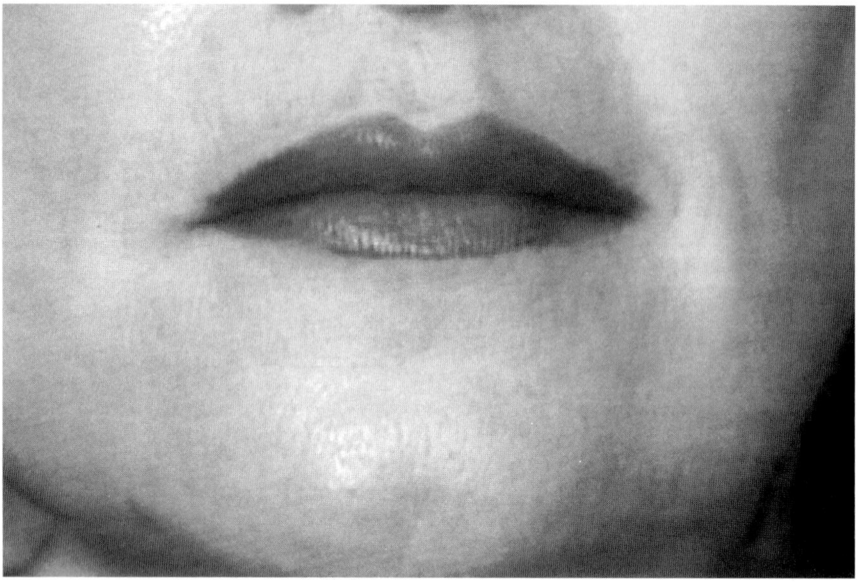

FIGURE 5 Continued

reported side effects have included transient hyperpigmentation overlying treatment sites and milia-like lesions attributable to placement of the material too superficially. No other side effects have been observed in clinical trials including 130 patients [26].

The major disadvantages of Dermalogen include patient concern regarding safety and discomfort associated with injection. A thorough explanation of the safety precautions and excellent track record of AATB-accredited facilities should be provided to patients.

AlloDerm

AlloDerm is an acellular dermal graft (homograft) derived from tissue banks. The allograft skin is processed into an immunologically inert dermal graft by removing the epidermal and dermal cells which serve as the antigenic targets of cell-mediated rejection. The graft is then freeze-dried, avoiding damage to the dermal architecture. After implantation, the dermal matrix provides a template for migration, repopulation, and revascularization by the patient's fibroblasts and endothelial cells [27–29]. Postsurgical biopsies have confirmed that AlloDerm tissue matrix is repopulated by the patient's cells and that functional tissue is regenerated. The material has been used in the treatment of burns and as an oral graft in periodontal and oral surgery [30]. Soft-tissue augmentation applications include depressed scars, revision rhinoplasties, rhytides, and lip augmentation (Fig. 6).

AlloDerm Grafts are processed from human allograft skin obtained from donors screened in accordance with all requirements of the FDA's regulation on human tissue (CFR Title 21, Part 1270). This includes donor blood testing for hepatitis B and C, human immunodeficiency virus 1 and 2, human T-lymphotropic virus type I, and syphilis, as well as extensive medical and social history screening for risk factors

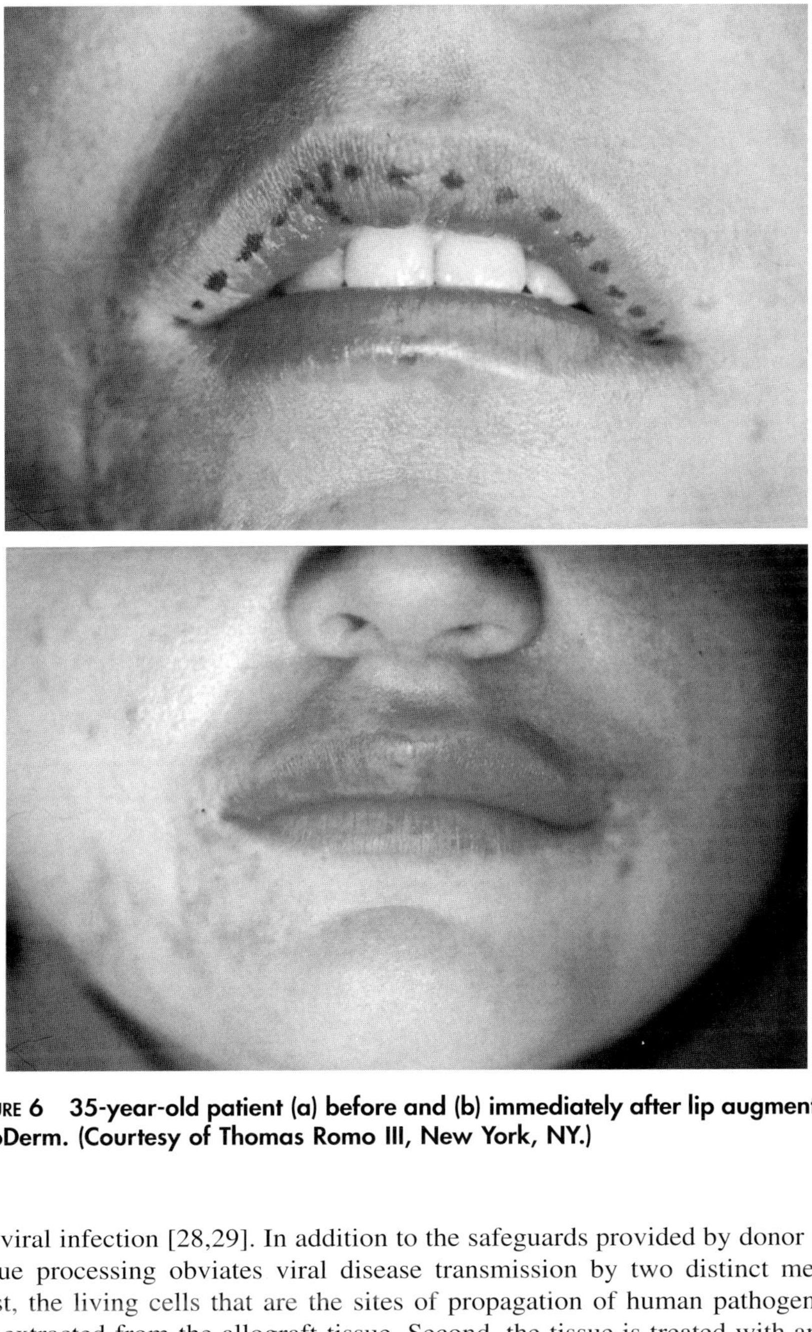

(a)

(b)

FIGURE 6 35-year-old patient (a) before and (b) immediately after lip augmentation with AlloDerm. (Courtesy of Thomas Romo III, New York, NY.)

for viral infection [28,29]. In addition to the safeguards provided by donor screening, tissue processing obviates viral disease transmission by two distinct mechanisms. First, the living cells that are the sites of propagation of human pathogenic viruses are extracted from the allograft tissue. Second, the tissue is treated with an effective antiviral agent that has been shown to inactivate the human immunodeficiency virus (HIV). There have been no reported cases of viral disease transmission in any patient treated with AlloDerm since its introduction in 1992. Immunohistochemical staining for major histocompatibility Class I and Class II antigens confirms the absence of antigens that induce rejection [31]. In contrast to conventional cryopreservaton and freeze-drying, the patented processing method preserves both the biochemical and structural integrity of the dermal matrix. The acellular dermal grafts can be stored under refrigeration for up to 2 years [30].

Technique

AlloDerm is reconstituted approximately 10 minutes before its use. The insertion of AlloDerm requires the use of local anesthetic, including nerve blocks and local infiltration. For lip augmentation, incisions are placed 1 cm medial to the oral commissure on the mucosal surface perpendicular to the vermilion border, superficial to the orbicularis oris muscle. After rehydrating the graft in saline, the 1- to 2-mm thick tissue is rolled and trimmed to the appropriate length. A tunnel is then created and an instrument is used to pass the tissue through the tunnel to the opposite end, where it is grasped and sutured in place. AlloDerm is implanted in a similar manner for the correction of depressed scars. The material has also been used in rhinoplasty revisions, glabellar contouring, rhytids, depressed scars, and nasolabial folds. In addition, it may be useful in the correction of iatrogenic depressions resulting from liposuction [30].

Results

Tobin and Karas performed 12 cases of lip augmentation for correction of thin and ptotic lips using AlloDerm grafts. They reported a 15 to 20% shrinkage rate, which stabilized after 4 to 6 weeks [31]. They hypothesized that factors responsible for resorption include graft compression after insertion and the ingrowth of tissue during the remodeling phase of wound healing. Postsurgical edema was mild to moderate, with most cases resolving within 1 week. The lips were initially indurated, but developed a natural feel within 3 months after surgery. At 12 months, all patients were pleased with their results and there was no evidence of graft rejection, hardening, or displacement. Other investigators have reported no evidence of rejection, resorption or extrusion [30]. Infection at the sutured sites of the graft has been reported and is attributed to abscess formation around the suture, unrelated to the graft itself [30,31]. After initiation of appropriate antibiotic therapy, the involved areas healed without scar formation. Tobin reported that two patients developed herpes labialis after graft insertion [31]. Complete resolution was achieved after a course of oral acyclovir. The investigators now routinely prescribe prophylactic antiviral therapy in patients with a history of herpes labialis and have noted no further incidence of herpetic infection.

SUMMARY

The recent development of human-derived filling agents heralds a new era in soft-tissue augmentation. Many of the disadvantages of xenogenic and exogenous materials have been overcome with the advent of these autologous and allogeneic alternatives. Early reports using human-derived filling agents have shown good results with no significant complications and prolonged duration of correction. It is too early, however, to assess long-term efficacy. Future investigations should include histological examination of these human-derived materials after facial implantation to document their long-term effects.

REFERENCES

1. Clark DP, Hanke CW, Swanson N. Dermal implants: safety of products injected for soft tissue augmentation. J Am Acad Dermatol 21:992–998, 1989.
2. Stegman SJ, Chu S, Armstrong RC. Adverse reactions to bovine collagen implant: clinical and histologic features. J Dermatol Surg Oncol 14(suppl 1):39–48, 1988.
3. Cooperman LS, MacKinnon V, Bechler G, et al. Injectable collagen: a six-year clinical investigation. Aesth Plast Surg 9:145–152, 1985.
4. Swanson NA, Stoner JG, Siegle RJ, et al. Treatment site reactions to Zyderm collagen implantation. J Dermatol Surg Oncol 9:377–380, 1983.
5. DeVore DP, Kelman DC, Fagien S, Casson P. Autologen: autologous, injectable dermal collagen. In: Bosniak S, ed. Ophthalmic Plastic and Reconstructive Surgery. Philadelphia: W.B. Saunders, 1996, Ch. 65.
6. Hanke CW, Coleman WP III. Collagen filler substances. In: Coleman WP III, Hanke CW, Alt TH, Asken BC, eds. Cosmetic Surgery of the Skin—Principles and Techniques. Philadelphia: BC Decker, 1991, p. 89.
7. Kligman AM. Histologic responses to collagen implants in human volunteers: comparison of Zyderm collagen with Zyplast implant. J Dermatol Surg Oncol 14(suppl 1):353–358, 1988.
8. Robinson JK, Hanke CW. Injectable collagen implant: histopathologic identification and longevity of correction. J Derm Surg Oncol 11:124–130, 1985.
9. Klein AW. Injectable collagen. In: Moschella SL, Hurley HJ, eds. Dermatology. Philadelphia: W.B. Saunders Company, 1992, pp. 2455–2461.
10. Stegman SJ, Chu S, Bensch K, Armstrong R. A light and electron microscopic evalution of Zyderm collagen and Zyplast implants in aging human facial skin: a pilot study. Arch Dermatol 123:1644, 1987.
11. Stegman SJ, Tromovitch TA. Injectable collagen. In: Stegman SJ, Tromovitch TA, eds. Cosmetic Dermatologic Surgery. Chicago: Year Book Med Pub, 1984, p. 131.
12. Siegle R, McCoy J, Shade W, et al. Intradermal implantation of bovine collagen: humoral response associated with clinical reactions. Arch Dermatol 120:183–187, 1984.
13. Mandy SH. Tretinoin in the preoperative and postoperative management of dermabrasion. J Am Acad Dermatol 15:878–879, 1986.
14. Boss WK, Marko O. Isolagen. In: Klein AW, ed. Tissue Augmentation in Clinical Practice: Procedures and Techniques. New York: Marcel Dekker, Inc., 1998, pp. 335–347.
15. Beekhius GJ. Saddle nose deformity: etiology, prevention and treatment: augmentation rhinoplasty with polyacrylamide. Laryngoscope 83:368, 1989.
16. Nunnery WR, Hetzler KJ. Dermal fat graft as a primary enucleation. Ophthalmology 92:1256, 1985.
17. Ilouz YG. Present results of fat injection. Aesthet Plast Surg 12:175, 1988.
18. Fredericks S. Fat-grafting injection for soft-tissue augmentation. Plast Reconstr Surg 84: 935, 1989.
19. West TB, Alster TS. Autologous human collagen and dermal fibroblasts for soft tissue augmentation. Dermatol Surg 24:510–512, 1998.
20. Alkek DS. Isolagen, a new autologous collagen. Cosmetic Derm Oct: 30–32, 1998.
21. Watson D, Keller GS, Lacombe V, Fodor PB, Rawnsley J, Lask G. Autologous fibroblasts for treatment of facial rhytids and dermal depressions. Arch Facial Plast Surg, 1999, accepted for publication.
22. Alster TS, West TB. New options for soft tissue augmentation. Skin & Aging July:32–36, 1998.
23. Fagien S. Autologous collagen injections to treat deep glabellar furrows (Letter). Plast Reconstr Surg 93:642, 1994.
24. Beran SJ, Rohrich RJ. The potential role of autologous, injectable dermal collagen (Au-

tologen) and acellular dermal homograft (AlloDerm) in facial soft tissue augmentation. Aesth Surg J 17:420–422, 1997.
25. DeVore DP, Hughes E, Scott JB. Effectiveness of injectable filler materials for smoothing wrinkle lines and depressed scars. Med Prog Tech 20:243, 1994.
26. Elson ML. Soft tissue augmentation with allogeneic human tissue matrix. Cosmetic Derm June:24–28, 1998.
27. Livesey SL, Herndon DN, Hollyoak MA, Atkinson YH, Nag A. Transplanted acellular allograft dermal matrix: potential as a template for the reconstruction of viable dermis. Transplantation 60:1–9, 1995.
28. Wainwright DJ. Use of an acellular dermal matrix (AlloDerm) in the management of full-thickness burns. Burns 21:243–248, 1995.
29. Wainwright DJ, Madden M, Luterman A, et al. Clinical evaluation of an acellular allograft dermal matrix in full-thickness burns. J Burn Care Rehabil 17:124–136, 1996.
30. Jones RJ, Schwartz BM, Silverstein P. Use of a nonimmunogenic acellular dermal allograft for soft tissue augmentation: a preliminary report. Aesth Surg Quarterly 16:196–201, 1996.
31. Tobin HA, Karas ND. Lip augmentation using an AlloDerm graft. J Oral Maxillofac Surg 56:722–727, 1998.

APPENDIX 1: ISOLAGEN INFORMATION AND CONSENT FORM

Isolagen is a process by which your own skin cells can grow collagen in a laboratory and then be injected back into your skin for filling in lines or scars, or for lip augmentation. Other collagen currently on the market is made from cows (bovine collagen), *not* your own cells. Because many people are allergic to foreign substances in their bodies, they may develop an allergic reaction to bovine collagen. With **Isolagen**, your own protein repair system is used to grow your own collagen and, thus, it is highly unlikely that you will be allergic.

Isolagen can provide immediate results in reducing the depth of wrinkles, correcting facial depressions, and augmenting lips. There is little, if any, recovery period. Immediately after treatment, you can reapply make-up and return to work or your regular activities.

Bovine collagen typically lasts for only three months, at which time the therapeutic benefits of wrinkle or scar correction have disappeared. With **Isolagen**, a single treatment typically can last for a longer period, with therapeutic benefits up to 1 year. **Isolagen** may even be superior to fat injections because fat cells do not have the rejuvenating or long-lasting effect on your skin that **Isolagen** does. After **Isolagen** treatment, you may have a little swelling in the area, but this quickly disappears, as your own cells and collagen are blended together for a natural look and feel.

You can safely use **Isolagen** even if you are using Retin A, Renova, or glycolic acid products. In addition, you can use **Isolagen** before or in conjunction with chemical peels or laser treatment to further enhance your facial rejuvenation results.

Since Isolagen is a process utilizing your own dermal cells, the FDA has ruled that this process does *not* require approval or registration. A similar technology is currently being utilized to grow cartilage for knee repair, bone marrow for transplants, and skin for burn victims.

Isolagen Technologies has the ability to store your protein repair system and grow more collagen when you desire additional treatments. Your dermal cells can be stored for an indefinite period of time. There is a modest annual storage fee for this service.

Procedures To Be Followed:
The first step in the **Isolagen** procedure will require an office visit at which time the physician will remove, via a small incision behind the ear, some of your own collagen-containing skin cells, known as fibroblasts. This incision will require closure with one stitch. You may experience some minimal pain and discomfort during the healing process from the incision for which you can take Tylenol.

The skin removed during this procedure will be transferred to a laboratory where your fibroblast and collagen-producing cells will be grown and the quantity of these cells increased.

Once your fibroblasts are grown (or harvested), you will return to the physician's office (usually 4 to 8 weeks later) in order to have your fibroblasts (collagen-producing cells) injected into the desired areas.

Prior to injecting the fibroblasts, the physician will test your skin to determine whether or not you are allergic to the harvested collagen or to any of the chemical agents that have been used to grow your fibroblasts. Thereafter, you will be followed on a regular basis by the physician's staff to determine how long the results last and whether there are any adverse reactions.

INFORMED CONSENT

I have completely read and understand the above information. All my questions have been answered to my complete satisfaction. I give my consent to obtain a skin punch biopsy and to undergo further Isolagen skin tests and injections. I understand that allergic reactions, though rare, can occur and that undercorrection, overcorrection, bleeding, infection, scarring, and skin irregularities could also occur. I give my consent for photographic documentation which will remain a part of my medical chart.

____________________________ __________________
Patient Signature Date

____________________________ __________________
Witness Date

APPENDIX 2: ALLODERM® ACELLULAR DERMAL GRAFT PATIENT INFORMATION SHEET

AlloDerm has been used extensively for trauma patients since 1992 and for elective surgery since 1994. No case of disease transmission has ever been reported.

AlloDerm grafts are processed from human tissues recovered exclusively within the United States. The tissue banks comply with both the United States Food and Drug Administration (FDA) regulations and the American Association of Tissue Banks (AATB) guidelines. These tissue banks rigorously screen all tissue donors, including their medical and social histories. In addition, blood samples from each tissue donor are tested and must be negative for viruses, including HIV (AIDS) and hepatitis, and bacteria, including syphilis, that could be transmitted to the graft recipients. During the processing of AlloDerm, the cellular components that would be necessary for viral transmission and survival are removed. In addition, AlloDerm grafts are screened to confirm the absence of bacterial contamination. AlloDerm grafts also undergo microscopic and other analytical testing to promote the uniform quality of processing.

When an AlloDerm graft is implanted into a patient, the patient's cells repopulate the graft, blood vessels grow into the graft, and the graft becomes part of the patient's own tissue. This process generally takes several weeks to several months. An AlloDerm graft implanted below the skin may feel firm for the first 2–3 months, then it will soften until it can no longer be felt by the patient. This will indicate that the normal healing process is complete. If a graft must subsequently be removed, some surgical dissection may be required.

In preparation for____*(procedure)*, I have had the opportunity to discuss various treatment options with my physician. One of the options explained to me by Dr. ______________________________________ is the use of AlloDerm acellular dermal graft. I have read and fully understand all of the information provided above discussing the source, characteristics and potential risks associated with the use of AlloDerm grafts. I have had all of my questions regarding this product answered by my physician to my satisfaction.

______________________________ ______________________

Patient signature Date

______________________________ ______________________

Witness signature Date

White copy - physician
Pink copy - patient

Notice to Physician: This Patient Information Sheet is not intended for use as, does not constitute, and should not be used in substitution for, your own patient informed consent form for the applicable procedure.

Rev. 8/97 008

15

Gortex

Naomi Lawrence
Cooper Health System, Marlton, New Jersey

INTRODUCTION AND HISTORY

Gortex is expanded polytetrafluoroethylene (ePTFE) (Fig. 1). The four highly electronegatively charged fluorine atoms protect the carbon atoms from interaction with various chemical substances and are responsible for the inertness and stability of the ePTFE polymer [1]. Gortex, invented in 1969 by Robert W. Gore, was first designed to be used as a vascular prosthesis in 1975 [1,2]. The molecular structure of ePTFE consists of solid nodes of PTFE interconnected by longitudinally oriented fibrils. In the original ePTFE (available in suture and patches), the node fibril structure occupies only 15 to 20% of the total volume of the material (Fig. 2). The remainder is air. In the new ePTFE the percentage volume by air is 90% (R. VonSeggern and W. L. Gore, personal communication) (Fig. 3).

The average fibril length and pore size is 22 μm. Gortex has high tensile strength, minimal deformation under load, good suture retention properties, no tumorigenicity or toxicity, and is chemically inert. All these properties make Gortex an ideal implantable substance. Since the introduction of Gortex as a vascular graft material, it has been used for vascular access grafts (in dialysis, total parenteral nutrition, cancer chemotherapy) and in ophthalmic, plastic, urogynecologic, and gastrointestinal reconstructive surgery [4–14].

ADVANTAGES AND DISADVANTAGES AS A SOFT-TISSUE FILLER

In the past 15 years, cosmetic surgeons have used Gortex in the form of patches and suture material for cosmetic augmentation of the nasolabial fold, lip, and glabella area. Gortex has the advantages of a long safety record in human use (since 1975) and chemical stability with minimal inflammatory response. In addition, the porosity of the Gortex material encourages fibrous ingrowth, which anchors its placement and leads to greater augmentation than one would expect with the material alone [3]. In any material, a pore size greater than 15 μm increases fibrous ingrowth.

After the recall of silicone breast implants, most physicians are understandably cautious about implantation foreign substances. There is a certain percentage of the cosmetic population that will reject Gortex on the basis that it is an artificial "non-

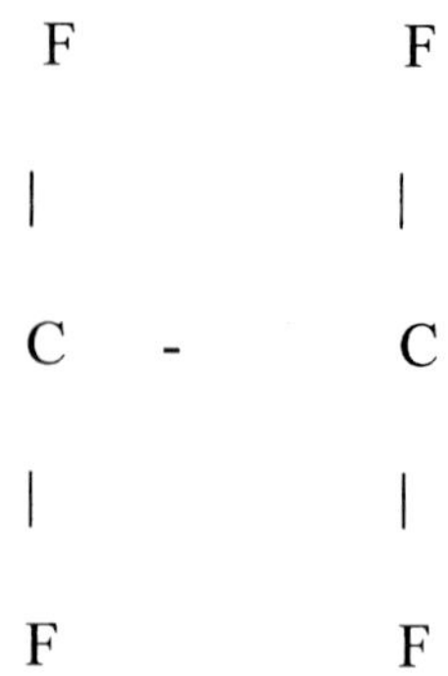

FIGURE 1 Chemical structure of polytetrafluoroethylene.

self'' material. The fact that Gortex is permanent is both an advantage and a disadvantage. Most patients are willing to accept the higher initial cost outlay for a permanent result. However, if the patient is not happy with the material, it must be removed which requires a second procedure that is technically more difficult than implantation.

The use of Gortex implants for cosmetic augmentation received Food and Drug Administration (FDA) approval in December 1993. It is available through two companies under the trade names SAM (Subcutaneous Augmentation Material; WL Gore and Associates, Elkinton, MD) and SoftForm Facial implant (Collagen Corp., Palo Alto, CA). Both companies specifically devised their new Gortex products for cosmetic soft-tissue augmentation. The Gortex used for cosmetic augmentation before

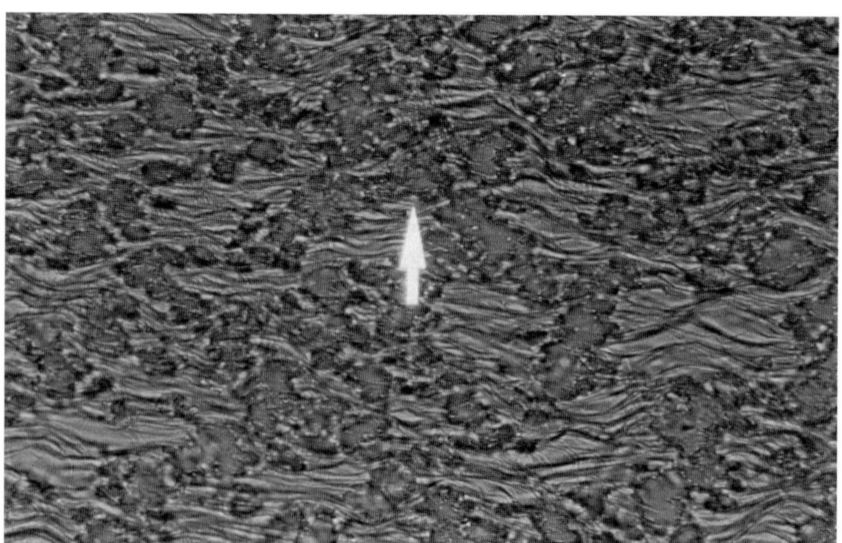

FIGURE 2 Histopathology of Gortex suture.

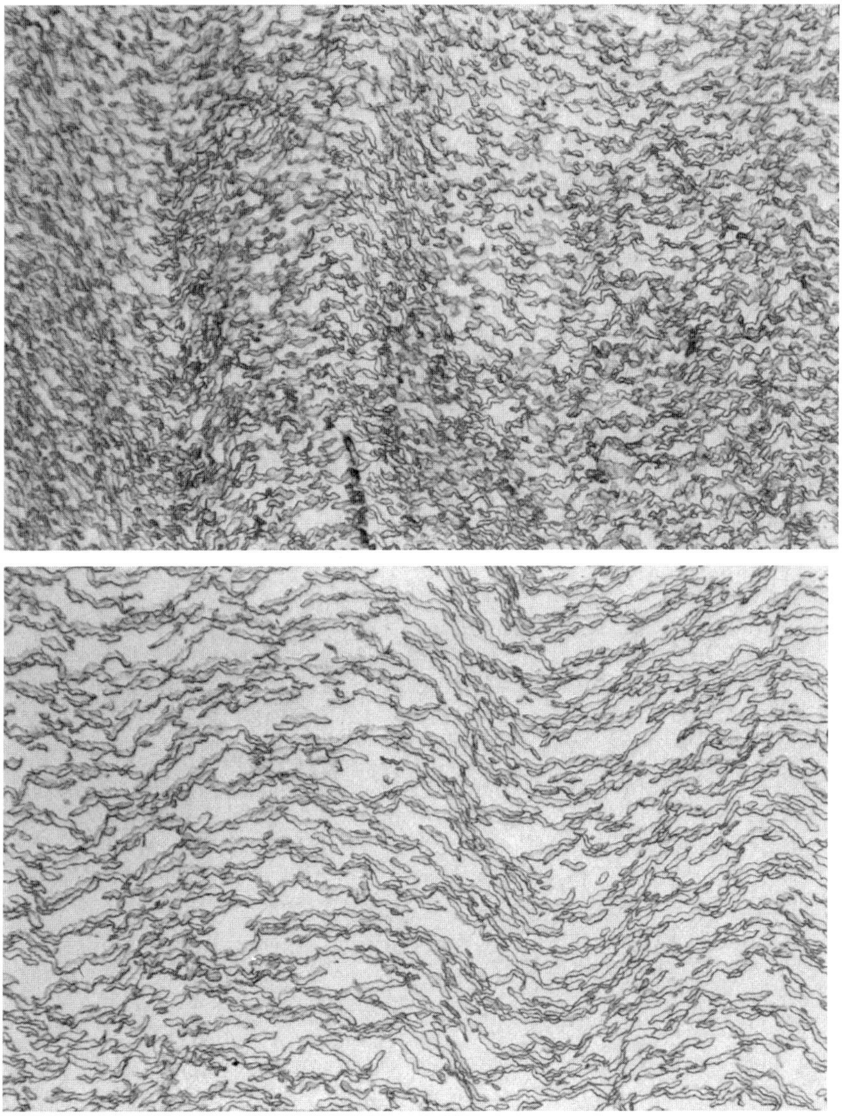

(a)

(b)

FIGURE 3 (a) Histopathology of SAM (Gore Corporation). (b) Histopathology of SoftForm (Collagen Corporation.)

these products—"old" Gortex—was less expanded by air. The patch had the disadvantage of needing special cutting and "tailoring" to the location. The 0-suture was small and required several passes to cause augmentation. The strands formed a palpable ridge. With layering of suture there was a risk of picking up another strand and causing a lump or knot (creating a nidus for suture extrusion). Movement of the implanted suture could occur particularly in a patient that manipulated the area. As with any implant there was a risk of infection.

ADVANTAGES OF "NEW" GORTEX

One caveat before this area is addressed: there is considerable bias in the literature available on Gortex. The two corporations that produce Gortex for cosmetic augmentation have completely different viewpoints on the appropriate form of the implant and method of implantation that are variably supported by scientific literature. These are new products and are still developing.

The literature from SAM claims that the greater porosity of the new Gortex leads to better fibrous ingrowth improving the percentage augmentation and anchoring the implant. With better anchoring there is less risk of movement of the implant and less risk of extrusion. Collagen Corporation has developed a tubular implant (SoftForm) based on research that showed greater stabilizing and less risk of extrusion with tubes than other configurations of implants [15,16]. Greene et al. implanted 396 Gortex pieces in a porcine model. They found extrusion and persistent infection rates were .85% for ePTFE tubes and 4.4% for the strips ($p < .05$). No extrusions occurred after 6 months (longest follow-up was 12 months). They concluded that the difference in stability between the strips and tube was attributable to fibrous ingrowth into the lumen of the tube. They also maintain that the fibrous ingrowth into the Gortex material itself is minimal and therefore does not provide sufficient stabilization [16]. Clearly there is some ingrowth into the material (Fig. 4). However, because the growth is minimal it does not impede the removal of the implant. According to the SoftForm product literature, the implant is "easy" to remove because the growth into the lumen provides stability but the external surface is relatively free of tissue ingrowth (Fig. 5). According to Maas, another advantage of the tubular configuration is that the convex surface creates greater surface augmentation [16].

AVAILABLE PRODUCTS AND MATCHING DIAMETER OF IMPLANT TO DEFECT

Collagen Corporation has 3 sizes of SoftForm now available (see Table 1). The delivery system and the shortened length (7 cm) necessitate two pieces to augment most areas (e.g., lip, nasolabial folds). The SAM product comes in two forms: single and multistranded (see Tables 2 and 3). The cross-sectional dimension (strands) and the nominal bundle diameter measurements (multistrand) are the most important information for the amount of augmentation provided. All of the strands are 15 cm in length so that only one strand is necessary to augment bilateral nasolabial folds or the lip area. Multistrand products are provided two to a packet. Because of this, SAM is more economical than SoftForm, averaging about half the cost. Gore company recently discontinued their tubular form.

When determining the size of the implant for the area to augment, it is important to be conservative around the lips. The implants are more palpable here and provide definition rather than volume. I most commonly use the SAM002 and 003 or the SoftForm 3.2 in the lips. In the nasolabial folds and marionette lines, the smaller sizes are really not adequate. The SAM003 or 004, the multistrands 108-210, or the SoftForm 3.2 are best for these locations.

(a)

(b)

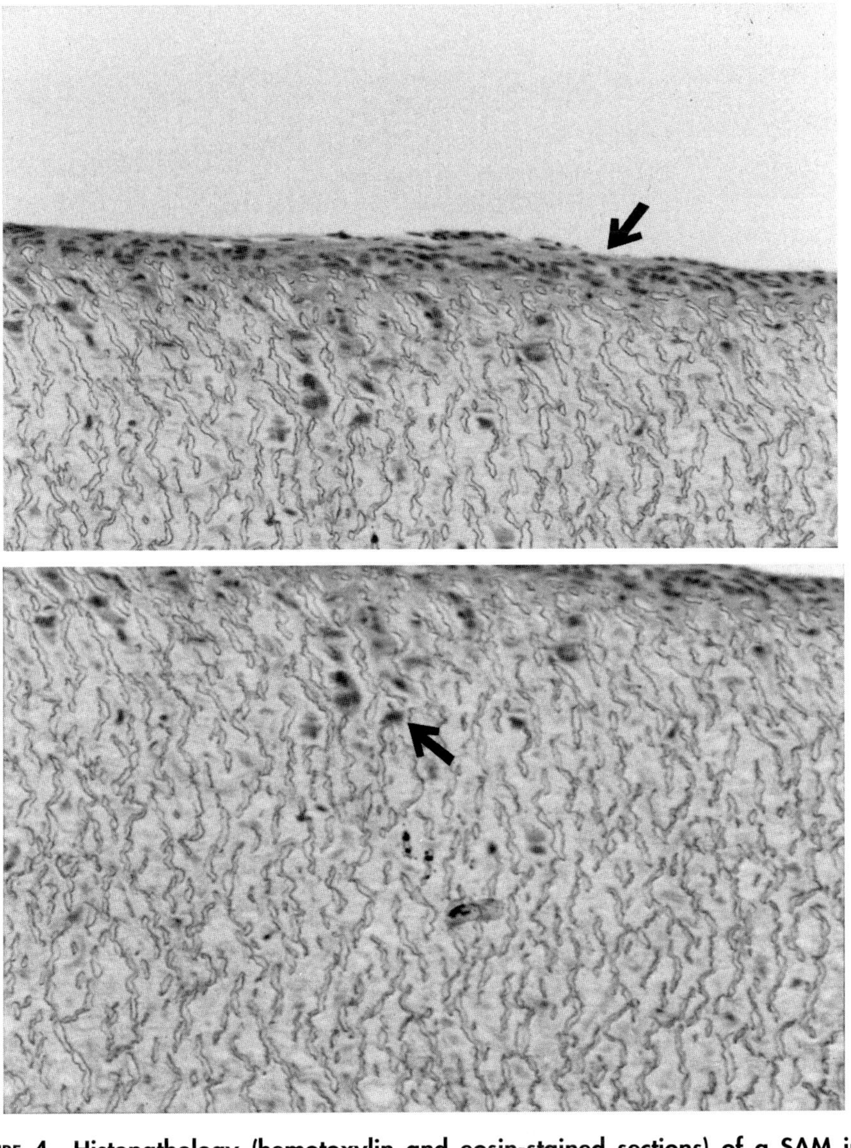

FIGURE 4 Histopathology (hemotoxylin and eosin-stained sections) of a SAM implant showing fibroblast and collagen ingrowth. This specimen was removed 4 months after SAM implantation. (a) Interface with tissue. (b) Fibroblasts and within implant.

INDICATIONS FOR COSMETIC USE

Facial rejuvenation can be divided into upper and lower face (Fig. 6). For the upper face, we have available both surgical and nonsurgical (botulinum toxin injections) methods of correction that are superior in result and have greater longevity than soft-tissue augmentation. In the lower face, soft-tissue augmentation still plays a large

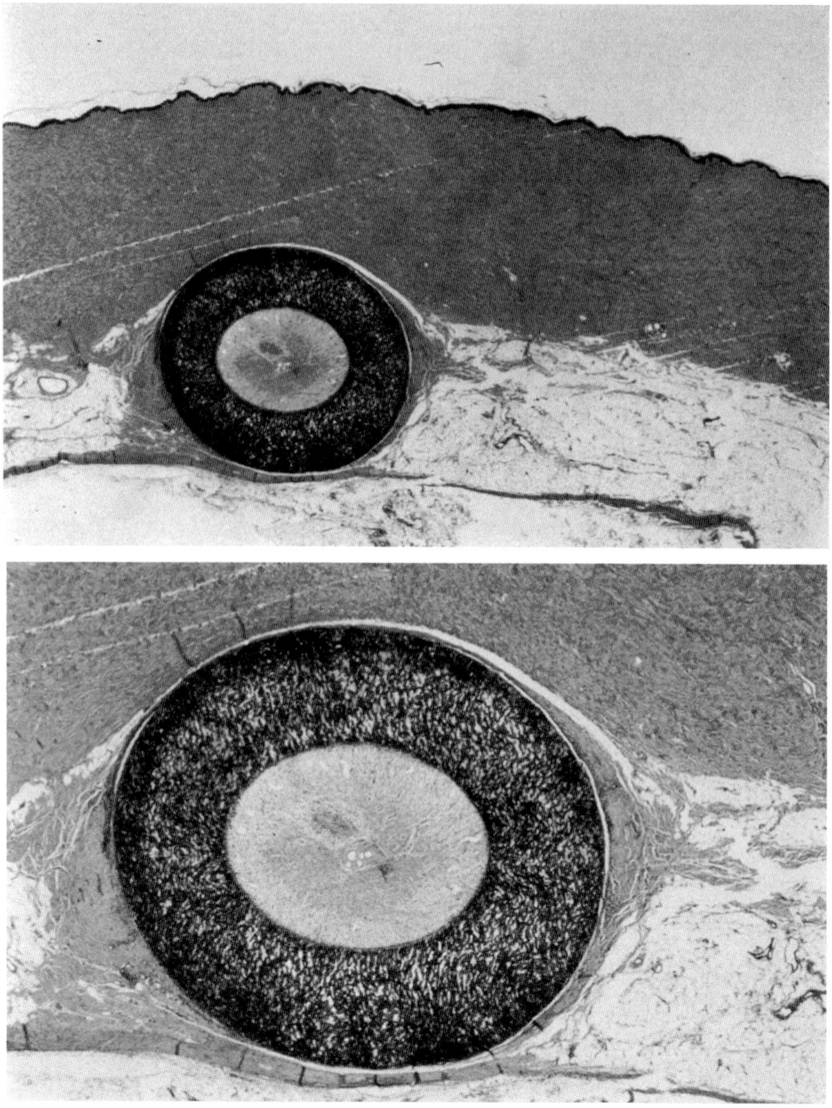

(a)

(b)

FIGURE 5 SoftForm implant with collagen into lumen (Courtesy of Collagen Corporation). (a) Low magnification of SoftForm implant after fibrosis in the lumen. (b) High magnification of SoftForm implant after fibrosis in the lumen.

role in facial rejuvenation. The injectable soft-tissue augmentation materials (bovine collagen is the prototype) are very short lived in the perioral area because of the high mobility in this location. Gortex can be used in this area to give definition to the lips and soften the nasolabial folds and marionette lines. Many of the patients who come in for augmentation in the nasolabial folds or marionette lines are not willing to accept the morbidity of a face lift or are trying to delay a face lift.

TABLE 1 SoftForm (Collagen Corp.)

Inside diameter	Outside diameter	Length
1.2	2.4	50 mm
1.2	3.2	70 mm
1.2	4.0	90 mm

THE CONSULTATION

The patient history is taken with particular attention to any bleeding abnormalities, predisposition to infection, and autoimmune disease. Every physician's approach to risk management is individual. My approach is to not take patients off aspirin for surgical procedures if they are on it for cardiac or neurological disorders. They are apprised of their increased risk of hematoma. Patients on Warfarin sodium (Coumadin; Dupont, Wilmington, DE) require medical clearance for removal off their medication. Immunosuppression is a relative contraindication to an implant because of the increased risk of infection. Autoimmune disease may also be considered a relative contraindication because of theoretical risks of auto-antibody stimulation.

As with any cosmetic consultation, it is important to make sure that the patient has realistic expectations. The key to consultation for Gortex implantation is to downplay the results. For the nasolabial fold and marionette line areas it is important to explain that there will be a 30 to 40% improvement with a softening of the line (Fig. 7). In the lips, Gortex gives definition but not volume (as a large injection of collagen would) (Fig. 8). The patient should be educated about the postsurgical course because there can be a measure of disappointment as they pass through the healing phases.

Initially in the first week after surgery, the fold can appear to be almost completely gone secondary to the tissue swelling from the implantation procedure. Patients are very pleased with this but they must be warned that the tissue swelling will resolve by 1 month and what will be left is the augmentation from the Gortex.

TABLE 2 SAM Single-Stranded Available Implants

Part no.	Nominal W × L × T (cm × cm × mm)	Nominal bundle diameter (mm)
1SAM107	.6 × 6.1 × 1	2.8
1SAM108	.9 × 6.1 × 1	3.4
1SAM109	1.5 × 7.3 × 1	4.4
1SAM112	1.5 × 5.5 × 1	4.4
1SAM113	1.5 × 6.1 × 1	4.4
1SAM114	1.5 × 6.7 × 1	4.4
1SAM209	1.5 × 7.3 × 2	6.2
1SAM210	1.5 × 6.7 × 2	6.2

Note: One unit = two multistrands at $215.00 each. Three or more units = $195.00 each.

TABLE 3 SAM Multistranded Available Implants

Cross-sectional dimension (mm × mm)	Length (cm)	Product number
1.8 × 1.8	15	1SAM001
3.2 × 2	15	1SAM002
4.2 × 3	15	1SAM003
6.5 × 3.5	15	1SAM004

As fibrous ingrowth occurs they will get anchoring and additional augmentation for 6 months to 1 year.

Presurgical instructions are relatively simple. The patient should come to the office with no make-up and wash their face with an antibacterial soap. Patients take a single dose of antibiotic such as Cephalexin hydrochloride (Keflex; Eli Lilly Industries, Indianapolis, IN), Cefadroxil (Duricef; Bristol Meyers Squibb, Princeton,

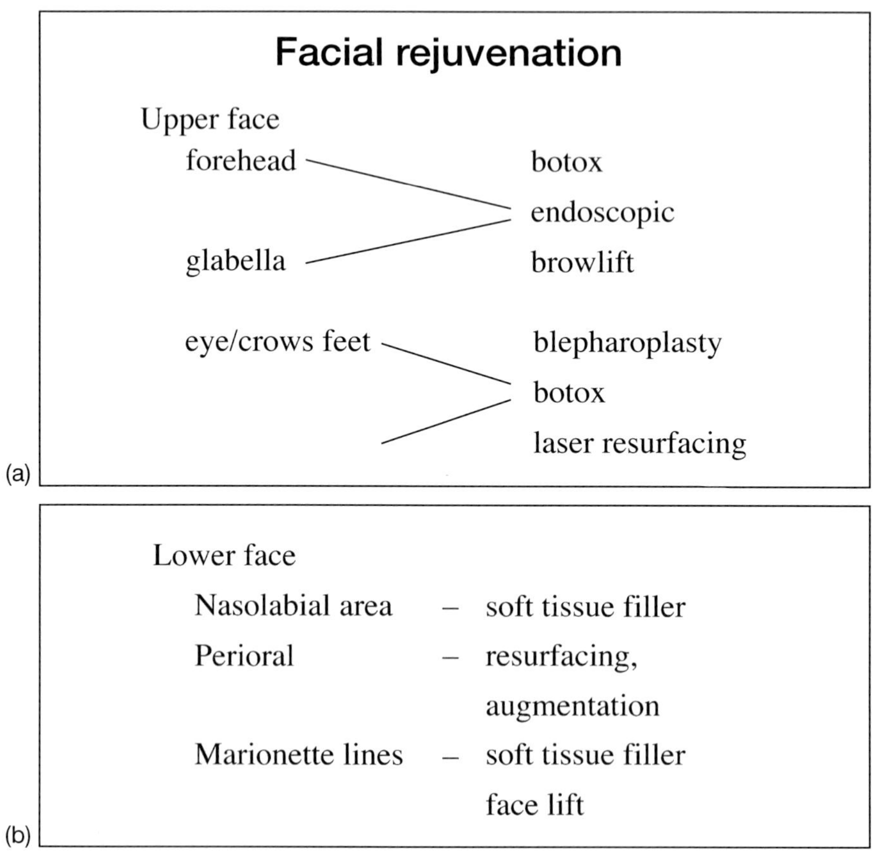

FIGURE 6 (a,b) Options for upper and lower facial rejuvenation.

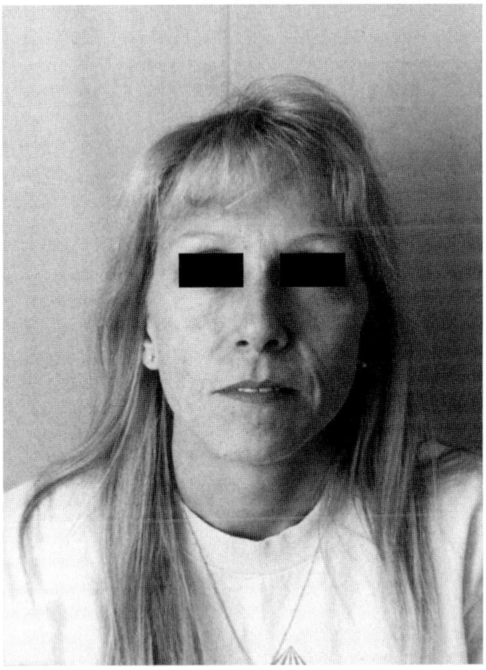

(a)

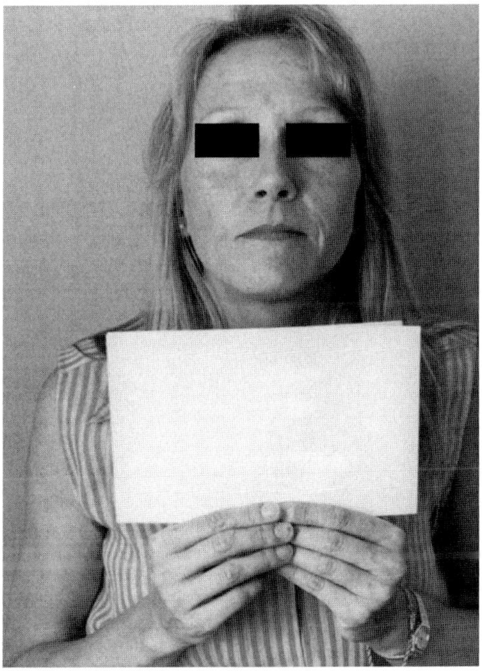

(b)

FIGURE 7 (a) Pre-implantation of Gortex to nasolabial/perioral lines. (b) After second implantation of two 3 mm tubular Gortex SAM (second implantation performed 8 months after original because of suboptimal augmentation). Note: this tubular form is now discontinued.

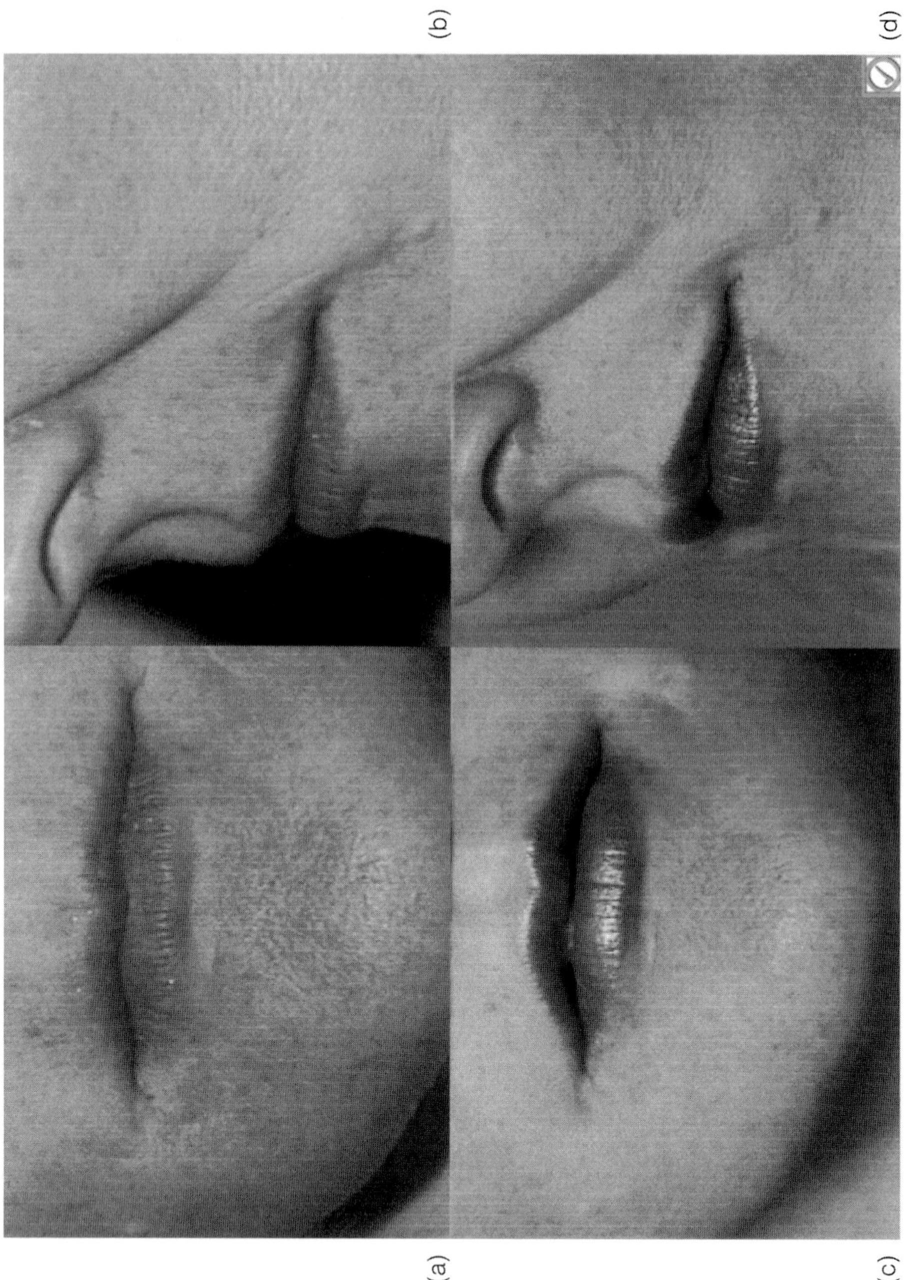

Figure 8 (a,b) Pre-implantation of SoftForm in the upper and lower lip. (c,d) Postimplantation of SoftForm in the upper and lower lip.

NJ), Amoxicillin/Clavulante potassium (Augmentin; Smithklein Beecham Pharmaceuticals, Philadelphia, PA) 1 hour before the procedure and continue on a week course of antibiotic after the procedure.

THE SURGICAL IMPLANTATION: PROCEDURE

The patient is prepared in a sterile fashion and marked with a sterile marking pen. With both forms of Gortex, proper placement is the key to a satisfactory procedure. It is important to take good pre- and postsurgical photographs. In a procedure such as Gortex placement where the defect is not completely obliterated but instead has a percentage improvement, the patient appreciates the photographic evidence of a positive change.

In both the nasolabial fold and the lip area it is possible to choose entrance and exit sites that can be camouflaged by cosmetic junctions. For the nasolabial folds and marionette lines it is important to mark the placement with the patient sitting up. Placement should be on the medial aspect of the depression. The lip placement is at the vermillion border. Although one strand can be used for the upper lip, the cupid's bow is better accentuated when two strands are used. This requires entrance site at the angle of the mouth and an exit site at the crest of the cupid's bow. The length of the implant to fill the defect is determined by measuring the length of the fold (or lip line) before injection with anesthesia.

For anesthesia, a combination of nerve blocks and local anesthesia work best. For both the upper lip and nasolabial fold area, an infraorbital block is performed. Cetacaine (Benzacaine Tetracaine; Cetylite Industries, Pennsauken, NJ) topical anesthetic is wiped on the upper gum line. Anesthesia is introduced first through a 30-gauge needle, and then a 25 $1\frac{1}{2}$ in. gauge needle is directed towards the infraorbital foramen and 1 to 1.5 ml are injected. In addition to the block, the area for implantation is also injected locally with anesthetic.

For the SAM material the surgical tray should contain two 14-gauge angiocatheters, a straight (Keith) needle, two 0-Silk suture, a straight iris, and a needle

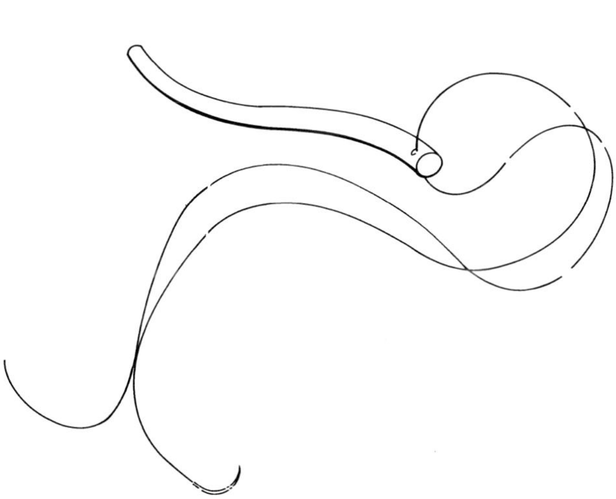

FIGURE 9 The SAM material is sauged onto a 0-silk suture.

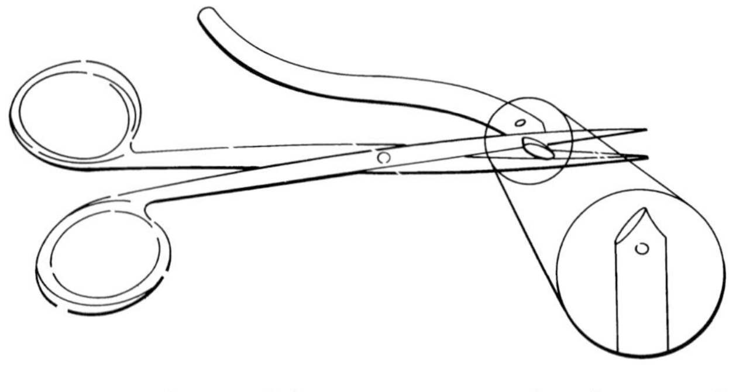

FIGURE 10 The tip of the SAM is trimmed with a straight Iris scissor.

driver. The piece of Gortex (cut to fit the defect) is threaded with the 0-silk (Fig. 9). The tip of the implant is trimmed to taper (Fig. 10). The needle is then cut off the 0-silk and double armed in the Keith needle (Fig. 11). This is left on the tray while the site is made ready for implantation. For the nasolabial folds, an insertion site is marked 2 to 3 mm inferior to the base of the fold and on the medial aspect. The 14-gauge angiocatheter is introduced into the subcutaneous plane through the area marked for insertions (Fig. 12). The stylet is removed and plastic catheter trimmed (Fig. 13). The Keith needle is inserted in the distal tip of the angiocatheter towards the proximal hub (Fig. 14). Once through the hub, the Keith needle can be removed. The angiocatheter is also removed (Fig. 15). A small scissors is used to enlarge the entrance wound slightly. The Gortex is then introduced into the subcutaneous plane by pulling the attached suture (Fig. 16). This takes steady pressure but should advance fairly easily (ie, smoothly). The suture is removed by cutting one end from its attachment. To ensure the tips are well buried, one can use the tips of the Iris scissors or the Keith needle to further bury the ends (Fig. 17). It is not necessary to suture the entrance and exit sites. A small bandage with Vaseline or an antibiotic

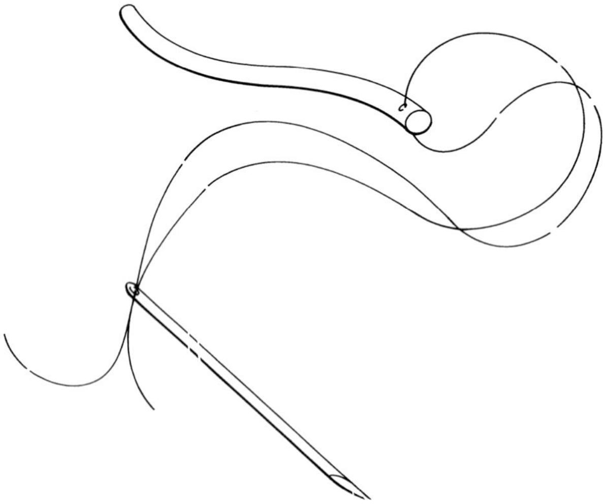

FIGURE 11 The Keith needle is double armed with the 0-silk suture.

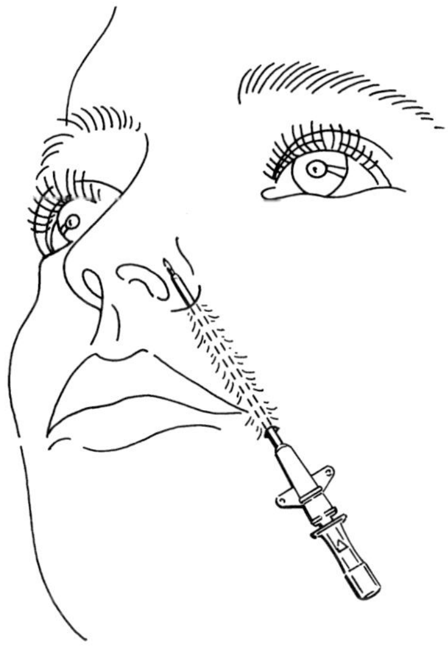

FIGURE 12 Pretunneling is accomplished with a 14-gauge angiocatheter. For the nasolabial fold, the entrance is placed near the corner of the mouth and advanced (2-4 mm) medial to the fold.

ointment is placed and the patient is given instructions on how to clean and change daily.

For the lips the same procedure is adhered except for the following variations. The insertion site is at the corner of the mouth. The area is not pretunneled with the angiocatheter. The Keith needle (with 0 silk suture and Gortex attached) is advanced

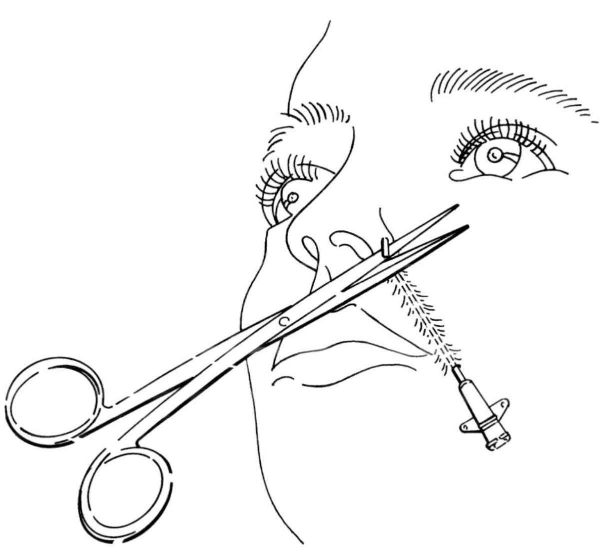

FIGURE 13 The stylet is removed from the angiocatheter and the plastic sleeve is trimmed with a straight Iris scissor.

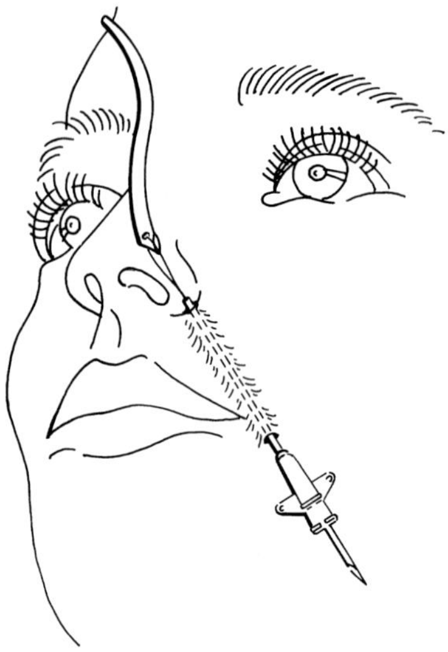

FIGURE 14 The Keith needle is inserted into the plastic sleeve and advanced towards the hub of the angiocatheter. A hemostat is used to pull the needle from the hub.

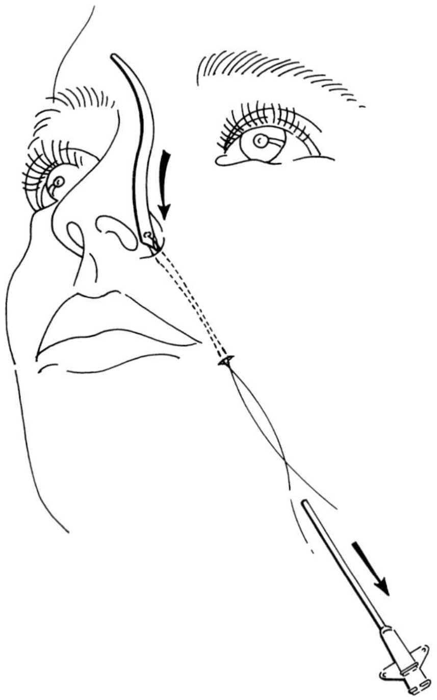

FIGURE 15 The angiocatheter is removed and the opening in the alar/cheek crease is enlarged with dissecting scissors. The Keith needle is removed.

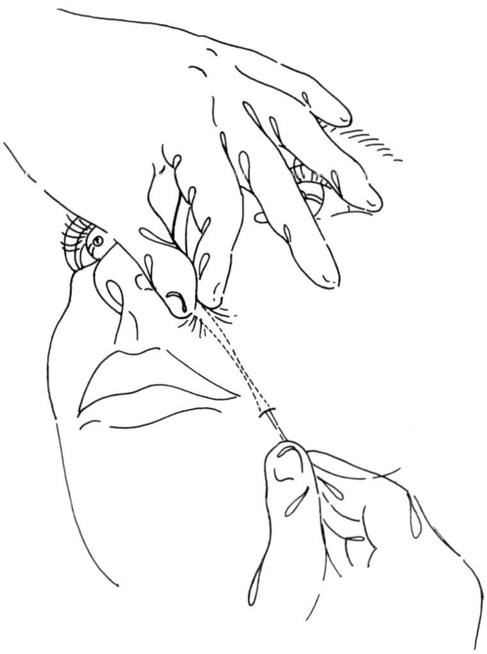

FIGURE 16 The skin is stabilized while the SAM is pulled into a subcutaneous plane.

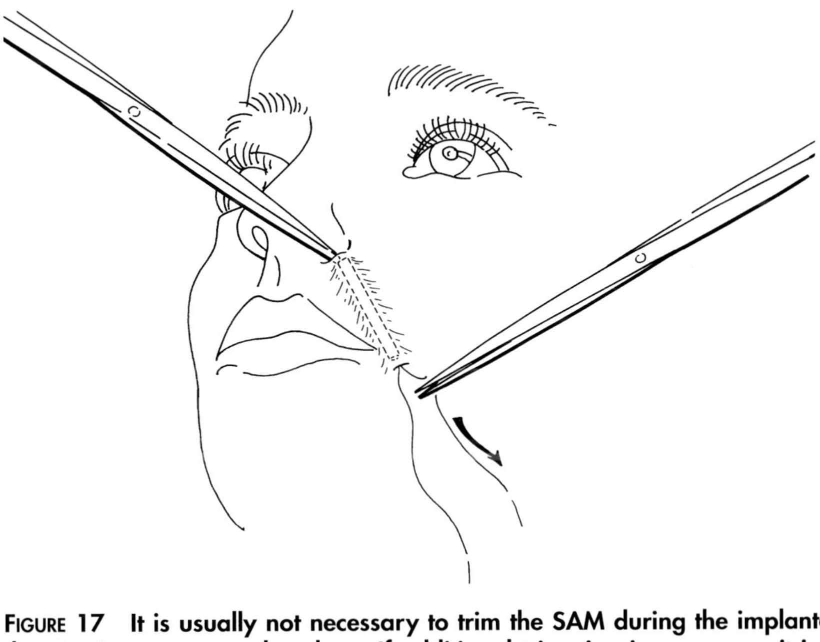

FIGURE 17 It is usually not necessary to trim the SAM during the implantation because the size is premeasured and cut. If additional trimming is necessary, it is performed at the alar/cheek end at this time. The tips of the implant are buried with the tips of a straight Iris or the Keith needle.

along the vermillion border to the top of the Cupid's bow on the same side and exited here (Fig. 18). The same procedure is performed on the other side of the upper lip. The lower lip is treated less commonly but here the pass can be made from one corner to the other.

SoftForm IMPLANTATION

Collagen Corporation has recently written a revised procedure guide for SoftForm implantation. The following text combines my experience and the new guidelines.

The surgical set up includes the following:

General Supplies
- Antiseptic for presurgical regional skin preparation (eg, Betadine, Hibiclens)
- Sterile powderless gloves
- Skin-marking pen
- Material for nerve block and local anesthetic (1% lidocaine)
- Two 6 ml syringes with 30-gauge needle

Sterile Set-up
- One to three sterile barriers (eg, towels, drapes, disposables)
- Gauze 4 × 4s
- No. 11 scalpel blade and handle
- Needle driver
- 6-0 sutures (clear nylon sutures may be less noticeable)
- Small sharp scissors
- Small toothed forceps
- Small hemostat (if pretunneling is desired)
- Steri-strips

The SoftForm implant is provided preloaded on a trocar (Fig. 19). The cannula has a notched window to allow you to view the implant. Before the procedure is begun it is important to check the implant and make sure that it is visible through the window and also check that the trocar is properly seated and engaged (Fig. 20). The green adhesive dot on the package of the implant device indicates that appropriate sterilization is intact.

A stab incision is made with a No. 11 blade at the predetermined entrance site (.3-.6 cm in diameter). Pretunneling with a 12- or 14-gauge liposuction cannula can make the advancement of the trocar much easier. Pinch the tissue between the thumb and index finger and insert the trocar to a subdermal plane at a 45° angle (Fig. 21). Once the depth of the tip reaches the appropriate plane, orient the trocar parallel to the surface of the skin and advance in the subdermal plane according to the skin markings (Fig. 22). A slight rotating motion may be used when advancing the trocar. If excessive resistance is encountered, the placement is probably too superficial. When approaching the exit site, there will be greater resistance as the tip goes through the dermis to pierce the skin. Place a hemostat or forceps to protect the surrounding facial anatomy from the emerging tip. While the cannula is still in place, redrape the skin over the device to eliminate puckering (Fig. 23). Next the cannula and trocar must be removed. It is important to stabilize the trocar tip before releasing the pin lock and pressing the plunger as the trocar can be forcefully projected from

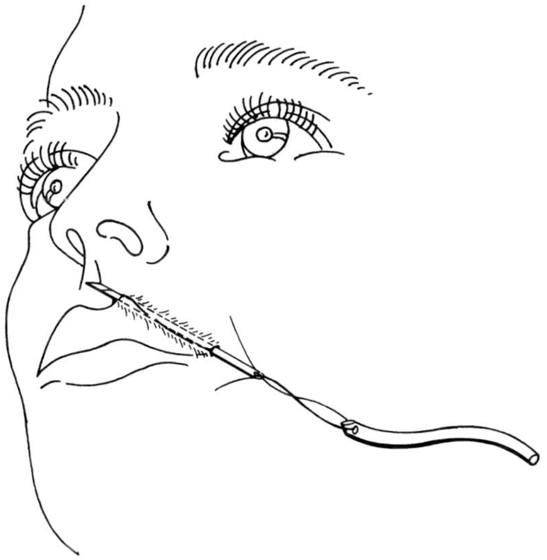

FIGURE 18 For the lip, implantation placement is directly at the vermillion border. In this area do not pretunnel with angiocatheter but instead use the straight Keith needle alone.

the cannula (Fig. 24). Once the cannula is removed, the trocar is removed (Fig. 25, 26).

Smooth the skin overlying the implant again (Fig. 27). Use an angle of 30 to 45° to cut the implant excess and leave a beveled edge (Fig. 28). The Collagen Corp. guidelines emphasize reopening the lumen before final implantation to maintain patency, which will ensure fibrous ingrowth and subsequent stabilization. The significance of that step remains to be determined. It seems that if the lumen were closed by minor pressure, the pressure of the overlying skin or the patient touching the area in the postsurgical period could potentially close the lumen.

Once the ends are subdermally placed, the entrance and exit sites are sutured closed with nonabsorbable 6.0 suture (Fig. 29).

WHAT TO EXPECT IN THE POSTSURGICAL PERIOD

Patients will have some bruising and swelling secondary to the local anesthetic injections and the surgical implantation procedure. It is important to tell the patient

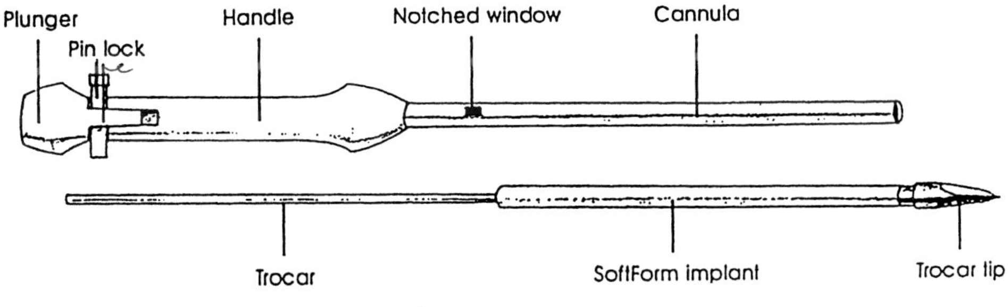

FIGURE 19 SoftForm implantation device.

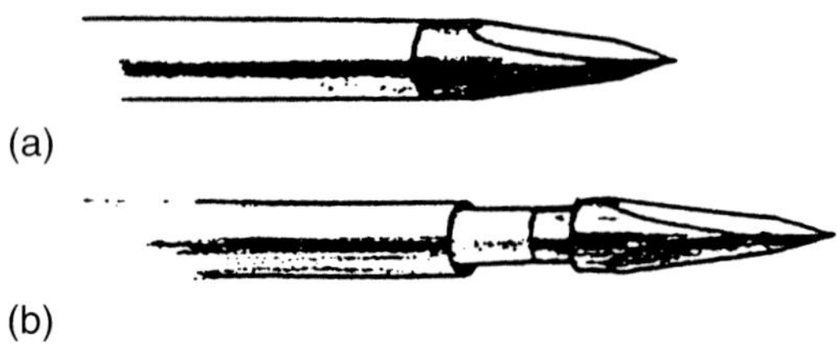

FIGURE 20 (a) Trocar tip correctly seated. (b) Trocar tip incorrectly seated.

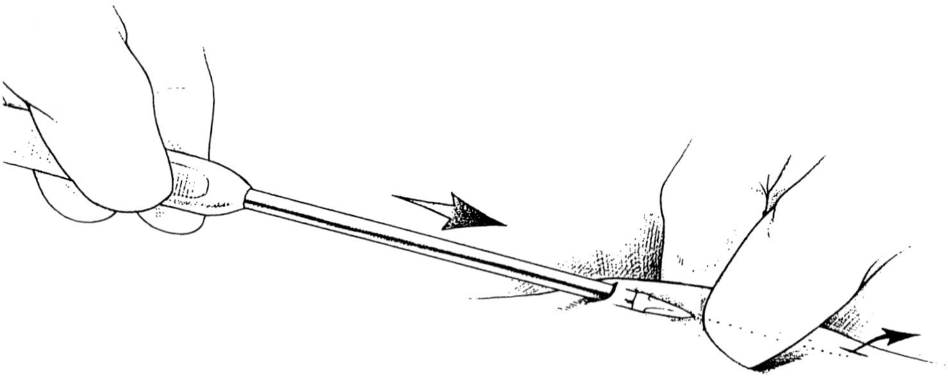

FIGURE 21 Inserting the device.

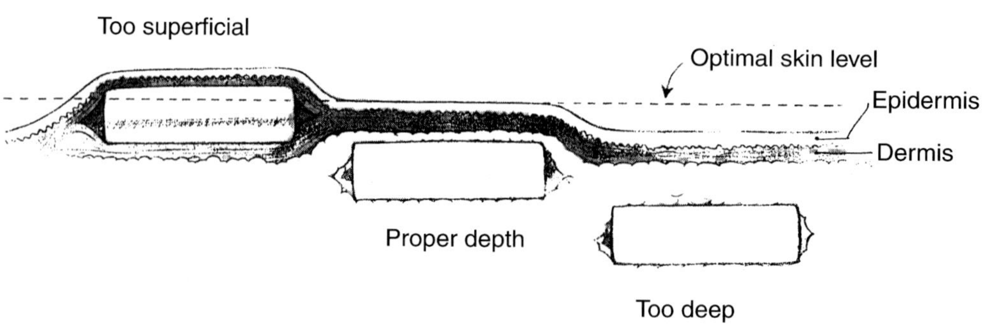

FIGURE 22 Proper placement in the subdermal plane.

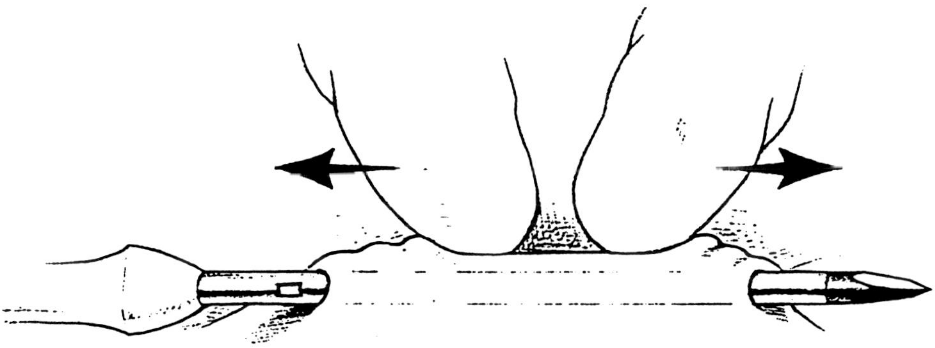

FIGURE 23 Draping the skin over the cannula.

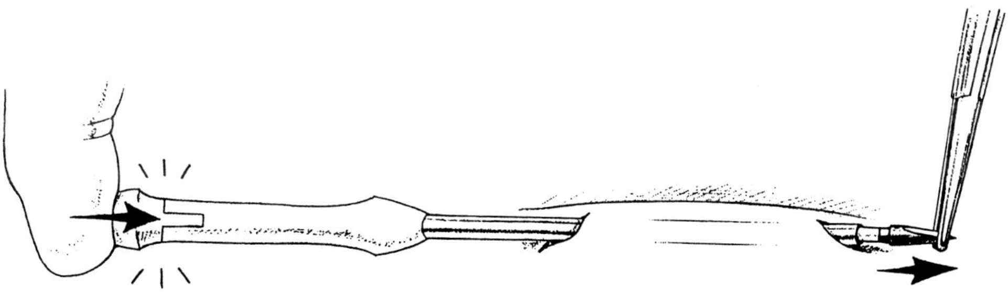

FIGURE 24 Grasp trocar, then release pin press plunger to disengage trocar.

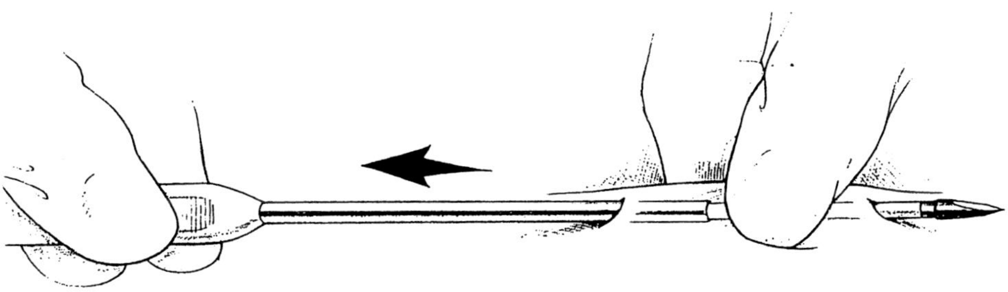

FIGURE 25 Cannula is extracted.

that there can be great individual variability in the amount of swelling. Application of ice packs in the first 24 hours will decrease the swelling. Acetaminophen is recommended for any discomfort. Patients are instructed not to take any aspirin or nonsteroidal (except for medical purposes). They are told to minimize mouth movement (talking, laughing, vigorous chewing) for 2 weeks. Patients are to refrain from manipulating the implant with their fingers (or tongue for lip implants) to "check" placement because this could cause movement (Appendix 1).

The implant has three clinical healing phases in the immediate postsurgical period. Patients are initially very pleased with their implant because the swelling from the procedure augments the defect well. Any assessment at 1 week will over-

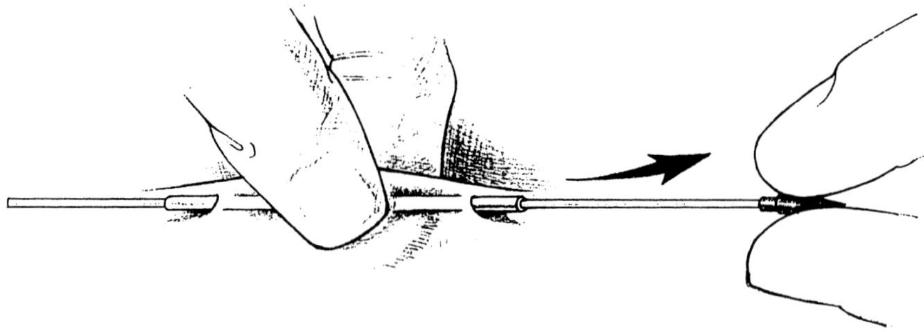

FIGURE 26 Trocar removed with implant in place.

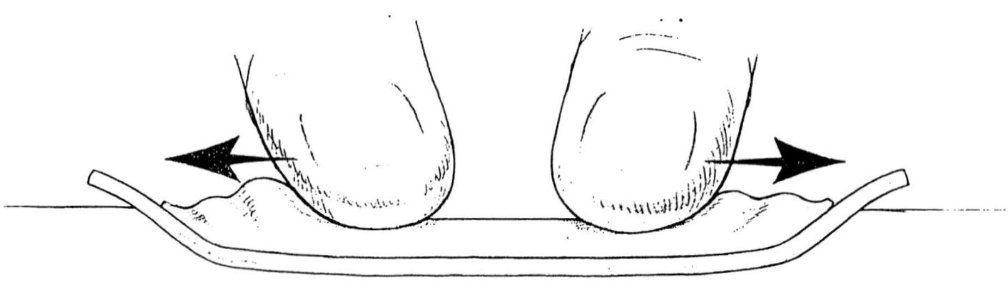

FIGURE 27 Redrape skin over implant.

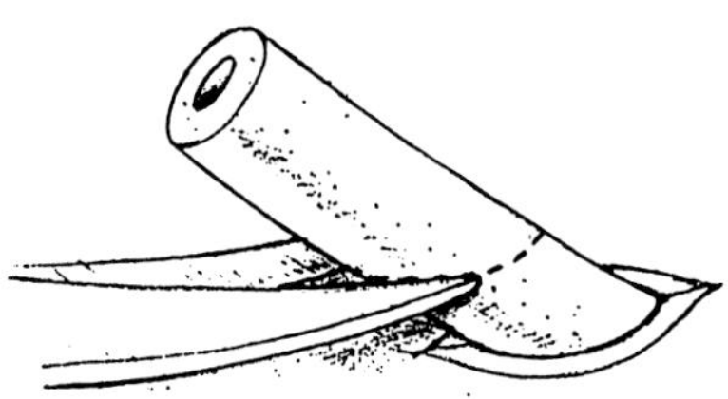

FIGURE 28 Cut tips of implant at 30-45° angle.

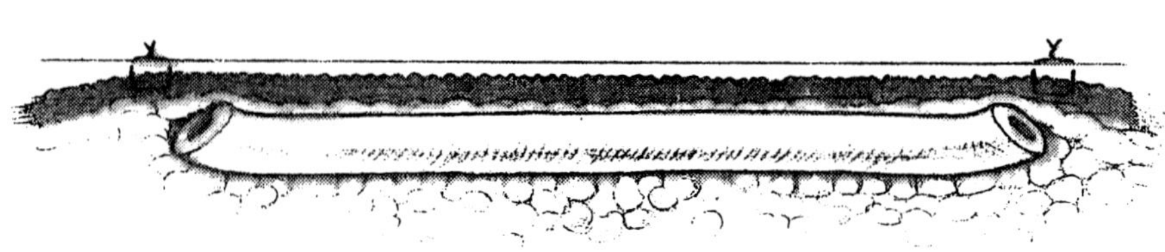

FIGURE 29 SoftForm in place in subdermal plane.

estimate the true correction afforded by the implant. After the swelling resolves, the augmentation from the implant alone is left. This can cause disappointment if the patient is not warned about the healing phases. Over the next 6 to 12 months fibrous ingrowth occurs. During this period the SoftForm implant may go through a phase in which it feels firm. It then softens again over time.

COMPLICATIONS AND MANAGEMENT

Infection, Extrusion, and Movement

Infection of the implant should be treated with removal and antibiotics. Extrusion of the implant is treated with complete removal as well. Extrusion is usually a consequence of placement that is too superficial. Movement of the implant is handled on a case-by-case basis. If the implant is on the lip, movement usually requires removal because the implant is more palpable and visible here. If the implant is in the nasolabial fold, often the implant moves laterally and is not easily palpable. If this is the case, most patients opt for a second placement alone rather than removal of the original implant and placement.

Removal of the Implant

The instruments necessary for removal of the implant are a small mosquito hemostat, fine dissecting scissors, and a No. 11 blade. In the lip area it is easier to stabilize and palpate the implant. The surgical assistant can roll the lip out for exposure and stabilize the implant by holding the mid lip and the angle of the mouth the surgeon makes a stab incision (over the area of greatest palpability) with a No. 11 blade on the mucosal surface and grasps the implant with the hemostats and gives a firm tug.

The nasolabial fold area is more difficult to stabilize and the implant more difficult to palpate. The least visible access on the external surface is the junction of the nasal ala with the cheek. Remember the tip of the implant is medial and 3 to 4 mm inferior to the crest of the nasolabial fold. With the SoftForm implant, it is recommended that the dissecting scissors are used to free the tip (1997, personal communication, C. Maas).

As with any procedure, it is important to be comfortable with managing the complications. With Gortex in particular, most difficulties require removal so it is important to have familiarity with its removal.

SUMMARY

Gortex is a useful addition to the cosmetic surgeon's soft-tissue augmentation armamentarium. It has a long track record of safety in human use. It is best used in the lower face, particularly in nasolabial folds, lip enhancement, and marionette lines. It does not provide 100% correction so it is important to prepare the patient for improvement of folds in the 40% range. The placement of the material in the correct plane is not technically difficult if the surgeon is familiar with the subcutaneous plane (ie, as in liposuction surgery). More difficult is correct placement (medial) in relation to the fold. When the implant is improperly oriented to the fold or when it moves, it results in inadequate augmentation. On the lips it can cause a palpable or visible ridge. Removal of the implant (SAM or SoftForm) is more difficult than placement. Because it is a new substance there are some issues that remain to be resolved, such as the optimum shape and size of the implant, the time to tissue ingrowth adequate to prevent early movement, and the percentage increase in augmentation from fibrous ingrowth.

REFERENCES

1. Boyce B. Biological and synthetic vascular prostheses, physical characteristics of expended polytetrafluoroethylene grafts. In: Stanley JC, ed., PA: Grune and Stratton, 1982, pp. 553–561.
2. US Patent 3,962,153. June 8, 1976 to WL Gore and Associates. Very highly stretched polytetrafluoroethylene and process therefor. 1976, pp. 1–24.
3. Anderson JM, Bennert KW, Johnson JM. The pathology and healing responses of expanded polytetrafluoroethylene vascular access grafts. In: Wilson SE, ed. Vascular Access Surgery, 2nd ed. Chicago: Year Book Medical Publishers, 1988, pp. 213–231.
4. Steinkogler FJ, Kuchar A, Huber E, Arocker-Mettinger E. Gore-Tex soft-tissue patch frontalis suspension technique in congenital ptosis and in blepharophimosis-ptosis syndrome. Plast Reconstr Surg 1057–1060, 1993.
5. Hanson LF, Donovan MG, Hellstein JW, Dickerson NC. Experimental evaluation of expanded polytetrafluoroethylene for reconstruction of orbital floor defects. J Oral Maxillofac Surg 52:1050–1055, 1994.
6. Karesh JW, Fabrega MA, Rodrigues MM, Glaros DS. Polytetrafluoroethylene as an interpositional graft material for the correction of lower eyelid retraction. Ophthalmology 96(4):419–423, 1989.
7. Karesh JW. Polytetrafluoroethylene as a graft material in ophthalmic plastic and reconstructive surgery. Ophthalmic Plastic Reconstr Surg 3(3):179–183, 1987.
8. Godin M, Waldman R, Johnson C. The use of expanded polytetrafluoroethylene (Gore-Tex) in rhinoplasty: a 6 year experience. Arch Otolaryngol Head Neck Surg 121:1131–1136, 1995.
9. Rothstein SG, Jacobs JB. The use of Gore-Tex implants in nasal augmentation operations. Entechnology 40, 42, 44–45, 1989.
10. Waldman SR. Gore-Tex for augmentation of the nasal dorsum: a preliminary report. Ann Plast Surg 26(6):520–525, 1991.
11. Bauer JJ, Salky BA, Gelernt IM, Kriel I. Repair of large abdominal wall defects with expanded polytetrafluoroethylene (ePTFE). Ann Surg 206:765–769, 1987.
12. Jenkins SD, Klamer TW, Parteka JJ, Condon RE. A comparison of prosthetic material used to repair abdominal wall defects. Surgery 94:392–398, 1983.
13. Wool NL, Strauss AK, Roseman DL. Clinical experience with Gore-Tex soft tissue patch in hernia repair. Proc Inst Med Chicago 38, 1985.
14. Pairolero PC, Arnold PG. Thoracic wall defects: surgical management of 205 consecutive patients. Mayo Clin Proc 61:557–563, 1986.
15. Greene D, Pruitt L, Maas CS. Biomechanical effects of e-PTFE implant structure on soft tissue implantation stability: a study in the porcine model. Laryngoscope 107:1–6, 1997.
16. Mass CS, Eriksson T, McCalmont T, et al. Evaluation of ePTFE as a soft tissue filling substance: an analysis of design-related implant behavior employing the porcine skin model. Plast Reconstr Surg 101(5):1307–1314, 1998.

APPENDIX

POST GORTEX INSTRUCTIONS

* Apply ice to areas during the first 24 hours. Twenty minutes out of each hour.

* Take antibiotics as directed until they are gone.

* Take pain medication (as needed) as directed. Remember that they may make you sleepy and can constipate you. Try to switch to extra strength Tylenol when possible.

* Minimize mouth movements. Eat soft foods in small bites.

Do not manipulate area.

Avoid putting your tongue to the inside of your cheek or lips.

* If you constantly touch, feel or push on area involved, you can move the implant and prevent it from knitting itself underneath.

* Keep insertion sites crust free by cleaning daily with soap and water and applying Vaseline to 6-8 times a day until they are healed. This usually takes 5-7 days, or until sutures are removed.

* It is possible that you may have some local bruising.

* Follow up in one week.

16

New Filling Substances on the Horizon

Arnold William Klein
University of California at Los Angeles School of Medicine, Los Angeles, California

INTRODUCTION

Early in my practice, I realized that patients frequently come to dermatologists in search of cosmetic improvement. As was standard for that era, I was much more schooled in recognizing and treating pathological processes than in providing image improvement and enhancement. Aesthetic augmentation was certainly not new territory, having been occupied by many fillers in the past—it was simply new to me. Since then, I have certainly learned much about soft-tissue augmentation and enhancement. I have also learned about the media, the FDA, and cosmetic hysteria.

What has caused the reinterest in filling agents? In part, this phenomenon is related to the breakthroughs and novel techniques that have revolutionized the field of cosmetic surgery over the past 15 years. First of all, we have to thank the BOTOX injection pioneers because they have shown us how to magically address the upper face—and you cannot have a young upper face and an old lower face. BOTOX has revolutionized many aspects of facial cosmetic surgery and has rapidly become an indispensable tool in the fight against the ravages of time and sun. It is certainly the best advice we can give our patients now that we have this terrific treatment for the glabellar complex. It not only corrects the problem for the majority of patients, but also treats the root cause of the rhytide simultaneously, i.e., the dynamic movement of muscles, usually preventing further progression.

Another reason is the concept of the two-dimensional look of the overpulled face. People understand that they want a more filled look. The youthful face has a much fuller look, not a pulled, flat look. Filling has replaced pulling—it's a very central part of rejuvenation.

And, additionally, we talked in the 1980s about lip enhancement. Subtle lip enhancement is something that is here to stay. In fact, it is the number one indication for injectable fillers.

Affordable outpatient surgery has replaced much of the expensive hospital-based surgery, and less-invasive techniques now provide patients and their physicians with a whole repertoire of therapeutic options.

Finally, more and more physicians are becoming trained in cosmetic surgery and are offering cosmetic services as part of their office practice. Dermatologists, plastic surgeons, ophthalmologists, otolaryngologists, and others have all entered the arena of cosmetic surgery. Medical meetings are filled with standing-room only presentations on cosmetic surgery techniques.

And with these facts in mind, we have seen a rekindling of interest in tissue augmentation. Today, physicians have a much larger armamentarium of tools and implant materials with which to improve facial contours, ameliorate wrinkles, and stall the telltale signs of the aging face. However, at the time of this writing we are still looking for the perfect filling substance.

Baby Boomers are now reaching the age where their once-youthful bodies are starting to show the signs of wear and tear so common in the middle-aged group. Hair is thinning, and wrinkles, stomachs, thighs, and love handles are ever more prominent.

Naturally, the most common reasons for patients to seek cosmetic surgery include the aging face and treatment of facial rhytides. It is the part of the body most visible to others and, typically, next to the hands it is the most reliable way to determine a person's age. The effects of time, smoking, the sun, and gravity tend to appear rather early on facial skin, and individuals are bombarded with media messages telling them they can use creams, injections, and surgery to erase these tattletale signs of their advancing age. Age-related changes of the lips and mouth include atrophy of both the upper and lower lips, actinic changes of the mucosal surface and vermilion border, and atrophy at the corners of the mouth, causing a downturn of the corners of the mouth and a resultant aged appearance.

Subtle improvements in the lips and their surrounding structures can produce astounding results, rebuilding the perioral structure and regaining a more youthful, rested visage.

One of the earliest signs of aging is an increase in prominence of the nasolabial folds. This, too, is one of the most important areas to be treated with filler substances in order to obtain the aesthetic results that we and the patients seek.

Soft-tissue augmentation has become increasingly important because more individuals seek aesthetic improvement without major surgical procedures. The choice of an appropriate subcutaneous implant, whether solid or injectable, requires a thorough understanding of the materials available. Filler substances are indispensable tools to be used when treating the face as stand-alone treatment or in conjunction with laser resurfacing, botulinum toxin (BOTOX), and chemical peels. The difficulty comes in choosing the proper treatment techniques and meeting patient expectations.

Kaminer and Krauss (1) note that there are two basic types of wrinkles (rhytides): dynamic and static. Dynamic rhytides are produced by muscle action and include glabellar, nasolabial (in part), and forehead wrinkles. Static rhytides are caused by an exogenous source, such as smoking, gravity, and sun. Dynamic and static wrinkles can be seen together in areas such as the crow's feet, forehead, and cheeks.

Dynamic rhytides in the upper one third of the face are best treated by BOTOX injections. It is impossible to properly discuss rhytide therapy without BOTOX as a central component. It has replaced filler substances as the treatment of choice for crow's feet, and glabellar and forehead lines. An understanding of the anatomy of wrinkles will help the physician to determine whether BOTOX alone will do the job. Combining BOTOX therapy with resurfacing or filler substances can dramatically improve efficacy. Long-term therapy with BOTOX can help to preserve the results once they are obtained. It is essential to determine the cause of rhytides if one is to design the proper treatment protocol for the patient.

Kaminer and Krauss (1) also comment that wrinkles come in various shapes and sizes, and treatment needs to be specifically tailored to the anatomy of the individual region. Failure to accurately determine the precise cause and depth of a wrinkle will place the physician at a disadvantage before treatment is ever initiated. Fine, superficial rhytides respond best to therapy at the intradermal level. Deeper, more substantial wrinkles typically have a subcutaneous component, with or without a facial-muscular element, and are best approached from the subcutaneous space. Oftentimes a wrinkle will have both a superficial and deep component, such as the nasolabial fold, and both of these components need to be addressed to obtain optimal results. It must be stressed that the precise evaluation of the patient and his or her wrinkles is one of the most important determinants of treatment success. A few minutes spent assessing the anatomy of wrinkles will almost always pay off many times over once therapy is begun.

HISTORY OF SOFT-TISSUE AUGMENTATION

The history of modern soft-tissue augmentation dates to the late 1800s. Since then, many implantable substances and devices have been used to cosmetically enhance soft-tissue defects and deficiencies. Injectable fat is the oldest material used for tissue augmentation (2–12). More than 100 years ago in Germany, Neuber reported on results from small adipose grafts transplanted from the arm for reconstruction of a soft-tissue defect on the face (2). In the early part of this century, free-fat grafts were used for tissue augmentation until the technique was replaced by the use of pedicle flaps and the subsequent use of paraffin or silicone as filling agents.

The use of injectable paraffin became quite popular during the early 1900s. However, it became evident that the injection of paraffin and other oils was associated with a high incidence of undesirable foreign body granuloma formation. In the United States and Europe, the use of paraffin for soft-tissue augmentation was largely abandoned before 1920. However, in the Orient, the subcutaneous injection of paraffin was still widely used well into the 1960s (13–17).

On the other hand, the injection of some substances, such as pure injectable-grade liquid silicone, although historically extremely useful and beneficial in the skilled hands of certain experienced physicians, has been declared illegal by the Food and Drug Administration (FDA) and is not available to the practitioner.

Injectable bovine collagen, Zyderm Collagen Implant, has been in use in the United States since 1977 (18). In 1979, the product became widely available to interested physicians in the United States under a Phase III protocol. In July of 1981, after $6\frac{1}{2}$ years of development, clinical trials, and testing by 728 physician investigators, Zyderm Collagen Implant ultimately received FDA approval. This was the first time an FDA-approved injectable device was available for soft-tissue augmentation. This approval renewed interest in the entire field of filling substances and, since then, well over 1.9 billion patients have received injectable collagen treatments.

In the years since approval of the first form of injectable collagen, information regarding new products, technique, and indications has continued to evolve. This process is ongoing and will continue as newer formulations become available and the existing products are re-evaluated.

The duration of correction with any injectable filling substance depends on multiple factors. Implantation technique, the amount implanted, the type of defect, and mechanical stresses at the implantation sites all influence persistence of correction. We must heed the lessons of the past, however, when choosing what should and should not be implanted in our patients.

THE PERFECT FILLING SUBSTANCE

Since the earliest experiments with paraffin in 1899, physicians have searched for an ideal bioinjectable material. A good understanding of implant materials is necessary for any physician who performs soft-tissue augmentation procedures. No matter the origins of implant material, there are important qualities necessary for achieving the goals of a given procedure while minimizing potential adverse effects.

In general, for a substance or device to be used for soft-tissue augmentation by the medical community, it must have certain intrinsic properties. It must have both a high "use" potential, producing pleasing cosmetic results with a minimum of untoward reactions, and a low "abuse" potential, such that widespread and possibly incorrect or indiscriminate use should not result in significant morbidity (19).

Whatever is used, it must be easy to obtain or fabricate. It has to be biodegradable or retrievable, because whatever you put in someone's face, things are going to go wrong. Either you want it to go away, or you want to be able to get it out. Additionally, it must be nonteratogenic, noncarcinogenic, and nonmigratory. Moreover, the agent must provide proven, predictable, and persistent correction through reproducible implantation techniques. That's what has caused the reinterest in filling agents. Reproducible implantation techniques should be easy to learn, produce results predictably, and be persistent. The substance should be biodegradable or retrievable if things do not go well. Obviously, it should require infrequent visits to maintain correction. It must be noninflammatory, nonmigratory, and multipurpose. Naturally, it should be cost effective and have minimal malpractice potential. Finally, if not autologous, the substance, agent, or device must be FDA approved. FDA approval of an agent or device assures purity and accessibility, as well as providing information regarding use.

The search for the perfect material to eradicate rhytides, smooth scars, and fill traumatic defects continues. New products appear, sometimes with great fanfare, that fail to fulfill the promise of a better alternative to what we use now. For this reason, an in-depth understanding of implant materials is necessary for any physician performing soft-tissue augmentation procedures.

Although no currently available implant fulfills all these criteria, many options exist that are adequate for a given task, satisfy patients, and offer excellent safety profiles. Natural materials for soft-tissue augmentation include human autografts and allografts as well as xenografts derived from animals. Autografts are materials collected from a patient for use only in that individual. There is no risk of rejection or nosocomial viral or retroviral infection as from human allografts or animal xenografts. Disadvantages include donor site morbidity and a limited available quantity, as well as resorption of implanted material. Commonly used autografts include fat and dermis.

Semisynthetic implants include altered human-derived materials as well as animal-derived materials. This latter category also includes bioengineered molecules that mimic the natural. With new technological advances, the distinction between these categories is becoming obscured. Synthetic substances are distinct chemically from those found in human tissue.

If I had shown you the list of available filling substances 10 years ago, there may have been 5 of them, but now its a veritable encyclopedia of agents that are available to the practitioner for use (sec Table 1). Determine the defect and this will define the substance. If you are working with a very deep defect for example, fat will work. But if you're working with a more superficial defect, you use Zyderm I or II, or for mid dermal defects, a material like Zyplast. So, often the defect that you are addressing will determine the substance that you will use.

But also remember that if all you have is a hammer, the whole world looks like a nail. Of course, the gold standard—bovine collagen— has been around for

TABLE 1 Available Filling Agents

Alloderm
Artecoll
Arteplast
Autologen
Biocell Ultravate
Bioplastique
BOTOX
Dermal Grafting
Dermalive
Dermalogen
Endoplast–50*
Fascian
Fat
Subcutaneous microlipoinjection
Lipocytic dermal augmentation
Fibrel
Gore-Tex
Human Placental Collagen*
Hylaform Gel*
Isologen
Koken Atelocollagen*
New Silicone Products
Permacol
*Pro*fill*
Recombinant Human Collagen†
Restylane*
Resoplast*
Silicone‡
Softform
Subcision
Zydern and Zyplast Collagen

*Not available in the United States.
†To become available.
‡Illegal in the United States.

20 years. In a very clever manner, physicians at Stanford dissected off the telopeptides with the end portion of the collagen molecule using pepsin digestion, suspended it in lidocaine, and injected it, and, lo and behold, it worked predictably to produce persistent correction. We now have 20 years experience, and 1.9 million patients worldwide have been treated. My love for collagen goes beyond that, and I often use collagen or injectable Zyderm or Zyplast for things that you would not normally use this agent. I am not familiar with the application of certain other fillers, so I do not have a high comfort level with them. Since I have adopted BOTOX as my "child," along with my other "child," bovine collagen, I find that BOTOX and Zyderm I work superbly in concert. The optimum tissue augmentation combination for me is collagen and BOTOX. Again, as I have already pointed out, if all you have is a hammer, the whole world looks like a nail.

Physicians should counsel patients on the risks and benefits of injectable substance therapy. Each physician should inform prospective patients about skin testing, the treatment procedure, and treatment expectations.

Currently, in the United States the most popular available injectable filling agents are autologous fat and Zyderm®/Zyplast® collagen (Collagen Aesthetics, Palo Alto, CA), of which the most popular substance used for soft-tissue augmentation is injectable bovine collagen.

SUBSTANCES NOT COVERED IN THIS CHAPTER

Many of the more widely known injectable filling agents and techniques are fully discussed in other chapters and thus will be briefly described here.

Allodern® is an acellular freeze-dried human cadaver dermis processed for purity. It has been used since 1992 on more than 3500 patients. Currently it is available as sheets of material for use in grafts and implanting. However, Life Sciences Corp. (Woodlands, TX) is working on an injectable form of Alloderm that will be a great addition to what we do.

Autologen™ has been around for a good while, and is an interesting product. It is a sterile suspension of intact collagen fibers prepared from the patient's own tissue. One square inch of tissue will yield 3 mL of material at a 3.5% concentration, which is about all you will get through a 30-gauge needle. It is applicable for fine lines, wrinkles, depressions, and lip augmentation. It is very difficult to inject. The physician's hand tires quickly because it does not have the flow characteristics of Zyderm or Zyplast. The new form is much more injectable than earlier forms of Autologen. It does give you persistent predictable correction, but is also very difficult. In addition, if you place it deep as you would Zyplast, it is going to go away quickly. It must be placed as superficially as possible, and you will not be able to place this material as superficially as you can place Zyderm I. You will be able to place it somewhere between where you place Zyderm I and Zyplast. With Autologen, you collect the specimen, store it in the freezer up to 2 weeks and ship the skin to Collagenesis (Beverly, MA). There is no charge for the first 6 months of storage. You order the material, receive the syringes, and refrigerate at 2 to 8° C. The syringes are stable for 6 months. The cost is $500 for the first syringe. It is applicable with a 27–30-gauge needle and, again, I use it only with a 30-gauge needle. It has been used in 1100 individuals. It is said that there is a greater longevity of correction than with bovine collagen because of the impact of the autologous composition. I do not use it with a nerve block. I believe the reason they had to use nerve blocks is that some people were very aggressive in the manner in which they injected it. I only use the eutectic mixture of local anesthetic when I inject Autologen.

As I have stated, BOTOX is the greatest advance in the minimally invasive treatment of the aging face to come along in the last 10 years. It is definitely effective in the upper third of the face, and has reawakened interest in other fillers for use in the lower face (20).

Dermal grafting is a unique technique whereby you take a punch graft of dermis from the back of the ear and put it in facial scars. It's a really unique and interesting technique for soft-tissue correction. Much of the work on dermal grating has been performed by James Swinehart (21).

I have also used Dermalogen, a human tissue collagen matrix from the dermal layer of donor skin specimens. It is suspended in a neutral pH buffer and is predominately composed of collagen fibrils. It contains other matrix proteins such as elastin. Extensive donor screening is undergone including interviews with next of kin. It is sterilized and undergoes viral inactivation procedures and a prion inactivation step. HIV and hepatitis tests are performed. The source of the donor skin, the American Association of Tissue Banks, is an accredited institution, and nearly 2 million tissue and organ transplants have been performed without any cases of communicable disease. How do you implant it? Well, first of all you have to skin test with it. People have been positive to the skin test. Now how could they be positive to a product that is human collagen? Because, possibly, it is a preservative or some agent that is present in the batch. And the incidence of erythema and problems with the skin tests of the old batch are much less with the new batch. The material is produced in a 3.5% concentration with no local anesthetic added. The company says to use it with EMLA or a nerve block. I use it only with EMLA. I do not use nerve blocks. The company also claims that implantation is associated with new vessel formation and host collagen deposition. Patients have been followed for up to 6 months, and some greater increase of longevity was seen with Dermalogen than with bovine collagen. At 12 months they were equal. I think it is a useful product for people who are allergic to bovine collagen. It is also much more difficult to inject. Again, put Dermalogen somewhere between the level you inject Zyderm and Zyplast. That is as superficial as you can get with this agent while using it with a 30-gauge needle.

Autologous fat transplantation is the oldest method for tissue augmentation, dating back 100 years. In the 1980s, with the advent of liposuction, a dramatic change occurred. Many investigators felt it was possible to return viable fat to the body. Nevertheless, the best mode of fat removal and the best mode of fat implantation may still elude us. Whereas many individuals prefer to gently collect fat in a syringe, others prefer to remove fat by liposuction and then return it to the body. Whether the size of the lipocyte, the metabolic rate, the site of removal, or washing and stabilizing agents are important in the application of fat transplantation remains unclear. Similarly, no one has yet defined the most amenable sites for transplantation. Controversy regarding longevity still exists, as well as controversy regarding the practice of freezing fat for subsequent use. The viability of fat cells that have been frozen and thawed has been questioned.

Additionally, we now have a new product called Isolagen™. Isolagen comes from Isolagen Technologies (Paramus, NJ) and is cultured autologous fibroblasts just as are used for the skin for burns, cartilage repair, and marrow transplants. It is applicable to fine lines, depressions, and lip augmentation. Basically, you take a 3 mm punch biopsy of skin. It was suggested initially postauricularly, although some use the back of the neck and I take it from the buttock. You ship it in an iced thermos, receive a test dose in 6 weeks, and begin treatment at 8 weeks. Two to three treatments are required and the cost is about $500 per treatment. I ice the area to be injected and use EMLA. It is a multilevel injection for most wrinkles and scars. You inject it in the superficial dermis, the mid dermis, and dermal and subcutaneous junction. Remember the concept, which is that you are placing fibroblasts there. It requires four treatments when you want to perform lip enhancement. The advantages are that there is an unlimited supply, there is no lumpiness, and it can be used in concert with Zyderm (but not Zyplast). The contraindications are that you cannot use it on a person with autoimmune disease or a malignancy, is older than 70 years, has systemic disease, or is unrealistic in expectations. What is the experience with Isolagen? It has been reported that it has existed for 5 years in a human wrist, and it has existed for 22 months therapeutically in patients. It has also been reported by William Boss that there was no resorption and results were apparent 3 to 10 months after the injection. He saw continual, gradual improvement over 16 to 18 months, and all patients acknowledged results with 92% satisfaction and no overgrowth, lumps, or allergy. Other investigators have not been able to duplicate these results. All they observed were improvements in two of 12 patients. I have been unable to duplicate this result. There is currently a temporary halt in this product because of the concept that they are using growth factors where it may be a medical device and not simply a transplant of autologous substance. It may be necessary to obtain FDA approval for the product.

Koken Atelocollagen implant is a 2% monomolecular solution of collagen of Japanese origin. It is supplied in cartridges to be injected with a dental syringe through a 30-gauge needle. The indications, contraindications, and injection techniques are the same as those for Zyderm collagen implant. Unlike Zyderm, Koken Atelocollagen does not contain lidocaine. It is a 2% aqueous solution of monomolecular collagen molecules, whereas Zyderm is a dispersion containing molecules, fibers, and fibrils of collagen. It is manufactured by the Koken Co., Ltd. of Japan but is not available in the United States.

Softform™ was developed from the work of Maas et al. with Gore-Tex (see Chapter 15). It is manufactured by Collagen Aesthetics, Palo Alto, CA.

Subcision is a process wherein the skin is traumatically undermined with, theoretically, subsequent new collagen deposition. This process was pioneered by David Orentreich (22).

Injectable bovine collagen, Zyderm/Zyplast collagen implants, have been in use in the United States since 1977. In 1979, the product became widely available to interested physicians in the United States under a Phase III protocol. Ultimately, in July of 1981, Zyderm collagen implant received FDA approval, representing the first time an FDA-approved injectable device was available for soft-tissue augmentation. Since the approval of injectable bovine collagen (Zyderm® I Collagen Implant (ZC-I); Collagen Aesthetics, Palo Alto, CA) for clinical use in 1981, an estimated 1,900,000 patients worldwide have been treated. After approval of the first injectable form, the FDA cleared two other formulations, Zyderm II Collagen Implant (ZC-II) and the Zyplast® Implant (ZP), also from Collagen Aesthetics. Additionally, a special packaging of ZC-I that contains a 32-gauge needle is available. The barrel of the syringe for this product—Zyderm I with Fine Gauge Needle (Z-FGN)—is specifically suited for use with the supplied 32-gauge, metal-hub needle.

Artecoll™ (Non-FDA Approved)

There is a material called Resoplast, which is monomolecular bovine collagen, and another material called Arteplast, which is plexiglass beads. If you combine the two, you have Artecoll. This is polymethylmethacrylate microspheres (PMMA) suspended in bovine collagen. The collagen serves as a bridge for the deposition of the PMMA beads. PMMA, commonly called Plexiglas or Lucite, is used extensively in medicine for bone cement, dentures, and artificial eye lenses. Polymerized PMMA is formed into smooth-surfaced spheres 30 to 40 μ in diameter and then suspended in the collagen vehicle. The collagen is degraded after injection with permanent deposition of PMMA. Company literature claims that these microspheres will be encapsulated by 2 to 4 months after injection, and that the nonbiodegradable particles are too large and smooth to be phagocytized and thus cannot migrate.

Artecoll is injected deeply with a 27-gauge needle, not in the dermal space but at the junction between dermis and subcutaneous fat, and can be molded with fingertip pressure. According to the manufacturer, it is indicated for deeper wrinkles and furrows, perioral lines, lip and philtrum augmentation, scar revision, and other subdermal and osseous defects. Patients must be skin tested for allergy to bovine collagen before use. It is contraindicated in patients who form keloids, have atrophic skin diseases, and those who have very thin, flaccid skin because of the risk of permanent superficial irregularities.

Gottfried Lemperle published results of a prospective study in 118 patients (23). Overall, 90% of patients who answered a survey were satisfied with the result of treatment, with 64% reporting striking and lasting improvement (follow-up approximately 2 years). Ten percent reported no improvement or adverse side effects. Swelling, redness, and moderate pain were common over the first few days. Longer-lasting redness occurred when the injection was too superficial. Itching in an unspecified number of patients subsided within weeks or months. Some patients with lip augmentation reported pain in the cold and lip tightness. Two patients required surgical removal of hypertrophic scars after dorsal lip augmentation. Other studies (24,25) have disputed Lemperle's results, and some investigators claim that particles of this size are able to be phagocytized, with the subsequent death of the engulfing macrophage and release of enzymes leading to a chronic inflammatory response. Lemperle (23) states that this is less likely given the smooth surface of PMMA microspheres.

There have also been problems reported with the collagen vehicle used for this product (24). The collagen was found to have nonhelical molecules subject to rapid degradation in vitro. Other impurities were also found in the vehicle.

The product is distributed by Rofil Medical International B.V., 4811 DH Breda, The Netherlands 011-31-76-520-9537. They also have a representative in Laguna Hills, California.

Arteplast™ (Non-FDA Approved)

This is polymethylmethacrylate (PMMA) beads and Tween 80. Arteplast is basically Plexiglas beads. It was part of the initial research before Artecoll was developed. It is no longer used, its applications having been replaced by Artecoll. It is distributed by Rofil Medical International B.V., 4811 D H Breda, The Netherlands 011-31-76-520-9537.

Biocell Ultravate™ (Non-FDA Approved)

This material is also called Biopolymere III. It is a biopolymer developed in Switzerland and contains Silicium (a derivative of silicon). According to the manufacturer, there is no need for allergy tests before treatment, and results may be permanent. It is distributed by Biocell Laboratoires, CH 593 Vaduz, Lichtenstein.

Bioplastique™ (Non-FDA Approved)

This material is a suspension of textured silicone rubber particles from 100 to 400 mm in size in a carrier vehicle. It is an investigational material for soft-tissue augmentation with a controlled foreign body response. Because of the controversy and resultant bad press surrounding silicone gel implants, it is unlikely to be FDA approved and thus studies have largely been abandoned.

Dermalive™ (Non-FDA Approved)

Dermalive is composed of hyaluronic acid and acrylic hydrogel fragments. It is produced by Dermatech in France.

Endoplast–50™ (Non-FDA Approved)

This is a new product of elastin solubilized peptides with collagen (bovine, US). Two skin tests are performed at 15-day intervals before treatment. There is a rare possibility of hypersensitivity. After treatment, inflammation is expected for 24 to 48 hours. The material influences proliferation of fibroblasts to produce collagen. Duration of correction is said to be 8 to 12 months. It sounds a lot like Fibrel, and is distributed by Laboratories Filorga, Paris.

Fascian™

Preserved, particulate fascia lata derived from screened human cadavers has recently become available. This injectable form of the material, sold under the trade name Fascian, can be injected when soft-tissue augmentation is desired. Historically, preserved fascia grafts have proven efficacy and an excellent safety record over the past 73 years. In a recent clinical trial, Burres (26) followed 81 subjects for 6 to 9 months after implantation without incidence of infection, allergic reaction, or acute rejection. Soft-tissue augmentation was evident 3 to 4 months after grafting or longer in most cases. The material is freeze-dried and typically preirradiated. Injected material was supplied in particle sizes of <0.25 mm, <0.5 mm, or <2.0 mm. The Fascian particles are hydrated in 3 to 5 ml of 0.3% lidocaine solution before injection. The injected area was preundermined with a 20-gauge needle, and the material injected into the preformed tunnel with a 16- to 25-gauge needle, depending on the size of the particles used.

According to Burres, histologic studies have shown (26) that, as in other locations with larger grafts, small pieces of fascia lata implanted intradermally were digested as an extraneous tissue and replaced with native collagen. This later reinvestment of the allograft matrix by the host fibroblast response generated a vascularized sheet of collagen that essentially restored the original elements found in native fascia and was titled recollagenation.

The product is available from Medical Aesthetics International, Inc., Redmond, Washington.

Fibrel™

Bailey and Ingraham first used "fibrin foam" as a surgical hemostatic agent in 1944. In 1957, Spangler reported the efficacy of "fibrin foam" in treating depressed scars in 23 patients. Subsequently, he reported good to excellent results in treating 7000 patients with this substance (27). The composition and fabrication of Fibrel, the modern descendant of fibrin foam, was further delineated by Gottlieb (28). In a very sophisticated manner, he described the "GAP" repair technique, in which plasma, gelatin, and aminocaproic acid were used in combination to stimulate collagen synthesis and elevate depressed scars.

Essentially, Fibrel works by creating a clot that becomes colonized. In this situation, the patient's plasma serves as a supplemental source of clotting factors. The gelatin provides the framework on which a clot forms, and aminocaproic acid is added to prevent lysis of this clot. The clotting process is believed to then stimulate fibroblasts near the site to synthesize collagen, and the resulting synthesized collagen replaces the clot formed by the implantation of Fibrel. Thus, the mechanism of action of Fibrel is in essence evocation of clot formation with subsequent substitution of this clot by host collagen. Unlike collagen where the material remains as a relatively inert implant, Fibrel is believed to induce a local wound-healing response that ultimately leads to new host collagen formation with replacement of the initial implanted product.

In that Fibrel produces a healing response or a clot at the site of implantation, it is to be expected that a certain degree of swelling and inflammation will occur with its application. Thus, bruising, swelling, redness, pain, or induration are expected local effects. Additionally, the use of Fibrel can be uncomfortable, and local anesthesia before its application is frequently used by those experienced in its use (29). Fibrel was manufactured by the Mentor Corporation and is no longer available.

Gore-Tex™

Gore-Tex subcutaneous augmentation material (SAM) is expanded polytetrafluoroethylene (ePTFE) created by extrusion of the material known as Teflon™ (Dupont, Wilmington, DE). Nodules of ePTFE are interconnected by a multidirectional fibril structure to make a soft, pliable polymer. Sheets, patches, sutures, and tubes are some of the forms created by the manufacturer. Gore-Tex has been in medical use in general, cardiovascular, urological, and reconstructive surgery since 1971. It is inert, nonallergenic, and exhibits low tissue reactivity with minimal capsule formation. The longevity of ePTFE when implanted in human tissue results from the body's inability to break down carbon-fluorine bonds. Its excellent safety record in cardiac and vascular surgery as well as hernia repair provides three decades of historical data in over 3.5 million patients. The 22 to 30 mm pores also allow fine-tissue incorporation. Gore-Tex is not so porous, however, that its removal in cases of infection becomes difficult because of extensive tissue integration.

In 1991, Lassus (30) reported the use of ePTFE for nasolabial fold and rhytide correction with only one infection in 100 patients. The infection cleared with oral antibiotics without removal of the implant. The same investigator later described combining liposuction lateral to the nasolabial fold with insertion of a rolled Gore-Tex Triangle under the nasolabial fold. This method yielded 50 to 60% improvement over a 5- to 9-year follow-up in three patients (31). Walter (32) followed another series of 400 implants for both reconstruction and aesthetic improvement for 5 years. He reported seven of the 400 required removal because of infection. Sherris and Larrabee (33) followed 24 patients for 2.5 to 4.5 years after augmentation of the nasolabial folds and marionette lines, among whom one patient experienced implant malposition and two patients required more augmentation.

Gore-Tex is best suited for very specific subsets of rhytides. These include nasolabial fold wrinkles that have a broad depression as their main component, glabellar lines with a prominent furrow, and atrophic areas at the corners of the mouth. The implants are inserted in the subcutaneous space and therefore are best used for augmentation of rhytides that have a subcutaneous or deep dermal component.

Techniques for the nasolabial fold, marionette lines, and glabellar area generally involve the use of a trochar or other instrument to tunnel subcutaneously. Sutures sewn to the implant can then be pulled through the insertion area, trimmed, and the incisions closed if necessary. Many investigators caution placement only in the fat, because dermal positioning leads to irregularities and extrusion. The use of pre- and postsurgical antibiotics is frequently advised. Patients should be cautioned that suboptimal correction may result and that revisions may be necessary. Despite excellent aesthetic results, patients may be able to palpate the implant indefinitely and should be forewarned. Adverse reactions can include infection (0–3.6%), foreign-body extrusion, and three-dimensional elevations.

Superficial rhytides are unlikely to improve much with ePTFE implants, and the physician and patient must be aware of this when choosing the proper soft-tissue augmentation technique. Proper patient selection appears to be the main criterion in obtaining good results. In addition, layering bovine collagen over ePTFE always remains an option for future correction enhancement.

Cisneros and Singla (34) first advocated the use of ePTFE suture in the vermilion border to augment lips. Ellis and Trimas (35) later described the use of 2- to 3-mm wide Gore-Tex strips threaded through the vermilion border and philtrum. One of 11 patients required removal of implant because of infection. Sherris and Larrabee (33) reported on 21 patients with lip augmentation with ePTFE. One patient's seroma required treatment. No infection, extrusion, inflammation or capsule formation, or loss of sensation in the lips resulted. Case reports in the literature have described necrosis of the lip mucosa requiring reconstruction and debridement just 24 hours after placement of ePTFE threads in the lips. Another report of disfiguring scarring attributable to an "inflammatory reaction" after implantation in the lips was reported (36). Active forces and constant motion of the oral region make this a challenging location for a synthetic implant.

Gore-Tex and Softform are constructed of essentially the same ePTFE material. Their differences derive from their engineering.

Maas et al. (37) performed studies in the procine model comparing the implantation of solid strips, rolled sheets, and tubular implants of ePTFE. There was a distinct reduction in the extrusion and persistent inflammation rates in the tubular implant sites (1.0%) as compared with the rolled or strip implants (4.4%). Fibroblastic ingrowth was seen filling the lumen of the tubular implants by 6 months after surgery, perhaps anchoring this type of implant more effectively than the other shapes. Removal of the implant remained simple and easy, however, after dividing the fibrous ingrowth at the ends of each tubular implant.

Gore-Tex is distributed by W. L. Gore and Assoc., Inc., 1500 N. Fourth St., Flagstaff, Arizona [(800) 396-4673].

Hylaform Gel™ (Non-FDA Approved)

Hyaluronic acid derivatives are exciting new materials for soft-tissue augmentation with great future potential. Hyaluronic acid is a mammalian polysaccharide found naturally in the dermis. Its ability to bond water assists in hydration and provides skin turgor. Unlike collagen, it is identical across all species and is produced by many types of cells.

Hylan gels are composed of cross-linked hyaluronan polymer molecules with very high molecular weights. Hyaluronic acid itself is broken down quickly within the dermis, then eliminated by the lymphatics and eventually the liver. Hylan gels have longer dwell times in tissues, but are eventually broken down into their original molecules and eliminated in the same fashion (38).

Piacquadio (39) reported the use of cross-linked hyaluronic acid (Hylan B gel) in 150 patients enrolled in a multicenter clinical study initiated in 1991. Patients with distensible scars or wrinkles received an initial treatment and a touch-up at weeks 2 to 4. At week 12, 84% showed moderate (33% or greater) improvement and 80% of patients reported moderate or higher satisfaction. Adverse reactions were rare, including persistent erythema and ecchymosis. Using a guinea pig model, Hylan gel was seen histologically in 87% of sites at week 26, whereas bovine collagen was present in only 25%.

Hylaform gel, also known as Hylan B gel, (Biomatrix, Inc., Ridgefield, NJ), is processed from the cock's combs of domestic fowl. Hylaform is used for facial augmentation throughout most of the world. It is especially popular for volume augmentation of the lips. However, it is not available for this purpose in the United States, although everyone else seems to have it. It is available in Canada, England and continental Europe, and Australia. It is a very interesting product. It is available in America to be used in osteoarthritis of the knee. There is reportedly no immunological activity, although there have been some reports of redness that persisted at the sites of implantation. Nick Lowe, in England, now skin tests people before he uses it. He has injected a great deal of the product. Adverse reactions have been less than 2% with some redness, ecchymosis, and acne. Again, the major problem has been a certain degree of redness that has occurred. And, again, some individuals are going on to skin test people before they use this product. Hylaform gel is manufactured by Biomatrix, Inc., of Ridgefield, New Jersey and is distributed in Europe by Collagen International, Inc., Avenue Gratta-Paille 2CP430, CH-1000 Lausanne 30 Grey, Switzerland.

Human Placental Collagen

Gamma-irradiated amnion collagen from human placentae has been suggested as an injectable soft-tissue augmentation material and tested in animal studies (40). This is collagen that is manufactured from human placentae. Placentae are readily available, and although there have been clinical trials on the material, it will probably never come to market. I did studies on human placenta collagen that was obtained from France. It was human collagen that they obtained from placentae, and although it worked extraordinarily well, the study was not continued.

Permacol™ (Non-FDA Approved)

Permacol is a permanent, cross-linked solid porcine collagen implant (not injectable). It is only presently available in sheets. It allows ingrowth of host tissue cells and blood vessels. No US studies exist on this porcine product. Hopefully, soon, it will come in injectable form. It is a new product and is distributed by Tissue Sciences and Laboratories, Ltd., Hants, United Kingdom.

*Pro*fill™ (Non-FDA Approved)

Provided as a translucent gel, *Pro*fill is a copolymer of polyoxyethylene and polyoxypropylene with mineral salts, amino acids, and vitamins. It is provided as a liquid that turns to gel on implantation. Several hours of redness are expected after implantation. Correction reportedly lasts 6 to 9 months. *Pro*fill is frequently used in concert with Endoplast. It, like Endoplast, is distributed by Laboratories Filorga, Paris.

Recombinant Human Collagen

Research efforts are underway to create a recombinant human collagen. Recombinant human collagen would eliminate the risk of donor viral or prion contamination, eradicate the need for proteolytic cleavage of animal collagen with its attendant degradation, and have no potential for allergy. This material will hopefully be available in the future. It is human collagen that is grown in the cow and separated from the cow's milk. This is the future—this is not reality for now.

Cohesion Technologies (Palo Alto, CA) has recently reported the ability to produce human collagen in the laboratory. Obviously, if this product comes to market, it would obviate the allergenicity problems associated with a bovine product.

Resoplast™ (Non-FDA Approved)

This is bovine *monomolecular* collagen in *solution*. Concentrations of 3.5 and 6.5% are available. Indications and techniques of implantation are similar to Zyderm collagen. A skin test is provided. It is distributed by Rofil Medical International B.V., 4811 D H Breda, The Netherlands 011-31-76-520-9537.

Restylane™ (Non-FDA Approved)

The hyaluronic acid derivative Restylane has been available for soft-tissue augmentation in Europe for over 4 years. Restylane is partially cross-linked hyaluronic acid created via bacterial fermentation and, thus, does not require an animal source.

It is biocompatible and biodegradable. It contains a higher concentration of hyaluronic acid (20 mg/ml of stabilized hyaluronic acid) than predecessors, which increases the filler's solubility. It is indicated for rhytides, depressions, and lip augmentation.

This is also a stabilized hyaluronic acid gel material like Hylaform. But whereas Hylaform gel comes from cock's combs, this product comes from streptococci bacteria. It has a higher concentration of hyaluronic acid than hylaform gel. Although there is a higher concentration, this material has a lower molecular weight, so it is like comparing apples and automobiles.

One clinical study involved 113 European patients receiving injections of Restylane to 285 facial wrinkles. Two thirds of the patients received a touch-up injection at 2 weeks. Physicians rated the degree of correction to be 82% at 3 months and 66% at 1 year, with similar patient opinion. Side effects were minimal, including erythema (when injected too superficially) and technique-related unevenness. There were no reported allergic reactions.

Another study consisted of 112 patients treated at 256 facial sites once or twice at weekly intervals. Fifty-two of 112 had immediate swelling, redness, or burning. So it is not the type of thing you can have and go out right away oftentimes. Sixteen had mild sporadic reactions during follow-up involving intermittent swelling of the lips. Patient/physician satisfaction was reported as 60% at 52 weeks. If you really study dermatologic surgery, you'll understand one thing. There was an 18% incidence of intermittent swelling of the lips. And this product was majorly interesting for lip augmentation. This was the first generation. If you want one in five of your patients to call you to tell you their lips are swollen up, you really may not want to use this first generation material. But, with the second generation of the product, they are reportely not having the problems with intermittent swelling of the lips that they had with the first generation.

Restylane is provided in 0.7 ml preloaded syringes containing 20 mg/ml of stabilized hyaluronic acid. Initially they recommended a linear threading, not a serial puncture technique, but now they are also using a serial puncture technique. It is used with a 30-gauge needle and no overcorrection is necessary.

They have shown indications all over the face for this product, but they say the best indication is for lip augmentation, putting it into the potential space and then actually the mucosa itself. It is distributed by Q-Med AB, Seminariegatan 21, S-752 28 Uppsala, Sweden (011 46 18 50 42 10, Fax: 011 46 18 50 31 35, Internet: http//www.q-med.se).

Silicone

Silicones are synthetic compounds and do not occur naturally. The liquid silicones used for medical purposes are long polymers of dimethylsiloxanes. Siloxane is an acronym used to describe compounds containing repeating units of silicon, oxygen, and methane. During the 1940s there was a large German, Swiss, and Japanese experience with injectable silicone.

There have been two major American protocols involving the use of highly refined, liquid silicone. In 1965, Dow-Corning conducted a trial involving seven investigators and 1334 patients. This trial was halted by the FDA in 1967 because of concerns about product quality, use methodology, and inadequate animal toxicity data. A second trial was conducted by Dow-Corning in 1978 involving 27 investigators and 144 patients.

Silicone has a very high use potential, providing pleasing aesthetic results in many patients, but unfortunately it also has a high abuse potential, such that many cosmetic disasters have been caused by the widespread and indiscriminate use of the material. Numerous disastrous complications have resulted from the use of adulterated or impure silicones. Foreign body type silicoma can occur up to 11 years after implantation, even with the highly refined, medical grade Dow-Corning MDX4-4011 and microdroplets. Other adverse reactions that have been reported are movement or drift of the implant, Peau D'Orange, beading, discoloration, site reactions in 12 to 14% of patients, and immunological reactions.

Dr. Norman Orentreich claims that silicone injections are permanent (41), whereas other investigators have reported a loss of material from the injection site. Aronsohn, with 20 years of experience, reports that it is applicable only for nose, lips, cheeks, and hands (42). Milojevic, with experience in 1677 patients, claims that it is contraindicated in lips and eyelids (43). Orentreich, on the other hand, maintains that it is applicable for all facial sites (41).

Techniques also vary from injector to injector. Some prefer fanning, some serial puncture with microdroplets, some tattooing or superficial placement, and some threading.

Although injectable silicone has a long history of use in the United States, its application for soft-tissue augmentation was declared illegal by the FDA. Nevertheless, two forms of silicone—Adatosil-5000 and Silikone-1000—were recently approved for injection into the eye for retinal detachment (see Jan. 13, 1999 transcript of the FDA Opthalmic Device Panel). These are highly viscous agents. The numbers associated with the products refer to the viscosity in centistokes (cs). Water has a viscosity of 100 cs. Mineral oil has a viscosity of 350 cs. There have been some recent indications that some physicians may be reducing these agents through chromatography to lower viscosity (350 cs) for soft-tissue application. Whether this is being performed, whether this is legal, or whether an Investigate New Drug (IND) protocol has been processed for this is unknown to me.

Other Materials

In addition to the aforementioned agents there are numerous products and techniques whose position in the field of soft-tissue augmentation have not yet been fully defined. Some of these agents are FDA-approved. Others lack approval or require testing.

ANTICIPATING THE FUTURE AND CONCLUSION

Efforts to develop the perfect soft-tissue augmentation material continue. New products and techniques are constantly evolving and appearing. Obviously, these techniques and substances for soft-tissue augmentation are being introduced at an accelerated rate. However, it behooves us, as physicians and guides for our patients, to resist jumping on the bandwagon of every new fad or implant material.

There are many substances available for soft-tissue augmentation. Although one must be familiar with all of the techniques, materials, and options, we feel that it is best to become proficient in two or three different methods so that you can provide your patients with options while still being experienced in the techniques that you use. You do not want to be a jack of all trades and a master of none. The choice of implant material should be based on the location of the defect, potential for hypersensitivity reaction, desire for permanency, and the patient's feelings about the need for a "natural feel" or the implant. You have a whole encyclopedia of substances to choose from. Of course, safety should be the primary concern when using any implant material.

But if you are going to use any of these products, and God knows there's enough of them, remember that if you sand wood, you are going to get splinters. Things are going to go wrong. If you plan to use any or all of these materials, remember to be honest with your patients, with your colleagues, and, above all, with yourself.

But I have one thought to leave you with and this is it. It is really not what you use that is most critical; it is really how you use it. As newer products develop, the methods of soft-tissue enhancement will continue to change, hopefully bringing improved results to patients.

REFERENCES

1. Kaminer M, Krause M. Filler substances in the treatment of facial aging. Med Surg Dermatol 1998; 5:215–221.
2. Neuber F. Fettransplantation. Chir Kongr Verhandl Dsch Gesellch Chir 1893; 22:66.
3. Neuhof H. The Transplantation of Tissues. New York: Appleton & Company, 1923.
4. Bames HO. Augmentation mammoplasty by lipotransplant. Plast Reconstr Surg 1953; 11:404.
5. Peer LA. Loss of weight and volume in human fat grafts with postulation of "cell survival theory." Plast Reconstr Surg 1950; 5:217.
6. Boering G, Huffstadt AJ. The use of derma-fat grafts in the face. Br J Plast Surg 1968; 20(2):172.
7. Roy JN. War surgery: plastic operations on the face by means of fat grafts. Laryngoscope 1921; 31:65.
8. Stevenson TW. Fat grafts to the face. Plast Reconstr Surg. 1949; 4:458.
9. Peer LA. The neglected "free fat graft," its behavior and clinical use. Am J Surg 1956; 92:40.
10. Katocs AS, Largis EE, Allen DO. Perfused fat cells: effects of lipolytic agents. J Biol Chem 1973; 248:5089.
11. Sidman RL. The direct effect of insulin on organ cultures of brown fat. Anat Rec 1956; 124:723.
12. Gurney CE. Studies on the fate of free transplants of fat. Proc Staff Meet Mayo Clin 1937; 12:317.
13. Matton G, Amseeuw A, De Keyser F. The history of biomaterials and the biology of collagen. Aesth Plast Surg 1985; 9:133–140.
14. Khoo Boo-Chai MB. Paraffinoma. Plast Reconstr Surg 1965; 36:101–110.
15. Millard DR. Oriental peregrinations. Plast Reconstr Surg 1955; 16:319–336.
16. Urback F, Wilne SS, Johnson WC, Davies RE. Generalized paraffinoma (sclerosing lipogranuloma). Arch Dermatol 1971; 103:277–285.
17. Klein JA, Cole G, Burr RJ, Bartlow G, Fulwider C. Paraffinomas of the scalp. Archiv Dermatol 1985; 121:382–385.

18. Knapp TR, Kaplan EN, Daniels JR, et al. Injectable collagen for soft tissue augmentation. Plast Reconstr Surg 1977; 60:389.
19. Klein AW, Rish DC. Injectable collagen: an adjunct to facial plastic surgery. Facial Plast Stira 1987; 4:87.
20. Klein AW. Cosmetic therapy with botulinum toxin. Dermatol Surg 1996; 22:757–759.
21. Swinehart JM. Pocket grafting with dermal grafts: autologous collagen implants for permanent correction of cutaneous depressions. Am J Cosmet Surg 1996; 12(4):321–331.
22. Orentreich D. Subcutaneous incisionless (subcision) surgery for the correction of depressed scars & wrinkles. J Dermatol Surg 1995; 21(6):543–549.
23. Lemperle G, Hazan-Gauthier N, Lemperle M. PMMA microspheres (Artecoll) for skin and soft tissue augmentation. Part II: clinical investigations. Plast Reconstr Surg 96: 627–634, 1995.
24. McClelland M, Egbert B, Hanko V, et al. Evaluation of Artecoll polymethylmethacrylate implant for soft-tissue augmentation: Biocompatibility and chemical characterization. Plast Reconstr Surg 1997; 100:1466–1474.
25. Constantino PD, Friedman CD. Soft-tissue augmentation and replacement in the head and neck. General considerations. Otolaryngol Clin N Am 1994; 27:1–12.
26. Burres S. Preserved particulate fascia lata (Fascian™) for injection: a new alternative. Dermatol Surg 1999; 25:790.
27. Spangler AS. (1975). Treatment of depressed scars with Fibrin foam—seventeen years of experience. J Dermatol Surg Oncol 1975; 1:65–69.
28. Gottlieb S. (1977). GAP Repair Technique. Poster exhibit. Annual Meeting of the American Academy of Dermatology, Dallas, Texas, December, 1977.
29. Milliken L. (1989). Long term safety and efficacy with Fibrel in the treatment of cutaneous scars. J Dermatol Surg Oncol 1989; 15(8):837–844.
30. Lassus C. Expanded PTFE in the treatment of facial wrinkles. Aesth Plast Surg 1991; 15:167–174.
31. Lassus C. A surgical solution to the deep nasolabial fold. Plast Reconstr Surg 1996; 97: 1473–1478.
32. Walter C. Aspects of facial correction and reconstruction by using transplants (composite grafts and implants) with special reference to surgical membrane implants. Arch Otolaryngol Head Neck Surg 1994; 110:524–529.
33. Sherris DA, Larrabee WF Jr. Expanded polytetrafluoroethylene augmentation of the lower face. Laryngoscope 1996; 106:658.
34. Cisneros JL, Singla R. Intradermal augmentation with expanded polytetrafluoroethylene (Gore-tex) for facial lines and wrinkles. J Dermatol Surg Oncol 1993; 19:539–542.
35. Ellis DAF, Trimas SJ. Gore-tex implants for the correction of thin lips. Laryngoscope 1995; 105:207–209.
36. Levine B, Berman WE. The current status of expanded polytetrafluoroethylene (Gore-tex) in facial plastic surgery. Ear Nose Throat J 1995; 74:684.
37. Maas CS, Eriksson T, McCalmont T, et al: Evaluation of ePTFE as a soft tissue filling substance: an analysis of design-related implant behavior employing the porcine skin model. Plast Reconstr Surg 1998; 101:1307–1314.
38. Balazs EA, Leshchiner EA. Hyaluronan, its crosslinked derivative hylan, and their medical applications. In: Inagake H, Phillips GO, eds. Cellulosics Utilization: Research and Rewards in Cellulosics. New York: Elsevier Applied Science, 1989, pp 233–241.
39. Piacquadia D. Crosslinked hyaluronic acid (hylan gel) as a soft tissue augmentation material: a preliminary assessment. In: Elson ML, ed. Evaluation and Treatment of the Aging Face. New York: Springer-Verlag, 1994, pp 304–308.
40. Spira M, Liu B, Xu Z, et al. Human amnion collagen for soft tissue augmentation—biochemical characterizations and animal observations. J Biomed Mat Res 1994; 28: 91–96.

41. Orentreich NO. Soft tissue augmentation with medical-grade fluid silicone. In: Rubin LR, ed. Biomaterials in Reconstructive Surgery, St. Louis: C.V. Mosby Co., 1983:859–881.
42. Aronsohn RB. A 22-year experience with the use of silicone injection. Am J Cosmet Surg 1984; 1:21–28.
43. Milojevic B. Complications after silicone injection therapy in aesthetic plastic surgery. Aesth Plast Surg 1982; 6(4):203–206.

17

Botulinum A Exotoxin

Alastair Carruthers and Jean Carruthers
University of British Columbia, British Columbia, Canada

INTRODUCTION

Botulinum A Exotoxin (BTX-A) has been used for cosmetic purposes for over a decade. During that period it has created a place for the management of facial lines, wrinkles, and expressions by the use of a paralytic agent. The effect of the underlying musculature has become much more important than before the availability of this agent.

For some individuals, BTX-A has produced a safe, simple solution to a problem. For others it has not been satisfactory, either because the effect achieved was not the effect desired because of complications or because of poor duration of effect. In this chapter we will summarize the experience of ourselves and others with this new agent and discuss the appropriate indications for BTX-A as well as the dosage and the avoidance and management of complications.

BACKGROUND

We have previously reported much of the information in the following paragraphs [1] and original references can be found in that publication.

BTX-A is produced in anaerobic culture by the A subtype of Clostridium botulinum. Subtypes A to G all produce neurotoxins. Subtype A is in the soil of North America west of the Mississippi and subtype B to the east. Subtype E is found in Alaska and the Arctic and is implicated in cases of botulism in that area. BTX-B and BTX-F have been clinically investigated and although not as effective as BTX-A, are of use in individuals who are resistant to BTX-A.

TOXICOLOGY

The neurotoxin is a dichain protein linked by a disulfide bond. It prevents release of acetylcholine (ACh) from the presynaptic neuron of the neuromuscular junction (NMJ). It achieves this by a four step process:

1. Binding to the cell membrane of the presynaptic neuron
2. Endocytosis of the neurotoxin molecule attached to the cell membrane

3. Release of the neurotoxin into the cytosol
4. Interference with peptides necessary for ACh release

Binding of the toxin occurs via the long chain of the neurotoxin and can occur relatively rapidly. This is presumed to take 1 to 2 hours in vivo which has clinical relevance because this is the period during which the ultimate effect of the neurotoxin can be affected.

The intracellular effect of the neurotoxin is accomplished by the short chain, and in the case of BTX-A this interferes with a peptide termed Synaptobrevin. The paralytic effect of BTX-A may be observed within minutes in in vitro experimental models and clinically within hours after exposure to large doses. However, with the clinical use of BTX-A, the onset of effect is usually evident at 24 to 48 hours. The ultimate effect is not apparent for 2 weeks. For example, side effects such as ptosis may not appear until 2 weeks after injection, indicating that the full effect of the toxin is not achieved until this time. Interestingly, if ptosis appears at 10 to 14 days after injection, it usually disappears after a further 2 to 4 weeks, indicating that a weak effect of the neurotoxin can be overcome or compensated for by mechanisms other than the usual repair process.

Recovery from BTX-A paralysis usually begins at 3 to 4 months after injection but may not be clinically complete for several more months. Disruption of ACh release at the NMJ produces a nonfunctional NMJ that is catabolized. There is a normal ongoing process of catabolism and replacement of NMJs that is enhanced after BTX injection. Sprouts appear proximal to the NMJ on the presynaptic neuron and reinnervate the myofibril. A disordered pattern of reinnervation is seen histologically up to 3 years after BTX injection despite clinically normal function many months earlier.

The above description pertains to the cholinergic neuromuscular junctions that determine the clinical effect usually desired. However, with the use of BTX-A to treat hyperhidrosis, we are now dealing with a cholinergic junction that is not an NMJ. The cholinergic junction at the relevant sweat glands is interfered with by BTX-A via the same mechanism as the NMJ. However, the dose of BTX-A seems to be larger to produce a desired effect than that effective at the NMJ.

COMMERCIALLY AVAILABLE BTX-A

The first commercially available product, produced by Schantz in 1979 [2] and developed by Scott and others, was known as "Oculinum." When it was acquired by Allergan Inc. (Irvine, CA) in 1989 and it became apparent that BTX-A was going to have extensive use outside ophthalmology, they renamed the toxin "BOTOX."

The original 150 mg batch of BOTOX produced by Schantz in 1979 was finally exhausted in early 1998 in Canada. Europe had switched to a batch of toxin produced in 1988 a few years earlier and the United States switched to a new batch, "New BOTOX" in late 1997. There were initial concerns that this batch had either greater potency or a greater ability to diffuse than the 1979 toxin; however, these fears have not been substantiated and most users of large amounts of BTX are now using the same dose of "New BOTOX" as of the old toxin. At the time of this writing, the United States is the only market using "New BOTOX"; the rest of the world is using the 1988 batch of toxin.

Soon after the clinical use of BTX-A was described by Scott [3], ophthalmologists in the United Kingdom stimulated a British group with a BTX-A to produce a clinically useful toxin. This was subsequently marketed as "Dysport" (Speywood Pharmaceuticals, Maidenhead, Berkshire). Whereas BOTOX is purified by a process of repeated acid precipitation followed by redissolution, Dysport is purified by column-based methods. This difference is reflected in a difference in potency of the two toxins such that, although both are measured in identical mouse units (1 unit is the LD_{50} of a standardized mouse model), the BOTOX unit is approximately four times more effective than the Dysport unit in humans [4]. Because Dysport may become available in the United States and other markets, the difference in the clinical effectiveness of the two toxins is of great importance. One investigator who uses both interchangeably has described his technique to address the difference by appropriate dilution of the vials [5].

DILUTION

BTX-A comes in lyophilized vials and should be reconstituted with nonpreserved saline. The company recommends the avoidance of foaming during the process, although clinically we have not found that this affects the potency of the reconstituted toxin.

There is considerable disagreement as to the volume of diluent which should be used. This subject has been addressed by Klein [6]. He advocates a dilution of 2 to 3 ml/100 unit vial of BOTOX. Increasing this volume by 25% will give the same clinical effect for a 500 unit vial of Dysport. The dilution discussion is based on a number of conflicting issues.

1. The injected volume must be sufficiently small to provide accurate delivery of the toxin to the intended target without excessive volume effect (lumpiness after injection) or increased risk of hematoma.
2. The volume must be sufficiently large to permit accurate injection of a required dose and to avoid wastage in the amount of toxin lost in the vial, in the syringe/needles that are discarded, and during drawing up in the syringe.
3. If too great a volume is used, it may be impossible to deliver a required dose with sufficient accuracy. For example, if it were intended to inject 10 units of BOTOX into procerus using a 10 ml/vial dilution, the injected volume would be 1 ml and the simple volume of fluid apart from being unsightly would probably deliver the toxin to muscles other than procerus.
4. If the injecting physician regularly used EMG, this requires a syringe and separate needle. The "dead space" in this combination is .05 to .08 ml or 5 to 8 units if a 1 ml/vial dilution is used or approximately 2 to 3 units if a 3 ml/vial dilution is used.
5. It is our preference to use 0.3 ml syringes with an attached 1/4″ 30 gauge needle (Becton-Dickinson). These syringes are extremely precise and accurate and have almost no dead space. For facial areas they give excellent accuracy of injection with very little volume effect.

To conclude, there is no single dilution that is right for all clinicians and all clinical uses and each of us must try different dilutions to find that which works best.

STORAGE

According to the manufacturers, unreconstituted vials of BOTOX should be transported and stored frozen. Vials of Dysport can be transported at room temperature and can be stored at domestic refrigerator temperatures. It is possible that the same is true for BOTOX, but we are unaware of any evidence about this. In our experience, short periods (up to 1–2 days) at temperatures above freezing appear to have no clinically detectable adverse effect on potency.

Once the vial is reconstituted with nonpreserved saline, Allergan recommends that the portion not used within 4 hours should be discarded. However, Garcia and Fulton [7] show little loss of effectiveness over a month. On the other hand, if unpreserved saline is used as a diluent, there is the potential for contamination by microorganisms to occur, and we have heard of one anecdotal case of cellulitis occurring after injection of BTX-A that had been stored for 1 week after reconstitution.

It is our practice to use toxin for up to 3 to 4 days after reconstitution. If a vial is reconstituted carefully to avoid contamination and then stored for 1 week in a refrigerator (not a freezer) without multiple withdrawals during that period, the current clinical experience suggests that the toxicity of the BTX-A in that vial will be close to its original toxicity. Further studies are needed in this area.

SYSTEMIC COMPLICATIONS AND RESISTANCE

The doses of BTX-A used in its cosmetic use are so small and the ability of the toxin to bind to its receptors so great that very little gets into the general circulation. In consequence we see virtually no systemic complications. The human LD_{50} is estimated to be 40 u/kg [8] and we use typically up to 2 u/kg for cosmetic indications and would therefore not expect to get generalized weakness. Doses of 5 u/kg are not uncommon in neurology and up to 15 ug/kg are common in the treatment of spasticity. With these doses there is a small incidence of "transient rashes," and more importantly the development of secondary resistance to the toxin.

BTX-A is an immunogenic protein and exposure to a sufficient dose of the toxin causes the development of IgG blocking antibodies which prevent further clinical effect of the toxin. Antibodies develop in 3 to 5% of neurological patients but is dose dependent. Doses of less than 100 u per treatment session and avoidance of reinjection within 2 weeks will reduce the likelihood of antibody development. With approximately 25,000 injection sessions, we have not had any significant generalized reaction to the toxin and are not aware of the development of secondary resistance to the toxin in any of the individuals treated.

GLABELLA

In Western society, when we communicate we look at one another's eyes. Failure to do this is regarded as failure to communicate, to understand. Because we look at one another's eyes, we use the muscles in this area to express our emotions in very complex ways. Lifting our eyebrows makes our eyes more open and signifies honesty or openness. Pulling down our eyebrows partially masks our eyes and reduces communication. It also can signify anger, dominance, fatigue. However, we can lift the central brow (a quizzical look), depress the medial brow, elevate the lateral brow and appose the eyebrows all at the same time, expressing concern.

Many individuals use their brow muscles inappropriately and this sends the "wrong message." The most common example of this is the individual who apposes and depresses the medial brow when concentrating, producing an angry appearance and causing remarks such as "are you angry/mad?," "lighten up!," etc. In addition, years of use of these muscles can cause a degree of brow ptosis and the appearance of glabellar lines—giving an aged or angry expression. All these can be corrected by paralysis of the muscles that appose the brow and the central depressors of the brow.

ANATOMY

We [9] along with other investigators [10] have addressed the relevant anatomy in this area. There is considerable individual variation and it is important to individualize the treatment. Corrugator supercilii is the most obviously important muscle in this area and must be adequately treated. However, in individuals with a procerus line, a large dose to procerus and depressor supercilii is necessary. For those with an arched brow, treatment in the midpupillary line is unnecessary whereas those with a more horizontal brow (the majority of females requesting treatment and all males) require treatment in this location.

DOSE AND TECHNIQUE

We have recently described our technique in some detail [11]. The initial decision relates to the total dose. In a female we use 25 units of BOTOX as a starting dose, in a male, 35 units. However, if the individual has larger muscles than usual or deep glabellar lines, we may use 35 units in a female, 50 units in a male. We and others have arrived empirically at this dose but scientific backing for this has recently been published [12].

This should be distributed approximately 20% into procerus, 15% into each corrugator and the remaining 50% into orbicularis oculi in four separate sites (Figs. 1, 2). In a female with a high arched brow, the injection in the midpupillary line is omitted (Fig. 3). In these figures, please note that the curving line represents the bony orbital margin and not the eyebrow, which is very variable in location. We recommend protection of the orbital rim with the thumb of the noninjecting hand in order to avoid injecting into the orbit. If the area above the midpupil is injected, it is important to be at least 1 cm above the orbital rim. In our experience, injecting closer to the orbital rim in this location is the greatest cause of ptosis.

PROBLEMS

The most likely cause of an incomplete response is inadequate dosage. The above injection technique has been developed by using EMG guidance in individuals who have not achieved a complete response. We still prefer to use this technique if we have not achieved the anticipated result. The optimum method is more painful for the subject but will give answers that can be used to tailor subsequent treatments. We use the Allergan 1½ inch 27-gauge Teflon coated needle, inserting it above the

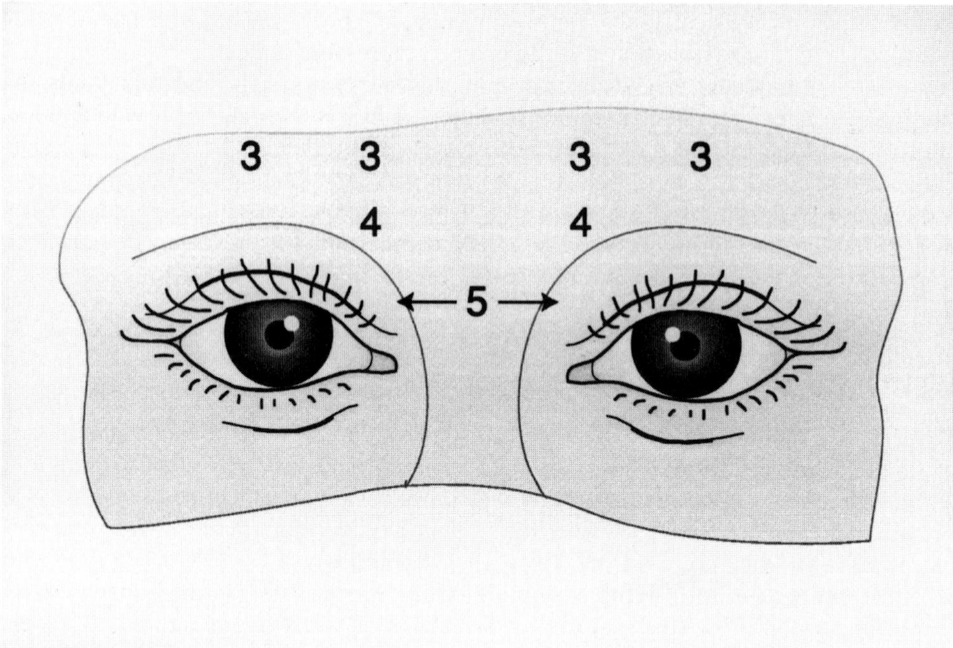

FIGURE 1 Botulinum toxin dose used to treat glabellar frown lines in a woman with a more horizontal-type brow.

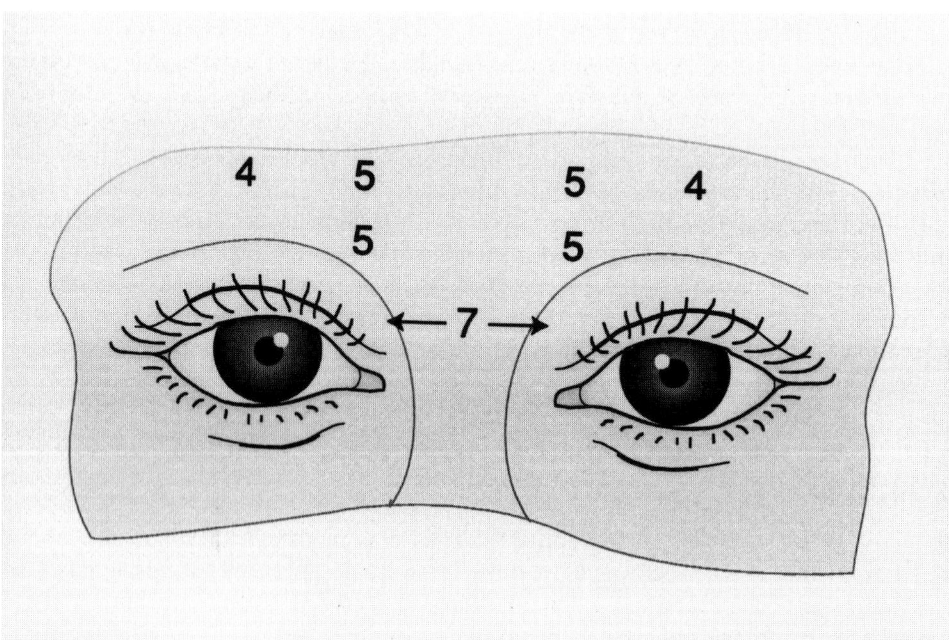

FIGURE 2 Botulinum toxin dose used to treat glabellar frown lines in a man.

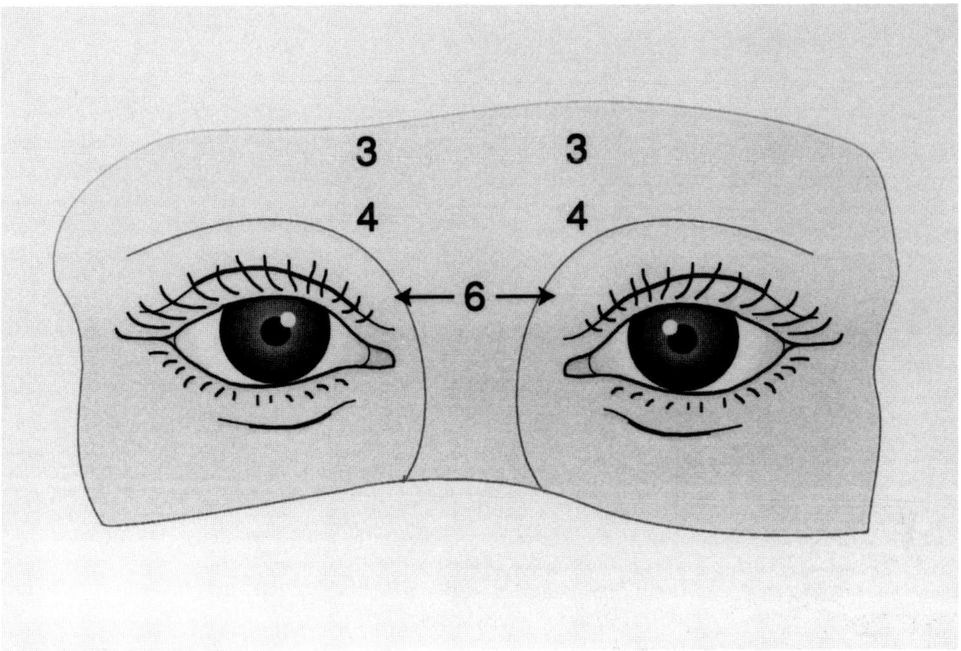

FIGURE 3 Botulinum toxin dose used to treat glabellar frown lines in an individual with an arched brow. Note the arch represents the bony rim, not the eyebrow.

central glabella and then using it fanwise to assess all the relevant muscles (Fig. 4) [13]. Using our current injection technique, less than 5% of individuals fail to achieve a satisfactory response and they usually require an increased dosage to corrugator supercilii.

The development of a complication is the other major problem. Minor complications include temporary bruising, but the development of ptosis is almost always significant. We believe that ptosis is the result of poor technique rather than overdosage. In particular, injection below or too close to the orbital rim is the most likely cause, and using a technique designed to prevent this is the best preventative. Neither of us has produced significant eyebrow ptosis in any of our cosmetic BTX-A patients in the past 4 years.

If ptosis occurs, it can be treated by stimulation of Muller's muscle. This lies beneath the upper lid levator and is adrenergically innervated. Using an alpha-adrenergic agent will stimulate this muscle, elevating the lid. Alpha-1-adrenergic agents such as Neo-synephrine (phenylephrine HCl; Sanofi Winthrop, Collegeville, PA) are effective but also produce mydriasis, dilating the pupil and causing photophobia, loss of accommodation, and possibly precipitating acute closed angle glaucoma. A partially selective alpha-adrenergic agent, apraclonidine 0.5% eyedrops (Alcon Inc., Dallas, TX) are usually successful at treating the ptosis without mydriasis.

FOREHEAD

Elevation of the eyebrows will "open" the eyes, indicating greater communication, openness, or honesty. In younger individuals, habitual elevation of the eyebrows

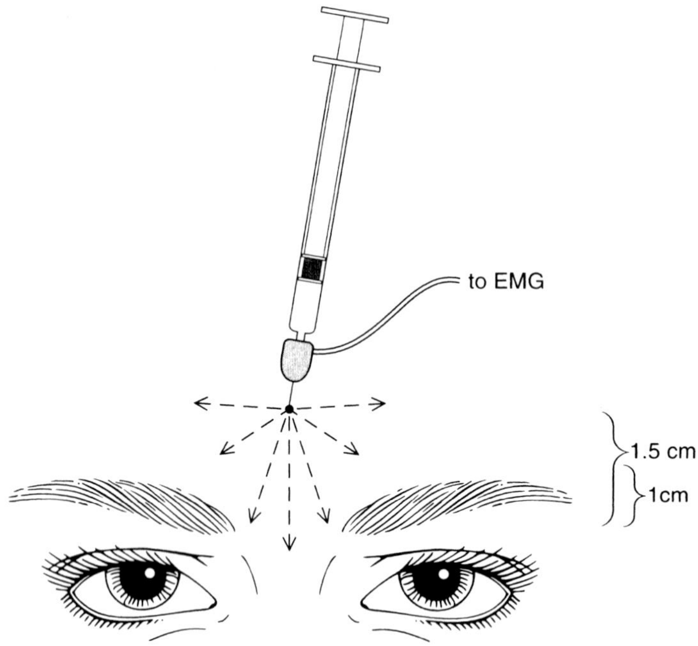

FIGURE 4 Diagram of electromyography-guided injection into the area using a fanwise injection technique.

produces horizontal forehead lines and tension headaches. Horizontal forehead lines are more common in males both because of their heavier brows and their thicker sebaceous skin.

With advancing years, brow ptosis will necessitate greater use of frontalis to "open" the eyes and to even keep the eyebrows out of the field of vision. Treatment of frontalis with BTX-A to get rid of expressionistic horizontal forehead lines gives a very satisfactory result, but there are a number of potential pitfalls:

1. Treatment of an individual with brow ptosis who requires frontalis action to lift the eyebrows out of the line of sight is contraindicated.
2. Treatment of an individual with minimal brow ptosis with BTX-A will change the balance of forces such that the brow depressors will overact, producing brow ptosis. This situation requires concomitant treatment of the brow depressors (see section on brow depressors).
3. Paralysis of all of frontalis produces an inexpressive face. In particular, we believe that retention of a small amount of frontalis, especially laterally (but avoiding the "Spock" look) is very valuable. We do not initially inject lateral to the midpupillary line, but will get the individual to return in 2 weeks and will add a few units laterally if requested.

In summary, it is better to undertreat frontalis and to add extra BTX-A than the reverse. Our current technique (Fig. 5) is to inject along a line in the mid forehead and to massage each injection site (reducing bruising and spreading the result). In

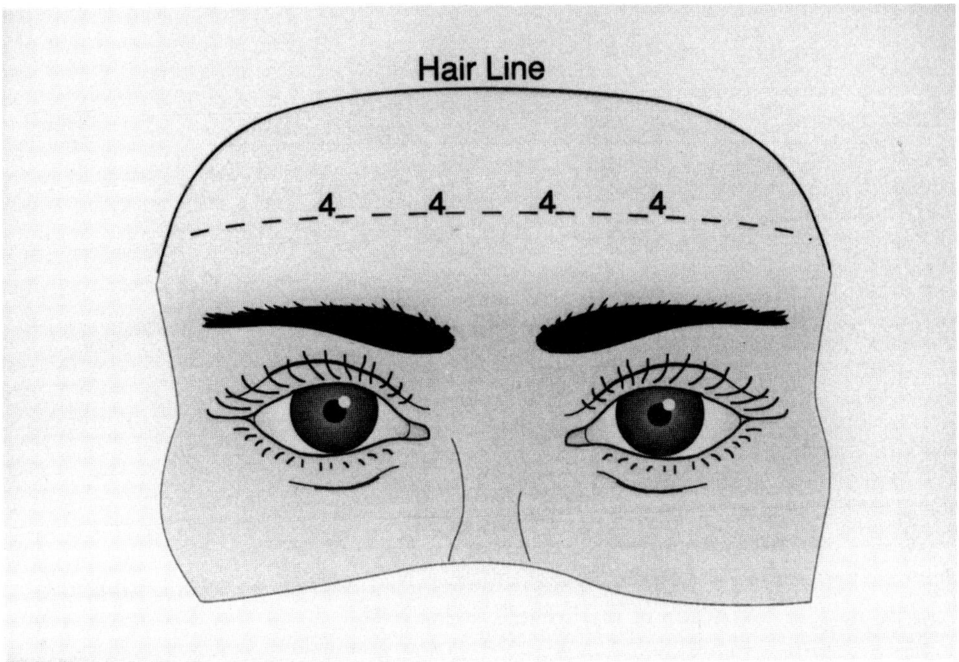

FIGURE 5 Botulinum toxin dose and injection sites for treating horizontal forehead lines in a young individual. The injection sites are spaced equally on a line midway between the orbital rim and the hairline.

individuals with a high forehead, a second row of injections can be used, but we do not inject closer than 2 cm above the eyebrow.

PROBLEMS

Loss of expressivity and brow ptosis have been discussed already and are integral to the selection of subjects suitable for this procedure and to the injection technique.

Occasionally these individuals complain of headaches for a few hours or a day after injection. We have seldom encountered this problem. It has been suggested that headache is attributable to small subperiosteal hematomas, and we attempt to avoid touching the periosteum as much as possible. Others describe going into the periosteum, then pulling the needle back a little. We do not recommend this technique both because it is more painful in the short term and because of the possibility of precipitating headaches.

The other possible cause of these brief headaches is spasm of frontalis. Such spasm is certainly seen occasionally during the onset of action of the toxin, during its action, and as it is wearing off. Most individuals will describe this as spasm and can differentiate it from headache although we could anticipate spasm generating the headache as an alternative mechanism to that previously described. Asymmetric treatment of the brow is described below. One of the complications of asymmetric treatment of the forehead, intentional or not, is the cocked eyebrow, quizzical eyebrow, or one-sided "Spock" eyebrow (Fig. 6). This is attributable to overaction of untreated

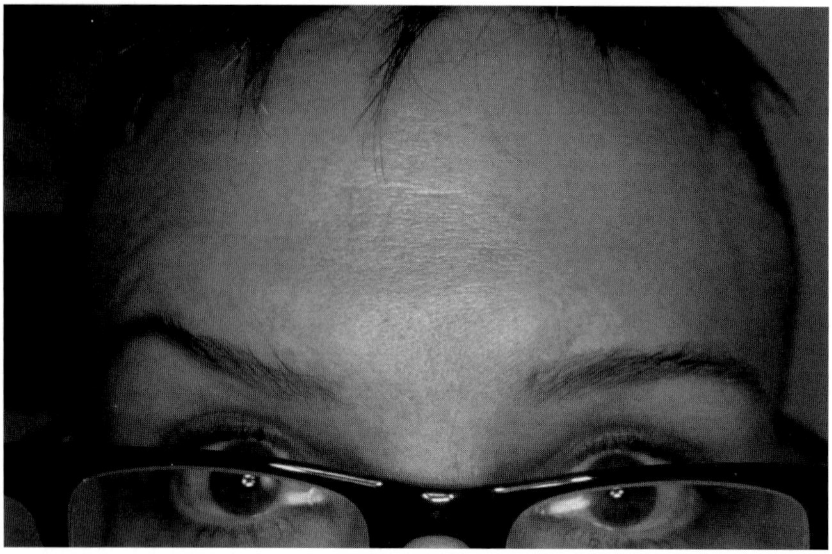

FIGURE 6 "Cocked" or "Spock" eyebrows showing marked elevation of the lateral eyebrow because of overaction of the frontalis in this area.

frontalis producing lateral elevation of the eyebrow. Treatment is simple—2 to 3 units of BOTOX into the active muscle.

BROW DEPRESSORS

We have recently reported [14] a small study of the treatment of brow depressors unassociated with other BTX-A treatment. The purpose of this study was to show the browlifting effect of treating the brow depressors and allowing unopposed action of the brow elevator (frontalis) to produce a browlift. The injection technique was to inject approximately 10 units centrally below a line joining the eyebrows and 2 to 3 units of BOTOX vertically above the lateral canthus just above the orbital rim (Fig. 7). Measuring from the center of the pupil to the lowest eyebrow cilium, five of the seven individuals showed central eyebrow elevation of up to 3 mm. This was manifest as improved "show" of the tarsal upper eyelid, greater openness of the orbit, and a more relaxed appearance. In these five individuals, the relatively large dose of BOTOX injected into procerus produced some clinical spread to corrugator with noticeable reduction in involuntary frowning and clinically reduced but not abolished ability to frown. The significance of this observation is:

1. It confirms the "browlift" that many of us have seen and our patients have reported associated with BTX-A treatment of the glabella.
2. It points out a way to improve treatment of horizontal forehead lines by concomitant treatment of the brow depressors to avoid brow ptosis.
3. It provides a new way of using BTX-A—a single central injection into the area of procerus. This will allow frowning and will produce central brow elevation. In other words, it will avoid the "BOTOXed" look. It is anticipated that this effect will be of reduced longevity, but it is a satis-

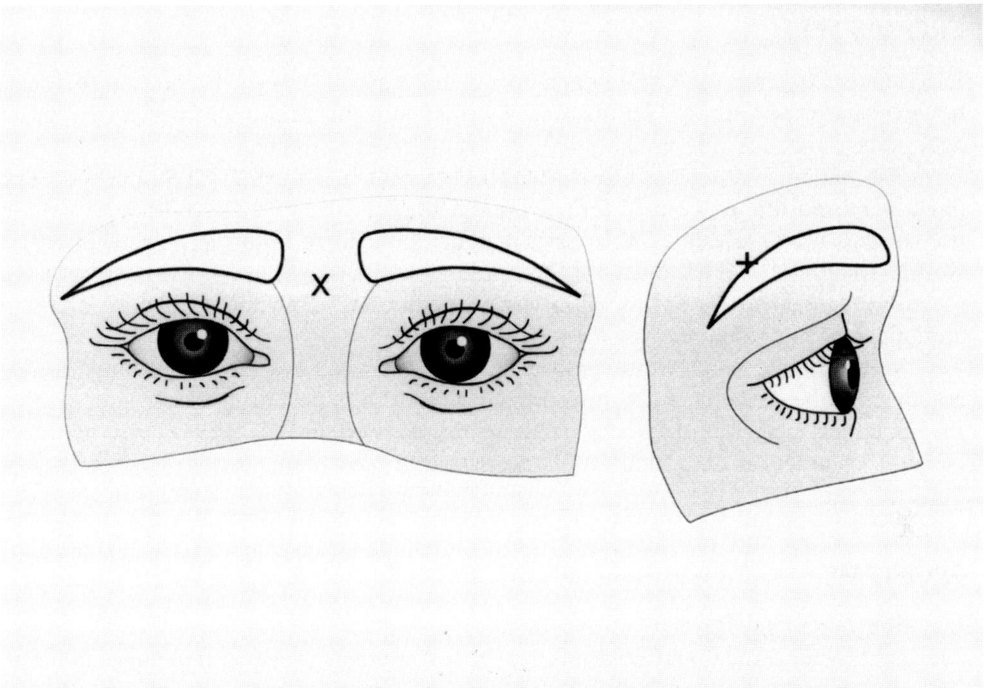

FIGURE 7 Placement of botulinum toxin into the glabella and superlateral eyebrow areas.

factory alternative form of treatment especially for those in the visual media.

BROW ASYMMETRY

Brow asymmetry is extremely common, and relatively small degrees of asymmetry (less than 2 mm) can become cosmetically obvious. Assessment of such asymmetry is an important part of the pretreatment evaluation of anyone before BTX-A treatment of frontalis.

In order to improve asymmetry, the simplest and best approach is to treat the brow depressors on the affected side. For example, 2 to 3 units of BOTOX injected into the tail of the eyebrow just above the orbital rim above the lateral canthus will give a 1 to 2 or more mm elevation of the lateral eyebrow.

After a surgical browlift, treatment of frontalis to drop the elevated eyebrow is more relevant. Again, relatively low doses (approximately 5 units of BOTOX) are usually sufficient to accomplish this.

A third way of treating brow asymmetry that may be indicated in some individuals is to weaken adjacent frontalis to produce overaction of the frontalis over the area requiring elevation. This is an elegant but risky solution because failure of the technique will probably exacerbate the problem.

Low doses, augmented at 2 week intervals are the best way of working out an appropriate treatment for brow asymmetry.

CROW'S FEET

Individuals 20-years-old or younger do not have wrinkling of the crow's feet area however hard they smile. Getting rid of wrinkles in this area will only get rid of an aged appearance as long as the smile is not otherwise affected.

We began treating the crow's feet area with 6 units of BOTOX per side and have increased this to 12 u in females and 15 u per side in males, although we are prepared to increase this as necessary in order to achieve both the desired effect as well as longevity. We have used a three injection site technique in the past but have recently changed to a two injection site technique although the total dose of toxin administered has remained the same (Fig. 8).

Interestingly, some individuals learn not to frown and so get prolongation of response in the glabella much longer than would be expected neurophysiologically. In our experience, this does not occur to the same degree in the crow's feet area because contraction of orbicularis is an essential part of the smile. Contraction of the smile muscles of the lower face without orbicularis produces a rictus or grimace.

PROBLEMS

Injection under the lower eyelid will produce a droop of the lower eyelid, an unacceptable appearance, and photophobia. It is important to avoid injecting medial to a vertical line through the lateral canthus.

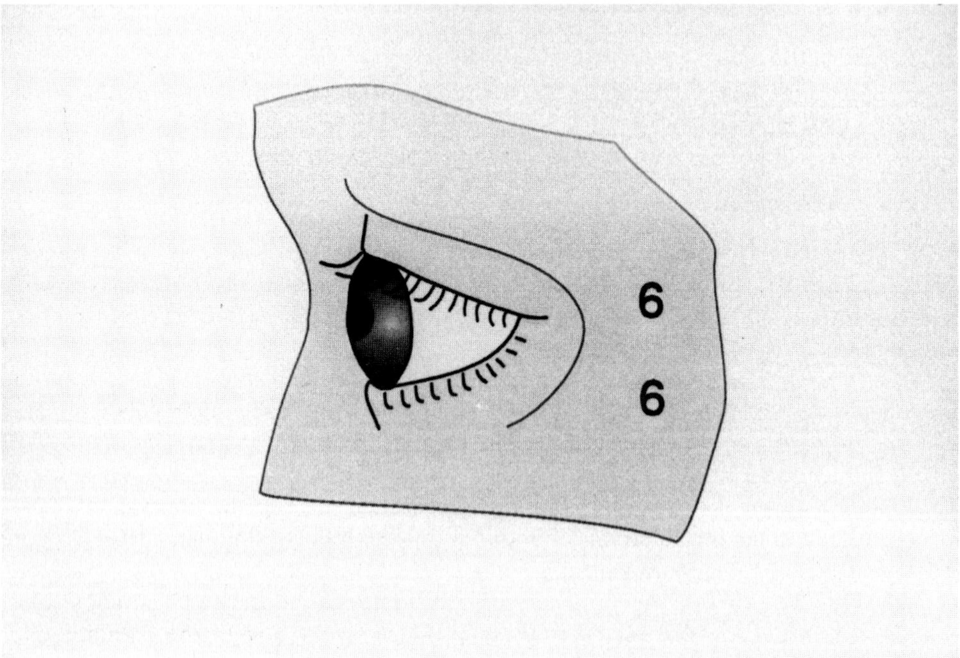

FIGURE 8 Botulinum toxin dose used to treat the crow's feet area. Note the curving arc around the eye represents the lateral orbital rim, and the injection sites should be 1 cm outside this.

Injecting too low in the cheek will affect risorius and perhaps zygomaticus major, causing a droop of the upper lip and an asymmetric smile. This can be avoided by staying well above the inferior margin of the zygomatic arch.

Finally, there is one reported [7] case of diplopia after injection into this area. This can be avoided by injecting at least 1 cm from the lateral orbital margin, avoiding excessive dilution of the toxin and only massaging away from the orbit.

OTHER FACIAL AREAS

Lower Lid Orbicularis Hypertrophy

Some individuals develop a ridge of muscle along the lower eyelid below the lash margin. Weakening of this muscle (1–2 u of BOTOX per side injected subcutaneously under the center of the lash margin) will soften this ridge, smoothing the area and improving the shape of the palpebral fissure. Again, avoid too-large doses and injecting too low or too lateral.

Nasolabial Folds

Levator labii superioris alaeque nasi inserts into the upper medial portion of the nasolabial fold and its contraction exaggerates the fold. Weakening this muscle will soften the upper part of the nasolabial fold. However, the effect is not dramatic and is accompanied by lengthening of the upper lip, an aging effect (Fig. 9). In individuals with a short upper lip this can be acceptable, but in our experience there are usually better ways of treating this indication.

Nasalis

Nasal flare is an embarrassment to some individuals. Typically the flare of the ala produces columella show, which is unappealing. Five to 10 u of BOTOX per side will ameliorate this problem [9].

Upper Lip Wrinkles

The lower face is extremely sensitive to the effect of BTX-A by comparison with the upper face. Treating anywhere around the mouth can affect the appearance and function of this area. Especially important are asymmetry of the mouth and incompetence or weakness of the lips and cheeks, which result in biting of the treated area. We always recommend using lower doses and symmetrical treatment in this area. Many individuals have wrinkling of the upper lip—typically three or four deeper wrinkles with numerous softer rhytides. Injecting 1 u of BOTOX under each wrinkle (repeating after 2 weeks if necessary) will soften these wrinkles. However, the individual may lose the ability to whistle and may not like the change in lip function. This treatment must be avoided in wind instrument players.

Depressor Anguli Oris (DAO)

By comparison with BTX-A treatment of other perioral indications, this is much more satisfactory but still not as dramatic as in the upper face. We tend to use this as an add-on to other BTX-A treatment rather than in isolation.

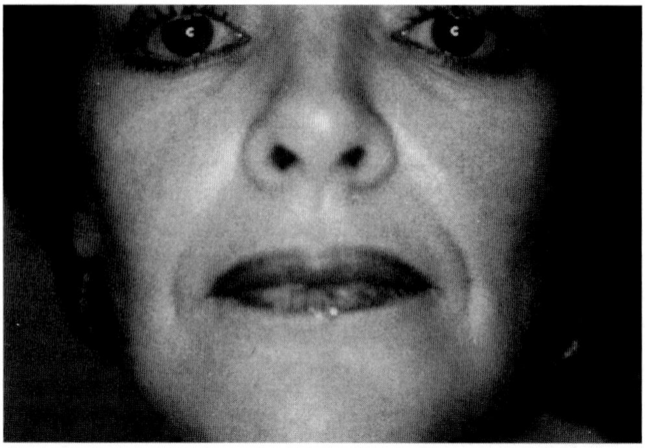

(a)

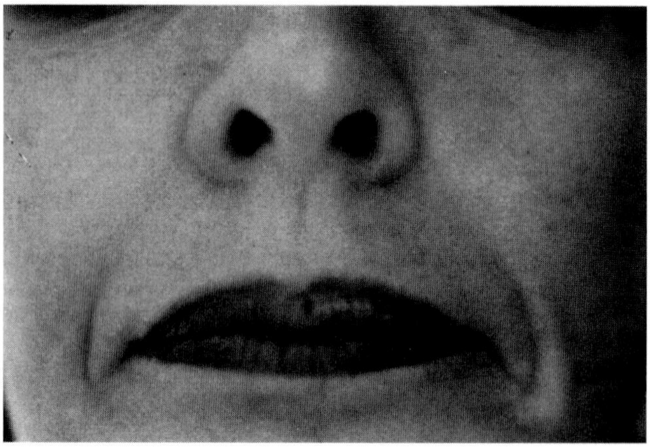

(b)

FIGURE 9 An individual before and after botulinum toxin treatment of levator labii superioris alaeque nais showing improvement in the nasolabial folds and lengthening of the upper lip.

DAO runs from the modeolus, lateral to the lateral commissure, inferomedially to the ramus of the mandible. Injection of 2 to 3 u of BOTOX 2 cm inferior to the lateral commissure where the tensed muscle can be palpated will produce elevation of the corners of the mouth (Fig. 10). Careful symmetry is important, and this is an area where EMG guidance can be valuable.

Mentalis

Contraction of mentalis will produce an irregular or bumpy appearance of the chin. This can be especially obvious after surgery or trauma to the area. Five to 10 u of BOTOX injected close to the point of the chin and allowed to diffuse to mentalis will soften this appearance. We have attempted to soften the mental fold but have had problems with asymmetry and drooling.

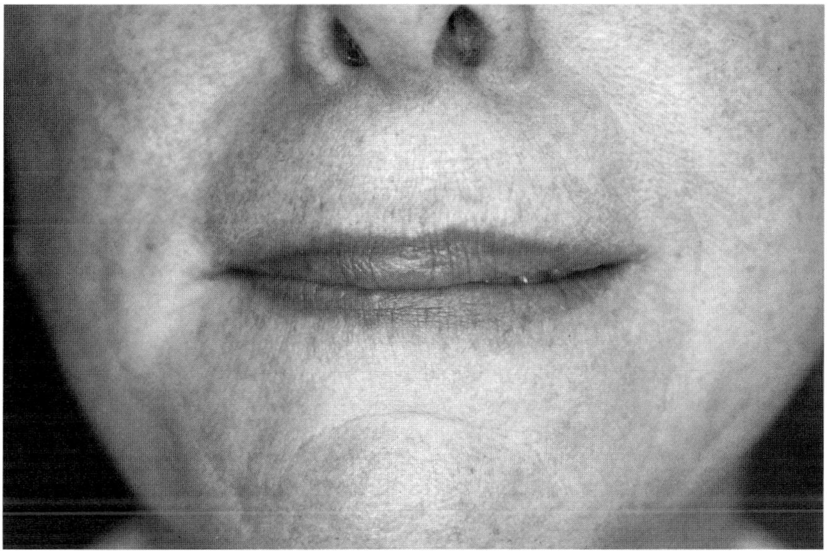

FIGURE 10 Unilateral BOTOX treatment of depressor anguli oris on the subject's left side. Note the upturn of the corner of the mouth on the left.

PLATYSMA

Some individuals use platysma as a muscle of expression. This may be manifest as vertical platysmal bands or as horizontal neck lines. Vertical bands may be especially noticeable after facelifting procedures that have not dwelt with the neck adequately. Treatment of vertical bands with BTX-A (approximately 15 u of BOTOX divided into three injection sites along the band) will produce satisfactory softening of the band. Usually the total dose is 30 to 60 u of BOTOX. Smaller doses every 2 cm along a horizontal neck line is similarly effective.

Recently, Brandt and Bellman [15] have been using larger doses of BOTOX to achieve greater weakening of platysma and greater improvement. In particular, they regard platysma as a depressor muscle of the face and they comment on the improvement in the lower face after BTX-A treatment of platysma. In some individuals they are using BOTOX doses of 100 to 200 u. When we have attempted to use doses of BOTOX of 100 u injected into platysma, we have had an unacceptably high incidence of side effects, particularly dysphagia and weakness of neck flexion. This may be a result of our technique and we look forward to further studies on platysma.

ADJUNCTIVE USE

We have recently summarized our experience of the use of BTX-A combined with other therapeutic modalities for cosmetic enhancement [16].

Laser Resurfacing

BTX-A has made a significant improvement in resurfacing treatment for wrinkles. The thesis is that allowing new collagen to be laid down and matured without repeated folding should give a significantly better long-term result. We have treated a number of individuals with the combination of BTX-A with CO_2 laser resurfacing, some of these with BTX-A on one side only. Our conclusion was that the BTX-A–treated side was better at least to 1 year with only a single injection of BTX-A 1 week before resurfacing. It is now our practice to maintain the results of CO_2 laser resurfacing with BTX-A to the glabella and crow's feet as much as the patients will allow.

BTX-A and Facial Surgery

BTX-A can be used to enhance the results of face and brow cosmetic surgery and also to improve some complications. Although we have little experience in this area, we believe that pretreatment of the brow muscles before browlift surgery and of platysma before facelift surgery should allow for an easier operation and for healing to occur without active muscles reducing the final result. Greater symmetry should be achievable because the intraoperative assessment will more accurately reflect the final result.

Our principal experience with the combination of BTX-A and facial cosmetic surgery has been in the treatment of suboptimal results. BTX-A is extremely valuable in the treatment of synkinesia after facelift surgery and malar implant surgery (Fig. 11). Cutting small branches of the facial nerve, which regrow in an aberrant manner, can produce uncomfortable results. Commonly blinking will produce twitching of muscles elsewhere on the face. This can be managed by small doses of BTX-A under EMG guidance.

In addition, BTX-A can be used to correct asymmetry produced by facial cosmetic surgery. Browlift surgery is particularly amenable to this form of therapy, and the abnormal appearance of the muscle in the brow which can occur in some browlift patients is very well treated by BTX-A.

HYPERHIDROSIS

Excessive sweating is a major social problem and can cause some affected individuals to either shun social contacts or go to great lengths to control the problem. Treatments range from the use of aluminum chloride preparations of varying degrees of effectiveness to sympathectomy.

Reports of the successful treatment of Frey's syndrome (gustatory sweating) by BTX-A appeared in 1995 [17]. This was soon followed by reports of the BTX-A treatment of axillary hyperhidrosis [18–20] and palmar hyperhidrosis [21–23]. This literature has been recently summarized [24].

Axillary Hyperhidrosis

Treatment of axillary hyperhidrosis is relatively simple and almost uniformly satisfactory for patient and physician. Studies show that a dose of 50 to 70 u per axilla is effective in almost all individuals. Varying dilutions are used from 1 to 5 ml/100 u vial. The number of injection sites used varies but is usually 2 cm apart. Injection is into the superficial subcutaneous tissue. We routinely use 50 u/axilla in 15 to 20 injection sites per axilla in a 5 ml/100 u vial dilution. The patients are reviewed at 2 weeks, and if the response is not clinically satisfactory the starch-iodine test is

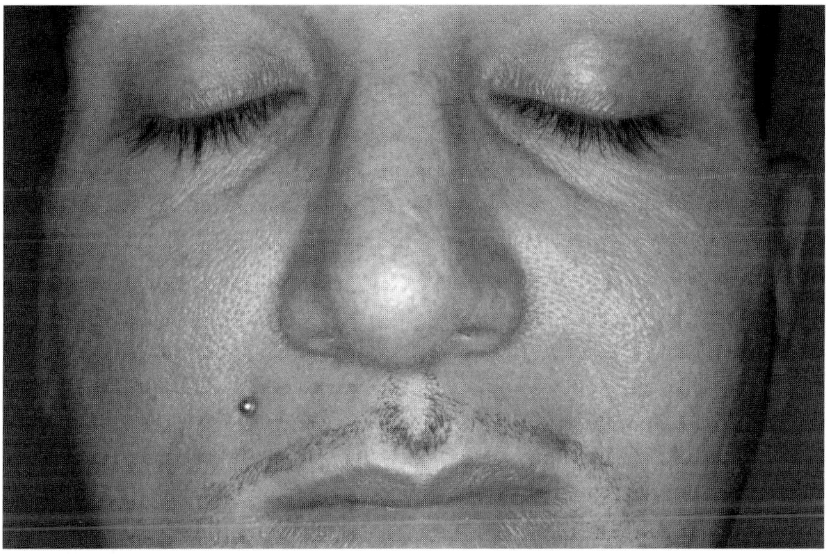

(a)

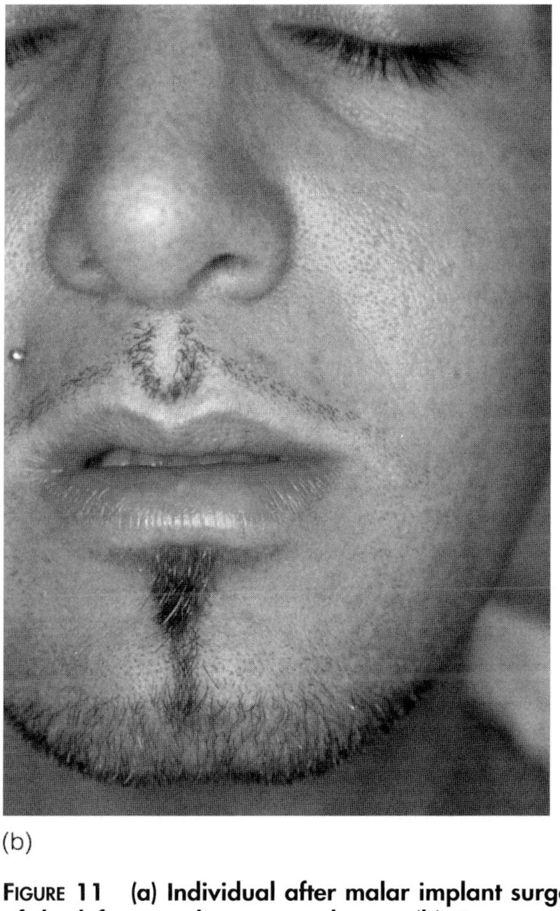

(b)

FIGURE 11 (a) Individual after malar implant surgery with synkinesis causing elevation of the left upper lip on eye closure. (b) One month after BOTOX treatment showing a normal upper lip on eye closure.

used to find the remaining areas of hyperhidrosis. A further 10 to 20 u is used in these areas.

In the majority of individuals, a clinical remission lasts 4 to 8 months or longer. Side effects apart from minor local effects are absent.

Palmar/Plantar Hyperhidrosis

Treatment of these areas is not as easy as treatment of the axilla. First, the area to be treated is larger and the effective dose required also larger, which may limit the availability of effective therapy. Second, the areas are sensitive and consideration must be given to the use of nerve blocks for the procedure. Some investigators use such blocks [23] whereas others do not [18]. An effective does will range from 50 to 100 u per palm or sole. Severe hyperhidrosis typically affects the skin on the sides of the toes/fingers, palms/sole, and distal wrist so there is often some residual sweating in these areas.

We prefer to use 50 u per palm or sole, diluted in 5 ml/100 u vial and injected through 50 injection sites. At present we use posterior tibial nerve blocks for the anterior sole but do not use nerve blocks for the palm, preferring to rely on the sharpness of frequently changed 30-gauge ½ inch needles and ice-induced hypoesthesia. We take particular care to put the peripheral series of injections around the sides of the palm and onto the distal fold of the wrist. Again we see patients at 2 weeks and use the starch-iodine test to accurately locate touch-up injection sites, injecting approximately 1 u per site. Dose required at this session is 0 to 50 u per palm/sole.

The major side effect of BTX-A therapy of the palms is weakness of the small muscles of the hand. This is usually manifest as difficulty with zippers, bottle tops, buttons, etc., and usually only lasts 2 to 4 weeks. Keeping the dose per injection site small will minimize this. However, because of this weakness we prefer to treat only one hand at a time, usually the right because this is the hand most frequently socially contacted. The patient is reviewed at 2 weeks, the first hand touched up and the second hand treated with a dose based on the response to the first hand treatment.

CONCLUSIONS

BTX-A is, molecule for molecule or weight for weight, the most toxic material known to humanity. Paradoxically and as a result of its effectiveness, it is also the safest medication available to us. It is administered in accurate doses exactly at the required treatment site. Little is available to go into circulation to cause generalized effects, certainly at the doses most commonly used cosmetically. Side effects are limited to local spread of the toxin to unwanted muscles, causing, for example, ptosis, and effects of the injection such as bruising and pain. This unparalleled safety profile combined with the effectiveness of treatment and the ease of administration have given great satisfaction to both physicians and their patients. In the future, manipulation of the molecule or its mode of delivery may further improve on the treatment and its longevity, but at the present time BTX-A is firmly established as an important part of the cosmetic physician's practice.

REFERENCES

1. Carruthers A, Kiene K, Carruthers J. Botulinum A exotoxin use in clinical dermatology. J Am Acad Dermatol 34:788–797, 1996.
2. Schantz EJ, Kautter DA. Microbiological methods: standardized assay for clostridium botulinum toxins. J Association Analytical Chemists 61(1):96–99, 1977.
3. Scott AB, Rosenbaum A, Collins CC. Pharmacologic weakening of extraocular muscles. Invest Ophthalmol 12:924–927, 1973.
4. Pearce LB, Borodic GE, First ER, et al. Measurement of botulinum toxin activity: evaluation of the lethality assay. Toxicol Appl Pharmacol 128:69–77, 1994.
5. Lowe NJ, Maxwell A, Harper H. Botulinum A exotoxin for glabellar folds: a double-blind, placebo-controlled study with an electromyographic injection technique. J Am Acad Dermatol 35:569–572, 1996.
6. Klein AW. Cosmetic therapy with Botulinum toxin: anecdotal memoirs. Dermatol Surg 22:757–759, 1996.
7. Garcia A, Fulton JE. Cosmetic denervation of the muscles of facial expression with botulinum toxin. Dermatol Surg 22:39–43, 1996.
8. Scott AB. Clostridial toxins as therapeutic agents. In: Simpson LL, ed. Botulinum Neurotoxin and Tetanus Toxin. New York: Academic Press, 1989, pp. 399–412.
9. Carruthers JDA, Carruthers JA. Treatment of glabellar frown lines with C. botulinum-A exotoxin. J Dermatol Surg Oncol 18:17–21, 1992.
10. Wieder JM, Moy RL. Understanding botulinum toxin: surgical anatomy of the frown, forehead, and periocular region. Dermatol Surg 24:1172–1174, 1998.
11. Carruthers A, Carruthers J. Clinical indications and injection techniques for the cosmetic use of botulinum A exotoxin. Dermatol Surg 24:1189–1194, 1998.
12. Hankins CL, Strimling R, Rogers GS. Botulinum A exotoxin for glabellar wrinkles: dose and response. Dermatol Surg 24:1181–1183, 1998.
13. Carruthers A, Carruthers J. The cosmetic use of botulinum A exotoxin. In: Dzubow LM, ed. Cosmetic Dermatologic Surgery. Philadelphia: Lippincott-Raven, 1998, pp. 1–18.
14. Huilgol S, Carruthers A, Carruthers J. Raising eyebrows with botulinum toxin. Dermatol Surg 25:373–376, 1999.
15. Brandt FS, Bellman B. Cosmetic use of botulinum A exotoxin for the aging neck. Dermatol Surg 24:1232–1234, 1998.
16. Carruthers J, Carruthers A. The adjunctive use of botulinum toxin. Dermatol Surg 24: 1244–1247, 1998.
17. Drobik C, Laskawi R. Frey's syndrome: treatment with botulinum toxin. Acta Otolaryngol (Stockh) 115:459–461, 1995.
18. Bushara KO, Park DM, Jones JC, Schutta HS. Botulinum toxin—a possible new treatment for axillary hyperhidrosis. Clin Exp J Dermatol 21:276–278, 1996.
19. Odderson IR. Axillary hyperhidrosis: treatment with botulinum toxin A. Arch Phys Med Rehabil 79:350–352, 1998.
20. Glogau RG. Botulinum A neurotoxin for axillary hyperhidrosis: no sweat Botox. Dermatol Surg 24:817–819, 1998.
21. Nauman M, Flachenecker P, Brocher EB, Toyka KV, Reiners K. Botulinum toxin for palmar hyperhidrosis. Lancet 349:252, 1997.
22. Schneider P, Binder M, Auff A, Kittler H, Berger T, Wolf K. Double-blind trial of botulinum A toxin for the treatment of focal hyperhidrosis of the palms. Br J Dermatol 136:548–552, 1997.
23. Shelley WB, Talanin NY, Shelley ED. Botulinum toxin therapy for palmar hyperhidrosis. J Am Acad Dermatol 38:227–229, 1998.
24. Odderson IR. Hyperhidrosis treated by botulinum A exotoxin. Dermatol Surg 24:1237–1241, 1998.

APPENDIX 1: LASER BLEPHAROPLASTY (LID-LIFT)

1. WHAT IS BLEPHAROPLASTY?

Blepharoplasty or lidlift is a delicate surgical procedure in which the laser beam is used as a means of removing excess skin and/or fat from both upper and lower eyelids. The eyes then have a more open, youthful, and bright appearance.

2. WHAT IS INVOLVED?

Dr. Carruthers uses the Sharplan $C0_2$ laser beam to perform the lidlift surgery. This laser beam is 1/5 mm in diameter and it seals tiny blood vessels as it cuts, so that there is very little swelling and bruising. This translates to a shorter recovery time and reduced discomfort for the patient. Most individuals are ready to go back to their normal activities in 5-7 days.

3. WHAT IS THE DIFFERENCE BETWEEN LASER AND TRADITIONAL "COLD-STEEL" SURGERY?

With previous "cold-steel" surgery, eyelids could be bruised-looking for two to three weeks after blepharoplasty. With the use of the laser beam as the cutting instrument, bruising is dramatically reduced and many individuals are able to be back at work with only slight residual swelling by the end of the first week after surgery.

4. WHAT ARE THE ADVANTAGES?

Usually, the upper lid fold starts to be hidden in the mid-thirties and this appearance can make one look tired, angry, and frustrated. Lifting the excess skin and fat away gives the sparkle back to the eyes and the expression. Lidlift surgery is a most effective way to restore an open, relaxed, and youthful appearance.

In the lower lid, the prominent fat pockets can be removed from the inside (transconjunctival blepharoplasty) so that there is no visible scar afterwards. We also resurface lower and upper eyelid skin right after the CO_2 laser incisional surgery, using the Erbium-YAG laser or CO_2 laser, because it dramatically changes tired, creepy skin to a new, youthful, smooth, translucent skin. Laser resurfacing is precise and the length of time to recover from the resurfacing parallels the time for recovery from the procedure, so it is most efficient to perform both procedures at the same surgical appointment.

5. WHAT IS THE RECOVERY TIME?

We recommend that individuals should take at least one week off their regular activities. With makeup, individuals can often go out a day or two earlier.

6. HOW LONG WILL IT LAST?

Blepharoplasty turns back the clock but we must continue with our ongoing skin maintenance program and sunscreen, AHA, and Vitamins A and C therapy. If the lid skin does become creepy again, instead of the blepharoplasty a resurfacing of the lid skin, using the Erbium-YAG laser or CO_2 laser, is an effective adjunctive procedure.

7. CAN OTHER PROCEDURES BE COMBINED WITH AN EYELID-LIFT?

Yes. As previously mentioned, laser resurfacing of the skin around the eyes helps produce a new, smooth, youthful look. Also, BOTOX to the forehead, brow furrows, and crow's feet results in a more youthful appearance.

APPENDIX 2: COSMETIC LASTER BLEPHAROPLASTY OPERATIVE CONSENT

I hereby authorize Dr. Jean Carruthers and her associates to perform a ____. I fully understand that this procedure has limited applications. No guarantees or assurances have been given to me by anyone as to the results that may be obtained.

Dr. J. Carruthers and assistants have carefully explained to me the nature, goals, limitations, and possible complications of this procedure and have discussed alternative forms of treatment.

By placing my initials next to these items, I clearly understand and accept the following:

INITIAL
HERE

___ 1. The potential benefits of the proposed procedure(s)
___ 2. The possible alternate medical procedure(s)
___ 3. The probability of success
___ 4. The reasonably anticipated consequences if the procedure is not performed
___ 5. The possibility of ancillary services/fees including, but not limited to, anesthesia, laboratory, medications, and/or surgical facility use.
___ 6. The goal of laser surgery, as in any cosmetic procedure, is improvement, not perfection. Satisfaction is based on realistic expectation.
___ 7. Although the procedure is intended to improve my appearance, in rare cases it may leave it unchanged or in some cases worsened.
___ 8. The final result may not be apparent for 3 to 12 months after the procedure.
___ 9. To achieve the best possible result, additional procedures may be required. There will be a charge for any additional procedure performed.
___ 10. Strict adherence to the postsurgical regimen discussed by Dr. J. Carruthers (i.e., medications, creams, postsurgical care instructions, and all other regimens discussed) is necessary in order to achieve the best possible results.
___ 11. The surgical fee is paid for the surgery itself and subsequent postsurgical office visits. There is no guarantee that the expected or anticipated results will be achieved.
___ 12. I give my permission for the administration of anesthesia, as deemed appropriate by the physician.
___ 13. Protective eye covering will be provided to protect my eyes from accidental laser exposure, but accidental exposure to laser is possible.

Although complications after these procedures are infrequent, by placing my initials next to the following I understand that they may occur and that other procedures may be needed to correct them:

INITIAL
HERE

___ 1. ORBITAL HEMORRHAGE: Can occur in one out of 2500 cosmetic blepharoplasty cases.
___ 2. BLINDNESS: Can occur in one in 40,000 cosmetic blepharoplasty cases.
___ 3. BRUISING/BLEEDING/SWELLING: In some cases, bruising/bleeding of the treated area may occur. Additionally, there may be some swelling noted.
___ 4. INFECTION: Infection is rare. Should it occur, treatment with antibiotics and/or surgical drainage may be required.
___ 5. SCARRING: Scarring is a rare occurrence, but it is a possibility when the skin's surface is disrupted. To minimize the chances of scarring, it is important that I follow all postsurgical instructions carefully.
___ 6. VISUAL changes, dry eyes, ulcerations, and cysts are rare.
___ 7. ALLERGIES: Allergic or toxic responses to anesthetic are extremely rare, but possible.
___ 8. GENERAL RISKS: In addition to these possible complications, I am aware of the general risks inherent in all surgical procedures and anesthetic administration.

My signature certifies that I have discussed the above material thoroughly with Dr. J. Carruthers and assistants. I understand the goals, limitations and possible complications of the above procedure(s), and I wish to proceed with them. I authorize and direct Dr. J. Carruthers and/or associates or assistants of his/her choice, to perform this procedure(s) on me and/or to do any other additional therapeutic procedure that his/her judgement may dictate to be advisable, reasonable, or necessary for my well being.

____
PATIENT SIGNATURE DATE

____
PATIENT PRINTED NAME

____
WITNESS DATE

____
PHYSICIAN SIGNATURE DATE

18

Moles, Cysts, and Lipomas: Surgical Treatment of Cutaneous Cysts

Vicki J. Levine
New York University School of Medicine, New York, New York

Epithelial cysts are common problems for the dermatologic surgeon. The most common type of epithelial cyst is the epidermal cyst, which is also known as the epidermoid inclusion cyst. The other less common cysts, such as pilar (tricholemmal) cysts, dermoid cysts, milia, steatocystoma multiplex, hidrocystoma, mucous cyst, and preauricular sinus and cyst, will also be discussed.

EPIDERMAL CYST

The vast majority of all cutaneous cysts are epidermal cysts [1]. They are asymptomatic, dome-shaped, skin-colored growths that are not erythematous or tender unless they are inflamed or infected. Although they are most common on the head, neck, and upper trunk, they can occur anywhere—even on the palms and soles [2]. Epidermal cysts commonly occur on the genitalia but are rarely present before puberty [3]. Although malignant transformation of these lesions is unusual, both basal cell carcinomas and squamous cell carcinomas have been found to arise from the wall of an epidermoid cyst [4]. Thus, it is important that whenever a cyst is excised, a portion of the wall should be submitted for histopathological examination.

Presurgical Considerations/Consultation

It is necessary to excise the entire cyst wall and punctum to prevent recurrence of the lesion. Thus, during the consultation the physician should inquire whether the cyst has ever been infected or removed in the past. This will help decide which method of removal is optimal. Previous infections will lead to fibrosis and scarring and will alter the decision regarding the technique that is chosen to remove the lesion. Several different techniques have been used to treat the noninflamed, noninfected cyst. To help determine the best technique, palpate to determine if the cyst is freely moveable. It is also helpful, if possible, to identify the punctum. The following methods have been used: (1) punch removal technique, (2) incisional surgical method, (3) fusiform excision technique, (4) electrosurgical technique, (5) excision with secondary intention healing technique, (6) cryosurgery technique, (7) chemical irritant technique, and (8) excisional surgical technique.

Skin Preparation

The skin should be prepared in a sterile manner. A marking pencil can be used to outline the planned incision before administration of the local anesthesia.

Anesthesia

The skin overlying and surrounding an epidermal cyst must be anesthetized before surgical removal. Local anesthesia is obtained by injecting 1% lidocaine with 1:100,000 epinephrine unless the cyst is located on a digit. The anesthesia should be injected between the cyst and the cyst wall so it will dissect around the cyst wall, separating it from surrounding tissue. This may make it easier to dissect the cyst out. Anesthetize the skin around the entire cyst and try not to inject into the cyst itself. If you do, there is the possibility that the cyst will rupture during the procedure. Finally, inject some anesthesia superficially into the skin directly overlying the cyst.

BIOPSY PUNCH METHOD

Freely moveable cysts can often easily be removed using a 2 to 4 mm dermatologic biopsy punch [5]. The other necessary instruments include a chalazion curette, a small curved hemostat, and a gradle scissors. If this method is used, the local anesthesia should be injected deeply into the sac of the cyst. The surgeon should then squeeze the cyst firmly with one hand and place the biopsy punch over the punctum and push it through the skin into the cyst cavity. The specimen of skin is removed with a gradle scissors and pressure is applied to extrude the cyst contents. A small chalazion curette is then inserted to remove the remaining cyst contents and free the cyst wall from the surrounding tissue. When the cyst wall is visible, it should be grasped with a small curved hemostat and removed. Pressure alone may be adequate to remove the wall from the surrounding stroma but one may have to dissect the wall away from the connective tissue with the gradle scissors. The surgical defect can then be closed with sutures or allowed to heal by secondary intention. A sutured wound will healed more rapidly and may give a better cosmetic result. While larger punches can be used to remove large cysts, this method is ideal for small cysts. It may be less successful if used on fibrosed cysts because one may not be able to remove the entire cyst wall. An advantage of this method is that it can be performed more quickly than an excision. In addition, the hole created by the skin punch affords the surgeon better visibility than a linear incision.

Incision and Drainage Technique

This method is another approach that can be used for the removal of small- to medium-sized freely moveable cysts. A single linear incision with a #11 scalpel blade is made along the relaxed skin tension lines over the cyst. If a punctum is present, the incision should be made through it or to one side of it. The punctum should then be removed. The incision should be made into the cyst cavity and pressure should be used to remove the cyst contents. The length of the incision should be smaller than the diameter of the cyst because it is possible to remove the cyst contents through a small wound. This will also result in a smaller surgical scar. The contents of the cyst can be removed with pressure. Many times a cyst wall is extruded along with the cyst contents. More often it will be necessary to extract the cyst wall using a hemostat. Before wound closure, visually inspect the cavity to be sure that no cyst wall remains. Cotton-tip applicators may be helpful in visualizing the cavity. If you find any cyst wall fragments, they can be removed with a small curette or forceps and gradle scissors. If a portion of the cyst wall remains, a new epidermoid cyst may develop. Retained cyst contents may also cause a foreign body reaction. To decrease the risk of these complications, irrigation with sterile saline before wound closure is helpful. The incision can then be closed with buried absorbable or percutaneous sutures.

DISSECTION TECHNIQUE

Medium- to Large-Sized Slightly Moveable Cysts

Make an initial slightly curved incision directly over the cyst. Then, if it is necessary, it can be converted to a fusiform excision. The incision should be made along the relaxed skin tension lines if possible. Make the incision lightly so that you allow the scalpel to penetrate the epidermis and only partially into the dermis so as not to puncture the cyst wall. The assistant should apply lateral traction to help visualize the cyst wall as soon as it is reached. The cyst wall is recognizable because it is glistening white in color compared with the dermis. When the cyst wall is reached, use either the scalpel or Iris scissors to extend the rest of the incision to that depth. Then, using the Iris scissors, separate the cyst wall from the surrounding tissues, being careful not to penetrate the cyst wall. Ideally, one should attempt to dissect around the entire cyst and remove it intact. Sometimes, however, during the dissection of the cyst, the wall may be inadvertently ruptured followed by the extravasation of the cyst contents into the wound. It may be helpful to remove the contents of the cyst before continuing dissection of the cyst wall. If significant fibrosis is noted, it may be impossible to totally dissect the cyst wall from the surrounding tissue. Once the cyst has been totally excised, examine the wound carefully to be sure all of the wall has been removed. If the cyst was moderately large in size, there will be a significant amount of dead space present. Thus, it is important to obtain adequate hemostasis to decrease the risk of development of a hematoma or seroma. The dead space can be closed by the placement of interrupted buried absorbable sutures. A technique that can be used to remove dead space is the "tie-down suture" (Figs. 1–4) [6]. The tie-down suture can be helpful to eliminate the dead space following the removal of the cyst. A nonabsorbable suture is placed at 0.5 to 1 cm from the margin of the wound down to the dead space. It is then passed through the deep wound margin to anchor it before going on to the other side of the wound. The ends of the sutures are not tied at this point but are clamped down until the other tie-down sutures are in place. Similar sutures should be placed along the entire length of the wound approximately 1½ cm apart. The wound is then closed with subcutaneous and cutaneous sutures. Antibiotic ointment is then applied along the wound edge. A tubular shaped piece of gauze (a dental roll can be used) is placed on the wound edge, and the tie-down sutures are tied over it obliterating the dead space. The suture

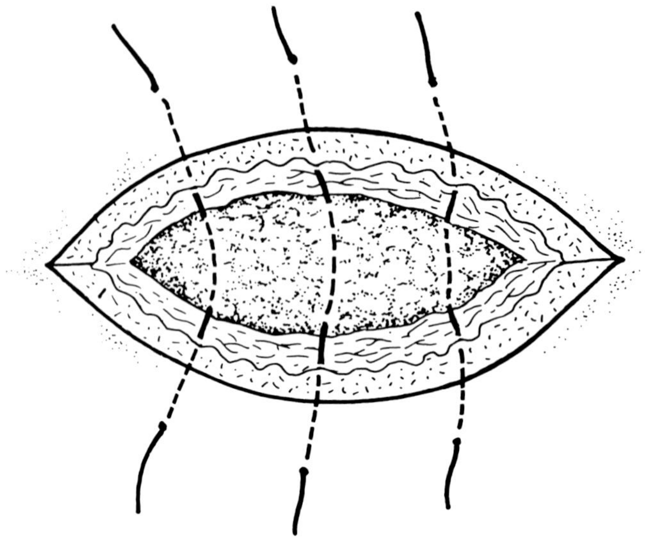

FIGURE 1 Graphic representation of tie-down sutures 1.5 cm apart in a symmetrical arrangement.

should not be tied too tightly to avoid tissue necrosis. The tie-down suture should be removed within 72 to 96 hours to prevent suture marks. Afterwards, normal suture removal should be performed. Another problem that must be dealt with after the removal of a large cyst is the excess skin that was overlying the cyst. There is often redundant atrophic skin that should be excised before the wound is closed.

Excisional Removal

If a cyst is clinically not moveable on examination, there are usually two causes: either the cyst was infected in the past and ruptured with resultant fibrosis, or the

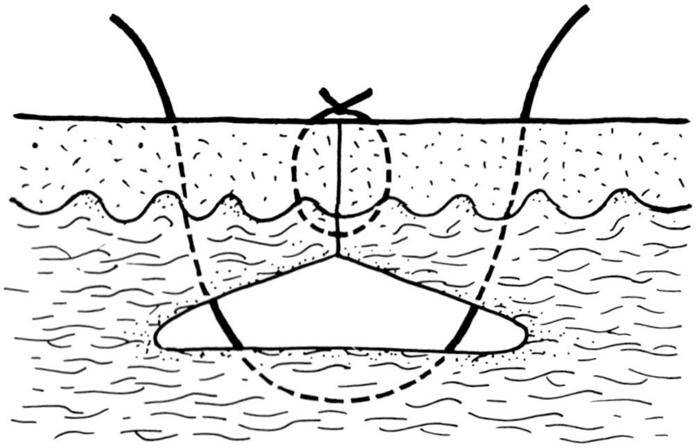

FIGURE 2 Graphic representation showing the epidermis already sutured, the residual partial cavity, and the tie-down suture.

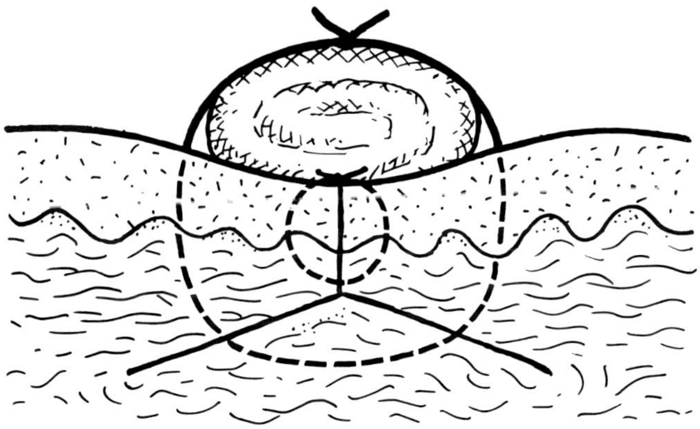

FIGURE 3 Collapsed dead space after tie-down sutures have been laced.

cyst was excised in the past and has recurred. In either case, it is preferable to remove the cyst by excising the cyst with the surrounding fibrous tissue. This will allow the cyst wall to be entirely removed. An ellipse should be drawn overlying the cyst so it is wide enough to encompass the entire cyst. One should then proceed with a standard excision of the elliptical area (Fig. 5).

Electrosurgical Technique

The Danna method of cyst removal was first described in 1945 [7,8]. This method is probably best used for cysts not adherent to the surrounding connective tissue. After the injection of local anesthesia, a diathermy needle is inserted through the skin overlying the cyst until it is just inside the cyst cavity. The electrodesiccating current is then used to create an opening into the cyst. If the cyst is under pressure, it will decompress immediately; otherwise, the cyst contents will slowly extrude on their own over the next few weeks. Manual extrusion of the cyst contents is not part of this technique. The cyst wall will shrink on its own over time. Because the cyst

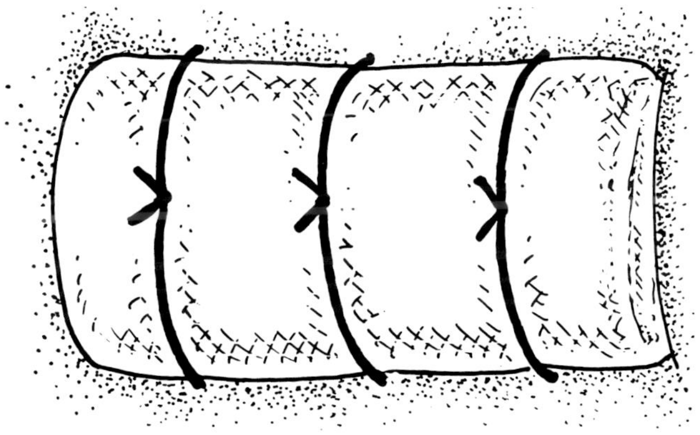

FIGURE 4 Top view. All tie-down sutures have been tied over the gauze.

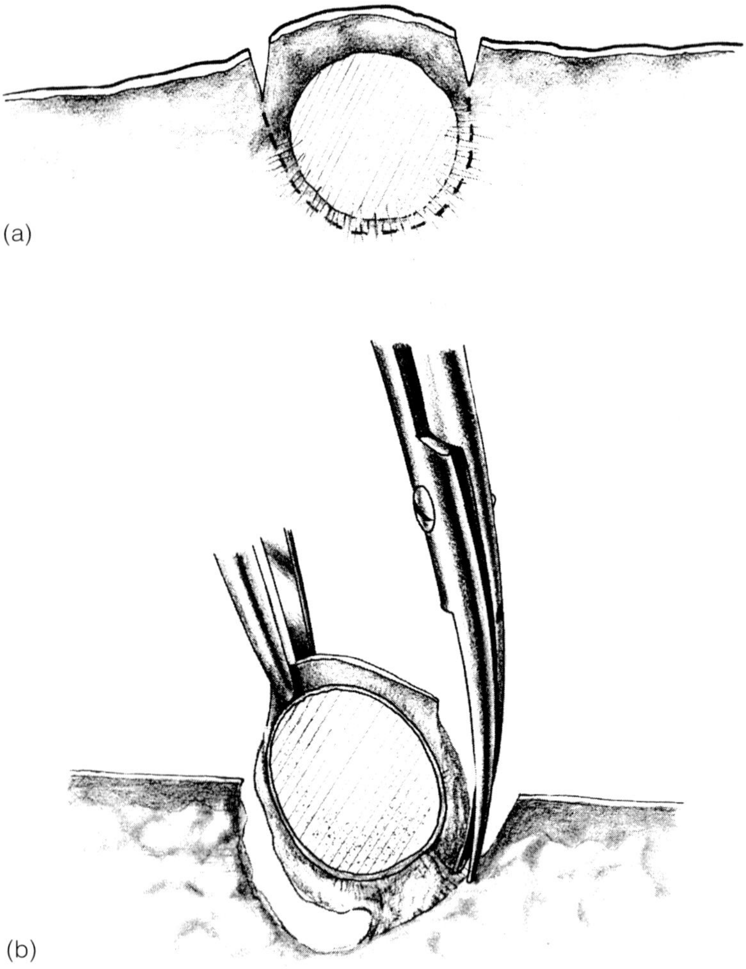

(a)

(b)

FIGURE 5 (a) Incisions to remove nonmoveable cyst. Note amount of epidermis incised is slightly smaller than fixed area shown by radiating lines. (b) Cyst and surrounding fibrous tissue are excised with scissors.

wall may not be totally removed with this method, it may be associated with a higher recurrence rate.

Complications

After any of the previously discussed techniques, complications may occur. If all of the cyst wall is not removed, the cyst may recur. Rupture of the cyst wall during the procedure associated with extravasation of the cyst contents may cause an inflammatory response. Thorough irrigation with saline before wound closure may prevent this complication. If the dead space is not obliterated during the wound closure, a depressed scar will result. Another complication that may occur if the dead space is not eliminated is the development of a hematoma or seroma. A pressure dressing applied after surgery may help prevent the development of a hematoma or seroma.

Pilar Cyst

Synonyms for pilar cyst include tricholemmal cyst, sebaceous cyst, or wen. Although the term sebaceous cyst continues to be used, it is not correct because the cyst wall contains no true sebaceous gland cells [9]. The clinical appearance of pilar cysts or epidermal cysts are identical. However, they are much less common and occur almost exclusively on the scalp. They are often multiple, especially in young to middle-aged women [10]. Because they may commonly become very large, there is often an area of alopecia overlying the scalp that may not be permanent after removal of the cyst. The walls of tricholemmal cysts are much thicker and firmer than epidermal cysts, which makes them much easier to remove. The treatment techniques that were discussed for epidermal cysts can also be used for pilar cysts. The biopsy punch and incision and drainage methods are good options for pilar cysts. After extrusion of the cyst contents, the cyst wall often pops out intact because it is thicker than that of an epidermal cyst. A curette or forceps can also be used to remove the cyst wall. Deep and cutaneous sutures can then be placed. It may be helpful to cut some of the hairs directly overlying the cyst to make suturing easier. The use of blue sutures in a dark-haired individual will make suture removal easier.

Proliferating Trichilemmal Tumor

The proliferating trichilemmal tumor is also referred to as a proliferative trichilemmal cyst, proliferating pilar tumor, and proliferating epidermoid cyst [11,12]. The vast majority (80%) of the patients are elderly women who present with a single lesion on the scalp. Clinically, the lesion initially appears identical to a pilar tumor; however, with time, the lesion may develop into a large ulcerated lobulated mass that can be difficult to distinguish from a squamous cell carcinoma. The tumor may present in association with one or more trichilemmal cysts of the scalp [13]. There have been several case reports of malignant transformation and metastases associated with proliferating trichilemmal tumors [14]. Given the risk of malignant transformation, the recommended treatment of these lesions is total excision with a margin of normal tissue to prevent a recurrence [15]. If what appears to be a pilar cyst is incised and drained, and histology reveals the lesion is a proliferating tricholemmal tumor, the area around the scar must be excised down to periosteum with 1 to 2 cm margins to prevent recurrence [16]. This tumor highlights the importance of submitting a specimen from all presumed cysts for histopathological examination.

Dermoid Cyst

Dermoid cysts present as subcutaneous nodules present at birth. They range in size from 1 to 4 cm and are not attached to the overlying skin but are commonly adherent to the underlying periosteum. These lesions are most commonly located on the head, usually in the region of the lateral third of the eyebrow [17]. They are commonly misdiagnosed as epidermoid cysts. The dermoid cyst is the most common periorbital mass of infants and children [18]. A dermoid cyst can also present in the nasal region from the glabella to the base of the columella. They may present clinically simply as a pit or a small papule. They may also present on the occipital scalp and with continued growth may actually indent the outer table of the skull. Because nasal and occipital dermoids can extend intracranially, it is important to consider this diagnosis when presented with a nasal or occipital mass in a child [19]. If a child presents with a subcutaneous nodule of the lateral eyebrow, the differential diagnosis includes dermoid cyst, epidermoid cyst, pilar cyst, and lipoma. Dermoid cysts are the only cysts that may be fixed to the periosteum. The differential diagnosis of nasal dermoid cysts include encephaloceles and extranasal gliomas. Before surgical excision of these lesions, it is prudent to obtain a computerized tomographic (CT) scan or magnetic resonance imaging (MRI) to evaluate the dermoid cyst and its intracranial extension. Lateral orbital dermoids are typically excised by making an incision over the bulk of the lesion [20]. In an attempt to camouflage the scar, the incision may be made at the inferior border of the eyebrow [21]. Another approach is to make an incision in the lateral eyelid crease below the lesion and to dissect superiorly and laterally to expose and remove the dermoid. Although the cyst is easily separated from surrounding tissues with blunt dissection, a sharp incision is often necessary to separate the lesion from the periosteum. In contrast with other methods of removal, the scar is hidden by the lid fold when the patient's eye is open. One should be familiar with the upper eyelid anatomy before attempting this approach [18].

Milia

Milia are superficial small (1 to 2 mm), whitish papules that are epidermal cysts. They are usually present in multiple numbers on the faces of middle-aged or older women, although they can be seen at any age. Milia are separated into two categories: primary and secondary [22]. Primary milia are facial lesions that develop without a cause. Histologically, they are small epidermal cysts. Secondary milia develop after trauma to the skin such as dermabrasion, subepidermal blistering diseases such as porphyria cutanea tarda, and burns and wounds that have been sutured or allowed to heal by secondary intention. They may contain some epithelial appendage such as a hair follicle, sweat duct, sebaceous duct, or epidermis [23]. However, sometimes no connection can be found to any skin appendage [24]. Milia may occur in wounds that have been sutured closed. They may be found in the incision wound or the point where the suture needle punctured the skin. These milia may be caused by an ingrowth of the epidermis along the suture track or a follicle that was transected by the scalpel during the procedure [25]. Milia can be simply treated by incision and drainage without local anesthesia. Several instruments can be used: a #11 scalpel blade, an 18- to 21-gauge needle, or a Hagedorn needle. While holding the skin around the milia taut, incise the roof of the milia and attempt to tease it out with the tip of the needle or scalpel. Alternatively, you can use a comedone extractor to express the lesion. After either method, the wound heals quickly without problem. Alternatively, a hot cautery fine-point tip can be used with success. Allow it to heat to just below red-hot and lightly tap the skin on top of the milia. Subsequently, the milia will drain spontaneously [26]. Other physicians prefer to use low-current electrodesiccation with a fine electrode or epilating needle. Multiple milia can be treated in a single session. Secondary milia after dermabrasion usually need no treatment because they resolve spontaneously.

Steatocystoma Multiplex

Patients with steatocystoma multiplex present in adolescence with multiple round cystic nodules (1 to 3 cm in size) that are adherent to the overlying skin [27]. There is a predilection to include the axilla, sternum, and arms. When the cyst is incised, an oily or creamy discharge is produced. The steatocystoma can also present as an isolated lesion in adults and is referred to as steatocystoma simplex [28]. Although isolated lesions of steatocystoma can be easily treated, when patients present with a multitude of cysts, there is no optimal surgical treatment. The surgical treatment of steatocystomas is the same as epidermoid cysts. However, given the fact that most of these lesions are located on the chest, which has a high propensity for hypertrophic or keloidal scarring, one must weigh the risks and benefits of attempting to remove a large number of lesions. Cryosurgery with the use of a cryoprobe has been advocated as an alternative form of therapy [29].

Hidrocystoma

Hidrocystoma is an uncommon cystic lesion that is of eccrine or apocrine origin. These lesions are small (1 to 3 mm), bluish in color, and occur only on the face, especially in the periorbital skin. Apocrine hidrocystoma presents as a solitary translucent nodule that can be as large as 1.5 cm. Eccrine hidrocystomas are usually also solitary lesions; however, occasionally a patient may present with a few or multiple lesions. These lesions can be excised if the patient desires. If the lesion is simply incised and drained, recurrence is likely. Thus, careful dissection should be performed to separate the clear cyst from the overlying epidermis. CO_2 laser vaporization has also been reported as another therapeutic option [30].

Digital Myxoid Cyst

Synonyms for myxoid cyst include mucous cyst, mucoid cyst, myxomatous cyst, synovial cyst, and focal mucinosis. There are two types of digital myxoid cysts [31]. One type is identical to focal mucinosis and is thus not a true cyst. It is located near the proximal nail fold. The cause of the second type is a herniation of the joint lining. It develops on the dorsal aspect of the distal interphalangeal joint. A myxoid cyst is a flesh-colored, slightly translucent, semifluctuant nodule that occurs on the fingers and the toes. They may be as small as a few millimeters or greater than 1 cm. Myxoid cysts can be tender and may cause longitudinal grooves of the nail plate. If the cyst is incised, a clear, thick gelatinous fluid may be expressed. Radiological examinations of the joint usually reveals osteoarthritis. There are several treatments for myxoid cysts, although recurrence is common. After the surface of the lesion is punctured with a 20-gauge needle, gentle pressure is performed to remove the cyst contents. Some advocate that the base of the lesion then be injected with triamcinolone acetonide (beginning with 5 mg/ml). This procedure needs to be repeated when the cyst becomes noticeable again. Epstein has reported a 70% success rate with the repeat needling and expression technique. He advocates teaching the patient how to perform this technique at home because no anesthesia is required [32]. This requires an intelligent and motivated patient because the procedure will need to be repeated anywhere from two to 10 times. Another treatment option involves electrosurgical destruction of the cyst after the contents have been expressed. Cryotherapy also has its proponents. First the cyst is incised and drained. The lesion is sprayed with a cryo gun until a halo of frost forms beyond the margin of the cyst. Freezing time varies between 15 and 20 seconds. The wound usually heals within a month. Although cosmetic results are usually good, one complication is notching of the proximal nail fold. If a double freeze/thaw cycle technique is used, the rate of recurrence is lower than with a single freeze/thaw cycle technique [33]. Salashche has described a surgical method for the removal of myxoid cysts of the proximal nail fold (Figs. 6, 7) [31]. It involves the en bloc removal of the proximal nail fold with the cyst and a portion of the lateral nail fold. The resultant wound is allowed to granulate. After a nerve block and antiseptic preparation, the proximal edge of the cyst is marked with a sterile surgical marker. The mark is extended to include symmetrical lateral portions of the proximal nail fold. A Freer sector elevator is introduced under the proximal nail fold into the proximal nail groove to protect the underlying nail matrix and extensor tendon. With the Freer elevator in place, the excision is carried out with a #15 surgical blade. A beveled rather than a vertical incision is made under the cyst to avoid damaging the extensor tendon insertion. Gel foam is used for hemostasis. The wound is allowed to heal by secondary intention, which will be complete in approximately 2 months. The cure rate of this technique is reportedly excellent.

CO_2 laser vaporization has also been successfully used in the treatment of myxoid cysts. After local anesthesia, the laser is used with a power of 5 watts in the defocused mode [34]. Finally, if the above methods fail, excision of the lesion may be necessary. Dissection of the cyst is performed, removing both the cyst and then

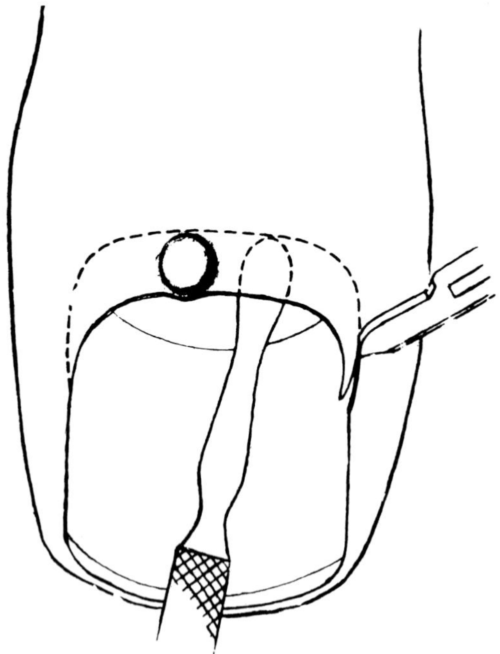

FIGURE 6 Illustration of incision design and Freer elevator in proximal nail groove.

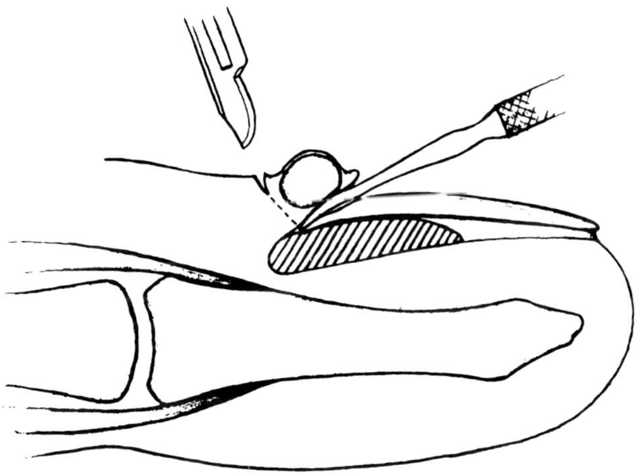

FIGURE 7 Beveled incision behind and under cyst to proximal margin of nail groove.

tracing its origin to the adjacent joint space. A portion of the joint capsule is also excised [35].

Mucous Cysts

Mucous cysts of the minor salivary glands are also referred to as mucous retention cysts and mucoceles. A mucous cyst is a solitary asymptomatic lesion that can range in size from 2 mm to 1 cm. Although they usually occur on the lower lip, they can be located in other areas of the oral mucosa such as the floor of the mouth. The lesions usually occur in the 11- to 30-year age range, and men and women are equally affected. Clinically, the lesion is a translucent whitish/bluish dome-shaped lesion that may be fluctuant or tense. If the lesion is incised, a sticky viscous fluid can be expressed. A mucous cyst is not a true cyst because it lacks an epithelial lining. The pathogenesis of this lesion consists of rupture of a mucous duct, which is followed by an outpouring of sialomucin into the tissue. Multiple cystic spaces develop surrounded by granulation tissue and a fibrovascular wall [36]. Current treatment of a mucocele involves the excision of the lesion and the underlying mucous gland down to the level of the orbicularis oris muscle. The resultant defect is then sutured with either silk suture or an absorbable suture. If the cyst is only incised and drained, it will usually recur because the underlying mucous gland was not destroyed [37]. If you try to dissect a mucous cyst as one might do for an epidermoid cyst, the lesion will usually rupture because there is no actual cyst wall. Cryosurgery is another treatment option with a reported cure rate of almost 100% [33]. First, the lesion is anesthetized with local anesthesia. The cyst is left intact. The lesion is sprayed with liquid nitrogen until there is a visible frost 2 mm beyond the margin of the lesion. The necessary freeze time varies between 15 and 30 seconds. After the lesion completely thaws, a second freeze/thaw cycle is performed. The patient is instructed to apply cold compresses every 8 hours to reduce edema. Wound healing is usually complete within 3 to 4 weeks.

SUMMARY

The average dermatologist and dermatolgic surgeon are confronted with a myriad of cystic lesions on a daily basis. In order to determine the appropriate presurgical evaluation and surgical treatment, it is vital to be familiar with the various cyst types and their distinguishing characteristics. This will help to ensure an optimal outcome for the patient as well as the surgeon.

LIPOMAS

Lipomas are one of the most common mesenchymal tumors [38]. Most lipomas are found in the fatty subdermal layer or occasionally can also be found in deeper locations such as the viscera or intramuscular. They may invade deeper tissue such as fascia, muscle, nerve, and even bone. Lipomas are most commonly located on the trunk, shoulder, posterior neck, and proximal extremities [39]. Less common sites include the scalp, face, lower legs, and inguinal area [40]. Occasionally lipomas have been found on the vulva [41], toe [42], and palm [43]. Lipomas in women are usually found on the shoulder and thigh. Men usually present with lipomas in the head, neck, and chest region [39]. Most solitary lipomas are less than 5 cm in size although they can be as small as a few millimeters and as large as several centimeters. Lipomas are rarely reported in infants and children, and usually develop in early adulthood [44]. They are usually asymptomatic, solitary, round, or oval subcutaneous tumors. On examination, they are usually nontender (except for angiolipomas), soft, and doughy.

TYPES OF LIPOMAS

Solitary

The vast majority of lipomas are solitary and encapsulated. They are usually small and superficially located.

Multiple

When a patient presents with multiple lipomas, it is helpful to determine the class of lipomatosis: benign symmetrical lipomatosis, diffuse congenital lipomatosis, familial multiple lipomatosis, adiposis dolorosa, and Gardner's syndrome.

BENIGN SYMMETRIC LIPOMATOSIS

Benign symmetric lipomatosis, also known as Madelung's disease, is a disorder that characteristically affects adult males. These patients develop severe lipomatous involvement of the head, neck, shoulders, and the proximal arms during middle age. Other associated conditions include excessive alcohol ingestion, hyperuricemia, obesity impaired by glucose tolerance, and liver abnormalities [45]. Benign symmetric lipomatosis is familial with an autosomal dominant inheritance [46]. The lipomatous tissue has been shown to have an increased lipoprotein lipase activity, which may explain the elevated high density lipoprotein (HDL) cholesterol levels found in these patients [47].

DIFFUSE CONGENITAL LIPOMATOSIS

The lipomas found in diffuse congenital lipomatosis are poorly demarcated and localized to the trunk. They spread between muscle fibers and may extend to the retroperitoneal space. Given the infiltrative nature of these lipomas, they usually recur after removal. This condition is not inherited [48].

FAMILIAL MULTIPLE LIPOMATOSIS

Familial multiple lipomatosis is an inherited condition that usually presents during adolescence with numerous small well-defined subcutaneous lipomas localized to the arms and trunk. Unlike benign symmetric lipomatosis, the neck and shoulders are not affected in familial multiple lipomatosis [49]. The lipomas are encapsulated, easily removed, and do not recur.

ADIPOSIS DOLOROSA

Adiposis dolorosa (Dercum's disease) is a rare syndrome first described in 1891 [50]. It consists of multiple painful lipomas, usually located on the extremities. The patient is usually an obese, postmenopausal woman, although men can occasionally be affected. Although Dercum's disease is usually sporadic, familial cases with an autosomal dominant pattern of inheritance have been reported [51]. Surgical excision of the lipomas only relieves the pain temporarily because new lesions usually develop [52]. Histologically, the lipomas found in Dercum's disease are of the encapsulated type seen in patients with ordinary asymptomatic lipomas. Occasionally, the lesion will prove to be an angiolipoma.

GARDNER'S SYNDROME

Patients with Gardner's syndrome will present with multiple lipomas of the skin. Other features of this condition include polyposis of the colon, multiple epidermoid cysts, osteomas, and desmoid tumors. The inheritance is autosomal dominant with variable penetrance. These patients need to be identified because they are at high risk of the development of colon cancer before the age of 30.

ANGIOLIPOMAS

Angiolipomas are painful, well-demarcated soft subcutaneous nodules that are usually found on the trunk and extremities. The pain will occur spontaneously or develop with pressure. The infiltrative angiolipoma is an uncommon variant that can affect children as well as adults. Unlike the more common solitary angiolipoma, they are painless and nonencapsulated masses. Although they are benign, they characteristically have an infiltrative growth pattern extending to skeletal muscle. This makes removal difficult and accounts for the 33% recurrence rate reported in the literature [53].

PLEOMORPHIC LIPOMAS

Pleomorphic lipomas are a variant that develop in the subcutaneous tissue of the posterior neck, shoulder, and back. They present in men during the fifth to seventh decade of life. Although they are benign lesions, histologically they can be confused with liposarcomas [54].

SPINDLE CELL LIPOMAS

Spindle cell lipomas are another variant of lipomas that, like pleomorphic lipomas, develop in elderly males. They are painless nodules that are also found on the neck, shoulder, or back [55]. These tumors also need to be differentiated from liposarcomas.

HISTOPATHOLOGY

Lipomas are a well-circumscribed collection of mature adipocytes that are surrounded by a thin connective tissue capsule. Angiolipomas also contain a variable number of small blood vessels with microthrombi in addition to mature adipose tissue.

DIAGNOSTIC CONSIDERATIONS

The most serious diagnostic consideration that needs to be entertained in the examination of lipomatous tumors is the liposarcoma. Liposarcomas classically present in middle-aged or elderly men as slowly enlarging diffuse nodular subcutaneous tumors. They develop in the intermuscular fascial planes with a characteristic predilection for the medial thigh, popliteal fossa, and shoulder. Liposarcomas have a high incidence of metastasis especially if they are poorly differentiated. The most common sites of metastasis are the lungs and liver. When examining a presumed lipoma, if the lesion is larger than 5 cm (especially if it is larger than 10 cm) and if the lesion is located deep in the soft tissue of the thigh, there is a statistically significant chance that the lesion is a liposarcoma rather than a lipoma.

SURGICAL TREATMENT OF LIPOMAS

Presurgical Evaluation

Most patients request the removal of lipomatous tumors for cosmetic reasons. Because lipomas are usually located in the subcutaneous tissue, the diagnosis can usually be made on a clinical examination. However, with deep-seated lesions that present in the subfascial tissue or intramuscular planes, it can be difficult to distinguish an infiltrating lipoma from a liposarcoma. Diagnostic imaging can be useful for the diagnosis of these deep soft-tissue tumors. In addition, because imaging can define the anatomic location of the lesion and the surrounding structures, it can be used to plan the surgical approach for biopsy and excision. CT is probably the best tool to differentiate benign fatty tumors from liposarcomas and is indicated in the evaluation of growing or painful lipomatous masses, especially when they are located in the subfascial tissues [56]. A CT scan of lipoma is homogeneous in density throughout and does not enhance with contrast. A liposarcoma, on the other hand, will have a nonhomogeneous appearance on a CT scan. In addition, with the use of intravenous contrast, liposarcomas will usually show peripheral enhancement, whereas lipomas do not. A classic CT scan may obviate the need for a biopsy. A CT scan, in addition, can also be used in the presurgical assessment to determine if a lipoma is infiltrating and its proximity to neurovascular structures. If fine needle aspiration is deemed necessary for diagnosis, a CT scan can be used to guide the physician in this procedure [56]. Usually if, on CT, the lipomatous lesion is well delineated, has no contrast enhancement, and has a homogeneous density throughout, no further evaluation is needed. Magnetic resonance imaging can also be used to help define the size of the tumor and its location with respect to vascular structures. Magnetic resonance imaging, however, is not helpful in differentiating benign from malignant lesions and bony involvement [57].

SURGICAL METHODS

The techniques reviewed below are best used in the removal of encapsulated lipomas. The removal of infiltrating lipomas can be problematic because of the fact that they are often nonencapsulated and have intra or intermuscular locations and have an infiltrative pattern often involving tendons, bones, and nerves. The removal of these infiltrative lipomas may be best left to surgeons with expertise in microdissection so vital vascular and neural structures will not be injured.

INCISION TECHNIQUE

Incision, commonly referred to as the "squeeze technique," is a simple method for the removal of superficial encapsulated lipomas through a small stab incision [58]. The margins of the lipoma are marked on the skin surface. A wheel of local anesthesia is made over the center of the lesion. Using a #11 scalpel blade, a 2 to 3 mm stab incision is made in the skin parallel to the relaxed skin tension lines. The incision is then deepened to penetrate the deep capsule of the lipoma. Using the first and second finger of the nondominant hand, the lipoma is then squeezed out of the incision. If the lipoma is large, it may be necessary to exert lateral pressure with both hands. If pressure alone is not adequate, dissection with a curette or blunt undermining scissors can be used to free the lipoma of any fibrous connections. When part of the lipoma has been extruded, it is then grasped with a forceps and pulled out [59]. The wound may be sutured or left to heal by secondary intention.

DISTANT INCISION TECHNIQUE

The distant incision technique is advantageous for lipomas that are located on cheeks, lower eyelids, forehead, lips, and chest. Instead of making the incision directly over the lesion, it is made in a site somewhat distant from it. Ideal sites for these incisions include the scalp, eyelids, preauricular area, nasolabial folds, oral mucosa, and inframammary folds. With this method, the resultant scar is located in a less conspicuous area [60]. Before injection of local anesthesia, the tumor and the site of the skin incision are marked. The length of the incision should equal the distance between the incision and the lesion. After the incision is made, the lesion is undermined and removed. Because the lipoma is removed from under a skin flap, adequate lighting and an assistant are necessary. Before wound closure, hemostasis must be obtained to prevent hematoma formation. Thorough knowledge of the anatomy of the facial nerves is a prerequisite for this technique. Although this is a time-consuming technique, it is gratifying to be able to place the scar in a less noticeable location.

EXCISION

The easiest method to remove moderate and larger sized lipomas is surgical excision. Before the injection of local anesthesia, the borders of the lesion should be marked on the skin surface. The surgeon should then make a linear incision parallel to the relaxed skin tension lines, approximately one third to one half the diameter of the lipoma. Because lipomas are natural tissue expanders, it may be advantageous to excise an ellipse of skin to remove excess skin. After the incision is made, the tumor should be dissected from the surrounding tissue with dissecting scissors such as Metzenbaum or Ragnell scissors [61]. It is helpful to grasp the lipoma with the hemostat and move the lipoma in several directions to make dissection easier. After the dissection is complete, the lipoma can be removed. If you find that the incision you made is too small to remove the lipoma, it can be enlarged during the procedure. The wound should be visually inspected and carefully palpated to ensure complete removal of the lipoma. Because a large potential dead space is created, hemostasis with electrocautery should be performed. A layered wound closure is then performed to prevent a depressed scar. A pressure dressing is then applied that should be left in place for 1 to 2 days. In addition, the patient should be advised to limit physical activity to prevent hematoma formation. During the early postsurgical period, excessive bruising and hematoma formation can be prevented with the use of an ice pack. A surgical drain may be placed if the wound is at high risk of developing a hematoma.

LIPOSUCTION

Liposuction is the most recent addition to the armamentarium in lipoma removal. It is most advantageous in the removal of large lipomas [62], multiple lipomas or angiolipomas [63,64], and benign symmetric lipomatosis (Madelung's disease) [65]. The reported complication rate after the removal of lipomas with liposuction surgery is very low. The advantage of lipoma removal using liposuction includes a smaller surgical scar, even with very large tumors and a lower risk of bleeding, postsurgical pain, and infection [66]. The technique used in the liposuction removal of lipomas is similar to that used in cosmetic liposuction. After the administration of local anesthesia, a 1 cm incision is made in the skin adjacent to the lipoma. A liposuction cannula is inserted into the lipoma cavity and the tubing is attached to the liposuction pump. The cannula is used to create multiple tunnels in a spoke-like array through the lipoma with the open portion of the cannula positioned away from the skin surface. Although the majority of the fat cells can be suctioned out, the remaining fibrous stroma must be removed with forceps and scissors. Manual pressure is often needed to remove the remaining adipose tissue. The wound is then closed with sutures and a pressure dressing is applied [67]. The previously described method sounds easy, but it may be more difficult. Pieces of the lipoma may break off and clog the suction apparatus, and removal of the fibrous stroma can be difficult. A small portion of the lipoma should always be submitted for histological examination (Fig. 8).

SUMMARY

Because lipomas are the most common soft-tissue tumor, dermatologic surgeons need to be knowledgeable in the various types of lipomas and their associated syndromes. This will help determine which lipomatous tumors need presurgical radiologic evaluation to help confirm the diagnosis and location of the lipoma. The most appropriate surgical technique for removal of the lesion can then be decided.

Acquired Melanocytic Nevi

Acquired melanocytic nevi are common benign lesions of the skin. Patients commonly request removal of these lesions for cosmetic reasons or because of repeated trauma caused by clothing or shaving. The average Caucasian may have an average of 15 to 39 acquired nevi [68]. On the average, men have 43.23 moles whereas women have 27.13 moles [69]. The number of nevi reaches a peak in the teens to early 20s. After the age of 40, the number of acquired nevi declines and reaches a nadir in people 80 years of age.

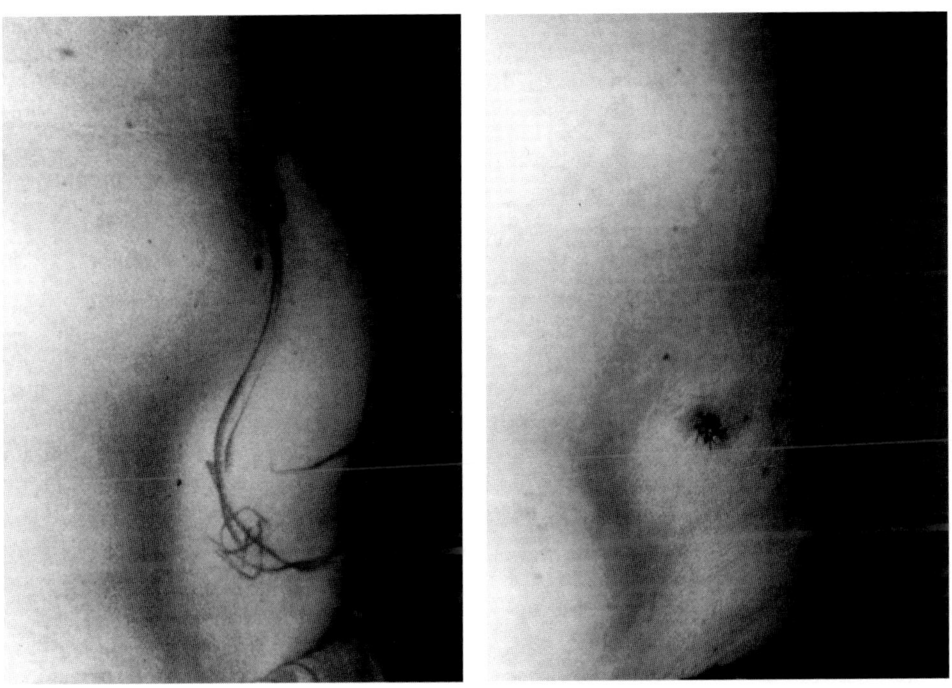

(a) (b)

FIGURE 8 (a) Large lipoma marked before liposuction. (b) Immediately after tumescent liposuction. (Courtesy of R. Ashinoff, New York, NY.)

CAUSAL ORIGINS

Ultraviolet exposure is related to the development of acquired nevi. The number of moles on sun-exposed areas will be greater than those on the sun-protected areas of the body. Although nevi of the face will appear in the first or second decade of life [70], nevi of other areas will develop later. For the same reason, there are usually more nevi on the lateral aspect of the arms than the medial aspects. There is a lower incidence of nevi in African Americans that may be explained by the protection or effect because of the greater pigmentation of their skin [71].

TYPES OF ACQUIRED MELANOCYTIC NEVI

There are three types of acquired melanocytic nevi: junctional, compound, and intradermal. Junctional nevi are flat and hyperpigmented. Compound nevi are raised and usually hyperpigmented. Intradermal nevi are raised and commonly skin colored. However, one may not be able to distinguish an intradermal nevus from a compound nevus on a clinical basis alone. The three types of acquired nevi are benign and rarely develop into a malignant melanoma. Acquired melanocytic nevi have a life history over the course of time. They usually develop in infancy or early childhood although they can occur at any age. However, it is unusual for a nevus to appear after the age of 40. Initially, a melanocytic nevus presents itself as a flat junctional nevus. During adolescence as the nevus cells proliferate, the compound nevus is formed. It is normal to develop multiple melanocytic nevi during pregnancy and preexisting moles may darken. Melanocytic nevi are usually light brown to black in color and the pigmentation is uniformly distributed throughout the lesion. The shape and borders of the lesion should be symmetric and regular. They range in size from 1 to 5 mm. Intradermal or compound nevi may have hairs protruding from their surfaces.

TREATMENT

Melanocytic nevi can be removed by an excision or a shave removal.

Excision

When the nevus is removed by an excision, the lesion is completely removed. One advantage of an excision is that the entire specimen is submitted for histologic examination making correct interpretation easier. Another advantage is that there is no risk of recurrence of the nevus. However, because most patients have melanocytic nevi removed for cosmetic reasons, an excision may provide an inferior cosmetic result because the scar will be larger than the original lesion. In addition, if suture marks develop, the cosmetic result will be further compromised. Finally, this method is irreversible, if the patient is unhappy with the cosmetic result, it is too late.

Partial Removal

Melanocytic nevi may be partially removed by a shave removal, electrocautery, or electrodesiccation. The advantage of incompletely removing the nevus is that a superior cosmetic result is usually obtained. However, accurate histological diagnosis

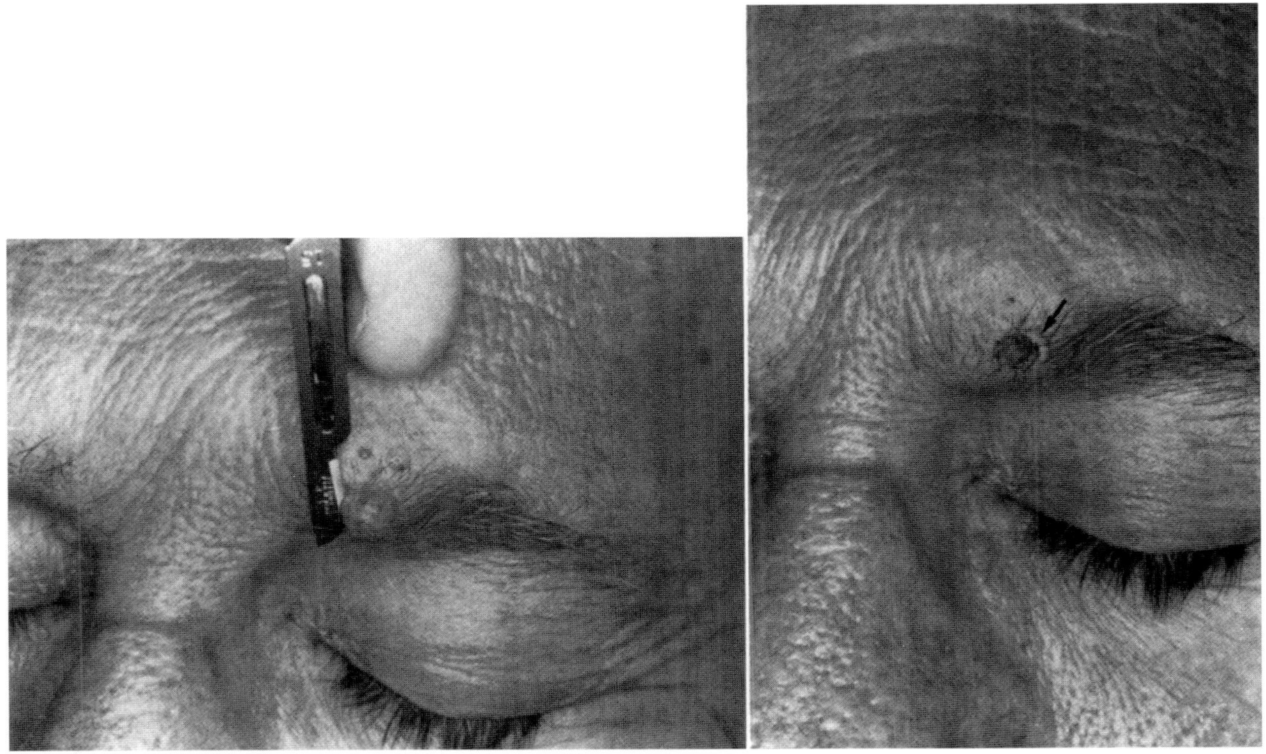

(a) (b)

FIGURE 9 (a) Incisional ("shave") removal of intradermal nevus. (b) Wound after removal. Small portion of nevus still remains (*arrow*), which was subsequently shaved off.

may be more difficult when the lesion is not totally removed. A nevus can recur after partial removal, and spotty repigmentation may occur, which may be of concern during future examinations. Even skin-colored intradermal nevi will occasionally leave a pigmented macule after shave removal. It is important to warn a patient that if the intradermal nevus contains hairs, they will continue to grow after shave removal of the lesion. These hairs can be removed by electrolysis or a laser after removal of the lesion. The technique for shave removal of the mole varies with the shape of the base of the lesion. If the mole is sessile or pedunculated, it can be removed with scissors after the injection of a small amount of lidocaine with epinephrine. The lesion is grasped with a fine tip forceps and snipped flush with the skin using curved Iris scissors. Aluminum chloride is usually adequate for hemostasis. If the nevus has a flat base, a #15 or #11 surgical blade or a carbon steel blade (safety razor blade) can be used. Each of these three instruments has their own proponents. If the mole has a flat base, the injection of local anesthesia may elevate the mole. To compensate for this, the skin is pulled taut using the first three fingers of one hand or with tension from an assistant. If a scalpel blade is used, multiple small sweeping strokes are used to remove the lesion. Forceps may be used to stabilize the mole. If a safety razor blade is used, it should be held at a horizontal angle over the skin. If necessary, one can curve the blade slightly; however, if it is excessively curved, a depressed scar may result. While the skin is held taut with the opposing hand, a back and forth swinging motion is used to excise the nevus. Sometimes it is helpful to use electrodesiccation to lightly "feather" the edges of the wound for a better cosmetic result. A low setting should be used to prevent hypopigmentation. Because the anesthetic elevates the nevus, it is possible to remove too much of the lesion during the shave removal. This will produce a slightly depressed scar. To prevent this from happening, one might choose to be more conservative during a shave removal, even if this means producing a slight elevation at the site of the nevus. After the wound heals, one can lightly electrodesiccate the residual for an optimal cosmetic result (Fig. 9). A topical anesthetic, such as EMLA cream, may be used before removal of an elevated nevus to prevent the development of a depressed scar. After the removal of the nevus, hemostasis is obtained with aluminum chloride or light electrodesiccation. The use of ferric subsulfate (Monsel's solution) is not recommended because if the lesion is re-excised in the future, the iron deposits from the solution may be misinterpreted as melanin pigment within dermal melanophages, causing the pathologist to confuse these cells with melanoma cells [72]. If electrocautery or electrodesiccation is used alone to remove a nevus, no tissue is available for pathological examination. Some physicians will remove a small portion of the nevus with a shave technique and then use electrodesiccation to flatten the remaining elevated portion of the nevus.

REFERENCES

1. McGavran MH, Binnington B. Keratinous cysts of the skin. Arch Dermatol 94:499–508, 1966.
2. Greer KE. Epidermal inclusion cyst of the sole. Arch Dermatol 109:251–252, 1974.
3. Love WR, Montgomery H. Epithelial cysts. Arch Dermatol Syph 47:195, 1943.
4. McDonald LW. Carcinomatous change in cysts of skin. Arch Dermatol 87:208–211, 1963.

5. Lieblich LM, Geronemus RG, Gibbs RC. Use of a biopsy punch for removal of epithelial cysts. J Dermatol Surg Oncol 8:1059–1062, 1982.
6. Ocampo J, Camps A. The applications of the tie-down suture to the excision of cutaneous tumors. J Dermatol Surg Oncol 14:1357–1360, 1988.
7. Danna J. A simple treatment for sebaceous cysts. N Orleans Med Sci J 98:5–8, 1945.
8. Calloway JL. A treatment for sebaceous cysts. S Med Surg 109:42, 1947.
9. Kligman AM. The myth of the sebaceous cyst. Arch Dermatol 89:253–256, 1964.
10. Leppard BJ, Sanderson KJ. The natural history of trichilemmal cysts. Br J Dermatol 94: 379–390, 1976.
11. Hanau D, Grosshans E. Trichilemmal tumor undergoing specific keratinization. J Cutan Pathol 6:463–475, 1979.
12. Brownstein MH, Arluk DJ. Proliferating trichilemmal cyst. Cancer 48:1207–1214, 1981.
13. Holmes EJ. Tumors of the lower hair sheath: the common histogenesis of certain so-called "sebaceous cysts," adenomas, and "sebaceous carcinomas." Cancer 21:234–248, 1968.
14. Saida T, Oahara K, Hori Y, et al. Development of a malignant proliferating trichilemmal cyst in a patient with multiple trichilemmal cysts. Dermatologica 166:203–208, 1983.
15. Chait GE, Shemen LJ, Robbins KT, et al. Pilar tumor of the scalp. Otolaryngo Head Neck Surg 93:116–119, 1985.
16. Morgan RF, Dellon AL, Hoopes JE. Pilar tumors. Plast Reconstr Surg 63:520–524, 1979.
17. Brownstein MH, Helwig EB. Subcutaneous dermoid cysts. Arch Dermatol 107:237–239, 1973.
18. Kersten RC. The eyelid crease approach to superficial lateral dermoid cysts. J Pediatr Ophthalmol 25:48–51, 1988.
19. Pensler JM, Bauer BS, Naidich TP. Craniofacial dermoid. Plast Reconstr Surg 82:953–958, 1988.
20. Grove AS. Dermoid. In: Fraunfelder FT, Roy FH, eds. Current Ocular Therapy Two. Philadelphia: W.B. Saunders, 1985, p. 192.
21. Sherman RP, Rootman J, Lapointe JS. Orbital dermoids: clinical presentation and management. Br J Ophthalmol 68:642–652, 1984.
22. Kirkham N. Tumors and cysts of the epidermis. In: Elder D, Elenitsas R, Jaworsky C, Johnson B Jr, eds. Levers. Histopathology of the Skin. Philadelphia: Lippincott-Raven 1997, pp. 685–745.
23. Epstein W, Kligman AM. The pathogenesis of milia and benign tumors of the skin. J Invest Dermatol 26:1, 1956.
24. Tsuji T, Suga T, Suzuki S. The mode of growth of eccrine duct milia. J Invest Dermatol 75:388–393, 1975.
25. Bennett R. Fundamentals of Cutaneous Surgery. St. Louis: C.V. Mosby, 1988.
26. Stegman SJ, Tromovitch TA, Glogau RC. Cosmetic Dermatologic Surgery. Chicago: Year Book Medical, 1990, pp. 20–21.
27. Contreras MA, Costello MJ. Steatocystoma multiplex with embryonal hair formation. Arch Dermatol 76:720, 1957.
28. Brownstein MH. Steatocystoma simplex: a solitary steatocystoma. Arch Dermatol 118: 409–411, 1982.
29. Notowicz A. Treatment of lesions of steatocystoma multiplex and other epidermal cysts by cryosurgery (cryo corner). J Dermatol Surg Onc 6:98–99, 1980.
30. Huerter CJ, Wheeland RG. Multiple eruptive vellus hair cysts treated with carbon dioxide laser vaporization. J Dermatol Surg Oncol 13:260–263, 1987.
31. Salasche SJ. Myxoid cysts of the proximal nail fold: a surgical approach. J Dermatol Surg Oncol 10:35–39, 1984.
32. Epstein E. A simple technique for managing digital mucous cysts. Arch Dermatol 115: 1315–1316, 1979.

33. Bohler-Sommeregger K, Kutschera-Hienert G. Cryosurgical management of myxoid cysts. J Dermatol Surg Oncol 14:1405–1408, 1988.
34. Huerter CJ, Wheeland RG, Bailin PL, Ratz JL. Treatment of digital myxoid cysts with carbon dioxide laser vaporization. J Dermatol Surg Oncol 13:723–727, 1987.
35. Young L, Bartell T, Logan SE. Ganglions of the hand and wrist. South Med J 81:751–760, 1988.
36. Lattanand A, Johnson WC, Graham JH. Mucous cyst (mucocele): a clinicopathologic and histochemical study. Arch Dermatol 101:673–678, 1970.
37. Laskin DM. Surgery of the oral cavity. In: Epstein E, Epstein E Jr, eds. Skin Surgery. Philadelphia: WB Saunders, 1987, p. 505.
38. Enzinger FM, Weiss SW. Benign lipomatous tumors. In: Soft Tissue Tumors. St. Louis: Mosby, 1983, p. 199.
39. Rydholm A, Berg NO. Size, site and clinical incidence of lipoma: factors in the differential diagnosis of lipoma and sarcoma. Acta Orthop Scand 54:929–934, 1983.
40. Salasche SJ, McCullough ML, Angeloni VL, Grabski WJ. Frontalis associated lipoma of the forehead. J Am Acad Dermatol 20:462–468, 1989.
41. Fukamizu H, Matsumoto K, Inoue K, Moriguchi T. Large vulvar lipoma. Arch Dermatol 118:447, 1982.
42. Erichsen B, Medgyesi S. Congenital lipoma imitating gigantism of a toe: a case report. Scand J Plast Reconstr Surg 17:77–78, 1983.
43. Froimson AI. Benign solid tumors. Hand Clin 3:213–217, 1987.
44. Adair FE, Pack GT, Farrior JH. Lipomas. Am J Cancer 16:1104–1120, 1932.
45. Economides NG, Liddell HT. Benign symmetric lipomatosis (Madelung's disease). South Med J 79:1023–1025, 1986.
46. Rubinstein A, Goor Y, Gazit E, Cabili S. Non-symmetric subcutaneous lipomatosis associated with familial combined hyperlipidemia. Br J Dermatol 120:689–694, 1989.
47. Enzi G, Favaretto L, Martini S, et al. Metabolic abnormalities in multiple symmetric lipomatosis; elevated lipoprotein lipose activity in adipose tissue with hyperalphalipoproteinemia. J Lipid Res 24:566, 1983.
48. Carlsen A, Thomsen M. Different clinical types of lipomatosis. Scand J Plast Reconstr Surg 12:75–79, 1978.
49. Leffell DJ, Braverman IM. Familial multiple lipomatosis: report of a case and review of the literature. J Am Acad Dermatol 15:275–279, 1986.
50. Dercum FX. Three cases of a hitherto unclassified affection resembling in its grosser aspects obesity but associated with special nervous symptoms—adiposis dolorosa. Am J Med Sci 104:521–535, 1892.
51. Lynch HT, Harlan WL. Hereditary factors in adiposis dolorosa. Am H Hum Genet 15: 184–190, 1963.
52. Held JL, Andrew JA, Kohn SR. Surgical amelioration of Dercum's disease: a report and review. J Dermatol Surg Oncol 15:1294–1296, 1989.
53. Puig L, Moreno A, DeMoragas JM. Infiltrating angiolipoma: report of two cases and review of the literature. J Dermatol Surg Oncol 12:617–619, 1986.
54. Shmookler BM, Enzinger FM. Pleomorphic lipoma: a benign tumor simulating liposarcoma. Cancer 47:126–133, 1981.
55. Brody HJ, Meltzer HD, Someren A. Spindle cell lipoma. Arch Dermatol 114:1065–1066, 1978.
56. Wolfe SW, Bansal M, Healey JH, Ghelman B. Computed tomographic evaluation of fatty neoplasm of the extremities: a clinical radiographic and histologic review of cases. Orthopedics 12:1351–1358, 1989.
57. Petasnick JP, Turner DA, Charters JR, et al. Soft tissue masses of the locomotor system. Comparison of MR imaging with CT. Radiology 160:125–133, 1986.

58. Powell B, McLean NR. The treatment of lipomas by the "squeeze" technique. JR College Surg Edinb 30:391–392, 1985.
59. Hardin FF. A simple technique for removing lipomas. J Dermatol Surg Onc 8:316–317, 1982.
60. Peinert RA, Courtiss EH. Excision from a distance: a technique for removal of benign subcutaneous lesions. Plast Reconstr Surg 72:94–96, 1983.
61. Fish F. Incisional Surgery. In: Ratz R, ed. Textbook of Dermatologic Surgery. Philadelphia: Lippincott-Raven, 1998, pp. 127–137.
62. Pinski KS, Roenigk HH. Liposuction of lipomas. Dermatol Clin 8:483–492, 1990.
63. Kanter WR, Wolfort FG. Multiple familial angiolipomatosis: treatment with liposuction. Ann Plast Surg 20:277–279, 1988.
64. Spinowitz AL. The treatment of multiple lipomas by liposuction surgery. J Dermatol Surg Oncol 15:538–540, 1989.
65. Carlin MC, Ratz JL. Multiple symmetric lipomatosis: treatment with liposuction. J Am Acad Dermatol 18:359–362, 1988.
66. Newman J, Dolsky RL. Evaluation of 5,458 cases of liposuction surgery. Am J Cosmet Surg 1:25–28, 1984.
67. Rubenstein R, Roenigk HH, Garden JM, Goldberg NS, Pinski JB. Liposuction for lipomas. J Dermatol Surg Oncol 11:1070–1074, 1985.
68. Pack GT, Lenson N, Gerber DM. Regional distribution of moles and melanoma. AMA Arch Surg 65:862, 1952.
69. Cooke KR, Spears GFS, Skegg DCG. Frequency of moles in a defined population. J Epidemiol Community Health 39:48–52, 1985.
70. Nicholls EM. Development and elimination of pigmented moles, and the anatomical distribution of primary malignant melanoma. Cancer 32:191–195, 1973.
71. Kopf AW, Lazar M, Bart RS, Dubin N, Bromberg J. Prevalence of nevocytic nevi, on lateral and medial aspects of arms. J Dermatol Surg Onco 4:153–158, 1978.
72. Duray PH, Livolsi VA. Recurrent dysplastic nevus following shave excision. J Dermatol Surg Oncol 10:811–815, 1984.

19

Flaps and Grafts

David A. Davis and Christopher J. Arpey
University of Iowa College of Medicine, Iowa City, Iowa

INTRODUCTION

An extensive literature has evolved regarding flaps and grafts used in dermatologic surgery. Many disciplines have made contributions to the current understanding of the management and closures of wounds. This chapter will discuss commonly used flaps and grafts and will address some of their various applications with an emphasis on cosmetic outcome.

A variety of possible repair options exist for most cutaneous defects. Some examples include secondary intention and granulation, primary closure, flaps, and grafts. Recognition of the concepts of tissue movement and techniques of wound closure is a constantly evolving and acquired skill. Secondary and primary closures of defects are generally easy to understand and design. Planning and designing random pattern flaps are often more difficult. Performing successful flap closures requires thorough understanding of neurovascular and cutaneous anatomy. Often, greater technical skill is required for attaining optimal results. Flaps require conceptualizing the three-dimensional fields of the cutaneous surface.

HISTORY

A patient's medical history must be considered before planning any repair. An individual with a history of a coagulopathy, alcohol abuse, hematological disease, or anticoagulants may be a poor candidate for flap reconstruction [1]. A history of tobacco use, chronic pulmonary disease, or poor peripheral vascularization may similarly present limited closure options. Persons with a history of chronic illness, immunosuppression, or previous radiation to the site may have impaired wound healing. Flaps require more incision lines and undermining, placing such patients at higher risk for complications.

In cutaneous surgery, the surgeon must understand the nature of the disease or lesion being treated. If a primary lesion is a malignancy, the expected biological behavior of that cancer must be assessed. In particular, the likelihood of recurrence must be evaluated and considered before the repair is undertaken. Flap and graft closures often mask tumor recurrences. Flap and graft repairs may enlarge the defect, alter tissue planes, and lengthen scars, making subsequent re-excisions difficult and more extensive if tumor recurrence arises. Patients with a history of multiple cutaneous malignancies, such as those with nevoid basal cell carcinoma syndrome or remote radiotherapy, should have a minimal number of complex repairs performed because of the tendency for multiple adjacent tumors [2].

It is unwise to close a defect with a flap or graft if there is a significant risk that residual tumor may be present. Some form of margin control must be obtained before such a complex closure. Acceptable forms of margin control include Mohs micrographic surgery and multiple frozen or permanent sections before the delayed closure. A flap or graft repair performed in the setting of a large, albeit benign, lesion carries less risk.

PRESURGICAL CONSIDERATIONS/CONSULTATION

Identification of the patient's expectations and fears regarding the surgical outcome is important. Although patients may state that they are not concerned about the scar, this is rarely the case. Many preconceived expectations regarding the outcome and appearance of a scar often may exist, and often may be unrealistic. A patient who is well informed about the expected range of surgical outcomes is generally more satisfied over the long term. Appropriate discussion of possible complications that may be encountered in a given procedure should be addressed before commencing.

Familiarity with superficial cutaneous anatomy and terminology is also important before proceeding with surgery. The most important of these are cosmetic units (Fig. 1), relaxed skin tension lines, and the superficial musculoaponeurotic system (SMAS). Cosmetic units refer to aesthetic regions of the face. Performance of surgery within a unit, or replacement of an entire unit, is often preferable to surgery that crosses multiple boundaries or distorts a given unit. Relaxed skin tension lines (RSTL) are natural folds and/or wrinkles in a given region. Generalizations exist by anatomic location, but individual variation is common and requires close observation and palpation. RSTL are parallel to the direction of a planned closure and cause the least visible and palpable tension. RSTL are usually perpendicular to the direction of contracture of the underlying muscle. The SMAS consists of a fibromuscular layer that envelops facial muscles. It extends into and blends with the galea of the scalp, superficial temporalis fascia, parotid fascia, and platysma muscle of the neck. Most major vessels and nerves course within or below the SMAS. Mobilization, reduction, and plication of the SMAS occur in most facelift procedures.

On the scalp, the subaponeurotic (subgaleal) region is relatively avascular and loosely attached to the underlying bone. This is the favored area for undermining, but is also at risk for hematoma formation from severed vessels in the subcutaneous layer above it if hemostasis is not achieved.

PRESURGICAL INSTRUCTION/TREATMENT

A wide variety of wounds and repair options exist in dermatologic settings. Thus, each patient should be thoroughly evaluated preoperatively in order to obtain the best possible result in each case. Assessment of the nature of each individual problem, evaluation of the health status of a patient, and determination of potential risk factors for a given closure must be made. An individual's ability to perform post-

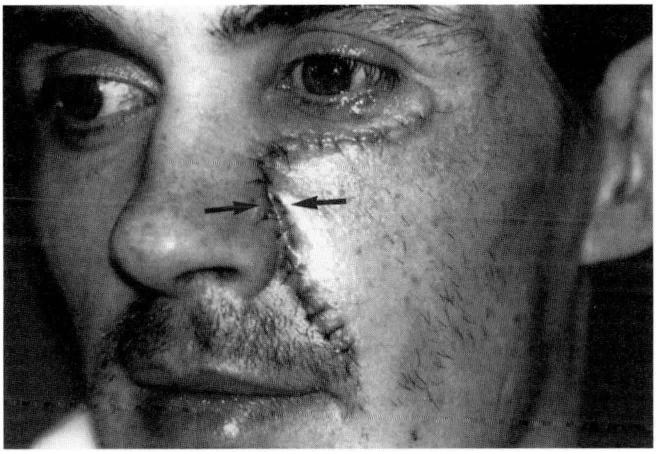

(c)

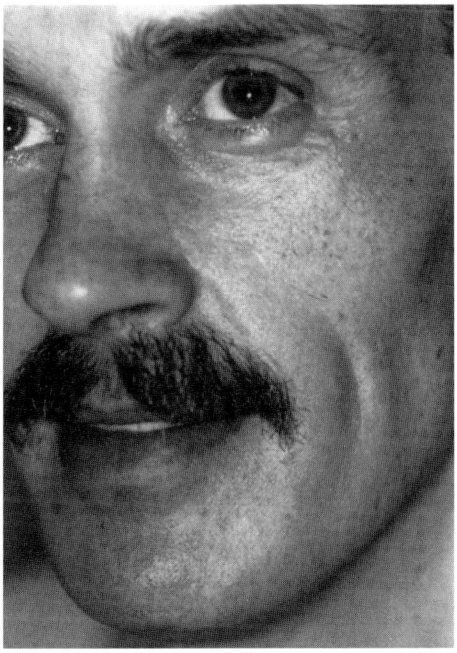

(d)

FIGURE 2 Continued

(Fig. 5). The incised tissue is freed from its base and surrounding skin, and lifted over adjacent intact tissue to fill the defect. This type of movement offers many benefits over advancement and rotation. A smaller tissue reservoir and less undermining are required compared with advancement or rotation flaps. The most common types of transposition flaps include those with rhombic shapes and their variants. This is accomplished by modifying the angles of the "rhombus" to adjust to the shape of the defect, or to plan for closure of the secondary defect within a cosmetic

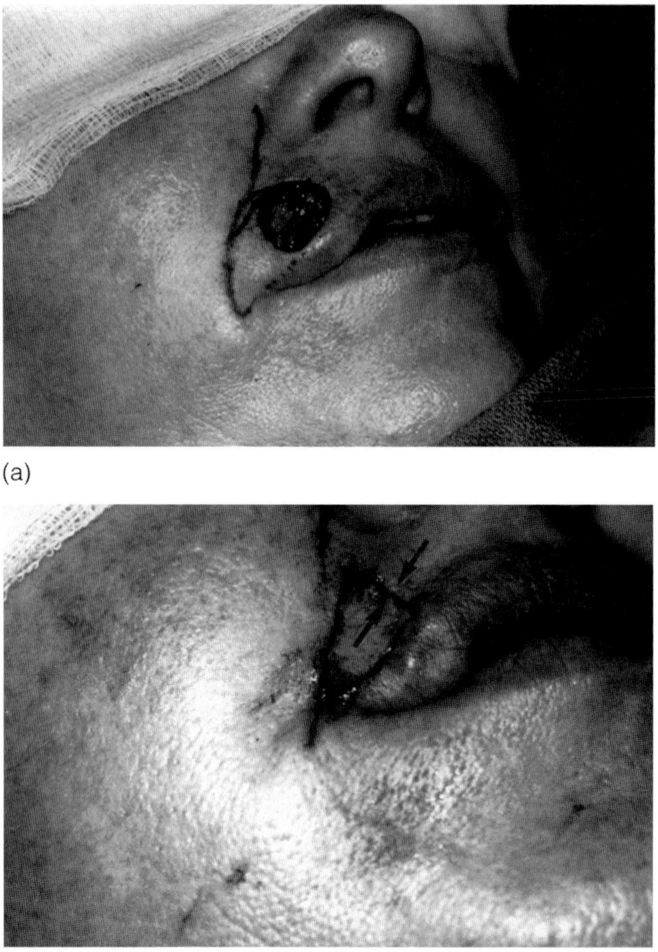

(a)

(b)

FIGURE 3 Island pedicle advancement flap. (a) Postsurgical defect with nasofacial sulcus outlined laterally. The flap will consist of incising the inferior portion of this line, as well as a line along the white roll of the lip deep into the subcutis. Caution is used to avoid undermining directly into the "stalk" of adipose nourishing the flap. (b) Appearance of the flap after placement of buried suture. The direction of highest tension is located between the arrows, thereby avoiding upward retraction of the vermilion. This incision line will parallel the radial furrows that exist around the mouth. (c) Final appearance of the flap with epidermal sutures in place. (d) Six-month postsurgical result.

unit. Alternatively, such adjustments may be made to place a closure line within a pre-existing fold.

A variation of the transposition flap is the bilobed flap (Fig. 6) or double transposition. This modification allows transferring tissue a greater distance while minimizing redundant tissue. The Z-plasty is essentially a transposition flap. This versatile flap shifts variable amounts of tissue as required for the procedure. The Z-plasty is primarily used in scar revisions to redistribute skin or movement vectors.

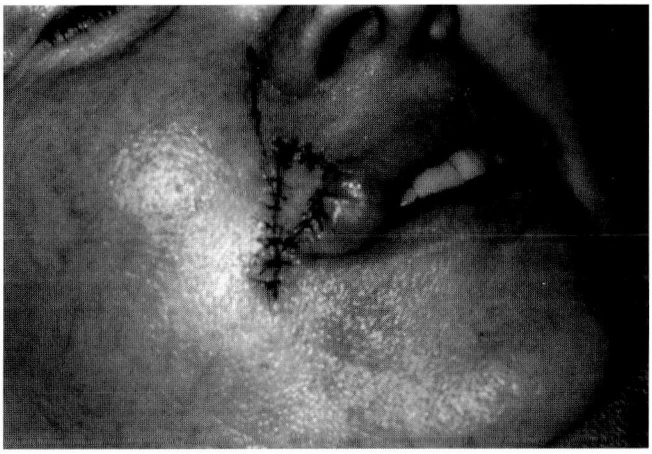

(c)

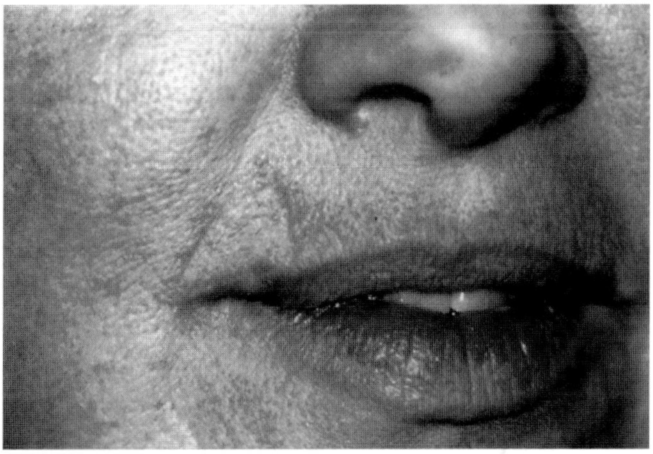

(d)

FIGURE 3 Continued

PAPERWORK

Given the variety of possibilities encountered in flap and graft surgery, a standardized consent form is not possible. Important items to discuss include the increased size of the surgical site, the possibility of a second surgical site (graft donor), additional scar lines, and the possibility of flap or graft loss. These items should be addressed in addition to those common to all incisional surgery: bleeding, pain, infection, motor or sensory alteration, and the possible need for an additional surgical procedure if the first fails or is inadequate in some way.

Presurgical assessment and counseling are addressed elsewhere in this chapter, although a single information sheet is not adequate to cover the variety of possibil-

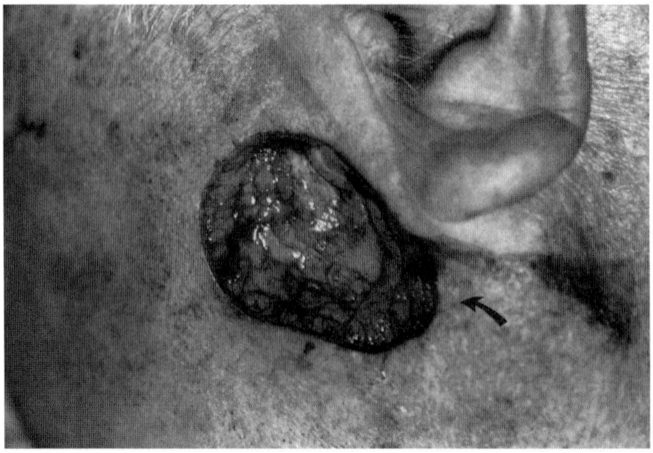

(a)

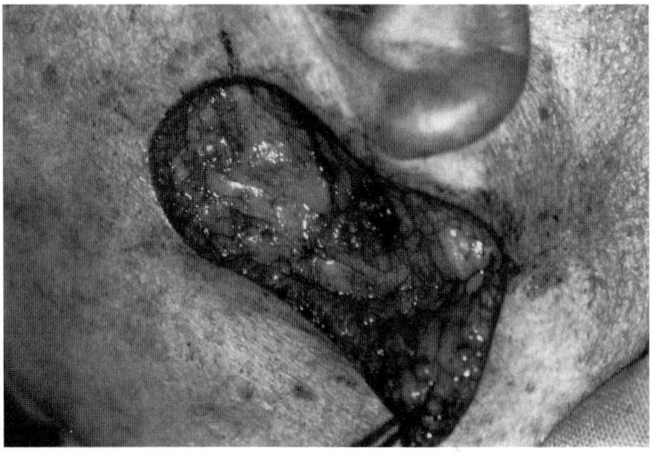

(b)

FIGURE 4 Rotation flap. (a) Preauricular surgical defect. Primary apposition in this case is difficult because the wound is large and the tragus is relatively immobile. The main reservoir of tissue is located in the loose inferolateral cheek region. The direction of planned tissue movement is illustrated with the curved arrow. (b) Flap incised, undermined, and reflected. The primary incision line is a slight arc inferior to the earlobe. (c) Initial apposition with buried suture. Tissue redundancies are evident in typical locations, at both ends of the arc of rotation. (d) Final appearance of the flap once epidermal sutures are placed. (e) Final result 2 months after surgery.

ities engendered by flap and graft procedures. Postsurgical care instruction sheets are shown in Appendixes 1 and 2.

EQUIPMENT

The majority of supplies necessary for flap and graft repairs are used in other types of cutaneous surgery. The equipment is summarized in Tables 1 to 3.

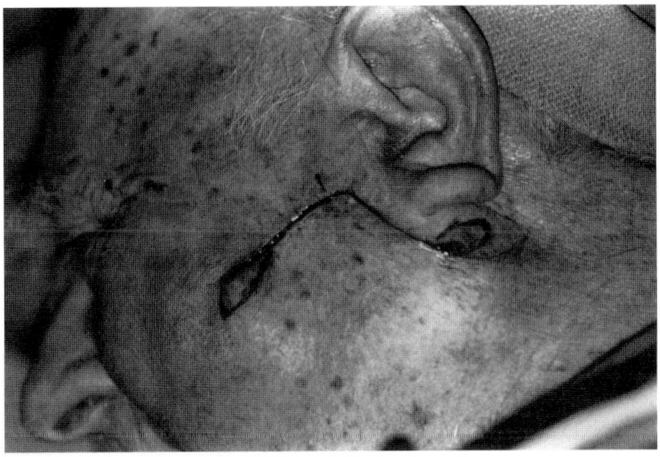

(c)

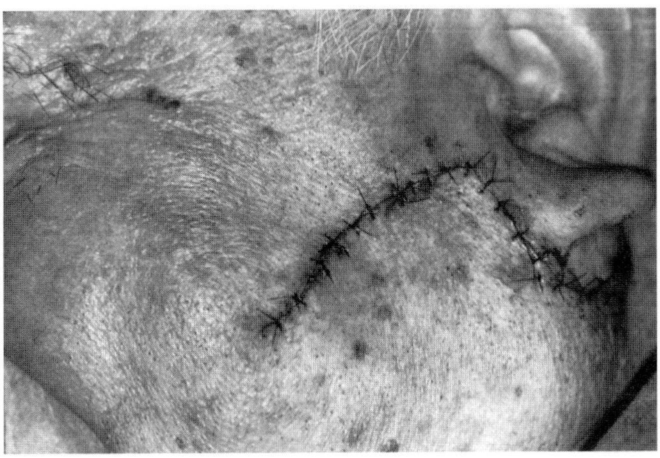

(d)

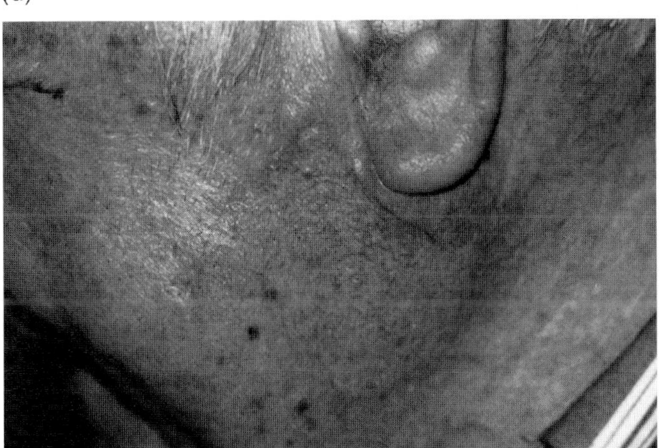

(e)

FIGURE 4 Continued

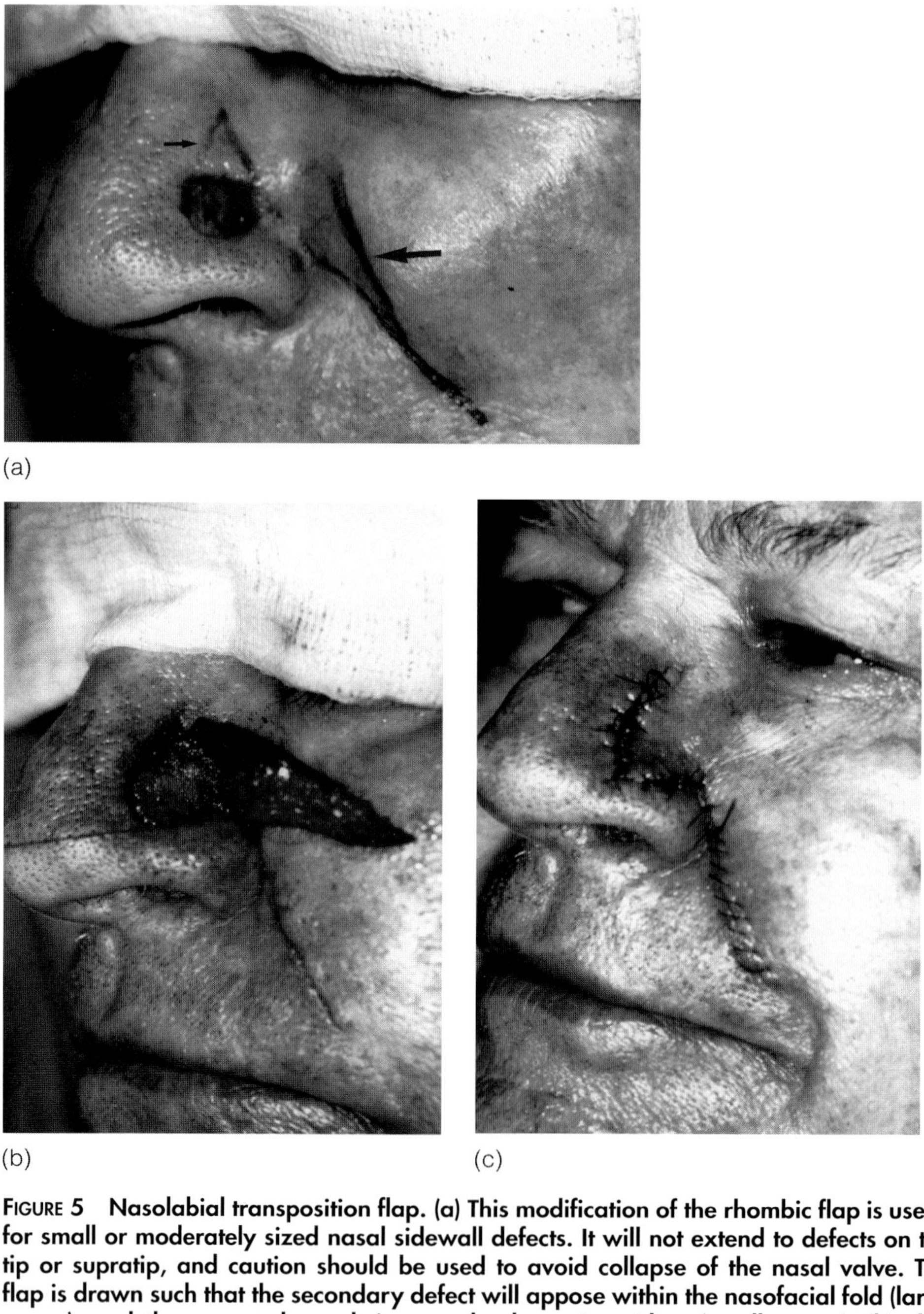

(a)

(b) (c)

FIGURE 5 Nasolabial transposition flap. (a) This modification of the rhombic flap is useful for small or moderately sized nasal sidewall defects. It will not extend to defects on the tip or supratip, and caution should be used to avoid collapse of the nasal valve. The flap is drawn such that the secondary defect will appose within the nasofacial fold (large arrow), and the expected nasal tissue redundancy is evident (small arrow). (b) Flap incised, lifted, and reflected. The secondary defect has been repaired with buried suture. (c) Postsurgical appearance with the flap in its final location, trimmed, and sutured with buried and epidermal sutures. (d) Result 6 months after surgery.

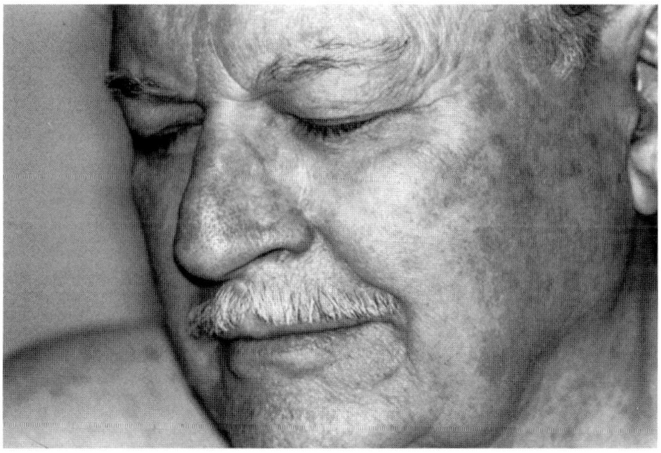

(d)

FIGURE 5 Continued

DAY OF SURGERY

Patients should shower or bathe with an antibacterial or deodorant soap the day of surgery. After informed patient consent, the surgical site should be scrubbed with povidone-iodine or chlorhexidine. Chlorhexidine should be avoided around the eyes because of potential ocular toxicity. Sterile draping with towels and clamps or with prefabricated paper drapes with a "window" for the surgical site may be used. The surgeon and assistants should use sterile gloves and maintain sterile technique during the procedure.

Patients with prosthetic joints, heart valves, or other internal devices occasionally require prophylactic antibiotics, although there is ongoing debate about this necessity in clean cutaneous surgery [12]. Consultation with the appropriate caregiver, eg, the cardiologist, orthopedic surgeon, or primary care physician, is helpful in such situations. The most commonly prescribed antibiotics for such patients are dicloxacillin, cephalexin, erythromycin, and clindamycin, which are typically given 1 hour before and 6 hours after surgery.

ANESTHESIA

A thorough discussion of topical, local, and regional anesthesia is included in Chapter 20. Similar to most cutaneous surgical procedures, local anesthesia is the preferable form of pain control for flaps and grafts. Local anesthesia offers less morbidity, greater ease of administration than general anesthesia, and aids in hemostasis when used with concomitant epinephrine.

Peripheral nerve block anesthesia is particularly useful for the large anatomic areas often required for flaps and tissue mobilization. Long-acting anesthetics are often beneficial in obtaining long-term pain control after reconstruction has been performed. Less distortion of operative site tissues is obtained with nerve blocks. However, nerve block anesthesia does not produce vasoconstriction of the operative

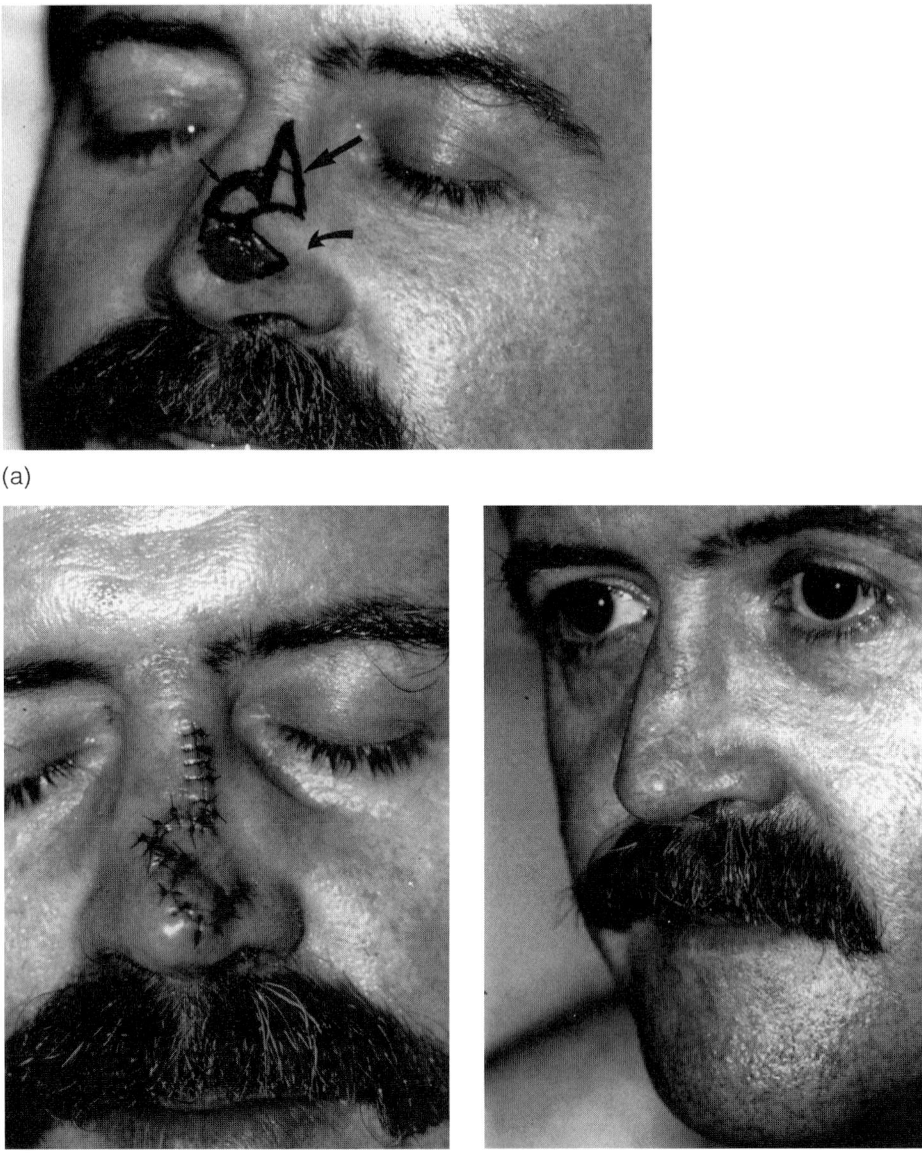

(a) (b) (c)

FIGURE 6 Bilobed transposition flap. (a) Supratip surgical defect. Primary repair would likely result in alar retraction or nasal valve dysfunction. The defect is unsuitable for a nasolabial flap because of its near-midline position. The largest tissue reservoir is located superiorly, and the skin will be "marched down" the nose by replacing the defect with the first lobe (small arrow), and replacing this lobe with the second lobe (large arrow). The direction of movement is shown with the curved arrow. (b) Postsurgical appearance with buried and epidermal sutures in place. The tertiary defect is apposed in a nearly vertical fashion. The sharing of tension over the nasal dorsum reduces the risk of alar retraction. (c) Final result 6 months after surgery.

TABLE 1 General Items Used in Flap and Graft Surgery

Sterile towels and clamps
1% lidocaine with epinephrine
30-gauge needle with 5–10 ml Luer-lok® syringe
Suture (absorbable, nonabsorbable, and silk for tagging/bolsters)
Iris scissors (curved and straight)
Suture scissors
Toothed forceps
Needle driver
Curved hemostat
Sterile gauze and cotton-tipped swabs
Antibiotic ointment
Sterile marking pen or gentian violet solution
Skin hooks (optional)

TABLE 2 Equipment for Grafts

General items (see Table 1)
Dish of sterile saline for temporary graft holding to form template for graft
Absorbable epidermal suture (eg, 5-0 mild chromic gut or 5-0 fast-absorbing gut)
Sterile mineral oil
Silk suture for bolster tie
Bolster material (eg, cotton balls, dental rolls, or foam)
Antibiotic ointment
Adaptic® gauze
Telfa® or suture packet foil

TABLE 3 Additional Equipment for STSG

Instrument for harvesting:
Air-driven or electric dermatome, or
Weck blade, or
#10 scalpel blade with handle
Instrument for meshing (optional):
Skin mesher
#11 blade for manual meshing

site that would otherwise be expected with local infiltration of an anesthetic with epinephrine. Thus, a combination of both nerve blocks and local infiltration may be desirable.

HOW-TO TECHNIQUES

Skin grafts and flaps may be performed in a variety of surgical settings. These include any setting where the defects cannot be closed primarily, or when poor healing, unacceptable cosmesis, or impaired function would likely be encountered with secondary intention healing [11].

The choice of grafting may be made in situations in which inadequate adjacent tissue is present for flap movement. Large defects are often best repaired with grafts [4]. Variably sized and shaped defects may be adequately closed with a graft. Grafts offer flexibility, relative ease of application, and reasonable predictability with regard to the size and ease of repair of the secondary defect. Essentially any defect with a vascularized base will accept a graft. The advantages and disadvantages of FTSG versus STSG were previously discussed. FTSG are favored cosmetically over STSG because adnexal structures and melanocytes are retained. STSG are best used in those areas with higher risk of graft failures [6]. These include areas of decreased vascularization such as lower extremities, and wounds overlying bone or cartilage. Imbibition, inosculation, and neovascularization are accelerated in STSG. These three stages of graft survival occur over the first 1 to 2 weeks. They refer to initial diffusion of nutrients in the critical early hours, subsequent ingrowth of nearby vessels, and eventual formation of new vessels, respectively. As such, better graft survival is expected with STSG because of lower nutritional requirements and easier diffusion of oxygen and nutrients from the wound base.

FTSG

When the decision for FTSG grafting has been made, a donor site must be selected. For small defects of the face, skin from the preauricular or postauricular sulcus are good choices for donating tissue. In general, tissue from the preauricular area is often thicker and more photodamaged than postauricular tissue (Fig. 7). Preauricular tissue works well for deeper defects and often provides better color match. A caution in this area, however, is to avoid collecting the sideburn hairs that would be transported to the new site. If larger areas are to be covered, sites that may provide an adequate reservoir include the supraclavicular region, neck, proximal arm, or thigh. These donor sites also offer acceptable cosmetic results or are camouflaged postsurgically. It is important to not select areas with extensive terminal hairs for donor sites unless a hair-bearing graft is specifically indicated.

Once the donor site is selected, it is scrubbed, prepared, and draped in the usual sterile fashion. A template of the defect is often constructed from a Telfa® pad or the foil packaging of suture material. It is important to oversize, typically by 10 to 15%, the template pattern to account for irregularities and tissue contraction. If the donor site is to be closed as an ellipse, an ellipse should be drawn around the pattern as desired and the entire ellipse taken en toto. Handling the donor tissue gently, preferably at the tips, will minimize trauma to the dermal tissue. It is important to

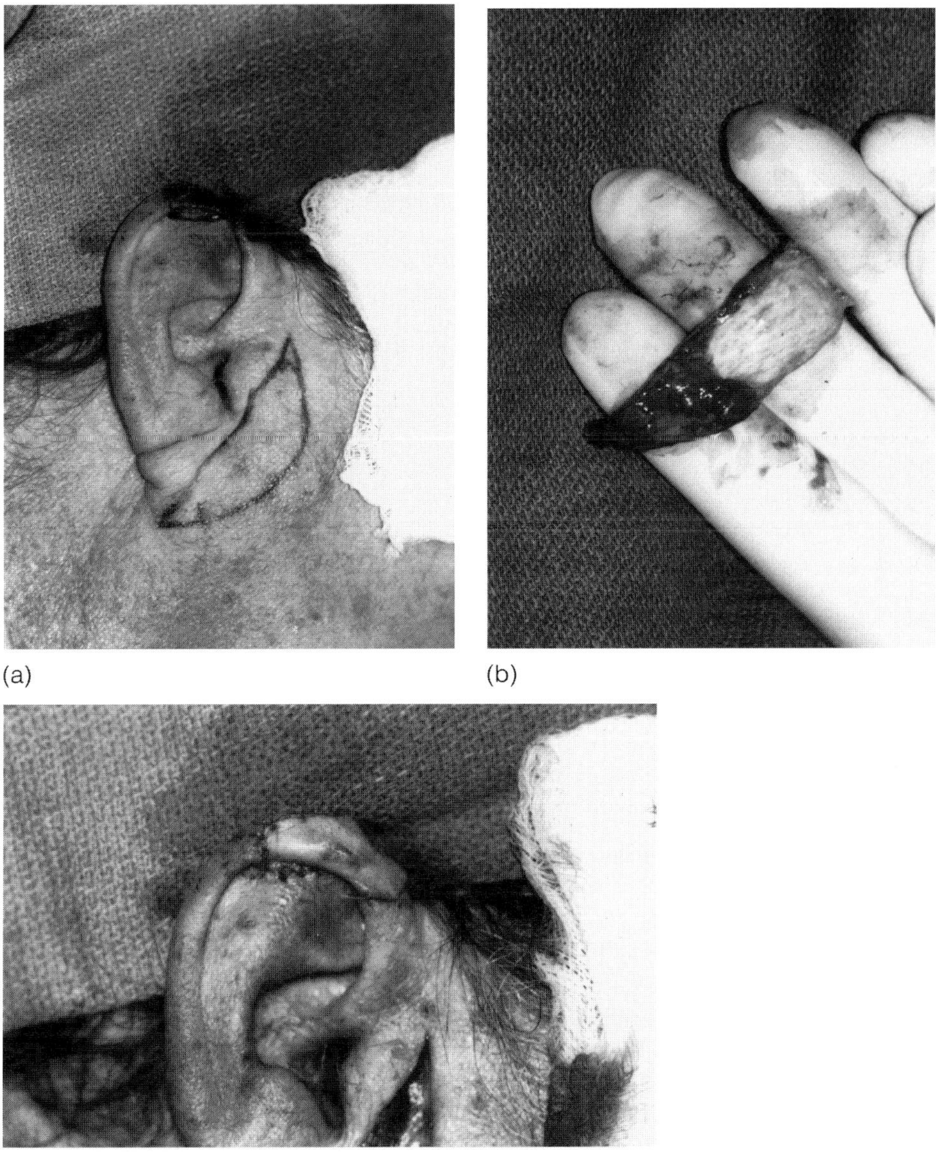

(a) (b) (c)

FIGURE 7 **Full-thickness skin graft. (a) Surgical defect of the superior helix, a difficult location to repair primarily or with a flap. Preauricular donor tissue has been identified, and an ellipse planned for its removal. (b) Elliptical donor tissue inverted and partially defatted. Note the glistening dermis visible in the region over the surgeon's third finger, while residual adipose remains to be trimmed over the second finger [2]. (c) Donor skin trimmed and sutured into place with absorbable epidermal sutures. Note the superior portion remains to be trimmed completely. (d) Bolster consisting of dental rolls and held in place with 4-0 silk suture. (e) Final outcome 1 year later.**

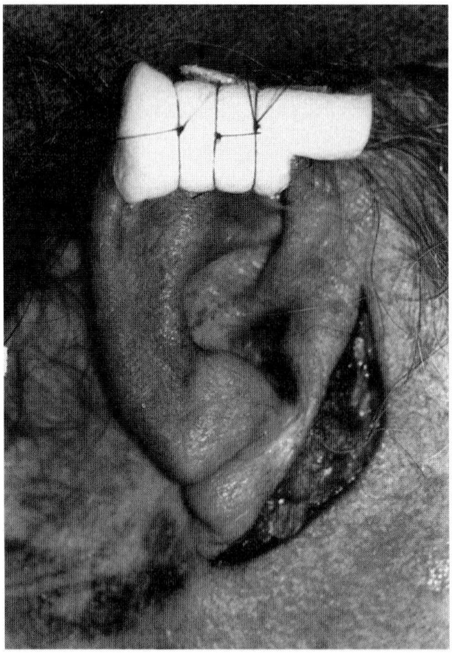

(d)

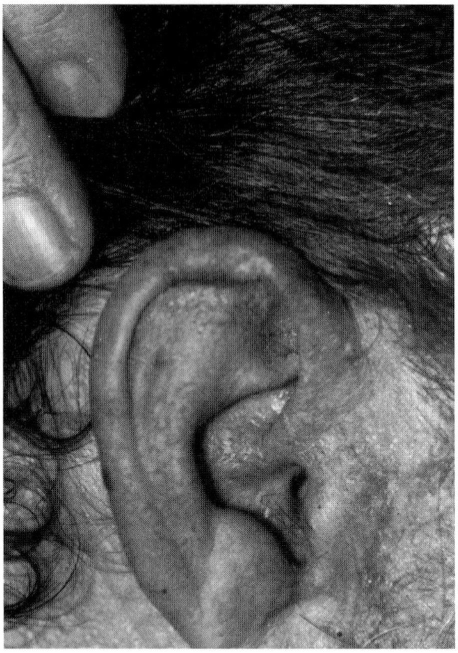

(e)

FIGURE 7 Continued

work efficiently to minimize trauma to the tissue and not deprive the donor tissue from nutrients longer than necessary.

The donor tissue is completely defatted. This is accomplished by grasping the inverted tissue between the fingers and removing subcutaneous tissue with curved iris scissors. This should be performed until the glistening white dermis is visible. Small, broad, tangential cuts are made. One finds that it is difficult to damage or remove the dermis with this approach. In fact, it is better to risk removal of small amounts of dermis than to allow adipose to remain behind. It is important to completely defat the tissue because added subcutis may rob the dermis of its diffusable nutrients. Exceptions to this exist with hair-bearing grafts. If hair is desired for the graft, the donor should be taken from similar hair type, ie, scalp, to replace scalp tissue. Minimal defatting should be performed to minimize damage to the hair follicles. These thicker grafts may be less viable than their defatted counterparts. If hair-bearing grafts are used, it is important to align the direction of donor hair follicles to parallel surrounding recipient hairs, especially before trimming the donor tissue to fit the site.

It is important to undermine the recipient site several millimeters before graft placement. Undermining decreases the risk of ''pin-cushioning'' of the lesion after surgery, and subsequently may allow for more uniform wound contraction and remodeling.

Once defatted, the donor tissue should be immediately placed onto the donor site or briefly in saline to prevent desiccation. The donor defect should be temporarily ignored except for judicious hemostasis, with the attention paid to the graft and its placement. The margin of the graft is sutured with precise apposition to a portion of the recipient site rim. Precise alignment of FTSG is required, although STSG may be allowed to overlap the defect slightly. The rationale is that FTSG will remain viable in their entirety, while STSG redundant edges almost always slough, leaving an appropriately sized graft. Sutures are typically placed approximately every 2 to 3 mm and usually consist of 5-0 mild chromic gut or fast-absorbing gut. As the donor tissue is tacked to the periphery, meticulous trimming of the donor tissue to the size of the recipient bed is required. Alternating trimming and suturing, the graft is completely apposed to the margins of the wound. If central tacking sutures are placed, it is important to do so at the outset so that hemostasis can be achieved from the margins if a vessel is inadvertently pierced. This should be performed under direct vision to avoid even mild bleeding. A small hematoma may cause necrosis of the graft because of nonadherence to the underlying bed.

Bolster placement overlying the graft improves apposition of the graft to the wound base. Bolsters help to avoid inadvertent trauma or manipulation of the graft. Bolsters may range from a layered pressure dressing for small grafts to large sutured bolsters for larger grafts. For sutured bolsters, pairs of 4-0 silk suture are placed at opposite poles of the graft margins. Small grafts may require only two pairs of silk sutures; larger grafts may need four or more pairs of silk sutures. The goal is to have as many pairs necessary to prevent tangential movement of the graft. For very large grafts (eg, >3 cm diameter), larger caliber silk suture may be required. These sutures are left with a short tail at one end, and a long tail of about 4 to 5 cm at the other end. In this manner, one is less likely to snap the suture. Bolsters may consist of a thick layer of antibiotic ointment overlying the graft site, followed by a nonadherent contact layer (eg, Adaptic® or Telfa®). A bulky material such as cotton balls, foam, or dental rolls serves as the top layer. This is sized slightly larger than the graft and applied. Saturating the bolster with mineral oil may aid in prevention of postsurgical desiccation of the graft. The bolster is then tied down with the previously placed silk sutures. Each pair is then tied by hand across the top layer of the bolster. An instrument tie is avoided because it may result in higher risk of snapping the suture.

STSG

Similar techniques are used for STSG grafting as are used in FTSG. Adequate donor sites must be chosen for the defect. Large defects are often best served with donor tissue from the anterior proximal thigh. Smaller defects are often closed with donor tissue from the superomedial arm. Both the thigh and arm are readily accessible, and the resultant donor scars easily concealed by clothing. In addition, these sites are easily compressed by the dermatome at collection.

As with FTSG, donor site anesthesia is achieved and a template of the defect is marked at the site. If extensive meshing is planned, the template may be undersized up to 30%. However, it is always best to have excess tissue if possible.

Collection may be manually performed with a #10 scalpel blade for defect sizes less than 4 cm^2. Hand collection (Fig. 8) is performed with a smooth back-and-forth sawing motion by using a scalpel, Weck blade, or mechanical dermatome. The blade should be visible through the epidermis as collection is carried out. The goal with manually collected STSG is to obtain as little dermis as possible without breaking through the epidermis. Small breaks are acceptable because they often granulate and allow small amounts of serum or blood to extrude from the wound base.

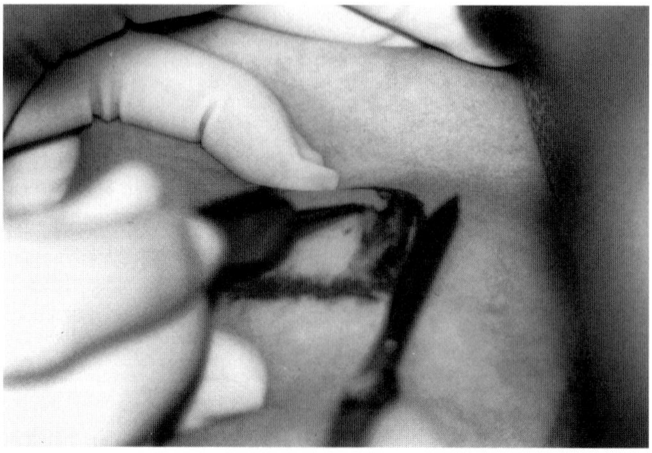

(a)

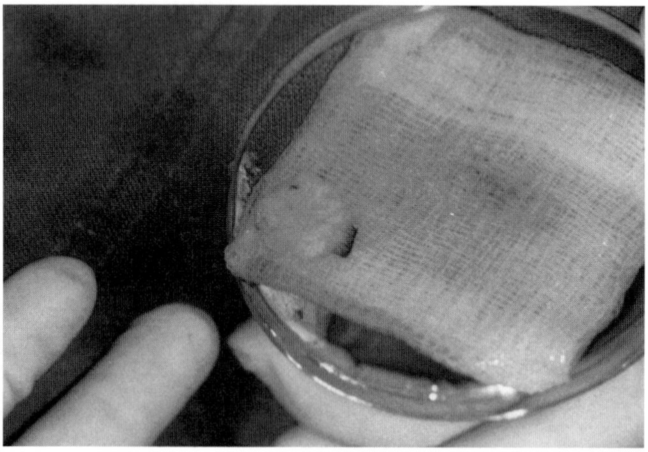

(b)

FIGURE 8 Hand-collected split-thickness skin graft. (a) Small square of tissue outlined with gentian violet. A #10 scalpel is oriented tangentially to obtain very thin donor skin for a lower extremity defect. (b) The collected donor is briefly placed on saline-soaked gauze to achieve focal meshing with a #11 scalpel blade. (c) Appearance of the graft 10 days after initial placement. (d) Outcome at 3 months. Note the "shiny" appearance, lack of hair, and relative hypopigmentation expected with split-thickness grafts. (e) Result 2 years after surgery.

Thickness of STSG may be varied when mechanically collected (Fig. 9). Settings range between $^{2}/_{1000}$ to $^{20}/_{1000}$ of an inch. Medium-thickness grafts (about $^{12}/_{1000}$ of an inch) are suitable for most defects, permitting for adequate coverage and cosmetic appearance.

A lubricant, such as antibiotic ointment or mineral oil, applied to the donor area facilitates graft collection by minimizing friction. Retraction of the donor skin emerging from the advancing dermatome are best achieved by an assistant who grasps the corners with toothed forceps. Once the dermatome has engaged the donor

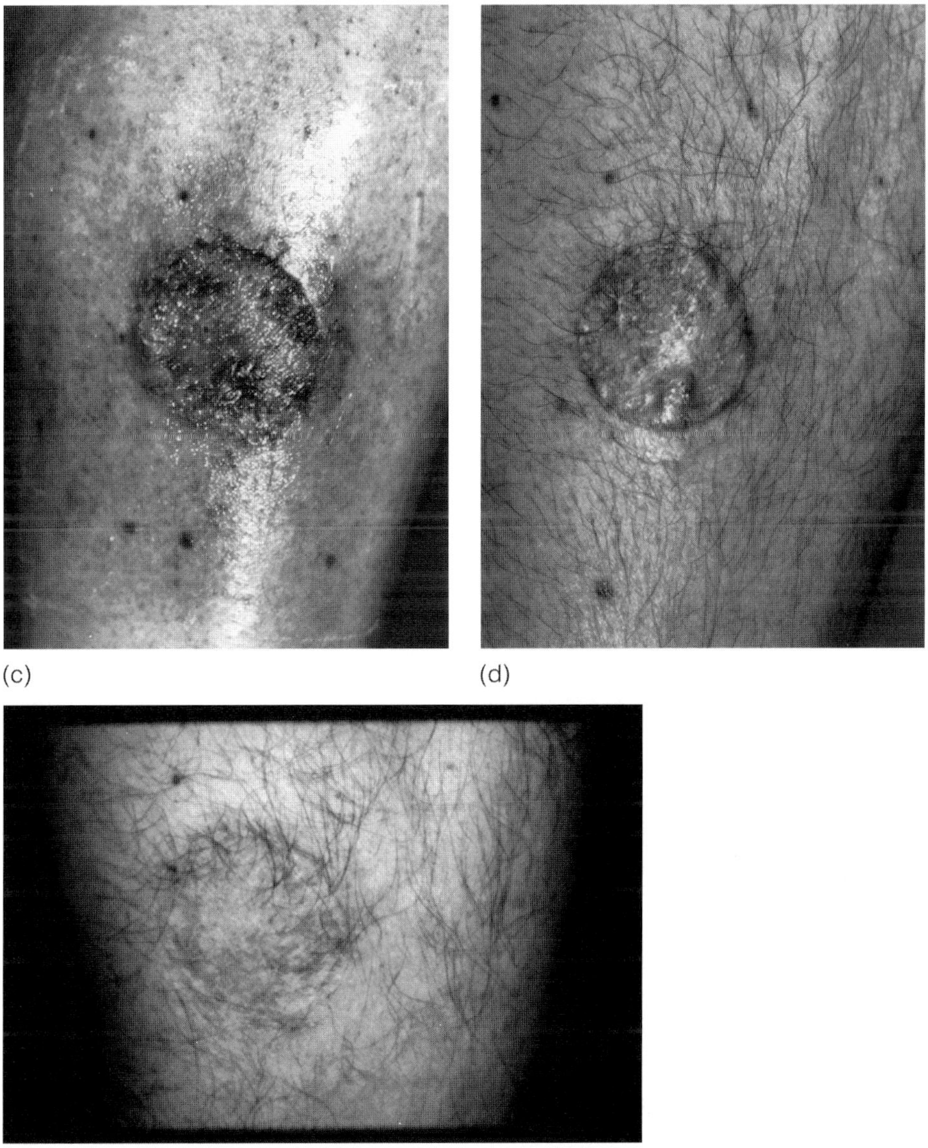

(c) (d)

(e)

FIGURE 8 Continued

tissue, it is essential to continue firm pressure throughout the procedure until the entire graft has been collected. As the free margin of donor tissue is expelled, an assistant gently "delivers" it from the device. When an adequate length of donor material has been collected, lifting up the operating dermatome will effectively free the rectangular donor tissue from the site. The transected donor specimen is immediately placed into a saline petri dish, preventing desiccation and curling of the graft onto itself. A gauze dressing soaked in 1% lidocaine with epinephrine placed tem-

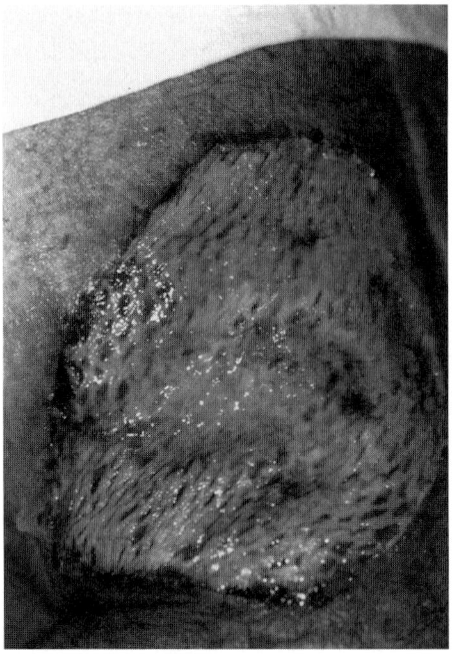

(a)

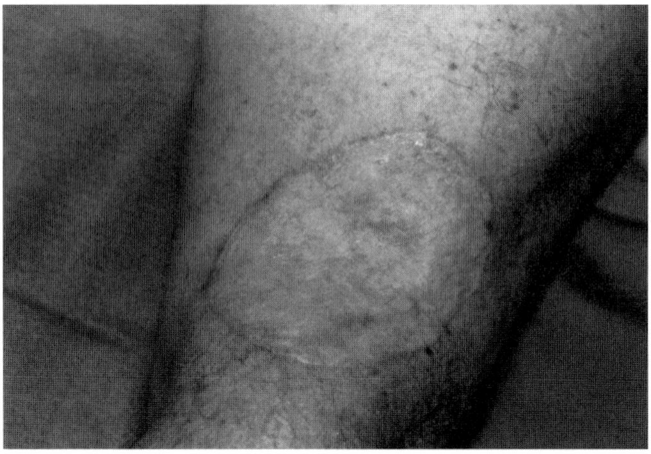

(b)

FIGURE 9 Mechanically collected split-thickness skin graft. (a) Large graft collected from the thigh with a Stryker® dermatome and placed on the upper arm. The graft has been mechanically meshed at a 1:2 ratio, resulting in the "honeycombed" appearance. (b) Outcome at 6 months. Note the hypopigmentation and the absence of meshed areas that have healed by granulation.

porarily over the donor site adequately accomplishes hemostasis while attention is paid to the graft and its placement.

Mechanical meshing is typically performed at a 1:2 ratio, especially for larger STSG. Meshing is especially useful for covering large areas or when wound drainage is likely. Manual meshing with a #11 blade is often easier and may achieve better cosmesis because a "honeycombed" appearance is frequently observed with mechanical meshers. Manual meshing is also simpler for smaller grafts and can be performed while the tissue is still in the petri dish.

Application of a STSG is the same as that of FTSG. Suturing and trimming is similar, although precise trimming and apposition are often not necessary as redundancies readily desiccate and slough. Bolster application is the same for small and medium STSG and FTSG. However, large STSG may require generation of a much larger bandage consisting of stacked gauze or foam held in place with tape and compression materials. The donor site generally requires moist occlusive wound care only. Typically, this consists of antibiotic ointment or petrolatum and a nonadherent dressing for 2 weeks which promotes re-epithelization and minimizes discomfort.

Porcine Xenografts

If a poor recipient bed exists, porcine grafts may be chosen to precede the FTSG or STSG. These inexpensive commercial biological dressings are sterile tissue specimens consisting of a dermis and overlying epidermis derived from pigs. Application is the same as for other grafts. Meticulous trimming and suturing is not necessary because the porcine graft will simply serve as a biological dressing for 1 to 2 weeks before permanent FTSG or STSG placement (Fig. 10). This allows for improved granulation tissue formation and contraction of the defect before permanent graft placement. Bolstering may be accomplished with either silk ties or carefully placed adhesive pressure bandaging. As with other bolsters, this will remain in place for approximately 1 week.

Flaps

Well-designed flaps are preferable to grafts for most patients because they often look and function better. Among repair options, the difficulty in choosing and appropriately applying flap closures is greatest. The use of free flaps requires adequate experience and familiarity with a variety of repair options for given anatomic locations and host circumstances. Various movements and their advantages, disadvantages, and expectations were discussed earlier in this chapter.

Skin mobility varies by anatomic location. In general, older patients have greater tissue laxity than younger patients. Relaxed skin tension lines and the cosmetic units of the face must be observed and considered in any closure. Thus, the effect of the donated tissue and the direction of its movement must be considered. Initial evaluation of RSTL should be made with gentle pinching and pulling with hands and/or skin hooks. Incisions are often best concealed if parallel to these lines when possible. Respecting cosmetic units and attempting to remain within these landmarks will assist in concealing surgical scars.

Application of gentian violet or marking pen should be used to outline proposed flap options. A variety of closures may be entertained for a defect before the optimal

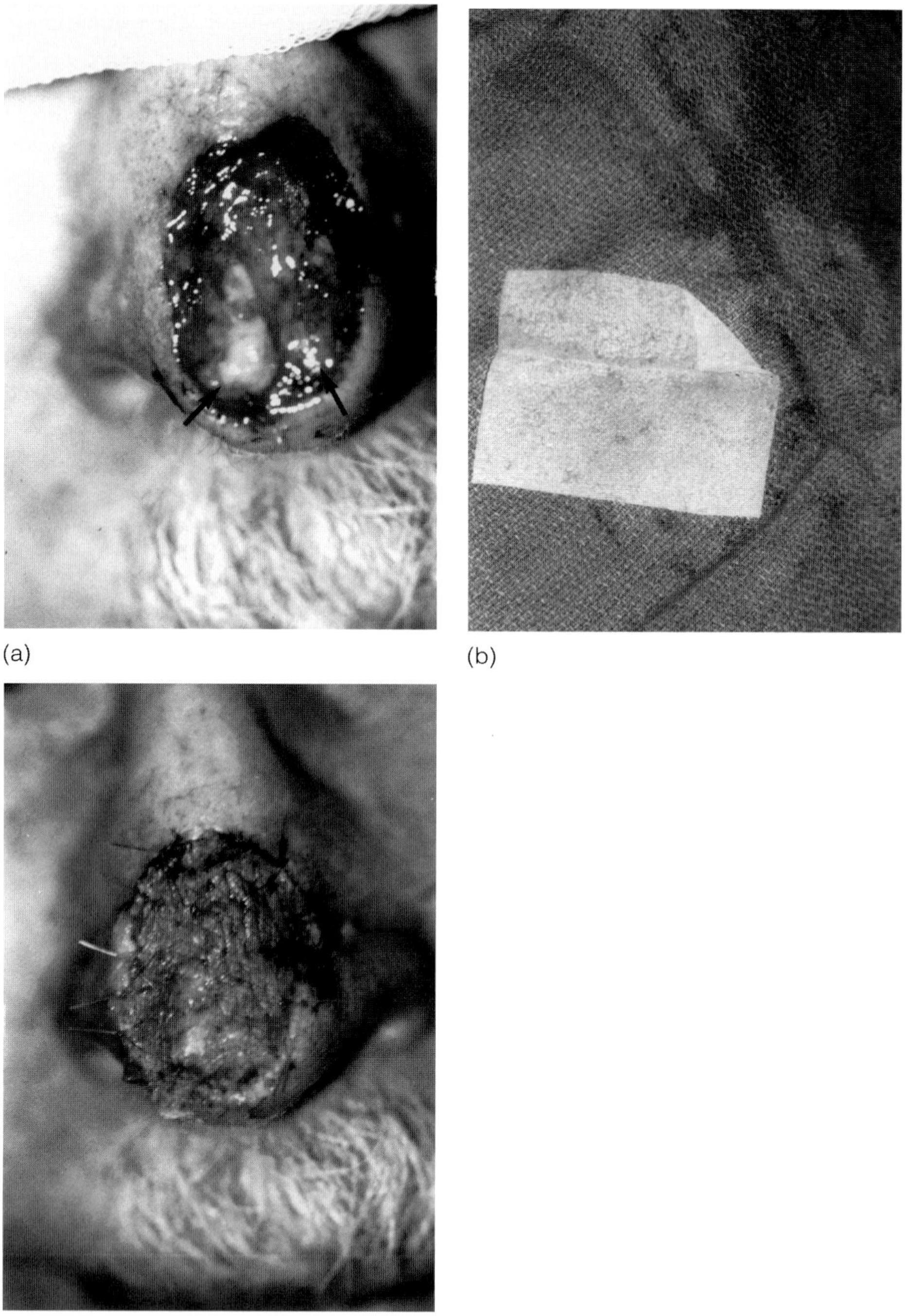

(a) (b) (c)

FIGURE 10 Porcine xenograft use. (a) Deep defect of the nasal tip, exposing the alar cartilages (arrows). Immediate repair with a graft might fail in the absence of a well-vascularized base, and the patient declined a paramedian forehead flap. (b) Thawed porcine skin on sterile field before placement. (c) Appearance of the graft 10 days after apposition with absorbable epidermal sutures. There is no evidence of necrosis or infection.

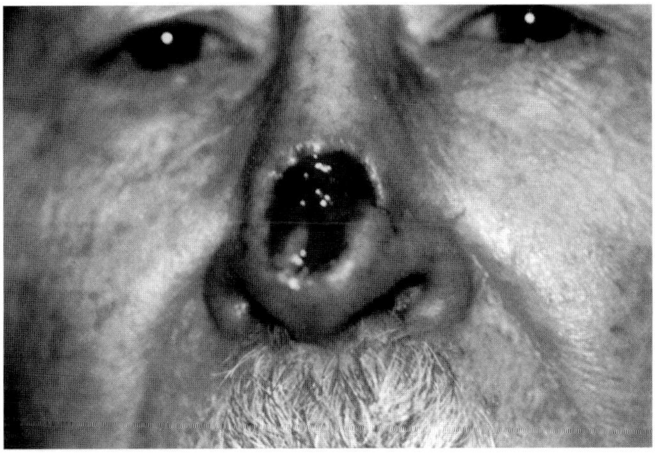

(d)

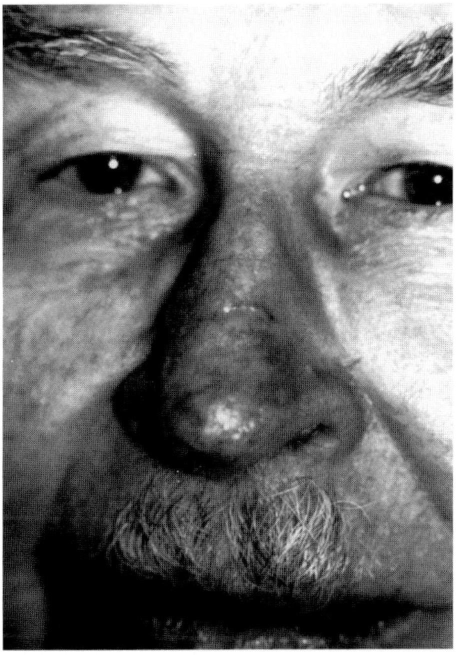

(e)

FIGURE 10 Continued (d) Once the graft is removed at 10 days, the base reveals extensive granulation tissue and the cartilage is largely covered. This base would likely successfully accept an autologous graft. (e) Postsurgical appearance at 2 months after placement of a full-thickness skin graft using supraclavicular donor tissue.

closure is decided and drawn. The flap and surrounding tissue should be reassessed throughout the closure to assess results of tissue movement.

Undermining of both the defect and the surrounding tissues is required. This not only frees up tissue for even redistribution but helps to relieve excess tension on the flap. Extensive undermining may be necessary, especially in larger rotation flaps. Undermining should be performed in the upper subcutis to leave adequate arteriolar and capillary supply to the flap. The thickness of adipose remaining on the undersurface of the flap is typically 2 to 3 mm. Excessive adipose will increase the risk of flap "bulkiness" and should be avoided. An exception to undermining is the previously discussed island pedicle flap. Undermining around the defect helps to prevent "trapdooring" of the flap. Meticulous hemostasis is mandatory to prevent hematoma formation under the flap.

Closure of the secondary defect, by convention, is initially performed. Placing these "key sutures" along the secondary/tertiary defect first helps to alleviate tension on the free portion of the flap, allowing it to be more gently placed into the defect with minimal tension. Next, one apposes the dermis and subcutis of the flap to the deep margins of the defect using an appropriate absorbable suture, such as Vicryl®, PDS®, or Dexon®. Subsequent epidermal apposition is performed with appropriate nonabsorbable suture. In areas of minimal skin thickness or tension, the smallest caliber suture appropriate for the site will improve the resultant scar. Careful suture placement with a slight wound margin eversion will likewise improve the appearance of the expected scar.

A bolster is not required for flaps because they possess their own blood supply, and imbibition is unnecessary. A firm, nonadherent dressing is usually adequate.

IMMEDIATE POSTSURGICAL CARE

Wound care for grafts is minimal during the first week. Bolsters should remain in place during this time period. Care should be taken to keep the bolster clean and dry. It is important to prevent any manipulation or trauma of the graft site during this time period to allow maximal neovascularization to occur.

Wound care for flap closures is similar to other primary closures of the skin. A light compression bandage, if possible, should remain in place for 48 hours. Wounds should be kept clean and dry. Gentle cleansing of the wound and removal of debris should be performed twice daily in most cases, generally with hydrogen peroxide. This should be followed by a liberal amount of antibiotic ointment or petrolatum.

Edema, ecchymoses, and discomfort may be observed for several days after surgery. Periorbital and neck ecchymoses are quite common when performing facial surgery. If extensive undermining was performed, an increased risk of hematoma exists. Judicious follow-up of such patients is important.

Analgesia, most often acetaminophen, should be used especially in the first several evenings after surgery. If large areas of tissue were undermined and displaced, or the wound is under some tension, greater analgesia may be required. Most commonly, acetaminophen with codeine is sufficient to alleviate this discomfort. Occasionally, for extensive surgery or tissue movement, stronger opiate analgesics may be required. Achieving pain control early is important in maintaining patient comfort. Aspirin-containing or nonsteroidal anti-inflammatory agents should be avoided. Most patients on therapeutic anticoagulation may restart their daily warfarin or aspirin 24 hours after surgery.

Patients should minimize activity for several weeks after surgery because fresh wounds have minimal tensile strength. Activities such as weight lifting, aerobics, or other moderate to extensive exercise should be terminated during the healing process. Such activities greatly increase risk of dehiscence or hematoma formation.

LONG-TERM POSTSURGICAL CARE

Remodeling of wounds continues to occur for 1 year or more after the procedure. FTSG will change in texture and contour during this time, although perhaps in a more subtle fashion after many months. Grafts may elevate, especially at the border, early in their course. Generally, these flatten as the graft matures and progresses [3].

Focal dermabrasion and CO_2 or Erbium laser ablation may be considered for raised or irregular borders of scars. Intralesional steroids may be of benefit for hypertrophic or keloidal scarring or bulkiness, although it is often best to wait at least 6 to 8 weeks to make such assessments with flaps or grafts. Some practitioners routinely abrade surgical sites at 6 to 8 weeks after surgery, whereas others may prefer to allow wounds to remodel more slowly and abrade only those sites that show irregularity after 6 to 12 months.

COMPLICATIONS AND TREATMENT OF COMPLICATIONS

For most surgical procedures, presurgical assessment, patient education, and postsurgical monitoring improve the likelihood of an uneventful recovery. However, complications will occasionally result from any surgery. Experience with multiple normal wounds is helpful in determining those that may show signs of infection, necrosis, or delayed or abnormal healing.

The anticipated appearance of skin grafts is often violaceous to frankly dusky, especially before blood supply is adequately re-established. Even when frank necrosis has occurred (black rather than violaceous), viable dermal tissue is often present. The temptation to debride graft tissue should be resisted. Education of the patient about this expected appearance should be made before surgery and again at bolster removal. A more normal color can be expected at about 4 weeks after surgery. Bandage replacement is made at this time and will remain in place for an additional 48 hours. Thereafter, gentle cleansing with topical antibiotic or petrolatum applications should be instituted at home twice daily. The patient should be reminded to use nonstick dressings and to remove them carefully so that the graft is not removed inadvertently. Slight superficial eschar or exudate often continues for 1 to 2 weeks. This material results primarily from epidermal slough and suture breakdown. Wound care is generally continued for 4 to 6 weeks, or longer as needed. In general, STSG heal sooner and achieve a healthy appearance more quickly than FTSG because of their lower nutritional requirements.

It is uncommon for grafts to fail. The most common cause of failure is secondary to compromised blood supply, which may occur for several reasons as previously discussed. Recognition and prevention of these causes is clearly important. Tobacco use should be discontinued or reduced as much as possible, at least on a temporary basis, preferably 2 weeks before and 2 weeks after surgery. Meticulous hemostasis should be performed to minimize the chance of hematoma forming under the graft. Blindly suturing the graft to the recipient bed risks hematoma formation.

It is important not to attempt grafts over exposed bone or cartilage. A blood supply from intact periosteum or perichondrium is essential. Where this lining of tissue with blood supply is absent, grafts cannot be expected to survive. It is best to allow granulation tissue to form and perform a delayed graft repair or flap repair initially.

Large wounds or those that require extensive surgery-room time may benefit from postsurgical staphylococcal and streptococcal coverage with antibiotics. Closures that are staged and performed days after the original wound creation should be placed on such antibiotic prophylaxis; typically, this is initiated 1 day before and 4 days after the surgical repair is performed.

Complete necrosis of a graft can occur; however, it is uncommon, especially for STSG. Although it may take several weeks of postsurgical follow-up to determine complete necrosis, watchful waiting is usually the best approach. Partial-thickness slough may occur but the dermis will usually survive and re-epithelialize. Even in the setting of frank necrosis, the dead graft serves as a biological dressing, allowing new granulation tissue and epithelialization to occur. Infection, likewise, is an uncommon complication of grafts. Treatment with antibiotics and similar watchful waiting is usually the best course. If purulent, a culture should be sent before instituting gram-positive antibiotics in the event that an atypical organism or *Candida* is involved.

Even with prudent planning and execution, occasional difficulties and complications can occur with any surgical procedure. The most common of these include bleeding, infection, and dehiscence [13].

Although ecchymosis is common, hematoma formation is not. Ecchymosis is most common in the periorbital region, cheeks, forehead, and neck. Edema is also common, but induration of a wound is worrisome. This is particularly true if swelling has occurred or progressed over a short period of time. Such signs are suggestive of accumulating blood.

If a hematoma or active bleeding is discovered or suspected within several hours of surgery, the wound should be reopened and examined. This may be performed focally along the wound at first, starting along the most dependent portion or most indurated region of the wound. Sites of active bleeding should be sought. If focal coagulation or ligation is possible, the entire repair need not be taken down. If a source is not immediately apparent, more of the wound should be opened and explored. Residual clot should be removed. After hemostasis has been achieved, the wound may be closed and prophylactic antibiotics should be instituted. Late-forming hematomas are occasionally encountered, usually presenting 1 to 3 days after surgery. Hematomas containing 2 to 3 ml of blood or more will generally require intervention and evacuation. It may be possible to evacuate fresh hematomas with a large bore needle and syringe suction. Generally, opening the most dependent or inferior portion of the wound must be performed to remove the gelatinous clot. Thorough, but gentle, irrigation should be performed and hemostasis regained. Secondary intention healing is best for these wounds.

Wound infections are a relatively uncommon complication of dermatologic surgery. Those patients at greater risk include the immunocompromised and diabetics. Although prophylactic antibiotics are generally not required for these or other patients, awareness of this risk may alter postsurgical assessment and management. Postsurgical wounds will often show signs and symptoms of erythema, mild edema, and tenderness. If these worsen after several days, and/or are accompanied by fever or serosanguineous drainage, a wound infection should be suspected.

The majority of postsurgical ambulatory infections are staphylococcal in origin. Thus, empiric coverage for *Staphylococcus* should be instituted pending culture. Similar to hematoma evacuation strategies, the wound should be compressed and perhaps partially opened to investigate and drain any abscess present. Cultures should be performed whenever purulence is present. One should be mindful of the occasional candidal or herpetic wound infection; appropriate antifungal or antiviral therapy is warranted in such instances.

Wound dehiscence may result from a variety of causes. The most common predisposing factors include hematoma formation or infection. Other frequent causes include poor suture placement or size selection and excessive tension on the wound margins. The management of hematoma and infection has been previously discussed.

Appropriate suture materials and placement are important for successful flap and graft outcome. Direct manual approximation and closure of the wound should be performed before suturing. The wound should not be under excess tension; otherwise alternative methods of closure should be entertained. Most wounds benefit from some form of buried suture for added integrity, dead-space elimination, and strength. Adequate numbers and size of buried suture should be selected for a given body area. Regions of the body at particular risk of dehiscence are those overlying joints (knees, elbows, fingers) or pressure or weight-bearing areas (feet, buttocks). Strict avoidance of stress should be emphasized to the patient during the healing process. Often, splints or slings may be appropriate to help eliminate these tension forces.

Dehisced wounds should be managed with moist occlusive wound care and allowed to heal secondarily. These should not be resutured because the risk of infection is greatly increased. If a known cause for the dehiscence is identified, such as infection or hematoma, it should be rectified. Supporting bandages or splints may aid in improved healing of the dehisced wound.

SUMMARY

Flaps and grafts are important repair options for many wounds encountered in dermatologic surgery. They are most useful for wounds that are not easily repaired by primary closure and where granulation is likely to result in a poor cosmetic or functional result. With adequate presurgical assessment, patient education, and intraoperative planning, excellent results can be expected.

REFERENCES

1. Leshin B, Whitaker DC, Swanson NA. Preoperative evaluation in dermatologic surgery. J Amer Acad Dermatol 19:1081–1086, 1988.
2. Arpey CJ, Whitaker DC, O'Donnell MJ. Cutaneous Surgery. Illustrated and Practical Approach. New York: McGraw Hill, 1997.
3. Johnson TM, Ratner D, Nelson BR. Soft tissue reconstruction with skin grafting. J Amer Acad Dermatol 27:151–159, 1992.

4. Branham GH, Thomas JR. Skin grafts. Otolaryngol Clin N Am 23:889–892, 1990.
5. Cronin TA, Cronin TA Jr. A classification of the island grafts. Dermatol Clin 13:483–488, 1995.
6. Skouge JW. Techniques for split-thickness skin grafting. J Dermatol Surg Oncol 13: 841–844, 1987.
7. Hill TG. Skin grafts. In: Wheeland RG, ed. Cutaneous Surgery. Philadelphia: W.B. Saunders Company, 1994:318–328.
8. Baker SR. Local cutaneous flaps. Otolaryngol Clin N Am 27:139–142, 1994.
9. Whitaker DC. Random-pattern flaps. In: Wheeland RG, ed. Cutaneous Surgery. Philadelphia: W.B. Saunders Company, 1994:329–352.
10. Summers BK, Siegle RJ. Facial cutaneous reconstructive surgery: facial flaps. J Amer Acad Dermatol 29:917–922, 1993.
11. Tromovitch TA, Stegman SJ, Glogau RG. Flaps and Grafts in Dermatologic Surgery. Chicago: Year Book Medical Publishers, 1989.
12. Haas AH, Grekin RG. Antibiotic prophylaxis in dermatologic surgery. J Am Acad Dermatol 32:155–176, 1995.
13. Salasche SJ, Grabski WJ. Complications of flaps. J Dermatol Surg Oncol 17:132–136, 1991.

APPENDIX 1: GRAFT POSTSURGICAL CARE INSTRUCTION SHEET

The dressing and bolster should remain dry and in place until you return to see your doctor.

Avoid tension to the area. Do not bend, stretch, lift heavy objects, or lie on the involved area. To reduce swelling, keep the area elevated as much as possible and apply an ice pack as needed.

Avoid taking aspirin or aspirin-containing products for the next 2 weeks because of the increased risk of bleeding. You may use acetaminophen, eg, Tylenol, as needed for pain.

Contact your doctor or clinic if the following occurs:

bleeding that saturates the dressing
increased redness or pus-like drainage
separation of the suture line
sudden firm clot or thickening occurs under the stitches

APPENDIX 2: FLAP POSTSURGICAL CARE INSTRUCTION SHEET

The dressing should remain dry and in place for 2 days.

After two days, wash your hands and remove the dressing. If the dressing sticks to the wound, soak dressing with tap water for 10–15 minutes. Clean the suture line twice a day. Put a small amount of hydrogen peroxide into a clean container. Dip cotton-tipped applicator into the hydrogen peroxide and roll the applicator over the suture line. Remove as much crust, scab, or drainage material from the wound as possible. It is very important to not allow a scab to form.

Apply a thin layer of antibiotic ointment with a cotton-tipped applicator to the suture line. It is important to keep the area moist with ointment at all times. Continue wound care until you return to see your doctor for wound check or suture removal.

Cover the suture line with a bandage or dressing as needed to protect from dust or irritation from clothing.

Avoid tension to the area. Do not bend, stretch, lift heavy objects, or lie on the involved area. To reduce swelling, keep the area elevated as much as possible and apply an ice pack as needed.

Avoid taking aspirin or aspirin-containing products for the next 2 weeks because of the increased risk of bleeding. You may use acetaminophen, eg, Tylenol, as needed for pain.

Contact your doctor or clinic if the following occurs:

bleeding that saturates the dressing
increased redness or pus-like drainage
separation of the suture line
sudden firm clot or thickening occurs under the stitches

20

Topical Anesthetics and Local and Regional Blocks

Tri H. Nguyen
Mayo Clinic Foundation, Rochester, Minnesota

INTRODUCTION AND HISTORY

Local anesthesia is defined as the pharmacologic induction of sensory loss in a regional anatomic site, which may be achieved by injectable or topical medications. It has many advantages over general anesthesia and is especially desirable in dermatologic and cosmetic surgery, where procedures are typically minimally invasive. The patient retains protective airway reflexes and is an interactive part of the procedure. Local anesthesia enables cosmetic procedures to occur in an outpatient setting with not only less morbidity and fast recovery but also substantially less expense. Elderly patients in particular benefit given that their attendant risks for general anesthesia and stresses of postsurgical recovery are greater.

The advent of local anesthesia occurred in 1860 when Niemann extracted crystals from the South American plant *Erythroxylon coca*, observed that it produced numbness of the tongue, and named the alkaloid substance cocaine [1]. Centuries before, the Indians of Peru considered the plant sacred and noted that it suppressed hunger, invigorated the weary and depressed, and remedied altitude sickness [2]. Sigmund Freud authored a review on cocaine in July 1884, lauding its effect on endurance and alleviating morphine addiction. Months later in September 1884, aspiring ophthalmologist Carl Loller applied cocaine to the cornea in the world's first locally anesthetic surgery, a glaucoma operation [2]. Koller's seminal work began an intensive search for other agents, which bore fruit in 1904 when Einhorn developed procaine. One year earlier, Braun had mixed epinephrine with cocaine and described its hemostatic effect [2]. In 1943, the efforts of Lofgren and his predecessor Erdtman produced lignocaine (lidocaine), the world's first amide anesthetic [1]. Since then, advances have consisted of modifications of the two primary classes, esters and amides.

CLASSIFICATION AND PHARMACOLOGY

Local anesthetics may be classified as esters and amides according to the structure of their intermediate chains. Both families have in common a benzene aromatic ring (lipophilic), the intermediate link chain, and an amine group (hydrophilic). Modifications in the aromatic ring or amine group may affect potency, onset, and duration of action. Whereas the intermediate chain determines whether an agent is an ester or an amide, the aromatic ring and the amine group reflect the lipophilic and hydrophilic properties respectively. Increasing lipid solubility facilitates diffusion across cellular membranes and hence increases potency. Duration of action, however, is dependent on protein binding affinity. Bupivacaine and etidocaine, for example, are strongly bound to plasma proteins and have the longest duration of action.

The active form of all anesthetics is in the cationic (positively charged) form. However, it is the base form (uncharged) that diffuses across cell walls. Lowering the pH raises the acidity and increases the ionized portion of local anesthetics, impairing effective diffusion and delaying onset of action. A lower pH will also aggravate the burning discomfort of local injection. Agents with a lower pKa (dissociation constant), on the other hand, will diffuse across lipid membranes more readily because of a higher proportion of the drug in an uncharged, nonionized form. In general, amides have a lower pKa than esters. Both esters and amides are components of injectable and topical formulations. Table 1 presents the most commonly used agents in both families.

MECHANISM OF ACTION

After tissue injury (incisional, thermal, crush, etc.), a neurohumoral cascade occurs to produce the sensation of pain. Peripheral nociceptive receptors in injured areas send afferent impulses centrally via small myelinated A fibers (fast) and unmyelinated C fibers (slow). Neurons generate impulses by the action potential or the depolarization of its resting potential by the opening of Na+/K+ channels. All local anesthetics effect sensory loss by stabilizing these Na+/K+ channels and preventing peripheral nerve depolarization.

While suppressing peripheral nerve impulses, local anesthetics may either stimulate or depress central nervous system function. Initial effects may include tremors, restlessness, and seizures (see Table 5a) followed by respiratory and central nervous system (CNS) depression. All local anesthetics, with the exception of cocaine, are vasodilators. They are negative cardiac inotropes and reduce cardiac output as well

TABLE 1 Injectable Anesthetics

Classification	Generic	Trade name
Esters	Procaine	Novocaine, neocaine
	Cocaine	None
	Chloroprocaine	Nesacaine
	Tetracaine	Pontocaine, pentacaine
Amides	Lidocaine	Xylocaine, seracaine
	Bupivacaine	Marcaine, sensorcaine
	Mepivacaine	Carbocaine
	Prilocaine	Citanest
	Etidocaine	Duranest

as inhibit conduction. This characteristic assumes vital importance in the suppression of cardiac arrhythmias.

METABOLISM

The metabolism of esters and amides differ significantly. Esters are degraded by plasma pseudocholinesterases into PABA metabolites. It is these metabolites that are often associated with allergic reactions. Cocaine, however, differs from other esters by being partially metabolized in the liver and excreted unchanged in the urine [4].

Amides are metabolized by hepatic microsomal enzymes and renally excreted. Lidocaine and mepivacaine additionally undergo enterohepatic circulation. Conditions that diminish liver function (cirrhosis, medications inhibiting microsomal enzymes) or reduce hepatic blood flow (congestive heart failure (CHF), dehydration, portal hypertension, the use of beta-blockers, and circulatory shock) will impair metabolism and potentially increase drug toxicity.

ESTER ANESTHETICS

Agents within this family have an ester linkage in their intermediate chain (Table 2). They are metabolized by the plasma enzyme, pseudocholinesterase. Patients with a genetic deficiency in this enzyme are at an increased risk for toxicity. Metabolized to para-aminobenzoic acid (PABA), esters are contraindicated in patients allergic to PABA and its related compounds (sulfonylureas, hydrochlorothiazide, procainimide). The use of esters decreases the effectiveness of sulfonamide antibiotics. The incidence of allergic reactions among esters is significantly higher than for amides and these agents are rarely used clinically.

Cocaine

The ancestor of all local anesthetics, cocaine is useful as a topical agent for mucosal surfaces of the nose or mouth. Its vasoconstrictive property is unique among the local anesthetics and has secured for it a role in the treatment of epistaxis. The onset of action is within 3 to 5 minutes with a 4% solution [3]. Cocaine is a stimulant to the CNS as well as systemically. It may produce hypertension and tachycardia and should be avoided in patients with severe cardiovascular disease or uncontrolled hyperthyroidism.

Procaine

Procaine was once a popular anesthetic but has now been rendered obsolete by lidocaine. It has a slow onset of action and short duration (30–60 min) and is not effective as a topical agent. Its primary role now is as a repository with penicillin G for intramuscular injections.

Tetracaine

Effective as a topical anesthetic, tetracaine has a rapid onset of action (3 min for mucosal surfaces), long duration of action, and is 10 times as potent as procaine. It is available in injectable, topical, and ophthalmic formulations, alone or in combi-

TABLE 2 Ester Anesthetics

Agent	Onset	Duration of action (min)		Maximum dose	Formulations	
		Without epinephrine	With epinephrine	(without epinephrine)	Injectable	Topical
Cocaine	Rapid	45	No data	No data	None	Table 5
Procaine*†	Slow	15–30	30–90	≤1 gm total	1, 2, 10%	None
Chloroprocaine†	Rapid	30–60	NA	800 mg	1, 2, 3%	None
Tetracaine*	Rapid	120–240	240–480	NA	0.2, 0.3, 1%	Table 5

*Available without preservatives.
†Contains sodium bisulfite.

nation with other topical anesthetics (lidocaine, adrenaline, tetracaine [LAT], tetracaine, adrenaline, cocaine [TAC]). Topical tetracaine has a high incidence of allergic contact dermatitis and has largely been replaced by topical lidocaine.

Chloroprocaine

With the shortest $T_{1/2}$ among local anesthetics, chloroprocaine has a quick onset of action. Intradermal injection of this agent is associated with an uncomfortable burning sensation attributable to its lower pH [3]. It is not effective as a topical agent and is rarely used in dermatologic surgery.

AMIDE ANESTHETICS

Agents in this family are preferred as local anesthetics (Table 3). Due to their lower pKa, more drug crosses cellular membranes as compared with esters. They are much safer because of their lower incidence of allergic reactions.

Lidocaine

As the first synthesized amide, lidocaine has become the workhorse of local anesthetics. Lidocaine may be delivered as an injection or topically and has a rapid onset of action and an intermediate duration of action (30–120 min without epinephrine). It is the primary agent for local infiltration or in topical formulations. Xylidide is an active albeit weaker metabolite of lidocaine degradation.

Mepivacaine

Comparable to lidocaine in clinical use, mepivacaine putatively has a shorter onset and longer duration of action. One practical advantage is its higher maximal dosing which allows for usage of greater quantities (maximal dose without epinephrine: 7 mg/kg for mepivacaine, compared with 5 mg/kg for lidocaine). It is not effective topically.

Prilocaine

With a slower onset of action but a longer duration than lidocaine, prilocaine is rarely used alone. It is often used in combination with lidocaine as the topical anesthetic EMLA (eutectic mixture of local anesthetics). Unfortunately, prilocaine is also known for its unique adverse effect of methemoglobinemia. Methemoglobinemia occurs with the oxidation of iron from the ferrous to the ferric state and diminishes hemoglobin's oxygen carrying capacity. Clinical cyanosis occurs when methemoglobin levels are 10% or higher. Infants less than 3 months old, patients with congestive heart failure and/or pulmonary disease, and those with G-6-PD deficiency are most at risk. Prilocaine should also be avoided in patients with methemoglobin-inducing medications (e.g., dapsone, nitroglycerin, nitrofurantoin, phenytoin, chloroquine, cyclophosphamide, acetaminophen, nitroprusside, and phenobarbitol).

Bupivacaine

This agent is a favorite for nerve blocks because of its long duration of action (up to 4 h without epinephrine) and greater potency than lidocaine. It theoretically has

TABLE 3 Amide Anesthetics

Agent	Onset	Duration of action (min)		Maximum dose (without epinephrine)	Formulations	
		Without epinephrine	With epinephrine		Injectable	Topical
Lidocaine*	Rapid	30–120	60–400	4.5 mg/kg (no Epi) 7 mg/kg (+Epi)	0.5, 1, 2%	Table 5
Mepivacaine*	Medium	30–120	60–400	7 mg/kg	1, 1.5, 2%	None
Prilocaine	Rapid	30–120	60–400	Up to 400 mg within 2 hr period	4%	Table 5
Bupivacaine*	Slow	120–240	240–480	2 mg/kg or 400 mg daily max	0.25, 0.5, 0.75%	None
Etidocaine*	Rapid	200	240–360	4 mg/kg		None

*Available without preservatives.

a slower onset than lidocaine, which would render it impractical for local infiltration alone. Spivey et al. showed, however, that the onset of bupivacaine is only 30 seconds longer than lidocaine. Furthermore, patients receiving bupivacaine required significantly less postsurgical analgesia. Bupivacaine is often combined with lidocaine to capitalize on the advantages of both agents, producing a potent mixture with a quick onset and long duration. In a randomized, prospective, double blind study by Valvano and Leffler, bupivacaine 0.25% was compared with a mixture of bupivacaine 0.25% plus lidocaine 1%. The investigators found no differences in regard to onset, duration, and complications. Bupivacaine is not frequently a first line agent, however, because of its higher cardiotoxicity profile and lower maximal dose (Table 3). Bupivacaine is not effective topically.

Etidocaine

Etidocaine is a long-acting anesthetic in the class of bupivacaine. Its long duration (up to 3.5 h without epinephrine) is complemented by a rapid onset of action and a higher maximal dose than bupivacaine (maximum of 300 mg/injection for etidocaine and 175 mg/injection for bupivacaine). Injecting etidocaine causes a painful burning sensation.

TOPICAL ANESTHETICS

Within both classes, individual agents have been formulated in topical preparations (Table 4a). Examples include topical lidocaine ointment and gel for cutaneous or mucosal application. Mixtures of individual agents are also available such as EMLA (Table 4b). Topical anesthetics are popular because of their painless application and effectiveness depending on the procedure, patient age, and anxiety level. Topical anesthesia may be adequate for laser photocoagulation of tattoos, for example, but is inadequate for CO_2 laser resurfacing or scalpel surgery. In these latter procedures, topical agents may be adjuncts in negating the discomfort of local infiltration or the placement of intravenous access. Numerous studies have confirmed their effective-

TABLE 4a Topical Anesthetics: Single Agents

Anesthetic	Cream	Ointment	Spray	Solution	Gel
Lidocaine* (xylocaine®)	NA	2.5% OTC 5% Rx	2% spray 0.5, 1.0, 5% aerosol	NA	0.5, 1% jelly 2.5% film forming gel
Dibucaine (Nupercainal®)	0.5%	1%	NA		NA
Tetracaine (pontocaine®)	1%	0.5% (ophth)	NA	0.25, 0.5%	NA
Benzocaine† (cetacaine®)	5%	5, 20%	2% spray 20% aerosol		7.5% oragel 10% oragel D 20% orabase

*Also available as patches in 5% and 20%.
†Maximum use of 2 days for the gel.

TABLE 4b Topical Anesthetics: Mixture of Agents

Preparation	Ingredients
EMLA cream (eutectic mixture of local anesthetics)	Lidocaine 2.5%, Prilocaine 2.5%
TAC	Tetracaine 0.5%, Adrenaline 1:2000, Cocaine 11.8%
MAC	Marcaine 0.5%, Adrenaline 1:2000, Cocaine 10%
LAT	Lidocaine 4%, Adrenaline 1:2000, Tetracaine 1%
TLE (topical lidocaine with epinephrine)	Lidocaine 5%, Epinephrine 1:2000
LET	Lidocaine 40 mg/ml, Epinephrine 2.25 mg/ml, Tetracaine 5 mg/ml

TABLE 4c Recommended Dosing of EMLA Cream on Intact Skin in Infants and Children

Age	Body weight (kg)	Maximum total dose of EMLA	Maximum application area
1–3 months	<5 kg	1 gm	10 cm^2
4–12 months	5–10 kg	2 gm	20 cm^2
1–6 years	>10–20 kg	10 gm	100 cm^2
7–12 years	>20 kg	20 gm	200 cm^2

TABLE 4d Contraindications to EMLA

Infants <1 month or <12 months but on methemoglobinemia-inducing medications*
Usage on or near tympanic membranes (ototoxicity)
Glucose-6-phosphate dehydrogenase deficiency or patients prone to methemoglobinemia, from underlying disease or medications

*Methemoglobinemia-inducing agents: dapsone, nitroglycerin, nitrofurantoin, antimalarials, sulfonamides, phenobarbitol, phenytoin, nitroprusside, acetaminophen.

TABLE 4e Depth of EMLA Anesthesia

Duration of application (occlusion)	Depth of dermal anesthesia
60 min	3 mm
90 min	4 mm
120 min	5 mm

ness as single agents for the repair of lacerations in both facial and extremity wounds [8–12].

Tetracaine (0.5%)-adrenaline (1:2000)-cocaine (11.8%) (TAC) was introduced in 1980 as the first mixture of topical anesthetics. Onset of action is within 30 minutes and anesthesia is sufficient to repair scalp and face lacerations. Its efficacy was overshadowed by the toxicity of its ingredient cocaine, which included seizures, hypertension, euphoria, and even death from mucosal absorption. Elimination of cocaine, however, resulted in a loss of efficacy. Attempts to reduce the toxicity of TAC included lowering the concentration of cocaine and substituting tetracaine for marcaine [10]. Cocaine, however, remained an expensive and toxic ingredient as a controlled substance. Lidocaine (40%-adrenaline (1:2000)-tetracaine (1%) (LAT) became an alternative that compared more favorably than TAC for topical anesthesia in face and scalp lacerations [8]. Other amide-ester combinations appeared such as LET (lidocaine-epinephrine-tetracaine), but all suffered from the sensitizing propensity of the ester component.

EMLA

In the early 1980s, the lidocaine-prilocaine mixture known as EMLA emerged and heralded the most effective topical anesthesia to date. EMLA contains 2.5% lidocaine and 2.5% prilocaine, is preservative free, and consists of an oil-in-water emulsion. Eutectic describes a substance that melts easily, or a mixture in which the melting temperature is lower than any of its ingredients. EMLA provides effective anesthesia in a variety of procedures (e.g., shave biopsies, laceration repairs in children, venipuncture, epilation, collecting split-thickness skin grafts, electrodessication, and curettage) [14–19]. The onset, duration of action, and depth of anesthesia is dependent on the duration and site of application (Table 4e). Cutaneous application, for example, requires a minimum application of 1 hour under occlusion, whereas mucosal application may require only 5 to 15 minutes. A thick layer of 1 to 2 gm/cm^2 under occlusion for 60 minutes (1/10) of a 5 gm tube) is recommended by the manufacturer. Peak anesthesia occurs within 2 to 3 hours and lasts 1 to 2 hours after cream removal. Dermal anesthesia may reach 5 mm after a 2-hour application. EMLA appears to be less effective in children less than 7 years old (Table 4c).

Expected effects include skin blanching (37%), erythema (30%), and edema, all of which are transient. Systemic absorption is minimal. In one study, a 24-hour occlusion with EMLA to intact, nonmucosal skin only resulted in systemic lidocaine concentrations at 1/20 toxicity levels. Prolonged usage on broken skin or mucosa, however, may result in significant systemic absorption with the risk of methemoglobinemia secondary to prilocaine. Contraindications to EMLA use are few (Table 4d).

As a single agent, the role of EMLA in cosmetic surgery may be limited to superficial procedures. After 120 minutes of occlusive application, dermal anesthesia is up to 5 mm (Table 4e). The effectiveness of EMLA in abolishing pain is highly individualized, as is duration. Van der Burght et al. showed that EMLA application to genital mucosa resulted in anesthesia within 10 minutes for all the study patients, but duration was variable, ranging from 5 to 46 minutes [29]. Effectiveness of anesthesia for laser therapy has also been variable. Egkervist et al. reported that after 120 minutes, both the EMLA patch and EMLA cream provided total and equal analgesia for Argon laser treatment [28]. The discomfort from pulse dye laser (PDL) treatment of port wine stains (PWS), however, may not be completely abolished, especially in young children. Sherwood et al. treated 73 children of ages 5 to 16 with the PDL for PWS. EMLA effected a pain-free experience in 40% of participants and significantly reduced discomfort in others [30]. These differences in efficacy may be more related to variations in study designs than to EMLA itself. Such factors as duration of application, anatomic site, and patient age will all influence pain perception. Additionally, surgical apprehension or anxiety will alter reactions to painful stimuli. Pain is a product of not only nociceptive fiber transmission but also supratentorial interpretations. A highly anxious patient will thus experience more pain from the same stimulus than a calm and relaxed patient. Procedures amenable to EMLA anesthesia may include laser photocoagulation of tattoos, telangiectasias, or other superficial vascular lesions. Superficial chemical peels are also appropriate for EMLA although most do not require any anesthesia. More destructive procedures such as CO_2 laser resurfacing, dermabrasion, and deeper chemical peels will require adjunctive anesthesia. Goodman reported pain-free full-face dermabrasions with tumescent anesthesia and EMLA cream. No intrasurgical cryogenic sprays or additional sedation was necessary in this report [25].

EMLA alone is generally inadequate for incisional surgery. For example, cervicofacial rhytidectomies (facelift), hair transplantation, blepharoplasties, scar revisions, brow plasties, and forehead lifts require deeper anesthesia with nerve blocks, local infiltration, and/or conscious sedation. Other procedures, such as liposuction and ambulatory phlebectomy, are also not amenable to EMLA alone. In these cases, EMLA may serve to minimize the discomfort of local anesthetic infiltration or intravenous access.

Anesthetic Patches

Anesthetic patches are also effective methods of topical anesthesia. Their utility is limited by the patch size. Amethocaine and Lido-Gel (10% lidocaine with an absorption promoter) patches are as effective as EMLA but are not currently available in the United States [21]. Liposome encapsulated topical anesthetics are novel delivery systems that enhance drug penetration and duration while controlling drug release by acting as a reservoir depot [21]. These agents are under study and not commercially available. EMLA is now available in a disk/patch form.

Iontophoresis

Iontophoresis is a method that applies an electric current to increase the penetration of medications (20-60–fold increase in penetration over topical application) [34]. The effectiveness of iontophoresis requires the following: (1) a drug is charged or in the ionized form, (2) the electrodes are in the same charge as the drug, and (3) the condition treated be at or near the skin surface. The ionized medications are applied to the skin, over which electrodes are placed. An electric DC current charges the electrodes and repels the ionized medication towards the opposite charge. Medications delivered by iontophoresis have included topical anesthetics, antivirals, epinephrine, antibiotics, methylprednisolone, dexamethasone, and 5-fluorouracil. Conditions such as laceration repair, postherpetic neuralgia, varicella and herpes simplex infections, and superficial basal cell and squamous cell carcinomas have all been effectively treated with iontophoresis-delivered medications.

TABLE 5d American Society of Anesthesiologists Physical Status Classification

Class	Description
1	Healthy patient
2	Patient with mild systemic disease
3	Patient with severe systemic disease that is not life-threatening
4	Life-threatening systemic disease
5	Moribund patient with little chance of survival

reactions to amides. Antioxidants are part of anesthetics containing vasoconstrictors and have rarely been reported to cause anaphylaxis.

A patient allergic to an ester should avoid all agents within this class, as cross-reactions within esters are common. Cross-reactions among amides do occur but are less common. A patient sensitive to one amide may have intradermal testing to other amides to determine reactivity or, alternatively, use an ester agent (Table 5e). Cross-reactions between esters and amides do not occur unless the hypersensitivity is to the preservatives found in both.

An evaluation of allergic reactions begins with the history and symptoms. Anaphylaxis presents as a systemic IgE-histamine release and is associated with urticaria and/or angioedema, wheezing, pruritus, and shock with loss of consciousness. The patient has a reflex tachycardia and the skin is warm and diffusely erythematous because of histamine-mediated vasodilation. Symptoms may be localized to the injection site but are usually systemic. Treatment may range from oral benadryl for minor reactions to resuscitation efforts with intravenous benadryl and corticosteroids, subcutaneous epinephrine, and intubation and airway support for systemic events.

Type IV delayed hypersensitivity reaction requires prior sensitization and may also present with erythema, edema, and pruritus, but systemic symptoms are absent. An allergic contact dermatitis to topical antibiotics may develop. Type IV reactions are by far more common than Type I mechanisms among reactions to local anesthetics [6] (Table 5e).

These immune-mediated symptoms contrast with vasovagal or autonomic events. Vasovagal reactions are typically associated with high anxiety and autonomic reflexes to pain states. Subjectively, the patient admits to being apprehensive and anxious. Objectively, syncope may occur with pupil dilation, and the skin is cold and clammy rather than warm and red. An initial tachycardia from anxiety is followed by a reflex bradycardia from vagal stimulation. No histamine symptoms are seen. Treatment is supportive because most reactions are transient. Prolonged symptoms may be reversed by atropine.

Toxicity from local anesthetics may be attributable to impaired metabolism, excessive dosages, or inadvertent intravascular injections. Symptoms correlate with serum levels (Table 5a) and may be biphasic, with an initial excitatory stage followed by CNS and respiratory depression. Local anesthetics by themselves are vasodilators and are negative inotropes to cardiac function. Hypotension with bradycardia may ensue with cardiovascular collapse. The longer-acting amides (bupivacaine, etido-

TABLE 5e Skin Testing in the Evaluation of Local Anesthetic Allergy

Type	Mechanism	Utility/comment*
Patch Test	Type IV: delayed type hypersensitivity	Determines allergic contact dermatitis to anesthetic agent, preservatives or antioxidants. Not reliable in evaluating type I anaphylaxis reactions. T.R.U.E. test (Glaxo) contains benzocaine, tetracaine, and dibucaine in its caine mixture allergen. Hermal Allergen Patch test kit (Hermal Dermatology group) contains benzocaine as its caine representative.
Prick Test	Type I: IgE/Histamine Anaphylactic reactions	Not reliable, high rate of false positive reactions
Intradermal Skin Test	May measure both Type I and Type IV reactions depending when injected areas are evaluated	Injections are in serial dilutions of the anesthetic agent, beginning with a 1:1000 solution. Each injected dilution is observed for 15–30 minutes for erythema and urticaria in evaluating for Type I reactions. The site may be re-evaluated in 48 hrs to assess Type IV delayed-type hypersensitivity.

*All testing are performed separately with a preservative-free local anesthetic agent, methylparaben preservative, and metabisulfite antioxidant. Histamine serves as a control for immunologic reactivity and saline for dermatographism.

TABLE 5f Alternatives to Allergic Constituents

Allergic component	Alternative
Ester Agent	Amide agent
Methylparaben Preservative	Preservative-free amides (esters should not be used as, like methylparaben, it is metabolized to PABA)
Metabisulfite Antioxidants	Local anesthetics without vasoconstrictors, or if vasoconstriction and hemostasis is essential, a single-dose preparation of preservative-free epinephrine may be used separately.
Amide Agent	Intradermal testing to other amide agents, or refer to ester agents (ensure that the reaction was to the amide itself and not to the methylparaben preservative)
Both Amides and Esters	Benadryl (anesthesia within 5 min, duration $\leq$30 min), saline (for brief procedures, i.e., shave biopsies), refrigerant sprays
	General anesthesia

caine) have a greater risk of cardiotoxicity. Treatment is supportive and benzodiazepines may be given to raise the seizure threshold lowered by local anesthetics.

Epinephrine's adverse effects are direct extensions of its pharmacologic properties. Local vasoconstriction may result in ischemic necrosis of vulnerable sites or damage to proximal nerve branches. Transient hypertension may follow if intravascular injections occur. β-agonist effects may produce tachycardia, palpitations, arrhythmias, and tremors and may exacerbate or unmask uncontrolled hyperthyroidism or pheochromocytoma.

History alone may not be able to distinguish the possible causes of a claimed "allergy." Skin testing may be helpful in clarifying the origins (Table 5e) [6]. Testing is performed separately with a preservative-free local anesthetic, methylparaben preservative, and metabisulfite antioxidant. Equipment and personnel trained in resuscitative efforts is mandatory should anaphylaxis occur. Medications that may modify reactions (systemic antihistamines, over-the-counter preparations containing antihistamines, tricyclic antidepressants, and steroids) should be discontinued 1 week before testing.

ADJUNCTS TO LOCAL ANESTHESIA

Sensory loss to pain alone may not be sufficient for a calm and cooperative patient. This may be especially applicable to cosmetic surgery where the expectations are high and the patient may be anxious about the procedure or results.

An informed patient is by far better prepared, both physically and emotionally, for surgery. The presurgical consultation is vital in educating the patient to the details of the procedure, its postsurgical course and realistic outcomes, and potential complications. Many visits may be necessary to adequately educate the patient.

A highly anxious patient may benefit from anxiolytics the night before and on the day of surgery. Benzodiazepines, with their anxiolytic and amnestic effects, are excellent adjuncts to local anesthesia. Adequate time must be given for their onset of action and varies with individual agents and methods of administration. Benzodiazepines also reduce the risk of seizures when large doses of local anesthetics are required. Monitoring for respiratory depression is essential, especially if narcotics are used concurrently.

Nitrous oxide may be helpful in effecting sedation and increasing the pain threshold. The onset of action of nitrous oxide is rapid, as is its loss of effect and recovery once inhalation ceases. The above medications, with or without narcotics, in addition to local anesthesia may be part of a program of conscious sedation for ambulatory cosmetic surgery.

In addition to adjunctive medications, the operative environment is also important to a successful procedure. Calming music and voices, a confident and knowledgeable surgeon and staff, and distracting conversations and soothing reassurances are all helpful and cannot be overemphasized.

DELIVERY METHODS OF LOCAL ANESTHESIA

For many patients undergoing cosmetic surgery, overcoming the initial anesthesia is the primary hurdle. "How much pain will there be?" is the invariable question asked in the cosmetic consultation. The technique of injecting local anesthesia with minimal discomfort is itself an art and an essential skill for the surgeon and ancillary staff.

Informing the patient of each step may eliminate one part of presurgical apprehension: fear of the unknown. Few patients, however, will prefer not to know and only wish to be informed when the procedure is finished. The discomfort of local infiltration is related to the following three factors: (1) the initial needle insertion, (2) the pH of the anesthetic solution, and (3) tissue distention. Neutralizing the pH of local agents to minimize discomfort was previously discussed. Following are practical suggestions that I find helpful in administering local anesthesia.

General Recommendations
Describe in general the process of local infiltration. Descriptive phrases may include a burning or stinging sensation, a mosquito bite or sting, etc., although individual reactions will vary significantly.
Massage the area to be infiltrated, in circular or kneading motions. This serves as a sensory distraction for the patient. Additionally, local anesthesia is more efficacious when tactile stimulation to the affected nerves occurs just before injection.

Needle Insertion
Use the smallest needle possible (30-gauge).
Slightly pinch the site at the moment of injection. This is especially useful in sensitive areas such as the nose or digit. Insert the needle quickly.
A 60-minute occlusive application with EMLA cream will permit a pain-free local infiltration.
An ice cube or cryogenic spray at the site may suffice if time does not permit for EMLA.
Always insert within an anesthetized area to inject a new area. Inject from proximal to distal.

Tissue Distension

Inject the anesthetic slowly, rubbing or kneading the area as one injects. Slow injection will minimize the rate of tissue distention and reduce pain. Occasionally, stimulating another separate skin area may be preferred as a distraction. Speak to the patient in soothing tones during the injection, and involve the patient in conversation.
The depth of injection will also influence pain. Intradermal injection, producing a wheal, will effect immediate anesthesia but with greater discomfort because of more tissue distention. Subcutaneous injection, however, is slower in onset but results in less discomfort.
A nerve block may minimize direct infiltration into the site and reduce the volume of anesthetic agent needed.

BLOCKS

Field or Ring Block

A field block occurs when an area surrounding the surgical site, rather than the site itself, is infiltrated with local anesthetics. Anesthesia is injected circumferentially to include the site and the anticipated surgical field. It is essential that injection be both superficial and deep to create a "wall" of anesthesia surrounding the entire site. Ring blocks are advantageous when the surgical area is large, or when distention of the site by direct infiltration is to be minimized. Affected nerves usually include the tributaries of more than one named sensory branch. Extensive procedures on the scalp, for example, may be performed after a circumferential ring block in a "headband" fashion (Fig. 1a, 1b). Affected nerves in this block include the supraorbital and supratrochlear of the ophthalmic nerve (V1), the zygomaticotemporal of the maxillary nerve (V2), the auriculotemporal of the mandibular nerve (V3), and the lesser and greater occipital nerves from the cervical plexus. Various field blocks are illustrated below (Figs. 1–8).

Nerve Block

By anesthetizing the proximal branch of a specific sensory nerve, a nerve block attempts to affect the distal areas of its sensory distribution. Nerve blocks are more targeted versions of field blocks and rely on a precise knowledge of anatomy. Only minute volumes of anesthetic are needed to anesthetize a large surface area. The disadvantage of a nerve block lies in its lack of hemostasis afforded by local infiltration with an epinephrine-containing agent.

Cosmetic surgery often uses combinations of field and nerve blocks, in addition to local infiltration for hemostasis. Because most cosmetic procedures occur on the face, blocks affecting this area will be discussed in greater detail.

Sensory innervation of the face originates from the three divisions of cranial nerve V, the trigeminal nerve (CN V). These three divisions are the ophthalmic, maxillary, and mandibular nerves or V1, V2, and V3 respectively, and they give rise to smaller sensory branches. The major branches of V1, V2, and V3 are the supraorbital, infraorbital, and mental nerve, and they emerge from foramina of the same name. These foramina are classically depicted as lining up vertically along the mid-

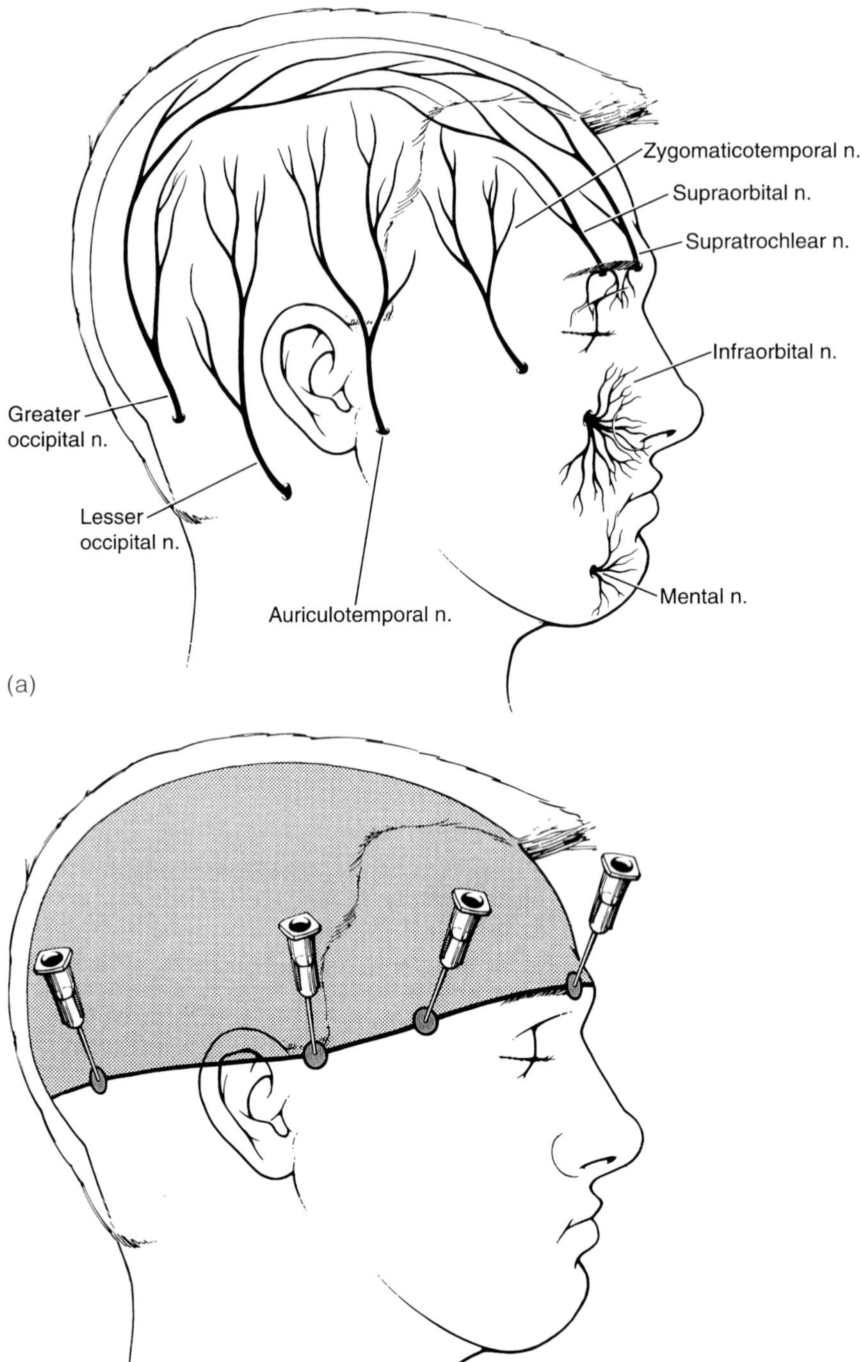

FIGURE 1 (a) Sensory nerves of the scalp. (b) Ring block anesthesia of the scalp.

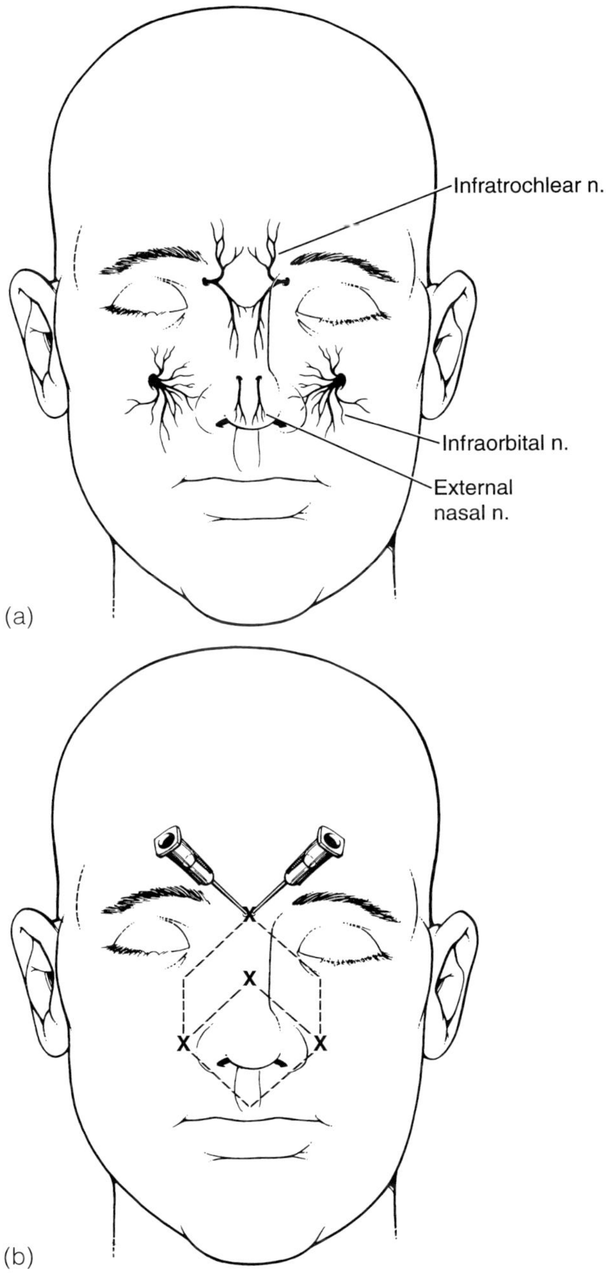

FIGURE 2 (a) Sensory nerves of the nose. (b) Ring block of the nose.

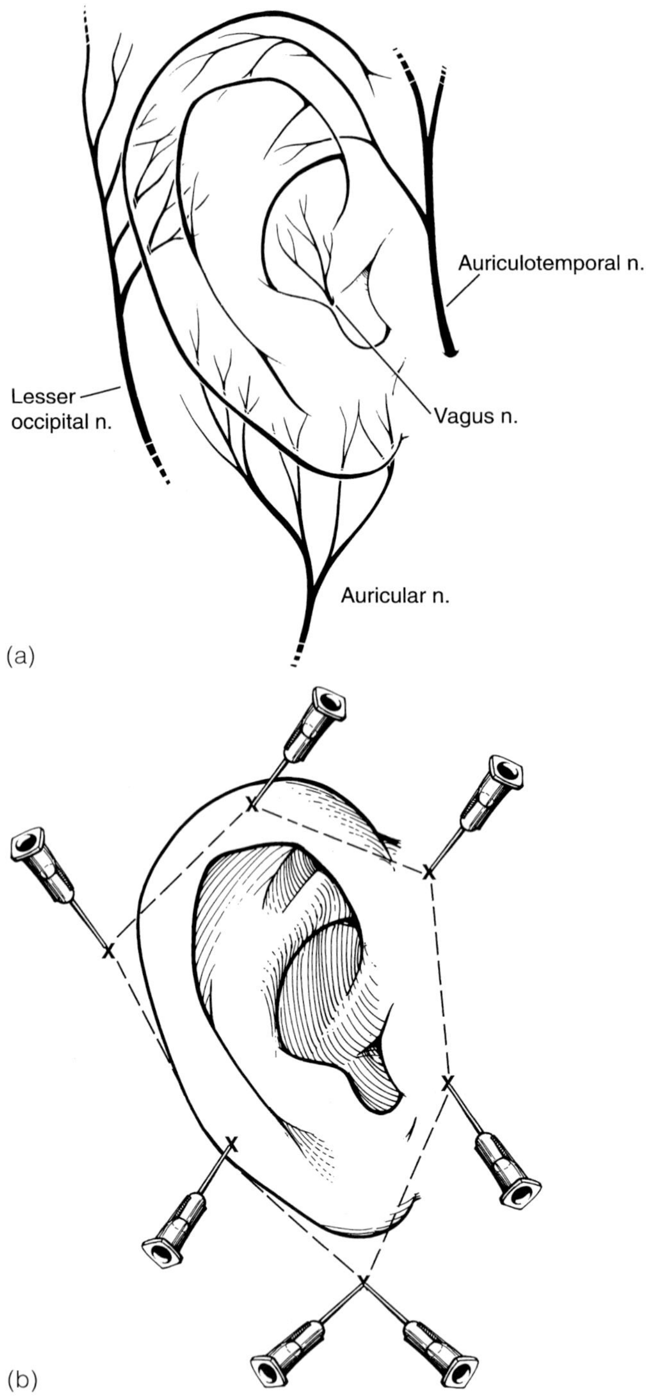

FIGURE 3 (a) Sensory nerves of the ear. (b) Ring block of the ear.

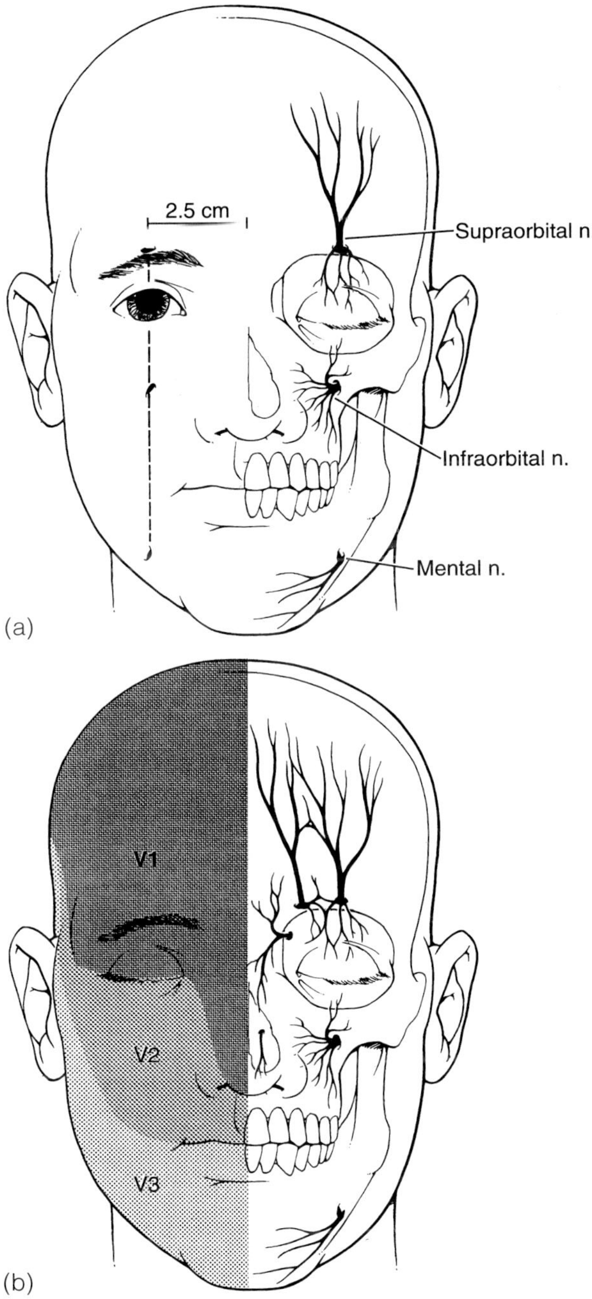

FIGURE 4 **(a) Midpupillary line location of the supraorbital, infraorbital, and mental nerves. (b) Anterior view, sensory zones V1, V2, and V3. (c) Lateral view, sensory zones V1, V2, and V3.**

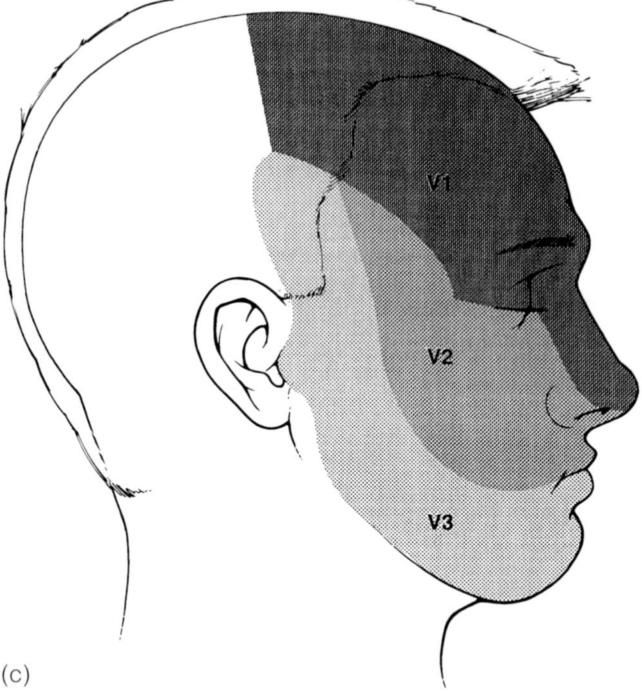

(c)

FIGURE 4 Continued

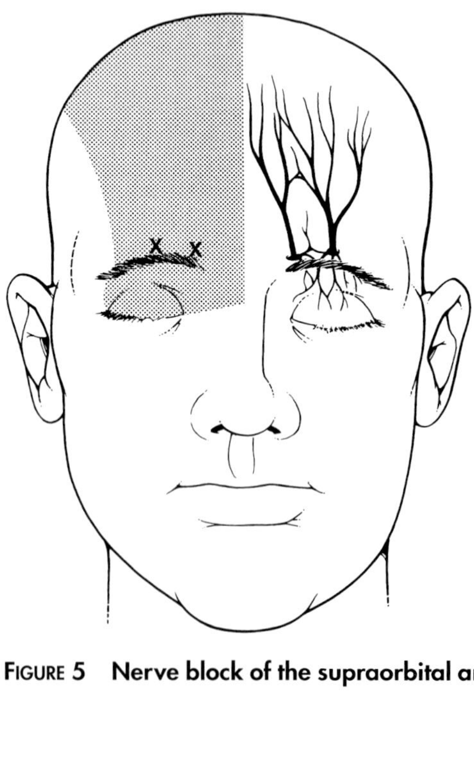

FIGURE 5 Nerve block of the supraorbital and supratrochlear nerves, zone of anesthesia.

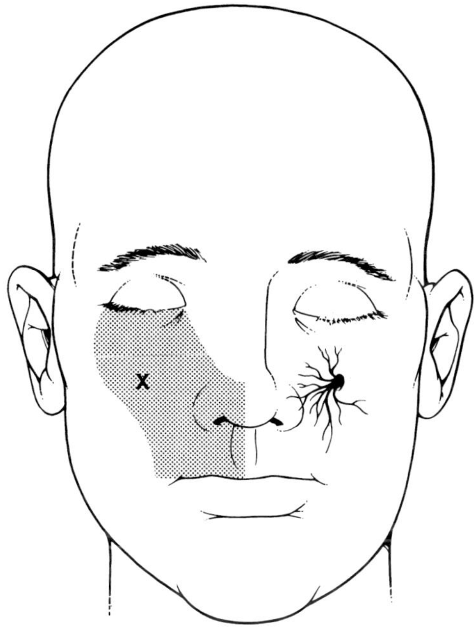

FIGURE 6 Nerve block of the infraorbital nerve, zone of anesthesia.

pupillary line, approximately 2.5 cm lateral to the facial midline (Fig. 4a). Cadaver dissections, however, reveal that they are millimeters slightly medial to the midpupillary line.

General Comments on Nerve Blocks

One must remember that sensory nerves travel in a neurovascular bundle. Any aspiration of blood or symptoms of paresthesia or shooting pain may indicate intravascular or direct nerve infiltration, in which case the needle should be withdrawn partially and redirected. This caution applies to all nerve blocks.

Applying EMLA or lidocaine gel 5 minutes before needle insertion will eliminate any minor discomfort of intraoral nerve blocks. Cutaneous approaches will require 60 minutes of EMLA cream application under occlusion or the EMLA patch.

Supraorbital Nerve Block (Fig. 5)

The opthalmic division (V1) enters the orbit via the superior orbital fissure. It consists of the lacrimal, supraorbital, supratrochlear, and infratrochlear nerves. These branches supply sensory innervation to the forehead and anterior scalp skin, the superior eyelid, and nasal root, dorsum, and tip and mediates the afferent limb of the corneal reflex. These nerves may be anesthetized by direct infiltration at their exit points into the skin. Injections must be deep to be effective.

Technique

1. Use a ½ inch, 30-gauge needle, on a 5 ml syringe.
2. Standing behind the patient's head affords the optimal position. One spares the patient from seeing the needle and can palpate the supraorbital ridge

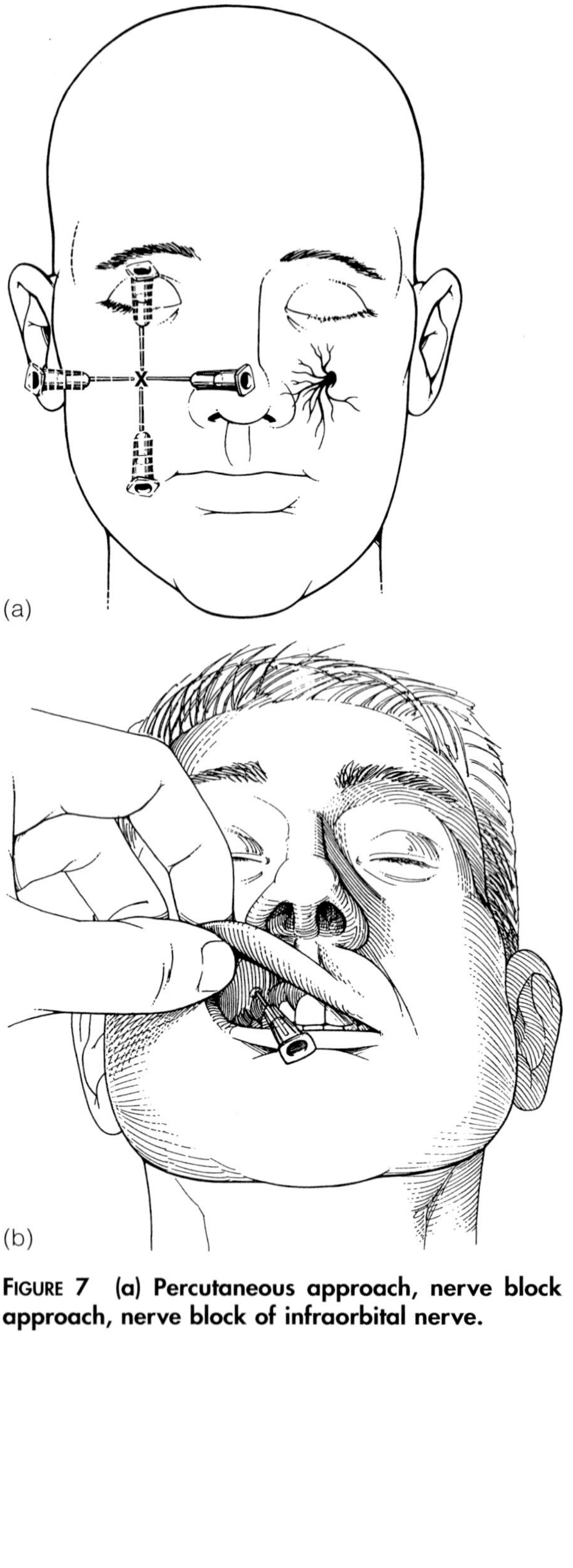

(a) (b)

FIGURE 7 (a) Percutaneous approach, nerve block of infraorbital nerve. (b) Intraoral approach, nerve block of infraorbital nerve.

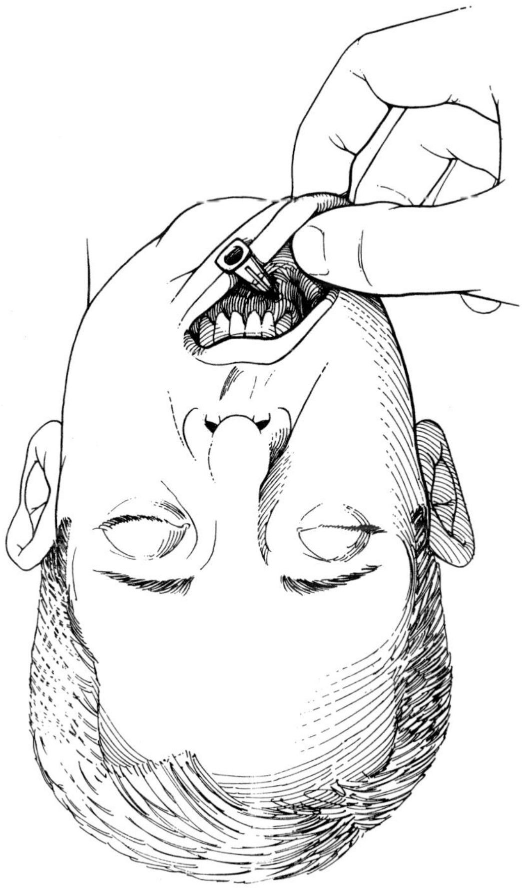

FIGURE 8 Intraoral approach, nerve block of mental nerve.

and notch easily. At the supraorbital bony ridge, raise a bleb of anesthesia at the skin over the desired nerve site. While aspirating, insert the needle perpendicularly to the skin until one reaches the periosteum. If periosteum is not reached after inserting half the length of a ½ inch needle, then withdraw and redirect the needle. This may indicate insertion into the foramen itself or past the orbital rim into the orbital cavity. Care must be taken to not inject past the infraorbital rim as the local anesthesia may affect the motor nerves and produce a transient ptosis.

3. Withdraw 1 to 2 mm from the periosteum and slowly inject 1 to 2 ml of the local anesthetic. One should avoid excessive volumes of anesthesia, as this may gravitate inferiorly and cause unnecessary albeit temporary periorbital edema and ecchymosis.
4. Massaging the injected area will spread the solution and enhance anesthesia.
5. Allow 15 minutes for maximal anesthesia.

Infraorbital Nerve Block (Figs. 6, 7)

The maxillary division (V2) enters the skull via the foramen rotundum. It consists of the infraorbital, zygomaticofacial, and zygomaticotemporal nerves and innervates sensation for the lower eyelid, upper lip and cheek, lateral lower nose, and the anterior temple. Its major branch, the infraorbital nerve, may be blocked from both a cutaneous and an intraoral approach, whereas the latter two can only be anesthetized by cutaneous infiltration. An intraoral approach is preferred for the infraorbital nerve for two reasons: (1) less discomfort with mucosal or intraoral injection, and (2) optimal access to the infraorbital foramen. The infraorbital foramen opens at the maxilla not directly anteriorly, but angles medially towards the nose. An intraoral approach angles towards the foramen direction, and thus enables optimal infiltration of the anesthetic solution.

Technique

1. Tilt the patient's head backwards and turn the patient's head slightly to face you. Identify the location of the infraorbital foramen. It lies at the midpupillary line and approximately 1 cm below the infraorbital rim. Place the fourth or third (middle) finger of the free hand here. With the index finger and thumb of the same hand, lift up and out the ipsilateral lip.
2. Use a 1-inch, 30-gauge needle on a 5 ml syringe. With the opposite hand, insert the needle at the gingival-labial sulcus above the upper canine fossa (third tooth laterally). Raise a bleb at the mucosa and insert superiorly and laterally (northwest) towards the finger marking the infraorbital foramen. The needle should traverse in a plane deep to the subcutaneous fat to reach the infraorbital nerve.
3. Slowly inject 2 to 4 ml of anesthetic surrounding this site. With the finger at the skin over the foramen, one will sense the slow swelling deep below from the anesthetic infiltration. If swelling is noted too superficially (i.e., in the subcutaneous fat or dermis), then withdraw the needle and insert in a deeper plane. Stop injecting if swelling is palpable superior to the marking finger. This may indicate injection above the infraorbital rim and into the orbital cavity.
4. Again massage the area and allow 15 to 20 minutes for adequate anesthesia.

Mental Nerve Block (Fig. 8)

The mandibular division (V3) includes the mental and auriculotemporal nerve and exists the skull via the foramen ovale. V3 provides sensory innervation to the lower lip and chin, posterior temple, external auditory meatus, and anterior external ear. Like the infraorbital nerve, the mental nerve is the primary branch of V3 and is best anesthetized from an intraoral approach.

Technique

1. Stand behind the patient's head and locate the mental foramen. The foramen lies at the midpupillary line, midway between the superior and inferior edge of the mandibular bone. Place the fourth or third (middle) finger of

the free hand here to mark the site. With the index finger and thumb of the same hand, retract up and out the ipsilateral lip.

2. Use a 1 inch, 30-gauge needle on a 5 ml syringe. With the opposite hand, insert the needle at the gingival-labial sulcus below the second bicuspid. Raise a bleb at the mucosa and insert inferiorly towards the finger marking the foramen.
3. Slowly inject 2 to 4 ml of anesthetic surrounding this site. With the finger at the skin over the foramen, one will sense the slow swelling directly below the anesthetic infiltration.
4. Again massage the area and allow 15 to 20 minutes for adequate anesthesia.

PROCEDURE-ORIENTED ANESTHESIA

Anesthesia for specific cosmetic procedures may combine local infiltration, ring and/or nerve blocks, or even tumescent anesthesia. Certain procedures, however, deserve special comment.

Facial Resurfacing

Resurfacing small cosmetic subunits, whether by dermabrasion, chemical peels, or CO_2 laser, may be accomplished by direct local infiltration or nerve blocks. If a full face or a large area is to be resurfaced, one must not forget the periphery of the nerve-blocked regions. Feathering procedures under the mandibular rim and angle will require additional local infiltration. The nose at the alar grooves and the base of the columella, and the commissures of the lips often require additional anesthesia as well. Although general anesthesia is usually not needed, adjunctive anxiolytics or conscious sedation is especially useful for extensive resurfacing. Some surgeons use Wydase® (hyaluronidase) in the anesthetic mixture (1:10 ratio, 0.5 ml hyaluronidase to 5 ml anesthetic) to aid in the extension of local anesthesia. Wydase® not only facilitates diffusion by spreading the anesthetic mixture but may also minimize edema. Alternatively, tumescent anesthesia is effective in large regions such as the cheeks. Tumescent anesthesia is especially advantageous in dermabrasion by providing both a firm skin surface as well as minimizing the bleeding associated with dermabrasion.

Blepharoplasty

Particular attention must be paid to the volume of anesthetic injected in this procedure. As mentioned, excessive volumes may result in unnecessary periorbital edema and bruising, which may last 7 to 10 days after surgery. Intra-arterial injection during supraorbital nerve blocks may have devastating consequences of visual loss, and mandates aspiration before injection. Anxiolytics are essential in all blepharoplasty procedures because of the anxiety associated with periorbital surgery.

Upper-lid blepharoplasty requires direct local infiltration. Local anesthetic is injected in the mid preseptal eyelid. From here, the needle may be directed medially and laterally to achieve total eyelid anesthesia.

Anesthesia for lower-lid blepharoplasty may vary depending on the percutaneous or transconjunctival approach. In the traditional cutaneous approach, local anesthesia is injected in two planes. The first injection is below the obicularis oculi muscle and above the orbital septum to create a plane of hydrodissection. The second injection is placed deeper, below the orbital septum to anesthetize the infraorbital fat pad. For the transconjunctival approach, these planes also apply, with extension of injections superiorly to the lower eyelid and conjunctiva.

Cervicofacial Rhytidectomies (Facelifts)

Like facial resurfacing, facelift procedures require a program of conscious sedation and anxiolysis if general anesthesia is not elected. Some investigators favor tumescent local anesthesia to facilitate a plane of hydrodissection intrasurgically, minimizing the risk of injury to facial nerves as well as the risk of lidocaine toxicity. Tumescent infiltration should not be too deep or transient motor nerve paralysis may occur, to the distress of both the surgeon and patient.

CONCLUSION

Wide options are available to the cosmetic surgeon for effective local anesthesia. No one method alone is sufficient for every patient. All patients require an evaluation of their pain threshold, anxiety level, and previous experiences. Cosmetic surgery is by nature elective and tailored to improve appearances. In no surgery, however, should our patients experience undue discomfort from our endeavors to do no harm.

REFERENCES

1. Wildsmith JAW, Strichartz GR. Local anaesthetic drugs—an historical perspective. Br J Anaesth 56:937—939, 1984.
2. Finks BR. Leaves and needles: the introduction of surgical local anesthesia. Anesthesiology 63:77–83, 1985.
3. Grekin RC, Auletta MJ. Local Anesthesia for Dermatologic Surgery. Churchill Livingstone Inc., 1991.
4. Eggleston ST, Lush LW. Understanding allergic reactions to local anesthetics. Ann Pharmacother 30:851–857, 1996.
5. Dzubow LM. The interaction between propanalol and epinephrine as observed in patients undergoing Mohs surgery. J Am Acad Dermatol 15:71, 1986.
6. Eggleston ST, Lush LW. Understanding allergic reactions to local anesthetics. Ann Pharmacother 30:851–857, 1996.
7. Vance JC. Anesthesia. In: Roenigk RK, Roenigk Jr HH, eds. Roenigk & Roenigk's Dermatologic Surgery. New York: Marcel Dekker Inc., 1996, pp. 31–41.
8. Ernst AA, Marvez-Valls E, Nick TG, Weiss SJ. LAT (lidocaine-adrenaline-tetracaine) versus TAC (tetracaine-adrenaline-cocaine) for topical anesthesia in face and scalp lacerations. Am J Emerg Med 13;151–154, 1995.
9. Kuhn M, Rossi SOP, Plummer JL, Raftos J. Topical anesthesia for minor lacerations: MAC versus TAC. MJA 164:277–280, 1996.
10. Blackburn PA, Butler KH, Hughes MJ, Clark MR, Riker RL. Comparison of tetracaine-adrenaline-cocaine (TAC) with topical lidocaine-epinephrine (TLE): efficacy and cost. Am J Emerg Med 13:315–317, 1995.
11. Vinci RJ, Fish SS. Efficacy of topical anesthesia in children. Arch Pediatr Adolesc Med 150:466–469, 1996.
12. Spivey WH, McNamara RM, MacKenzie RS. A clinical comparison of lidocaine and bupivacaine. Ann Emerg Med 16:752–757, 1987.

13. Valvano MN, Leffler S. Comparison of bupivacaine and lidocaine/bupivacaine for local anesthesia and digital nerve blocks. Ann Emerg Med 27:490–492, 1996.
14. Hjorth N, Harring M, Hahn A. Epilation of upper lip hirsutism with eutectic mixture of lidocaine and prilocaine used as a topical anesthetic. J Am Acad Dermatol 25:809–811, 1991.
15. Juhlin L, Evers H, Broberg H. A lidocaine-prilocaine cream for superficial skin surgery and painful lesions. Acta Dermato Venereol 60:544–546, 1980.
16. Rosdahl I, Edmar B, Gisslen H, Nordin P, Lillieborg S. Curettage of molluscum contagiosum in children: analgesia by topical application of lidocaine/prilocaine cream (EMLA). Acta Dermato Venereol 68:149–153, 1988.
17. Hallen B, Uppfeldt A. Does lidocaine-prilocaine cream permit pain free insertion of IV catheters in children? Anesthesiology 57:340–342, 1982.
18. Lahteenmaki T, Lillieborg S, Ohlson L, Olenius M, Strombeck JO. Topical analgesia for the cutting of skin grafts: a multicenter comparison of two doses of a lidocaine/prilocaine cream. Plast Reconstr Surg 82:458–462, 1988.
19. Zempsky WT, Karasic RB. EMLA versus TAC for topical anesthesia of extremity wounds in children. Ann Emerg Med 30:163–166, 1997.
20. Frayling IM, Addison GM, Chattergee K, Meagin G. Methemoglobinemia in children treated with prilocaine-lignocaine cream. Br Med J 301:153–154, 1990.
21. Lener EV, Bucalo BD, Kist DA, Moy RL. Topical anesthetic agents in dermatologic surgery. Dermatol Surg 23:673–683, 1997.
22. Bjerring P, Arendt-Nielson L. Depth and duration of skin analgesia to needle insertion after topical application of EMLA cream. Br J Anesth 64:173–177, 1990.
23. Covino BG. Local anesthesia (first of two parts). N Engl J Med 286(18):975–983, 1972.
24. Covino BG. Local anesthesia (second of two parts). N Engl J Med 286(19):1035–1042, 1972.
25. Goodman G. Dermabrasion using tumescent anesthesia. J Dermatol Surg Oncol 20(12): 802–807, 1994.
26. Barrasso R. Effectiveness of local anesthesia using EMLA cream for laser treatment of cervical and vulvar lesions. Contraception, Fertilite, Sexualite. 25(11):861–864, 1997.
27. McCafferty DF, Woolson AD, Handley I, Allen G. Effect of percutaneous local anesthesia on pain reduction during pulse dye laser treatment of port wine stains. Br J Anesth 78(3):286–289, 1997.
28. Egekvist H, Bjerring P. Comparison of the analgesic effect of EMLA cream and EMLA patch on normal skin evaluated with laser-induced pain stimuli. Acta Dermato Venereol 77(3):214–216, 1997.
29. Van der Burght M, Schonemann NK, Laursen IK, Arendt-Nielson L, Bjerring P. Duration of analgesia following the application of eutectic mixture of local anesthetic (EMLA) on genital mucosa. Acta Dermato Venereol 73(6):456–458, 1993.
30. Sherwood KA. The use of topical anesthesia in removal of port wine stains in children. J Pediatrics 122(5):836–840, 1993.
31. Meyer D, Linberg J. Iontophoresis for eyelid anesthesia. Ophthalmic Surg 21:845–848, 1990.
32. Kassan DG, Lynch AM, Stiller MJ. Physical enhancement of dermatologic drug delivery: iontophoresis and phonophoresis. J Am Acad Dermatol 34:657–666, 1996.
33. Ernst AA, Pomerantz J, Nick TG, Limbaugh J, Landry M. Lidocaine via iontophoresis in laceration repair: a preliminary study. Am J Emerg Med 13:17–20, 1995.
34. Gangarosa LP, Ozawa A, Ohkido M, Shimomura Y, Hill JM. Iontophoresis for enhancing penetration of dermatologic and antiviral drugs. J Dermatol 22:865–875, 1995.

21

The Pharmacology of Tumescent Liposuction

Jeffrey A. Klein
University of California at Irvine, Irvine, California

The essence of the tumescent technique is the direct infiltration of very dilute lidocaine (typically less than or equal to 1.5 g/L = 0.15%) with epinephrine into an area of subcutaneous fat resulting in an unprecedented slow rate of systemic lidocaine absorption. The secret to the success of tumescent local anesthesia is the synergistic interplay between the unprecedented slow rate of lidocaine absorption and the well-known rapid rate of lidocaine metabolism by the liver and subsequent renal excretion of less toxic metabolites.

The fact that tens of thousands of tumescent liposuction patients have received 35 mg/kg to 50 mg/kg of lidocaine with no know reports of deleterious effect gives proof to the safety of tumescent local anesthesia for liposuction. An understanding of the pharmacokinetics of tumescent lidocaine is necessary for safe tumescent liposuction surgery [1].

In this chapter, the word *dosage* implies the total amount of a given drug relative to the patient's weight in kilograms (mg/kg); a *dose* is a quantity of a medicine given at one time measured in milligrams (mg).

SAFETY WARNING

Safe dosages of tumescent (very dilute) lidocaine and epinephrine are not the same for "out-of-the-bottle" commercial (considerably more concentrated) lidocaine. Whereas the safe maximum dosage of tumescent (dilute) lidocaine (with epinephrine) at concentrations of between 0.05% and 0.15% is between 45 mg/kg to 50 mg/kg, the traditional dosage limitation for commercial lidocaine (with epinephrine) at concentrations of 0.5%, 1%, or 2% remains valid at 7 mg/kg. All physicians should be extremely careful to recognize this vital distinction.

PHARMACOKINETICS OF TUMESCENT LIDOCAINE

For tumescent local anesthesia, pharmacokinetics provides a basis for predicting safe dosages and for understanding the factors that might increase the risk of lidocaine toxicity. An accurate prediction of the maximum plasma lidocaine concentration (C_{max}) after a specific dose of tumescent lidocaine, and the time (T_{max}) when the peak concentration will occur, requires an accurate kinetic model.

The pharmacokinetics of lidocaine is based on the time course of concentrations of lidocaine measured at intervals in samples of peripheral blood. This is reasonable because of the close correlation between lidocaine concentrations in blood and in other tissues. Although lidocaine concentration in the blood is not the same as in other tissues, at steady state conditions the concentrations differ only by a constant factor.

Irrational Dosage Limits

The large doses of lidocaine used for tumescent liposuction appear excessive to physicians who are not familiar with the pharmacokinetics of tumescent lidocaine. There is a legitimate concern about the risk of toxicity. Fear and caution are the usual responses expressed by surgeons and anesthesiologists how have learned the "standard dose limitation of lidocaine" by rote memorization. Without a rational scientific basis, such dose limitations are literally irrational.

The traditional lidocaine dose limitation of 7 mg/kg remains a reasonable estimate of a maximum safe dose of lidocaine with epinephrine for commercial "out-of-the-bottle" lidocaine (concentrations that range from 1% to 2%) when injected into highly vascular tissue, such as for an intercostal block. However, this dosage limitation is unreasonably conservative for subcutaneous infiltration of very dilute lidocaine into fat. Because of the 7 mg/kg dosage restriction, surgeons and surgical training programs around the world have been compelled to subject patients to general anesthesia for procedures that are more safely and less painfully accomplished by tumescent local anesthesia.

Bulk Spread of Tumescent Anesthetic Solution

The process of tumescent infiltration involves the spread of the local anesthetic solution through the intestinal space by a process known as bulk flow. This is simply the flow of liquid through a porous substance such as the interstitial gel substance. The optimal distribution and spread of the tumescent anesthetic solution throughout the targeted compartment of fat is not instantaneous. Even with an optimal infiltration technique, it requires many minutes for local anesthesia and hemostasis to become optimal.

Upon incising the skin and examining the gross appearance of tumescent fat, one appreciates the marbled appearance of pale yellow lobules of fat embedded between the grey, glistening, diaphanous sheets of collagen and within the supersaturated interstitial tissue gel. The consistency of tumescent fat is gelatinous, soft, and jelly-like. This is literally the interstitial colloidal gel. Grape-sized puddles of anesthetic solution are loculated within and between connective tissue septa. The overall pattern is reminiscent of porous Swiss cheese or a honeycomb. These lakes of anesthetic solution act as physical reservoirs of lidocaine. As the liquid is dispersed through the substance of the interstitial tissue it is likely that some of the lidocaine is absorbed locally into the lipids contained within the adipose tissue.

Lidocaine Diffusion

True chemical diffusion only becomes important once the anesthetic solution is within a few millimeters of a targeted neural axon, or a capillary wall.

The tumescent lidocaine, consisting of free and tissue-bound lidocaine, is slowly absorbed into the intravascular compartment by a process of diffusion. The unbound (free) fraction of tumescent lidocaine arrives in the systemic circulation by the process of chemical diffusion across fibrous membranes and cells of the adipose tissue, through capillary endothelium and vascular walls, and into the intravascular space for transport throughout the circulation.

Profound Delay of Lidocaine Absorption

The absorption of tumescent lidocaine is exceptionally slow because

1. By elevating interstitial hydrostatic pressure above capillary intraluminal pressure, a large volume of tumescent infiltration compresses and collapses capillaries and venules. With virtually no blood flowing through the capillaries within the tumescent tissue, the rate of lidocaine absorption is minimized even before the onset of beta-adrenergic vasoconstriction. A small volume (e.g., 100 mL) of tumescent infiltration might not significantly compress local capillaries over an extended interval of time.
2. The formation of the dilute lidocaine subcutaneous reservoir produces a physical separation of the lidocaine from the blood vessels, thus increasing the distance over which lidocaine must diffuse before it reaches a blood vessel.
3. The dilution of lidocaine reduces the lidocaine concentration gradient across the capillary endothelial wall, thereby minimizing its rate of absorption.
4. The profound epinephrine-induced capillary vasoconstriction minimizes capillary perfusion and thus decreases transcapillary absorption.
5. The relative avascularity of adipose tissue limits vascular absorption.
6. Because of the high lipid solubility of lidocaine, the subcutaneous fat acts as a reservoir for lidocaine and limits the amount of lidocaine available for absorption. The sum of these additive effects account for the unprecedented profound slow rate of systemic lidocaine absorption.

The combination of very slow systemic absorption of tumescent lidocaine and rapid hepatic metabolism and swift renal elimination result in significantly low lidocaine blood levels and thus minimal risks of lidocaine toxicity.

Slow-Release Oral Tablet Analogy

The absorption of lidocaine from the subcutaneous deposit of tumescent anesthesia is analogous to the absorption of a slow-release tablet taken by mouth. When the anesthetic solution is in the subcutaneous tissue, it is isolated from the systemic circulation. Similarly, the drug contained within a slow-release tablet is not immediately absorbed into the systemic circulation. In both instances, the drug is contained within an isolated reservoir, and is released only gradually and absorbed into the systemic circulation incrementally.

One may regard the infiltrated subcutaneous fat containing the deposit of tumescent lidocaine as being analogous to the stomach or GI tract containing a slow-release tablet administered by mouth. Although the drug is technically inside the body, the anatomic site of drug absorption is kinetically distinct and isolated from the rest of the body. Under this assumption, the kinetics of lidocaine after tumescent delivery is analogous to the one-compartment model for oral administration of a "slow-release" tablet.

Absorption Rate Determines Peak Concentration (C_{max})

The maximum lidocaine plasma concentration (C_{max}) is directly affected by any factors that alter either the rate of lidocaine absorption or the extent of lidocaine absorption (systemic bioavailability).

For any given dose of subcutaneous lidocaine, anything that accelerates the rate of lidocaine absorption will result in both a shorter time interval necessary to achieve the peak plasma lidocaine concentration (C_{max}) and increase the magnitude of C_{max}. Not surprisingly, anything that slows lidocaine absorption will also delay the time (T_{max}) of occurrence of the peak concentration (C_{max}) as well as diminish the magnitude of C_{max}.

Absorption Rate Determines Duration of Toxicity

The rate of lidocaine absorption affects the length of time that the plasma lidocaine concentration remains above any specified concentration. When lidocaine absorption is rapid, the peak level is achieved rapidly and then the plasma concentration decreases rapidly. If a relatively small dose of lidocaine associated with rapid systemic absorption produces plasma concentrations that exceed the toxic threshold (6 μg/ml), then toxicity will be brief.

If toxic threshold concentration is exceeded after a prolonged absorption, then peripheral tissues will already be in equilibrium with the blood lidocaine, and there will be no rapid decrease in lidocaine blood levels. However, if toxicity does occur after a slow lidocaine absorption, then toxicity will persist for a relatively longer time.

Dilution Slows Absorption

A study with a volunteer showed 1% lidocaine was absorbed faster and had a higher peak than did 0.1% lidocaine, with total dose and infiltration rate held constant. In each instance, the total dose of lidocaine was 1000 mg, and the total dose of epinephrine was 1 mg. In each instance, the time allowed for infiltration was exactly 45 minutes. For 1% lidocaine, the magnitude of the peak plasma concentration was $C_{max} = 1.5\ \mu g/mL$, which occurred at time $T_{max} = 9$ hours. For 0.1% lidocaine, the $C_{max} = 1.2\ \mu g/mL$ and $T_{max} = 14$ hours.

Vascularity Affects Absorption Rate

Tissue vascularity affects the rate of lidocaine absorption. Absorption is slower from relatively avascular fat compared with highly vascular tissue of the gingiva or epidural space. A high blood flow rate through highly vascular tissue maintains the high concentration gradient across the vascular wall.

Vasoconstriction Slows Absorption

Epinephrine-induced vasoconstriction slows the rate at which blood can transport lidocaine away from the site of injection. The vasoconstriction induced by epinephrine is as vital for the safety of the tumescent technique as is the dilute nature of tumescent local anesthesia. Vasoconstriction not only prolongs the duration of local anesthesia, but more importantly vasoconstriction slows the rate of systemic absorption of lidocaine and thereby significantly reduces the magnitude of the maximum plasma lidocaine concentration.

Elimination after Tumescent Delivery

The rate of elimination of lidocaine after tumescent delivery is significantly different from the process of elimination after an IV bolus dose. An obvious difference is the total amount of lidocaine in a tumescent dose, up to 50 mg/kg is significantly larger than the typical IV bolus dose of 1 mg/kg to 2 mg/kg.

After tumescent infiltration, the lidocaine elimination process is prolonged by the continuous slow systemic absorption of tumescent lidocaine that persists for up to 48 hours. Elimination of lidocaine after tumescent infiltration is not greatly different from the rate of absorption of lidocaine from the tumescent fat. In fact, when the rate of lidocaine absorption is exactly equal to the rate of lidocaine elimination, the plasma lidocaine concentration is constant. When lidocaine absorption and elimination are equal, the concentration of lidocaine as a function of time will be a constant plateau.

The Concept of Drug Bioavailability

Bioavailability of a drug is defined as the fraction of a given dose that ultimately reaches a particular targeted tissue.

The concept of bioavailability is different from the concept of absorption. The study of drug absorption is concerned with the fraction that is absorbed from the site of administration and the rate at which a drug diffuses away from its site of administration and into the body's systemic circulation. The study of bioavailability is concerned with the fraction of dose that actually makes it to the site of action. In other words, a drug's bioavailability depends on both its absorption and its ability to penetrate certain barriers, and avoid metabolism or elimination on its journey to the site of the drug action.

Bioavailability of Tumescent Lidocaine

Tumescent liposuction is unusual in that the site of action is the local subcutaneous fat targeted for liposuction. Optimal local bioavailability requires a certain time for the tumescent solution to be dispersed by bulk flow throughout the targeted compartment and for lidocaine to diffuse into sensory nerves. In order to minimize lidocaine toxicity, one must minimize systemic bioavailability by minimizing systemic absorption.

Lidocaine toxicity is reduced by minimizing the amount of lidocaine that is absorbed into the systemic circulation. Thus, lowering the systemic bioavailability of tumescent lidocaine reduces the risk of lidocaine toxicity. it is our goal with tumescent liposuction to maximize local bioavailability and to minimize the systemic bioavailability of lidocaine.

Liposuction removes a percentage of lidocaine, and thus reduces the systemic bioavailability of lidocaine. Without liposuction, the systemic bioavailability of lidocaine after a tumescent infiltration would be 100%.

Open drainage and bimodal compression reduces the amount of systemic lidocaine absorption still further by increasing the amount of lidocaine that drains out of the body after surgery. Accelerated drainage of residual tumescent anesthetic solution is accomplished by using adits (punch biopsy holes of 1.5 or 2.0 mm in diameter) instead of incisions. If incisions are used, the drainage will be maximized by allowing incisions sites to remain open (not closing incisions with sutures). Finally, applying a high degree of uniform compression over the treated areas encourages a maximum volume of drainage.

A Maximum Safe Dosage Must Assume 100% Bioavailability

In determining the maximum safe dose of lidocaine for tumescent liposuction we must assume that liposuction may be canceled at the last minute, and that there will be 100% systemic absorption of lidocaine. After tumescent infiltration has been completed and before liposuction can be initiated, there is always a possibility that the patient or the surgeon will decide to cancel the surgery. In this unusual scenario, there will be 100% lidocaine bioavailability and an increased risk of systemic toxicity.

Thus, any estimate of a maximum safe dose of lidocaine for tumescent liposuction, must assume that there will be 100% systemic bioavailability. It would be foolishly naive to assume that liposuction will always be accomplished after tumescent infiltration is completed, and that the systemic bioavailability will be substantially less than 100%.

The 35 mg/kg Estimate

The first reasonable estimate of the maximum safe dose of tumescent lidocaine was 35 mg/kg and was published in 1990 in the Journal of Dermatologic Surgery and Oncology [1]. The dosage of dilute lidocaine at concentrations of 500 mg/L (0.05%) to 1,000 mg/L (0.1%) with dilute epinephrine at (1 mg/L = 1:1,000,000) ranged from 11.9 to 34.1 mg/k with associated peak plasma lidocaine concentrations that ranged from 0.8 to 2.7 μg/ml. This report also showed for the first time that T_{max}, the peak plasma lidocaine concentration for tumescent lidocaine, is achieved after the initiation of the infiltration. We now know that T_{max} typically occurs 8 to 14 hours after initiation of the infiltration.

Importance of Sentinel Cases

For the pragmatist, finding a reasonably safe dose of lidocaine for tumescent liposuction must involve caution and common sense as well as objective statistical logic. Sentinel cases of toxicity are a most important consideration. For example, there have been at least two liposuction-related deaths that occurred in patients who received general anesthesia and lidocaine doses of 95 mg/kg and 105 mg/kg. A surgeon who used general anesthesia has reported that more than 70% of his tumescent liposuction patients experienced nausea and vomiting after lidocaine doses in the range of 80 mg/kg. Yet another surgeon has reported that 30% of his patients had nausea and vomiting at average doses of 70 mg/kg. In my personal experience with several thousand patients, approximately 0.5% of patients have nausea or vomiting at doses below 50 mg/kg, and at doses between 55 to 60 mg/kg there have been about a 5 to 10% incidence of nausea and vomiting. From this information alone, it is reasonable to expect that the maximum safe dose of tumescent lidocaine to be in the range of 45 to 55 mg/kg.

To the best of my knowledge, at doses below 55 mg/kg the only reports of plasma lidocaine concentrations in excess of 6 μg/ml have been in association with adverse drug interactions mediated by the inhibition of cytochrome P450 3A4. Nevertheless, at doses of 50 mg/kg to 55 mg/kg of tumescent lidocaine there are occasional patients who experience nausea and vomiting approximately 12 hours after the tumescent infiltration. In these patients, whenever the plasma lidocaine concentration has been measured, it has never exceeded 3.5 μg/ml. To minimize the risk of this bothersome symptom, it is preferable to not exceed 45 mg/kg of tumescent lidocaine. Furthermore, the surgeon must not forget that these dosage limitations assume that there are no drug interactions and no unimpaired function of hepatic Cytochrome P450 3A4.

Except in unusual circumstances, 50 mg/kg should be regarded as a reasonable and safe dosage of tumescent lidocaine.

Formulation of Tumescent Anesthetic Solutions

There is no standard, official, rigidly prescribed, or canonical recipe for the tumescent anesthetic solutions. The optimal concentration of lidocaine and epinephrine in an anesthetic solution varies according to the clinical requirements. There is no "correct" or sanctioned concentration of lidocaine or epinephrine for tumescent local anesthesia. The recommendations in this chapter with respect to the concentration of tumescent lidocaine for liposuction of various areas of the body has been developed empirically. Years of experience and careful observation have helped define an estimate of the optimal concentrations. The goal is to determine the minimal concentration for each component of the anesthetic solution that consistently permits painless liposuction. Areas that are especially fibrous, such as the upper abdomen, the breast, and the back, also tend to be associated with increased surgical bleeding. The more fibrous areas tend to require a higher concentration of lidocaine and epinephrine. Less fibrous and less sensitive areas require lower concentrations. Recommended concentrations are simply guidelines and are always subject to modification (Table 1).

The use of smaller cannulas is associated with less discomfort and a smaller probability of encountering an area of painful liposuction. Thus the use of smaller cannulas allows the use of lower drug concentrations. The use of a careful deliberate surgical technique that initiates liposuction using the smallest cannulas and then increases cannula size sequentially causes less discomfort than beginning liposuction with relatively large cannulas.

Cumbersome Definitions of Dilutions

Commercially available formulations of local anesthetics usually specify lidocaine concentration in somewhat archaic terminology of "grams per 100 mL" or "grams

TABLE 1 Recommended Concentrations for Effective Tumescent Anesthesia for Liposuction

Areas	Lidocaine (mg/L)	Epinephrine (mg/L)	Sodium bicarb (meq/L)
Basic/checking	500	0.5	10
Hips Lateral Thighs Medial Thighs Anterior Thighs Knees Abdomen, Lateral	700 to 750	0.65	10
Back Male Flanks Arms	1000	0.65 to 1.0	10
Female Abdomen, Medial	1000 to 1250	1.0	10
Male Abdomen, Medial Male Breasts	1250	1.0	10
Female Breasts Chin/Cheek/Jowls	1500	1.5	10
CO_2 Laser Facial Resurfacing	600 mg/250 ml	1 mg/250 ml	5 meq/250 ml

percent." Thus a 1% lidocaine solution contains 1 g lidocaine per 100 mL of solution, which is equivalent to 10 mg/mL. Similarly the traditional, if somewhat quaint, specification for epinephrine concentration is defined as a ratio of 1 g solute to the number of milliliters of solution required to provide the desired concentration. For example, a 1:1,000 solution of epinephrine contains 1 g epinephrine in 1,000 ml solution, or equivalently 1 mg per 1 ml. Thus a tumescent solution having an epinephrine concentration at 1:1,000,000 contains 1 g per 1,000,000 ml, or 1 mg per 1,000 ml. These old-fashioned designations are sufficient when a surgeon simply needs to specify which of two or three possible off-the-shelf bottles of local anesthetics are being ordered. However, when ordering the formulation of customized solutions for tumescent local anesthesia, the antiquated method of specifying dilutions, as described above, require mathematical calculations that are cumbersome and prone to error.

Efficient Definitions of Dilutions

Formulations of tumescent lidocaine and epinephrine solutions should be specified in terms of milligrams per liter (mg/L). Similarly, the amount of sodium bicarbonate is specified in terms of milliequivalent per liter (meq/L). This method of specifying the formulation of a dilute solution of local anesthesia is easy for staff to use and understand. When multiple bags of anesthetic are used on one patient, this also provides a clear method for keeping track of the total dose (mg) of lidocaine that has been given.

Signed Written Orders

It is absolutely essential that the surgeon provide explicit written orders for the formulation of the tumescent local anesthetic solution. It should be standard policy that no solutions are to be mixed unless the surgeon has signed the orders and the orders are in the patient's chart. All orders for tumescent anesthesia should include: (1) documentation of patient's weight in kg, (2) the maximum desired dosage expressed in mg/kg, and (3) the exact amount of each drug to be included in the tumescent solution expressed in mg/L or meq/L.

I am aware of at least three cases where surgeons were charged, but not convicted, with criminal negligence because of apparent errors in lidocaine dosing that were attributable to imprecise or ambiguous written orders.

Avoid Medication Errors

It is preferable that a surgeon's formulary only stock 1% lidocaine commercial vials of lidocaine. The risk of a inadvertent overdose is vastly increased when 2% vials of lidocaine are available. I know of more than one incident where a patient received double the intended dose of lidocaine because a 2% lidocaine solution was used instead of the intended 1% solution. There are no dermatologic surgical procedures that cannot be accomplished with 1% lidocaine or a more dilute lidocaine solution.

Furthermore, it is preferable that well-trained licensed personnel do the actual preparation, that is, do the mixing of the ingredients for the tumescent solution. Unlicensed personnel may be more likely to make errors in the interpretation of anesthetic orders, or the actual mixture of the tumescent anesthetic solution. The actual mixing of the tumescent local anesthetic solution requires the immediate "eyes-on or hands-on" supervision of licensed medical personnel.

In order to avoid medication errors, it is probably safer to prepare the tumescent anesthetic solution in the surgical room at the time of surgery. Preparing the tumescent anesthetic solution in large batches, and far in advance of the individual surgery, may increase the risk of unrecognized contamination or inadvertent dosage errors. Concerns about safety, in particular, the avoidance of unanticipated mix-ups would appear to outweigh the possible convenience of preparing tumescent solutions intended for multiple patients far in advance of the time of surgery. From this perspective, any questions about the "shelf-life" of tumescent anesthetic solutions appear irrelevant.

All empty vials of lidocaine and all empty vials of epinephrine should be temporarily saved until the surgical procedure is completed. This precautionary strategy, or plan of action, will enable anyone to double-check the total lidocaine or epinephrine dosage. If there is a discrepancy between an intended dosage and the number of empty vials of lidocaine or epinephrine, then all the remaining tumescent anesthetic mixtures must be discarded and new mixtures prepared.

The safety of a surgical patient is ultimately the responsibility of all physicians, surgeons, and anesthesiologists in the surgical operating room. If an anesthesiologist is providing systemic anesthesia, the anesthesiologist must be completely informed about and concur with the total dosage of tumescent lidocaine. An anesthesiologist who is not cognizant of the lidocaine dosage (mg/kg) or the volume of subcutaneously infiltrated tumescent fluid may be unable to avoid adverse drug interactions or systemic fluid overload. When providing anesthesia for tumescent liposuction, any anesthesiologist who is unfamiliar with the pharmacology and pathophysiology of tumescent liposuction is not in compliance with the standards of the American Society of Anesthesiologists [2].

Postsurgical Sedatives

Patients should be told that the use of sedatives in the immediate postsurgical period may cause undesirable side effects. Sedative drugs such as diazepam (Valium®) should be avoided for the first 24 hours after tumescent liposuction. The side effects of benzodiazepines and other sedative-hypnotic medications produce symptoms that are easily mistaken for mild lidocaine toxicity, such as confusion, dysarthria, and unsteadiness or an ataxic gate, excessive sleepiness, and even nausea or vomiting. First, sedatives are not necessary in the immediate postsurgical period. Second, there is a high probability of an adverse drug interaction that increases the risk of toxicity, perhaps mediated by a mutual inhibition of the hepatic enzymes, such as cytochrome P450 3A4, that is responsible for the elimination of lidocaine and benzodiazepines. Third, a patient may self-medicate or overmedicate with sedatives or narcotic analgesics, and then, when unpleasant symptoms appear, the patient may vehemently deny taking any extra medication. Last, the preemptive use of diazepam under the mistaken assumption that the diazepam will reduce the risk of lidocaine-induced seizures is contraindicated. The postsurgical use of diazepam may actually increase the risk of lidocaine toxicity.

The common misperception that premedication with a benzodiazepine such as Valium will prevent lidocaine-induced seizures after tumescent liposuction is an erroneous concept. Postsurgical sedation is usually unnecessary and is a potentially dangerous practice. The preemptive use of diazepam is contraindicated and is unsupported by objective clinical studies. Diazepam can depress the respiratory drive and impair ventilation, as well as result in respiratory acidosis that predisposes to lidocaine-induced seizures. A dose of diazepam that is sufficient to treat a seizure can also be expected to suppress respiration. The use of intravenous diazepam to treat seizures always presupposes the presence of trained medical personnel to provide adequate respiratory support.

Avoid Bupivacaine

Bupivacaine is a larger and less soluble molecule than lidocaine. For example, adding 5 meq of sodium bicarbonate to 50 ml of bupivacaine (0.75%) will result in the immediate precipitation of the bupivacaine. Injecting such a suspension intradermally or subcutaneously has caused full-thickness dermal necrosis.

EPINEPHRINE

Epinephrine is responsible for the profound vasoconstriction and consequent hemostasis for which the tumescent technique is famous. Significant toxicity attributable to tumescent (very dilute) epinephrine is extremely rare. Nevertheless, postsurgical sinus tachycardia can occur. Minimizing the concentration of epinephrine will minimize the incidence of transient sinus tachycardia. Clonidine also reduces the incidence of epinephrine-associated tachycardia.

Adverse Reactions to Epinephrine

Simple adverse reactions to therapeutic epinephrine can be caused by either a pharmacologic hypersensitivity or an immune-medicated allergic reaction to an additive. More complex adverse reactions involve adverse drugs interactions in which therapeutic doses of epinephrine interact with other therapeutic agents.

Despite the fact that life is impossible without endogenous epinephrine, there are patients who have a true clinical hypersensitivity to therapeutic doses of epinephrine. In some patients tachycardia is precipitated by a routine therapeutic dose of epinephrine; it is the result of a labile or hypersensitive cardiac sinus pacemaker, sino-atrial node, or myocardial conduction systems. Other patients may have an allergic-like hypersensitivity to bisulfate, an antioxidant often added to pharmacologic preparations containing epinephrine.

The most common adverse reaction to epinephrine is simply the predictable normal pharmacologic response to the rapid absorption of a therapeutic dose of epinephrine. For example, a rapidly absorbed dental injection of lidocaine with epinephrine will induce a pharmacologic supraventricular tachycardia. It is not unusual for patients to be incorrectly told that a pharmacologic tachycardia is an allergic reaction.

Epinephrine Interaction with Beta-Blockers

In my experience there have been no adverse events when patients on propranolol are given tumescent local anesthesia. Nevertheless, there are a few case reports in the literature of severe hypertension after an injection of out-of-the-bottle commercial concentrations of local anesthetics containing relatively high concentrations of epinephrine.

It is common to encounter prospective liposuction patients who are taking propranolol or another beta-blocker for either migraine headaches or hypertension. Relatively large doses of very dilute epinephrine in the clinical setting of tumescent anesthesia have not shown any clinically apparent adverse drug interactions with the concomitant use of beta-blocker drugs such as propranolol. My patients are not asked to discontinue propranolol before tumescent liposuction. Although clinical judgment must be used, it is generally not necessary to interrupt propranolol treatment of migraine headaches or hypertension as a prerequisite to tumescent liposuction. Presumably the rate of systemic absorption of epinephrine from tumescent subcutaneous fat is too slow to permit any significant adverse interaction.

Other Epinephrine–Drug Interactions

Clinically significant drug interactions with local anesthetics usually involve either lidocaine metabolism via hepatic cytochrome P450 3A4, or epinephrine adrenergic agonist effects with other vasoactive drugs. Epinephrine is contraindicated in patients with significant cardiovascular disease, peripheral vascular disease, hyperthyroidism, pheochromocytoma, and in any patients taking the drugs listed below.

Monoamine oxidase inhibitors (MAOI), tricyclic antidepressants, butyrophenones such as droperidol (Inapsine®), and phenothiazines may interact adversely with epinephrine to produce severe hypotension or hypertension.

Oxytocin-like drugs that induce labor interact with epinephrine-like drugs to produce malignant hypertension and cerebrovascular accidents.

Cocaine, which blocks the reuptake of norepinephrine, interacts adversely with lidocaine by reducing the seizure threshold and with epinephrine by augmenting systemic vasoconstriction and tachycardia.

Hyperthyroidism, induced either endogenously, iatrogenically, or by intentional drug abuse, can interact adversely with epinephrine to precipitate supraventricular tachycardia.

CLONIDINE

Clonidine (Catapres®) is a highly selective alpha-2 adrenergic agonist that has a number of desirable attributes as an oral sedative for surgery by local anesthesia. Clonidine 0.1 mg and the benzodiazepine lorazepam 1 mg, both given orally, are now the preferred persurgical sedatives for tumescent liposuction totally by local anesthesia.

Clonidine is an antihypertensive especially effective for treating severe or malignant hypertension. Many patients with malignant hypertension who are given 0.1 mg of clonidine while in the emergency room respond so well that by the time they are admitted to the intensive care unit they do not require intravenous treatment therapy. Because of its "bothersome" sedative effect, clonidine is usually not acceptable among ambulatory patients for the long-term therapy for hypertension.

Clonidine Sedation

Sedation is the most consistent central effect of $\alpha 2$ adrenergic agonists [3]. Although sedation is an undesirable pharmacologic side-effect for an antihypertensive drug, it is a most desirable effect in conjunction with outpatient surgery by local anesthesia. Clonidine synergistically increases the potency of benzodiazepines such as lorazepam and midazolam [4]. Clinical doses of $\alpha 2$ andrenoreceptor agonists do not depress respiratory drive and are not associated with hypoxia or hypercapnia. The lack of respiratory depression is one of the principal benefits of clonidine as a sedative.

Clonidine Anxiolysis

Anxiolysis is process of eliminating or alleviating anxiety and worry. Clonidine has been shown to have anxiolytic effects independent of its sedative effect [5]. The $\alpha 2$ agonists reduce anxiety to a degree that is comparable with the benzodiazepines [6]. Clonidine can suppress panic disorder in humans [7]. Clonidine attenuates the stress response to surgical trauma, and decreases the sympathoadrenal outflow [8].

Clonidine, Bradycardia, and Hypotension

The cardiovascular effects of clonidine include bradycardia, hypotension, and an antiarrhythmia effect, all of which are advantageous in the clinical setting of tumescent liposuction. The $\alpha 2$ agonists can prevent epinephrine-induced arrhythmias [9].

By inhibiting the release of norepinephrine from peripheral sympathetic presynaptic nerve endings, $\alpha 2$ agonists lower the heart rate, or at least counteract the tachycardia associated with epinephrine. Although the ability of clonidine to lower pulse rate and lower blood pressure is desirable, excessive degrees of bradycardia and hypotension are potentially dangerous side effects.

Clonidine and Tumescent Liposuction

The sedative effects of $\alpha 2$ adrenoceptor agonists are ideal for tumescent liposuction totally by local anesthesia. The use of clonidine has significantly reduced the incidence of intrasurgical tachycardia that had previously been encountered as a result of the epinephrine absorption after tumescent infiltration. It is not uncommon for patients with a history of hypertension to arrive in the surgical room with elevated blood pressure despite ongoing treatment for hypertension. In this situation, clonidine, in a 0.1 mg dose, has proved to be valuable in lowering the blood pressure to acceptable levels, thereby avoiding a cancellation of the scheduled surgery. Clonidine acts synergistically with benzodiazepines to produce excellent sedation.

For outpatient tumescent liposuction surgery, clonidine is given as a single 0.1 mg oral dose. Hypotension or bradycardia are rarely a problem at a dose of 0.1 mg. One should avoid giving more than 0.1 mg of clonidine to any tumescent liposuction patient. On the one occasion that a patient was given a second 0.1 mg of clonidine, the result was a 3-hour delay before discharge because of a prolonged episode of orthostatic hypotension. If a patient requires additional sedation, it would be preferable to give a benzodiazepine such as lorazepam 1 mg by mouth, or alternatively a small dose of intravenous midazolam in 1 mg to 2 mg increments.

REFERENCES

1. Klein JA. Tumescent Technique: Tumescent Anesthesia and Microcannular Liposuction. St. Louis: Mosby, 2000.
2. American Society of Anesthesiologists. Standards, Guidelines and Statements. 1998, p. 21.
3. Doze VA, Chen BX, Maze M. Dexmedetomidine produces a hypnotic-anesthetic action in rats via activation of central $\alpha 2$-adrenoreceptors. Anesthesiology 71:75, 1989.
4. Salonen M, Reid K, Maze M. Synergistic interaction between $\alpha 2$-adrenergic agonists and benzodiazepines in rats. Anesthesiology 76:1004, 1992.
5. Handley SL, Mithani S. Effects of alpha-adrenoceptor agonists and antagonists in a maze-exploration model of 'fear'-motivated behaviour. Naunyn-Schmiedebergs Arch Pharmacol 327:1–5, 1984.
6. Ferrari F, Tartoni PL, Margiafico V. B-HT 920 antagonizes rat neophobia in the X-maze test. Arch Int Pharmacodyn Ther 298:7–14, 1989.
7. Uhde TW, Stein MB, Vittine BJ, et al. Behavior and psychologic effects of short-term and long-term administration of clonidine in panic disorder. Arch Gen Psychiatry 46:170, 1989.
8. Langer EZ. Presynaptic regulation of catecholamine release. Biochem Pharmacol 23: 1793, 1974.
9. Hayashi Y, Sumikawa K, Maze M, et al. Dexmedetomidine prevents epinephrine-induced arrhythmias through stimulation of central $\alpha 2$ adrenoceptors in halothane-anesthetized dogs. Anesthesiology 75:113, 1991.

22

Laser Removal of Vascular Lesions, Scars, Warts, and Poikiloderma

Robin Ashinoff
New York University, New York, New York

INTRODUCTION

The laser removal of vascular lesions has progressed greatly over the last twenty years (Table 1). Initially, research efforts were directed towards treating congenital lesions such as portwine stains and then infantile hemangiomas [1–3]. It soon became apparent that these lasers were useful in the removal of facial telangiectasias [4–11], rosacea erythema [12–15], poikiloderma of Civatte [16], warts [17], scars [18,19], and perhaps striae [20]. Lasers have become a more efficient, less destructive method of treatment in the therapy of many skin lesions and the treatment of choice in the removal of others.

The first lasers developed for the treatment of vascular lesions were continuous wave lasers such as the argon and argon-pumped tunable dye laser. These lasers, in general, carry a greater risk of scarring because of nonselective heating of surrounding tissue. Other lasers used to treat vascular lesions include quasicontinuous wave lasers such as the copper vapor [21–25], copper bromide [26], krypton [11], and potassium titanyl phosphate (KTP) lasers [27–29]. In addition, the Photoderm VL (ESC Medical Systems, Haifa, Israel) is not a laser but an intense pulsed light source that emits light at variable pulse durations, intervals, and wavelengths [30–35].

The greatest milestone in clinical laser development was the proposal of the theory of selective photothermolysis which paved the way for the development of the flashlamp-pumped pulsed dye laser [1,2]. This revolutionized the treatment of vascular lesions especially in children, where the use of argon or other continuous wave lasers was complicated by an unacceptable rate of scarring or permanent pigmentary alteration.

The trend today is for laser manufacturers to develop systems that combine capabilities such as removal of vascular and pigmented lesions to become more cost effective for physicians.

In this chapter, we will first discuss the lasers and light sources commonly in clinical use and then, in detail, their use in the treatment of vascular lesions, poikiloderma, scars/striae, and warts.

TABLE 1 Vascular Lasers

	Wavelength (nm)	Best Rx	Features	Concerns
Argon	488–514/cw	Mucosal venous malformations Large facial vessels	Can use with scanner/ gated small spot ≤1 mm	Scarring permanent hypopigmentation
CW Dye	488–630/cw	Discrete facial vessels	Can use with scanner, gated No purpura	Scarring pigmentary alterations
Copper Vapor Copper Bromide	511/578/cw	Discrete facial vessels	Can use with scanner —No purpura	Scarring pigmentary problems
Krypton	521–530/568/cw	Discrete facial vessels	.1-1 mm spot No purpura	Scarring pigmentary problems
KTP	532/cw	Discrete facial vessels	Can use scanner—No purpura	Scarring, pigmentary problems
Photoderm VL	Light source 500–1100, 515, 550, 570, 590	Deeper vessels, leg veins/ resistant PWS	Variety of fluences, modes and pulse durations, 8 × 35 mm spot size No purpura	Scars; many parameters to choose/difficult to master
Versapulse	532/cw	Facial/leg veins	No purpura	Scars/pigmentary problems
PDL	585/Pulsed	PWS/Rosacea Erythema	User friendly ≤10 mm spot	Purpura/Temporary pigmentary alterations
Sclerolaser	585, 590, 595, 600 Pulsed	Leg veins Resistant PWS	User friendly Large 2 × 7 mm spot	Purpura/ hyperpigmentation

ARGON LASER

The argon laser is a continuous wave laser that emits visible blue-green light with six absorption peaks between 488 and 514 nm. The laser energy can be gated or shuttered to emit a pulse duration of 50.0 ms to 0.3 seconds through a fiberoptic cable, with powers of 0.8 to 2.9 watts and spot sizes of 0.1 and 1.0 mm [15,36–44]. The emission wavelengths of the argon laser are absorbed by oxyhemoglobin as well as melanin. This can cause permanent pigmentary changes in dark skin as well as being less effective in these patients [43]. In addition, because the length of laser exposure exceeds that of the typical cutaneous vessel, thermal injury can spread to surrounding tissues and cause scarring [9,15,45–48]. Histological analyses of vascular lesions treated with the argon laser have shown that clearance occurs because of perivascular fibrosis which occurs over time [21,47–49]. Therefore, it is important not to retreat an area with argon laser too quickly because perivascular fibrosis could take several months to occur.

The argon laser was the first vascular laser used to treat port wine stains in children. However, this resulted in an almost 20% incidence of hypopigmentation and an unacceptable degree of hypertrophic scarring, especially on the neck and upper lip [9,45–49]. This laser has also been used in the treatment of telangiectasias [40,42,50,51], cherry angiomas [36], venous lakes [52], pyogenic granulomas, Kaposi's sarcoma, angiokeratomas, and angiofibromas [37,40,43,50]. The argon laser has also been used successfully in the treatment of keloids and hypertrophic scars [53]. One would also want to make sure that a patient is not on isotretinoin before performing argon laser treatment because as with dermabrasion, this has resulted in an increased incidence of keloid and hypertrophic scar formation [54–56]. Retinoids have been shown to inhibit collagenase synthesis in fibroblast cultures, and therefore this may account for the higher incidence of abnormal healing after isotretinoin use [56]. Scarring as long as 9 months after use has been seen in patients undergoing dermabrasion and argon laser treatment [54,55].

The use of the argon laser requires more training and skill than many of the pulsed lasers in use today. I still find it useful for larger-caliber vessels on the alae as well as mucosal venous malformations where the excess thermal injury is needed in order to coagulate larger vascular channels. In general, the use of the argon laser has fallen out of favor since the development of more selective lasers.

ARGON-PUMPED TUNABLE DYE LASER

The argon-pumped tunable dye laser contains a fluorescent organic dye like rhodamine that absorbs light at one wavelength and emits light of another wavelength [36,57–59]. This laser emits a band of wavelengths ranging from 488 nm to 638 nm [58]. To treat most vascular lesions, including port wine stains, this laser is most often used at a wavelength of 577 or 585 nm. The laser light is produced in a continuous fashion but can be mechanically or electronically shuttered to produce shorter pulses. The argon-pumped tunable dye laser can be used to treat facial telangiectasias, rosacea-associated erythema, poikiloderma of Civatte, and port wine stains (Fig. 1) [4–6,15,41,60]. Port wine stains have been treated with a very tedious tracing technique using a .1 mm spot size at 0.1 to 0.4 watts [4,58,61]. When using the flexible fiberoptic cable on this laser one must use loop magnification of 3 to 8× to trace out vessels or to cover a port wine stain. One observes blanching of the treated site with mild edema and crusting afterwards. Although most laser surgeons would prefer not to use this laser in this fashion, excellent results have been achieved with minimal morbidity such as scarring or pigmentary alterations [7].

Robotized scanning devices can also be used with the argon-pumped tunable dye laser in an attempt to automate the delivery of laser energy and produce greater selectivity and reproducibility of results. These devices has resulted in faster, less painful treatments and more homogenous lightening than treatments done by tracing [8,62,63]. One would choose a fluence of 18 to 20 J/cm^2 and a pulse duration of 30 to 100 ms for smaller vessels and a fluence of 20 to 22 J/cm^2 for larger vessels [4,10,11].

I have had the opportunity to use this laser with and without a robotized scanner. I found no advantage of the scanner over using a pulsed dye laser at 1 Hz for port wine stain therapy. I use this laser for larger-caliber facial, especially nasal, vessels, or when a patient does not want the purpura associated with the pulsed dye

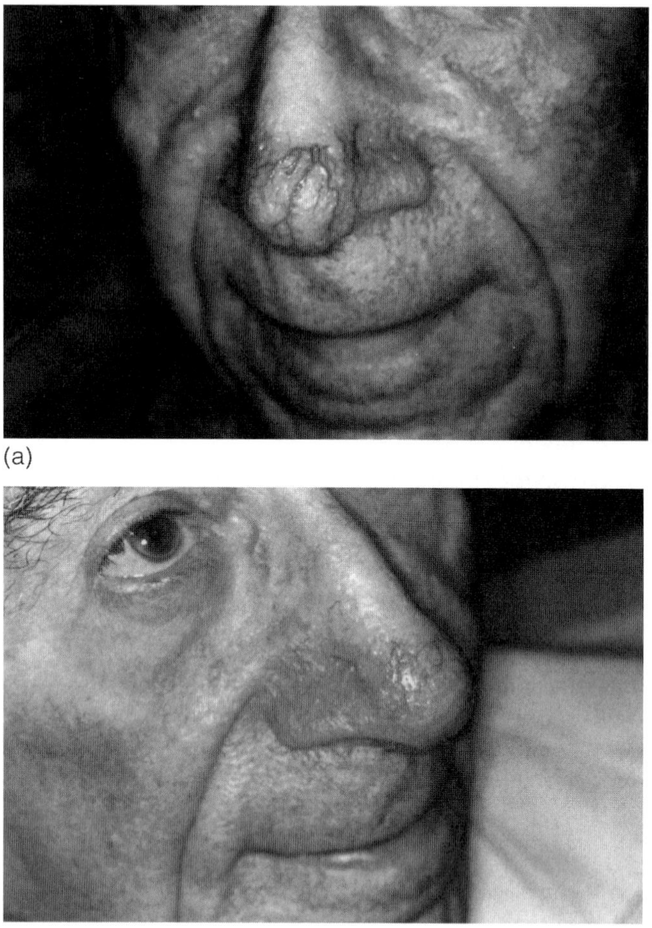

(a)

(b)

FIGURE 1 (a) Numerous large-caliber vessels on the nose before treatment with the argon-pumped tunable dye laser using 1 watt of power and a 1 mm spot. (b) Two months after one treatment to the larger vessels on the nose there is significant clearing without scarring.

laser. Because it is a continuous wave laser, more experience is needed to safely treat patients and the incidence of scarring and hypopigmentation are greater than pulsed lasers [5].

COPPER VAPOR LASER/COPPER BROMIDE

Both the copper vapor and copper bromide lasers emit at two wavelengths, 511 nm (green) light for the treatment of pigmented lesions and 578 nm (yellow) for the treatment of vascular lesions [23,58]. These lasers both heat elemental copper or copper salts in the optical cavity of the laser to produce a chain of short 20 to 40 nanoseconds pulses at a very high frequency of 10 to 15 kHz. To the naked eye this beam appears continuous; however, it can be electronically shuttered to produce pulses of 0.075 to 0.3 seconds in duration, or even attached to an optical scanner to produce larger geometric patterns [22–24,26,64–68]. These lasers are useful for larger caliber facial telangiectasias, mucosal venous malformations, cherry and spider angiomas, angiokeratomas, and pyogenic granulomas [23,25,26,64,66,67].

The copper vapor uses a 150 um handpiece with 450 to 500 mW with 0.2-second intervals of exposure. One needs loop magnification with this laser as well because of the small spot size [4]. The laser is used to trace out the vessel and the clinical endpoint is disappearance of the vessel without purpura. Minimal crusting occurs which lasts 1 to 2 weeks, during which time the patient is instructed to keep the area moist with ointment.

The copper bromide laser can produce a quasipulse as short as 7 microseconds at 16 kHz through a fiberoptic cable with a 0.7 mm spot size [4,26].

My experience with the copper vapor laser was not very rewarding. The laser is large, requires a long start-up time, emits a great deal of heat, and is not very comfortable to use. Oftentimes patients needed to be treated more than once for eradication of a vessel. Temporary postinflammatory hyperpigmentation and scarring have been reported [65].

KRYPTON

The krypton laser is another continuous wave laser that emits yellow (568 nm) and green (520 nm) light that can be shuttered to make a quasicontinuous wave [4,15,69]. The laser light goes through a fiberoptic cable using a 100 um collimated or a 1 mm handpiece. The laser is set at 0.4 to 0.6 watts with a 0.2-second pulsed or continuous wave and 0.7 to 0.9 watts with a 0.2-second pulsed or continuous wave when using a 1 mm handpiece [4]. This laser can also be attached to an automated scanner [70]. The treatment endpoints are similar to the other continuous wave lasers: disappearance of the vessel followed by some edema, erythema, and mild crusting.

KTP LASER

The potassium titanyl phosphate laser, or KTP laser as it is commonly referred to, uses a neodymium:yttrium-aluminum-garnet (Nd:YAG) crystal (1064 nm) that is frequency-doubled with a potassium titanyl phosphate crystal, producing a wavelength of 532 nm [4,15]. It is another continuous wave laser that can be shuttered or used with an automated scanner. This laser offers 100, 150, and 250 um handpieces that have been used primarily for facial telangiectasias [27–29]. Again, the clinical endpoint is blanching of the vessel followed by erythema, edema, and crusting for several days. The patients are instructed to keep these areas moist with ointment. The largest spot size is used at 0.5 to 0.7 watts and a repeat pulse of 0.1-second on and 0.1-second off times. This laser can have similar complications to the other continuous wave lasers such as scarring and pigmentary changes.

VERSAPULSE

Laser companies are trying to combine multiple wavelengths and capabilities so that physicians are able to treat a multitude of abnormalities with one purchased machine. The Versapulse laser (Coherent Medical Group, Palo Alto, CA) is a product of this endeavor. It has four different wavelengths in one laser: a variable pulse 532 nm, Nd:YAG laser for vascular lesions; a Q-switched Nd:YAG laser for pigmented lesions and tattoos at 532 nm and 1064 nm; and an alexandrite 755 nm laser. There are, to date, little published data on the efficacy of this laser. Reports have shown the utility of the variable pulse 532 nm Nd:YAG laser for facial telangiectasias ranging from 0.2 to 1.5 mm. Up to 95 of 100 patients treated twice with his laser achieved clearance of the treated vessels [71]. A 4 mm spot with a 10 microsecond pulse and a fluence of 9 to 12 J/cm^2 were used to trace out the vessels with 1 to 4 passes until the vessel disappeared. This laser also uses a water-cooled chill tip at 4 to 5.5°C. There is transient edema and erythema and patients report minimal discomfort.

The Versapulse laser at 532 nm with a 3 or 4 mm spot, a 10 microsecond pulse, and fluences of 9.5 to 16 J/cm^2 has also been used to treat 20 port wine stains [72]. The area of treatment is covered by 1 to 3 passes of the laser. Papular port wine stains and even those resistant to the traditional pulsed dye laser seem to respond especially well. Advantages of the Versapulse laser include lack of purpura, patient comfort, and reduced postsurgical recovery times [73].

PHOTODERM VL

Photoderm VL (ESC Medical Systems, Ltd, Haifa, Israel) is not a laser, but a pulsed light source that produces a noncoherent beam that includes a wide spectrum of wavelengths from 500 to 1100 nm [4,30,34]. Cutoff filters at 515, 550, 570, and 590 nm are used for the treatment of telangiectasias. One can also choose a variety of fluences in single, double, or triple-pulse modes. The pulse duration can be varied as can the time between pulses [15]. Larger areas can be treated with the large 8 × 35 mm spot size. The longer wavelengths used in this light source should increase depth of injury. In one study of leg veins, it was able to achieve more than 50% clearance in 94% of cases with minimal side effects [30]. The Photoderm VL has also been reported useful for facial telangiectasias and port wine stains [31]. One study found that the Photoderm VL can be used effectively for facial and leg telangiectasias but that longer pulse durations yielded better clearing of vessels, which was associated with a higher rate of complications including hyperpigmentation [35].

DIODE LASERS

The introduction of semiconductor-based laser designs is going to revolutionize the reliability and size of most lasers. Light energy from these lasers can be emitted continuously or in a pulsed fashion [58]. There are several diode lasers available for the treatment of vascular lesions, including a diode-pumped frequency doubled solid state 532 nm laser (Diolite; Iriderm, Mountain View, CA) which I am about to begin using on some of my patients. The major advantage presented to the physician is the small size and transportability of these diode lasers. Studies in the future will reveal their efficacy and safety as compared with older laser systems.

FLASHLAMP-PUMPED PULSED DYE LASER

The flashlamp-pumped pulsed dye laser (PDL) was the first laser designed around the concept of selective photothermolysis proposed by Anderson and Parrish in 1983

[1,2,15,37,58]. Initially, the wavelength was set at 577 nm to correspond to one of the oxyhemoglobin absorption peaks, but was then increased to 585 nm which provides a deeper depth of vascular injury without loss of selectivity [4,74–76]. Selective injury by lasers will occur when the duration of the pulse of light is shorter than the thermal relaxation of that vessel. This allows the thermal damage to remain confined to the vessel without spread to adjacent structures and therefore greatly decreases the chances of cutaneous scarring. A typical cutaneous vessel has a thermal relaxation of 1 to 5 ms [1,4,75]. The PDL has a pulse duration of 450 microseconds which is transmitted down a fiberoptic cable, and so each pulse ends before there is transmission of heat to surrounding cutaneous structures.

Unlike that which occurs with continuous wave lasers, histology of vessels treated with the PDL do not reveal perivascular fibrosis, but rather agglutination of erythrocytes and vessel wall degeneration in the papillary and superficial reticular dermal vessels to a depth of about 1.2 mm [1,4,75–77]. At 1 week there is a replacement of the vessels with granulation tissue and at 1 month there is normal histology of epidermis, dermis, vasculature, and adnexal structures without evidence of fibrosis. Clinically this is the rationale behind spacing treatments with the PDL in at least 1-month intervals.

The PDL is available in 2, 3, 5, 7 and 10 mm beam sizes and can operate at 1 Hz by continuous depression of the foot pedal. The maximum fluence is 10 J/cm^2 but most vascular lesions are treated in the 6 to 7.5 J/cm^2 range with the 5 mm spot. When decreasing the spot size one must accordingly increase the fluence to maintain the same energy [4,15,22].

The PDL was first developed to treat port wine stains [13,78–85], but is also an excellent treatment choice for telangiectasias [22,86–92], telangiectasias associated with rosacea [12], actinic damage and chronic corticosteroid use [4], pyogenic granulomas [88,93], cherry angiomas [15,90,94], venous lakes [88], and hemangiomas [3,95]. The PDL is also effective for the treatment of angiofibromas [14,96], hypertrophic scars [18,19,97–101], and poikiloderma of Civatte [16,102]. It has also been used to treat the cutaneous lesions of Kaposi's sarcoma [103], telangiectasias after plastic surgery [104], striae [20,105], and warts [17,106].

The side effects of the PDL are minimal. Scarring is seen in less than 1% of cases, and if it occurs is usually transitory [77,107,108]. One large study of 500 patients found less than 0.1% incidence of atrophic scarring and no hypertrophic scars. Hypertrophic scarring has been seen when PDL has been used on the anterior chest and shoulders where one should decrease the fluence about 10 to 20% [109]. Keloid formation has also been reported after PDL treatment of a patient who was on isotretinoin [110]. A 16-year-old Asian female with a port wine stain on her neck and chest was treated with a fluence of 6.0 J/cm^2 for 5 years without any problems. Then another physician put the patient on isotretinoin for acne between PDL treatments, and she then developed keloids in the treated sites. I suggest that before laser treatment, one should inquire about isotretinoin use. Isotretinoin alters the pilosebaceous unit, which is important in wound healing. This alteration can last for several months after stopping isotretinoin. Even after periods of 9 months after cessation of isotretinoin there have been reports of scarring in areas treated with dermabrasion and argon laser [54,55]. Therefore, it may be prudent to wait 12 to 18 months before performing PDL on those patients who have taken isotretinoin [110].

Hyperpigmentation is the most frequent complication occurring in as many as 10 to 15% of cases [77,107]. Hyperpigmentation occurs more frequently in darker-skinned or tanned patients, in the spring or summer months when the patient is not careful about sun protection, and also when excess fluences are used [107]. The PDL is ineffective in black patients because of the competition with epidermal melanin [111,112]. Hypopigmentation has been seen in 2.6 to 5% of patients and is also usually temporary [105]. Hypopigmentation can persist especially on the neck, chest, and legs [15,57].

Patients' major complaint about the PDL is the purpura they must endure for 1 to 2 weeks (Fig. 2a). This often prompts them to consider another laser or modality of treatment. I will go into the details of PDL treatment, including pre- and post-surgical instructions and fluences, when discussing the lesions being treated in the next section.

SCLEROLASER AND SCLEROLASER PLUS (Candela Corp, Wayland, Mass.)

Recently, a new PDL has been developed with longer wavelengths of 585, 590, 595, and 600 nm that has been used on resistant port wine stains and leg veins [4,15,57]. The longer wavelengths allow for deeper depth of injury and the longer pulsewidth of 1.5 microseconds allows for longer heating and more effective clearing of larger caliber vessels. It has spot sizes of 2, 3, 5, 7, and 10 mm circles and an elliptical 2 $\times$ 7 mm spot size with fluences of 2 to 30 J/cm^2 with 15 to 20 J/cm^2 commonly used. Purpura still occurs as does postinflammatory hyperpigmentation when used for leg veins, but purpura is not a clinical endpoint for facial vessels. Anecdotal reports of scarring and hypopigmentation have also been noted.

LASER TREATMENTS

Facial Telangiectasias

Telangiectasias are divided according to their configuration and size [86]. Linear telangiectasias as well as arborizing telangiectasias occur especially on the nose, midcheeks, and chin. These are 0.1 to 1.0 mm in diameter and represent a dilated capillary, venule, or arteriole [6,15]. Spider telangiectasias are also common in both children and adults. Usually one can press on the central arteriole and cause the lesion to blanch and disappear. Papular telangiectasias may be seen in collagen vascular disorders or generalized essential telangiectasia [4].

All of these telangiectasias can be caused by a variety of factors, such as: excessive actinic exposure; posttraumatic caused by neovascularization during healing [49]; diseases such as rosacea; patients with flushing disorders who complain of severe heat and burning; and collagen vascular diseases such as CREST syndrome and lupus erythematous.

The size and configuration of the telangiectasia will determine the optimal laser or lasers for its treatment. However, for most of these lasers patients may be given similar presurgical instructions and precautions. Patients should be screened as to a history of postinflammatory hyperpigmentation, excessive scarring, and even use of

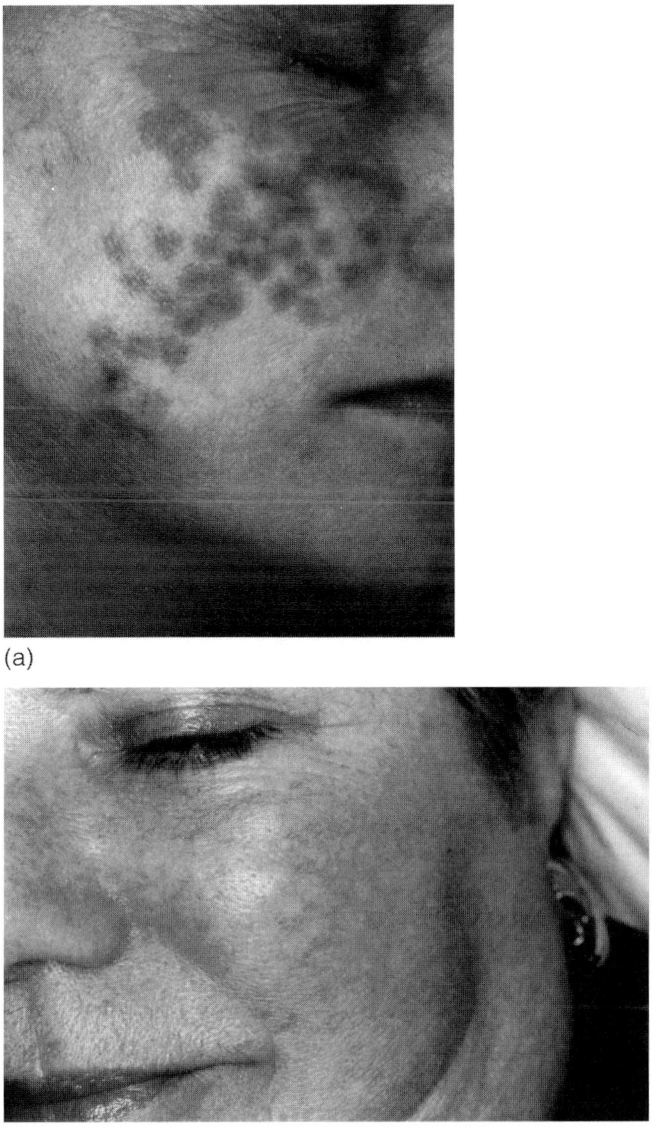

FIGURE 2 (a) Purpura is visible on the cheek immediately after pulsed dye laser (PDL) treatment of facial telangiectasias. (b) A lattice pattern is seen during the course of a series of PDL treatments.

isotretinoin. Patients should be advised to avoid excessive sun exposure before, during, and after laser treatments, which could contribute to postinflammatory changes or limit the effectiveness of their treatments. It is wise to give patients written information about the laser with which they will be treated that described discomfort, any discoloration such as purpura, swelling, and crusting, and how they will treat these. In my office I also keep a portfolio of patient pre- and postsurgical photographs so that patients can actually see expected results. The most useful photograph is one of a patient immediately after PDL so that the purpura is quite evident (Fig. 2a). This will save the physician from a great number of fearful telephone calls. I also show a photograph of a patient in the middle of treatments, such as for rosacea-associated erythema or a port wine stain where I am treating a confluent area of erythema, in order to show them the lattice pattern that occurs because of spaces between laser pulses (Fig. 2b).

The pain associated with laser treatment of telangiectasias varies according to the laser used and how large an area is treated. For children and fearful adults, EMLA cream can be applied under occlusion. We have found EMLA can provide adequate anesthesia if applied for 1.5 to 2 hours to an area that is degreased well with acetone before application. Regional blocks with xylocaine can also give pain relief from the pinprick or "rubber band" sensation of PDL or the burning sensation of continuous wave lasers. Recently, lasers have become available that use a cryogen spray for immediate presurgical anesthesia [113–115]. Millisecond cryogen spurts immediately before laser irradiation can reduce the epidermal surface temperature to 30 to 40°C, therefore, reducing treatment discomfort and protecting the epidermis from thermal injury.

A number of laser options are available for treatment of facial telangiectasias. Larger-caliber linear telangiectasias, especially those around the nose, can be treated with continuous wave lasers such as the argon-pumped tunable dye laser, copper vapor/copper bromide lasers, KTP, and krypton lasers. One study [5] found that a majority of patients preferred the argon-pumped tunable dye laser over the PDL even though the tunable dye laser was not as effective in clearing the telangiectasias. Patients often find the purpura associated with the PDL a barrier to its use. The tunable dye laser, however, along with the other continuous wave lasers, requires more skill and is more time consuming in tracing out vessels. Another study again compared PDL with the tunable dye laser and found that 100% of the PDL-treated areas showed excellent clearing compared with only 47% of the argon-pumped tunable dye laser. The parameters used were fluences of 6 to 6.75 J/cm^2 with a 5 mm spot size using the PDL and 26 to 27 J/cm^2 with a hexagonal treatment area of 13 mm using the argon-pumped tunable dye laser and a computerized scanner. Although the PDL was more effective in clearing the telangiectasias, patients again preferred the tunable dye laser because of the purpura and the postinflammatory hyperpigmentation which is more severe after PDL treatment [8].

PDL has achieved good-to-excellent clearing of linear and spider facial telangiectasias using fluences of 6 to 7.75 J/cm^2 and a 5 mm spot [89]. In one series, 97.5% of patients had more than 50% vessel clearance after 1 to 2 treatments with best results using fluences above 7 J/cm^2 [57]. I generally treat facial telangiectasias with fluences of 7 to 7.5 J/cm^2 depending on how large they are and their locations. Telangiectasias near the eye may be treated at lower fluences, or I may switch to a smaller spot size and then compensate with a higher fluence of 8.5 to 10 J/cm^2 in order to decrease the incidence of purpura. I agree with studies that have shown that larger blue vessels do not respond as well as smaller red ones [88].

The copper vapor laser has also been compared with the PDL for the treatment of facial telangiectasias. One study [25] found them equally effective with no scarring. Another study found that 18 of 20 patients treated with the copper vapor laser responded well, but one patient suffered a small scar and three patients developed temporary postinflammatory hyperpigmentation [65]. The copper vapor laser, along with the copper bromide, KTP, and krypton lasers, produces fine linear crusting rather than purpura after treatment.

In summary, for the removal of isolated facial telangiectasias, continuous wave lasers offer the advantage of no purpura and less postinflammatory hyperpigmentation but are best at treating larger-caliber vessels, whereas the PDL is better suited for smaller vessels. Photoderm VL and Sclerolaser may also be appropriate for larger vessels because their pulse durations are longer.

Rosacea Associated-Erythema and Telangiectasias

Erythema, telangiectasias, and flushing are also symptoms and signs of rosacea. Topical and systemic treatments are often ineffective in eradicating these components of the disease. Lowe et al. [12] reported good-to-excellent reductions in erythema and telangiectasia in 24 of 27 patients who received one to three treatments with the PDL with fluences of 6 to 7.5 J/cm^2 and a 5 mm spot size. Fifty-nine percent of the patients also noted a decrease in papules and pustules, and those patients who did respond in this way required lower doses of both topical and systemic antibiotics. No scarring or pigmentary changes were seen (Fig. 3).

In addition, patients with actinic damage or chronic corticosteroid use can also have excellent cosmetic results with the PDL. Patients should be advised to expect to see a lattice develop as clearing of the redness occurs, which will require additional treatments.

The argon-pumped tunable dye laser used with a 0.2 or 0.3 mm spot size and 0.2-second pulses has also been used successfully in the treatment of patients with rosacea with minimal complications [60]. The copper vapor laser has also been used but one report claimed poor responses [65] and another claimed good clearing with a number of patients suffering from hyper- and hypopigmentation and scarring [66].

Another alternative to the PDL for rosacea is the KTP laser, which showed satisfactory results after one to two treatments in 70% of patients with no purpura, scarring, or pigment changes [28].

Spider Angiomas

The continuous wave copper bromide/copper vapor, krypton, and KTP lasers can give good results in the treatment of spider telangiectasias and angiomas. However, of these lasers there are only published studies using the copper vapor and copper bromide lasers. Key and Waner [65] treated 20 patients, and 18 of these showed satisfactory results, 3 developed transient postinflammatory hyperpigmentation, and one developed an atrophic site. The copper bromide laser has also been used for spider angiomas, with a depressed scar reported in one patient [26].

I personally prefer the PDL for the treatment of spider telangiectasias/angiomas. Certainly in children it is the safest laser to use. Geronemus [92] reported 100% clearing in 12 children using fluences of 6 to 6.5 J/cm^2 with a 5 mm spot size. The only complication reported was transient hyperpigmentation in 4 patients. Goldman et al. [6,57] reported on 23 children treated at fluences between 6.5 to 7.5 J/cm^2 and

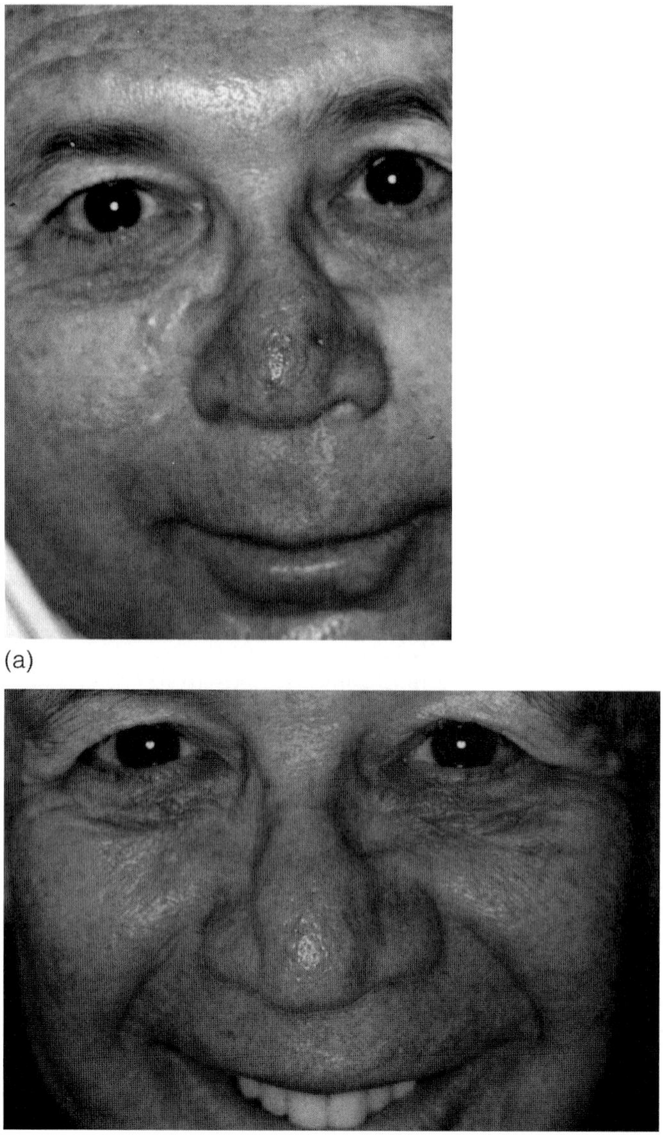

(a)

(b)

FIGURE 3 (a) Rosacea-associated erythema and telangiectasias on the nose before PDL treatment. (b) After two PDL treatments to the nose using a fluence of 7.5 J/cm^2 and a 5 mm spot size.

showed 70% clearing after one treatment and 12 lesions cleared after a second treatment. In adults, 93% resolution after one treatment using fluences of 6.5 to 7.0 J/cm^2 has also been reported [57].

Using the PDL for spider telangiectasias/spider angiomas usually involves giving one or two pulses to the central punctum; two are used especially if this area is raised or thick, and are followed by additional pulses with 10% overlap to the feeder vessels surrounding the punctum. Usually no anesthesia is required and postsurgical antibiotic ointment or petrolatum is used for any scabbing or crusting.

Cherry Angiomas

The continuous wave lasers such as the argon [50], copper vapor [23], argon-pumped tunable dye laser [60], and the KTP laser [27] have all been used to treat cherry angiomas. However, textural changes and scarring are more likely especially if too much energy is used. The PDL is rapid, safe, and very effective [90,94]. I generally double pulse a thick cherry angioma and will typically treat using fluences of 7 to 7.5 J/cm.^{2} Patients are given postsurgical antibiotic ointment for crusting. Usually these lesions require one treatment, unless they are large or thick, and clearing is usually seen over the course of 1 month.

Pyogenic Granuloma

These often-eroded, bleeding papules can be treated with a variety of methods including electrodesiccation, surgical, excision, and more destructive lasers such as CO_2, and argon [15,57]. PDL has also been used to treat these lesions using fluences between 6.5 to 8 J/cm^2 after one or more treatment sessions [88,93]. Scarring after PDL has also been reported [93]. Thicker lesions may not respond and either need to be surgically debulked first or treated with multiple overlapping pulses, which does not adhere to the principle of selective photothermolysis but rather causes nonselective thermal injury [57]. Some physicians claim that compression with a glass slide is useful to get penetration to the deep component of the lesion, with then removal of the slide to treat the superficial vessels.

I have treated several pyogenic granulomas with both the CO_2 and PDL and I find that the CO_2 laser, although carrying a greater risk of scarring, is more effective than repeated treatments with the PDL.

Venous Lake

Venous lakes, if small, can easily be treated with the PDL after one or two treatments. Gonzalez et al. [88] found clearance of venous lakes after one to three treatments with the PDL. He used multiple overlapping pulses at 6 to 8 J/cm.^{2}

If the PDL does not work I often turn to the argon laser. Usually one treatment at 1 watt or less is sufficient to seal off the dilated venule. One group using argon laser noted slight scar formation in a few patients [52]. When treating large-caliber lesions with more power, argon laser can cause textural changes and hypopigmentation which can be permanent. I also give an injection of xylocaine into the lip or do a mental nerve block before doing argon laser for a venous lake.

POIKILODERMA OF CIVATTE

Laser treatment of nonfacial skin is much more likely to have complications such as scarring and pigmentary changes. Chronic ultraviolet light exposure has numerous adverse effects on the skin, including premature aging, fragility, purpura, and pigmentary irregularities [116,117]. Poikiloderma of Civatte is a condition that is attributable to chronic sun exposure and is more common in women [118]. It presents with telangiectasias, atrophy, and hyper- and hypopigmentation on the sides of the neck, upper chest, and even the sides of the cheeks, but usually spares the submental area.

Treatment of the neck in this condition can be fraught with problems. Electrocautery can remove some of the larger vessels, but will not affect the atrophy or pigmentary problems and carries a high risk of textural changes [16]. The argon laser has also been used for this purpose but has resulted in scarring and permanent hypopigmentation [39,50].

The PDL is the most frequently used laser for the treatment of poikiloderma because of its limited thermal injury and great selectivity (Fig. 4) [16,102,119]. Most physicians do not use anesthesia in adults when treating this condition with PDL because they experience a mild sunburn sensation, although EMLA cream can be used presurgically with good anesthesia achieved in the skin of the neck and chest. One physician reported 95% clearance rates in three patients after an average of four treatments using fluences between 6.5 to 7.0 J/cm^2 [102]. Wheeland and Applebaum [16] used even lower fluences of 5 to 6 J/cm^2 and saw good responses, without complications. One can apply a cool soothing dressing after the procedure, such as polyethylene oxide dressings or cool compressions, to decrease the burning sensation. It is important to perform on a small test area, using a lower fluence than one would use on other areas. I would be very cautious in using fluences greater than 7.0 J/cm^2 on the neck using a 5 mm spot, because this area can easily develop hypopigmentation and textural changes. The treatments are spaced at 6 to 8 week intervals to allow full healing between treatments. Patients must avoid sun exposure between sessions because of the likelihood of postinflammatory changes, although hydroquinones can be useful at the first signs of hyperpigmentation. On retreatment, one often does not have to relaser the entire area, but only those areas not treated in the prior sessions, because of the lattice pattern left by the laser.

Other poikilodermatous conditions such as Rothmund-Thomson syndrome have been successfully treated with the PDL without adverse side effects [119]. One recent study, however, followed 20 patients over 4 years treated with the PDL for Poikiloderma of Civatte [120]. Contrary to previous reports, these investigators report hyperpigmentation which was most often transient, but permanent hypopigmentation and depigmentation was seen in a majority of patients. They saw slight improvement in some patients but scarring was also evident. They advise extreme caution in the poikiloderma in the neck and chest area.

SCARS

Many treatments have been proposed for hypertrophic scars and keloids, including intralesional steroids [121–124], radiation [125,126], pressure therapy [99,127], and excision and grafting [121,128]. These therapies usually resulted in recurrence of larger scars and keloids. Topical silicone dressings have recently been tried but with limited success as a solo treatment [129,130]. Lasers have also been tried in the amelioration of scars and keloids, including the CO_2 laser [131–134], Nd:YAG laser [135–137], and argon lasers [138,139]. All of the aforementioned lasers are destruc-

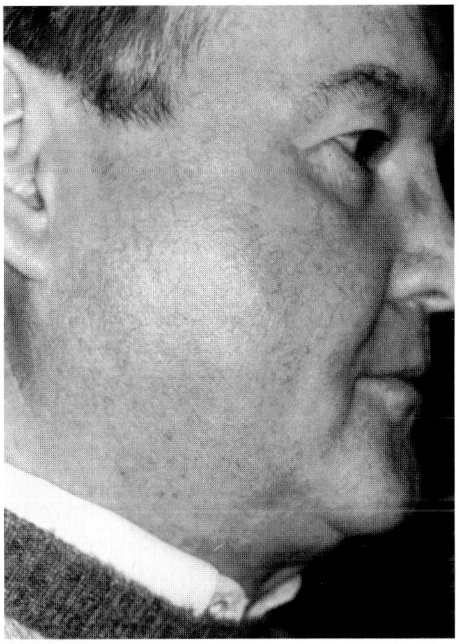

(a)

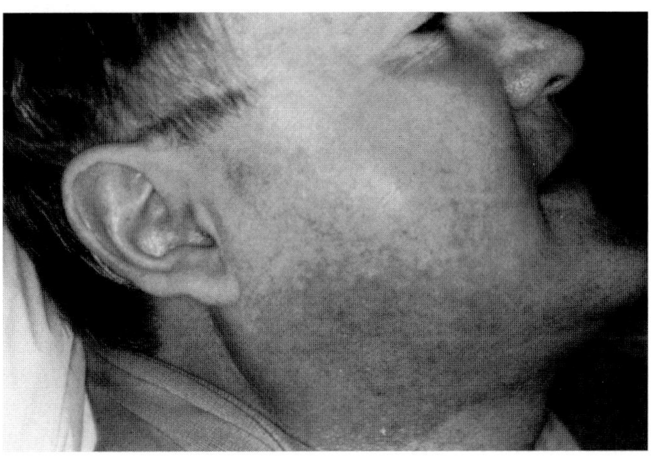

(b)

FIGURE 4 (a) Actinic poikiloderma before PDL treatment. (b) After two PDL treatments to the cheeks using a fluence of 7.5 J/cm^2 and a 5 mm spot size. Before treatment of the neck one can notice a line of demarcation.

tive or ablative and may cause additional injury, fibrosis, as well as recurrences usually within 2 years [99,140]. Earlier attempts to limit thermal injury seemed promising but still can cause additional scarring [141]. The PDL is the only laser used for the treatment of scars that does not work by cutting or ablating the tissue [99,142]. The PDL is thought to work by inducing a state of relative hypoxia because of its selective uptake by blood vessels. This increase in lactic acid may stimulate collagenase which causes collagen turnover and remodeling with the result being a flatter, nonerythematous scar.

The first report using PDL for erythematous hypertrophic scars was Alster (18) who reported on 14 patients who were treated with one to two PDL treatments at 585 nm over a 2-month period. She had first shown improvement of scars that were the result of previous argon laser treatment after an average of five PDL treatments of the residual port wine stain [19]. Histologic evaluation showed that the dilated vascular channels present in scar tissue were cleared after laser treatment in eight of 10 patients treated. In her next study, optical profilometry was performed on five of the 14 patients evaluated. Fluences of 6.5 to 6.75 J/cm^2 were used with a 5 mm spot size, and the two treatments were separated by 6 weeks. A 57% improvement was seen after one PDL treatment and an 83% improvement after two treatments. At the end of the 6-month follow-up period, no patient showed worsening or increased erythema. Optical profilometry was consistent with the results evaluating clinical improvement. Another study of 15 patients with hypertrophic erythematous scars treated with the PDL showed an average improvement of 77% after an average of 1.8 treatments and 47% of the patients had 100% improvement after one to three treatments [101]. They used fluences that were slightly higher of 6.0 to 7.5 J/cm^2 with a 5 mm spot size. Unlike Alster's initial study, these patients had all failed previous attempts at scar revisions with surgery, radiation, CO_2 and argon laser, as well as corticosteroid injections. Maximal improvement was seen after 4 to 8 weeks. In this study there was no significant difference in treatment outcome versus the fluence of the laser. Less than 1-year old and facial scars were the most responsive to treatment (Fig. 5). They also postulated additional mechanisms for how selective vascular injury can improve scars. Type V collagen has been found to be increased in hypertrophic scars which have numerous capillaries. PDL-induced removal of capillaries may decrease endothelial stimulation of type V collagen production which leads to flattening of hypertrophic scars [101]. Also mentioned was that superheating of collagen fibers may cause disassociation of their disulfide bonds, allowing the fibers to reassociate in a more parallel, less haphazard array as is seen histologically.

A controlled study of hypertrophic and keloidal median sternotomy scars resulting from heart surgery was then performed on 16 patients [101]. Half of the scar was treated with the PDL at fluences of 6.5 to 7.25 J/cm^2 on two successive sessions at 6 to 8 weeks apart. Histology and optical profilometry were also used to evaluate results. Eleven of 12 patients noted a decrease in pruritus. Mean scar height, pliability, and skin surface topography improved significantly after one and two treatments. Erythema decreased but was not eliminated by two treatments. Histologically there was a decrease in the number of fibroblasts and replacement of thick collagen bundles by looser, less-coarse collagen fibers, and an increase in the number of mast cells. It is also thought that this increase in mast cells may explain why the PDL stimulates collagen remodeling, because histamine may stimulate normal and keloid fibroblast growth [99]. Another study of erythematous acne scars treated with the PDL at an average fluence of 6.5 J/cm^2 also showed significant clinical improvement [143].

I have used the PDL for many hypertrophic and even some keloidal scars (Figs. 5, 6). I find that it is quite effective for facial hypertrophic, erythematous scars after one to four treatments. These patients do not require anesthesia, although I find that icing the area both before and after treatment makes the patient more comfortable.

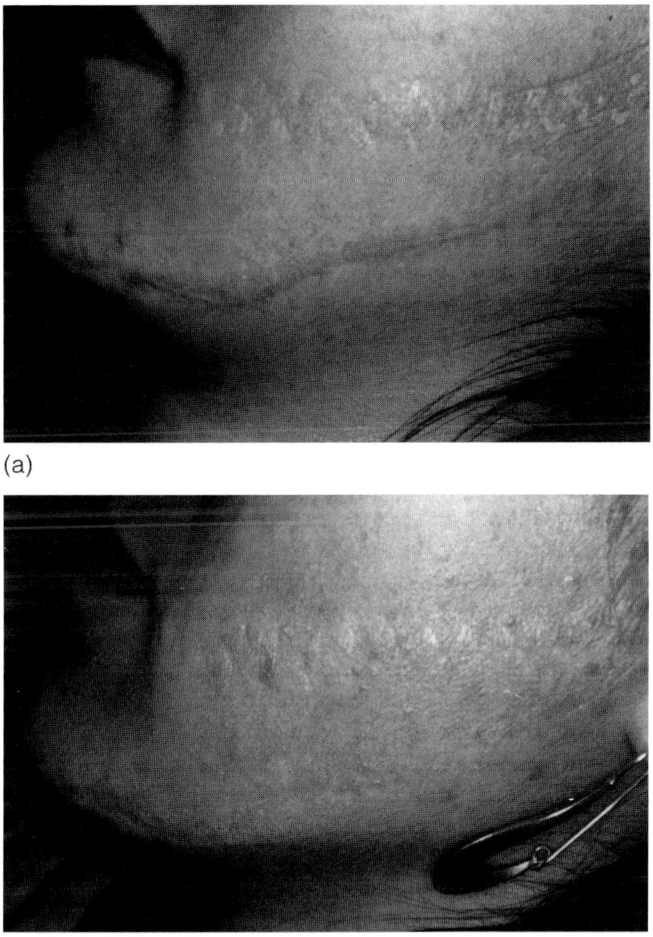

(a)

(b)

FIGURE 5 (a) Erythematous and raised scars on the left cheek after being slashed with a razor blade during the commitment of a robbery. (b) After two PDL treatments using a fluence of 6.75 J/cm^2 and a 5 mm spot.

If they experience any crusting postsurgically they are given an antibiotic ointment to apply at home twice a day. Immediately after the treatment, a cool polyethylene oxide dressing is applied. Patients are also instructed to use sunscreen and avoid excessive sun exposure so that postinflammatory hyperpigmentation does not occur. I use fluences of 6.0 to 7.5 J/cm^2 with the 5 mm spot which is decreased to 6.0 to 6.5 J/cm^2 if the 7 mm spot size is used. The patients are advised that the area will be purpuric for 10 to 14 days. I usually treat at 6 to 8 week intervals. I have had great success in treating facial scars resulting from resurfacing procedures, Mohs micrographic surgery for skin cancer, and violent knife attacks. I have been disappointed with the improvement seen in very hypertrophic scars resulting from breast reduction and augmentation procedures, and those scars that are older than 1 year.

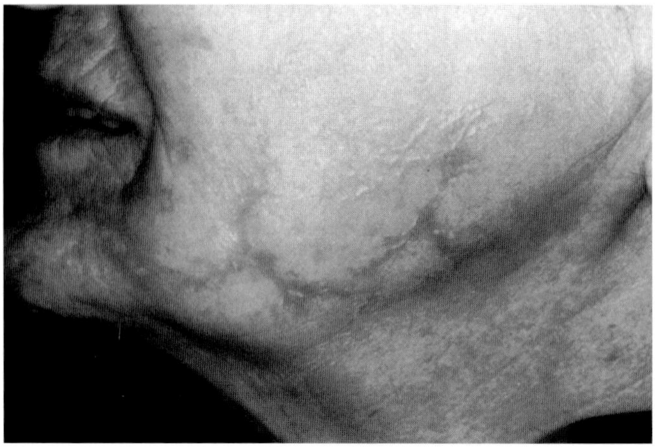

(a)

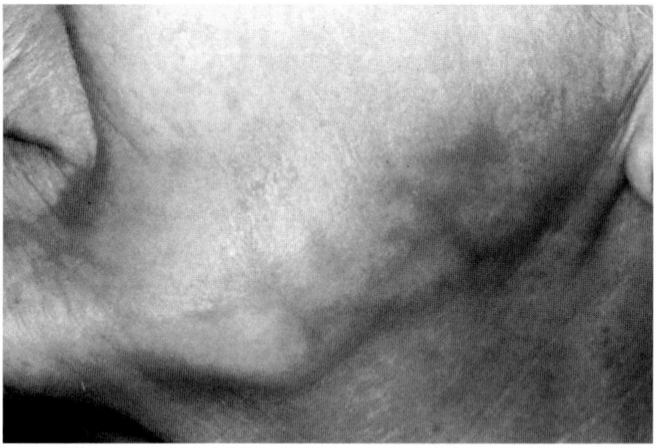

(b)

FIGURE 6 (a) Erythematous and raised scars that were the result of a bacterial infection complicating healing after a medium depth 35% trichloroacetic acid/Jessners solution peel. (b) After two PDL treatments using a fluence of 7.0 J/cm^2 and a 5 mm spot, there is noted improvement.

STRIAE

Striae distensae or stretch marks are very distressing to patients whether they occur as a result of rapid growth, pregnancy, or corticosteroid use [144]. Some investigators describe them as simply caused by stretching and thinning of the supporting structures of the skin, whereas others describe them a type of dermal scarring [145]. Clinically, early striae are flat and faint pink in color, which then darkens to a violaceous color. Fully mature striae are white and atrophic. Mast cell degranulation is seen in early striae which apparently results in damage of collagen and destruction of elastin [146]. With time, mature striae have some regeneration of collagen and elastin with orientation of the fibers along the direction of stress. Histologic studies support the idea that striae are a form of dermal scarring. Histologically, striae lack both hair follicles and other appendages, and there is an absence of rete ridges which results in a flattening of the epidermis [147]. The collagen bundles are densely packed horizontal to the surface in a parallel fashion. The absence or abnormal elastic fibers in striae again confirm that striae are a dermal scar [148]. Tretinoin, which has been useful in photoaging and has been shown to increase collagen and stimulate fibroblasts, has been used in the treatment of early striae. Fifteen of 16 patients treated with tretinoin showed clinical improvement in their early striae [149].

Studies have shown that low-level energy from lasers such as the argon-pumped tunable dye laser in human skin fibroblast cultures can increase the secretion of growth factors from fibroblasts and stimulate cell proliferation, in vivo, in mice [150]. The PDL has also shown significant improvement of erythematous and hypertrophic scars [18,19,98–101,143]. It has also been used successfully in the hypoplastic areas in Goltz syndrome [151]. Because striae are dermal scars, PDL was then used to treat mature striae [20]. Thirty-nine striae were treated with a variety of fluence. The response to therapy was evaluated with sequential photography, optical profilometry, and biopsies in two patients. Optical profilometry showed that all treatment protocols improved the striae. The 10 mm spot size using 3.0 J/cm^2 seemed to yield the best clinical response. The two biopsies showed increased elastin and normalization of histologic architecture. A longer-term study seemed to confirm these results but clinical photographs did not really show significant improvement [152].

I recently reported on five patients with mature striae on the abdomen, hips, and thighs. I treated them every 2 months for two to seven treatments [105]. The follow-up period was 1.5 years. The results were not consistent with the previous report. Optical profilometry suggested a mild improvement in skin surface markings, but clinically there was no improvement noted even after several treatments, and histologically there was no increase in elastin or significant normalization of striae collagen. Patients were somewhat happy with the treatment, but they were receiving the treatment gratis. In addition, when doing biopsies on striae it is sometimes difficult to be certain that you are taking exactly the same area of the striae as one did in the presurgical site. The only complication noted was temporary hyperpigmentation, with no scars or erosions seen postsurgically. No anesthesia was necessary because very low fluences such as 4.25 J/cm^2 with a 10 mm spot was used. I try to discourage my patients from treating mature striae in this fashion because I feel that the improvement is not significant.

WARTS

Warts are common benign lesions of the skin caused by human papillomavirus infection, and their incidence approaches 10% [153]. Many modalities have been used in the attempt to eradicate warts, including the applications of caustics and keratolytics, cryosurgery [154–156], electrosurgery [157,158], chemotherapeutic agents such as bleomycin and 5-fluorouracil [159], surgical excisions, and some laser treatments. These methods are all nonselective, cause unnecessary destruction of adjacent tissue, and still have high recurrence rates.

The first laser used for the treatment of warts was the CO_2 laser. This laser emits in the infrared region with a wavelength of 10,600 nm, and its energy is absorbed by the water present in skin. It works by vaporizing tissue infected with the virus [160–164]. The CO_2 laser can lase through the nail plate and can be used

TABLE 2 Laser Protocol for Warts

Periungual or subungal warts. Digital block using 2% lidocaine.
Pare down hyperkeratotic lesions and/or remove overlying nail.
PDL-585 nm and a 5 or 7 mm spot size using 9-10 J/cm^2 and 450 microsecond pulse at 1 Hz. Lowered fluences for flat facial warts—7 to 8 J/cm^2.
Use 3-9 pulses per wart area to achieve uniform gray discoloration.
Treat every 3 weeks until there is no clinical evidence of wart or regrowth.
Follow patients at monthly intervals for 6 months or more to monitor for recurrences.

for periungual and plantar warts. It has a reported success rate of 57 to 95% in the treatment of nongenital warts [160–163]. However, CO_2 laser can cause permanent scarring and prolonged healing, delayed bleeding, infection, and discomfort. In addition, one must take precautions with the plume which may contain infectious viral particles [165]. When performing CO_2 laser for plantar or periungual warts, one must administer regional anesthesia or a digital block with xylocaine without epinephrine, which can be painful in and of itself. The patient is left with an open granulating wound for several weeks to several months, requiring wound care with an antibiotic ointment and covering or perhaps an expensive synthetic dressing. And, unfortunately, even after all of this the wart has a rather good chance of recurring.

The next laser that was used in wart therapy was the copper vapor [166]. Genital and body warts were successfully treated with a very low risk of scarring. It was thought that the laser light was targeting the virally afflicted epidermis which contained pigment. Tan [106] was the first to report use of the PDL for the treatment of warts. Her reasoning was that a characteristic histologic feature of all verrucae was the presence of dilated, prominent blood vessels in the dermal papillae. The PDL had been shown to selectively injure blood vessels [167]. The PDL could then be used to abolish the nutritional blood flow to the keratinocytes infected with papillomavirus and/or to destroy the basal layer of the epidermis, which contained virus and the most rapidly dividing cells. Tan [106] first evaluated 39 patients with warts on the neck, face, legs, and knees, as well as 14 with finger and hand verrucae, six with plantar warts, and seven with periungual warts. Periungual and plantar warts tend to be the most recalcitrant types to any mode of treatment. Her protocol was to pare down any hyperkeratosis over the wart with a #15 scalpel blade until there was visualization of bleeding points. In the case of a periungual wart, as much of the overlying nail as possible was removed. A 5 mm spot size and fluences of 6.25 J/cm^2 to 7.5 J/cm^2 with single pulses to the wart were used. Postsurgically either a dry dressing or an antibacterial ointment and a cold pack was applied. The patients were retreated at 1- to 3-week intervals. The patients reported minimal discomfort during or after the PDL treatments. They usually developed an adherent black eschar that was still present when they returned for their follow-up treatments and was then removed according to their protocol. Twenty-eight of 39 patients, or 72% were cleared of their wart after an average of 1.68 treatments. In 18% there was a reduction in wart size by 80 to 95% and four patients had their warts reduce in size by 50% after one laser treatment. Eighty-six percent of patients with periungual warts cleared after 1.85 treatments, and 50% of plantar warts cleared after 1.5 treatments. The average follow-up period of the 28 cases cleared of their warts was 5 months.

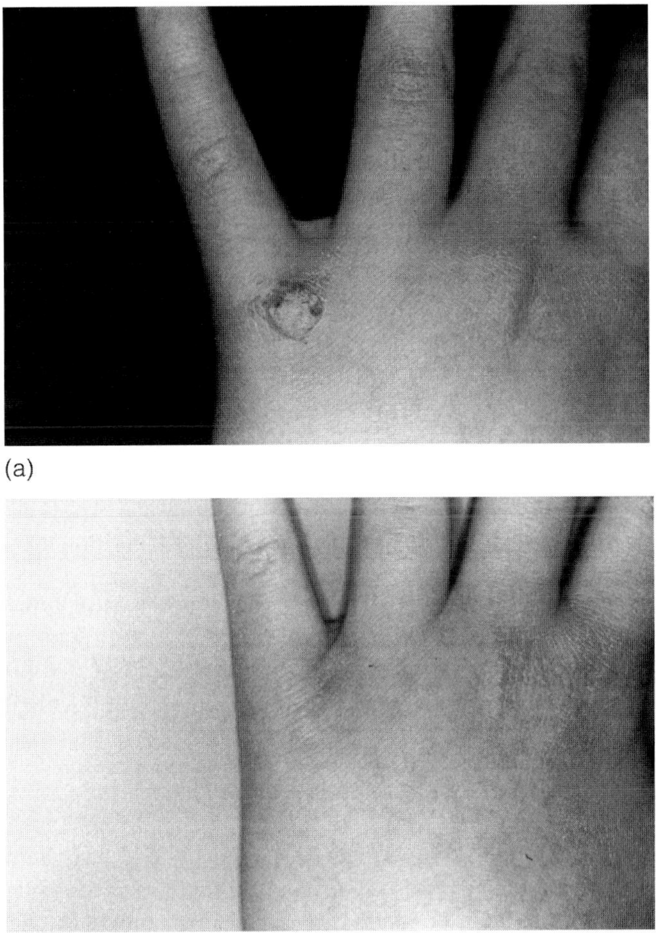

(a)

(b)

FIGURE 7 (a) Recalcitrant, hyperkeratotic wart on the dorsum of the hand. (b) After five PDL treatments and 3-week intervals the wart has resolved. The fluence was 9.5 J/cm^2 and a 5 mm spot. The wart was pared down with a #15 blade before treatment.

Another study reported on 54 patients with recalcitrant warts who were treated with the PDL. Warts were not debrided or pared before treatment [168]. They used fluences of 6.75 to 10 J/cm^2 and treated a rim of several millimeters of normal adjacent tissue. Flat warts were most responsive, followed by palmar/plantar, common, as well as periungual warts. Periungual warts, which can be the most difficult to treat, also had greater than 50% improvement in 58% of patients, with 33% clearing. Most warts required several treatments. These investigators claim that PDL offers the advantage of little or no pain associated with therapy, and that it is also bloodless.

Other recent studies report lower response rates. Huilgol et al. [169] found a 0% clearance for recalcitrant warts, all of which were periungual and plantar in location. Jacobson et al. [170] reported clearance rates as low as 47% for primary, never-before-treated lesions and 68% for recalcitrant warts. Most of these warts were on the extremities and follow-up was only 2 months.

I performed my own study of 33 patients with 96 warts which were all previously treated [171] (Table 2). The warts were located on the body, face, plantar, periungual, subungual, and digital locations (Fig. 7). Forty-eight percent of patients had complete clearance; 45% partially cleared. Sixty-five percent of those who cleared remained wart free for an average of 11 months. Mean fluence used was 9.5 J/cm^2 with a 5 mm spot size and an average of 3.4 treatments. The warts on the palm, body, and face responded the best, with plantar warts being the most resistant. When necessary, I administered digital blocks with 2% lidocaine or locally infiltrated with lidocaine. Hyperkeratotic warts were pared to the level of the wart vasculature with a #15 blade. Nails were trimmed or avulsed as necessary. Sequential pulses were delivered until the area developed a gray discoloration. A 1 Hz repetition rate was used and a surrounding rim of 2 mm of normal-appearing tissue was treated as well. Most patients developed a black eschar. Patients were given topical antibiotic ointment to apply twice daily. The number of necessary treatments ranged from one to 12 at 3 to 4 week intervals. Patients were followed for as long as 21 months with an average of 11 months.

Palmar warts had a high clearance rate of 75%. Digital, peri-, and subungual lesions responded in 50% of cases. Plantar lesions responded worst; only 20% of cases were cleared. The only side effects were transient pain in two patients and erythema in two patients. No scars, pigmentary changes, nail dystrophy, or persistent pain were noted.

This study indicates that PDL treatment of recalcitrant warts may have variable response rates. Unlike some of the previous studies, mine used only recalcitrant warts which may account for decreased clearing, as well as the fact that most of the lesions were not in favorable locations like the face or body. The PDL does have an excellent side-effect profile with only four patients reported with hyperpigmentation and one patient with scarring [17,169]. Although pain after treatment is limited, most patients do require local anesthesia, and postsurgically they may experience soreness, especially for plantar warts.

Patients who are immunosuppressed for whatever reason do not respond well to any known treatment, and this includes laser removal. As I explain to patients, they need an intact immune system in order to work alongside any treatment modality. However, there was a recent report of a patient with acquired immunodeficiency syndrome, had innumerable molluscum contagiosum, and responded well to PDL treatment [172]. He was reportedly cleared of his facial lesions and this was maintained for at least 4 months.

SUMMARY

Vascular lesions such as telangiectasias, spider angiomas, and rosacea are very commonly seen in the office. Lasers and other light-based systems offer the advantages of minimal pain, lower risks of scarring, and great efficacy. It is up to the trained laser surgeon to appropriately choose the correct laser for his/her patient. Larger-caliber vessels, especially around the mid face, can be treated with the PDL or continuous wave lasers such as the copper vapor/copper bromide, KTP, or krypton lasers. Some of these lasers are effective in one treatment session but some may require more than one treatment routinely. Diffuse erythema such as seen in rosacea or poikiloderma are more effectively treated with the PDL with a lesser risk of scarring. New systems are constantly being developed and need to be compared scientifically with established laser systems.

Scars can be dermabraded, laser abraded, injected with corticosteroids, and have silicone dressing applied to them. However, the PDL can be used to flatten hypertrophic, erythematous scars, especially those on the face without significant postsurgical morbidity or further risks of worsening the scar. I have found the PDL a great asset in treating facial scars attributable to Mohs micrographic surgery, overzealous chemical peeling, traumatic injury, dog bites, as well as CO_2 laser resurfacing.

Mature striae, which do represent a form of dermal scarring, can also be treated with the PDL. Clinically, I believe it is not a very effective therapy, although some investigators do feel that it is a worthwhile treatment.

Warts can be one of the most difficult problems for a dermatologist to treat. They often are multiple and tend to recur, and one does not want the patient to suffer any permanent morbidity or scar from the therapies used to treat the wart. CO_2 laser carries the risk of permanent scarring, whereas the PDL can be effective without the risk of prolonged wounds and possible scarring, even after multiple treatments.

Lasers may be the first line of treatment for certain cutaneous lesions such as port wine stains, or the treatment that allows greater selectivity and ease for both the patient and the physician such as in the treatment of spider telangiectasias and angiomas. Laser technology continues to improve and broaden. The future will provide us with vascular lesion lasers that maintain selectivity but are more able to treat larger/deeper vessels without significant scarring or permanent pigmentary changes.

REFERENCES

1. Anderson RR, Parrish JA. Microvasculature can be selectively damaged using dye lasers: a basic theory and experimental evidence in human skin. Lasers Surg Med 1: 263–276, 1981.
2. Anderson RR, Parrish JA. Selective photothermolysis: precise microsurgery by selective absorption of pulsed radiation. Science 220:524–527, 1983.
3. Ashinoff R, Geronemus RG. Capillary hemangiomas and treatment with the flashlamp-pumped pulsed dye laser. Arch Dermatol 127:202–205, 1991.
4. Waldorf HA, Lask GP, Geronemus RG. Laser treatment of telangiectasias. In: Alster TS, Apfelberg DB, eds. Cosmetic Laser Surgery. New York: John Wiley and Sons, 1996, pp. 93–109.
5. Broska P, Martinho E, Goodman M. Comparisons of the argon tunable dye laser with the flashlamp pulsed dye laser in the treatment of facial telangiectasia. J Dermatol Surg Oncol 20:749–754, 1994.
6. Goldman MP, Weiss RA, Brody HJ, Coleman WP, Fitzpatrick RE. Treatment of facial telangiectasia with sclerotherapy, laser surgery, and/or electrodesiccation: a review. J Dermatol Surg Oncol 19:899–906, 1993.
7. Ofrenstein A, Nelson JS. Treatment of facial vascular lesions with a 100um spot 577-nm pulsed continuous wave dye laser. Ann Plast Surg 23:310–316, 1989.
8. Ross M, Watcher MA, Goodman MM. Comparison of the flashlamp pulsed dye laser with the argon tunable dye laser with robotized handpiece for facial telangiectasia. Lasers Surg Med 13:374–378, 1993.

9. Tan OT, Carney M, Margolis R, Seki Y, Boll J, Anderson RR, Parrish JA. Histologic responses of portwine stains treated by argon, carbon dioxide and dye lasers: a preliminary report. Arch Dermatol 122:1016–1022, 1986.
10. McDaniel DH. Clinical applications of lasers for skin disorders: comparisons and contrasts. Skinlaser Today 5–13, 1992.
11. McDaniel DH. Cutaneous vascular disorders: advances in laser treatments. Cutis 45: 339–359, 1990.
12. Lowe NJ, Behr KL, Fitzpatrick R, Goldman M, Ruiz-Esparza JR. Flashlamp pumped dye laser for rosacea-associated telangiectasia and erythema. J Dermatol Surg Oncol 17:522–525, 1991.
13. Garden JM, Tan OT, Boll J, Parrish JA. The pulsed dye laser for the treatment of port wine stains. J Dermatol Surg Oncol 12(abstr):757, 1986.
14. Hoffman SJ, Walsh P, Morelli JG. Treatment of angiofibroma with the pulsed tunable dye laser. J Am Acad Dermatol 29:790–791, 1993.
15. Ross BS, Levine VJ, Ashinoff R. Laser treatment of acquired vascular lesions. Clin Dermatol 15:385–396, 1997.
16. Wheeland RG, Applebaum J. Flashlamp-pumped pulsed dye laser therapy for Poikiloderma of Civatte. J Dermatol Surg Oncol 16:12–16, 1990.
17. Kauvar ANB, McDaniel DH, Geronemus RG. Pulsed dye laser treatment of warts. Arch Fam Med 4:1035–1040, 1995.
18. Alster TS. Improvement of erythematous and hypertrophic scars by 585-nm flashlamp-pumped pulsed dye laser. Ann Plast Surg 32:186–190, 1994.
19. Alster TS, Kurban AK, Grove GL, Grove MJ, Tan OT. Alteration of argon laser-induced scars by the pulsed dye laser. Lasers Surg Med 13:368–373, 1993.
20. McDaniel DH, Ash K, Zukowski M. Treatment of stretch marks with the 585-nm flashlamp-pumped pulsed dye laser. Dermatol Surg 22:332–337, 1996.
21. Neumann RA, Knobler RM, Leonhartsberger H, Gebhart W. Comparative histochemistry of port-wine stains after copper vapor laser (578 nm) and argon laser treatment. J Invest Dermatol 99:160–167, 1992.
22. Alster TS. Laser treatment of vascular lesions. In: Manual of Cutaneous Laser Techniques. Philadelphia: Lippincott-Raven, 1997, pp. 44–70.
23. Dinehart SM, Waner M, Flock S. The copper vapor laser for treatment of cutaneous vascular and pigmented lesions. J Dermatol Surg Oncol 19:370–375, 1993.
24. Dinehart SM, Waner M. Comparison of the copper vapor and flashlamp-pulsed dye laser in the treatment of facial telangiectasia. J Am Acad Dermatol 24:116, 1991.
25. Waner M, Dinehart SM, Wilson MB, Flock ST. A comparison of copper vapor and flashlamp pumped dye lasers in the treatment of facial telangiectasia. J Dermatol Surg Oncol 19:992–998, 1993.
26. McCoy S, Hanna M, Anderson P, McLennan G, Repacholi M. An evaluation of the copper-bromide laser for treating telangiectasia. Dermatol Surg 22:551–557, 1996.
27. Keller GS. Use of the KTP laser in cosmetic surgery. Am J Cosmetic Surg 9:177–180, 1992.
28. Silver BE, Livshots YL. Preliminary experience with the KTP/532 nm laser in the treatment of facial telangiectasia. Cosmetic Derm 9:61–64, 1996.
29. Apfelberg DB, Bailin P, Rosenberg H. Preliminary investigation of KTP/532 laser light in the treatment of hemangiomas and tattoos. Lasers Surg Med 6:38–42, 1986.
30. Goldman MP, Eckhouse S. Photothermal sclerosis of leg veins. Dermatol Surg 22:323–330, 1996.
31. Raulin C, Hellwig S, Schonermark MP. Treatment of a nonresponding port-wine stain with a new pulsed light source (Photoderm VL). Lasers Surg Med 21:203–208, 1997.
32. Taylor MB. Photoderm treatment of resistant port wine stain vascular malformations. Lasers Surg Med 8(suppl):39–40, 1996.

33. Weiss RA, Weiss MA, Goldman MP. Photothermal sclerosis of resistant telangiectatic leg and facial veins using the Photoderm VL. Lasers Surg Med 8(suppl):40–41, 1996.
34. Narurkar VA, Vidimos AT. Cutaneous lasers and incoherent light sources: new applications. Cosmetic Derm 9:11–21, 1996.
35. Kovak SJ. A comparison in the treatment of leg and facial telangiectasias with the Photoderm VL system using long and short pulse durations. Lasers Surg Med 10(suppl):175, 1998.
36. Alster TS, Kohn SR. Dermatologic lasers: three decades of progress. Int J Dermatol 31:601–610, 1992.
37. Geronemus RG. Argon laser for the treatment of cutaneous lesions. Clin Dermatol 13: 55–58, 1995.
38. Garden JM, Geronemus RG. Dermatologic laser surgery. J Dermatol Surg Oncol 16: 156–168, 1990.
39. Apfelberg DB, Maser MR, Lash H. Expanded role of the argon laser in plastic surgery. J Dermatol Surg Oncol 9:145–149, 1983.
40. Apfelberg DB, Maser MR, Lash H, Rivers J. The argon laser for cutaneous lesions. JAMA 245:2073–2075, 1981.
41. Key D. Argon-pumped tunable dye laser for the treatment of cutaneous lesions. Clin Dermatol 13:59–61, 1995.
42. Ashinoff R. Introduction to lasers. Semin Dermatol 13:48–59, 1994.
43. Spicer MS, Goldberg DJ. Lasers in dermatology. J Am Acad Dermatol 9:1–25, 1996.
44. McBurney E. Clinical usefulness of the argon laser for the 1990s. J Dermatol Surg Oncol 19:358–368, 1993.
45. Cosman B. Experience in the argon laser therapy of port wine stains. Plast Reconstr Surg 65:119–129, 1980.
46. Dixon JA, Huether SE, Rotering RH. Hypertrophic scarring in argon laser treatment of portwine stains. Plast Reconstr Surg 73:771–780, 1984.
47. Finley JL, Barsky SH, Geer DE, Kamat BR, Noe JM, Rosen S. Healing of portwine stains after argon laser therapy. Arch Dermatol 117:486–489, 1981.
48. Apfelberg DB, Kosek J, Maser MR, Lash H. Histology of portwine stains following argon laser treatment. Br J Plast Surg 32:232–287, 1979.
49. Noe JM, Barsky SH, Geer DE, Rosen S. Portwine stains and the response to argon laser therapy: successful treatment of the predictive role of color, age and biopsy. Plast Reconstr Surg 65:130–136, 1980.
50. Arndt KA. Argon laser therapy of small cutaneous vascular lesions. Arch Dermatol 118:220–224, 1982.
51. Apfelberg DB, Maser MR, Lash H. Treatment of nevus araneus by means of an argon laser. J Dermatol Surg Oncol 4:172–174, 1978.
52. Landthaler M, Haina D, Waidelich W, Braun-Falco O. Laser therapy of venous lakes (Bean-Walsh) and telangiectasias. Plast Reconstr Surg 73:78–81, 1984.
53. Hulsbergen-Henning JP, Roskam Y, van Gemert MJ. Treatment of keloids and hypertrophic scars with an argon laser. Lasers Surg Med 6:72–75, 1986.
54. Rubenstein R, Roenigk HH, Stegman S, Hanke CW. Atypical keloids after dermabrasion of patients taking isotretinoin. J Am Acad Dermatol 15:280–285, 1986.
55. Zachariea H. Delayed wound healing and keloid formation following argon laser treatment or dermabrasion during isotretinoin treatment. Br J Dermatol 118:703–706, 1988.
56. Bauer EA, Seltzer JL, Eisen AZ. Inhibition of collagen degradative enzymes by retinoic acid in vitro. J Am Acad Dermatol 6:603–607, 1982.
57. Goldman MP, Fitzpatrick RE. Treatment of cutaneous vascular lesions. In: Goldman MP, Fitzpatrick RE, eds. Cutaneous Laser Surgery: the Art and Science of Selective Photothermolysis. St. Louis: Mosby-Year Book, 1993, pp. 19–105.
58. Wheeland RG. Clinical uses of lasers in dermatology. Lasers Surg Med 16:2–23, 1995.

59. Greenwald J, Rosen S, Anderson RR, Harris T, MacFarland F, Noe J, Parrish JA. Comparative histological studies of the tunable dye (at 577 nm) laser and argon laser: the specific vascular effects of the dye laser. J Invest Dermatol 77:305–310, 1981.
60. Apfelberg DB. Argon-pumped tunable dye laser. Ann Plast Surg 32:394–400, 1994.
61. Scheibner A, Wheeland RG. Argon-pumped tunable dye laser for port-wine stain hemangiomas in adults: a new technique using small spot size and minimal power. J Dermatol Surg Oncol 15:277–282, 1989.
62. Dover JS, Geronemus RG, Stern RS, O'Hare D, Arndt KA. Dye laser treatment of port-wine stains: comparison of the continuous-wave dye laser with a robotized scanning device and the pulsed dye laser. J Am Acad Dermatol 32:237–240, 1995.
63. Apfelberg DB, Smoller B. Preliminary analysis of histological results of hexascan device with continuous tunable dye laser at 514 (argon) and 577 (yellow). Laser Surg Med 13:106–112, 1993.
64. Pickering JW, Walker EP, Butler PH, van Halewyn CN. Copper vapour treatment of port-wine stains and other vascular malformations. Br J Plast Surg 43:273–282, 1990.
65. Key JM, Waner M. Selective destruction of facial telangiectasia using a copper vapor laser. Arch Otolaryngol Head Neck Surg 118:509–513, 1992.
66. Neumann RA, Leonhartsberger H, Bohler-Sommeregger K, Knobler R, Kokoschka EM, Honigsman H. Results and tissue healing after copper-vapour laser (at 578 nm) treatment of port wine stains and facial telangiectasias. Br J Dermatol 128:306–312, 1993.
67. Wheeland RG. Copper vapor and dye laser therapy for cutaneous vascular disorders. West J Med 151:650–651, 1989.
68. Goldman L. New developments with the heavy metal vapor lasers for the dermatologist. J Dermatol Surg Oncol 13:163–165, 1987.
69. Thibault PK. A patient's questionnaire evaluation of krypton laser treatment of facial telangiectasias. A comparison with the copper vapor laser. Dermatol Surg 23:37–41, 1997.
70. McDaniel DH, Mordon S. Hexascan: a new robotized scanning laser handpiece. Cutis 45:300–305, 1990.
71. Tanghetti EA, Adrian RM. Long-pulsed 532 nm laser treatment of facial telangiectasias. Lasers Surg Med 10(suppl):212, 1998.
72. Tanghetti EA, Adrian RM. Long-pulsed 532 nm laser treatment of port wine stains. Lasers Surg Med 10(suppl):176, 1998.
73. Narurkar V, Haas A. Comparison of variable pulse width and wavelength pulsed dye laser with the variable pulse with 532 nm laser for the treatment of facial vascular lesions. Lasers Surg Med 10(suppl):210, 1998.
74. Tan OT, Murray S, Kurban AK. Action spectrum of vascular specific injury using pulsed irradiation. J Invest Dermatol 92:868–871, 1989.
75. Garden JM, Tan OT, Kerschmann R, Boll J, Furumoto H, Anderson RR, Parrish JA. Effect of dye laser pulse duration on selective cutaneous vascular injury. J Invest Dermatol 87:653–657, 1986.
76. Tan OP, Morrison P, Kurban AK. 585 nm for the treatment of port-wine stains. Plast Reconstr Surg 86:1112–1117, 1990.
77. Glassberg E, Lask GP, Tan EML, Uitto J. The flashlamp-pumped 577-nm pulsed tunable dye laser. Clinical efficacy and in vitro studies. J Dermatol Surg Oncol 14:1200–1208, 1988.
78. Tan OT, Sherwood K, Gilchrest BA. Treatment of children with port-wine stains using the flashlamp-pulsed tunable dye laser. N Engl J Med 320:416–421, 1989.
79. Alster TS, Lewis AB. Dermatologic laser surgery: a review. Dermatol Surg 22:797–805, 1996.

APPENDIX 1: CONSENT TO OPERATION FOR LASER SURGERY, COSMETIC, OR OTHER PURPOSES

Date:________________________

1. I hereby request and authorize **ROBIN ASHINOFF, M.D.** to perform an operation upon me on or about the ____________________________ of _______________, 19___ for the purpose of attempting to improve the appearance with respect to the following conditions:

   ____ _____________

   ____

2. The effect and nature of the operation to be performed, risks involved, as well as possible alternative methods of treatment have been fully explained to me.

3. I also authorize the operating surgeon to perform any other procedures which she may deem necessary or desirable in attempting to improve the condition(s) stated in paragraph 1, or any unforeseen condition(s).

4. I also agree that the operating surgeon may use my photograph for medical publication and teaching purposes.

5. I know that the practice of medicine and surgery is not an exact science and, therefore, that the reputable practitioners cannot properly guarantee results. I acknowledge that no guarantee has been made by anyone regarding the operation which I have requested and authorized.

Signed:____
(Patient or person authorized to give consent)

Witness:____

23

Laser Treatment of Pigmented Lesions and Tattoos

David J. Goldberg
New Jersey Medical School, Newark, New Jersey

PIGMENTED LESIONS

In 1958, Schawlow and Townes, who were working with microwaves, first proposed a technique for the generation of monochromatic radiation by stimulated emission. They produced monochromatic radiation in the infrared optical region of the electromagnetic spectrum with an alkali vapor used as the active medium. Maiman, using a ruby crystal in 1960, developed stimulated emission of a red-light beam with a wavelength of 694 nm. It is from this prototype that today's lasers are derived. Since 1960, research and technical advances have adapted lasers to dermatology. In 1963, Goldman [1] first experimented with a normal-mode (500 microsec pulse duration) 694 nm ruby laser pulses on human skin. The darker the skin color, the more the laser was absorbed. Based on these observations, he speculated that melanin selectively absorbs laser light. In later studies, Goldman [2–4] used a Q-switched ruby laser (50 microsec pulse duration) and found that the damage threshold of pigmented lesions was independent of skin color. This suggested a more selective effect, perhaps at the level of the melanosome. Early work with the ruby laser consisted of ablation techniques. Little bleeding was noted after nonspecific damage to the superficial dermal layers. Small areas of skin could be treated with high-intensity radiation with few complications.

Some 20 years later, Polla [5] and Dover [6] in separate studies showed that the Q-switched ruby laser targeted individual melanosomes. Electron microscopic analysis of these thermally damaged targeted melanosomes revealed membrane disruption and disorganization of the internal contents. The destruction of melanosomes is pulsewidth dependent; both pulse durations of 40 nanoseconds and 750 nanoseconds disrupt melanosomes, but longer pulse durations such as 400 microseconds do not damage the melanosomes. This is consistent with the theory of selective photothermolysis, which states that the pulse duration of an emitted laser wavelength must be less than the thermal relaxation time of the targeted object. A typical 1.0-micron melanosome has a thermal relaxation time somewhere between 0.5 to 1.0 microseconds.

The cause of melanosomal destruction is unknown. Plasma formation probably does not occur. The peak powers produced, with lasers used to interact with melanosomes, are quite low for such an occurrence. Shockwave and/or cavitation damage, the photomechanical physical effects produced from thermal expansion, and/or the extreme temperature gradients created within the melanosome are the more likely explanations. Studies of acoustic waves generated by pulsed irradiation of melanosomes and pigmented cells support these possibilities [7]. Melanin absorbs and localizes the high intensity irradiation from Q-switched lasers, thereby creating a sharp temperature gradient between the melanosome and its surrounding structures. This gradient leads to thermal expansion and the generation and propagation of acoustic waves, which can mechanically damage the melanosome-laden cells.

Tissue repair after laser-induced melanosomal disruption shows a two-staged initial transient cutaneous depigmentation followed by subsequent repigmentation weeks later [8]. Black guinea pig skin irradiated with 40 nanoseconds Q-switched ruby pulses at radiant exposures of 0.4 J/cm^2 or greater whitens immediately, fades in 20 minutes, depigments 7 to 10 days later, and then repigments 4 to 8 weeks after treatment. Guinea pig skin exposed to radiant exposures less than that of threshold exposure (<0.3 J/cm^2) undergoes paradoxical melanogenesis. This may be due to either a sublethal change in the melanosome (interfering with the normal feedback inhibition of melanogenesis) or simply postinflammatory hyperpigmentation. Further studies are required to evaluate the therapeutic implications of this paradoxical reaction.

Laser irradiation leads to histologic melanosomal disruption and vacuolization of pigment-laden cells in the basal layer. Human keratinocytes and melanocytes exhibit pigment and nuclear material condensation at the periphery of laser irradiated cells. This leads to a characteristic "ring-cell" appearance. Epidermal necrosis and regeneration of a pigmented epidermis follow over the next 7 days [9]. Transient hypopigmentation is followed by gradual repigmentation to the normal constitutive color. Other short-pulsed, high-fluence specific pigmented lesion lasers produce similar clinical and histologic findings in human skin.

Three action spectrum studies have analyzed the ability of different wavelength pulsed lasers to disrupt cutaneous pigment. Anderson et al. [10] evaluated the effects of a Q-switched Nd:YAG laser with pulse duration of 10 to 12 nanoseconds, at three distinct emitted wavelengths (355 nm, 532 nm, and 1064 nm), on guinea pig skin. The threshold exposures for immediate skin whitening, the sign of laser-induced melanosomal changes, required energy fluences of 0.11 J/cm^2, 0.20 J/cm^2, and 1.0 J/cm^2 at 355 nm, 532 nm, and 1064 nm respectively. These findings show that the threshold exposure dose is wavelength dependent. Furthermore, longer wavelengths (which are less well absorbed by melanin) require higher energy fluences to induce these changes. At all evaluated wavelengths, electron microscopic examination revealed disrupted melanosomes within keratinocytes and melanocytes. Histologically, irradiated basal cells showed the characteristic "ring cell" appearance. As expected, the transient immediate whitening of the laser-treated area exhibited delayed epidermal depigmentation followed by repigmentation back to the constitutive skin color.

Flashlamp-pulsed tunable lasers [11] with pulse duration of 750 nanoseconds also show the relationship between wavelength and whitening threshold. Threshold fluences were found to be 0.44 J/cm^2, 0.62 J/cm^2, 0.76 J/cm^2, and 0.86 J/cm^2 at 435 nm, 488 nm, 532 nm, and 560 nm, respectively.

Finally, Sherwood et al. [12] performed an action spectrum study of guinea pig skin using a flashlamp-pulsed tunable laser with pulse duration of 300 nanoseconds at four different wavelengths (504 nm, 590 nm, 720 nm, and 750 nm). They found the 504 nm wavelength produced the most pigment-specific injury because the longer wavelengths caused disruption of the basement membrane with pigmentary incontinence.

Today, there are numerous lasers that can specifically target pigmented lesions, including red light lasers (694 nm ruby and 755 nm alexandrite), green light lasers (510 nm pulsed dye and 532 nm frequency-doubled Nd:YAG), and near infrared lasers (1064 nm neodymium:yttrium-aluminum-garnet [Nd:YAG]). The wide range of lasers that can be used to treat pigment is a result of the broad absorption spectrum of melanin. Even so, other less pigment-specific lasers have been used to treat pigmented lesions, including the argon, krypton, copper, CO_2 and, most recently, Erbium:YAG lasers. The CO_2 laser exerts its effect on tissue by simple vaporization of water-containing cells. Textural skin changes and scarring may result from this nonselective destruction. A very low wattage CO_2 laser appears to reduce the risk of scarring and has been used effectively to treat superficial epidermal pigmented lesions, such as solar lentignes. The Erbium:YAG laser also vaporizes water-containing cells and may more precisely ablate superficial layers of skin than does the CO_2 laser.

It should be noted that wavelengths not selectively absorbed by melanin indiscriminately destroy pigmented as well as nonpigmented structures in the skin. Alternatively, as alluded to previously, lasers with wavelengths which are both preferentially absorbed by melanin over other cutaneous chromophores (such as hemoglobin) and penetrate to the depth of the targeted pigment can be used to more selectively target cutaneous pigment. Thus, lasers emitting wavelengths between 630 nm and 1100 nm may provide selective melanosome damage, good skin penetration, as well as selective absorption by melanin over hemoglobin.

Pulsed lasers with appropriate wavelengths have a distinct theoretical advantage over continuous wave devices in the selective destruction of cutaneous pigment. The green and blue light (488 and 514 nm, respectively) of the argon laser is specifically absorbed by melanin. The problem with the system is that it functions as a continuous wave laser. Thus, although this laser selectively targets the melanin chromophore, the heat produced dissipates from the absorbing melanosomes, causing thermal damage to surrounding tissue with resultant hypopigmentation and potential scarring. Similar findings can ensue after use of the krypton (520–530 nm), copper (511 nm), and variable pulse width KTP (532 nm) quasicontinuous wave lasers.

Pigment-specific lasers can be divided into three categories: green, red, and near infrared. Green light lasers are further subdivided into both pulsed and nonpulsed systems. Red light lasers are subdivided into short pulsed (Q-switched) and long pulsed (normal-mode) systems. The currently available near infrared laser is short pulsed (Q-switched). Green light lasers do not penetrate as deeply into the skin as do the red and near infrared lasers because of their shorter wavelengths. Green light lasers are therefore effective only in the treatment of epidermal pigmented lesions (Table 1).

TABLE 1 Pigmented Lesions

	Epidermal	Dermal
Q-switched ruby (694 nm)	++++	++++
Q-switched Nd:YAG (1064 nm)	++	++++
Frequency doubled Q-switched Nd:YAG (532 nm)	++++	+
Pigmented lesion pulsed dye (510 nm)	++++	+
Alexandrite (755 nm)	+++	+++

+ Poor
++ Fair
+++ Good
++++ Excellent

Green Light Pulsed Lasers

These lasers produce energy with pulses shorter than the thermal relaxation time of melanosomes. Examples of these lasers are the flashlamp-pumped pulsed dye and frequency-doubled Q-switched Nd:YAG lasers. The flashlamp-pumped pulsed dye laser produces a 510 nm wavelength and 300 nanoseconds pulse of energy, whereas the frequency-doubled Q-switched Nd:YAG laser produces a 532 nm wavelength and a 5 to 10 nanoseconds pulse of energy. Both lasers produce excellent results when used to treat epidermal-pigmented lesions (Figs. 1, 2). Because the green wavelength of these lasers is also well absorbed by oxyhemoglobin, purpura formation may occur after laser irradiation. The purpura resolves in 1 to 2 weeks after treatment, with resolution or lightening of the clinical lesion in 4 to 8 weeks after treatment. Occasionally, purpura leads to postinflammatory hyperpigmentation.

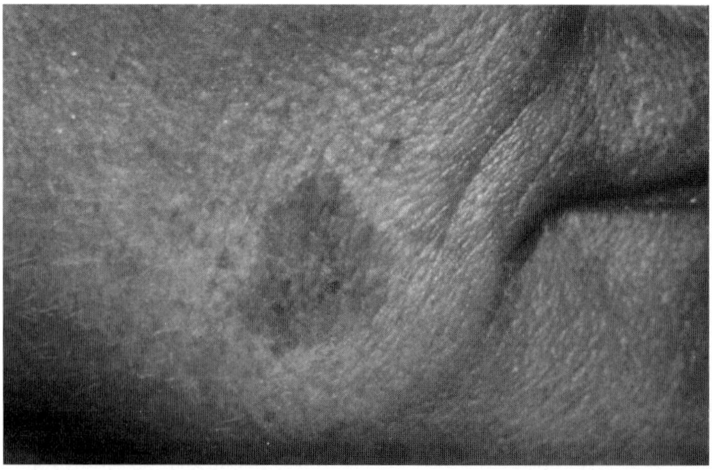

FIGURE 1 Solar lentignes before treatment with the frequency doubled Q-switched Nd: YAG laser.

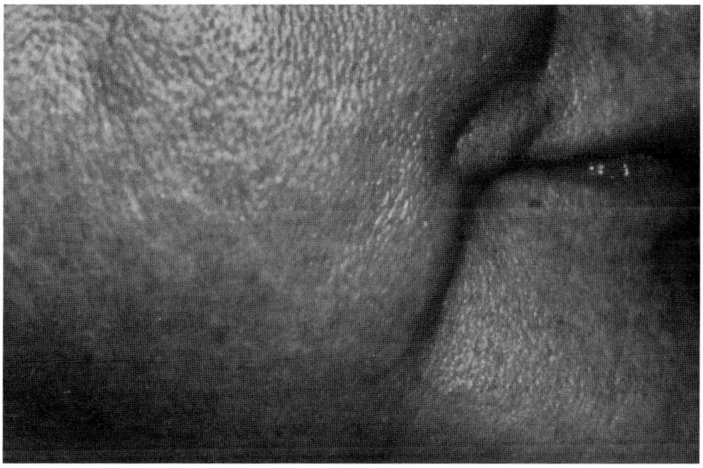

FIGURE 2 Clearance after one treatment with the frequency doubled Q-switched Nd:YAG laser.

Flashlamp-pumped pulsed dye laser treatment results in excellent clearing of epidermal pigmented lesions such as lentignes, ephilides, seborrheic keratoses, and café-au-lait macules. In a study of 492 benign epidermal pigmented lesions in 65 patients, 50% of the treated lesions cleared completely after one treatment when treated at a fluence of 2 to 3.5 J/cm^2. Another 33% of the treated lesions were lightened considerably [13]. Ninety percent of treated epidermal pigmented lesions can be cleared after three treatments [14]. Treatment results can be affected by anatomic location. Although up to 90% of hand and facial lentignes may be cleared, less favorable results are usually seen after treatment of trunk or leg epidermal pigmented lesions [14]. A typical treatment response included purpura lasting 5 to 7 days, followed by subsequent sloughing of the treated lesion at 7 to 14 days [15]. The underlying new skin was pink for 2 to 3 days but faded to normal skin color with rare textural changes or scarring. In another study, 25 patients with solar lentignes showed excellent laser-induced clearing after 1 to 2 treatments [16]. Fourteen patients with café-au-lait macules showed complete clearing after 3 to 6 treatments. Two patients with nevus spilus and two patients with Becker's nevi showed clearing with up to six treatments. As a general rule, this laser produces a variable response in some epidermal-pigmented lesions such as café-au-lait macules, Becker's nevi and epidermal melasma. Epidermal postinflammatory hyperpigmentation may also respond. Predominantly dermal pigmented lesions show little to no response. Because some lesions show a variable clinical response, testing the treatment areas of the respective lesion may be prudent before engaging in a full treatment. Even when café-au-lait macules and Becker's nevi show resolution after treatment, recurrences have been reported. Recurrences may occur because of the impact of these lasers on melanosomes, with little effect on the pigment-producing melanocytes. Careful sun protection may retard, but not prevent, recurrence. Because melasma occurs secondary to a combination of genetic, sun-induced, and hormonal factors, successful laser treatment is the exception rather than the rule with the use of this laser.

The Q-switched Nd:YAG laser is a solid state high-fluence, short pulsed (10–20 nsec) laser that emits at a wavelength of 1064 nm. By placing doubling crystals in the laser beam's path, frequency doubling halves the wavelength to 532 nm. Epidermal lesions such as lentignes and café-au-lait macules, can be lightened considerably by the frequency-doubled Q-switched Nd:YAG. In one study, 84% of 17 lentignes lightened by at least 50% after several treatments at 2 to 5 J/cm^2 [17]. Postsurgical purpura developed in all patients and 25% of treated individuals showed transient hyperpigmentation. The degree of response to the laser at this wavelength is proportional to the amount of pigment chromophore present at the treatment site. When high fluences are delivered through small spot sizes, whitening of the skin is noted. This is then followed by pinpoint bleeding leading to a hemorrhagic crust, which falls off in 7 to 10 days.

Green Light Nonpulsed (Quasicontinuous Wave) Lasers

Nonpulsed, quasicontinuous wave green light lasers such as the copper vapor, krypton, and variable pulse width KTP lasers share some characteristics with the aforementioned pulsed lasers. However, because the thermal relaxation time of the melanosome is exceeded using these lasers, they do not produce the same consistent clinical results. Although small epidermal pigmented lesions may be successfully cleared, more treatment sessions are usually necessary to achieve similar results to those seen with pulsed green light lasers. We have tried robotized scanning devices to allow occasional effective treatment of larger lesions such as café-au-lait macules. These lasers are not useful in the treatment of dermal pigmented lesions such as Nevus of Ota. It should be noted that the epidermal pigmented lesion response after treatment with a noncoherent flashlamp intense pulsed light source is somewhere between that of the pulsed laser and nonpulsed laser systems.

Red Light Pulsed Lasers

The two currently available red light pulsed pigmented lesion lasers are the Q-switched ruby and Q-switched alexandrite lasers. The Q-switched ruby laser emits a 694 nm beam with a 20 to 50 nanoseconds pulse duration. The Q-switched alexandrite laser emits a 755 nm wavelength with pulse duration of 50 to 100 nanoseconds. The longer wavelengths of these lasers allow deeper penetration into the dermis. Their mechanism of action on melanin-containing melanosomes and melanocytes involves selective photothermolysis, photoacoustical mechanical disruption, and chemical alteration of the target tissue. Photoacoustic mechanical disruption is caused by rapid thermal tissue expansion, creating pressure waves that fragment pigment particles in the dermis. Within the dermis, absorption of the laser energy by melanin-rich stage III and IV melanosomes causes selective pigment destruction.

Q-Switched Ruby Laser

The Q-switched ruby laser is made with a ruby (aluminum oxide) crystal which has been grown in the presence of chromium. This combined crystal is surrounded by a helical flash lamp. The laser, in its natural state, produces a train of nonuniform pulses. In the Q-switched mode, very high peak powers can be attained with each pulse (over 1×10^8 W/cm^2 per pulse).

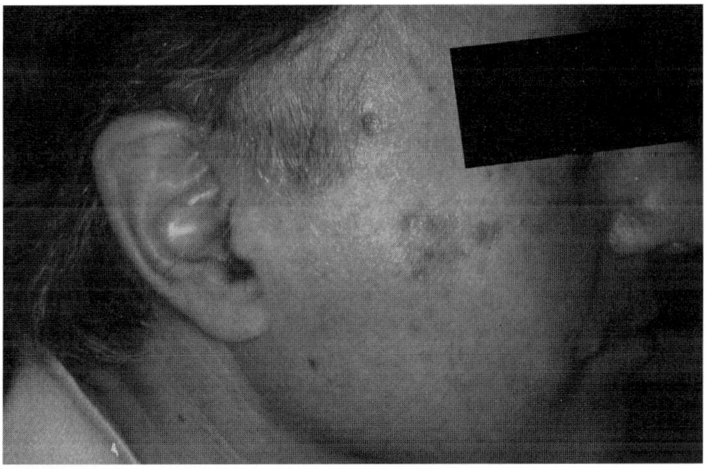

FIGURE 3 Solar lentignes before treatment with the Q-switched ruby laser.

Ruby laser light penetrates about 1 mm into the skin, is well absorbed by melanin, and is minimally absorbed by hemoglobin. Thus, this laser can be used for dermal pigmented lesions while avoiding vascular dermal structures. Epidermal pigmented lesions, such as lentignes and ephilides usually clear after one to four treatments with the Q-switched ruby laser. Taylor et al. reported 29 lentignes that totally cleared after only one treatment. Café-au-lait macules, nevus spilus, and Becker's nevi may also respond to treatment with this laser [18]. Ashinoff et al. treated 15 café-au-lait macules and found significant lightening after an average of six treatments. Frequent recurrences are the general rule after treatment of café-au-lait macules, nevus spilus, and Becker's nevi (Figs. 3–6) [19].

The Q-switched ruby laser is highly effective in treating dermal pigmented lesions such as the Nevus of Ito and Ota [20]. The long wavelength successfully

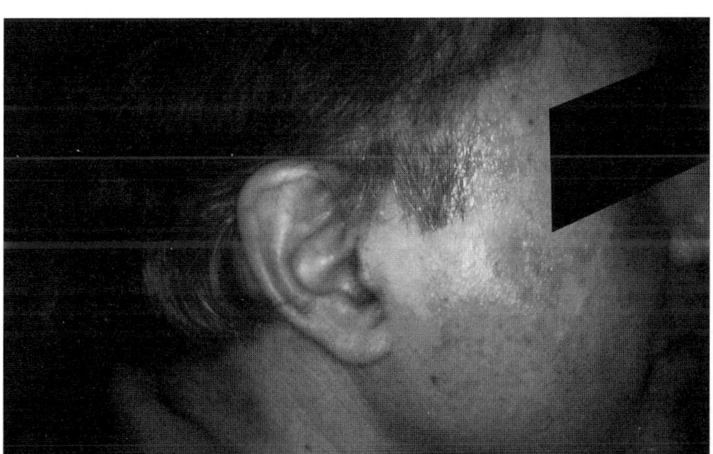

FIGURE 4 Clearance after one treatment with the Q-switched ruby laser.

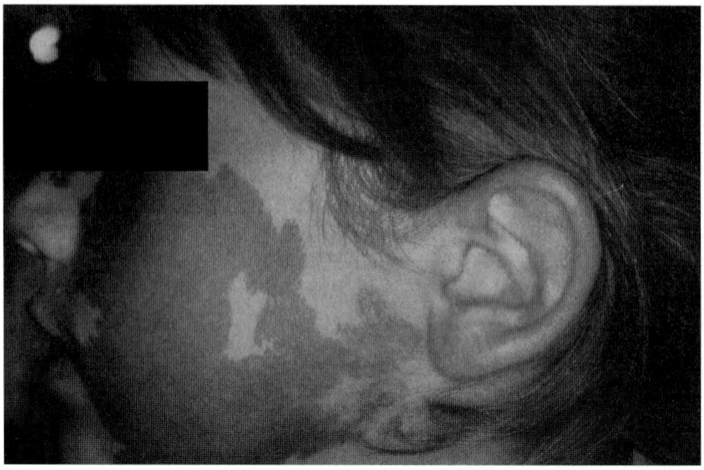

FIGURE 5 Café-au-lait macule before treatment with the Q-switched ruby laser.

targets the deep spindle cell-shaped dermal melanocytes. Histologically, they appear to be destroyed [21]. Geronemus et al. treated 15 patients with Nevus of Ota up to seven times with the Q-switched ruby laser. They noted complete clearing in four patients with significant lightening in the others [22]. In a large Japanese study, over 100 individuals were treated with the Q-switched ruby laser. In this study, the degree of lightening was related to the number of treatments. Total clearing was seen in all individuals treated at least four times (Figs. 7, 8) [23].

Lower eyelid hyperpigmentation, secondary to dermal pigmentation, may respond to treatment with the Q-switched ruby laser. Several treatments are usually required [24]. Mixed epidermal and dermal lesions, such as postinflammatory hyperpigmentation and melasma, respond better to this laser than the green pulsed lasers. However, the results remain somewhat variable (Figs. 9, 10) [25].

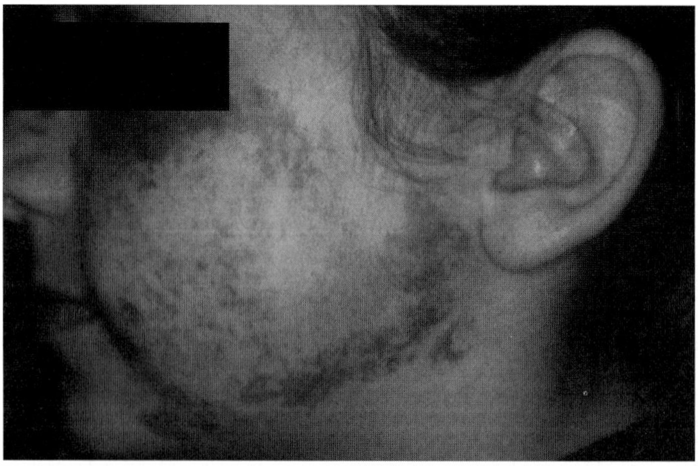

FIGURE 6 Improvement after three treatments with the Q-switched ruby laser.

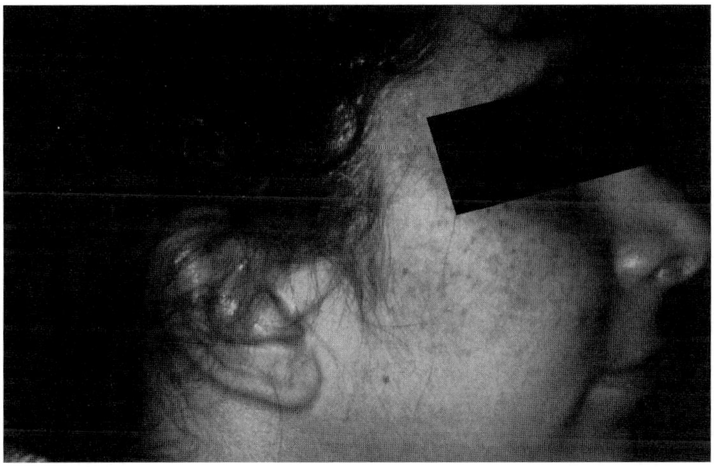

FIGURE 7 Nevus of Ota before treatment with the Q-switched ruby laser.

The Q-switched ruby laser may be used in the treatment of congenital nevi [26]. Although occasional significant clinical lightening may occur, recurrence of pigmentation is the general rule. Histologically, residual nevomelanocytes were seen in the deeper dermis (Figs. 11, 12).

The Q-switched alexandrite laser is a solid state laser, which emits light at 755 nm with pulse duration of 50 to 100 nanoseconds. There is less published data about this laser as compared with the Q-switched ruby laser. However, because the wavelength and pulse durations are similar to those of the Q-switched ruby laser, results should be somewhat similar. A good response has been seen in the treatment of lentignes and café-au-lait macules (Figs. 13, 14) [27]. Dermal pigmented lesions, such as Nevus of Ota, also respond [28]. In one study, the Q-switched alexandrite laser was compared with the Q-switched Nd:YAG laser (1064 nm) in the treatment

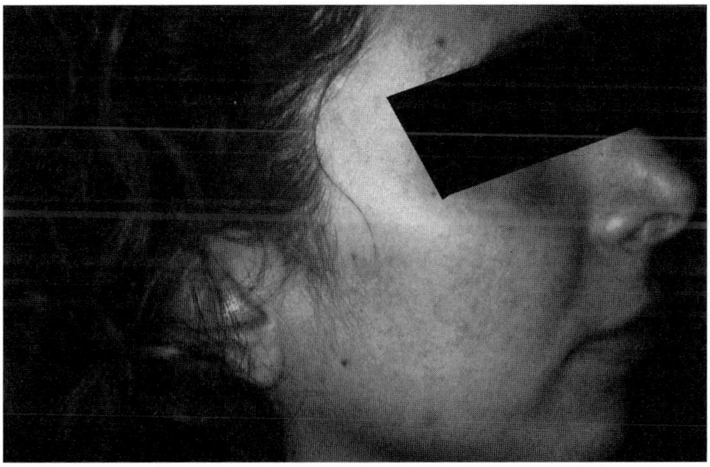

FIGURE 8 Clearance after treatment with the Q-switched ruby laser.

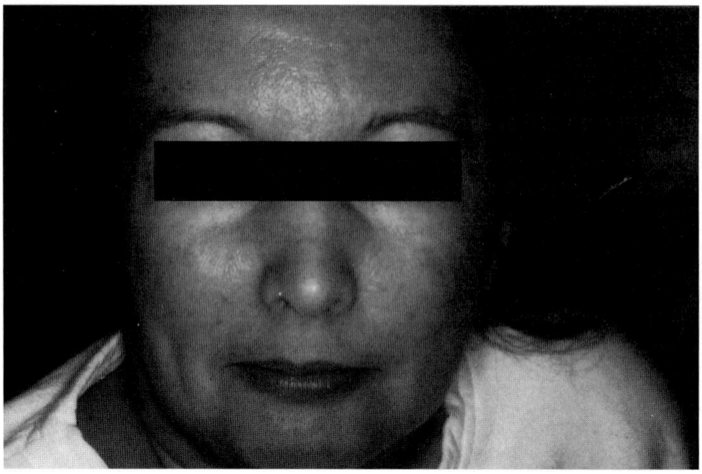

FIGURE 9 Melasma before treatment with the Q-switched ruby laser.

of benign melanocytic nevi in 19 patients [29]. Both lasers produced significant improvement after three treatments although the Q-switched alexandrite laser was slightly more effective. Twelve-month follow-up of 12 of the 18 treated patients showed no evidence of recurrence or pigment darkening.

Normal Mode Alexandrite and Ruby Lasers

Recently, long-pulsed ruby (300–3000 microsec) and alexandrite (2–20 msec) pulses have been shown to be effective in the treatment of Q-switched ruby-laser–resistant congenital nevi and other pigmented lesions. These lasers may also be of use in laser-assisted hair removal.

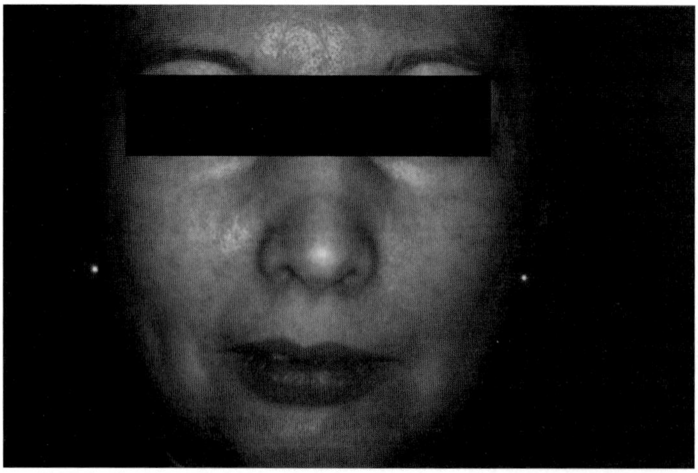

FIGURE 10 Improvement after treatment with the Q-switched ruby laser.

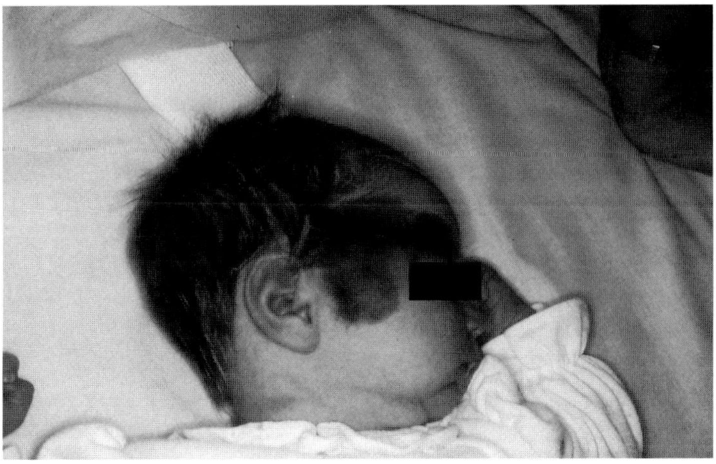

FIGURE 11 Congenital nevus before treatment with the Q-switched ruby laser.

The normal-mode alexandrite laser emits light at a wavelength of 755 nm with 2 to 20-millisecond pulse durations. This laser is effective in removing pigmented hair. There are no published data on its use in pigmented lesions.

The normal-mode ruby laser is also highly effective in removing pigmented hair. The Japanese have the only published experience with the use of long pulsed lasers for pigmented lesions. Congenital nevi treated four times showed significant clearing of pigmentation. Treated skin was almost indistinguishable from the normal surrounding skin.

Near Infrared Pulsed Lasers

The Q-switched Nd:YAG laser produces a 1064 nm wavelength beam with pulse duration of 10 nanoseconds. Melanin does not absorb the 1064 nm wavelength well.

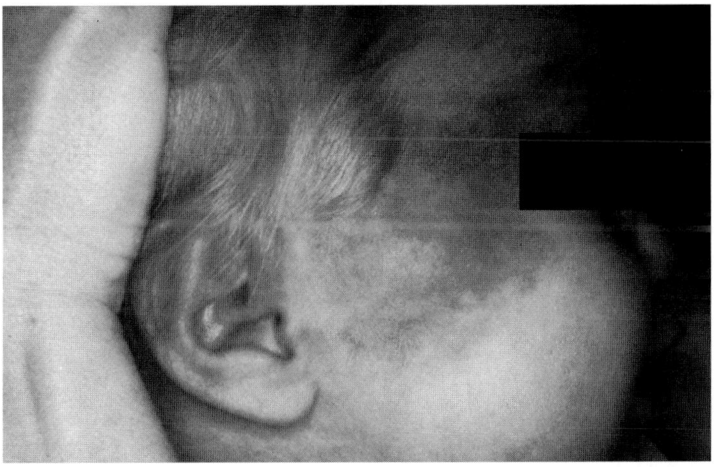

FIGURE 12 Improvement after four treatments with the Q-switched ruby laser.

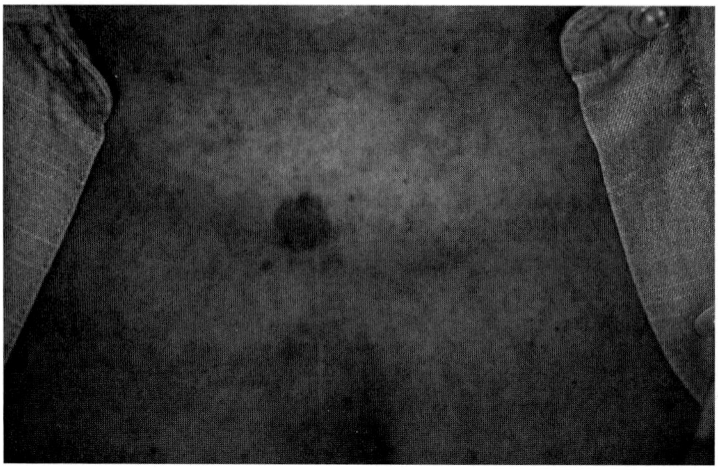

FIGURE 13 Solar lentignes before treatment with the Q-switched alexandrite laser.

Thus, the 1064 nm wavelength is not ideal for the treatment of benign pigmented lesions. Despite less absorption of this wavelength by melanin compared with the green and red light lasers, its advantage lies in its ability to penetrate more deeply in the skin (up to 4–6 mm). This laser may be more useful in the treatment of lesions in individuals with darker skin tones (Figs. 15, 16). Like the Q-switched ruby and alexandrite lasers, the Q-switched Nd:YAG laser is highly effective in clearing of Nevus of Ota. Histologically, the findings at 1064 nm are identical to that of the Q-switched ruby laser. "Ring cells" representing vacuolated pigmented cells with peripheral condensation of pigment are detected in the epidermal basal cell layer.

Nonselective Laser Techniques—CO_2/Er:YAG Lasers

The CO_2 laser (10,600 nm) and the Er:YAG laser (2940 m) emit infrared laser energy, which is. The Er:YAG laser produces much less thermal damage than is seen with the CO_2 laser. Nevertheless, even the CO_2 laser, when used with low fluences, produces only limited epidermal thermal damage [31].

In a study evaluating CO_2 laser treatment of 146 solar lentignes, 10% cleared completely and two thirds lightened considerably. Thermal damage occurred in the basal cell layer (vacuolization and spindling of the melanocytes and keratinocytes). This damage led to epidermal necrosis 24 hours later with subsequent dermal-epidermal separation. There was minimal dermal thermal damage. Sloughing of the damaged epidermis was followed by subsequent re-epithelialization [31]. Similar improvement can be seen after Er:YAG laser treatment (Figs. 17, 18).

TATTOOS

Leon Goldman was the first to experiment with laser tattoo removal in 1964. Despite his reported success, the method became popular only during the last decade. Reid [32,33], in a Scottish study, was the first to show that the Q-switched ruby laser effectively treated both amateur and professional blue-black tattoos. Treatment could be undertaken with minimal to no cutaneous textural changes or scarring. In the Reid

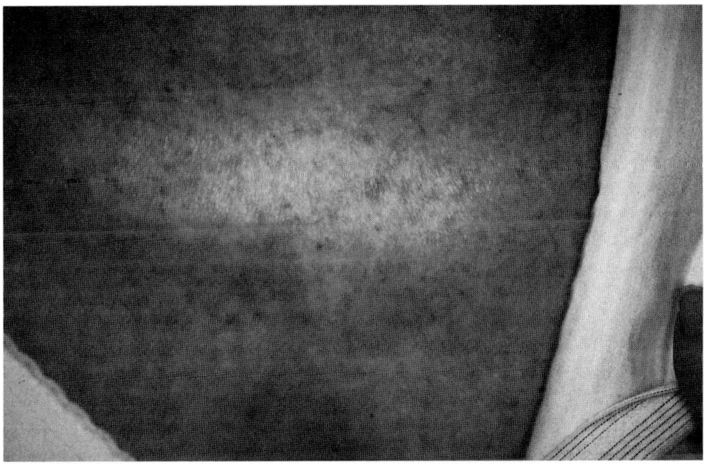

FIGURE 14 Clearance after one treatment with the Q-switched alexandrite laser.

study, amateur tattoos cleared after an average of four to six treatments; professional tattoos required 1 to 3 additional treatments. U.S. studies evaluating Q-switched ruby laser treatment of amateur and professional tattoos revealed similar findings [34].

Q-switched ruby laser treatment of a tattoo leads to a gray-white appearance of the treated site which is more marked in the tattooed areas than in the adjacent normal skin. This is thought to occur because of rapid steam formation around the treated pigment particles. Over the next 7 to 10 days, crusting may occur in the treated area. Tattoo pigment may be seen within this wound. After several treatments, tattoo lightening often occurs with little to no textural change.

After treatment, tattoo pigment is found within membrane-bound intracellular granules in perivascular fibroblasts, macrophages, and mast cells [35]. After Q-switched ruby laser treatment, the usual melanosome-targeted injury to melanocytes

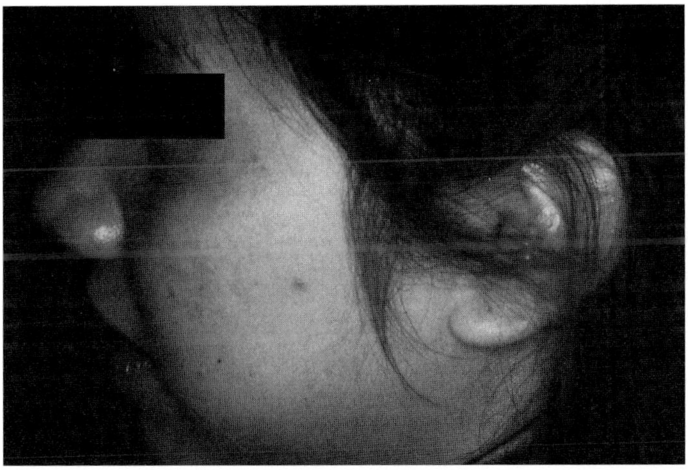

FIGURE 15 Nevus of Ota before treatment with the Q-switched Nd:YAG laser.

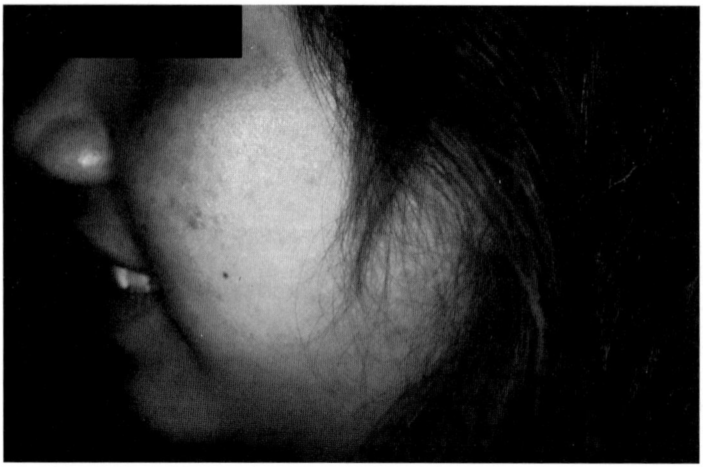

FIGURE 16 Improvement after treatment with the Q-switched Nd:YAG laser.

and keratinocytes is evident. In addition, there is cellular debris adjacent to altered tattoo-pigment particles. By day 11 after treatment, all the altered pigment particles are repackaged within cells into the same types of perivascular cells. Despite residual histologic persistence of tattoo pigment, 80% of amateur tattoos show clinical clearance in four to six treatments; 65% of professional tattoos are lightened significantly within six to eight treatments [34].

The mechanism by which a Q-switched ruby laser removes dermal tattoo pigment is unknown. External elimination of tattoo pigment with simultaneous phagocytosis of the altered pigment particles reduces or eliminates the unwanted tattoo pigment. However, as mentioned, posttreatment histologic studies still show considerable residual tattoo pigment. It is likely that other tattoo treating lasers lead to similar results.

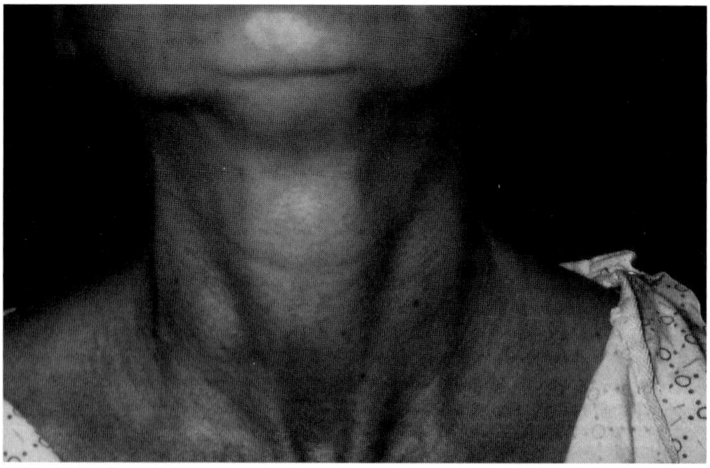

FIGURE 17 Solar lentignes before treatment with the Er:YAG laser.

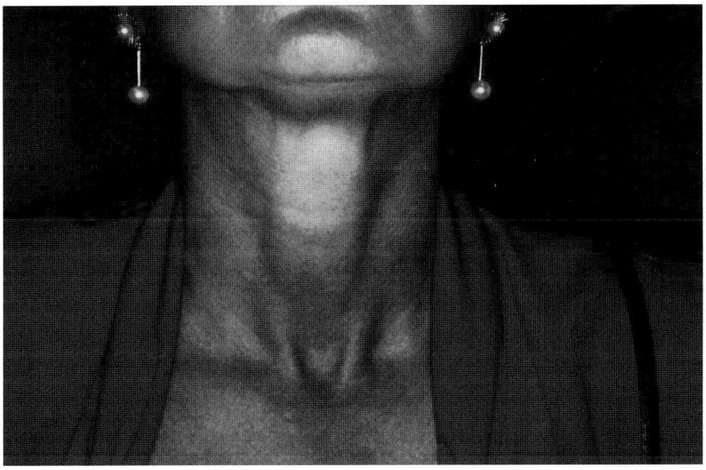

FIGURE 18 Clearance after one treatment with the Er:YAG laser.

Q-Switched Ruby Laser

The Q-switched ruby laser is highly effective for amateur tattoos and moderately successful for the treatment of black professional tattoos. Brightly colored professional tattoos show a variable response. Eighty-five percent of amateur tattoos are completely removed in an average of three treatments. Professional tattoos are more difficult to treat. Ten percent are completely removed, 70% are partially removed, and 20% are minimally improved after an average of six Q-switched ruby laser treatments [36]. Dark blue and black ink shows the greatest response. Green has a variable response, but 65% of treated green tattoos clear with six to eight treatments. Red and yellow tattoo pigments do not respond [37]. Yellow tattoos do not respond because the spectral absorbance of yellow ink drops dramatically in this range (Figs. 19–22).

Q-Switched Alexandrite Laser

The alexandrite laser shows some similarities to the Q-switched ruby laser. Alexandrite laser (755 nm, 100 nsec pulse duration) treatment of tattooed pig skin [38] leads to the removal of blue-black tattoo pigment. Similar results are seen when human tattoos are treated [39]. Histologically, fragmentation of pigment granules is observed after laser treatment. The Q-switched alexandrite laser is best at the removal of green tattoo but is less effective than either the Q-switched ruby laser or the Q-switched Nd:YAG laser in removing blue, black or brightly colored tattoos (Figs. 23, 24) [40–43].

Q-Switched ND:YAG

The Q-switched Nd:YAG at 1064 nm clears most amateur blue-black tattoos with the greatest response after the first treatment [44]. Previously untreated amateur blue-black tattoos fade by 50% on the first treatment and are 95% cleared by the fourth treatment (Figs. 25, 26).

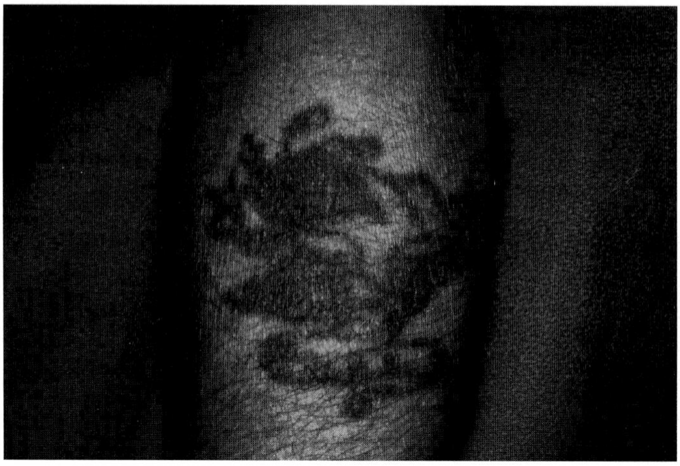

FIGURE 19 Amateur tattoo before treatment with the Q-switched ruby laser.

Twenty-eight patients with blue-black tattoos, resistant to a long pulse duration (approximately 40 nsec) experimental Q-switched ruby laser, had 30% lightening of their tattoos after the first treatment with the Q-switched Nd:YAG laser; 85% cleared by the fourth treatment [45].

The 1064 nm wavelength is not highly effective in removing colored tattoo pigment: yellow, green, and red tattoos clear less than 25% after four treatments. At a wavelength of 532 nm, the frequency-doubled, Q-switched Nd:YAG laser is the treatment of choice for red tattoo pigment. Red pigment may clear up to 75% of the time with three treatments (Figs. 27, 28) [37].

The 510 nm wavelength of the pulsed dye laser, with its shallow dermal depth of penetration, is ineffective in removing most tattoo pigments. However, like the

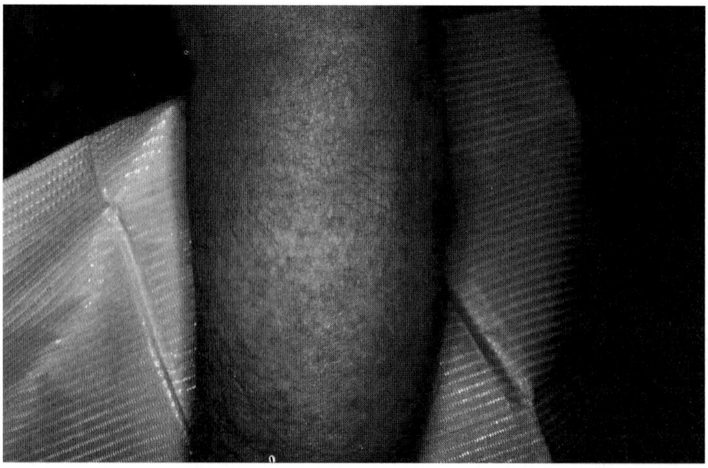

FIGURE 20 Clearance after four treatments with the Q-switched ruby laser.

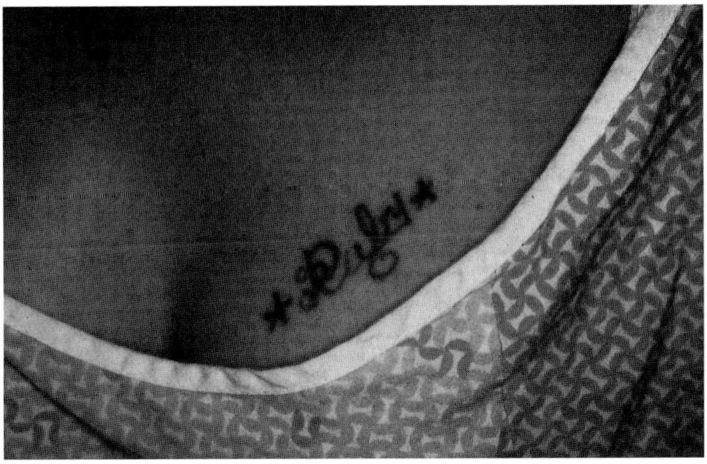

FIGURE 21 Professional tattoo before treatment with the Q-switched ruby laser.

frequency doubled Q-switched Nd:YAG laser, the pulsed dye laser effectively removes red tattoo colors.

Several comparative studies have evaluated Q-switched ruby laser tattoo removal as compared with the Q-switched Nd:YAG and Q-switched alexandrite lasers (Table 2). Levine and Geronemus [46] compared the Q-switched ruby laser (694 nm, 25 nsec pulse duration, 8–10 J/cm^2) with the Q-switched Nd:YAG laser (1064 nm, 25 nsec pulse duration, 10–14 J/cm^2). One half of each of 48 tattoos (39 professional, nine amateur) was treated with each laser type. After one treatment, they found that the Q-switched ruby laser produced better results in 18 tattoos; the Q-switched Nd:YAG laser led to more lightening in four tattoos. Seventeen tattoos showed similar results with both lasers.

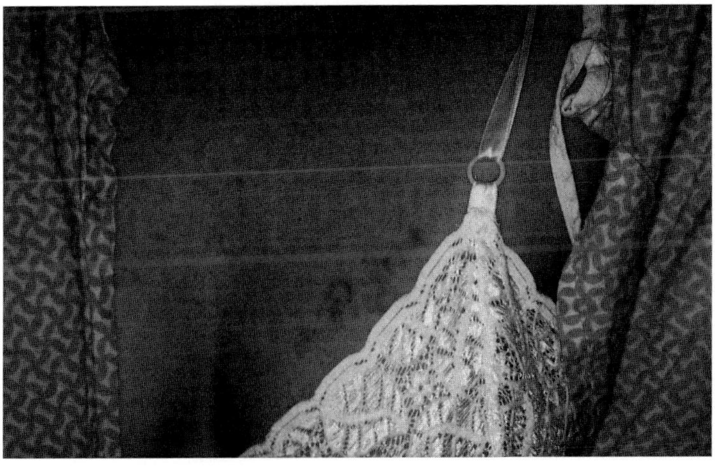

FIGURE 22 Clearance after eight treatments with the Q-switched ruby laser.

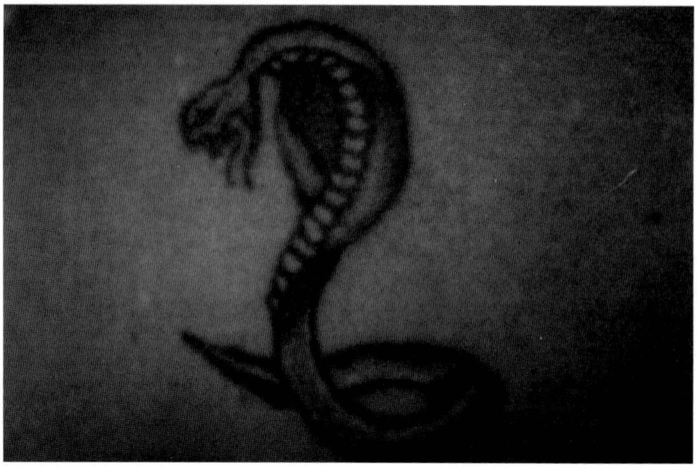

FIGURE 23 Professional tattoo before treatment with the Q-switched alexandrite laser.

McMeekin [47] compared the Q-switched ruby laser (694 nm, 25 nsec, 6 J/cm^2) to the Q-switched alexandrite laser (694 nm, 100 nsec, 6 J/cm^2) in the treatment of 10 black amateur tattoos. He found that the Q-switched ruby laser produced better clearing in all treated tattoos.

Zelickson [48] performed a comparative study of the three laser types in which he injected 14 commonly used tattoo pigments into guinea pig skin and then compared amount of lightening produced by the Q-switched ruby (694 nm), the Q-switched Nd:YAG (532 nm and 1064 nm), and the Q-switched alexandrite (755 nm) lasers. He found that the Q-switched ruby laser was the most efficacious in removing blue-black tattoos. The Q-switched alexandrite laser worked best for blue and green tattoos and the frequency doubled Q-switched Nd:YAG laser was most useful for

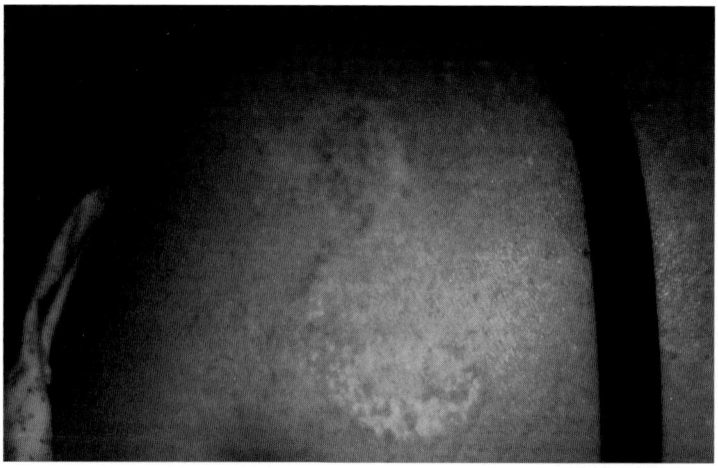

FIGURE 24 Improvement after eight treatments with the Q-switched alexandrite laser.

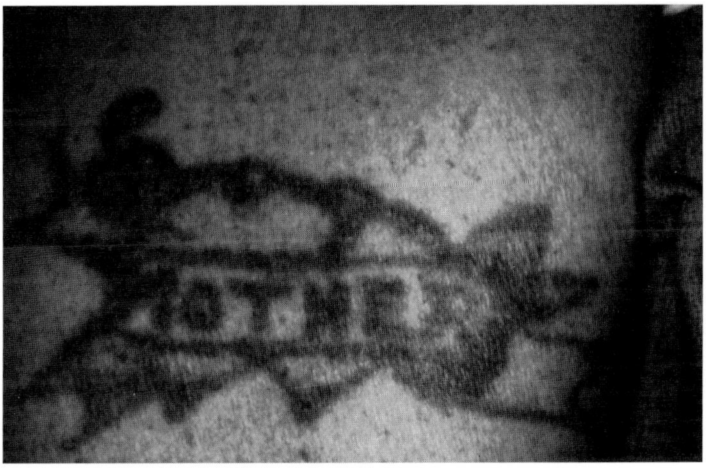

FIGURE 25 Professional tattoo before treatment with the Q-switched Nd:YAG laser.

the red tattoo pigment. The longer Q-switched Nd:YAG laser 1064 nm wavelength allows for deeper penetration and less absorption by melanin, as compared with the 694 nm Q-switched ruby laser. It has a higher efficacy in removing black tattoo ink [40, 49].

In a series of 410 tattoos [50], transient hypopigmentation occurred in 184 Q-switched ruby laser-treated tattoos, six combined Q-switched ruby and Nd:YAG laser-treated tattoos, and only one Q-switched Nd:YAG laser-treated tattoo. Scarring is uncommon (<5% of patients) and appears to occur in professional tattoos more often than amateur tattoos. Incomplete tattoo removal occurs more frequently in professional tattoos and is seen in 20 to 40% of patients. Color tattoos are more treatment refractory than blue-black tattoos.

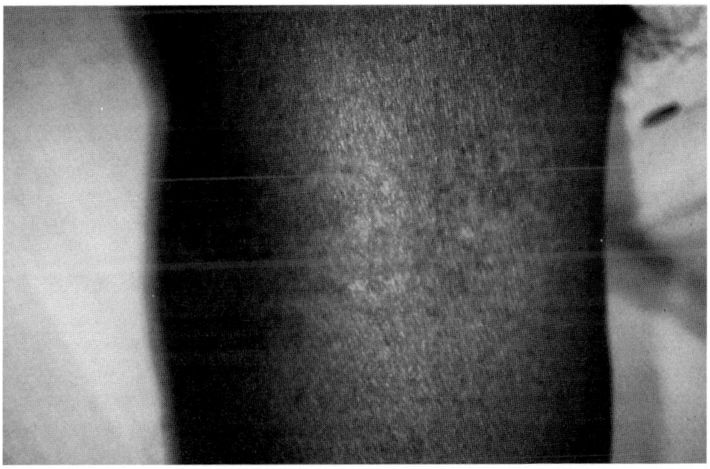

FIGURE 26 Improvement after six treatments with the Q-switched Nd:YAG laser.

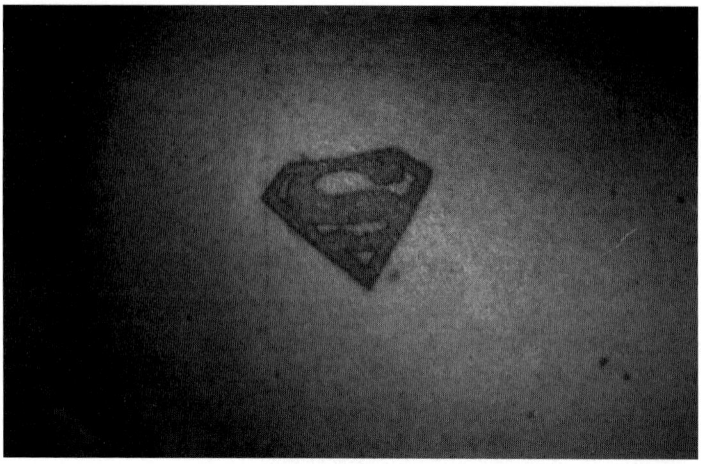

FIGURE 27 Red tattoo pigment before treatment with the frequency doubled Q-switched Nd:YAG laser.

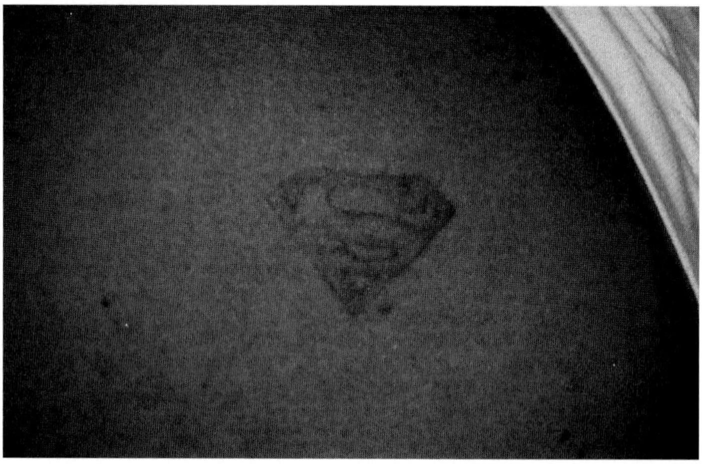

FIGURE 28 Improvement in red tattoo pigment after two treatments with the frequency doubled Q-switched Nd:YAG laser.

TABLE 2 Tattoos

	Amateur	Professional
Q-switched ruby laser (694 nm)	++++	++++ (except red, yellow, and some bright colors)
Q-switched Nd:YAG (1064 nm)	++++	++++ (except red, yellow, and green)
Frequency doubled Q-switched Nd:YAG (532 nm)	+	+++ (highly successful with red)
Pigmented lesion pulsed dye (510 nm)	+	+++ (highly successful with red)
Alexandrite (755 nm)	+++	+++ (except red and yellow)

+ Poor
++ Fair
+++ Good
++++ Excellent

In Levine's study, 1064 nm Q-switched Nd:YAG laser induced side effects included textural changes (more frequently than with the Q-switched ruby laser) and hypopigmentation (less frequently than the Q-switched ruby laser) [46].

Cosmetic tattoos that are flesh-colored, white, pink, or varying shades of brown frequently blacken after laser treatment. This blackening is attributable to laser-induced high temperatures changes with resultant reduction of Fe_2O_3 to the black FeO. Repeated Q-switched ruby laser treatments have occasionally been successful in eradicating the blackened skin tone tattoos [51].

CONCLUSION

Several pigment-specific lasers can effectively treat epidermal and dermal pigmented lesions. Lasers are most effective in treating pigmented lesions such as lentignes and ephilides. Variable responses can be expected in café-au-lait macules, Becker's nevi, nevus spilus, and melasma. Nevus of Ota is unique in the near-total clearance often seen after laser treatment. New, long-pulsed pigment-specific lasers may prove to further enhance the clinical results obtained in resistant pigmented lesions. Future pigmented lesion lasers may selectively target melanocytes, rather than melanosomes. Q-switched lasers are highly effective in treating blue, black, green, and red tattoos. Future lasers will provide the ability to treat other colors and with less treatment sessions.

REFERENCES

1. Goldman LBD, Kindel DJ, Richfield D, Franke EK. Pathology of the effect of the laser beam on the skin. Nature 1963; 197:912–914.
2. Goldman LIJ, Richfield DF. Impact of the laser on nevi and melanomas. Arch Dermatol 1964; 90:71–75.
3. Goldman LWR, Hornby P, et al. Radiation from a Q-switched ruby laser. J Invest Dermatol 1965; 44:69–71.
4. Goldman L. Optical radiation hazards to the skin. In: Sliney DW, ed. Safety With Lasers and Other Optical Sources: A comprehensive Handbook. New York: Plenum Press, 1983: 167–169.
5. Polla L, Margolis R, Dover J, et al. Melanosomes are a primary target of Q-switched ruby laser-irradiation in guinea pig skin. J Invest Dermatol 1987; 89:281–286.
6. Dover J, Polla L, Margolis R, et al. Pulse width dependence of pigment cell damage at 694 nm in guinea pig skin. SPIE 1987; Vol. 712.
7. Ara G, Anderson R, Mandel K, Ottesen M, Oseroff A. Irradiation of pigmented melanoma cells with high intensity pulsed radiation generates acoustic waves and kills cells. Lasers Surg Med 1990; 10:52–59.
8. Dover JS, Margolis RJ, Polla LL, et al. Pigmented guinea pig skin irradiated with Q-switched ruby laser pulses. Morphologic and histologic findings. Arch Dermatol 1989; 125:43–49.
9. Hruza GJ, Dover JS, Flotte TJ, Goetschkes M, Watanabe S, Anderson RR. Q-switched ruby laser irradiation of normal human skin. Histologic and ultrastructural findings. Arch Dermatol 1991; 127:1799–1805.
10. Anderson RR, Margolis RJ, Watenabe S, Flotte T, Hruza GJ, Dover JS. Selective photothermolysis of cutaneous pigmentation by Q-switched Nd:YAG laser pulses at 1064, 532, and 355 nm. J Invest Dermatol 1989; 93:28–32.

11. Margolis R, Dover J, Polla L, et al. Visible action spectrum for melanin-specific selective photothermolysis. Lasers Surg Med 1989; 9:389–397.
12. Sherwood K, Murray S, Kurban A, Tan O. Effect of wavelength of cutaneous pigment using pulsed irradiation. J Invest Dermatol 1989; 92:717–720.
13. Grekin RC, Shelton RM, Geisse JK, Frieden I. 510-NM pigmented lesion dye laser. Its characteristics and clinical uses. J Dermatol Surg Oncol 1993; 19:380–387.
14. Fitzpatrick R, Goldman M. Laser treatment of benign pigmented lesions using a 300 nanosecond pulse and 510 nm wavelength. J Dermatol Surg Oncol 1993; 19:341–346.
15. Tan O, Morelli J, Kurban A. Pulsed dye laser treatment of benign cutaneous pigmented lesions. Laser Surg Med 1992; 12:538–542.
16. Alster T. Treatment of benign pigmented epidermal lesions with the 510 nm pulsed dye laser: further clinical experience and treatment parameters. Laser Surg Med 1993; 5(suppl):55.
17. Goldberg D. Treatment of pigmented and vascular lesions of the skin with the Q-switched Nd:YAG laser. Lasers Surg Med 1993;13(suppl 5):55.
18. Taylor CRFT, Michaud N, Jimbow K, Anderson RR. Q-switched ruby laser of benign pigmented lesions: dermal vs. epidermal. Laser Surg Med 1991; 3(suppl):65.5.
19. Ashinoff RGR. Q-switched ruby laser treatment of benign epidermal pigmented lesions. Laser Surg Med 1992; (suppl 4):73.
20. Goldberg DJ, Nychay SG. Q-switched ruby laser treatment of nevus of Ota. J Dermatol Surg Oncol 1992; 18:817–821.
21. Goldberg D. Benign pigmented lesions of the skin: treatment with the Q-switched ruby laser. J Dermatol Surg Oncol 1993; 19:376–379.
22. Geronemus RGAR. Q-switched ruby laser therapy of nevus of Ota. Laser Med Surg 1992; (suppl 4):74.
23. Watanabe S, Takahashi H. Treatment of nevus of Ota with the Q-switched ruby laser. N Engl J Med 1994; 331:1745–1750.
24. Lowe N. Infraorbital pigmented skin: preliminary observations of laser therapy. Dermatol Surg 1995; 21:767–770.
25. Grevelink JMLH, Taylor CR, Anderson RR. Update on the treatment of benign pigmented lesions with the Q-switched ruby laser. Laser Surg Med 1992; (suppl 4):73.
26. Goldberg DJ, Nychay S. Q-switched ruby laser treatment of congenital nevi. Arch Dermatol 131-621-623, 1995.36.
27. Stafford TJ, Tan OT. 510-nm pulsed dye laser and alexandrite crystal laser for the treatment of pigmented lesions and tattoos. Clin Dermatol 1995; 13:69–73.
28. Alster TS, Williams CM. Treatment of nevus of Ota by the Q-switched alexandrite laser. Dermatol Surg 1995; 21:592–596.
29. Rosenbach A, Williams CN, Alster TS. Comparison of Q-switched alexandrite (755 nm) and Q-switched Nd:YAG (1064 nm) lasers in the treatment of bergen melanocytic nevi. Dermatol Surg 1997; 23:239.
30. Veda S, Imayama S. Normal-mode ruby dates for treating congenital nevi. Arch Dermatol 1992; 133:355.
31. Dover JS, Smoller BR, Stern RS, Rosen S, Arndt KA. Low-fluence carbon dioxide laser irradiation of lentigines. Arch Dermatol 1988; 124:1219–1224.
32. Reid W, McLeod P, Ritchie A, Ferguson-Pell M. Q-switched ruby laser treatment of black tattoos. Br J Plast Surg 1983; 36:455–459.
33. Reid WH, Miller ID, Murphy MJ, Paul JP, Evans JH. Q-switched ruby laser treatment of tattoos; a 9-year experience. Br J Plast Surg 1990; 43:663–669.
34. Taylor CR, Gange RW, Dover JS, et al. Treatment of tattoos by Q-switched ruby laser. A dose-response study. Arch Dermatol 1990; 126:893–899.
35. Taylor C, Anderson R, Gange R, Michaud N, Flotte T. Light and electron microscopic analysis of tattoos treated by Q-switched ruby laser. J Invest Dermatol 1991; 97;131–136.

36. Wheeland R. Q-switched ruby laser treatment of tattoos. Laser Surg Med 1991;
37. Kilmer S, Lee M, Anderson R. Treatment of multi-colored tattoos with the Q-switched Nd:YAG laser (532nm): a dose response study with comparison to the Q-switched ruby laser. Laser Surg Med 1993; (suppl 5):54.
38. Fitzpatrick R, Goldman M, Ruiz-Esparza J. Use of the alexandrite laser (755 nm, 100 nsec) for tattoo pigment removal in an animal model. J Am Acad Dermatol 1993; 28: 745–750.
39. Fitzpatrick R, Goldman M. Alexandrite laser removal of tattoos: a clinical and histological study. Lasers Surg Med 1993; 13(suppl 5):54.
40. Kaufmum R, Boehncke W, Konig K, Hibst R. Comparative study of Q-switched Nd: YAG and alexandrite laser treatment of tattoos. Lasers Surg Med 1993; 13(suppl 5):54.
41. Alster T. Q-switched alexandrite laser treatment (755 mn) of professional and amateur tattoos. J Am Acad Dermatol 1995; 33:69–73.
42. Rosenbach A, Alster T. Comparison of the Q-switched alexandrite (755 nm) and Q-switched Nd-YAG (1064 nm) lasers in the treatment of benign congenital nevi. Lasers Surg Med 1996; (suppl. 8):31.
43. Stafford TJ, Lizek R, Tan OT. Role of the alexandrite laser for removal of tattoos. Lasers Surg Med 1995; 17:32–38.
44. Kilmer S, Lee M, Grevelink J, Flotte T, Anderson R. The Q-switched Nd:YAG laser (1064 nm) effectively treats tattoos: a controlled, dose-response study. Arch Dermatol 1993; 129:971–978.
45. Kilmer S, Lee M, Farinelli W, Grevelink J, Anderson R. Q-switched Nd:YAG laser (1064 nm) effectively treats Q-switched ruby laser resistant tattoos. Laser Surg Med 1992; (suppl 4):72.
46. Levine V. Tattoo removal with the Q-switched ruby laser and the Q-switched Nd:YAG laser: a comparative study. Cutis 1995; 55:291–296.47.
47. McMeekin T, Goodwin D. A comparison of the alexandrite laser (755 nm) with the Q-switched ruby laser (694 nm) for the treatment of tattoos. Lasers Surg Med 1993; 13(suppl 5):54.
48. Zelickson B, Mehregan D, Zarrin A, et al. Clinical, histologic, and ultrastructural evaluation of tattoos treated with three laser systems. Laser Surg Med 1994; 15:364–372.
49. Kilmer S, Anderson R. Clinical use of the Q-switched ruby and the Q-switched Nd: YAG (1064 nm and 532 nm) lasers for treatment of tattoos. J Dermatol Surg Oncol 1993; 19:330–338.
50. Grevelink J, Casparian J, Gonzalez E, et al. Undesirable effects associated with treatment of tattoos and pigmented lesions with Q-switched lasers at 1064 nm and 694 nm. Laser Surg Med 1993; (suppl 5):53.
51. Anderson R, Geronemus R, Kilmer S, Farinelli W, Fitzpatrick R. Cosmetic tattoo ink darkening: a complication of Q-switched and pulsed laser treatment. Arch Dermatol 1993; 129:1010–1014.

24

Treatment of Varicose and Telangiectatic Veins: Sclerotherapy, Ambulatory Phlebectomy, and Laser

Robert A. Weiss and Margaret A. Weiss
Johns Hopkins University School of Medicine, Baltimore, Maryland

INTRODUCTION

One of the most deceptively simple procedures for cosmetic dermatologic surgeons is that of elimination of abnormal leg veins and telangiectasias. The skill required to place local anesthesia in the skin has very little application to the placement of a needle into a vein for sclerotherapy. Additionally, telangiectasias presenting on the leg are often manifestations of abnormal physiology of its venous system. However, because 50% of the patients we already treat for other conditions have abnormal leg veins to some extent, it is imperative that we develop the necessary skills. Although patients seek treatment for cosmesis, they experience symptoms attributable to pooling of stagnant blood within extensive reticular networks. The volume of blood sequestered and stagnant in these reticular veins and associated telangiectatic webs may cause enough pressure to produce symptoms [1]. It is our belief, from observing nearly 14,000 patients, that reticular varicosities associated with telangiectatic webs are the most underdiagnosed causes of leg pain and fatigue in young and middle-aged women.

Sclerotherapy and ambulatory phlebectomy allow treatment of virtually all large truncal varicose veins, myriad reticular varicose veins, and most telangiectasias. Once venous pressure is addressed, telangiectasias can also be treated by the newest lasers and intense pulsed light devices. Except for the situation in which an incompetent valve occurs at the main valve of the greater saphenous vein (GSV) at the junction of the femoral vein, virtually all patients may be treated in the office by the techniques described in this chapter.

Diagnosis

The first skill to acquire is the ability to diagnose origins of varicose or reticular veins associated with telangiectasias. It is reverse flow through incompetent valves that frequently leads to abnormal veins on the leg. The tools used are Doppler ultrasound (analogous to a stethoscope), digital photoplethysmography (analogous to an electrocardiogram), and Duplex ultrasound (analogous to an echocardiogram).

In order to use these noninvasive diagnostic tools properly, a familiarity with basic anatomy is important. The three important superficial venous systems include the GSV, lesser saphenous vein (LSV), and the lateral subdermic venous system (LSVS). The dermatologist's goal is to determine whether telangiectatic webs or varicose veins seen on the surface during physical examination originate from venous pressure in at least one of these three segments of venous anatomy. It is most helpful to think in terms of zones of influence during observation of the patient's leg (Fig. 1). More advanced techniques allow diagnosis of deep venous system disease and are detailed elsewhere [2].

For patients presenting to us in their twenties, thirties, or forties, most telangiectatic webs originate from reverse flow or reflux in the LSVS. When a positive family history for large varicose veins is noted, reflux originating from the GSV or LSV must be suspected. Detailed history along with physical examination is therefore useful to select those patients requiring further noninvasive diagnostic evaluation [3].

Detection and elimination of the larger sources of reflux must be accomplished before the leg will respond to treatment of smaller reticular veins and associated telangiectasias. This is to prevent treatment failure by recanalization in a higher venous flow setting and to minimize postsclerosis pigmentation, which occurs when treated telangiectasia become packed with red blood cells from high-pressure reflux into a treated site [4]. Many telangiectatic webs are actually manifestations of moderate to severe venous hypertension. A recent duplex study on patients presenting for treatment of "cosmetic" leg veins show a relatively high incidence of early associated axial or truncal reflux in the GSV [5].

Arborizing networks of telangiectasias have been shown to be dilated cutaneous venules with intrinsic connections to underlying larger veins of which they are direct tributaries [6,7]. Valves are found throughout the postcapillary venous system regulating flow within the smallest of venules [8].

The microanatomy responsible for the transmission of venous hypertension into telangiectasias via reticular varicosities was documented by high-resolution Duplex ultrasound [9]. A reticular vein is a thin-walled blue superficial venulectasia thought to be part of a network of subcuticular veins communicating with the venous system via direct connections to the saphenous system or by small perforating veins that can course through superficial and or deep fascia. These reticular veins are commonly called "feeder" veins because the assumption is that reflux through them causes the groups of telangiectasias, although when not diseased these veins drain blood from the telangiectasias.

FIGURE 1 Zones of influence of anatomy of the three major divisions of the superficial venous system. (a) Greater saphenous vein runs along the medial aspect of the thigh. The critical site for detection of reflux is the saphenofemoral junction. (b) Lesser saphenous vein. Saphenopopliteal reflux is important to detect as well. (c) Lateral venous system. Multiple perforating veins connected to reticular veins transmit pressure to the telangiectatic webs on the thigh and calf.

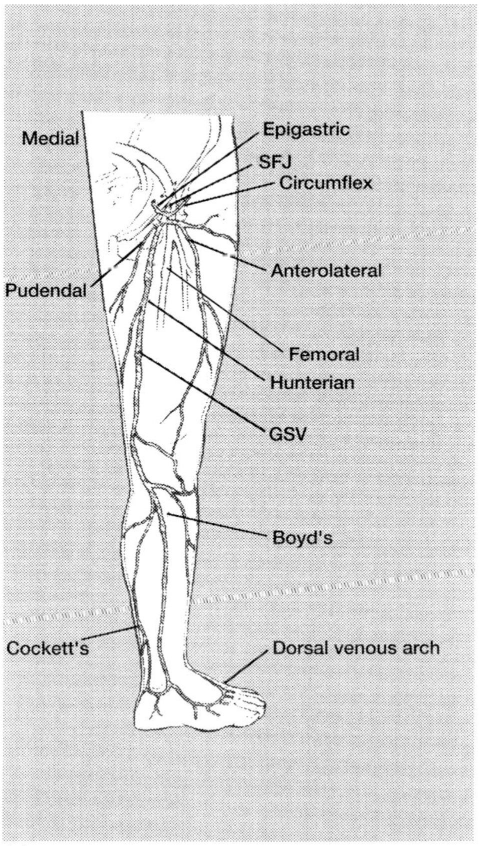
Medial
Epigastric
SFJ
Circumflex
Anterolateral
Pudendal
Femoral
Hunterian
GSV
Boyd's
Cockett's
Dorsal venous arch

(a)

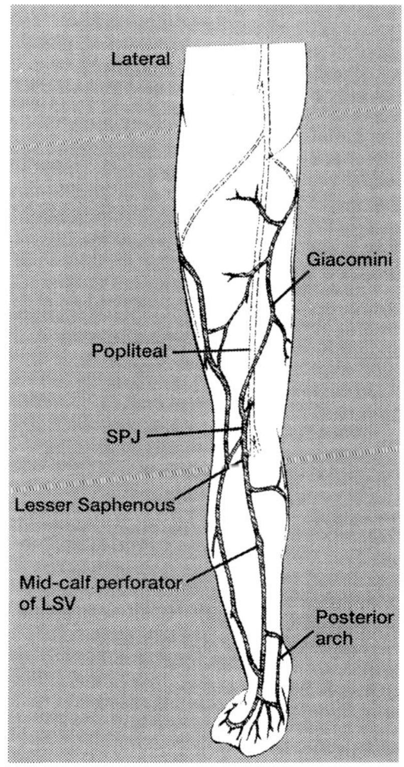
Lateral
Giacomini
Popliteal
SPJ
Lesser Saphenous
Mid-calf perforator of LSV
Posterior arch

(b)

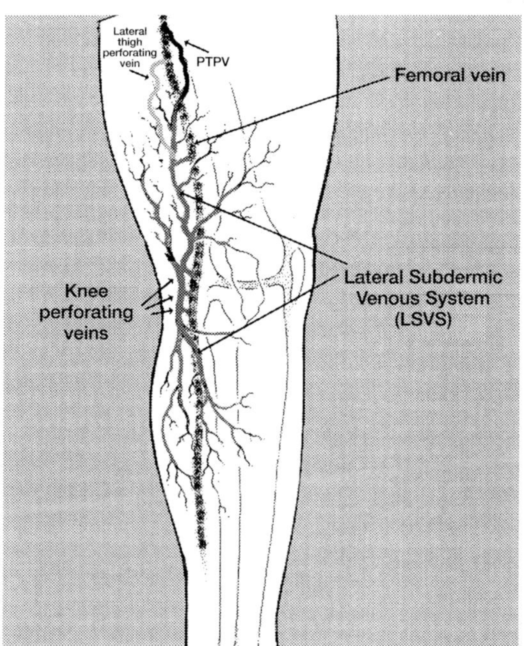
Lateral thigh perforating vein
PTPV
Femoral vein
Knee perforating veins
Lateral Subdermic Venous System (LSVS)

(c)

Doppler ultrasound findings on thousands of patients confirm that reflux through the lateral subdermic venous system is very frequently associated with large areas of painful telangiectatic webs on the lateral and posterior thighs [9,10]. This reticular plexus also extends down the calf and is often responsible for telangiectatic webs on the lateral and posterior calf as well (Fig. 2).

The handheld Doppler ultrasound is the main tool used to detect reverse flow or reflux in the superficial venous system. Optimal frequencies for examining superficial vessels (1–2 cm below the skin) are 8 to 10 MHz, whereas deeper vessels require a lower frequency of 4 to 5 MHz [11,12]. In order to generate or augment an audible signal of flow, a maneuver such as manual compression of the calf to simulate muscle contraction must be performed by the examiner. When compression is released, gravitational hydrostatic pressure causes reverse flow to cease within 0.5 to 1.0 seconds when valves are competent, but a long flow sound is audible when valves are incompetent (Fig. 3).

A simpler test to master is plethysmography, a technique to measure volume changes. Photoplethysmography measures changes in blood volume in the subcutaneous venous plexus by the use of a light-emitting diode (940 nm). Volume changes are measured by the amount of near infrared light absorbed by red blood cells. Although PPG reflects regional venous volume changes, it may be interpreted to represent the entire venous volume of the leg [13].

PPG permits quantification of the physiological significance of doppler findings, whereas venous doppler ultrasound is used to detect originating sites of reflux or reverse flow. PPG is independent of examiner experience unlike the skill required for accurate doppler ultrasound examination [14,15]. Recent advances have led to even greater reliability and quantitative results with digital PPG (ELCAT, GmbH, Wolfratshausen, Germany) in which a dedicated microprocessor standardizes the signal so that measurements are reliable regardless of skin color or edema [16].

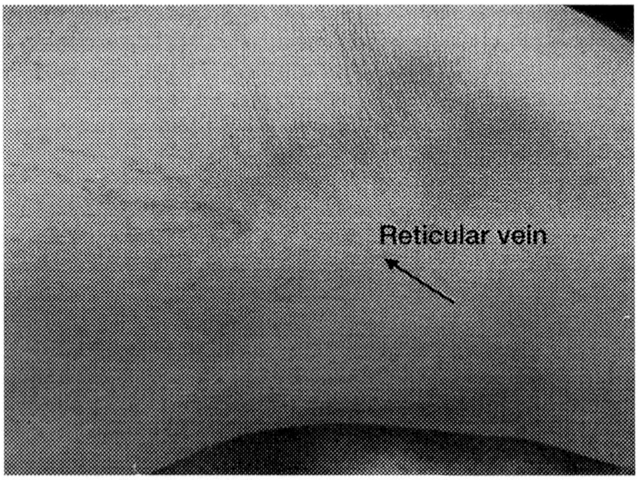

FIGURE 2 Reticular plexus and associated telangiectasias associated with the lateral venous system. Telangiectasias connect to reticular veins of the lateral venous system or can be directly connected to the deep venous system. Reticular veins may also connect directly to other major superficial veins such as the greater saphenous vein.

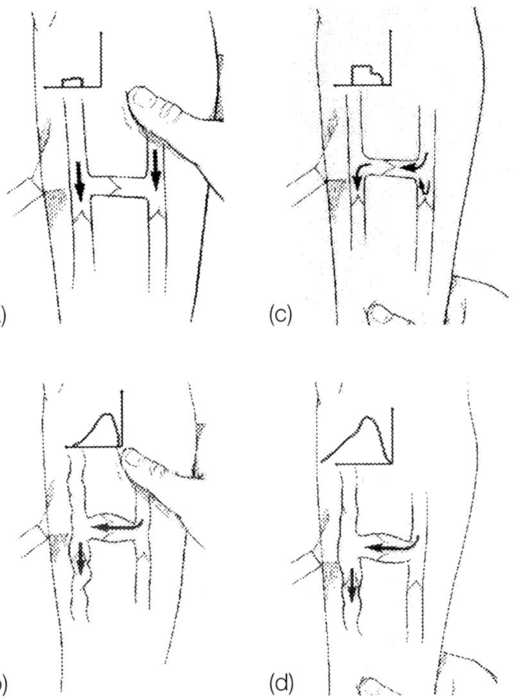

FIGURE 3 Doppler ultrasound examination. Reflux may be elicited by manual compression maneuvers with the leg dependent. (a) Compression proximal to the Doppler transducer induces a long flow sound as long as compression is maintained. In this case an incompetent perforating vein transmits reflux to surface varicosities. (b) Compression distal to the Doppler transducer induces a flow sound with compression and a long sound of reflux when distal compression is released. The leg must be dependent to hear reflux on release. (c) Competent valves reveal very little sound when proximal compression is applied. (d) Normal forward flow is heard with distal compression, but a sound no longer than 1 second occurs with release of compression in a vein with competent valves.

For PPG examination, the patient sits relaxed with the knees bent at a 110° to 120° angle. By convention, a small probe containing light-emitting and sensing diodes is taped to the medial aspect of the lower leg about 8 to 10 cm (four finger widths) above the medial malleolus. After resting the leg for several minutes to establish a smooth baseline tracing, the patient then dorsiflexes the foot eight to 10 times, activating the calf muscle pump and effecting drainage of the venous system. As the skin venous plexus empties, it causes increased reflectance of light. A tracing is made of the changes in reflected light from the skin under the probe (Fig. 4). After the calf muscle pumping ceases, blood refills the superficial venous skin plexus which absorbs increasing amounts of light as venules fill. Excellent correlation of vessel surface filling time (PPG refill time) with direct invasive pressure refill time has been shown [17]. The PPG tracing returns to its initial resting value as the calf venous system refills. A refill time shorter than 25 seconds indicates significant venous valvular insufficiency. Longer refill times indicate normal venous valve function. Table

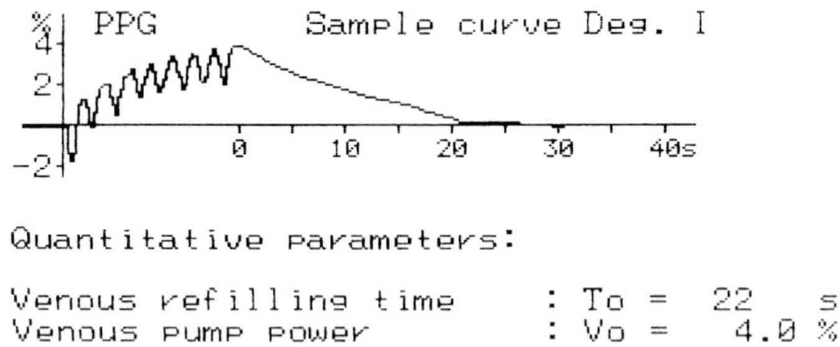

FIGURE 4 Digital PPG. A small handheld unit is attached to a printer. The diode from the handheld unit receives a reflected light signal dependent on capillary filling. This is graphed as shown in the inset. Pumping of the leg removes blood from the capillary network, causing an upward deflection of the graph. At point 0 seconds the calf pumping has stopped and blood starts to refill the leg. This patient shows a refill time of only 19 seconds showing mild venous insufficiency. Digital PPG is the only quantitative PPG. The area under the curve represents percent volume of blood ejected during pumping which in this case is 5.7%. Normal is greater than 3%. In general, when pump power is low Duplex ultrasound may be required to rule out DVT or obstruction.

1 shows suggested standard interpretations of PPG refill times. An abnormal PPG requires further investigation by Doppler, Duplex, or other means before treatment by sclerotherapy, ambulatory phlebectomy, or laser/light source is initiated.

Once the evaluation of the patient is complete, the presence and source of significant venous reflux should have been identified. If the patient has significant saphenofemoral reflux, treatment may include surgical control of that origin point of reflux before sclerotherapy or ambulatory phlebectomy of more distal branches. Although success rates for sclerotherapy of the SFJ have been reported as high as 93% [18–20], this has not been our experience. A classic comparison of surgery and sclerotherapy caused Hobbs to conclude that saphenous vein insufficiency is best managed by surgery whereas sclerotherapy is superior for treatment of isolated perforator incompetence [21].

Once the patient is judged to be a candidate for treatment, it is necessary to obtain informed consent. In our office, a video is shown detailing causes of varicose and spider veins; all treatments, including laser and intense pulsed light; and possible complications such as hyperpigmentation, matting, and ulceration. The necessity for

TABLE 1 Interpretation of PPG Refill Times

Insufficiency grade*	Refill time	Conclusion
Normal	>25 sec	Healthy veins
Grade I	24–20 sec	Mild venous insufficiency
Grade II	19–10 sec	Moderate venous insufficiency
Grade III	<10 sec	Severe venous insufficiency

*This grading applies only to the "sedentary dorsal extensions" movement routine.

multiple treatment sessions is emphasized. Once the patient understands the risks and signs the consent form, digital images using the Sony Mavica FD91 (Sony Corp, 1999) are recorded. The Sony system allows a floppy diskette with the images to be placed immediately in the patient's chart. These readily accessible images serve to evaluate treatment progress and allow patients to recognize improvement. Many patients have great difficulty distinguishing partial resolution from no improvement. The "before" treatment images are therefore invaluable to improve patient satisfaction and ultimately the physician's satisfaction with the procedure.

Patients are told to wear shorts and not to use moisturizers or shave their legs on the day of treatment. Shaving may cause erythematous streaks, making it difficult to visualize patterns of reticular and telangiectatic veins. Use of moisturizers causes poor adhesion of tape, which is used to secure compression after injections, as well as slower evaporation of alcohol, which is used to prepare the leg. Additionally, alcohol remaining on the skin causes heightened stinging sensations during skin puncture.

The room in which sclerotherapy is performed is kept cool to minimize vasovagal reactions; however, a warm room would cause vasodilatation and easier visualization of telangiectasias. The initial treatment session is usually limited to one or two sites. This allows observation of allergic reactions, ability to tolerate burning or cramping of a hypertonic solution, judge the result using the weakest concentrations of sclerosing agents, and to observe any reactions to the tape or wrap used for compression. The patient returns 4 to 6 weeks to compare the test site with pretreatment digital images. The patient is now familiar with the procedure, a response to sclerosing solutions can be predicted, and more areas can be treated with the patient less fearful and muscles relaxed.

Sclerotherapy may be used to treat any size of varicosity as long as certain conditions are met and certain principles followed (Table 2). Injection of telangiectasia should not be undertaken until larger diameter reflux sources flowing into the telangiectatic area are eliminated. Reflux from larger vessels may originate proximally or distally. The order of treatment is varicose veins, reticular veins, purple venulectases, telangiectatic webs or networks, and finally treatment of the smallest and most isolated telangiectasias. Final treatments may be performed with laser or intense pulsed light sources because many of the "stragglers" are streaky blushes too small to cannulate with a 30-gauge needle.

The use of transillumination may help identify the sources of reticular veins connected to telangiectatic webs (Fig. 6). Once the common patterns of the LSVS become second nature, use of Doppler or transillumination is reserved for cases in which the reticular veins are difficult to visualize. When no clear feeder vessel is identified by Doppler or transillumination, then the point at which the telangiectasias begin to branch out is the site at which to begin injection. Alternatively, one may use the "arrowhead sign" as a guide for initiating injections (Fig. 7). This saves time by decreasing the number of injection sites per telangiectatic group. It is best to perform the injection of telangiectasias simultaneously with injection of reticular veins. We believe that this decreases the total number of treatments [4,22].

To begin the injection process of larger veins, the patient is recumbent. A 3 mL syringe with a 27- to 30-gauge needle bent to an angle of 10 to 30° is inserted into the reticular vein, which is usually superficial and visibly blue. When the sensation of piercing the vein is felt, the plunger is pulled back with the thumb of the

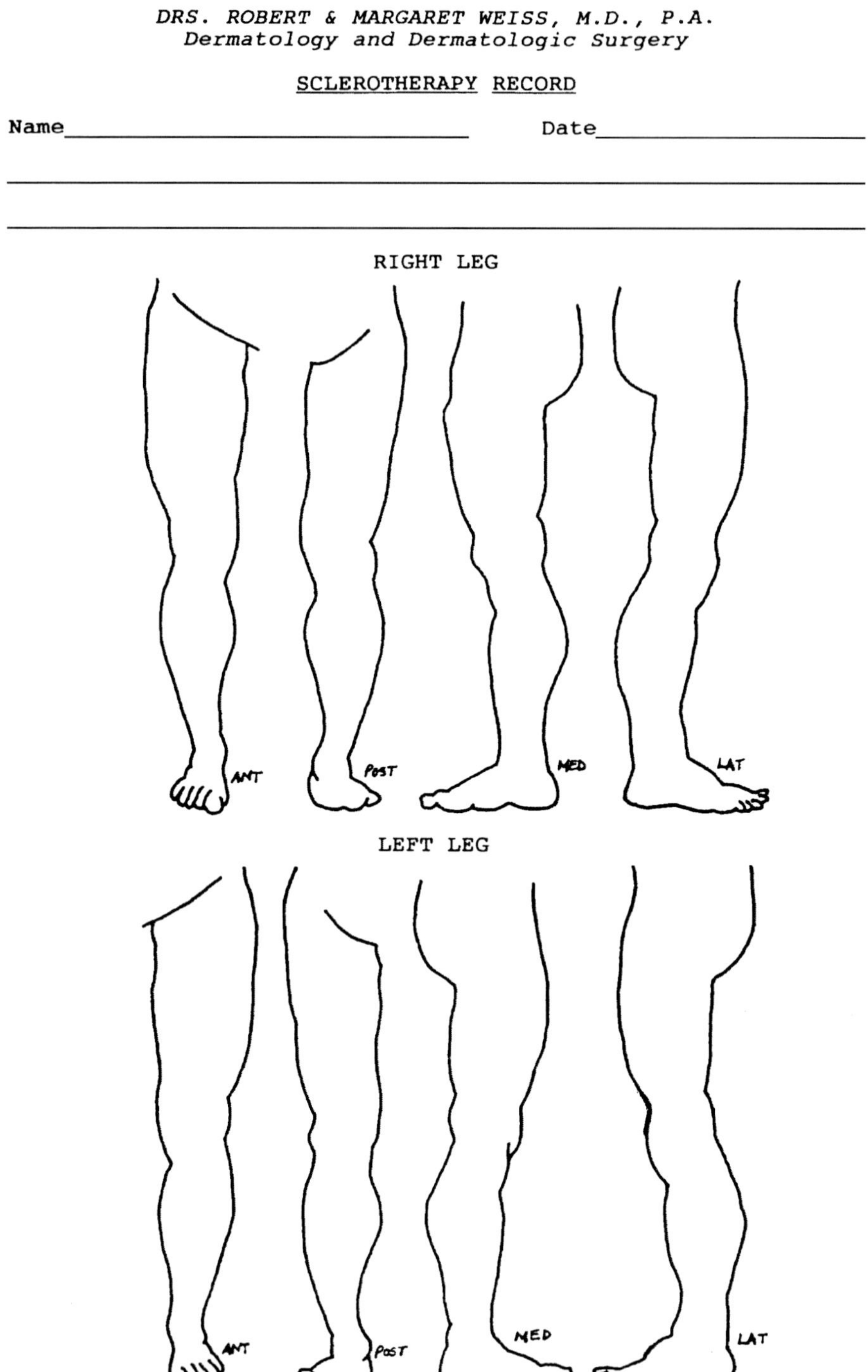

DRS. ROBERT & MARGARET WEISS, M.D., P.A.
Dermatology and Dermatologic Surgery

SCLEROTHERAPY RECORD

Name____________________ Date____________

RIGHT LEG

LEFT LEG

FIGURE 5 Sclerotherapy record. Anatomic diagram for recording of injection sites during a single treatment session. Four views are necessary for each leg. Areas in which each sclerosing solution have been used are clearly marked using a separate color for each concentration and/or type of sclerosant. Total volume injected can easily be seen or calculated.

TABLE 2 Principles of Varicose-Vein Sclerotherapy

Larger veins treated prior to smaller veins
Reflux at the SFJ is eliminated surgically
Reflux points determined initially and treated specifically
Vein must be emptied of blood by various maneuvers before injection
Direct finger pressure in a spreading and compressing motion following injection
Immediate and adequate compression until sustained vein contraction is observed

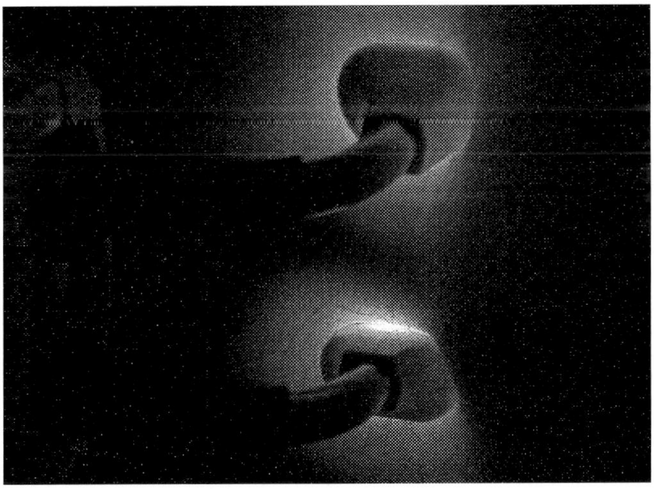

FIGURE 6 Transillumination allows visualization of a 'feeding' reticular vein as a dark shadow against a red background.

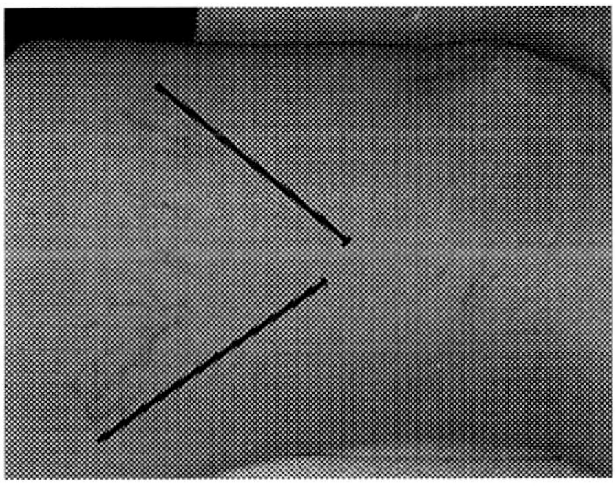

FIGURE 7 Arrowhead sign denotes the drawing of intersecting vectors from each end of a telangiectatic web. The point of intersection marks the location of the associated reticular vein.

dominant hand gently until blood is seen beginning to back up into the transparent plastic hub. If the wall of the reticular vein is very thin, the suction created by pulling back on the syringe may cause the wall to adhere to the needle bevel and prevent aspiration of blood. In this case one can move the needle gently forward and backward and if no resistance is felt, the vein has probably been cannulated and the injection may proceed very cautiously.

Reticular veins will undergo contraction after a cannulation attempt or when the skin temperature is cool. If this occurs, another injection site along the reticular vein must be sought. The cannulation of a reticular vein can be more difficult than protuberant venulectases or telangiectasias. Usually the volume per injection site is no more than 0.5 mL, but the capacity of long reticular veins may even exceed 1 mL. The progress of solution may be followed visually and the injection stopped when the entire reticular vein has cleared of blood.

The strength of sclerosants for treatment of reticular veins are as follows: 0.2 to 0.5% sodium tetradecyl sulfate (STS-Sotradecol), 0.5 to 1% policanol (POL-Aethoxysklerol (not FDA-approved), or 23.4% hypertonic saline HS or hypertonic saline and dextrose Sclerodex (not FDA-approved) (Table 3) [23,24]. Until the physician gains experience cannulating reticular veins, cautious injection is the rule. Resistance to injection will be felt when the reticular vein has not been properly cannulated, and then will be followed by a small hematoma. After injection, all sites treated are noted in anatomic diagrams in the chart. Concentration and volumes of all sclerosing solutions are recorded.

INJECTION OF TELANGIECTASIAS

The patient is recumbent as for the larger veins. The dermatological surgeon must have access to a typical sclerotherapy tray setup, which includes the following: (1) cotton balls soaked with 70% isopropyl alcohol, (2) protective gloves, (3) 3 mL disposable syringes, (4) 30 g disposable transparent hub needles, (5) cotton balls or STD pads for compression, (6) Transpore and/or paper tape, and (7) nitroglycerine paste (for prolonged blanching of an injection site). The sclerosing solutions used are:

1. Sodium tetradecyl sulfate (concentrations 0.1–0.5%)
2. Hypertonic saline (11.7–23.4%)
3. Hypertonic saline (10%) and dextrose (25%); mixed by local pharmacy
4. Polidocanol (concentrations 0.25–1%); pending FDA approval

As for reticular veins, the patient is placed in either the prone or supine position. Treatment sites are repeatedly wiped with cotton balls heavily saturated with 70% isopropyl alcohol. Not only does this reduce infection risk, but better visualization of the vessels by increasing light transmission through otherwise reflective white scale on the epidermal surface occurs. After complete evaporation of the alcohol, a 30-gauge needle, bent to an angle of 10 to 30° with the bevel up, is placed on the skin so that the needle is parallel to the skin surface. A 3 mL syringe filled with 1.5 to 2 mL of solution is held between the index and middle fingers while the fourth and fifth finger support the syringe against the leg in a fixed position facilitating accurate penetration of the vessel (Fig. 8). The nondominant hand is used to stretch the skin around the needle and may offer additional support for the syringe.

TABLE 3 Commonly Used Sclerosing Solutions in the United States

Chemical name	Brand names	Category	Advantages	Disadvantages
Sodium tetradecyl sulfate	Sotradecol Fibro-Vein Thrombovar	Detergent—rapid dissolution of endothelium	Painless intravascular Painful extravascular Strong for varicose veins Effective at low concentration	Skin necrosis with extravasation of concentrations >0.25% Expensive Pigmentation—postsclerosis
Polidocanol	Aethoxysklerol Sclero-Vein	Detergent	Always painless Cutaneous necrosis low Effective at low concentration	Urticaria (immediate) at injection site Skin necrosis from painless ateriolar injection Not FDA approved*
Hypertonic Saline (23.4%)	None	Hyperosmolar—slow crenation of endothelium	Low-risk allergic reaction Readily available Rapid action	Painful stinging and cramping Skin necrosis
Saline and Dextrose	Sclerodex	Hyperosmolar	High viscosity—remains in treated veins Low allergic risk Low-risk necrosis	Too weak for larger varicosities Slight stinging One concentration only Not FDA approved*

*Under review.

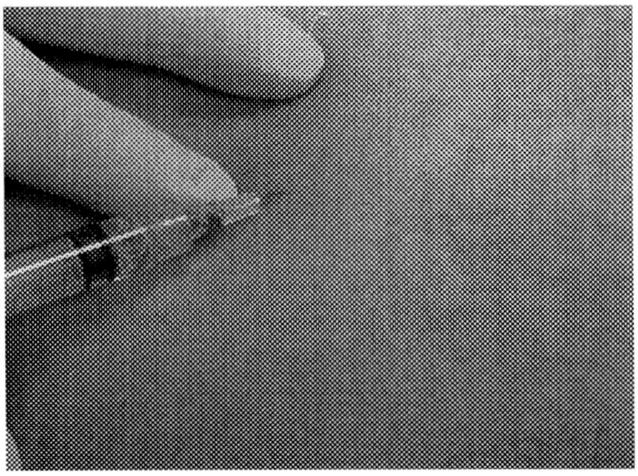

FIGURE 8 Correct position for sclerotherapy.

The firmly supported needle is then moved slowly 1 to 2 mm forward, piercing the vein just sufficiently to allow infusion of solution with the most minimal pressure on the plunger. Magnifying lenses on the order of 1.5 × to 3 × may help visualization of cannulation of the smallest telangiectasias particularly for physicians over 40 years old. Sclerotherapy technique requires a gentle, precise touch, as one learns to appreciate a subtle "pop" or "give" on entering the vessel. A very sharp needle is critical for this fine touch; the needle is changed as often as every three to four punctures to minimize tearing of the vessel. Similarly, one learns to visually recognize the appearance of the bevel of the needle within the lumen of the telangiectasia. The use of 32- to 33-gauge needles is not advised because they veer off course, tending not to move in the intended direction.

Injection of a tiny bolus of air (<0.05 mL) may be helpful to establish that the needle is within the vein, as slight clearing 1 to 3 mm ahead of the bevel can be seen. A larger air bolus theoretically allows the arborizing vessels to clear, instantly allowing greater spread of the sclerosing solution {223, 227}, but we and others have found this to occur infrequently and generally find a larger air bolus unnecessary [1,23,25].

STS will dissolve some of the rubber of the syringe plunger, causing difficulty moving the plunger and contaminating the sclerosing solution with rubber breakdown products (personal communication, Wyeth-Ayerst Laboratories). For this reason we strongly recommend the use of latex-free syringes (Terumo,). It is possible that most of the allergic reactions reported because of STS have been to latex contamination of the sclerosant.

Concentrations of sclerosants used for telangiectasias are less than for reticular veins: 0.1 to 0.2% STS, 0.1% to 0.5% POL (not FDA-approved), or 11.7 to 23.4% hypertonic saline HS or hypertonic saline and dextrose (not FDA-approved). The initial concentration is typically the lowest concentration listed above, termed the minimal effective sclerosant concentration [26]. Higher concentrations increase the risks of matting and pigmentation. The concentration may always be increased at subsequent treatments if ineffective sclerosis occurs. Increase of sclerosant concentration is safer than an increased volume per injection.

Injection of telangiectasias is performed extremely slowly by using drops of sclerosant (0.1–0.2 mL or less) with minimal or no pressure on a 3 mL syringe to maintain filling of the veins and contact with the vessel wall for approximately 10 to 15 seconds. Rapid flushing of the vessels with large volumes of sclerosant causes unnecessarily large quantities to be injected. Larger quantities increase risks of extravasation injury or entry into the deep system. This theoretically increases risks for necrosis and deep venous thrombosis, respectively.

To minimize skin necrosis, extravasation must be avoided. If resistance to the easy injection of sclerosant or the beginning of any "bleb" at the injection site is noted, the injection is immediately stopped. The physician needs to keep an eye on the injection site at all times in order to notice the bleb at the moment of its occurrence. Some physicians keep a syringe of 5 to 10 mL of normal saline nearby to flush and dilute any areas of extravasation that may develop. Sclerosant thought to have extravasated may also be diluted with 0.5 to 1.0% lidocaine without epinephrine (further vasoconstriction must be minimized). A prolonged time of blanching after injection indicates possible arteriolar compromise, and for this immediate use of topical nitroglycerine paste is recommended. Application is made in small dabs rubbed in until a faint blush replaces the blanch.

After massaging the injection site for 5 to 10 seconds, cotton balls are then secured over the injection sites by paper tape or Transpore tape. This is followed, particularly for protuberant telangiectasias or telangiectasias in association with reticular veins, with graduated 20 to 30 mmHg or 30 to 40 mmHg support hose for two weeks [27–29]. Patients are encouraged to walk and not restrict their activities, with the exception of heavy weightlifting with the legs or any activity that results in sustained contraction resulting in elevation of venous pressure.

Treatment intervals vary, but allowing 4 to 8 weeks between treatments helps to minimize the number of necessary sessions. This is true for laser or pulsed light treatment as well. Often telangiectasias will ultimately improve with at least partial clearing after exhibiting no initial response within the first 2 weeks. Typically a patient will undergo three to five treatments separated by 1 month each. After the initial series of treatments, a rest period of 4 to 6 months will allow pigmentation and matting to clear and cause remaining reticular veins to establish "new" routes of drainage. Approximately 80% of patients will clear satisfactorily during the first course of treatment. The physician may then judge and re-evaluate any remaining telangiectatic webs or new telangiectasias for the best approach for another round of sclerotherapy.

AMBULATORY PHELBECTOMY

For younger patients in particular, larger varicose veins may not be as responsive to sclerotherapy. Thicker vein walls in athletic individuals minimizes the likelihood that full-thickness injury of the vein wall will occur. Sclerotherapy is also less likely to be effective in areas of high flow such as in larger veins. Therefore, ambulatory phlebectomy should be an available modality for dermatological surgeons who treat varicose veins.

Ambulatory phlebectomy (AP) is a dermatological procedure, and was first attributed to Swiss dermatological surgeon Robert Muller [30,31]. He performed the technique in a private practice setting in Neuchâtel, Switzerland. Most veins can be treated with this technique except for reflux at the saphenofemoral and saphenopopliteal junctions. The decision to treat by ambulatory phlebectomy versus sclerotherapy is usually determined by anatomical location, patient preference, and estimated thickness of vein wall. One rough guideline is whether one observes a "blue" vein or flesh-colored varicose vein. Blue veins have walls thin enough to allow adequate damage by sclerosing solutions, but lead to easy shredding when trying to hook during ambulatory phlebectomy.

Anatomical locations amenable to AP are incompetent saphenous veins (except saphenofemoral and in most cases saphenopopliteal junctions), their major tributaries, perforators, or reticular veins, which supply telangiectasias with high-pressure reverse flow. Presurgical diagnosis with recognition of patterns of reflux is also critically important. As for sclerotherapy, expertise with the noninvasive diagnostic techniques previously discussed is required.

Once the origin point of reflux is diagnosed in truncal (axial) varicose veins, AP may be preferred over traditional surgery because little or no scar occurs compared with ligation incisions. AP also avoids possible complications of sclerotherapy for larger varicose veins, including intra-arterial injection, superficial thrombophlebitis, skin necrosis, and months of hyperpigmentation [32,33]. The recurrence rate of large varicose veins is also reduced, but again only when the major source of reflux has been eliminated.

Instrumentation requirements are quite basic (Fig. 9). Manufactured hooks include the classic Muller hook, available in four sizes, with a rather blunt tip, curves resembling a crochet hook, and a straight shaft designed to place under veins and pull out from below. Oesch's hook, available in three sizes, is characterized by a massive squared-off grip, and is designed with a small barb at the tip to pierce the vein from the lateral aspect and elevate. Ramelet's hook, available in two sizes, is a smaller, fine hook. The smaller of the two is designed to remove reticular or

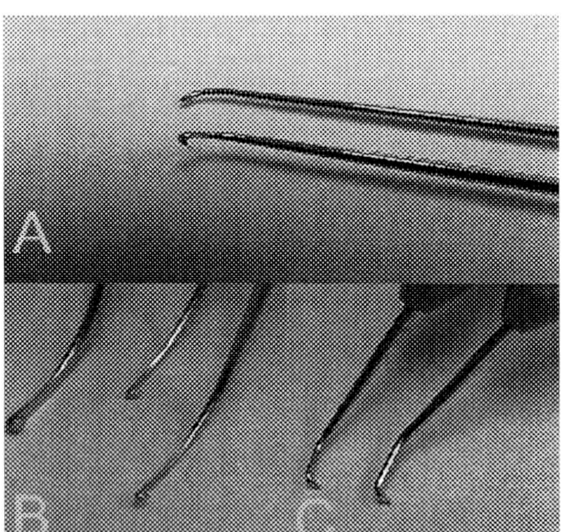

FIGURE 9 Types of ambulatory phlebectomy hooks. Usually all are placed on the tray. Shown are the Ramelet (set of 2 sizes), Muller (set of 4 sizes), and Oesch (set of 3 sizes) hooks. (a) Close-up of Ramelet tip. This hook allows "harpooning" of adventitia from above. (b) Close-up of Muller tip. This allows the surgeon to grasp the vein from below. (c) Close-up of Oesch tip, which has small wide-hooking surface. This allows the vein to be grasped from a lateral approach.

TABLE 4 Phlebectomy Supplies

Skin-marking pen
Iodine prepping solution
Disposable face mask, sterile gloves
Local anesthetic, syringes, needles
Ambulatory phlebectomy hooks: Muller, Oesch, Ramelet
Clamps, sterile 4 × 4 gauze pads
Needle 18-G, scalpel Nr 11
Mosquito forceps (one dozen)
Hydrogen peroxide for postsurgical washing of the leg
Absorbent dressings
Inelastic compression wrap
Elastic-graduated compression stockings

medium-sized truncal varicose veins. The larger one has a thicker stem, which is useful for large truncal and perforating veins. The cylindrical shape of the grip permits a gentle rolling of the hook between the fingers, diminishing the amount of rotation of the wrists and minimizing wrist and hand stress during the procedure. The shaft is short, allowing precise and close work as well as moderate traction. The hook angulation facilitates vein dissection while the sharp tip grips the vein by the perivenous collagen bundles and tunica externa, allowing lifting from above and limiting the damage to the surrounding tissues and lymphatics.

Other necessary equipment includes a number 11 scalpel or 18-gauge needle to perform the incisions or punctures (Table 4). A half dozen or more mosquito clamps or curved clamps should be on the tray with the phlebectomy hooks. A surgical table allowing rotation in the Trendelenburg position and good overhead lighting is necessary. The presence of an assistant to help hand over and remove clamps and provide compression at sites of oozing is very helpful.

Sedation, if required, consists only of an oral benzodiazepine. Varicose veins are carefully delineated with a skin marker pen on the standing patients. Special marks are made over the most superficial portions of the vein. The patient is then placed supine and the vein position is re-examined using a transilluminator. Areas that are deeper and will be more difficult to hook are then specially marked. Local anesthesia using a tumescent anesthesia technique requires a higher concentration than tumescent anesthesia for liposuction. Typically, 0.2% lidocaine with 1:500,000 epinephrine in normal saline is prepared. Injection is with a 22-gauge spinal needle that dissects the tissue just under the varicose veins to be avulsed. Usually no more than 200 mL is required for fairly long segments. Anesthesia of the leg often persists for 10 hours. When working in the popliteal fold, patients may experience a temporary foot drop from anesthesia of the peroneal nerve and require help for ambulating home.

Cutaneous incisions (with number 11 scalpel blade or 18-gauge needle) should be vertical along the thigh and lower leg and follow the skin lines at the knee or the ankle. The distance between the incisions varies from 2 to 15 cm, but is typically 3 to 4 cm. Once the AP hook is inserted into the puncture site, the targeted vein is gently dissected by undermining with the shaft of the phlebectomy hook. Attempts to pull vein through the puncture site may initially result in shreds of adventitial fibroadipose attachments. This process loosens them, and ultimately after the third or fourth attempt at lifting, a loosened vein segment can then be elevated with the sharp tip of the hook. As the vein loop is exposed and pulled through the small incision, the hook is moved to the nondominant hand. Mosquito forceps are then used to clamp the vein loop and traction is maintained by pulling as far as the vein slides easily. Too much tension will result in breakage.

Slight tension allows a subcutaneous palpable cord indicating the course of the vein adjacent to this incision site (Fig. 10). This cord is then used as a guide (along with skin markings) for the next incision. The whole varicose vein is then extracted progressively from one incision to the other. Attachments to perforating veins and points of bi- or trifurcation are carefully dissected and eliminated by gentle traction or torsion. These points of convergence of veins can be difficult to extract. Breakage of the veins often occurs at these junctions.

Difficult areas not to be tackled by the beginning surgeon include the popliteal fossa, dorsum of the foot, peripatellar or pretibial, and recurrent varicose veins after phlebitis or sclerotherapy. Hemostasis is achieved with intra- and postsurgical local compression and by Trendelburg positioning of at least 10°. Venous ligation is not necessary because stretching of the vein causes rapid hemostasis, most likely attributable to more exposed endothelial sites for platelet aggregation. Avoiding ligation avoids all the additional complications of foreign material left just below the skin. Ligation may occasionally be performed in a proximal portion of the GSV when subterminal SFJ valve reflux is present with a competent terminal valve.

A typical session lasts 30 to 60 minutes with the major portion of a varicose vein extending from thigh to midcalf. Additional branches may require additional sessions unless concomitant sclerotherapy is performed. At the conclusion of the procedure, the leg is carefully cleansed with hydrogen peroxide. Persistent bleeding of one incision is easily controlled with additional local compression held by an assistant for 10 minutes. Puncture/incision sites are typically closed with Steri-strips only, although some believe tumescent anesthesia drains more easily and complications are reduced when puncture sites are left unsealed. Occasionally incision sites in the midthigh may stretch with removal of large truncal veins and require one 5-0 suture. Postsurgical pain seldom occurs because of long action of the tumescent

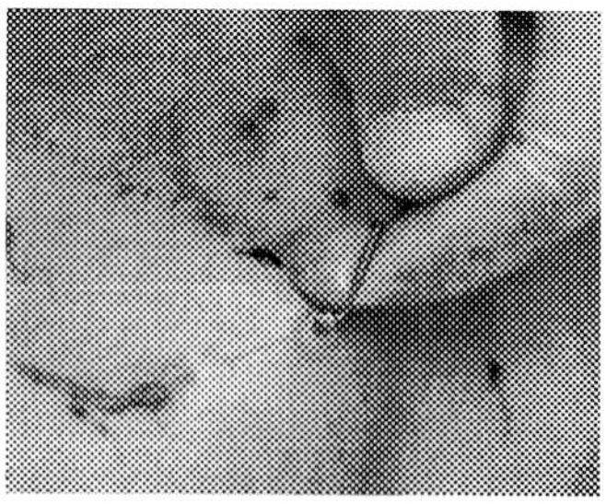

FIGURE 10 A palpable cord is seen stretched with tension between two puncture sites. This palpable cord serves to reassure the physician that the vein is being properly grasped and dissected. This cord-like appearance often provides guidance in choosing the next puncture site.

TABLE 5 Complications of Ambulatory Phlebectomy

Frequent
Skin: transient pigmentation, vesicles from pressure dressing
Vascular: hematoma
Rare
Skin: contact dermatitis, infection, scar, tattoo from marking pen, silicon (foreign body) granuloma
Vascular: postsurgical bleeding, telangiectatic matting
Neurological: postsurgical pain, transitory sensory defect, neuroma
Extremely Rare
Superficial thrombophlebitis
Lymphatic pseudocyst

anesthesia, but some patients have reported a slight burning at the site of incisions during the first postsurgical night. Analgesia is easily achieved by acetaminophen. Immediate ambulation reduces risks of deep venous thrombosis to a negligible rate.

Hematoma and bleeding are the most likely complications (Table 5). Therefore, meticulous postsurgical compression bandaging is required. The entire course of the removed varicose vein is covered with four layers of gauze pads or a single layer of the most absorbent sanitary napkins. These are secured with a low-stretch bandage (such as Comprilan) stretched to 80% of maximal stretch to obtain a low resting pressure dressing. Hematomas are minimized by placing compression at least 4 cm beyond the most proximal point of incision. An elastic graduated compression stocking is then placed over this to obtain high resting pressure. The patient walks for 10 minutes in the office and the dressing is observed for any signs of bleeding. If the dressing remains dry, the patient may drive home without assistance as long as local anesthesia has not compromised motor function.

Dressings are changed after 24 hours, the incision sites visually inspected. A less bulky dressing of gauze and inelastic compression is applied, and the compression stocking is placed over this again. The inner dressing may be removed at 48 hours, but daytime elastic graduated compression stockings are mandatory for 7 to 14 days.

Short showers are allowed 2 to 3 days after surgery. Surgical puncture sites are usually totally invisible after 3 to 6 months, but may persist much longer in younger patients with tighter skin. Hematomas rapidly disappear and pigmentation usually fades within 2 weeks. Long-term results are excellent as long as the source of venous reflux has been correctly eliminated (Fig. 11). As opposed to sclerotherapy of large varicose veins, one treatment session suffices for removal by AP. Because susceptibility to varicose veins is genetic, patients need to be warned about recurrences or new varicosities in the future, even with definitive eradication by AP.

LASERS/INTENSE PULSED LIGHT

Even when provided by expert hands, sclerotherapy has a number of potential adverse effects. Inherent to sclerotherapy is an inflammatory reaction leading to a relatively high incidence (30%) of postsclerosis pigmentation [34] and/or telangiectatic matting [35]. Lasers and IPL destroy endothelial cells through thermal damage that is believed to produce less inflammation compared with the chemical irritation of the vessel wall through sclerotherapy. Although many of the same side effects as sclerotherapy are common with all the laser and light devices. The optimal light source would have a wavelength specific for the vessel treated and be able to penetrate to the depth and diameter of the vessel through its entire course.

As with all the other treatment techniques, reverse pressure from associated reticular or varicose veins must be recognized or treatment will be doomed to failure. In many patients a combination of treatments will be necessary as most lasers or IPL will not treat associated reticular and varicose veins. In one of 26 biopsy specimens of leg telangiectasia, the origin has been shown to be a terminal arteriole or arteriovenous anastomosis [6]. In this situation alone, telangiectasias can be treated without consideration of underlying forces of hydrostatic pressure and lasers or pulsed light may be used without further problem.

The choice of wavelength(s), degree of energy fluence, and pulse duration of light exposure are all related to the type and size of target vessel treated. Deeper vessels require a longer wavelength to allow penetration to their depth. However, even at a penetrating wavelength, pulse duration must be matched to vessel size. As depth and size of vessel changes so do the absorption characteristics [36], and the problem with leg veins is that they course at different depths with different sizes. Large-diameter vessels require a longer pulse duration to allow sufficient time for diffusion of heat evenly throughout the cylindrical vessel lumen [37]. Various lasers have been used in an effort to enhance clinical efficacy and minimize the adverse sequelae of telangiectasia treatment. Unfortunately, most have also been associated with adverse responses far in excess of those associated with sclerotherapy. This is related both to the nonspecifity of the laser used and the lack of treatment of hydrostatic pressure from the "feeding" venous system.

As leg telangiectasias course along at different depths [38], they may require different wavelengths for complete treatment. Wavelengths between 600 and 900 nm have been predicted to be most useful for vessel depth [39]. During the process of delivering a sufficient quantity of energy to thermocoagulate the target vessel, the overlying epidermis and perivascular tissue should be unharmed. This requires minimal interaction with melanin and/or some form of epidermal cooling. A number of different laser and IPL systems have been developed towards this end.

FIGURE 11 Before and after views. (a) Example of clinical condition in which sclerotherapy is ideal with multiple telangiectatic webs arising from a prominent reticular vein of the lateral venous system. Results at 6 months are photographed after four treatments. A small insignificant group persists near the popliteal fossa. The most resistant area to treatment is typically around the knee. (b) Ambulatory phlebectomy is indicated for this large flesh-colored vein which comprises an anastomoses between the anteriolateral tributary of the greater saphenous vein and the lateral venous system (a common occurrence). The postsurgical appearance as photographed at 2 months is superimposed electronically adjacent to the presurgical view. Note clearing of most of the smaller varicosities originally associated with the large one.

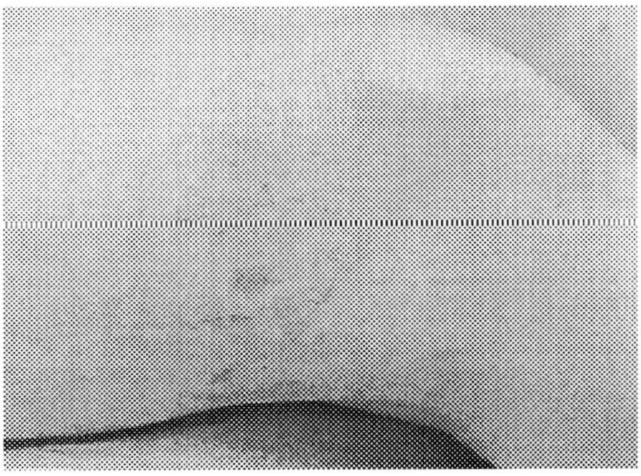

(a)

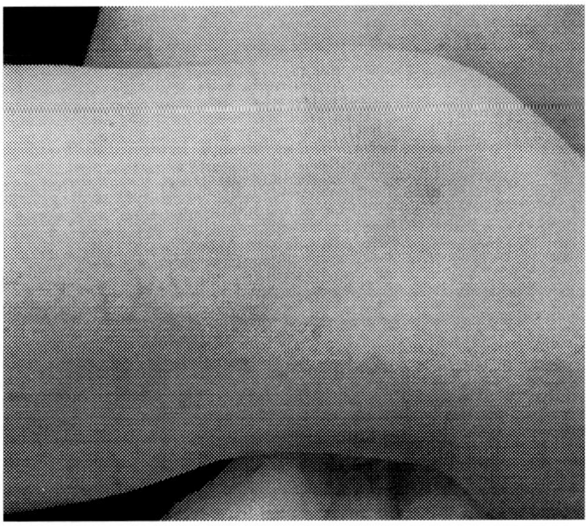

(b)

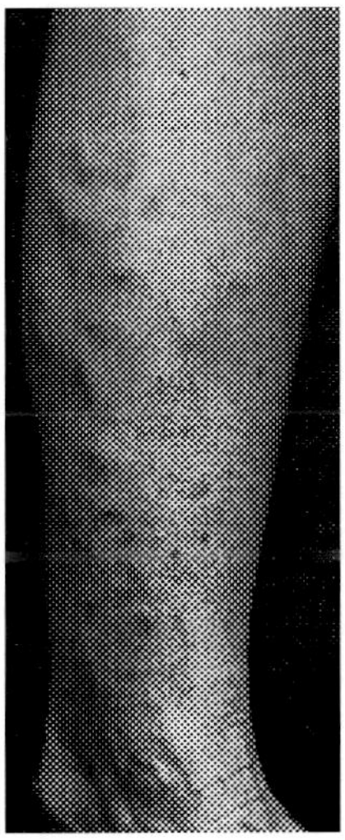

(c)

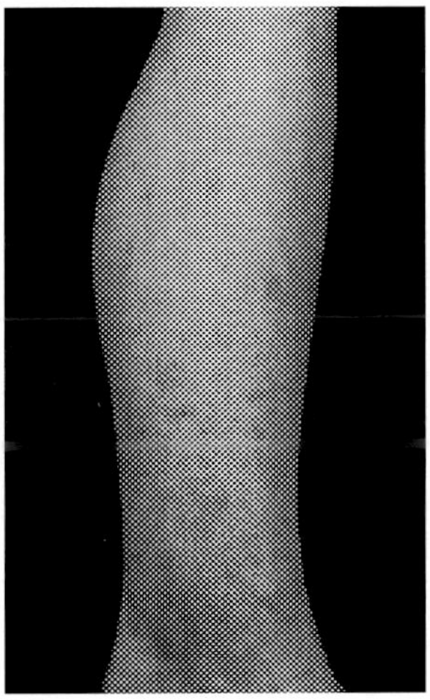

(d)

Nd:YAG (1064 nm)

The Nd:YAG (1064 nm) laser has been used to treat telangiectasia since over a decade ago [40]. The average depth of penetration in human skin is 0.75 mm and reduction to 10% of the incident power occurs at a depth of 3.7 mm [41]. This laser should theoretically be well suited to treat blood vessels within the mid-dermis. The 1064 nm wavelength is absorbed by both hemoglobin and water but to a much lesser degree by melanin. Paradoxically, the primary benefit for treatment of larger vessels is penetration because hemoglobin does not effectively stop 1064 nm absorption. However, high energies must be used for adequate penetration. Only with sufficient fluence and facilitation of heat dissipation, the posterior wall of a larger diameter (1–2 mm) vessel filled with deoxygenated hemoglobin can be reached and heated.

Newer 1064 nm lasers with pulse durations between 1 and 50 msec have recently been developed (Vasculight; ESC Sharplan Medical Systems, Needham, MA, and CoolTouch-V; Laser Aesthetics, CA). Our initial studies have found this wavelength to be effective with fluences of 60 to 120 J/cm^2 and pulse durations of 10 to 30 msec [42]. Epidermal cooling may be provided through cold gel, cryogen spray, or a skin-chilling device at 1 to 4°C. As interaction with melanin is extremely small, the use of the 1064 nm wavelength allows treatment of skin types up to Fitzpatrick V, which is not possible with the other lasers. An example of results using the 1064 nm Vasculight, which allows pulses of up to 16 msec to be synchronized with specific thermal relaxation intervals (10–30 msec), is shown in Figure 12. Vessels up to 3 mm can be treated with this wavelength and pulse duration.

KTP and Frequency Doubled Nd-YAG (532 nm)

Modulated Krypton triphosphate (KTP) lasers have been reported to be effective at removing leg telangiectasia using pulse durations between 1 and 50 msec. The 532 nm wavelength is one of several hemoglobin absorption peaks. Although this wavelength does not penetrate deeply into the dermis (about 0.75 mm), relatively specific damage (compared with argon laser) can occur in the vascular target by selecting a better pulse duration, although absorption by melanin is still significant. KTP lasers, which use a 1 or 2 mm diameter beam, focus too much heat in one spot in the target vessel and thus have led to less than optimal results [43].

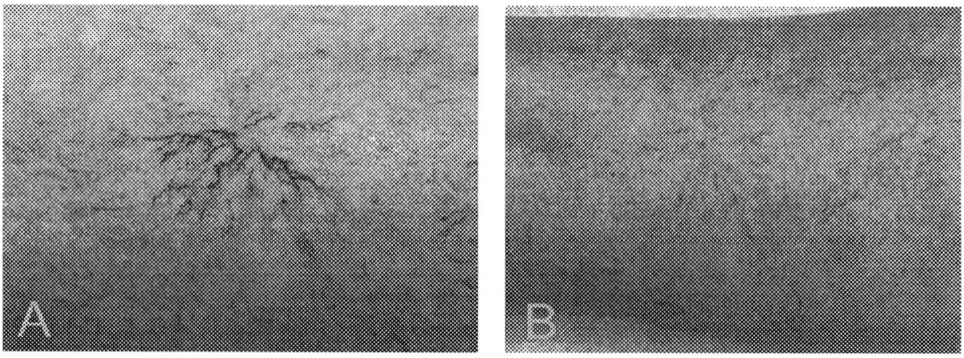

FIGURE 12 Ankle telangiectasias treated with 1064 nm. (a) Before, (b) 60 days after one treatment.

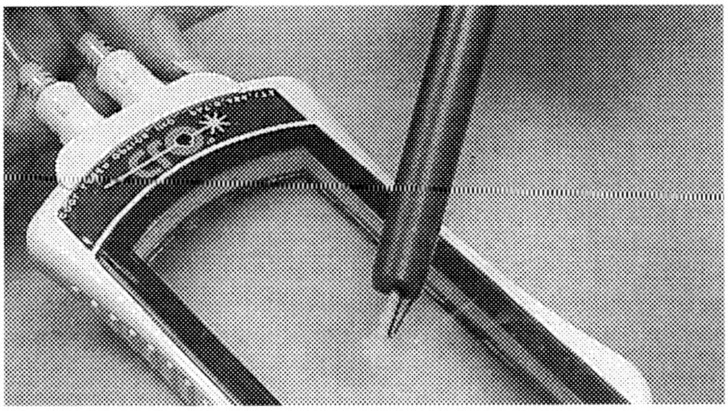

FIGURE 13 Treatment of a leg vein with the 532 nm.

A redesigned long-pulse 532 nm laser (frequency-doubled Nd:YAG) (Versapulse; Coherent, Inc., Palo Alto, CA) is more effective in treating leg veins because of the larger spot sizes and the use of epidermal cooling. Using fluences between 12 to 20 J/cm^2 delivered with a 3 to 5 mm diameter spot size, a train of pulses is delivered over the vessel until spasm or thrombosis occurs. For leg vessels less than 1 mm in diameter that are not directly connected to a feeding reticular vein, and with use of a 4°C chilled tip to protect the epidermis, this method can be quite effective. There is considerable variation in results reported by individual physicians. We found that two to three treatments were necessary for maximal vessel improvement although some have reported 100% resolution of the treated leg vein with one treatment (Fig. 13) [44]. We believe that this laser is best used for leg vessels recalcitrant to other laser, intense pulsed light, and sclerotherapy treatment. Patients with darker or tanned skin have a relatively high risk of temporary hypopigmentation.

Flashlamp-Pulsed Dye Laser (FLPDL), 585 nm

The FLPDL has been shown to be highly efficacious in treating cutaneous vascular lesions consisting of very small superficial vessels including PWS, hemangiomas, and facial telangiectasia [45]. The depth of vascular damage is estimated to be 1.5 mm at 585 nm. The pulse duration of the first generation of FLPDL was 450 μsec, optimal for the 50 to 100 μ diameter of PWS vessels. This pulse duration has been shown to be somewhat effective for treating leg telangiectasia less than 1 mm in diameter [46].

Vessels that should optimally respond to FLPDL treatment are predicted to be red telangiectasia less than 0.2 mm in diameter, particularly those vessels arising as a function of telangiectatic metting postsclerotherapy. This is based on knowledge of the type of thermocoagulation produced by this relatively short-pulse laser system. Two factors may minimize the induction of angiogenesis, which can be seen with sclerotherapy. These include the fact that FLPDL alters intravascular fibrin, which is believed to occur through thermal alteration of fibrin complexes of proteolytic cleavage of fibrinogen [46–48] with a relative decrease in perivascular inflammation [47,49].

FLPDL has led to long-term hypopigmentation in many patients with tanned skin, although 67% of telangiectatic patches completely faded within 4 months. In an effort to more safely thermocoagulate larger diameter blood vessels, the pulse duration of FLPDL has been lengthened to 1.5 ms and the wavelength increased to 600 nm [50]. This theoretically permits more thorough heating of a larger vessel. Studies using a 595 nm FLPDL at 1.5 msec found 50 to 75% clearance of leg veins [51–53]. Vessels ranged in diameter from 0.6 to 1 mm were treated with an elliptical spot size of 2 × 7 mm through a transparent hydrogel-based wound dressing.

Long-Pulse Infrared Alexandrite (LPIR, 755 nm)

In order to penetrate more deeply to treat larger vessels and to allow for greater thermal diffusion time, the alexandrite laser has been modified to allow pulse durations of up to 20 msec. This wavelength theoretically penetrates to 2 to 3 mm in depth. In its early clinical trials, this wavelength has been effective in clinical and biopsy studies. Optimal treatment parameters for LPIR appeared to be 20 J/cm^2, double pulsed at a repetition rate of 1 Hz. After three treatments at 4-week intervals, subjective grading indicated a 63% reduction in leg telangiectasias [54]. Medium-diameter vessels (0.4–1 mm) responded best with small vessel diameters responding poorly. This would match the theory that larger vessels have a larger thermal relaxation time, whereas smaller vessels absorb shorter pulses more readily. The best response in this study of LPIR was seen with sclerotherapy performed as a supplemental technique.

Diode Lasers

Diode lasers generate coherent monochromatic light through excitation of small diodes. Two methods of delivery for diode lasers are available. These include fiberoptic transmission of an 810 nm (gallium-arsenide) (LaserLite, Boston, MA) or an overlapping 800 nm diode array with a fixed spot size of 9 × 9 mm (Coherent Medical, Palo Alto, CA). These devices are therefore lightweight, reliable, and portable with a relatively small desktop footprint. Dierickx et al. evaluated an 800 nm diode array laser (Star Medical, Inc) on eight areas of leg veins [55]. The laser was used at 15 to 40 J/cm^2 given in 5 to 30 msec pulses as double or triple pulses separated by a 2-second delay time. Veins were treated every 4 weeks for three sessions and evaluated 2 months after the last treatment. One-hundred percent clearing occurred in 22%, 75% clearing in 42%, and 50% clearing in 32%.

Garden et al. [56] used an 810 nm diode laser with a 750 μm spot size at 40 watts and 50 msec pulses for a total of 453 J/cm^2 of fluence delivered. Twelve patients with 58 vessels 0.2 to 0.5 mm in diameter were treated with 3 to 4 passes until vessel spasm occurred. Patients were retreated every 2 to 4 weeks. There was a mean clearance of 60% after 2.2 treatments. Eighteen vessels had greater than 70% clearance after 3 treatments.

High-Intensity Pulsed Light (PhotoDerm VL)

The high-intensity pulsed light (IPL) source was developed as an alternative to lasers in an attempt to improve efficacy for treating leg veins, (PhotoDerm® VL; ESC Sharplan, Needham, MA). This device permits sequential pulsing of 1 to 12 msec duration separated and synchronized with 1 to 100 msec rest intervals using a filtered flashlamp to producing noncoherent wavelengths of 515 to 1000 nm. This primarily encompasses the yellow and red wavelengths with some infrared.

The therapeutic potential of IPL is explained by the optical properties of hemoglobin as the size and depth of its container (blood vessel) and state of oxygenation are changed. Figure 14 shows the oxyhemoglobin absorption and scattering coefficient depth of penetration into blood as a reflection of vessel size and depth. The main feature to note is the strong absorption at wavelengths below 600 nm with less absorption at longer wavelengths. However, as the size of the vessel increases 1 mm in diameter, it absorbs more than 67% of light even at wavelengths longer than 600 nm. This absorption band is even more significant for blood vessels 2 mm in diameter. Thus a light source above 600 nm should result in deeper penetration of thermal energy, thereby allowing much absorption of deoxyhemoglobin. This is because the absorption coefficient in blood is higher than that of surrounding tissue for wavelengths between 600 and 1000 nm.

A device that produces a noncoherent light as a continuous spectrum longer than 550 nm should theoretically have multiple advantages over a single-wavelength laser system. First, both oxygenated and deoxygenated hemoglobin will absorb at these wavelengths. Second, larger blood vessels located deeper in the dermis can be affected. Third, thermal absorption by the exposed blood vessels should occur with less overlying epidermal absorption because the longer wavelengths will penetrate more deeply.

Using these theoretical considerations, IPL emitting in the 515 to 1000 nm range was used at varying energy fluences (5–90 J/cm^2) and various pulse durations (2–12 msec) to treat venulectasia 0.4 to 2.0 mm in diameter. Clinical trials using various parameters with the IPL, including multiple pulses of variable duration, showed efficacy ranging up to 90% clearance in vessels less than 0.2 mm in diameter, 80% in vessels from 0.2 to 0.5 mm, and 80% in vessels 0.5 to 1 mm in diameter

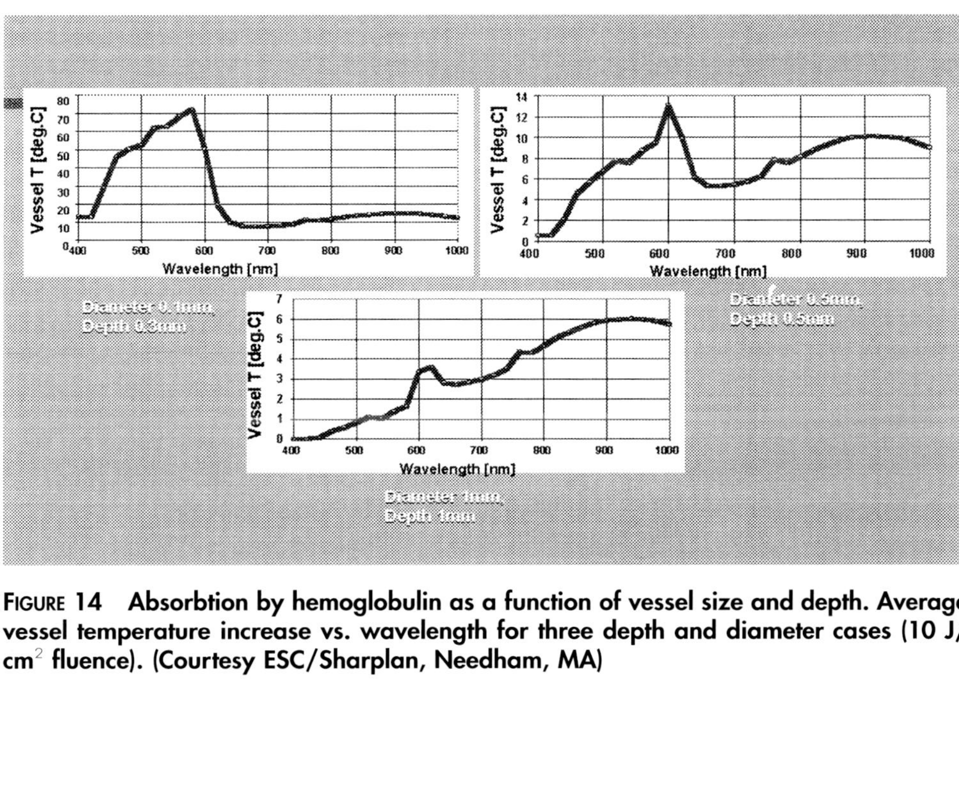

FIGURE 14 Absorbtion by hemoglobulin as a function of vessel size and depth. Average vessel temperature increase vs. wavelength for three depth and diameter cases (10 J/cm^2 fluence). (Courtesy ESC/Sharplan, Needham, MA)

[57–59]. The incidence of adverse sequelae was minimal with hypopigmentation occurring in 1 to 3% of patients resolving within 4 to 6 months. Tanned or darkly pigmented Fitzpatrick Type III patients were likely to develop hypo- and hyperpigmentation in addition to blistering and superficial erosions. These all cleared over a few months. Treatment parameters that were found to be most successful ranged from a single pulse to 22 J/cm^2 in 3 msec for vessels less than 0.2 mm or a double pulse of 35–40 J/cm^2 given in 2.4 and 4.0 ms with a 10 ms delay. Vessels between 0.2 and 0.5 mm were treated with the same double-pulse parameters or with a 3.0 to 6.0 ms pulse at 35–45 J/cm^2 with a 20 ms delay time. Vessels above 0.5 mm were treated with triple pulses of 3.5 to 3.1 to 2.6 ms with pulse delays of 20 ms at a fluence of 50 J/cm^2 or with triple pulse of 3 to 4 to 6 ms with a pulse delay of 30 ms at a fluence of 55 to 60 J/cm^2. The choice of a cut-off filter was based on skin color, with light-skinned patients using a 550 nm filter and darker-skinned patients using a 570 or 590 nm filter.

More recently, increased efficacy has been reported by increasing the pulse durations to a maximum of 12 msec in two consecutive pulses separated by a 20 to 30 msec delay with a 570 nm to 590 nm cut-off filter and fluences of 70 J/cm^2. Response rates of 74% in two treatments with an 8% incidence of temporary hypo- or hyperpigmentation has been reported [60]. By combining a shorter pulse (2.4–3 msec) with a longer pulse (7–10 msec), it is theoretically possible to ablate smaller and larger vessels overlying one another in the dermis. The shorter pulses theoretically are absorbed more selectively by smaller, more superficial vessels, whereas the longer pulses are absorbed by the larger-diameter vessels (Fig. 15). New epidermal cooling devices improve treatment results by allowing larger influences with less risks to the epidermis (Fig. 16).

CONCLUSIONS

Sclerotherapy, ambulatory phlebectomy, and/or laser of varicose, reticular veins, and telangiectasias is highly effective when approached in a systematic logical way. While sclerotherapy remains the gold standard, ambulatory phlebectomy is rapidly gaining acceptance as the preferred technique for larger varicose veins. The role of advanced techniques of laser and IPL are also emerging. Patients who are needle-phobic will tolerate the use of this technology even though the pain from laser/IPL may exceed that of sclerotherapy. Vessels below the ankle are particularly suitable for lasers or IPL because sclerotherapy has a relatively high incidence of ulceration in this area due to the higher frequency of arteriovenous anastamosis. Finally, patients who have vessels that are resistant to sclerotherapy are excellent candidates. Efficacy of 75% clearance with 2 to 3 treatments has been reported in sclerotherapy-resistant vessels [61]. Combination sclerotherapy plus laser or IPL treatments may also be more effective [49,62] (Fig. 14). Combination treatment allows sclerotherapy to treat the feeding venous system while laser or IPL effectively seals superficial vessels to prevent extravasation, thereby minimizing pigmentation, recanalization, and telangiectatic matting. Use of longer wavelengths, such as 1064 nm, with pulse durations of 10 to 20 msecs appears very promising to improve the capability of lasers to treat larger, deeper blood vessels of the leg and address the origins of hydrostatic pressure.

Clearing rates with sclerotherapy of 90% have been reported [1,26]. Experience gained over time greatly enhances results. Every patient should be approached with

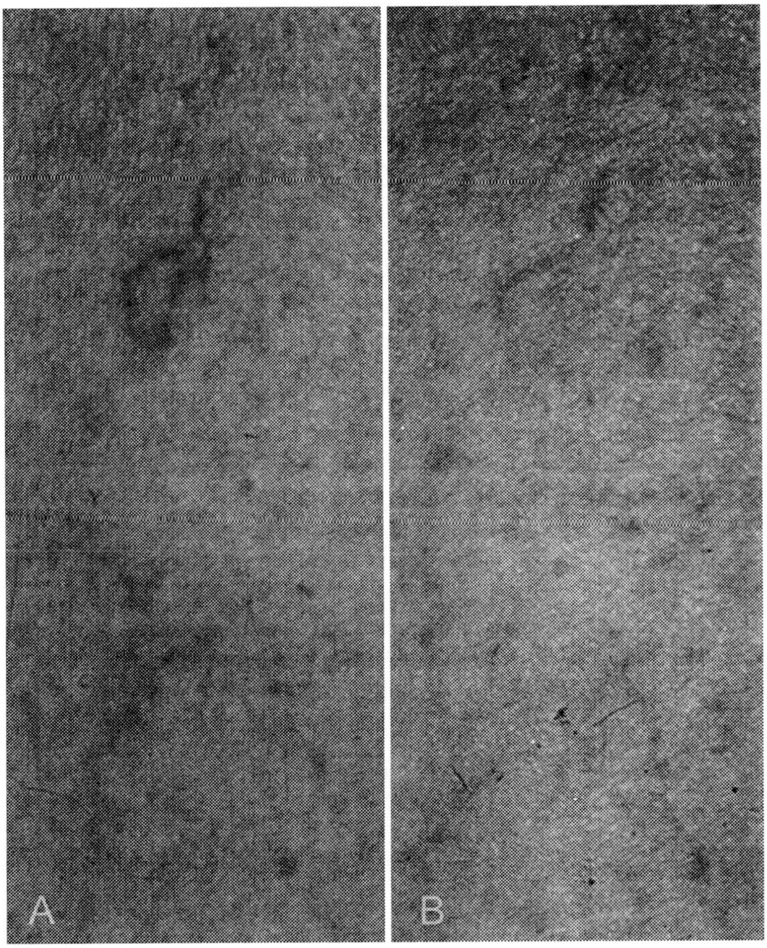

FIGURE 15 (a, b) Short- and long-pulse parameters yield highly specific results with associated clinical improvement.

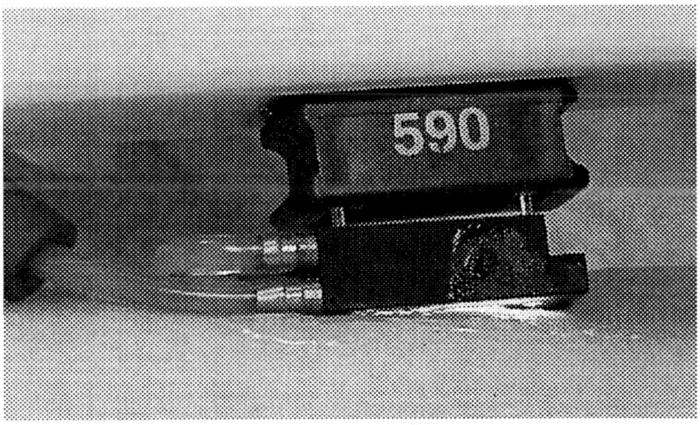

FIGURE 16 Epidermal cooling device for the IPL device.

knowledge of venous anatomy, understanding principles of reflux, thorough informed consent, photographic documentation, and familiarity with different sclerosing solution volumes and concentrations, in office surgical techniques and when laser or light therapy may be warranted. Treatment based on this foundation is highly likely to be successful.

REFERENCES

1. Weiss RA, Weiss MA. Resolution of pain associated with varicose and telangiectatic leg veins after compression sclerotherapy. J Dermatol Surg Onc 1990; 16:333–336.
2. Weiss RA. Vascular studies of the legs for venous or arterial disease. Dermatol Clin 1994; 12(1):175–190.
3. Goldman MP, Weiss RA, Bergan JJ. Diagnosis and treatment of varicose veins—a review. J Am Acad Dermatol 1994; 31:393–413.
4. Weiss RA, Weiss MA. Painful telangiectasias: diagnosis and treatment. In: Bergan JJ, Goldman MP, eds. *Varicose Veins and Telangiectasias: Diagnosis and Treatment.* St. Louis: Quality Medical Publishing, Inc., 1993:389–406.
5. Thibault P, Bray A, Wlodarczyk J, Lewis W. Cosmetic leg veins: evaluation using duplex venous imaging. J Dermatol Surg Onc 1990; 16:612–618.
6. deFaria JL, Moraes IN. Histopathology of telangiectasias associated with various veins. Dermatologica 1963; 127:321–321.
7. Wokalek H, Vanscheidt W, Martay K, Leder O. Morphology and localization of sunburst varicosities: an electron microscopic and morphometric study. J Dermatol Surg Onc 1989; 15:149–154.
8. Braverman IM, Keh-Yen A. Ultrastructure of the human dermal microcirculation. IV. Valve-containing collecting veins at the dermal-subcutaneous junction. J Invest Dermatol 1983; 81(5):438–442.
9. Somjen GM, Ziegenbein R, Johnston AH, Royle JP. Anatomical examination of leg telangiectases with duplex scanning [see comments]. J Dermatol Surg Onc 1993; 19(10): 940–945.
10. Weiss RA, Weiss MA. Doppler ultrasound findings in reticular veins of the thigh subdermic lateral venous system and implications for sclerotherapy. J Dermatol Surg Onc 1993; 19(10):947–951.
11. Partsch H. Primary varikose der vena saphena magna und parva. In: Kriessman A, Bollinger A, Keller H, eds. *Praxis der Doppler Sonographie.* Stuttgart: Thieme, 1982: 101–103.
12. Weiss RA. Evaluation of the venous system by Doppler ultrasound and photoplethysmography or light reflection rheography before sclerotherapy. Semin Dermatol 1993; 12:78–87.
13. Rosfors S. Venous photoplethysmography: relationship between transducer position and regional distribution of venous insufficiency. J Vasc Surg 1990; 11:436–440.
14. Weindorf N, Schultz-Ehrenburg U. Der wert der photoplethysmographie (licht reflexions rheography) in der phlebologie. Vasa 1986; 15:397–401.
15. McMullin GM, Coleridge Smith PD. An evaluation of Doppler ultrasound and photoplethysmography in the investigation of venous insufficiency. Aust N Z J Med 1992; 62:270–275.
16. Blazek V, Schmitt HJ, Schultz-Ehrenburg U, Kerner J. Digitale photoplethysmographie (D-PPG) fur die beinvenendiagnostik. Medizinisch-technische grundlagen. Phlebol Proktol 1989; 18:91–97.
17. Abramowitz HB, Queral LA, Flinn WR, et al. The use of photoplethysmography in the assessment of venous insufficiency: a comparison to venous pressure measurements. Surgery 1979; 66:434–441.

18. Vin F. [Echo-sclerotherapy of the external saphenous vein]. Phlebol 1991; 44:79–84, discussion 90–6.
19. Raymond-Martimbeau P. Two different techniques for sclerosing the incompetent saphenofemoral junction: a comparative study. J Dermatol Surg Onc 1990; 16:626–631.
20. Schadeck M. Sclerotherapy of great saphenous veins: a 48-month followup. J Dermatol Surg Oncol 1990; 16.87.
21. Hobbs JT. Surgery and sclerotherapy in the treatment of varicose veins. A random trial. Arch Surg 1974; 109:793–796.
22. Weiss RA, Weiss MA. Sclerotherapy. In: Wheeland RG, ed. *Cutaneous Surgery.* Philadelphia: W. B. Saunders Co., 1994: 951–981.
23. Weiss RA, Goldman MP. Advances in sclerotherapy. Dermatol Clin 1995; 13(2):431–445.
24. Goldman PM. Polidocanol (aethoxysklerol) for sclerotherapy of superficial venules and telangiectasias. J Dermatol Surg Onc 1989; 15:204–209.
25. Goldman PM. Sclerotherapy for superficial venules and telangiectasias of the lower extremities. Dermatol Clin 1987; 5:369–379.
26. Sadick NS. Sclerotherapy of varicose and telangiectatic leg veins. Minimal sclerosant concentration of hypertonic saline and its relationship to vessel diameter [see comments]. J Dermatol Surg Onc 1991; 17:65–70.
27. Struckmann J, et al. Venous muscle pump improvement by low compression elastic stockings. Phlebol 1986; 1:97–103.
28. Partsch H. Compression therapy of the legs. A review. J Dermatol Surg Onc 1991; 17: 799–805.
29. Goldman MP, Beaudoing D, Marley W, Lopez L, Butie A. Compression in the treatment of leg telangiectasia: a preliminary report. J Dermatol Surg Onc 1990; 16:322–325.
30. Muller R. [Ambulatory phlebectomy]. Ther Umsch 1992; 49:447–450.
31. Muller R. Traitement des varices par la phlebectomie ambulatoire. Bull Soc Franc Phlebologie 1966; 19:277–279.
32. Ramelet AA. La phlebectomie ambulatoire selon Mueller: technique, avantages, desavantages. Journal des Maladies Vasculaires 1991; 16:119–122.
33. Ramelet AA. Le traitement des telangiectasies: indications de la phlebectomie Selon Muller. Phlebol 1995; 47(4):377–381.
34. Goldman MP, Kaplan RP, Duffy DM. Postsclerotherapy hyperpigmentation: a histologic evaluation. J Dermatol Surg Onc 1987; 13:547–550.
35. Goldman MP, Sadick NS, Weiss RA. Cutaneous necrosis, telangiectatic matting, and hyperpigmentation following sclerotherapy, etiology, prevention, and treatment. Dermatol Surg 1995; 21(1):19–29.
36. Smithies DJ, Butler PH. Modeling the distribution of laser light in port-wine stains with the Monte Carlo method. Phys Med Biol 1995; 40(5):701–731.
37. Dierickx CC, Casparian JM, Venugopalan V, Farinelli WA, Anderson RR. Thermal relaxation of port-wine stain vessels probed in vivo: the need for 1-10 millisecond laser pulse treatment. J Invest Dermatol 1995; 105:709–714.
38. Braverman IM. Ultrastructure and organization of the cutaneous microvasculature in normal and pathologic states. J Invest Dermatol 1989; 93:28–32.
39. Kienle A, Hibst R. Optimal parameters for laser treatment of leg telangiectasia. Lasers Surg Med 1997; 20(3):346–353.
40. Apfelberg DB, et al. Study of three laser systems for treatment of superficial varicosities of the lower extremity. Lasers Surg Med 1987; 7:219–219.
41. Glassberg E, et al. The flashlamp-pumped 577-nm pulsed tunable dye laser: clinical efficacy and in vitro studies. J Dermatol Surg Onc 1988; 14:1200–1200.
42. Weiss RA, Weiss MA. Early clinical results with a multiple synchronized pulse 1064 nm laser for leg telangiectasias and reticular veins. Dermatol Surg (In press.)

43. West TB, Alster TS. Comparison of the long-pulse dye (590-595 nm) and KTP (532 nm) lasers in the treatment of facial and leg telangiectasias. Dermatol Surg 1998; 24(2): 221–226.
44. Adrian RM. Treatment of leg telangiectasias using a long-pulse frequency-doubled neodymium: YAG laser at 532 nm. Dermatol 1998; 24(1):19–23.
45. Garden JM, Bakus AD. Clinical efficacy of the pulsed dye laser in the treatment of vascular lesions. J Dermatol Surg Oncol 1993; 19(4):321–326.
46. Polla LL, Tan OT, Garden JM, Parrish JA. Tunable pulsed dye laser for the treatment of benign cutaneous vascular ectasia. Dermatologica 1987; 174(1):11–17.
47. Goldman MP, Martin DE, Fitzpatrick RE, Ruiz-Esparza J. Pulsed dye laser treatment of telangiectases with and without subtherapeutic sclerotherapy. Clinical and histologic examination in the rabbit ear vein model. J Am Acad Dermatol 1990; 23(1):23–30.
48. Nakagawa H, Tan OT, Parrish JA. Ultrastructural changes in human skin after exposure to a pulsed laser. J Invest Dermatol 1985; 84:396–399.
49. Goldman MP, Fitzpatrick RE. Pulsed-dye laser treatment of leg telangiectasia: with and without simultaneous sclerotherapy. J Dermatol Surg Oncol 1990; 16(4):338–344.
50. Edstrom DW, Ros AM. The treatment of port-wine stains with the pulsed dye laser at 600 nm. Br J Dermatol 1997; 136(3):360–363.
51. Hsia J, Lowery JA, Zelickson B. Treatment of leg telangiectasia using a long-pulse dye laser at 595 nm. Lasers Surg Med 1997; 20(1):1–5.
52. Hohenleutner U, Walther T, Wenig M, Baumler W, Landthaler M. Leg telangiectasia treatment with a 1.5 ms pulsed dye laser, ice cube cooling of the skin and 595 vs 600 nm: preliminary results. Lasers Surg Med 1998; 23(2):72–78.
53. Perez B, Nunez M, Boixeda P, Harto A, Ledo A. Progressive ascending telangiectasia treated with the 585 nm flashlamp-pumped pulsed dye laser. [In Process Citation]. Lasers Surg Med 1997; 21(5):413–416.
54. McDaniel DH, Ash K, Lord J, Newman J, Adrian RM, Zukowski M. Laser therapy of spider leg veins: clinical evaluation of a new long pulsed alexandrite laser. [In Process Citation]. Dermatol Surg 1999; 25(1):52–58.
55. Dierickx CC, Duque V, Anderson RR. Treatment of leg telangiectasia by a pulsed, infrared laser system. Lasers Surg Med 1998; 10(suppl):40.
56. Garden JM, Bakus AD, Miller ID. Diode laser treatment of leg veins. Lasers Surg Med 1998; 10(Supplement):38.
57. Goldman MP, Eckhouse S. Photothermal sclerosis of leg veins. ESC Medical Systems, LTD Photoderm VL Cooperative Study Group [see comments]. Dermatol Surg 1996; 22(4):323–330.
58. Schroeter C, Wilder D, Reineke T, et al. Clinical significance of an intense, pulsed light source on leg telangiectasias of up to 1 mm diameter. Eur J Dermatol 1997; 7:38–42.
59. Raulin C, Weiss RA, Schonermark MP. Treatment of essential telangiectasias with an intense pulsed light source (PhotoDerm VL). Dermatol Surg 1997; 23(10):941–945.
60. Weiss RA, Weiss MA, Marwaha S, Harrington AC. Non-coherent filtered flashlamp intense pulsed light source for leg telangiectasias: long pulse durations for improved results. Lasers Surg Med 1998; 10(supplement):40.
61. Weiss RA, Weiss MA. New treatment for telangiectases and venulectases: status of intense pulsed light therapy. Dermatol Surg 1996; 5(suppl):7.
62. Weiss RA, Weiss MA. Combination intense pulsed light and sclerotherapy: a synergistic effect. Dermatol Surg 1997; 23(10):969.

APPENDIX 1

DRS. ROBERT AND MARGARET WEISS
AND DERMATOLOGY ASSOCIATES

SCLEROTHERAPY FEE SCHEDULE

Patient's name ______________________________

Office Location ______________________________

Date ______________________________

Consultation with nurse ______________________________

Pre-Operative Testing:

Venous Doppler/PPG(93965) ______________________________

Venous Duplex Ultrasound (93970) ______________________________

First Visit with Doctor-

Office Visit ______________________________

Test Area (36470) ______________________________

Subsequent Treatments (36471) ______________________________

Duplex at time of treatment (93971) ______________________________

Equipment Tray ______________________________

Surgical Stockings ______________________________
Delilah/Venosan ______________________________
Samson Knee-highs (men) ______________________________

Photography Fee (one time) ______________________________

We make every effort to stay on schedule. Please call us if you will be delayed or cannot keep an appointment. There is a $50 charge for failure to cancel an appointment within 24 hours of its scheduled time.

Please remember that payment in full is due at the time of each treatment. We appreciate your cooperation with this policy.

An **average** session for many areas costs $250-350. Most patients need 2-4 sessions, spaced a month or so apart.

______________________ ______________________
Patient Witness

APPENDIX 2

DRS. ROBERT AND MARGARET WEISS
AND DERMATOLOGY ASSOCIATES

CONSENT FOR TREATMENT OF LEG VEINS

There have been many methods tried to remove unsightly "broken" or enlarged veins on the legs. Most do not work, and have been abandoned. The doctor uses a technique called sclerotherapy, which involves the following.

A tiny needle is threaded into the blood vessel and a small amount of a sclerosing agent is gently injected. This may sting for 20-30 seconds or cause a slight cramp. The injection "flushes" out the red blood cells temporarily, leading to an inflammatory reaction. This reaction causes "sclerosis", or the formation of fibrous tissue within the vessel, leading to the gradual disappearance of the vessel. This fading can take from a few weeks to a few months. Most areas will require between three to five treatments to fade.

A test area is injected first and observed for 4-6 weeks to see how well the procedure and particular solution achieves the desired result in that particular patient.

Some of the possible risks include:

1. The appearance of the veins may <u>not</u> improve. However, over 90% of patients see improvement.
2. Brown spots may appear that look like bruises or follow the path of the vein. These brown areas take several weeks to months to go away. It is rare for any discoloration to be permanent. Patients with naturally darker skin are more likely to experience this.
3. Blistering, redness, itching and irritation may develop as reaction to the adhesive tape used for compression.
4. Blistering, infection~ ulceration, and scarring may develop if someone is exceptionally sensitive to the tiny amount of solution that may leak out during the injection. This occurs in less than 1% of patients. An allergic reaction to some of the solutions is also a rare possibility.
5. Tenderness, bruising, or a firmness (especially along the larger vessels) in the treated area may last for varying periods of time. This can be minimized by the use of support hose after the treatment.
6. Some people (less than 10%) may develop a "matt", or pink blush of the skin, which comes from a temporary enlargement of the tiny capillaries. This is rarely permanent, and can be treated.
7. Sometimes blood may accumulate in the larger veins treated by sclerotherapy. These accumulations may be treated by the physician to decrease any discomfort. Strict use of support hose minimizes this possibility.
8. Rarely, this accumulation of blood may form a clot. Although this is usually trapped in the treated vein, an extremely rare possibility is the extension of this clot into a deeper vessel causing phlebitis. The risk of this occurring is much less than 1%.
9. People with significant circulatory problems , uncontrolled diabetes or pregnant women should not undergo this procedure.

<u>CONSENT</u>

By signing this form, I attest that I have read and understand the procedure and its risks, and that it has been explained to my satisfaction.

PATIENT ______________________________

WITNESS ______________________________

APPENDIX 3

DRS. ROBERT AND MARGARET WEISS AND DERMATOLOGY ASSOCIATES

SCLEROTHERAPY CONSENT AND FEE SCHEDULE

Name ____________________________ Date ____________________

- Sclerotherapy is the method for eliminating superficial telangiectasias ("spider veins") and some varicosities by the injection of a solution, called a "sclerosing agent", into the veins. The vast majority of patients who have sclerotherapy will have significant clearing of the veins with at least good improvement. There can by no guarantee, however, that it will be effective in every case. Less than 10% of patients undergoing sclerotherapy will have poor results, in which the veins do not improve despite multiple injections. It is extremely rare for anyone's condition to worsen because of treatment.

- It is important to realize that sclerotherapy does not prevent development of new spider veins and varicosities over the years. Many people will require treatments from time to time to keep their legs clear. Standing occupations, pregnancy, and estrogen increase this tendency.

- It is difficult to predict the number of treatments needed to clear or improve the condition. Each vein may need to be injected one to five or more times, over a period of several months. Improvement is usually seen over a period of months, not weeks. In each treatment session, multiple areas can be treated, thus reducing the total number of sessions required. The total number of treatment sessions needed depends on the amount and severity of the veins (the average is three to five), with severe cases requiring as many as ten or more.

- Side effects of sclerotherapy are detailed in another handout which you will receive.

- Sclerotherapy is not usually covered by your insurance company, depending on the size of the veins and whether or not they cause symptoms. When the veins are small, the treatment is considered cosmetic and not covered. When the veins are large and "varicose", or cause pain or discomfort, then there is a chance that the sclerotherapy will be covered. Each patient has the responsibility for payment at the time of service, whether or not the treatments are successful, and whether or not the treatments are covered by insurance.

- **All diagnostic testing and treatment must be paid for in full at the time the service is performed.** At your request, we will send a detailed letter, photographs, and vascular test results to your insurance company. Each patient must submit their receipt to his/her insurance company for reimbursement.

FEE SCHEDULE

- Each treatment session lasts 10-15 minutes and will treat multiple areas and will cost $_____.

- Each treatment session requires a "spider vein equipment tray" which cost $________.

- Some patients require prescription support hosiery, for which we charge $_________. This is approximately half the charge made by pharmacies. Other patients require light support hosiery, for which we charge $________.

- Because of long waiting times for appointments, we suggest scheduling several of your treatment sessions, a few weeks apart, at the same time. If your plans change, there is no charge for appointments canceled more than 24 hours in advance.

- **IMPORTANT**: There is a $50 charge for failure to cancel appointments within 24 hours of appointment time.

I understand and agree to these items.

Patient __________________________ Witness ________________________

APPENDIX 4

DRS. ROBERT AND MARGARET WEISS
AND DERMATOLOGY ASSOCIATES

Sclerotherapy Instructions

- Leave cotton balls, tape, and stockings on until bedtime.
- If itching or burning develops, then remove the tape immediately.
- If you have redness or irritation in the areas of the tape, please call the office for a prescription cream.
- When returning for treatment, do not put any lotion or oil on your legs for 2 days <u>before</u> each treatment session.
- Do not shave your legs the morning of your treatment.
- If you prefer, you may bring a pair of shorts to wear during the treatment- some patients feel this is more comfortable.
- After you remove the tape, wear prescription or Delilah/Venosan support hose for two weeks, except to sleep.
- After treatments, there is no restriction on activity, but to try not to bump the areas doing exercises, which can cause bruising. Weight lifting with the legs should be minimized for two weeks. We encourage walking.
- If something occurs (for example, illness or injury) that would interfere with normal walking, please postpone treatment.
- Please call us if you have any questions or problems.

OFFICES:

ASPEN MILL PROFESSIONAL CENTER
54 SCOTT ADAM ROAD, SUITE 301
HUNT VALLEY, MD 21030
(410) 666-3960
FAX (410) 666-3981

PERRY HALL PROFESSIONAL CENTER
9712 BELAIR ROAD, SUITE 200
BALTIMORE, MD 21236
(410) 529-0280
FAX (410) 529-0612

25

Tumescent Liposuction

Rhoda S. Narins

Dermatology Surgery and Laser Center, New York and White Plains, and New York University Medical Center, New York, New York

Since 1982, when it was first introduced in the United States, liposuction has evolved into the most commonly performed cosmetic surgical procedure. There have been marked changes in concept, application, instrumentation, and anesthesia during this time. I was introduced to liposuction by Drs. Yves Gerard Illouz and Dr. Pierre Fournier of France, and Dr. Giorgio Fisher of Rome in the clinic and office of Dr. Illouz in Paris, in 1982. Dr. Illouz made liposuction possible by designing a blunt cannula to go through the tissue easily with minimal bleeding [1,2]. He also used a "wet" technique and injected small amounts of a hypotonic saline solution into the tissue presurgically, which also markedly decreased bleeding. These two innovations made liposuction a safe procedure, allowing aspiration of the adipose bulk while preservating septae in which vessels, lymph channels, and nerves survive. The second important advance in liposuction occurred in 1986 with the development of the tumescent technique of local anesthesia by Dr. Jeffrey A. Klein, a dermatologic surgeon [3,4]. This technique allows the surgeon to perform liposuction in an office setting using local anesthesia alone. The tumescent anesthetic used is a dilute lidocaine/epinephrine solution. Over the last few years, cannulas and consequently incisions have gotten smaller, pumps have been developed to inject the tumescent fluid into the tissue, ultrasound has been used as an adjunct to regular liposuction, and the concept of how to do liposuction, including debulking procedures, the "hour-glass abdomen," and "the weekend alternative to the facelift," have improved the final result.

The demand for and public acceptance of such a technique for the removal of unwanted fat is great. Large accumulations of adipose tissue are considered unsightly among many of the world's peoples. Liposuction is a safe surgical means of changing genetically and hormonally controlled fat contours and has become a procedure of great importance. I have performed thousands of these procedures, and these techniques are reproducible, safe, and provide a great deal of physician and patient satisfaction.

PRESURGICAL CONSIDERATIONS/CONSULTATION

The most important part of any cosmetic procedure is the consultation. Although the best candidate for liposuction is young, slim, in good health and has good skin turgor, the applicability of this technique has steadily expanded to include young and old, male and female patients, and both aesthetic and reconstructive challenges. With a realistic patient, good results can be achieved in many nonobese patients. Liposuction has become appropriate for any individual with an indication for the procedure who can tolerate the pre-, intra-, and postsurgical stresses and risks and who accepts realistic limitations. Liposuction is not a treatment for obesity, and is a contouring —not weight-loss—procedure. In addition, there is not change in superficial skin lesions, such as striae, cellulite, pigmented lesions, spider veins, and so on.

At the consultation, the procedure is discussed with the patient in detail. It is important to know what the patient desires and expects. A physical examination is performed, concentrating on the location of fat as well as skin tightness. Any unusual deformities or unusual prominence of anatomic bony structures are evaluated and discussed with the patient as well. The benefits that can be achieved, along with the limitations and possible complications, are discussed. At the consultation, a photograph is taken and used in discussing the expected results. It can also be used to plan the procedure if the patient schedules at a later date. Medical history, including history of bleeding, medication, allergies, recent weight loss or gain, previous surgery, and illness, is taken at this time. The patient is shown photographs of other patients who have undergone this surgery, and the procedure is discussed in detail and all questions are answered at this time.

If the patient decides to go ahead with the surgery, blood tests are performed, including CBC with differential, Chem Screen 20, PT, PTT, Hepatitis C surface antibody, Hepatitis B surface antigen, and human immunodeficiency virus. Medical problems must be individually evaluated. Any patient taking systemic medication, having any illness, or over 50 years old needs an evaluation with an EKG and note on the chart from his or her family physician before this procedure. Presurgical instructions (see Appendix 1) are gone over and given to the patient at this time. Postsurgical instructions (see Appendix 2) are also gone over and given to the patient at this time. The patient is given a prescription for an antibiotic to be started the day before surgery, and warned to stop taking aspirin, aspirin-containing compounds, high doses of Vitamin E, and nonsteroidal anti-inflammatory drugs starting 2 weeks before surgery.

Most patients are extremely realistic about the results they can achieve. Liposuction gives extremely gratifying but not always perfect results with very little scarring or morbidity, and patients are happy to look better in clothing and have a nicer contour. Of course, there are always those patients that you can make perfect.

PRESURGICAL PROCEDURE: DAY OF SURGERY

When the patient comes in on the morning of surgery the vital signs are taken. Weight is measured so that I can calculate the total amount of lidocaine that is safe to use as well as the presurgical sedation. It also helps in the evaluation of postsurgical results. Consent forms are gone over and signed (see Appendix 3), and a medical history is taken. A physical examination is performed at this time, and the patient is then photographed with a Polaroid and a 35 mm camera. It is important to have photographic documentation so that future results can be compared. We also hang the photographs in the surgical room so that I can refer to them during the surgery. Any questions the patient may have are answered, and then I mark the areas with an indelible pen with the patient watching. This should be performed first with the patient standing, and then in varying positions so the surgeon can see how the fat falls. Possible incision marks are drawn at this time and then shown to the patient. After this, presurgical sedation is given.

SURGICAL PROCEDURE

Liposuction surgery involves the introduction of cannulas of varying lengths, widths, and designs through small incisions in the skin. A series of tunnels radiates out from each incision point and criss-crosses from various incision points and at different depths to give a nice, smooth result.

Anesthesia

IM and PO Sedation

For presurgical medication I use 0.1 mg catapres if the patient's blood pressure is over 120/80. I give 10 mg diazepam po as well as small amounts of mepridine, midazolam, and promethazine IM. No intravenous or intubation anesthesia is used at any time, and patients are awake during the procedure. The amount of sedation used depends on the patient requirements and takes into account the weight as well as the age and body type of the patient.

Tumescent Anesthesia

Since Klein first described the use of tumescent anesthesia, it has been used effectively and perfected by many other dermatologic surgeons in tens of thousands of cases [3–10]. The great benefits of this technique include markedly decreased bleeding, no risk from general anesthesia, patients feeling better after surgery, and being able to go back to work and exercise almost immediately. Patients can walk into and out of the surgical room, and can get into the exact position they need to have the fat removed. In addition, there is no need for transfusions or fluid replacement, and the anesthetic solution lasts for a long time, making this surgery basically pain free. The anesthetic solution is prewarmed to make the patient more comfortable.

Equipment

The equipment required for tumescent anesthesia includes the bags of tumescent anesthetic solution, a #11 blade to make the incisions, spinal needles and infiltrators to inject the solution, and syringes with 30-gauge needles to inject the incision sites. A pressure cuff or a Klein electric pump is used to push in the solution. In addition, tubing is needed to attach the bags of solution to the infiltrators.

Anesthetic Solution

The anesthetic solutions are made up using various percentages of lidocaine. I use 0.05% and 0.1% (Tables 1, 2) but many surgeons use a 0.075% solution as well. Solutions for smaller areas are made up in smaller bags (Table 3). Normal saline is the diluent with lidocaine used to provide anesthesia. The epinephrine is used to decrease the absorption of the anesthetic as well as to decrease the bleeding, and the bicarbonate buffers the solution and minimizes pain. Bicarbonate may also prevent infection. Triamcinolone acetonide, which may decrease the postsurgical operative

TABLE 1 Tumescent Anesthetic Solution (0.05%)*

	Solution	Concentration
1000	Normal Saline	0.9%
50	Lidocaine	1%
1	Epinephrine	1/1000
12.5	Bicarbonate	8.4%
1	Triamcinolone acetonide	10 mg/ml (optional)
Totals:	500 mg Lidocaine = .05%	
	1/1 million epinephrine	

*0.05% = 500 mg total Lidocaine.

swelling, is optional. The total amount of fluid used depends on the patient's size and age and the total amount of lidocaine used depends on the patient's weight, body type, and age. The safe dose of lidocaine has been reported as 55 mg/kg, but in heavy patients it may go up to 60 mg/kg and in thinner patients down to 45 to 50 mg/kg because lidocaine's reservoir is in the fatty tissue and thin patients do not have as much of this third space available [11,12].

If it is necessary to maximize the amount of tumescent solution because of the number of areas being treated, more of the 0.05% solution is used and less of the 0.1%. If I am doing a small area, then I use only the 0.1% solution. It is also necessary to take into account the total amount of fluid used. Because the total amount of lidocaine is predicated on the patient's weight, this gives us a natural safe limit for the number of areas that can be treated at one time. Patients should be treated in serial sessions if more anesthetic is needed than is safe. This natural limit accounts for the extreme safety of this procedure. It is easy to calculate the safe amount of anesthetic fluid that can be used [Table 4, Eq. (1)].

$$\frac{\text{Patient weight (lbs)}}{2.2} = \text{weight (kg)}$$

$$\text{Weight in Kg} \times 55 \text{ mg of Lidocaine/kg} = \text{number of mg of Lidocaine}$$

$$\frac{150 \text{ lbs}}{2.2} = 68 \text{ kg}$$

$$68 \text{ kg} \times 55 \text{ mg Lidocaine/kg} = 3740 \text{ mg Lidocaine}$$

TABLE 2 Tumescent Anesthetic Solution (0.1%)*

	Solution	Concentration
1000	Normal Saline	0.9%
50	Lidocaine	2%
1	Epinephrine	1/1000
12.5	Bicarbonate	8.4%
1	Triamcinolone acetonide	10 mg/ml (optional)
Totals:	1000 mg Lidocaine = 0.1%	
	1/1 million epinephrine	

*0.1% = 1000 mg total Lidocaine.

TABLE 3 Tumescent Solution for Smaller Areas

	Solution	Concentration
250	Normal Saline	0.9%
25	Lidocaine	1%
1/4	Epinephrine	1/1000
4	Bicarbonate	8.4%
Totals:	250 mg Lidocaine = 0.1% 1/1 million epinephrine	

Delivery of the Anesthetic Solution

I like to deliver the anesthetic solution in three stages. The incision areas are injected with the tumescent anesthetic solution with a syringe and a 30-gauge needle. Then a spinal needle is used radially through these incision sites with the Klein infiltration pump on very low, less than 2, to deliver anesthesia slowly which causes less pain [8]. Only after this preliminary anesthesia has been performed do you make the tiny incision with a #11 blade and then inject the tumescent solution at higher speeds, 4 to 7, through the infiltrators. The slower the infiltration, the more painless the infiltration [13]. It is important to inject the tumescent solution at all levels especially deeply through tunnels radiating from the incision sites. Raising a peau d'orange in the skin changes landmarks and should be avoided.

Equipment

I have an AAAHC-accredited facility, and procedures are performed using strictly sterile technique [14,15]. A pulse oximeter is used, as well as blood pressure, EKG, and pulse monitors during the procedure. I generally have a scrub nurse as well as a circulating nurse in attendance.

TABLE 4 Options for 1000 ml Bags of Tumescent Anesthetic Solution Based on 3500 mg Lidocaine Total

Number of bags	Concentration of Lidocaine		Total Lidocaine
$3\frac{1}{2}$	0.1%	=	3500 mg Lidocaine
3	0.1%	=	3500 mg Lidocaine
1	0.05%		
2	0.1%	=	3500 mg Lidocaine
3	0.05%		
1	0.1%	=	3500 mg Lidocaine
5	0.05%		
7	0.05%	=	3500 mg Lidocaine

Cannulas

Each surgeon has his or her favorite cannulas, which come in many sizes and shapes. Some are more aggressive than others and should be used only as surgeons become more experienced. I generally use between 8 and 15 cannulas per procedure [16]. My favorite cannulas are the Klein 10, 12, 14, 16, and 18 (needle sizes), as well as the Cook, Pinto, lamprey, and cobra in various lengths and sizes (generally sizes 2, 3, or 4 mm). I also use the Klein Capistrano cannula. Many of these cannulas can be seen at hands-on meetings, and you can pick your favorite. When I first started performing liposuction, I used Illouz blunt-tipped cannulas up to 10 mm in width, which now seem enormous [1]. When this cannula was used at deep levels, great results could be seen. With the smaller cannulas one can get more superficial and perform liposculpture as well (Fig. 1).

Aspiration Pump and Tubing

There are many manufacturers of aspiration pumps with a negative air pressure approaching 30″ (atmosphere of negative pressure) (Fig. 2). I have several of these pumps. The tubing, the bags and the viral filters are disposable and comply with OSHA regulations (Fig. 3).

Ultrasonic Machine

I have an ultrasonic machine that I use for larger, more fibrous areas and in patients who have had liposuction previously performed [17–20]. This is used as an adjunct to regular liposuction.

Monitors

As previously mentioned, a pulse oximeter is necessary to measure oxygen saturation in the bloodstream because toxicity to lidocaine is related to decreased oxygen.

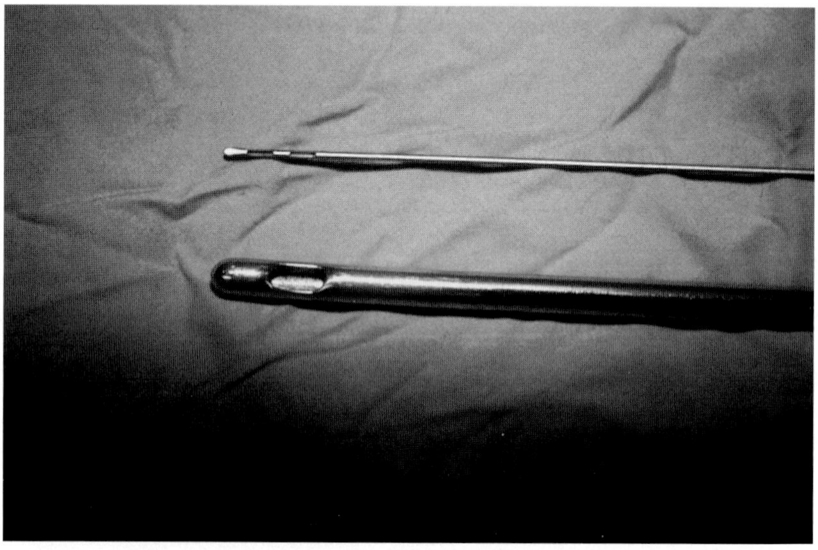

FIGURE 1 Old and new cannulas.

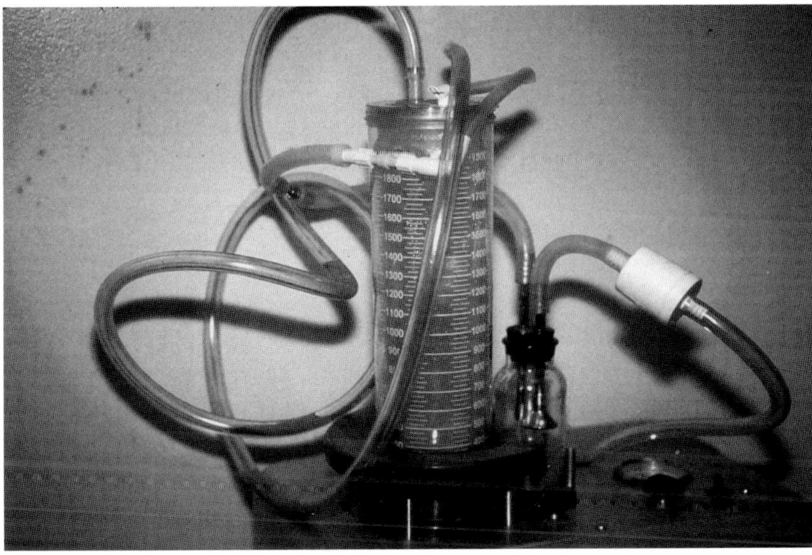

FIGURE 2 Aspiration with disposable bags and tubing.

Patients are awake and are told to take a deep breath if oxygen saturation diminishes. In addition, I use other monitors for the EKG, pulse, and blood pressure.

Back-up Equipment

If there is a problem with the equipment, the following options are available to the physician:

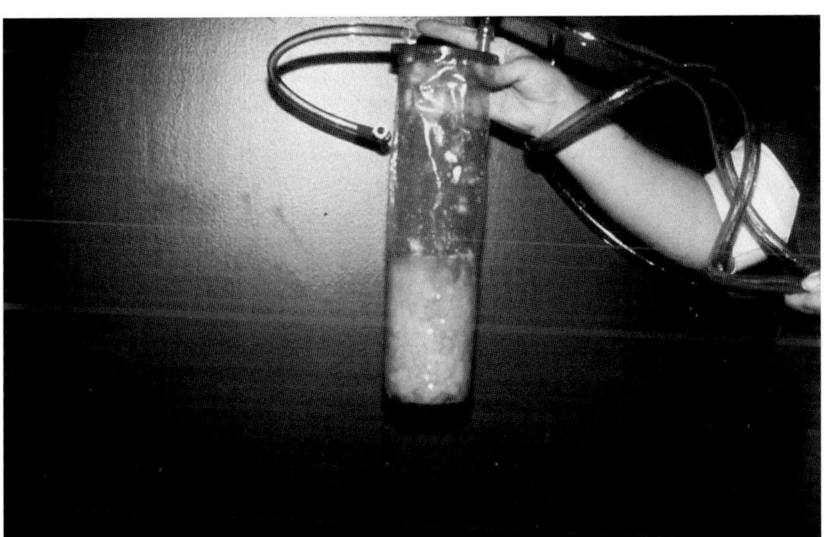

FIGURE 3 Disposable bags with fat asperate.

1. The patient can be sent home and the procedure performed safely on another day.
2. Back-up machines can be used.
3. If no back-up machine is available, the syringe technique works very well for taking out even large quantities of fat [21].

SURGICAL PROCEDURE

Presurgical Procedure

Have the patient go to the bathroom before the procedure; otherwise, because of the amount of fluid injected, the patient may have to go during the procedure. The patient is then washed with a bactericidal cleanser such as Betadine or Hibiclens. They are then placed on the surgery room table and draped with sterile sheets. The tumescent anesthetic is then injected, and I wait 15 to 30 minutes for the anesthetic to work and insure minimal bleeding and maximum anesthesia.

Technique

Internal Ultrasonic Liposuction

I use the internal ultrasonic machine for the first 30 seconds to 2 minutes in very fibrous or large areas. I use a Lysonix machine with a #4 or #5 mm cannula. It is necessary to use tumescent anesthesia in order to get results from ultrasonic liposuction, and so many of the benefits originally ascribed to ultrasonic liposuction are actually attributable to the use of tumescent anesthesia. These benefits include minimal bleeding, lack of pain after surgery, and rapid recovery after surgery. Surgeons who use general anesthesia—intubation or intravenous—and ultrasonic liposuction must use tumescent local anesthesia as well. Again, whether you are using general anesthesia with tumescent anesthesia or tumescent anesthesia alone there is a safety limit to the amount of fluid and lidocaine that can be used and this should be strictly adhered to [12,22].

Regular Liposuction

Whether or not ultrasonic liposuction is used, regular liposuction is always performed to refine the areas and to criss-cross through various incisions by using the hand that does not hold the cannula as a guide to tell you what depth the cannula is at. Fine gridwork that results from tunnels at different levels gives a nice, smooth result. The cannula moves with a steady piston-like motion to accomplish liposculpturing. Cannulas are never turned with the opening upward except in very difficult areas, such as male breasts just under the nipples and the neck area. In other areas, we try to preserve the neurovascular septae and thus diminish the risks of seroma, hematoma, infection, and postsurgical deformity. Several cannulas should be used in each area. A Toledo underminer can be used to lift scars.

Beginners should limit the amount of aspirate removed to under 2,000 ml. However, using larger amounts of anesthetic fluid, many surgeons routinely remove between 2,000 to 4,000 ml with 2,500 ml being the average removed at any one time. I do not suture the incisions after surgery. Much of the fluid drains out during the procedure and continues to drain easily after surgery as well. Incision marks slowly fade over time. If the surgeon is gong to suture the incision sites, this should not be performed until after surgery so that the drainage that occurs intrasurgically is allowed to occur.

Larger cannulas are generally used more deeply and smaller cannulas more superficially. Liposuction is a debulking procedure with immediate results, but the subsequent formation of fibrous tissue that retracts the skin enables the final result to be even better.

LIPOSUCTION AREA BY AREA

Neck, Jowls, and Face

Different options are offered to the patient who comes in for liposuction of the neck and jowls. The first is liposuction alone which is best for those people with tight to mildly loose skin and fat in the upper neck and jowl area [23]. The second is liposuction similar to the first option with an added excision of a little skin in the submental crease. This is good for those patients with some loose skin. The third option is The Weekend Alternative to a Face Lift, which includes some or all of the steps listed in Table 5 [24]. The fourth option is a necklift.

Liposuction of the Neck and Jowls

Liposuction of the neck and jowls is a relatively easy procedure. I use three incisions, one in the center of the submental crease and one under each ear. I use relatively small cannulas which I criss-cross over the area, removing the fat evenly and aggressively and allowing the neck to redrape. Patients can take 10 years off their appearance by having this procedure performed because it makes a tremendous difference in how they look. This is a great procedure to perform on an obese person because it is a limited procedure without removal of a great deal of fat and makes you look slimmer. For the person who just has a submental accumulation of fat without a good angle between the head and neck as well as the person who has a tremendous double chin that involves most of the neck from ear to ear liposuction of the neck works beautifully. A sharp jawline gives a very youthful appearance (Figs. 4, 5). The neck is one area where I use the cannula hole–side up to really defat the skin as much as possible. The area is taped for 2 to 3 days postsurgically, and generally there is no postsurgical bruising.

TABLE 5 Weekend Alternative to the Face Lift™

Liposuction of the neck and jowls and lower part of the face
Excision of a small piece of skin in the submental crease
Undermining of the neck
Defatting of the neck
Chin implant
Repair of platysma bands
CO_2 laser inside the skin
Suturing of the excision
Postsurgical wrapping

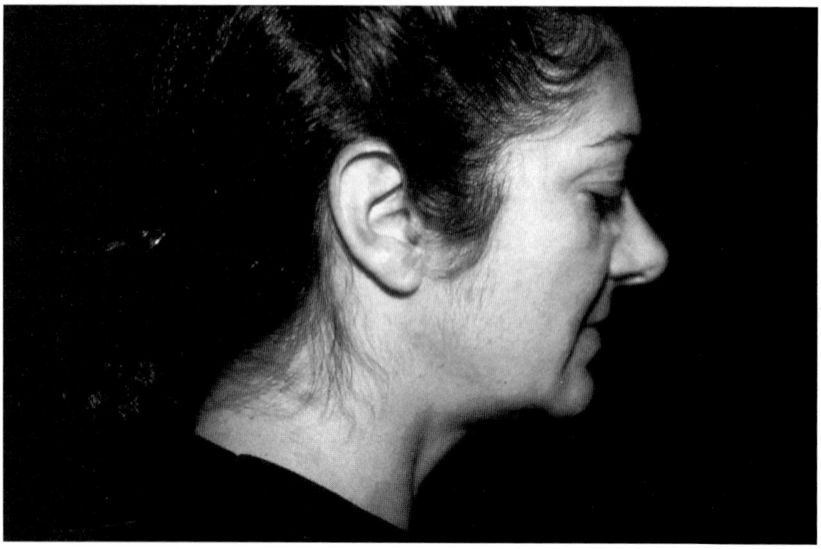

FIGURE 4 Presurgical liposuction neck.

Caveats

Liposuction will not take care of platysmal bands and patients should be warned that these may become visible. In addition, some patients' skin does not retract as well as others. Occasionally one can have vertical folds in the neck postsurgically which are temporary and can be helped by the use of external ultrasound. One can get some temporary trauma to the cervical mandibular branch of the facial nerve but

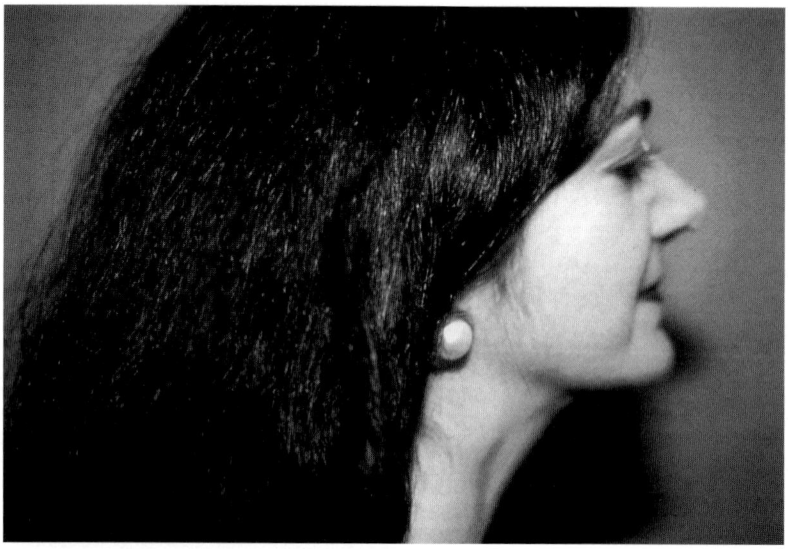

FIGURE 5 Postsurgical liposuction neck.

there has never been a report of permanent damage. I have seen a partial paralysis last for 2 months with complete recovery. It is usual for the area to get hard post-surgically, and again, this is temporary and if severe can be melted away with very dilute 1 to 2 mg/ml triamcinolone acetonide injections intralesionally. In the area of the face, liposuction should be performed with no bigger than a size 16-gauge cannula.

Liposuction of the Neck and Jowls Plus Excision

Liposuction of the neck with a small excision of skin is performed exactly the same as liposuction of the neck and jowls; however, after the liposuction, which effectively undermines the skin bloodlessly, a small excision of skin is performed in the sub-mental crease. It is important to make sure the excision does not extend over the line of the mandible and this should have been premarked presurgically. This procedure gives a nice result with very low morbidity, especially for those patients who do not want a necklift.

Liposuction of the Face

Liposuction of the face is routinely used as an adjunct to rhytidectomy and in fact has made the procedure much easier to perform. Liposuction of the face should be performed very carefully by an experienced surgeon with very small cannulas (i.e., 16- and 18-gauge Klein).

Weekend Alternative to the Face Lift

There are variations and modifications of this procedure (see Chapter 5) that I use that may include liposuction, ultrasonic liposuction, platysma repair, chin implant, excision of skin in the submental crease, and laser under the skin (Figs. 6, 7).

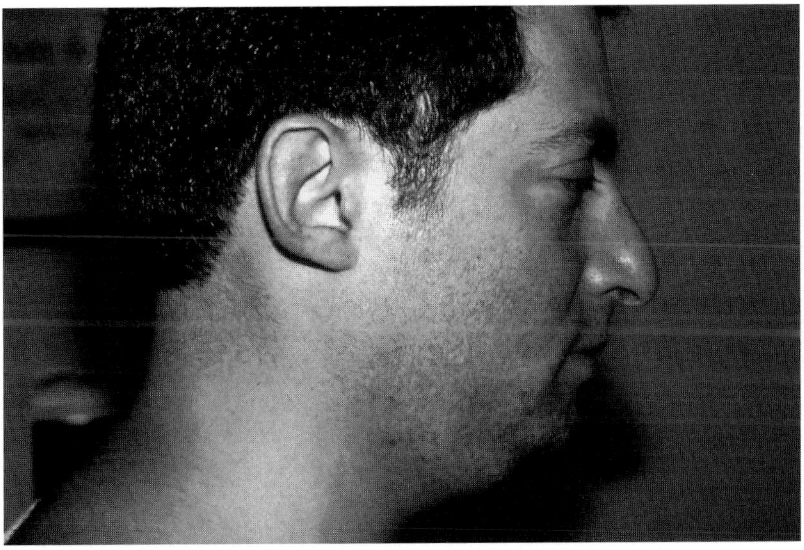

FIGURE 6 Presurgical liposuction, excision of skin, and laser neck.

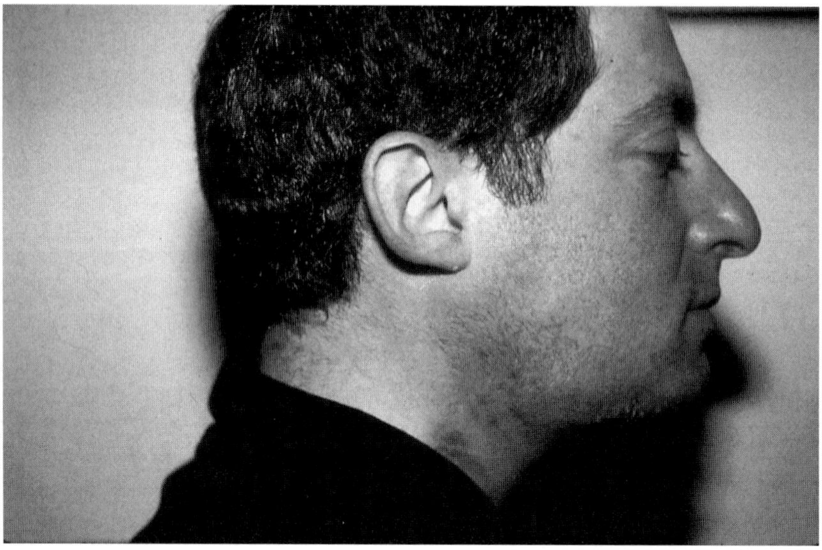

FIGURE 7 Postsurgical liposuction, excision of skin, and laser neck.

Liposuction of the Arms

Many women accumulate fat in the upper arms as a result of hereditary predisposition and obesity. It is important to perform the liposuction before the skin gets so loose that liposuction results in unsightly hanging skin necessitating an excision. In the usual patient, excellent results can be achieved using 1 to 3 incisions above the elbow (Fig. 8). Postsurgical wrapping is easily performed with support stockings or with special garments that are available and need only be used for 3 or 4 days.

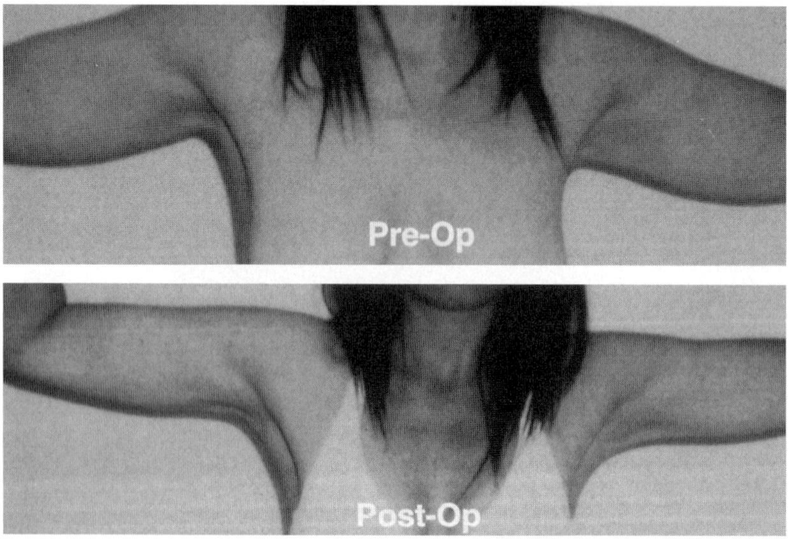

FIGURE 8 Pre- and postsurgical liposuction of the arms.

Bra Fat

Many women are bothered by unsightly accumulations of fat that hang over the bra either in front or back. These can be very easily removed through tiny incisions with cannulas size 12- or 14-gauge. Sometimes a Klein Capistrano cannula must be used because the area is very fibrous.

Pseudogynecomastia and Gynecomastia

Many boys as well as older men are bothered by pseudogynecomastia which makes them feel uncomfortable in public. Tumescent liposuction is a wonderful technique to remove this unsightly and upsetting fat accumulation. It gives tremendous improvement without scarring and without loss of time from school or work. Patients wear a bind for 1 to 4 days, and with a shirt on can appear perfectly normal even the day after surgery (Fig. 9).

For the surgeon, however, this is a very difficult area because of the amount of fibrous and glandular tissue that may be present under the nipples. Generally, liposuction in men is more difficult because they tend to be more fibrous. Incisions in the axilla are not visible and if you make small incisions elsewhere you can crisscross over the area. This is another area where the cannula can be turned upside down so that as much breast tissue as possible can be rasped out. This rasping is only performed in the areola and nipple areas. Tissue should always be sent for a biopsy. This is an area where very aggressive cannulas have to be used and where you want to remove as much fat as possible. Actually there are times when you have to go in through the axillary incision with a hemostat and pull some of the very fibrous tissue out from under the nipple. It is important to bind the area afterward and not suture the incisions.

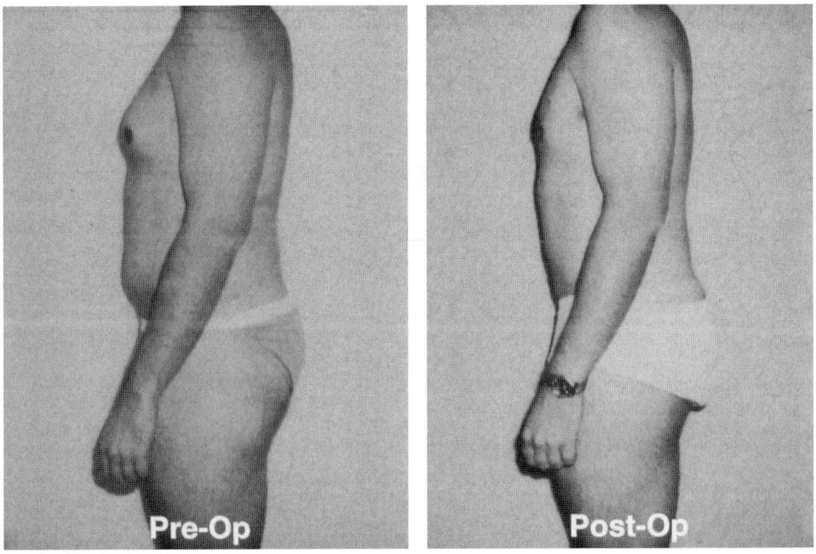

FIGURE 9 Pre- and postsurgical liposuction of pseudogynecomastia and gynecomastia.

Buffalo Hump

A "dowager's deformity," or buffalo hump, lends itself easily to liposuction surgery. Two tiny incisions allow the operator to criss-cross the area and easily remove this very soft fat which does not recur [25].

Flanks

Flanks are the most common area for men to lay down fat as they get older along with the abdomen. This is an area that does not always improve with weight loss and can be a problem even in men who are very slim. It responds very well to liposuction surgery. Retraction occurs in this area with significant contour results. Fat deposits almost always extend around to the back and the entire area should be addressed at the same time (Fig. 10).

Abdomen

It is necessary to evaluate the entire abdominal area before deciding on the best procedure to be performed. In general most people fall into four different groups:

1. The person in whom only the lower abdomen is a problem. This area responds very well to liposuction and the skin pulls back very well. This deformity is most common in younger people (Fig. 11).

2. The person in whom the upper and lower abdomen needs to be treated. Although the upper abdomen never pulls back as well as the lower abdomen where even an apron can disappear, liposuction in this area can also provide excellent results with a procedure of very low morbidity.

3. The person that needs an Hour-Glass Abdomen™ [26]. The Hour-Glass Abdomen™ addresses the problem of the upper and lower abdomen along with the waist, back, and hips (Figs. 12–14). In the older patient or the person who may have

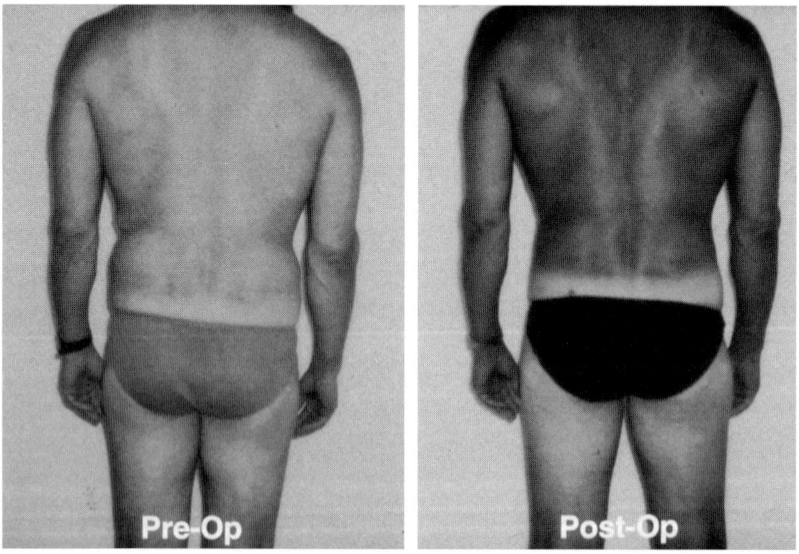

FIGURE 10 Pre- and postsurgical liposuction of "love handles" (flanks).

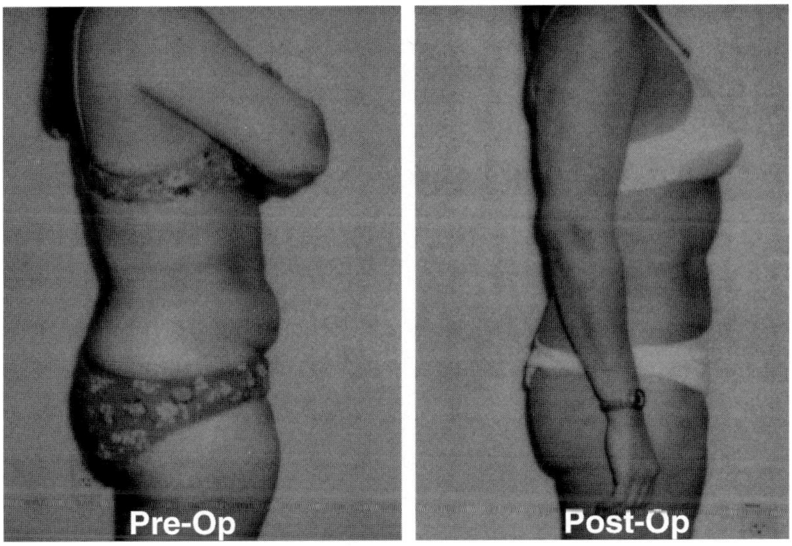

FIGURE 11 **Pre- and postsurgical liposuction of lower abdomen.**

a very square shape, this gives a more pleasing result than just treating the abdomen alone. If a large abdomen is removed and the patient does not lose weight, other areas such as large breasts, which already have a lot of fat, can become even larger as the fat in these cells increases. By the same token, people who do not have large breasts but have a lot of fat distributed on their waist and hip areas may actually increase their waist size and thus increase the size of clothing they need even though they now have a flat abdomen. This Hour-Glass procedure is especially needed in

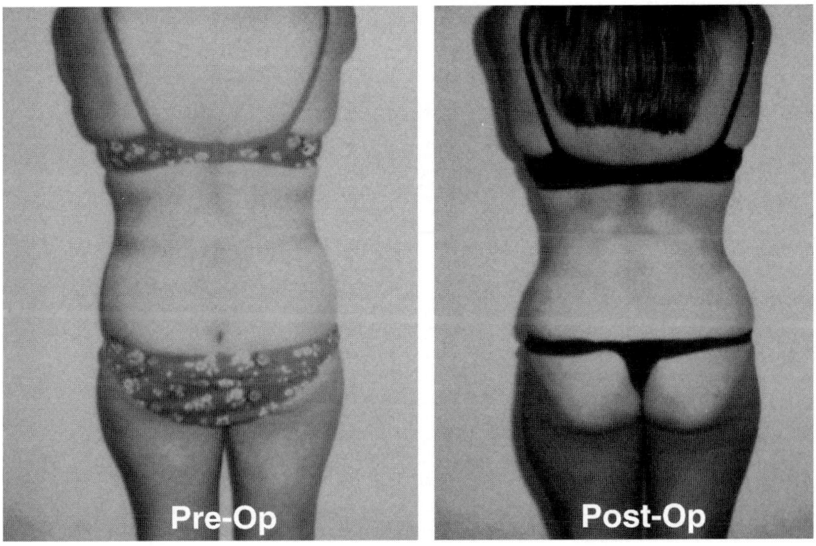

FIGURE 12 **Pre- and postsurgical liposuction Hour-Glass Abdomen™.**

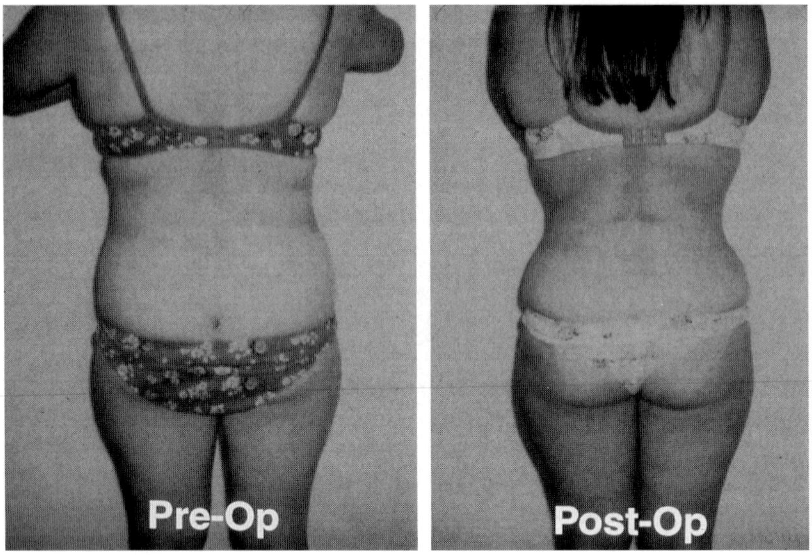

FIGURE 13 Pre- and postsurgical liposuction Hour-Glass Abdomen™.

women who may be on hormone replacement therapy or have gone through menopause. Some patients have this on a hereditary basis even from a young age. This procedure often works very well in men because men also lay fat down on the abdomen and flanks around to the bank as they get older.

4. The person who has fat behind the muscle. This is especially true in the upper abdomen of men with "beer bellies" and in some women with loose muscle

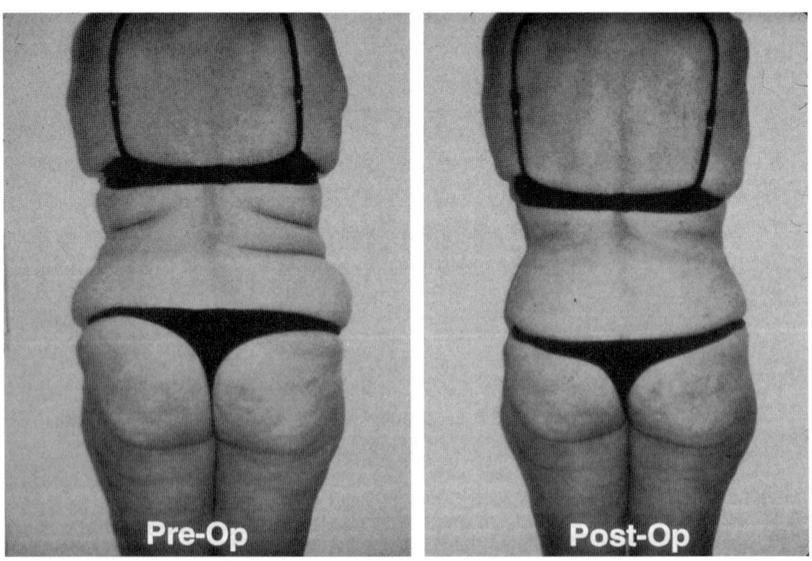

FIGURE 14 Pre- and postsurgical liposuction Hour-Glass Abdomen™.

after childbirth. Liposuction is not a procedure that will work for these people. Instead they should be evaluated for an open lipectomy with a rectus repair.

5. The patient who needs liposuction plus excision of skin. Women with some fat on the abdomen but a lot of loose skin generally after childbirth and men and women who have lost a lot of weight and have very loose skin fall into this category. These people generally have multiple striae and broken elastic tissue. The treatment of choice is liposuction plus excision of some of the loose skin in the suprapubic area. The muscle does not need to be repaired.

Caveats

The abdomen is an area where I often use ultrasonic liposuction as an adjunct to regular liposuction. It is very important for one to address the ring of fat immediately around the umbilicus where patients are most sensitive.

A hernia must be ruled out presurgically although with awake patients using the tumescent technique it would not be possible to go near or through the muscle because patients would let you know immediately that they feel pain. Both men and women sometimes have deposits in the mons pubis and this area should be treated at the same time as the abdomen. Incisions must be made and left open for drainage so that ecchymosis does not occur in either the scrotal area or labia.

Violin Deformity

This area includes the lateral thighs' "saddle bags," buttocks, and hips. Violin deformities are very common in women and can be seen at a very young age. These are hereditary deposits of fat and are very difficult to diet away completely without becoming anorexic. The entire area when present should be addressed at the same time. Eliminating this deformity can really change people's lives (Figs. 15, 16). Postsurgically they feel better about themselves and love wearing pants, skirts, and

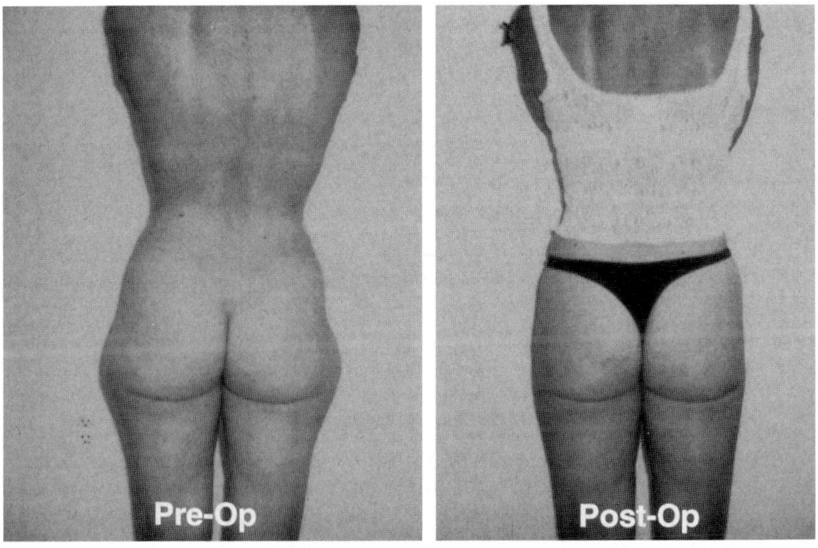

FIGURE 15 Pre- and postsurgical liposuction violin deformity.

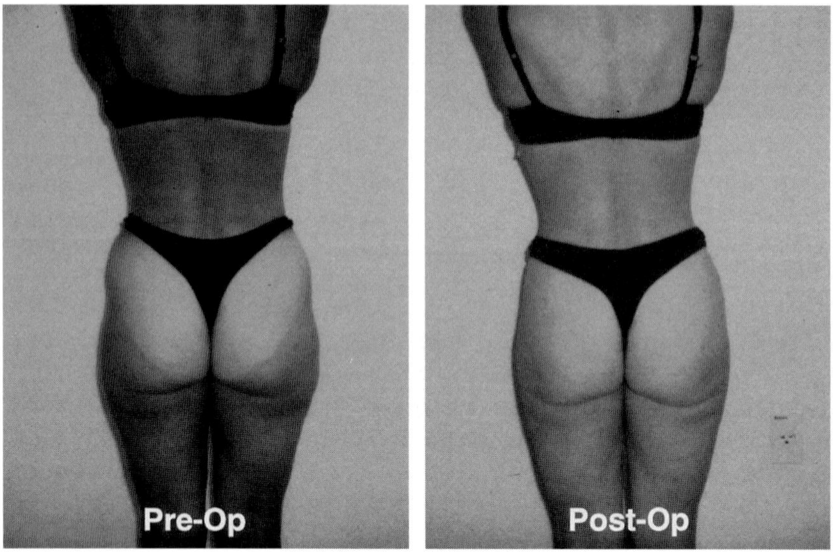

FIGURE 16 Pre- and postsurgical liposuction violin deformity.

bathing suits that they never allowed themselves to wear before in public. Women often have cellulite in this area and these little dimples are generally lessened by liposuction but cannot be eliminated. Make sure not to accentuate the trochanteric depression which most people have between the hip and outer thigh [27]. Some surgeons fill these depressions with injections of fat. Rare patients just need the buttock made smaller (Figs. 17, 18).

Caveat

This is an area where some fat should be left on the undersurface of the skin for a nice, smooth result.

Banana Roll

The banana roll, which occurs under the buttock, is caused by a protrusion of fat from the disintegration of the fascia in the upper posterior thigh and can be made smaller but may not be removed completely. This is support for the buttock and too much should not be done in this area because the buttock may fall and/or the banana roll can be accentuated if more of the fascia is destroyed, allowing deep fat to bulge out.

Inner Thighs

Inner thighs are easily treated with 80% of the procedure performed from incisions made in the posterior aspect and 20% from the anterior aspect. It should be explained to the patient that the surgery in this area is limited because we do not want to leave loose skin and/or empty the area completely. Sometimes what a patient is really looking for is a thighlift and it should be shown to a patient what can be achieved in this area by both a thighlift and just by liposuction alone so that they can make

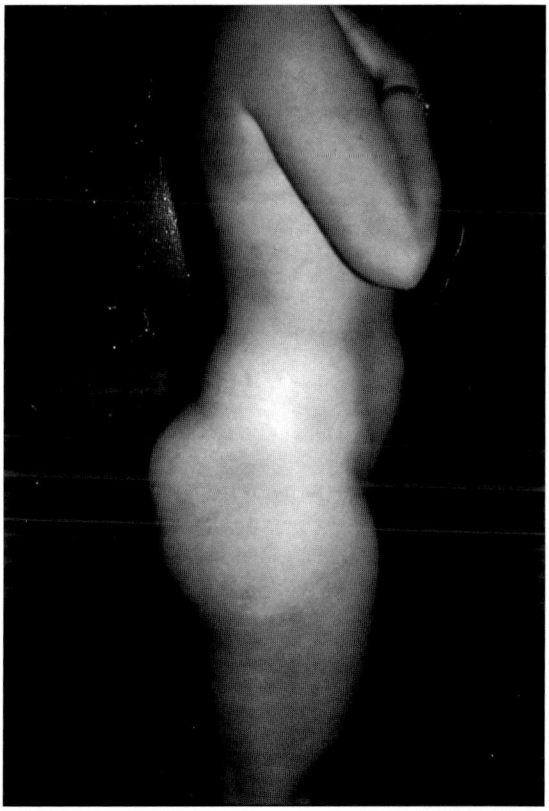

FIGURE 17 Presurgical liposuction buttock.

the proper decision. Liposuction of the inner thigh is a procedure with very low morbidity compared with an inner thighlift.

Circumferential Thigh Reduction and Knees

There are patients who are thin all over but have huge thighs all around. They have fat not only on the inner thigh, the outer thigh, and the knee, but the anterior and sometimes the posterior thigh as well. These areas are addressed very well by liposuction, but generally, this is the only area that can be treated at that time (Fig. 19). Entire thighs take a lot of local anesthesia and you will reach the limit of local anesthesia or come close to it [28]. The amount of improvement that can be expected should be adequately explained to the patient. Although I will address the knee as well at this time, including the upper medial calf, I will not treat the rest of the calf. The medial aspect of the knee and the medial aspect of the upper calf are easy areas in which to perform liposuction and debulk. It is more difficult to treat the area directly over the knee without treating the entire anterior thigh because one must be careful not to leave a shelf. Often what the patient wants is a lift of the skin, and this procedure will debulk the area but not lift the skin. Some patients actually need the lateral knee and suprapatella areas treated as well, and each of these little areas

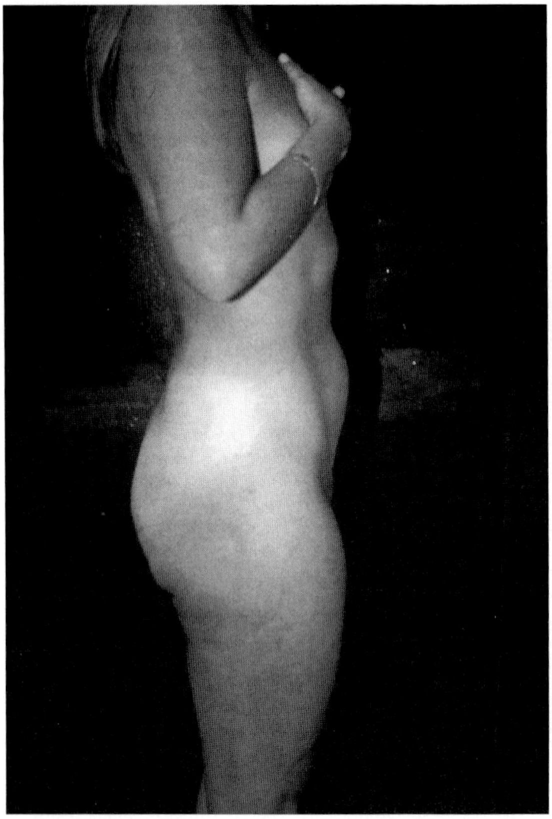

FIGURE 18 Postsurgical liposuction buttock.

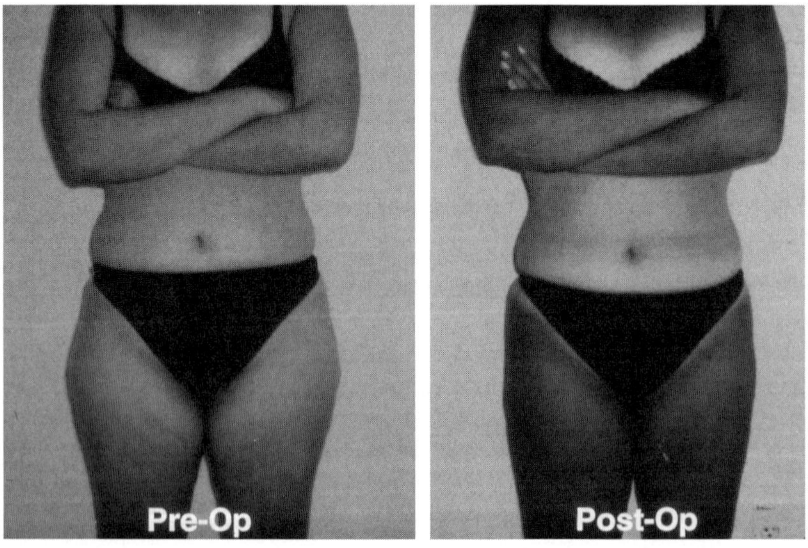

FIGURE 19 Pre- and postsurgical debulking thighs.

can be addressed and will give good results but will not give the excellent results that routinely are seen on a medial aspect of the knee.

Calves and Ankles

With the advent of smaller cannulas, liposuction surgery for the calves and ankles have become much easier. It is important to make sure that the patients actually have fat in this area and this is easily performed by having them stand on their toes. If it is just muscle it is easily palpated. The tiny cannulas and multiple tiny incisions enable the surgeon to carefully sculpt fat from these areas.

Lipomas

The removal of even massive lipomas in the subcutaneous tissue can be accomplished with very small incisions (Figs. 20, 21). However, the fibrous stroma in these benign tumors is very difficult to remove with liposuction alone, and often excision through the tiny liposuction hole is necessary with the fibrous tissue pulled out with hemostats. Tell the patient there is a 5% rate of recurrence and make sure before surgery that the lipoma does not project under and between the muscle.

Collection of Fat

Fat can be saved during liposuction with the use of collectors attached to the tubing during the procedure. This fat can be used at the same time for fat transplantation into the face or other areas and some can be frozen for use at a later date.

POSTSURGICAL PROCEDURE

After surgery our patient is moved to the postsurgical area where they are watched for a period of time. They are given something to eat at this time and told when to

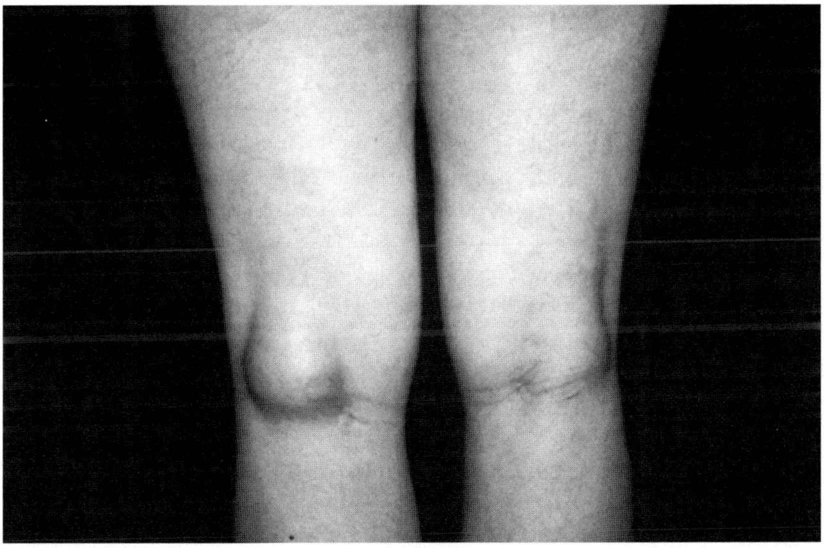

FIGURE 20 Presurgical liposuction of lipoma.

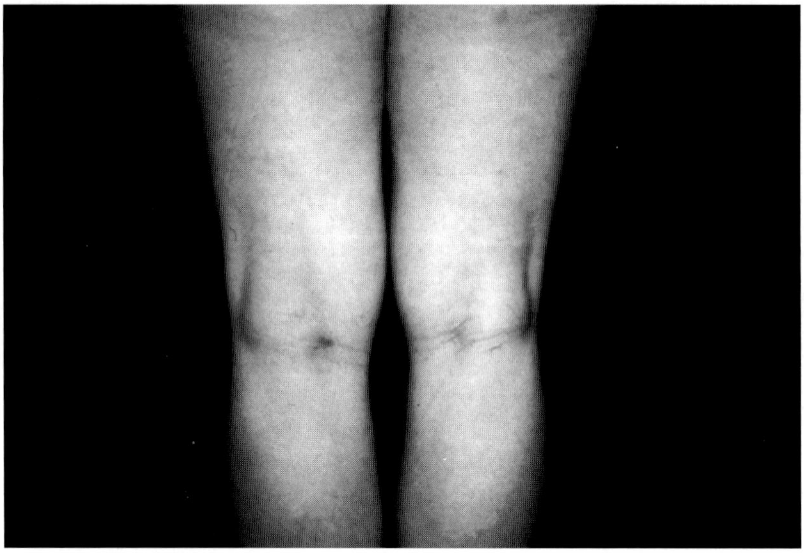

FIGURE 21 Postsurgical liposuction of lipoma.

remove the compression bandages that are placed on areas such as the neck, abdomen, and outer thighs. A new sheet of postsurgical directions (see Appendix 2) is given and gone over with the patient and the person who comes to pick them up. They are told how to care for the garment they have on and when to switch into support hose, bathing suits, onesies, etc. A follow-up appointment is made for them in 1 to 5 days depending on the surgery that was performed and their schedule.

I routinely give patients 2 ml of intramuscular celestone immediately after surgery and continue the prophylactic antibiotics until 1 or 2 days after any drainage stops.

Postsurgical Care

Patients continue wearing the pressure garment for 2 to 4 weeks depending on the looseness of their skin and the amount of fat removed. I think that postsurgical use of compression tape as well as compression garment makes patients feel better because the skin is stabilized and does not move, and I also think it prevents the formation of hematomas and seromas. Most people return to work in 1 to 3 days and can start exercise that is nonjarring and noncontact the day after surgery if desired.

Follow-up Care

If there are no problems, as is usually the case, patients are seen in 2 days, 1 week, 1 month, 3 months, and 6 months after surgery if their schedules allow it. At the third-, and sixth-month visits, photographs are taken and weight is measured so that the physician and patient can follow compliance and improvement. It is always amazing that patients who have lived with deformities for most of their lives cannot remember them 1 month later.

Complications

Tumescent liposuction is an extremely safe procedure with very rare complications [22,29–31]. Patients rarely get ecchymotic, and usual complaints consist of mild soreness, occasional dysesthesias, and slight ecchymosis, which may last 2 to 3 weeks. There have been reports of seromas especially with ultrasonic liposuction as well as burns, but infection, hematoma, seroma, fat embolism, and death are remarkably uncommon. Occasionally expected sequelae occur, such as skin waviness in people without very tight skin, etc. Small remaining deposits of adipose tissue can easily be removed in a touch-up procedure, which is more common on the larger person with larger fat deposits where refinement may be needed after surgery. This touch-up can be performed by machine if other areas are being treated or by hand. Occasionally the patient may have to stand up for these procedures so that the fat becomes more available for surgery. In the several thousand cases that I have treated, I have seen one seroma after removal of a large lipoma the size of a large grapefruit and one tiny seroma after performing ultrasonic liposuction. I have not seen any cases of hematoma, but I have seen a case of infection around an incision that responded to antibiotics by mouth.

When patients gain weight after surgery, they generally gain it all over their bodies and no longer just in the focally unsightly areas where surgery was necessary. If patients gain enough weight after surgery, they may be dissatisfied with the procedure. Additionally, there are those patients who have an excellent result where the procedure has not given them whatever it is they want. It is important to try to weed these patients out in the consultation. Most dire complications that are seen have been in hospitalized patients and those patients who have undergone other procedures or who have had general anesthesia of some type. The end results of tumescent liposuction are generally excellent with high patient and physician satisfaction.

SUMMARY

Liposuction is a safe, reproducible procedure that can remove unwanted fat deposits and change body contour. It does not treat obesity. Patients and surgeons are very happy with results.

REFERENCES

1. Illouz Y. Body contouring by lipolysis. A 5-year experience with over 3,000 cases. Plast Reconstr Surg 1983; 72:591.
2. Fournier P. Otteni F. Lipodissection in body sculpting: the dry procedure. Plast Reconstr Surg 1983; 72:598.
3. Klein JA. The tumescent technique for liposuction surgery. Am J Cosm Surg 1987; 4: 263.
4. Klein JA. Anesthesia for liposuction. J Dermatol Surg Oncol 1988; 14:1127.
5. Lillis PJ. Liposuction surgery under local anesthesia: limited blood loss and minimal lidocaine absorption. J Dermatol Surg Oncol 1988; 14:1145–1148.
6. Narins RS. Liposuction and anesthesia. Dermatol Clin 1990; 8:421.
7. Klein JA. Anesthesia for liposuction in dermatologic surgery. J Dermatol Surg Oncol 1988; 14:1124.
8. Narins RS, Coleman WP III. Minimizing pain for liposuction anesthesia. Dermatol Surg 1997; 23.

9. Klein JA. Tumescent liposuction: totally by local anesthesia. In: Principles and Practice of Dermatological Surgery. GP Lask, RL Moy, eds. New York: McGraw-Hill, 1993.
10. Klein JA. The tumescent technique: anesthesia and modified liposuction technique. Dermatol Clin 1990; 8:425.
11. Klein JA. Tumescent technique for regional anesthesia permits lidocaine doses of 35 mg/kg for liposuction: peak plasma concentrations are diminished and delayed 12 hours. J Dermatol Surg Oncol 1990; 16:248–263.
12. Ostad A, Kageyama N, Moy RL. Tumescent anesthesia with 55 mg/kg of lidocaine dose is safe for liposuction. Derm Surg 1996; 22:921.
13. Hanke CW, Coleman WP III, Lillis PJ, Narins RS, Michalak JA, et al. Infusion rates and levels of premedication in tumescent liposuction. Dermatol Surg 1997; 23:1131–1134.
14. Drake LA, et al. Guidelines of care for liposuction for American Academy of Dermatology. J Am Acad Dermatol 1991; 24:489–494.
15. The American Society for Dermatologic Surgery. Guiding principles for liposuction. Dermatol Surg 1997; 23:1127–1129.
16. Field L, Narins RS. Liposuction surgery. In: Skin Surgery, 6th ed. Epstein E, Epstein E, Jr, eds. Philadelphia: W.B. Saunders, 1987, pp. 370–378.
17. Coleman WP III, Brody H, Goldman M, Hanke CW, Lillis PJ, Moy RL, Narins RS. Statement on Ultrasonic Liposuction. Dermatol Surg 1998; 24:1035.
18. Zocchi M. Clinical aspects of ultrasonic liposculpture. Perspect Plast Surg 1993; 7:153.
19. Zocchi M. Ultrasonic liposculpting. Aesth Plast Surg 1992; 16:287–298.
20. Gilliland MD, Commons GW, Halperin B. Safety issues in ultrasound assisted large volume liposuction.
21. Fournier P, Otteni F. Lipodissection in body sculpting: The dry procedure. Plast Reconstr Surg 1983; 72:598.
22. Klein JA. Tumescent technique for local anesthesia improves safety in large volume liposuction. Plast Reconstr Surg 1993; 92:1085–1098.
23. Narins RS. Liposuction of the face and neck. Elson ML, ed. Evaluation and Treatment of the Aging Face. 1984, pp. 93–100.
24. Cook WR Jr. Laser neck and jowl liposculpture, including platysma laser resurfacing, dermal laser resurfacing, and vaporization of subcutaneous fat. Dermatol Surg 1997; 23:1143–1148.
25. Narins RS. Liposuction surgery for a buffalo hump caused by Cushing's disease. J Am Acad Dermatol 1989; 21:307.
26. Gilliland MD. Safe megavolume liposuction in the obese patient. Presented to the International Society of Aesthetic Plastic Surgery, 13th International Congress, New York, 1995.
27. Narins RS. Liposuction surgery of the lateral thigh. J Dermatol Surg Oncol 1988; 14:10.
28. Narins RS. Large volume liposuction, the hour-glass abdomen. Presented to the American Academy of Dermatology Meeting, New Orleans, 1999.
29. Hanke C, Bernstein G, Bullock S. Safety of tumescent liposuction in 15,336 patients. Dermatol Surg 1995; 21:459–462.
30. Coleman WP III, Lawrence N, Lillis PJ, Narins RS. The tumescent techniques (letter). Plast Reconstr Surg 1998; 101:1751–1752.
31. Hanke CW. Liposuction under local anesthesia (editorial). J Dermatol Surg Oncol 1989; 15:12.

APPENDIX 1. PRESURGICAL INSTRUCTIONS FOR LIPOSUCTION

1. Avoid aspirin, aspirin-containing compounds, and Ibuprofen for 2 weeks prior to surgery and 1 week after surgery.
2. Avoid Vitamin E as above.
3. Do not take Redux or Phentermine diet pills for 2 weeks prior to surgery.
4. Medications may be taken the morning of the surgery with a light breakfast.
5. Wash areas with Phisoderm or Hibaclens daily for 1 week prior to surgery.
6. Wash hair night before or morning of the surgery.
7. Shave hair if excessive in the areas of the surgery—2 days before surgery.
8. Arrange for a person to drive you home from the office.
9. Arrange for a person to stay with you overnight.
10. Start antibiotic as directed day before surgery.
11. Do not wear nail polish on the right index finger—if you have nail tips or acrylic nails, please remove them from the right index finger.
12. Wear loose, comfortable clothing (e.g., sweatsuit, black or dark colored) that is easy to put on after surgery.
13. Wear slip-on shoes (no laces or ties).
14. Bring girdle or binder in with you the day of the surgery.
15. Bring towels in with you the day of the surgery to put over car seats. Also bring a plastic bag to put directly over seat with towels on top to absorb fluid that is draining. Have both items ready on your bed as well.

APPENDIX 2. POSTSURGICAL INSTRUCTIONS FOR LIPOSUCTION

1. ANTIBIOTIC—Please take all as directed.
2. PAIN MEDICATION—Pain is usually minimal and usually consists of soreness. It improves markedly over the first 7 days. Extra-strength Tylenol is generally all that is required. If you have pain unrelieved by Tylenol, please call the office.
3. MEDICATIONS TO AVOID—Do not take aspirin or aspirin-containing compounds or nonsteroidal anti-inflammatory medication such as Ibuprofen for 2 weeks after surgery.
4. OTHER MEDICATIONS—______________________________
   ____
5. DIET—Meals are not restricted. Please do not be concerned if there is weight gain in the first few days from the fluid injected. We prefer you stay on a low fat diet. Please watch your weight. Try to stay 1–3 pounds lighter than your presurgical weight.
6. BATHING—Please sponge bathe until the tapes are removed. After that you may shower but replace the garment immediately after bathing. You may want to wash and dry the garment at the same time that you are showering.
7. REMOVAL OF TAPES—Remove the tapes on ________________. Soak in a tub of water with 1 cup of baby oil or mineral oil for 1/2 hour to

facilitate the removal. Remove dressing and immediately put the garment back on.

8. INCISIONS—Once tapes are removed, grease incisions 2× daily for 6 weeks with Bacitracin ointment or Vaseline.
9. GARMENT—Your special garment or binder should be worn for 3–4 weeks. Please wear the garment 24 hours a day for 2 weeks after surgery, except when it is being washed. (After washing garment put back on with seam on the outside). For the next 2 weeks the garment may be worn for 12–24 hours a day depending on your needs. The extent and location of your surgery will determine how long you need to wear the garment.
10. POSTSURGICAL APPOINTMENTS—Please make an appointment 2 days after surgery for a quick checkup. FOR THE FIRST POSTSURGICAL VISIT ONLY—please enter the office through the back door (to the left of the elevators), RING BELL, SPEAK INTO SPEAKER WHEN ANSWERED. At that time we will tell you when to come in for further follow-up.
11. DRAINAGE—Postsurgical drainage occurs after surgery and can last 1–7 days. Place a large plastic bag or rubber mattress cover over mattress with towels on top to absorb the fluid that is draining. Although the fluid is red tinged, there is very little blood in it, most of it being injected local anesthetic and tissue fluid. If there is excessive bleeding or swelling or pain unrelieved by medication, please call the office immediately.
12. BRUISING—Mild bruising may occur for 3 weeks after surgery.
13. NUMBNESS/SWELLING—Swelling will slowly disappear over 6 months. If mild numbness occurs it will usually disappear sooner. REMEMBER, ALTHOUGH YOU LOOK BETTER IMMEDIATELY AFTER REMOVAL OF THE DRESSING, IT WILL TAKE 6 MONTHS TO SEE THE FINAL RESULT.
14. EFFECTS—Your skin may be flushed 1–3 days after surgery—this is normal.
15. RETURN TO WORK—Most patients can return to work within 1–2 days after surgery.
16. EXERCISE—Patients can return to light nonjarring exercise as soon as they feel up to it. Jarring exercise, such as tennis, aerobics and running can be resumed in 3–4 weeks after surgery depending on the extent and area of the surgery. A regular exercise program is encouraged.
17. QUESTIONS—If you have any questions, please call the office.

APPENDIX 3. SURGICAL CONSENT FOR LIPOSUCTION SURGERY

I am aware that Dr. Narins has performed liposuction surgery since 1982. I have had the opportunity to ask questions about the procedure, its limitations and possible complications.

By placing my initials next to the following items, I clearly understand and accept the following:

_____1. The goal of liposuction surgery, as in any cosmetic procedure, is improvement, not perfection.

_____2. The final result will not be apparent for 3–6 months after surgery.
_____3. In order to achieve the best possible result, a "touch-up" procedure may be required. There will be a charge for any "touch-up" operation performed.
_____4. Areas of "cottage cheese" texture, i.e., cellulite, will be changed little by the liposuction surgery.
_____5. Liposuction surgery is a contouring procedure and is not performed for purposes of weight reduction.
_____6. Strict adherence to the postsurgical regimen discussed by Dr. Narins (i.e., wearing an elastic garment for several weeks or months, exercise, diet, and all other regimens discussed) is necessary in order to achieve the best possible results.
_____7. The surgical fee is paid for the operation itself and subsequent postsurgical office visits. There is no guarantee that the expected or anticipated results will be achieved.
_____8. The goal of liposuction surgery, as in any cosmetic surgery, is to improve the appearance. It does not guarantee the reduction of any measurements, including the neck, waist, and all other areas

Although complications after liposuction surgery are infrequent, by placing my initials next to the following, I understand that they may occur:

_____1. Bleeding is rare, and in rare instances could require hospitalization and blood transfusion. It is possible that blood clots may form under the skin and require subsequent surgical drainage.
_____2. Skin irregularities, lumpiness, hardness and dimpling may appear after surgery. Most of these problems disappear with time, but localized skin firmness, lumpiness, and/or irregularities may persist permanently. If loose skin is present in the treated areas, it may not shrink to conform to the new contour.
_____3. Infection is rare, but should it occur treatment with antibiotics and/or surgical drainage may be required.
_____4. Numbness or increased sensitivity of the skin over treated areas may persist for months. It is possible that localized areas of numbness or increase sensitivity could be permanent.
_____5. Objectionable scarring is rare because of the small size of the incisions used in liposuction surgery, but scar formation is possible.
_____6. Dizziness may occur during the first week after liposuction surgery, particularly on rising from a lying or sitting position. If this occurs, extreme caution must be exercised while walking. Do not attempt to drive a car if dizziness is present.
_____7. Allergic or toxic responses to anesthetic are extremely rare, but possible.
_____8. In addition to these possible complications, I am aware of the general risks inherent in all surgical procedures and anesthetic administration.
_____9. I have not taken "Phen-Fen", Redux or Phentermine diet pills in the past 2 weeks.

My signature certifies that I have discussed the above material thoroughly with Dr. Narins and I understand the goals, limitations and possible complications of liposuction surgery, and I wish to proceed with the surgery.

I hereby request, authorize, and give my consent to Dr. Rhode S. Narins, to perform on me ____

____

(Please initial above each area) and whatever surgeries, treatments, or technical procedures which may be deemed necessary or advisable in the diagnosis or treatment of my case. I further understand and agree that certain procedures may be performed by an associate of the stated doctor under his/her supervision or control. I also give permission to have such anesthetics administered as are deemed necessary or advisable.

I also give permission to use any of my radiographs or photographs in medical lectures or publications.

This particular surgery that I am about to undergo has been explained to me in detail and I understand in general what is to be done, that there are calculated risks, and that the doctor has not made any guarantee whatsoever.

Because Dr. Narins is internationally known for her pioneering work in liposuction, visiting doctors from around the United States and other countries are frequent observers. I grant permission for any non-local visiting physicians to observe the liposuction procedure.

Patient Signature:______________________________ Date:______________
Witness:___________________________________ Date:______________

26

Liposuction Using General Anesthesia: A Plastic Surgeon's Viewpoint

Mehdi N. Adham
University of Oklahoma Health Sciences Center, Oklahoma City, Oklahoma

Bahman Teimourian
Georgetown University Medical Center, Bethesda, Maryland

Michael Chiaramonte
University of Maryland, Baltimore, Maryland

INTRODUCTION

Liposuction has gained widespread acceptance over the last 20 years as the procedure of choice for the aesthetic removal of undesirable adipose tissue. The technique has evolved from one of skeptical acceptance to being one of the most commonly performed cosmetic procedures. Recent statistics reveal that over 100,000 liposuction procedures are performed annually in the United States [1].

Careful presurgical evaluation of patients and the establishment of realistic expectations will result in both patient and physician satisfaction. When these issues are not addressed the outcome can be disappointing for both.

It is of great importance to approach body contouring from the standpoint of balance. In order to obtain an ideal silhouette, fat is removed from some areas and added to others. Skin may also need to be released, anchored, or excised in adjacent areas [2]. It is important for the surgeon to be familiar with all of these techniques in order to obtain the best possible result.

History

Numerous techniques have been used by plastic surgeons to modify the body contour. Open procedures that removed skin and subcutaneous tissue en bloc improved the body's silhouette but resulted in long, unsightly scars [3]. J. Schrudde of Germany was one of the first plastic surgeons to perform a closed technique of fat removal

This work was supported in part by a grant from the Orthopaedic and Reconstructive Research Foundation.

using a curette. However, complications were frequent and included hematoma, seroma, infection, and focal necrosis of skin [4]. In 1976, G. Fischer and his father, A. Fischer, developed an instrument called the cellulosuctiontome to perform blunt closed liposuction. This instrument morsellized and extracted fatty debris after a planatome was used to undermine the adipose tissue [5]. Again, complications associated with blunt technique such as seromas, pseudobursa, and skin necrosis were noted.

Simultaneously, three surgeons working independently significantly improved on the concepts of Fischer. They were B. Teimourian in Washington, D.C.; U.K. Kesselring in Lausanne, Switzerland; and Y.G. Illouz in Paris, France.

Various modifications of smaller blunt tipped cannulas were introduced and a technique was developed for tunneling through multiple levels. This reduced the incidence of seromas, hematomas, and surface irregularities [6]. Illouz used a "wet technique" to soften the fat and facilitate its removal. A solution of normal saline, distilled water, and hyaluronidase was injected into the adipose tissue. The solution was thought to rupture cellular membranes and emulsify the adipose tissue to be aspirated [7]. Kline modified the "wet technique" by adding lidocaine and epinephrine to saline so that it could be used as the sole anesthetic agent. This resulted in minimal blood loss and decreased postsurgical pain [8]. This tumescent technique can be used for local anesthesia with sedation for liposuction [9].

PATIENT EVALUATION

Suction lipectomy is best suited for patients with good skin elasticity and muscle tone who have localized fat deposits that have not responded to diet and exercise [7,10–13]. Because the amount of skin is not reduced during liposuction, the best results are seen in younger patients whose skin contracts around their newly contoured frame. Localized fat deposits most frequently occur in the abdominal region of men and in the thighs and buttocks of women. Patients seek suction lipectomy to treat these areas when they are thought to be excessive. Surgery is not a substitution for weight loss through exercise and diet, but may serve as a stimulus to achieve better weight control.

Patients should have realistic expectations for the result from liposuction based on their presurgical body framework. Physicians should be cautious of patients requesting liposuction that are too young with minimal adipose tissue as well as those with generalized lipodystrophy that have had significant weight changes and have lost skin elasticity. Overweight patients are best treated with staged operations, approximately 4 to 6 months apart, using suction lipectomy and dermatolipectomy. This should be performed in combination with a weight-loss and exercise program [13].

A complete medical history should be obtained to assess the patient's surgical risk, especially if general anesthesia is to be used for large-volume liposuction. Any history of hypertension, coronary artery disease, previous myocardial infarction, diabetes mellitus, or COPD must be evaluated before surgery. Also, any history of keloid or hypertrophic scar formation should be noted, because this could obviously affect the outcome. An assessment of patient medications, especially those that affect hemostasis (i.e., aspirin, coumadin, NSAID), should be completed.

The surgeon should perform a complete physical examination with special attention to the patient's cardiopulmonary status. A careful assessment of any abdominal or inguinal hernias must be performed. Hernias are not an absolute contraindication to liposuction. The edges should be defined and contents of the hernia sac avoided in order to minimize the risk of bowel injury. Areas of lipodystropy should be examined for the presence of scars, asymmetry, underlying muscle development, and skin tone [14]. The assessment should document the patient's height and weight so that postsurgical changes can be monitored. Any disparities between the upper and lower body should also be noted [15].

It is important for the surgeon to obtain the patient's perspective as to the areas that are of greatest concern. While standing next to the patient, looking into a three-way mirror, the patient should point out the irregularities that they would like addressed. Distinguishing characteristics, such as dimples or ripples, should be pointed out to the patient to avoid the possibility of these first being noticed after surgery when patients have a heightened sense of awareness.

The patient's clothing preferences need to be investigated. For example, a patient who wears two-piece bathing suits in public would find a flat abdomen with loose skin unacceptable. Such a patient would benefit from combined suction-assisted lipectomy (SAL) and dermatolipectomy.

Presurgical Counseling

It is important for the surgeon to discuss with the patient the procedure and all risks associated with the surgery [16]. Some patients may be found to be unsuitable for surgery because they have unrealistic expectations or need psychological counseling before surgery. The following points should be made clear to the patient:

1. The operation will not remove fine skin wrinkles or dimples [17]. A certain amount of waviness will remain when suction lipectomy is the primary procedure.
2. Patients who are moderately overweight will have more contour irregularities and sagginess in exchange for better contouring in clothing after suction lipectomy.
3. Patients who are morbidly obese and have failed reduction by diet or exercise may benefit from suction lipectomy but may require a secondary skin resection. The same is true for older patients who have lost skin elasticity.

It is important that the patient be well informed with regard to the premedication that will be used, the different options for anesthesia available, duration of the surgical procedure, the typical postsurgical course, and expected recovery time. If a patient is to undergo large-volume liposuction (>15,000 ml) where there is a possibility that a blood transfusion may be needed, it is recommended that the patient make arrangements for autologous donation. Once the physician is comfortable that the patient has a full understanding of the procedure, that all questions have been answered, and that the patient has realistic expectations regarding the outcome of the surgery, the patient should be asked to sign a surgical consent form.

Photography

Precise photographic documentation is mandatory so that procedures may be planned appropriately and results communicated with the patient. The standards of basic photography must be followed with particular attention to uniform lighting, background, and distance. Patients should remove any jewelry, eyeglasses, or distracting undergarments for photos.

All the pictures taken in our office photography studio are shot with a 35-mm single-lens reflex camera and a 60-mm macro lens. A sky blue background works bests to achieve contrast and minimize shadowing. Thighs, hips, and abdomen are the most common areas for liposuction. These areas should be photographed from a distance of 5 ft, with the patient's feet separated by 12 in. When the feet are placed closer together, it gives the appearance of "photographic inner thigh liposuction." Also, the patient should have their hands folded on their chest because elevating the arms above the head will give the appearance of "photographic abdominoplasty." A focusing grid is used to reproduce alignment between presurgical and postsurgical photos [18]. It is important to review the presurgical photographs with the patient so that they have an understanding of the asymmetries that exist. This will enable the physician to better satisfy the patient with the body contouring technique. Photographs shown in this chapter may not necessarily follow these guidelines. Certain postsurgical photographs were taken to match presurgical positions. In addition, we have been using digital-imaging cameras for 3 years.

Presurgical Planning

The patient is instructed to shower with Betadine the night before surgery and on the morning of surgery. The patient is asked not to shave 48 hours before surgery to avoid causing scrapes or cuts. The patient is asked to try on the appropriate compression garment to ensure a proper fit for the postsurgical period.

Marking

A combination of visual inspection and viewing presurgical photographs is required to estimate the amount of fat to be removed. Pinching the skin over the iliac crest is also very useful in approximating how much liposuction is necessary in the abdomen [19,20]. With the patient in the standing position, the deformity to be contoured is marked along with an area 3 cm beyond the main area to ensure a smooth transition.

The patient's pictures are then posted in the surgery room. We have found this to be very helpful in identifying areas of asymmetry that require differential suctioning.

Surgical Preparation

The surgical field is prepared with Duraprep™ or a gel preparation, with special care taken to ensure the preservation of the markings. If liposuction is to be performed on the lower extremities, the patient is prepared from the waist down in the standing position and then placed in the supine position on a sterile drape.

Positioning of the Patient During Surgery

A majority of liposuction procedures can be performed in the supine position. However, if gluteal or calf liposuction is required, the patient may easily be turned to the prone position. Care should be taken to cover exposed areas with drapes that are not being liposuctioned to minimize hypothermia. When body procedures are combined with suction of the face and neck, the body procedure should be performed first to minimize face and neck swelling.

Anesthesia

Patients are premedicated in the waiting area with diazepam (Valium). A first-generation cephalosporin such as cefadroxil (Duricef) is given 1 hour before surgery and two doses are given after surgery. When only a small area is to be liposuctioned, anesthesia can be administered by using a propofol (Diprivan) drip and monitored anesthesia care. However, the majority of body contouring cases involve multiple areas and require general anesthesia.

After adequate general anesthesia is obtained, the patient is monitored with an automatic blood pressure, pulse oximeter and end tidal CO_2 monitor. The patient's body temperature is monitored. The room temperature is a minimum of 75°F and areas of the body that are not actively worked on are covered with towels to prevent hypothermia. Also, a bear hugger is used on the nonsterile areas if the room temperature is not adequately warm. A foley is inserted if the operation is expected to be greater than 3 hours, which is usually the case when abdominoplasty or lower-body lifting is planned.

Tumescent Solution

We routinely use tumescent solution [21,22]. The combination we most often use for body liposuction consists of 1000 ml NaCl, 10 ml NaBicarb, 25 ml 2% plain Xylocaine, and 1 Amp Epi (1:1000). For facial liposuction, we use 500 ml NaCl, 30 ml 1% Xylocaine, and 3 Amps Epi (1:1000). When using MAC, we add another 30 ml 2% plain Xylocaine [23].

All areas to be suctioned are symmetrically infiltrated with tumescent solution until tense. The ratio of tumescent solution to volume of fat to be suctioned is approximately 1:1. The estimated volume of tumescent solution is made just before surgery. A higher concentration of epinephrine may be used if continued bleeding is noted with suctioning, and quite often we will increase epinephrine to 2 Amps (1:1000) per liter.

SURGICAL TECHNIQUE

After the patient is anesthetized, the markings for liposuction are reinforced. A full-thickness skin incision, large enough to permit entry of the cannula, is made using a scalpel. The incision should be concealed in a skin fold or natural crease. Also, the skin incision should be located in the periphery of the area to be treated because this will allow greater maneuverability and avoid the difficult task of suctioning at the incision site.

The majority of liposuction is performed with the opening of the cannula directed away from the skin. It is important to always maintain the orientation of the cannula opening by noting the guide position on the cannula handle. Cannula tunnels should be created in the deep fatty layer using a forward and back motion, thereby preserving the blood vessels and collagen network. These tunnels can be cross-hatched through a separate incision to create a more even contour. The back and flanks are treated first in the lateral decubitus position. With the patient in the lateral decubitus position, both knees should be padded to protect against peroneal nerve injury.

If fat grafting is anticipated, a syringe is used to aspirate the fat, which is then centrifuged and kept in a closed, capped syringe for injection. Then, if ultrasonic-assisted lipectomy (UAL) is to be used, it is performed before SAL. When working on both sides of the body, the patient is rolled back and forth to maintain symmetry of shape by alternating sites. Also, the total amount of fat aspirated from each side is measured. It may be necessary to re-inject tumescent solution when alternating sides if the contralateral area is not tense. It is important to estimate the end points and to avoid oversuction, because correction is difficult.

After finishing the back and flanks, the patient is placed in the supine position. The chest, abdomen, and inner and anterior thigh and knee are then treated. At the end of the procedure, fat grafting is performed followed by massage in order to smooth the area. If fluid has collected in the flanks or the back during the procedure, the collections are aspirated and multiple closed drains are inserted. If required, dermatolipectomy is the final body contouring procedure to be performed. The patient is then taped and put into compression garments. Facial suctioning and contouring can be performed once the body contouring is complete.

Suction-Assisted Lipectomy (SAL) Equipment

There are a variety of syringes and suction machines available for use. We use the Lysonix system because both aspiration and injection systems are combined. The injection system is fast and powerful for quick infiltration. Also, this system can be used for UAL. For small areas, syringe suctioning may be adequate. However, for large-volume suctioning, the syringe is both time consuming and tiring and thus machine aspiration is recommended.

Ultrasound-Assisted Lipectomy (UAL) Equipment and Use

Although UAL is not necessary for body contouring, it can be helpful for the breasts and flanks. Potential complications exist for other areas, which will be mentioned later. The Lysonix system is also used for UAL. The power setting most frequently used for UAL is 5 to 6. The recommended guide for time in various areas is in Table 1. Some authorities recommend using UAL until there is no resistance [24]. Using this end point may cause a complication when performed by an inexperienced physician. The following areas should not be exposed to UAL: face, neck, inner thigh, and leg.

Cannula Use

When we started performing suction lipectomy in 1976, large cannulas, greater than 10 mm, were necessary to suction effectively. Now with more powerful aspirating machines and improved cannula tip design, the size of the cannulas has decreased.

TABLE 1 Average Time Spent on UAL Use*

Flank-Chest	6–7 min
Upper Quadrant Abdomen	3 min
Gynecomastia (Breast)	5–6 min
Buttocks	3–4 min
Upper-Outer Thighs†	3–4 min

*There may be some variation, depending on the size of the patient.
†Avoid face, neck, inner thighs, lower abdomen, and lower leg.

Cannulas ranging from 3 to 5 mm are adequate for the majority of body contouring procedures. The cannulas we most frequently use are the Becker cannula, keel cobra, Mercedes, and spatula for deep suctioning against muscles (Fig. 1).

For the neck area, we use a 2.5 mm cannula, and for the lower face, 2 mm and 1.8 mm cannulas are used. Generally, the smaller the cannula, the more time that is needed for fat aspiration. Inappropriate cannula use can result in complications such as dimpling, scarring, and discoloration of the dermis [25].

In general, we use a smaller cannula superficially and a larger cannula in deeper fat layers. Also, the aspirating port of the bigger cannulas is directed toward the deep tissue. When the goal is to create a depression or crease in the skin, the aspiration port is directed toward the dermis. This technique can be used to create the midabdominal line.

Blood Loss

In order to minimize blood loss during SAL, the tumescent solution should be infiltrated at least 3 cm outside the zone of suctioning. The physician should then wait at least 20 minutes for the epinephrine to take effect. During the procedure, it is important to ensure that the cannula does not go behind the anticipated area of suctioning because this may lead to unnecessary bleeding. If the aspirate becomes bloody and additional SAL is still required, more tumescent solution can be infiltrated. Whenever we expect to suction more than 15 L, the patient is asked to donate 2 units of autologous blood. This is usually given at the end of the procedure or in the recovery room.

POSTSURGICAL CARE

The majority of procedures can be performed in an outpatient surgery center with the first postsurgical visit the following day. If a suction lipectomy of more than 15 L is performed, the patient is kept overnight and discharged the next day. The patients are advised to continue wearing postsurgical compression garments for approximately 6 weeks. Three days after surgery, the tapes are removed and the patient is instructed to begin massaging treated areas. The patients are encouraged to begin walking the day after surgery and progress to light exercise as tolerated. Vigorous exercise is allowed with support after 3 weeks.

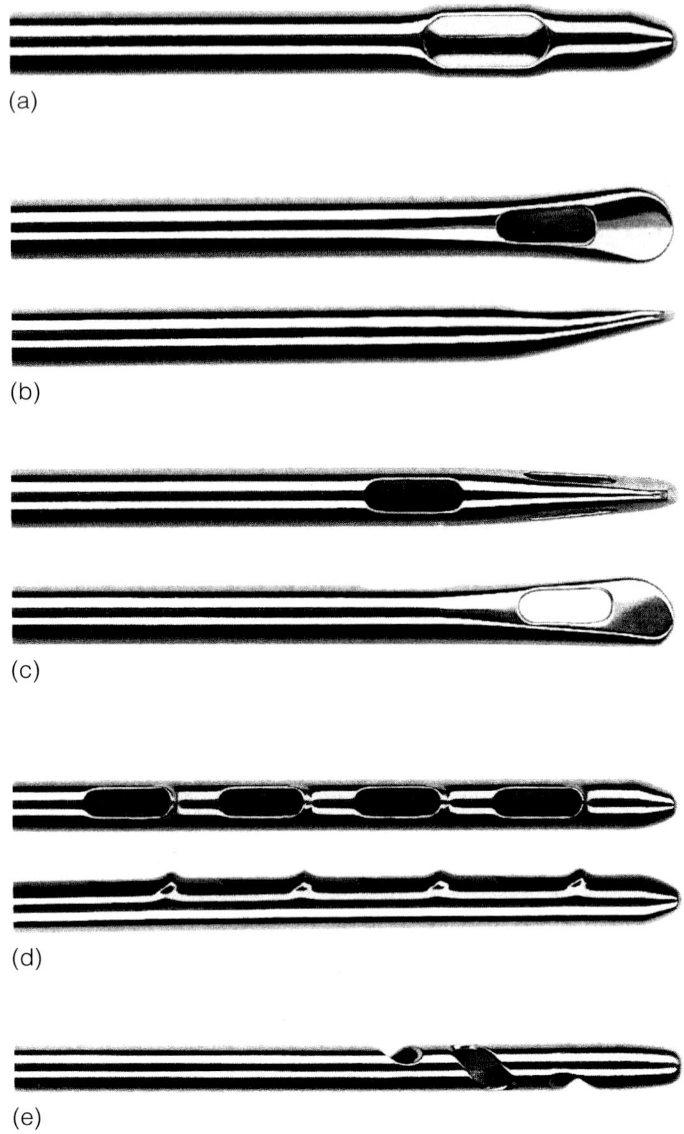

FIGURE 1 Various cannulas used by the authors.

Patients are given prescriptions for cephalexin (Keflex) 500 mg every 6 hours for 1 day, Percocet for pain, and diazepam (Valium) 5 mg every 8 hours for 3 to 5 days. The Valium is given to reduce spasm associated with muscle bruising and to prevent overactivity by the patient that may prolong the recovery phase.

Drains are removed when the output is less than 25 ml for 24 hours. The drainage is usually more with UAL use. The sutures or staples are removed at 1 week.

FACE AND NECK

Evaluation

Body contouring must be approached systematically. In order to obtain optimal results, a presurgical evaluation should be completed. The following should be assessed:

1. Skin laxity and turgor, facial rhytidies and jowls.
2. Fat distribution: face, neck, or face and neck.
3. Jawline anatomy: its presence or absence with face and neck blending together.
4. Shape of face: round, square, or oval.
5. Presence of a constricted and ptotic chin with depression lateral to it (witch's chin).
6. Presence of a nasojugular groove.
7. Flat malar eminence.
8. Hollowed cheek or prominent cheek.
9. Lip status.
10. Prominent nasolabial line or other facial grooving.
11. Presence or absence of platysmal band.
12. Presence or absence of subplatysmal fat.
13. Presence or absence of sternocleidomastoid outline.
14. Mobility of the neck.
15. Presence of dentures.
16. Length of the neck.
17. Occlusion.

These observations should be made in the sitting position. The patient should be observed from both the front and profile. A worm's eye view will allow one to see the nasojugular, nasolabial, and malar eminence. Then, the patient is placed in the supine position to observe the shift of the anatomy. This is important in planning the surgical procedure because it is essential to understand the soft tissue relationships in the face.

From a practical viewpoint, a young patient with a rounded face will usually require SAL in both the lower face and neck. SAL and plication of the platysma are required for patients with a fatty neck associated with a platysmal band. Patients with contour deformities and a fatty neck may need both liposuction and lipografting. A patient with an obtuse mentocervical angle with or without a hypoplastic chin may necessitate a chin implant and platysmal plication to correct the deformity. Some of these patients may not need SAL. Finally, patients with soft-tissue volume shift may only require soft-tissue repositioning rather than SAL. The patient with ptotic chin (witch's chin) may need a release with bone removal, central fat excision, and lateral fat graft [26].

Patients with poor skin health frequently benefit from skin preconditioning with Retin-A and glycolic acid that can improve the final result.

Marking and Surgery

Access sites should be selected so that the scar is well hidden and the potential for injury to important structures—such as a facial nerve or facial artery—is avoided while still obtaining adequate access. For access to the lower portion of the face, an incision is made anterior to the ear at the level of the tragus.

Adequate access to the neck can be obtained through an incision made at the ear lobule or in the retroauricular area. Incisions in the submental area work best for SAL of the anterior neck. An incision along the anterior border of the sternocleidomastoid muscle in midportion is best for an extremely obese patient. Piriform aperture incisions can be used for insertion of filler material. The corner of the mouth on the lower side can be used for suctioning the jowls area and tissue near the facial vessels and marginal mandibular nerve (Fig. 2) [27].

Suctioning of the face and neck can be performed by using either a syringe or machine aspirator. Also note that in an obese patient, a slight undercorrection is desirable because a postsurgical platysma band and contour deformity may appear, giving a suboptimal result. These patients should be aware of this before surgery.

Clinical Cases

Case 1. A 40-year-old female underwent suction lipectomy of the lower face and neck. The patient is shown 1 year after surgery. There is slight platysmal band anteriorly. There is definite separation of the face from the neck (Fig. 3). The patient could have benefited from neck plication and undermining.

Case 2. A 35-year-old female underwent lower face and neck SAL and plication of the platysma anteriorly and undermining of the neck extensively. The patient is shown 6 months after surgery (Fig. 4).

Case 3. A 40-year-old man with an obtuse cervicomental angle, overbite, fatty neck, and nasal obstruction. He underwent moderate suction lipectomy of the neck, neck plication, chin implant with 4 mm projection, lateral interlocking neck suture plication, and septorhinoplasty to correct the bifid tip [28]. The patient is shown 1 year after surgery (Fig. 5).

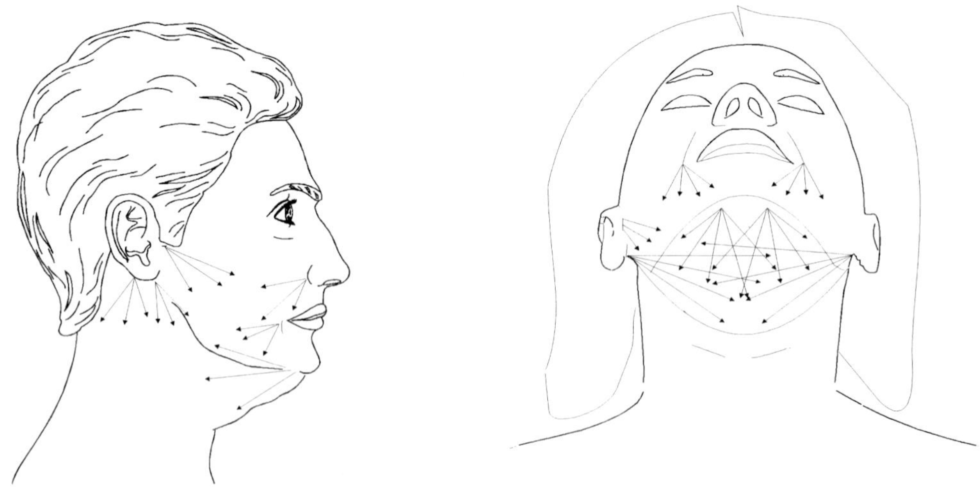

FIGURE 2 Access sites for liposuction of the face and neck.

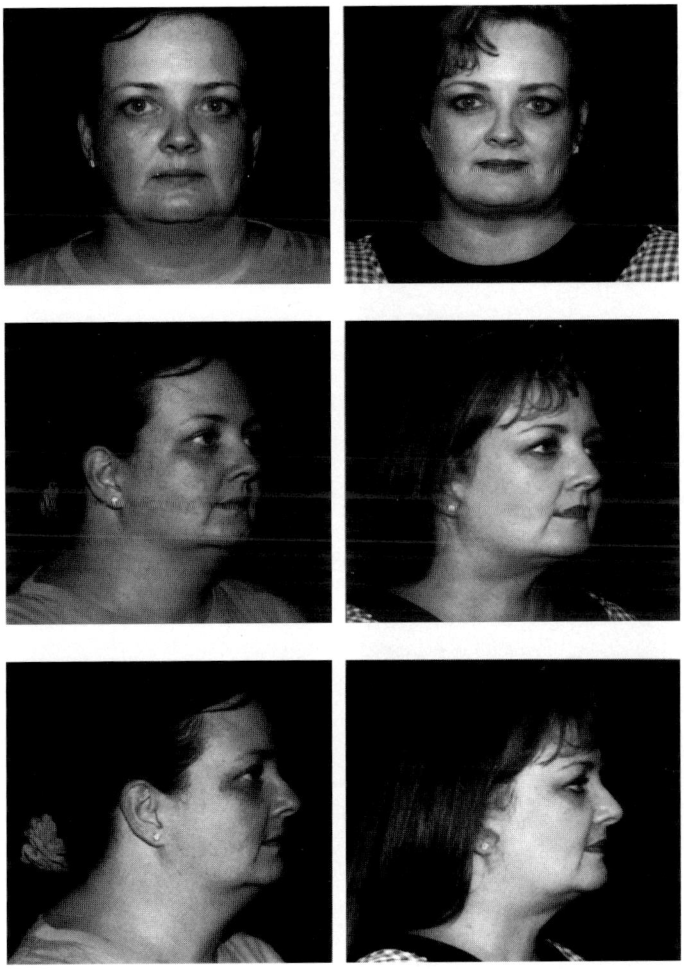

FIGURE 3 See p. 582 for details.

Case 4. A 34-year-old female with a hypoplastic chin and an obtuse neck who underwent mild suctioning of the neck, chin implantation, and plication. She has been followed for 1 year with good results (Fig. 6).

Case 5. A 63-year-old female with moderate loose skin of the face and neck in addition to a fatty face and neck. The patient underwent suctioning of the neck in combination with a facelift. This patient did not have a platysmal band and did not need midline plication (Fig. 7).

Case 6. A 58-year-old female with aging face, witch's chin, and pseudosubmental lipodystrophy underwent facelift with soft-tissue volume repositioning, fat graft, and skin redraping, with no suction lipectomy of the neck. Patient OGEE curve of youth is reproduced. The patient is shown 8 months after surgery (Fig. 8).

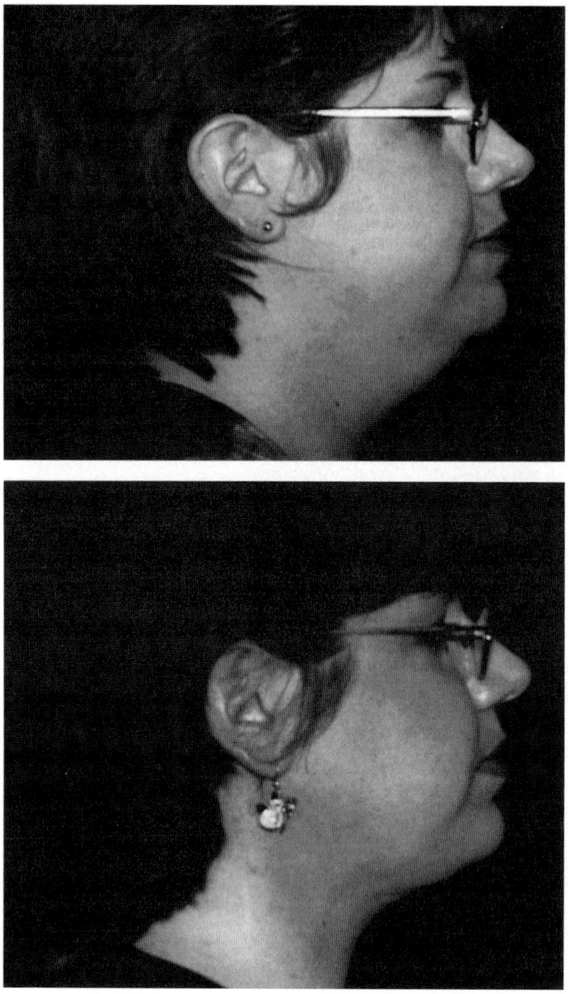

(a) (b)

FIGURE 4 **(a) Before surgery; (b) after surgery.**

Case 7. A 20-year-old female status postfacial fracture presents with "dish face," oral incompetence, and an obtuse metocervical angle. The patient was offered neck suctioning and chin implantation by another surgeon. The patient underwent piriform aperture augmentation with bone graft, upper-lip advancement, chin implant, minimal suction lipectomy of the neck, midline plication, and blepharoplasty. Her insurance refused rhinoplasty and she could not afford rhinoplasty. The patient is shown 1 year after surgery (Fig. 9).

MALE BREAST AND GYNECOMASTIA

Evaluation

Gynecomastia must be differentiated from chest lipodystrophy when evaluating male patients. The degree of gynecomastia needs to be determined in addition to the

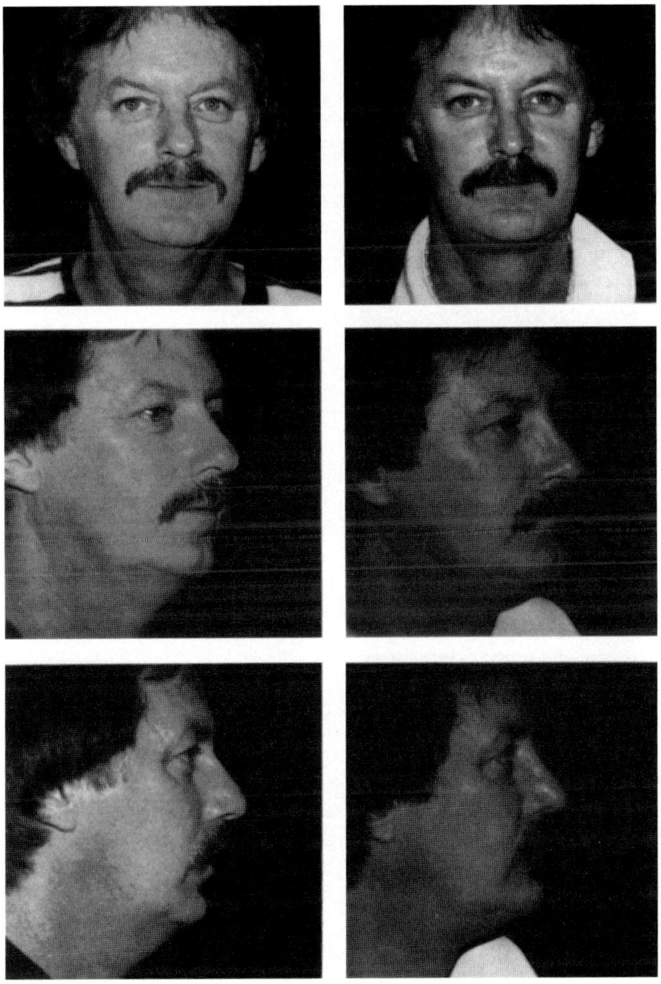

FIGURE 5 See p. 582 for details.

location and severity of the inframammary fold and its lateral extension [29]. The lateral border of the pectoralis muscle must also be identified. Excessive SAL or UAL of breasts in muscular patients may lead to an undesirable result by forming a depression below the pectoral line with contraction of the muscle. For patients with generalized obesity, suctioning should be performed uniformly over the chest, whereas patients with gynecomastia require suctioning mainly in the breast. Gynecomastia patients may also require release of the inframammary line [30]. The edge of latissimus dorsi and pectoralis muscles must be identified while the patient is flexing so that the amount of fat superficial to these muscles can be estimated.

Marking and Surgery

Access to the male breast and areola for suctioning can be obtained laterally in the anterior axillary line or inferiorly in the inframammary line (Fig. 10). Care must be

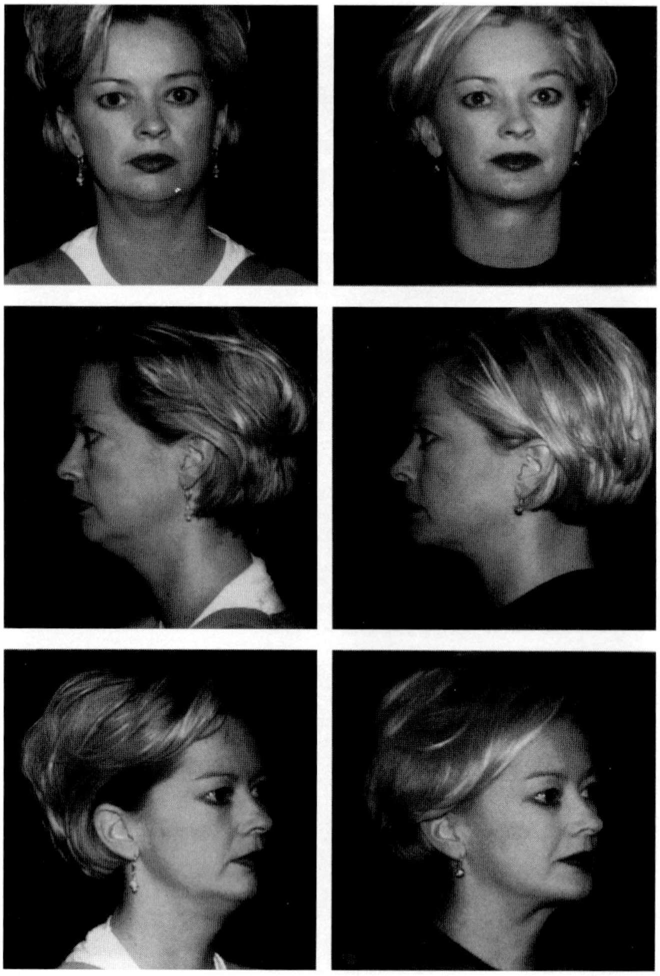

FIGURE 6 See p. 583 for details.

taken not to penetrate the latissimus dorsi muscle with the cannula during this approach. This is especially true for patients with firm skin and tight fibro-fatty tissue.

UAL through the inframammary incision seems to work best. There are several cannulas designed specifically for the SAL treatment of gynecomastia [31]. If the patient has a lot of loose skin after suctioning for gynecomastia, the inframammary line can be lowered to correct this defect. Male patients rarely require skin excision, as compared with female patients. However, if there is still too much glandular tissue after suctioning, it may be excised through an circumareolar incision [29].

Clinical Cases

Case 8. A 30-year-old male with left-sided gynecomastia. The patient underwent suction lipectomy of the left side. The patient is shown 1 year after surgery (Fig. 11).

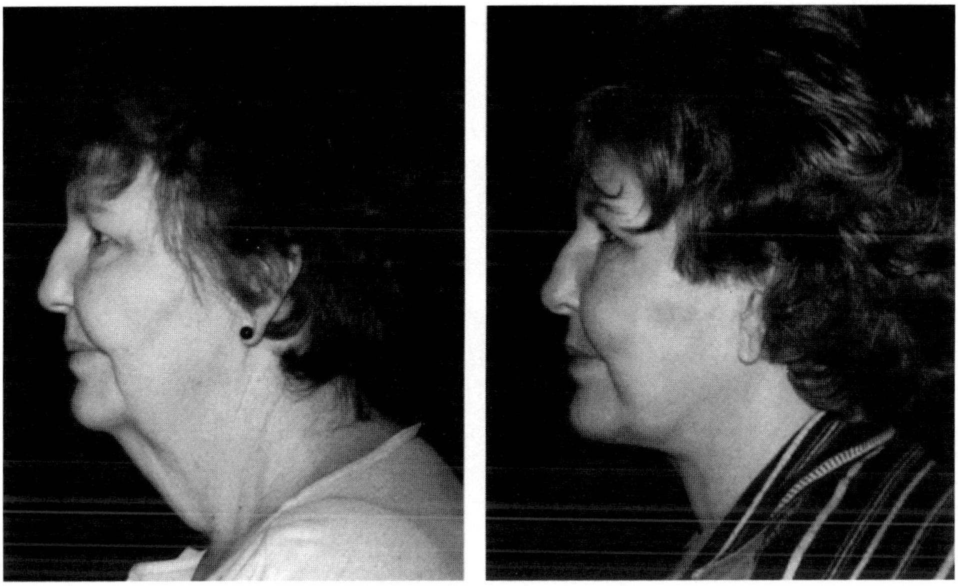

(a) (b)

FIGURE 7 (a) Before surgery; (b) after surgery.

Case 9. A 25-year-old male with bilateral gynecomastia. The patient underwent suction lipectomy and excision through a small areola excision. The patient required aspiration of seroma once after surgery (Fig. 12). The patient was followed up for 2 years.

Case 10. A 38-year-old male underwent SAL and excision of the breast tissue with lowering of the inframammary line (Fig. 13).

For additional clinical cases, see Figures 28 to 30.

FEMALE BREAST

Evaluation

In females, SAL can be used during breast reduction for lateral chest wall and axillary soft-tissue thinning. This procedure reduces lateral breast and chest wall scarring. However, for patients with loose skin, dermatolipectomy may be required to achieve optimal results. If the patient has mild to moderate hypertrophy without ptosis, SAL alone may be adequate.

Marking and Surgery

Because older female patients more commonly present for body contouring of the breasts, there is usually hypertrophy associated with some degree of ptosis. These patients most frequently require reduction mammoplasty. However, suction lipectomy can still be used in the lateral aspect of the breast to minimize the extension of the incision and subsequent scarring.

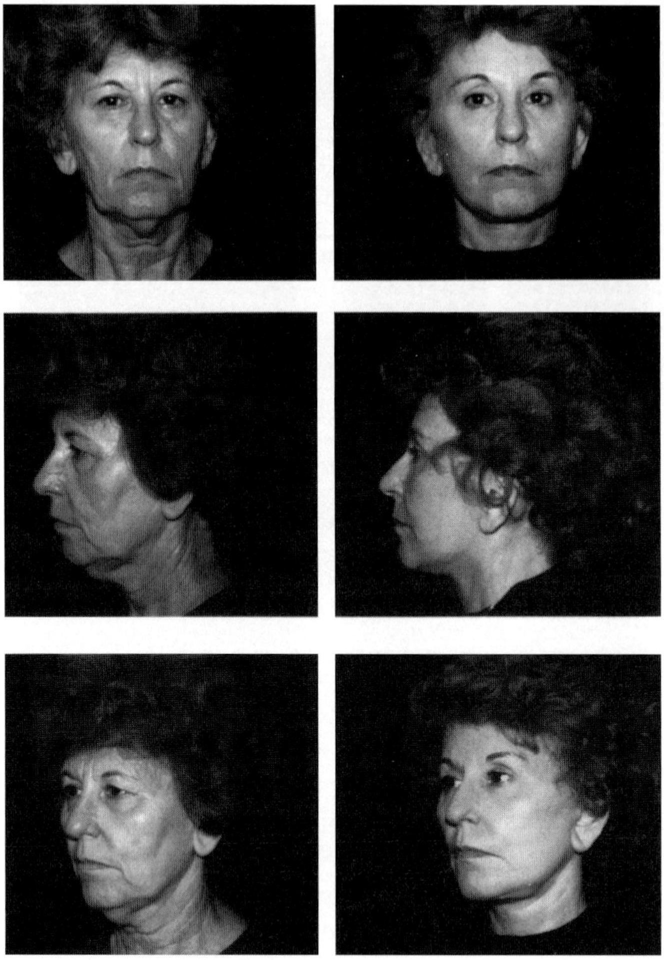

Figure 8 **See p. 583 for details.**

An extremely obese patient with loose skin will require excision of excess skin. As much as 600 ml have been removed by suction lipectomy from the lateral aspect of the breast (Fig. 14). Suctioning laterally also helps minimize the degree of undermining.

Clinical Cases

Case 11. A 46-year-old female underwent breast reduction and suctioning of 300 ml from the axillary tail of the breast and lateral chest wall with release of inframammary line laterally. The patient is shown 6 months after surgery. The folds in the axilla and upper back are reduced (Fig. 15).

Case 12. A 27-year-old white female underwent breast reduction and suctioning of the axillary folds. The patient is shown 1 year after surgery (Fig. 16).

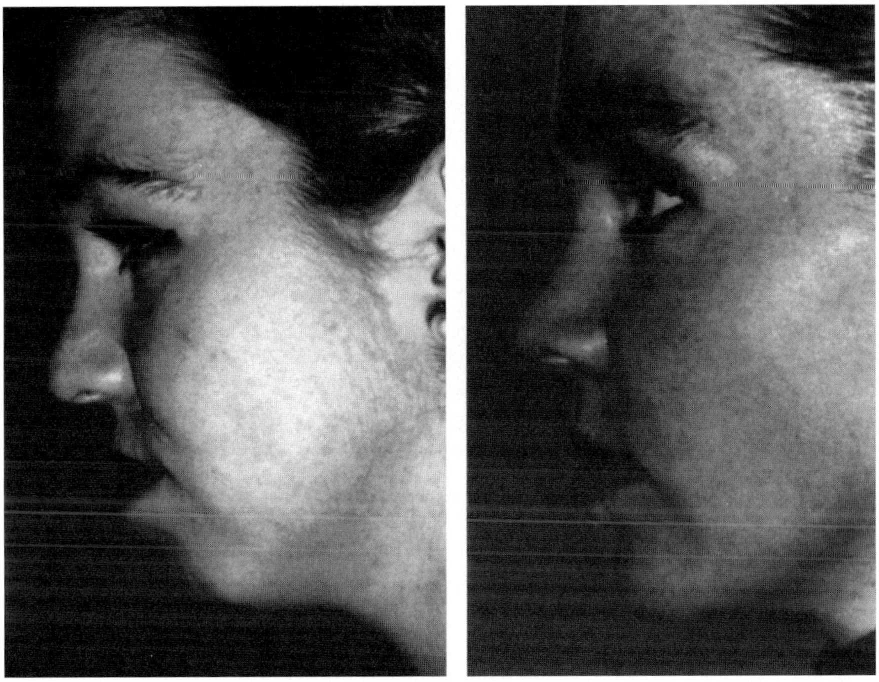

(a) (b)

FIGURE 9 (a) Before surgery; (b) after surgery.

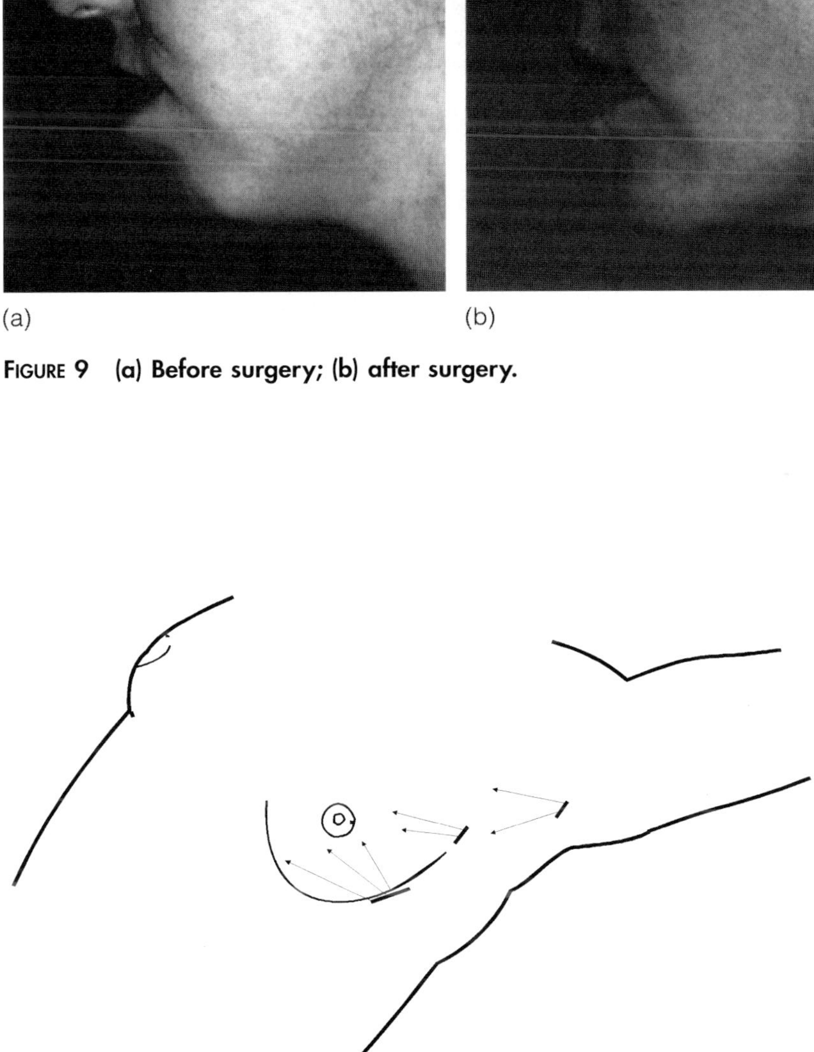

FIGURE 10 Access sites for liposuction of gynecomastia. Through the lower incision, UAL can be performed and the inframammary line can be released and lowered.

(a)

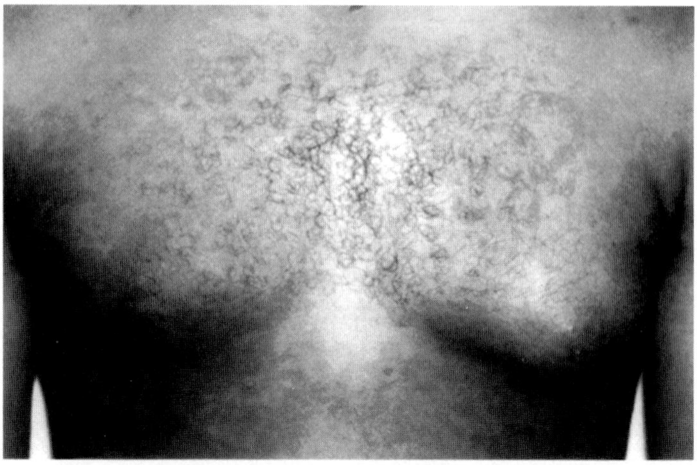

(b)

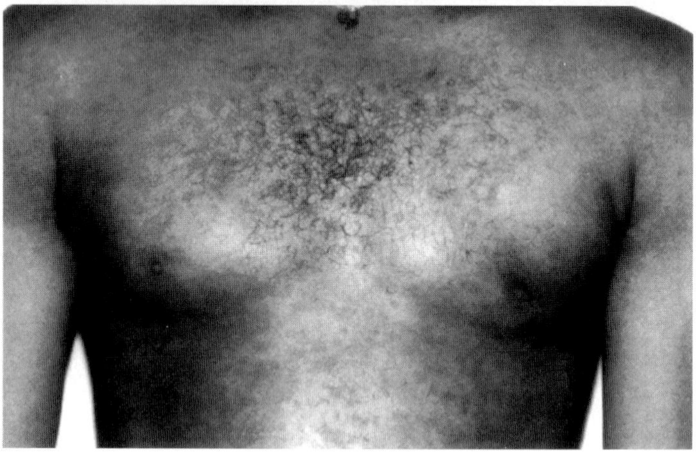

FIGURE 11 (a) Before surgery; (b) after surgery.

Case 13. A 50-year-old female underwent removal of ruptured silicon gel implant with mastopexy and suctioning of the lateral chest wall. The patient is shown 8 months after surgery (Fig. 17).

Case 14. A 40-year-old female underwent bilateral breast reduction and 250-ml suctioning of the lateral chest wall. The patient is shown 8 months after surgery (Fig. 18).

ARM

Evaluation

Many patients seeking reduction of their upper arms are concerned with the fat deposits, muscle mass loss, and laxity of the skin. Older patients who have undergone significant weight loss are likely to focus on the flabby skin that droops when they raise their arms, which are often referred to as "bat wings."

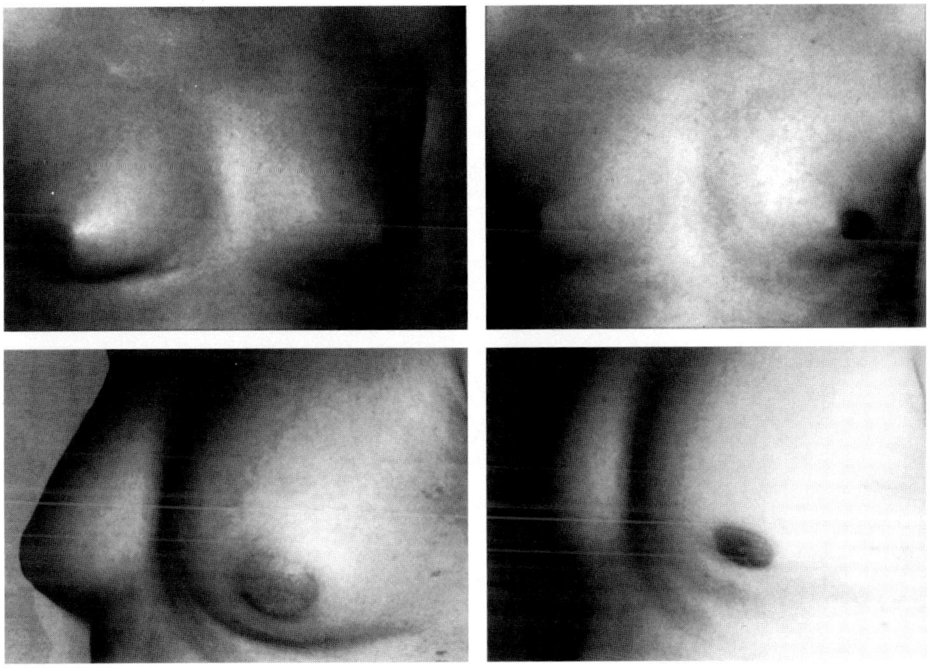

Figure 12 See p. 587 for details.

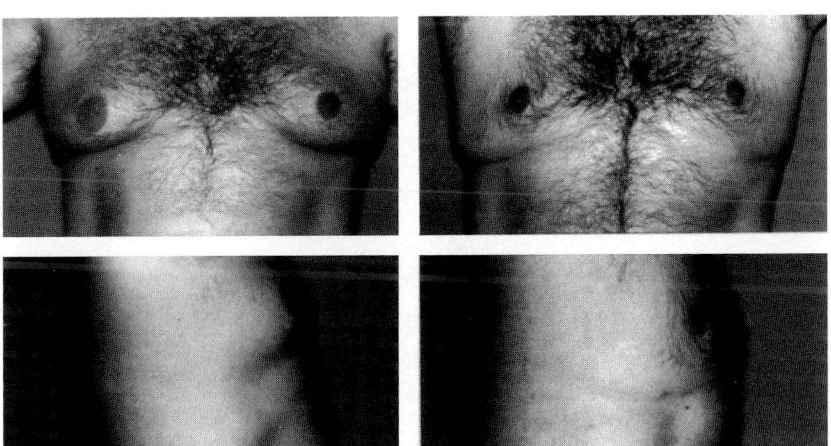

Figure 13 See p. 587 for details.

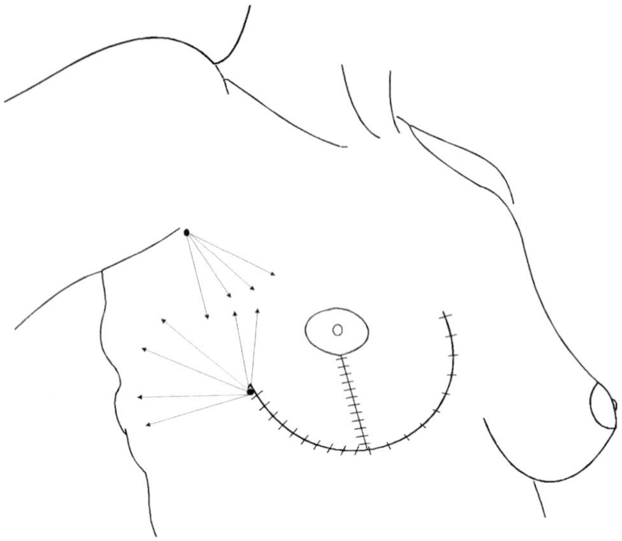

FIGURE 14 Access sites for liposuction of female breast during reduction mammaplasty. Laterally, through the corner of the inframammary line, the attachment of lateral axillary fold can be released and lowered.

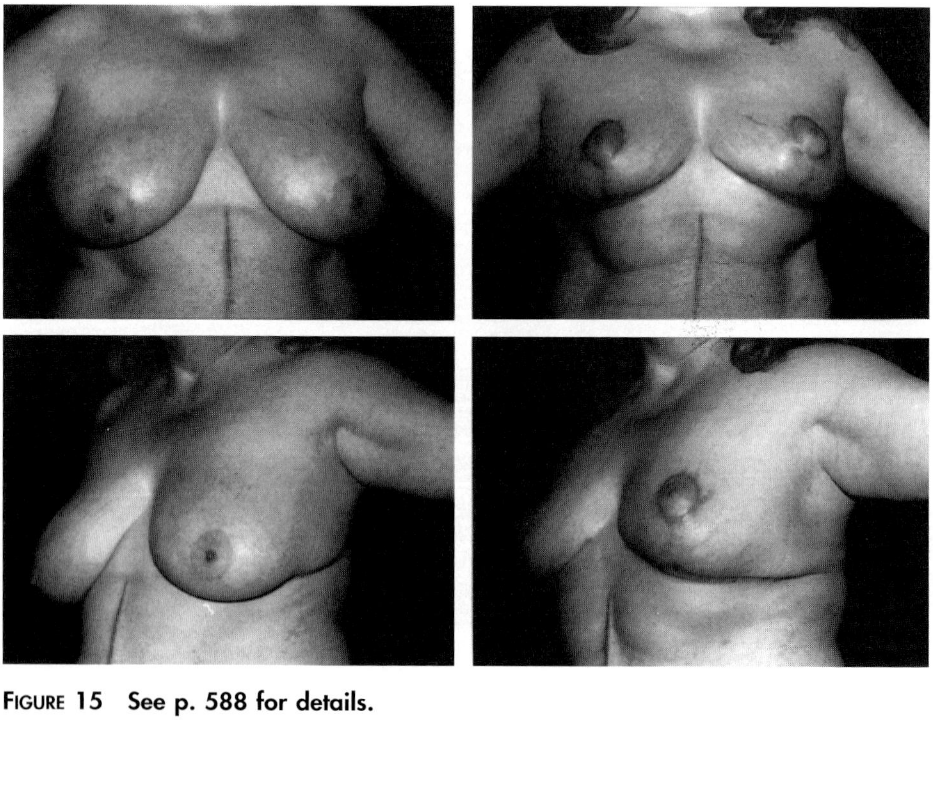

FIGURE 15 See p. 588 for details.

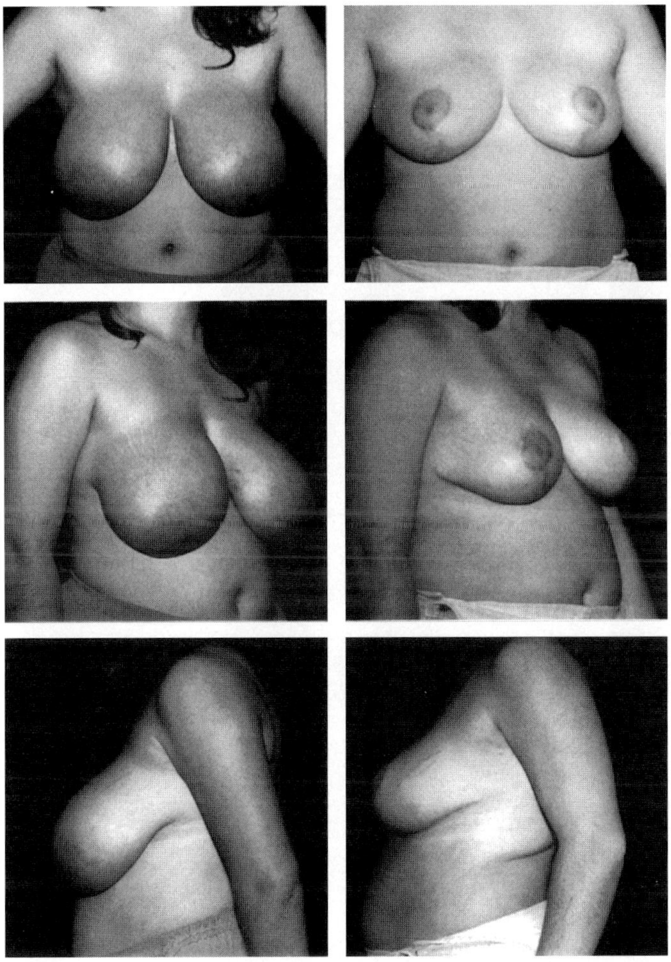

FIGURE 16 **See p. 588 for details.**

Marking and Surgery

The superior and medial aspect of the arm can be accessed from the anterior axilla. Suctioning of the inferior arm can be performed through an incision proximal to the medial epicondyle while care is taken to avoid the ulnar nerve. Laterally, the arm can be accessed through an incision in the posterior aspect of the axilla and lateral elbow (Fig. 19). Through the axillary incision, with the patient in supine or lateral decubitus position, the lateral chest can be suctioned as well [22].

Patients with excess skin and fat after SAL will need skin ridge plication in the axilla (Fig. 20) or skin resection in shape of an "L" or "T" from the inner arm (Fig. 21) [32].

The arm deformity has been classified by Teimourian into four groups for surgical treatment to obtain the best aesthetic result [33].

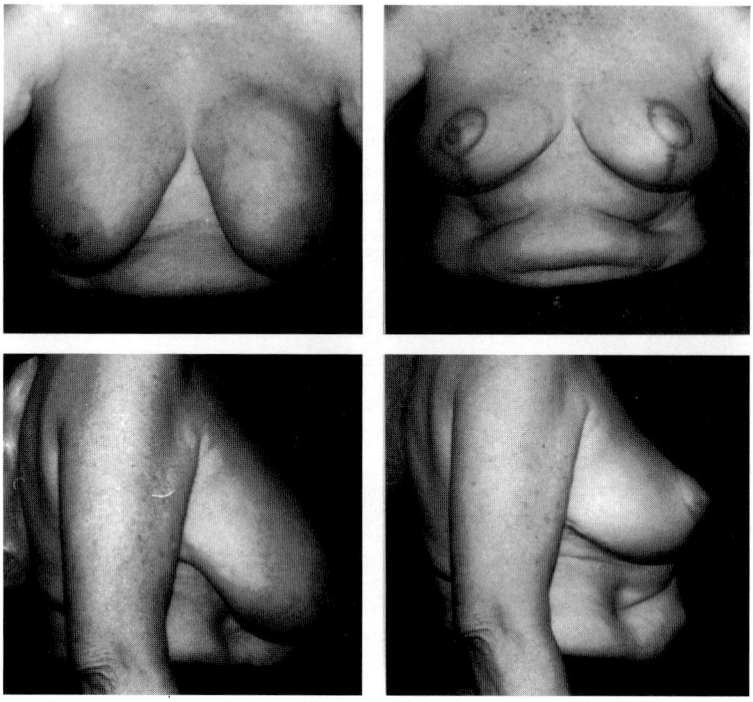

FIGURE 17 See p. 590 for details.

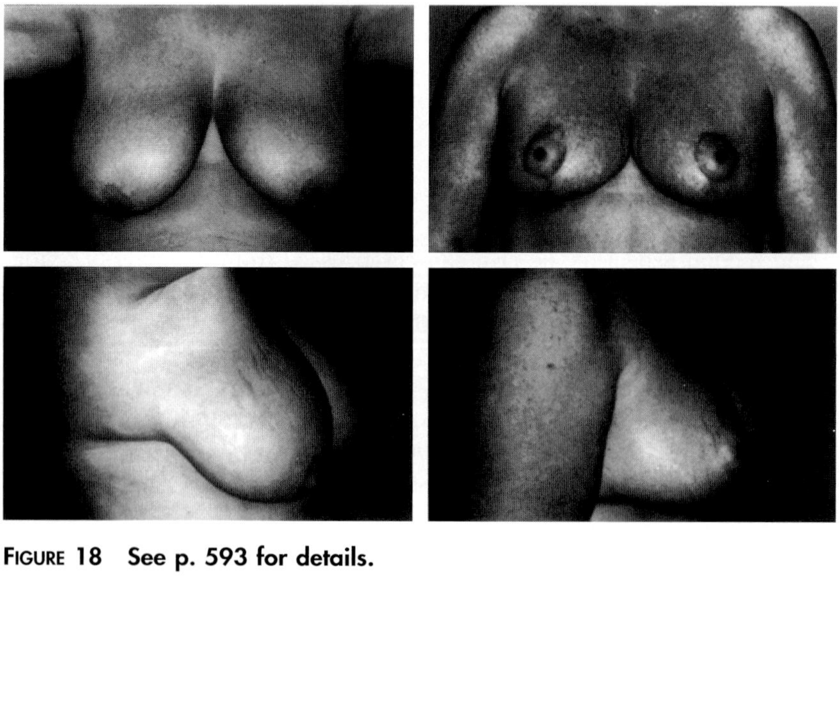

FIGURE 18 See p. 593 for details.

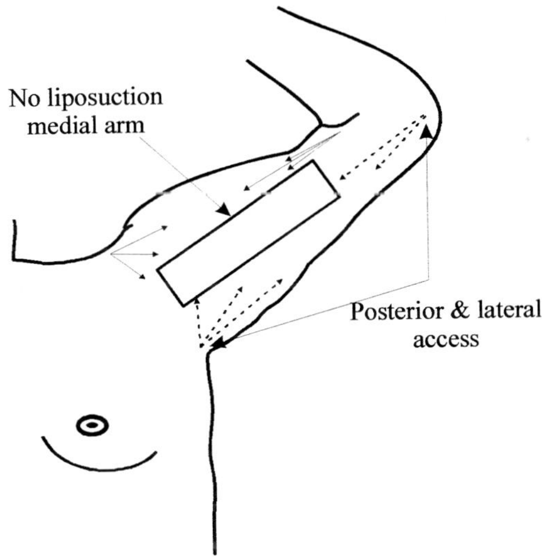

FIGURE 19 Access sites for suction lipectomy of the arm. In the middle part of the inner arm, skin is thin and loose and suction lipectomy of this area causes more looseness and should be avoided. Brachioplasty improves the contour, but causes scarring.

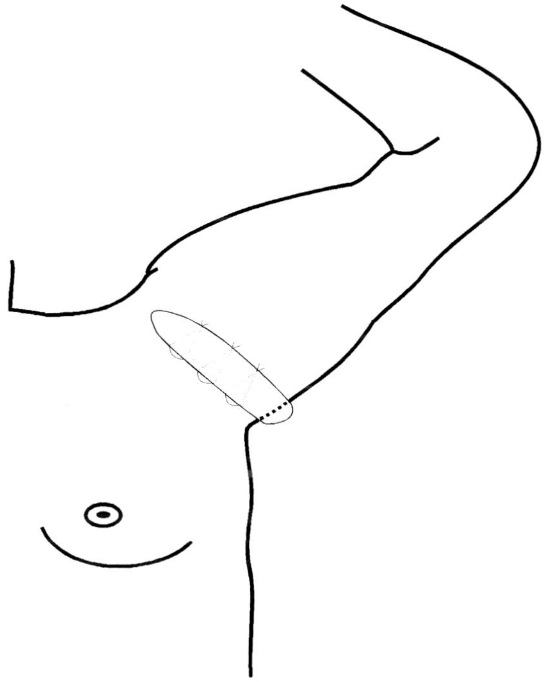

FIGURE 20 The "ridge" plication of the axilla after SAL with horizontal suturing.

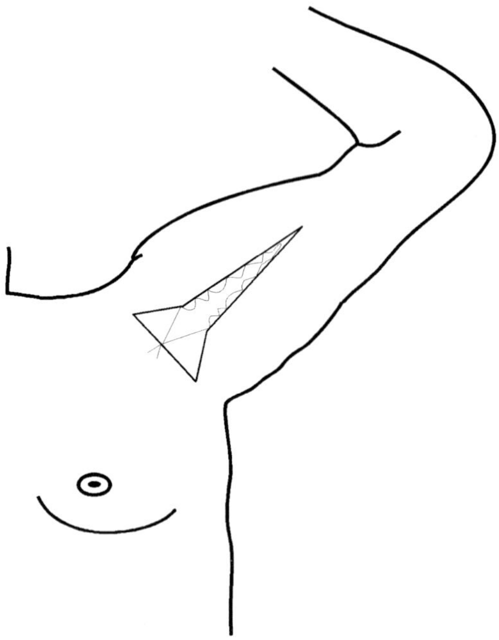

FIGURE 21 Short T-skin excision and purse-string suture closure to reduce the length of the scar.

Group I: Minimal to Moderate Subcutaneous Fat with Minimal Skin Laxity

Patients in this group have a circumferential increase in fat volume but adequate skin turgor and elasticity. These individuals can benefit greatly from circumferential suction lipectomy only.

Case 15. A 19-year-old woman who underwent SAL of the arm. The patient is shown 3 months after surgery (Fig. 22).

Group II: Generalized Accumulation of Subcutaneous Fat with Moderate Skin Laxity

These patients can be treated with suction lipectomy alone [22]. However, many patients may also desire some tightening of the skin, which can be performed in the axilla after the lipectomy. The scar that remains is then less visible and is usually acceptable to the patient. These patients can also be treated with axillary ridge plication without excision.

After the circumferential suction lipectomy, a series of absorbable sutures (usually 2-0 or 3-0 Vicryl) are used to create a "ridge" in the axilla. The placement of these sutures begins by roughly gauging the degree of skin laxity. The first stitch is placed in the medial axillary hair-bearing area and run subcutaneously to exit about 1.5 to 2 in distal to the axilla. The suture is then run back medially through the same

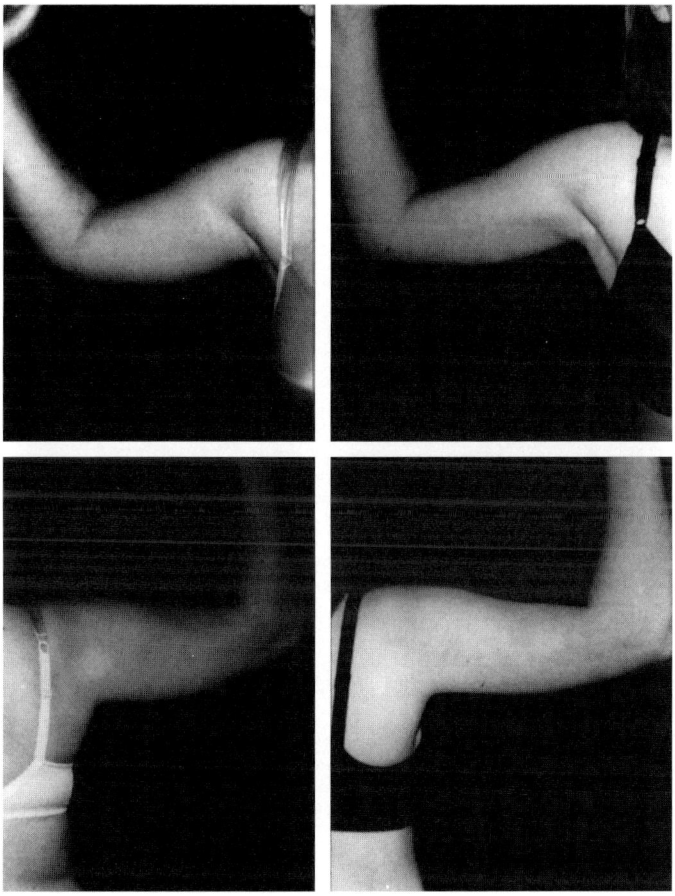

FIGURE 22 **See p. 596 for details.**

exit site. It emerges adjacent to the entry of the suture, much like a mattress stitch. Four to five stitches are placed along the axilla in this manner (Fig. 20). Once the sutures are removed or have dissolved (3–4 weeks), the ridge in the axilla flattens and becomes smooth.

In a subgroup of these patients, the ridge may remain very prominent. Excision of the ridge can be performed at the time of the first procedure if deemed necessary. More likely, it will become evident as a persistent edge, which may be excised under local anesthesia several weeks later. After excision, the wound is closed by using a routine subcuticular suture to avoid the hatch-markings of external sutures. In these cases, the scar is confined to the axilla that enables the patient to wear short-sleeve or sleeveless garments.

Case 16. A 33-year-old woman underwent suction lipectomy with "ridge plication." The patient is shown before surgery, immediately after surgery, and 5 months after surgery. The fold has flattened without skin excision (Fig. 23).

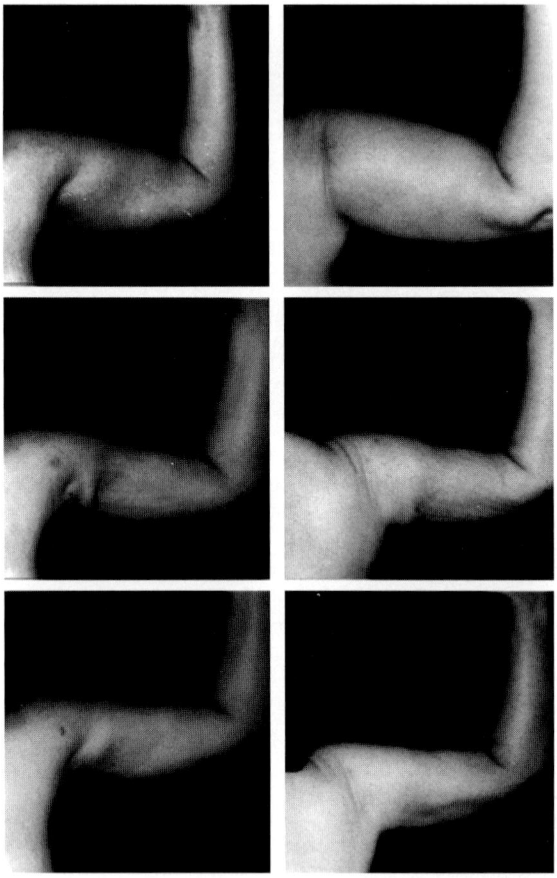

FIGURE 23 Frontal view of the axilla (left); posterior flipped image of the right arm for better and easier comparison (right). Top row shows before surgery. The middle row shows immediately after surgery with ridge plication. The bottom row shows 5 months after surgery.

Group III: Generalized Obesity and Extensive Skin Laxity

This group consists of patients who have excess fat and a substantial amount of loose skin (Fig. 24, top). In these cases, suction lipectomy will decrease the bulk of the tissue, but will not correct the ptosis. These patients will require an incision down the upper arm to achieve the best possible result. After performing circumferential suction lipectomy without any undermining, the skin of the medial upper one half to one third of the arm is resected. The resected skin defect is T-shaped with a widened base (Fig. 21). This defect is made considerably smaller by applying a purse-string suture that tightens the skin in the lower portion of the upper arm. A running subcuticular stitch of heavy absorbable suture is started in the medial axilla and taken around the incision back to the axilla and tied together. This maneuver reduces the length of the incision, thereby improving the aesthetic nature of the scar.

(a)

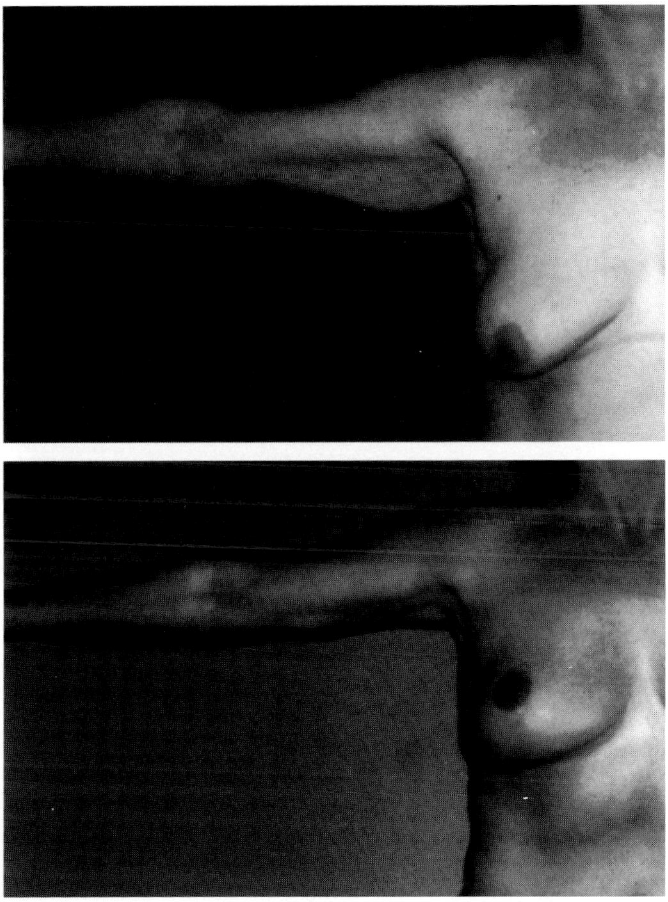

(b)

FIGURE 24 (a) Before surgery; (b) after surgery.

Case 17. A 40-year-old female with fatty arm, loose skin, and breast ptosis underwent bilateral mastopexy, arm SAL, T-skin resection, and purse-string suturing. The patient is shown 8 months after surgery (Fig. 24, bottom).

Group IV: Minimal Subcutaneous Fat and Extensive Skin Laxity

These patients are often older than those in the other groups. They show marked skin laxity and depletion of subcutaneous fat either as a result of the aging process or from massive weight loss, making brachioplasty the procedure of choice [32]. The objective is to decrease the excess skin and fat, while at the same time creating a cosmetically acceptable scar. Placement of the incision line in the brachial sulcus of the medial arm serves to hide the scar [34]. These patients must be advised of the necessity for skin tightening to avoid ptosis and of the possibility that the scars will remain visible after the brachioplasty. The surgeon should therefore establish that the patient is sufficiently motivated to accept the scarring. It is essential to inform the patient about the position and extent of the scars that will remain, because they will probably be visible when short-sleeved clothing is worn [27]. We use drains in these patients, because there is a tendency for seroma formation with extensive suctioning.

Case 18. A 42-year-old woman with marked laxity of the skin underwent brachioplasty. The patient is shown 8 months after surgery (Fig. 25).

ABDOMEN

In evaluating the abdomen, the following should be assessed:

1. Distribution of fat above and below the umbilicus.
2. Presence of a double bulge with depression at the belt line.
3. Determination of the edge of the rectus muscle.
4. Presence of a rectus diastasis or ventral hernia.
5. Abdominal scarring and any associated contraction.
6. Mons pubus ptosis or swelling.
7. Waist size.
8. Belt line location and area for desired reduction.
9. Determination of internal and external abdominal obesity.
10. Stretch marks and looseness of skin.

The patient's goals for abdominal liposuction must be established. It needs to be determined if a patient desires a smaller abdomen and waistline to improve their appearance in clothing or if they would like to have a firm abdomen that would be exposed to the public. Different goals require different procedures [35]. In addition,

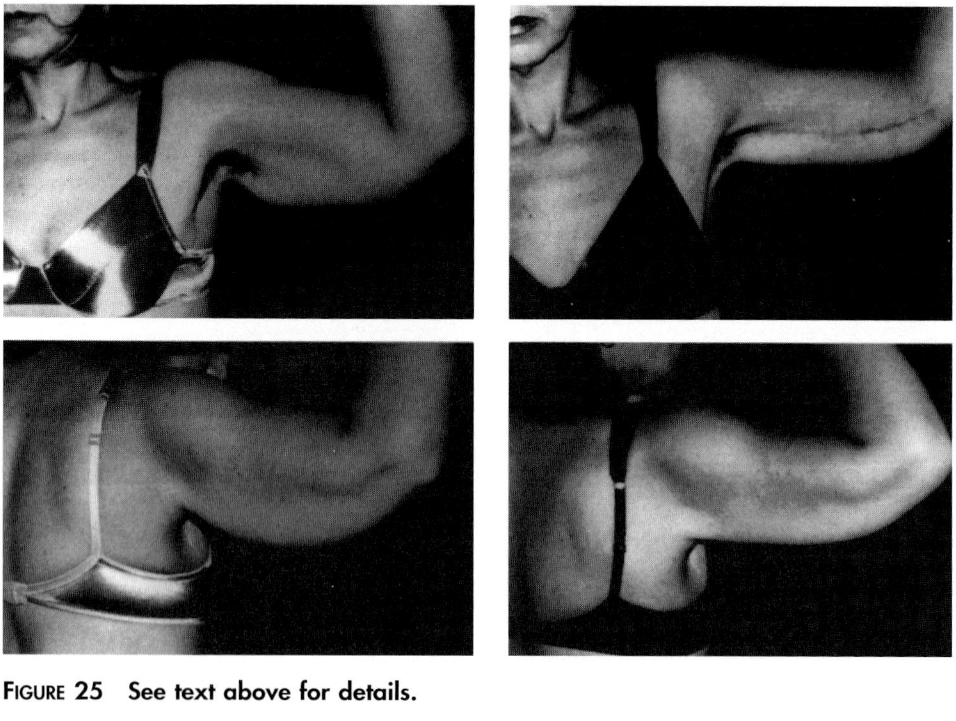

FIGURE 25 See text above for details.

male body builders frequently request cross hatching to create a semblance of rectus muscle contraction or "six-pack."

Scars on the abdomen may need release, fat augmentation, or revision. Finally, a patient with loose abdominal skin may require an abdominoplasty in addition to SAL. The type of abdomen has been divided into four categories by Matarasso [30]. In our experience, the treatment has been suction alone, suction with cincture, and suction and abdominoplasty or extended abdominoplasty. The scope plication, mini abdominoplasty, or lowering of the umbilicus has not been useful in the majority of our patients.

Marking and Surgery

The abdomen can be accessed through a variety of incisions: suprapubic, infraumbilical, supraumbilical, epigastric, iliac, and midlateral abdominal at the level of the anterior axillary line. Through the suprapubic and lateral abdominal incision, both UAL and SAL can be used (Fig. 26). Through a midline incision, superficial liposuction can be performed to create a midline groove. Through lateral incisions, horizontal superficial liposuction can be performed to create a semblance of tendinous

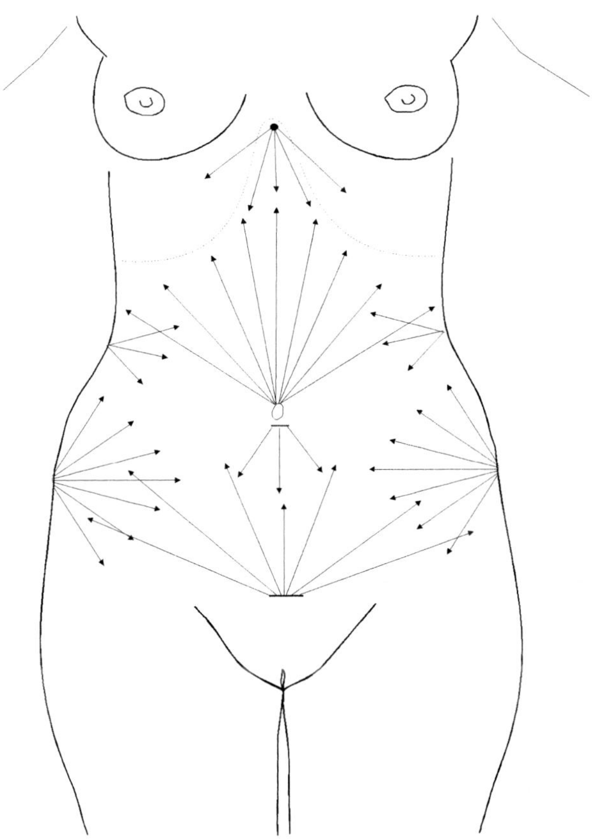

FIGURE 26 Access sites for suction lipectomy of the abdomen and flanks. Through flank and suprapubic incisions, UAL and SAL can be performed.

insertion of the rectus muscle to give a more muscular physique to an amorphous abdomen. Also, during presurgical marking, the waistline needs to be identified for possible suture cincture [6].

Clinical Cases

Case 19. A 30-year-old Hispanic patient s/p hysterectomy through a midline incision who desired a slimmer appearance in her clothing. She underwent suction lipectomy of the abdomen and flanks. The patient's body contour improved and she looks better in clothes (Fig. 27).

Case 20. A 32-year-old male underwent a 5,500-ml suction lipectomy of the breast, abdomen, and flanks with release of the inframammary line. The patient is shown 8 months after surgery (Fig. 28).

Case 21. A 38-year-old male underwent 9,000-ml SAL and UAL of the breast, abdomen, flanks, and back, with partial excision of the glandular breast after

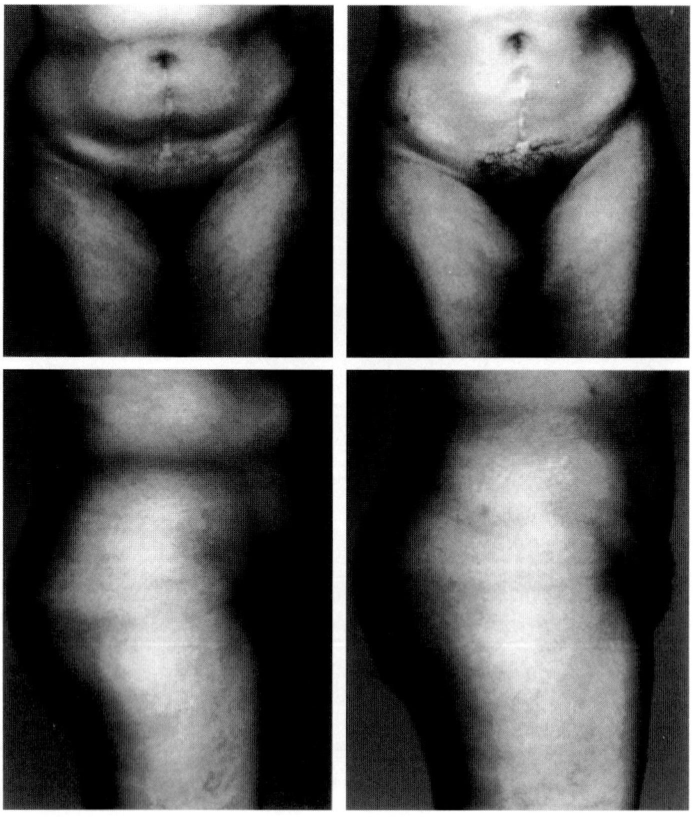

FIGURE 27 See text above for details.

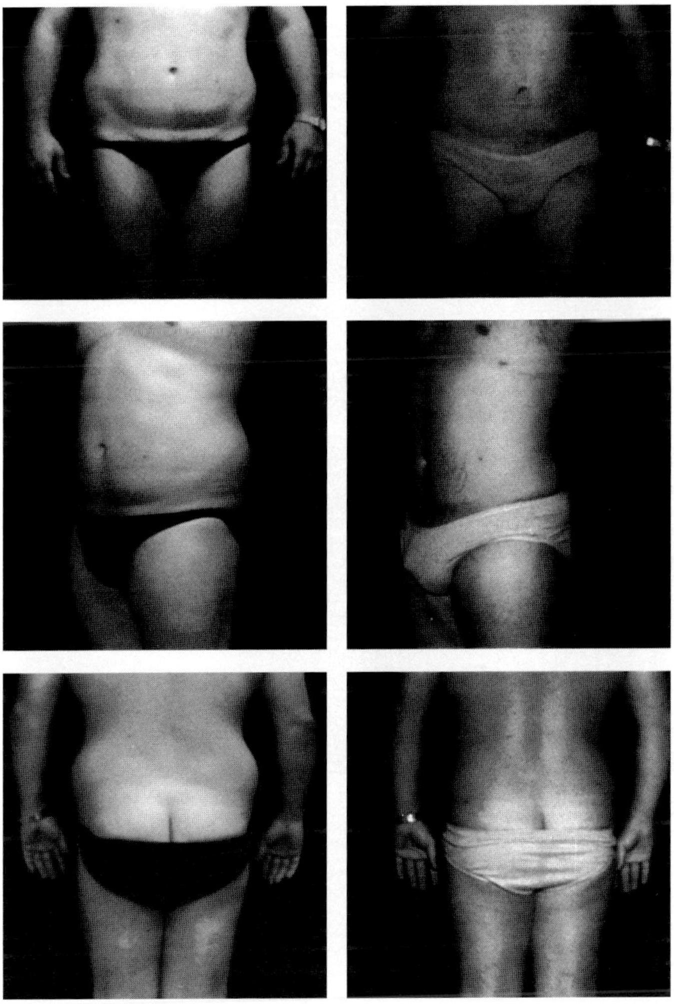

FIGURE 28 See p. 602 for details.

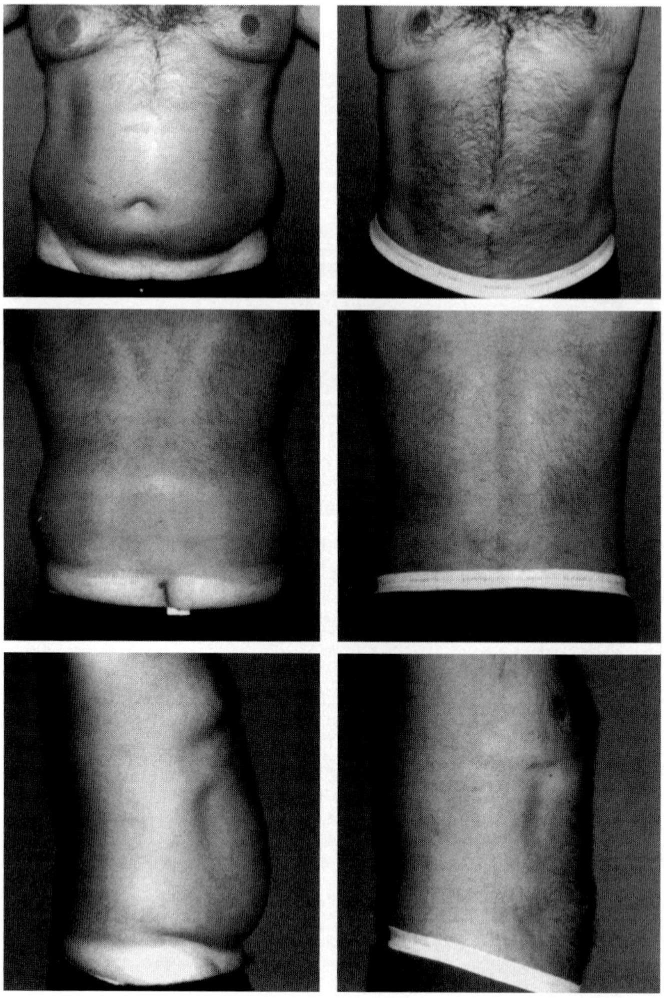

FIGURE 29 See pp. 602–604 for details.

SAL and UAL and release of inframammary line. The patient is shown 1 year after surgery (Fig. 29).

Case 22. A 30-year-old male with truncal obesity and asthma underwent 11-L SAL and UAL of the breast, abdomen, and flanks. The patient's asthma improved after surgery. The patient is shown 6 months after surgery. The patient refused abdominoplasty that could have improved the aesthetic result (Fig. 30).

Case 23. A 32-year-old female underwent suction lipectomy of the abdomen, flanks, and trochanter, with lipograft to the abdominal scar, infratrochanter, and scar release (Fig. 31).

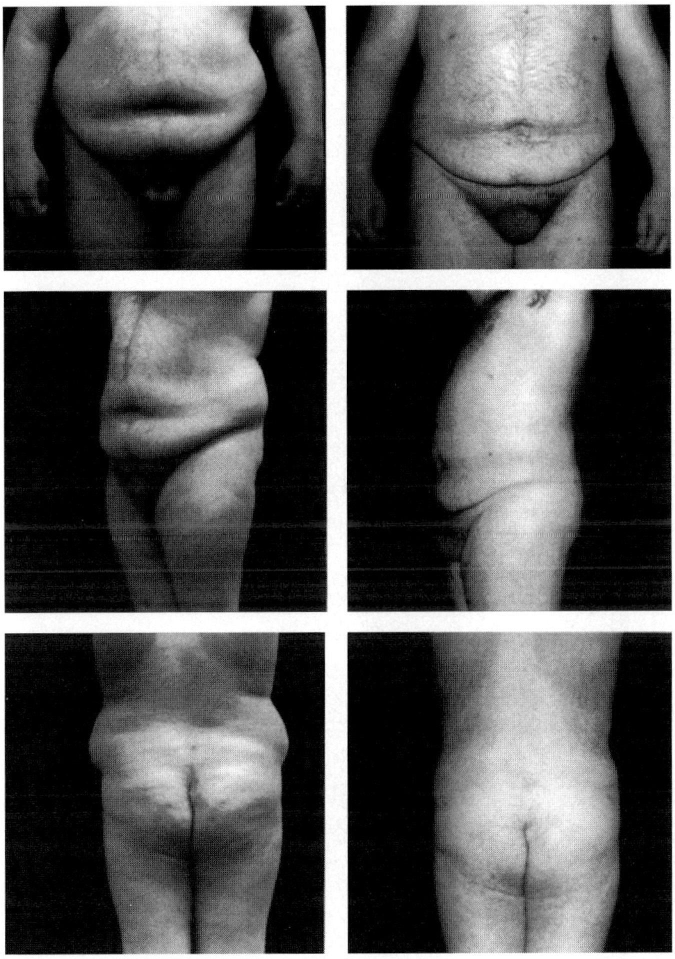

FIGURE 30 See p. 604 for details.

WAISTLINE CINCTURE

Frequently, patients with a wide waistline will desire a narrow torso without large skin incisions. This can be performed with waistline cincture [36]. The waist-narrowing technique may be performed alone but is usually performed in conjunction with other body contouring procedures.

Marking and Surgery

Presurgical marking is performed with the patient in the standing position. Problem areas are outlined, and sites of access incisions are determined and marked.

After general anesthesia is administered, the patient is prepared and draped in the standard manner for abdominoplasty [2]. The patient first undergoes ultrasound-

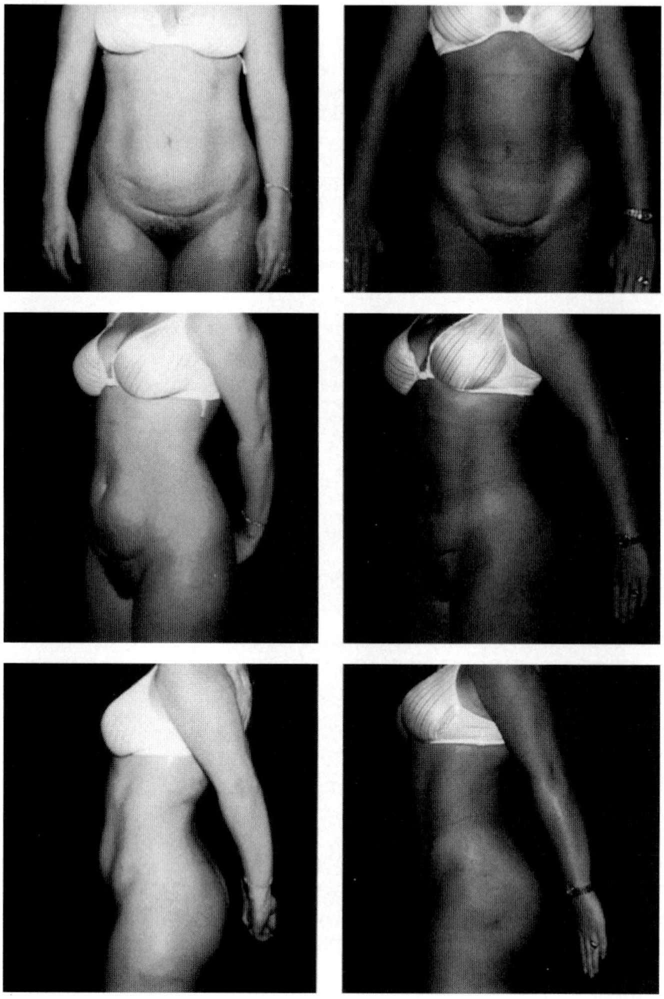

FIGURE 31 See p. 604 for details.

assisted lipoplasty and traditional tumescent liposuction of the abdomen, hips, and flanks as needed [37].

On completion of the UAL of the flanks and SAL of the flanks and abdomen, with the patient in the supine position, bilateral stab incisions are made in the previously defined waistline or desired "tension point." The incisions are less than 0.5 cm in length and are carried down through the subcutaneous tissue. A similar incision is made in the midline of the suprapubic area, at the hairline. Incisions from suctioning of the upper and lower abdomen will be present above and below the umbilicus (Fig. 32A). A slightly curved suction canula is passed through the upper umbilical incision toward the lateral waist incision on one side. After undermining of the cannula subcutaneously, a 0-Monocryl or comparable absorbable tie is passed

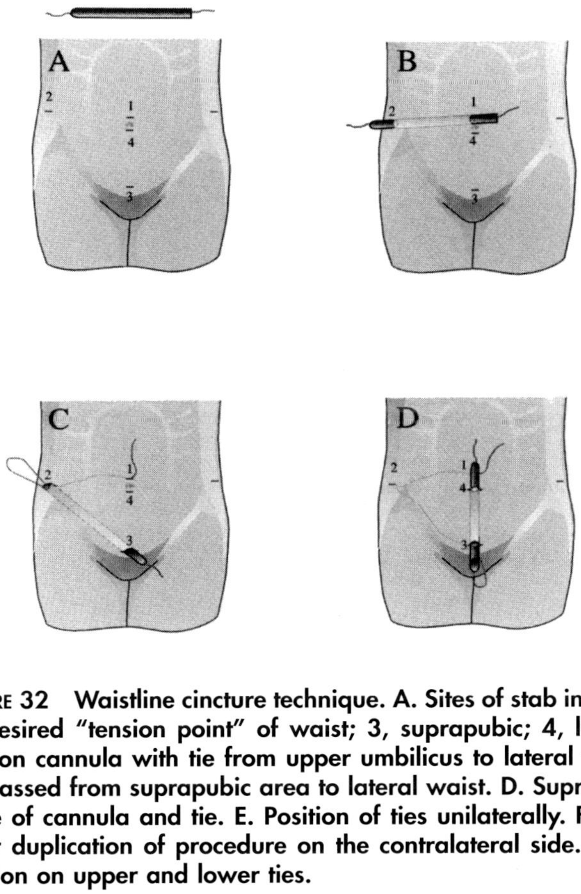

FIGURE 32 Waistline cincture technique. A. Sites of stab incisions are 1, above umbilicus; 2, desired "tension point" of waist; 3, suprapubic; 4, lower umbilicus. B. Passing of suction cannula with tie from upper umbilicus to lateral waist. C. Suction cannula and tie passed from suprapubic area to lateral waist. D. Suprapubic to lower umbilical passage of cannula and tie. E. Position of ties unilaterally. F. Final arrangement of all ties after duplication of procedure on the contralateral side. G. Result after application of tension on upper and lower ties.

through the cannula (Fig. 32B). The cannula is removed over the tie, and clamps are applied to each end of the tie.

In the same manner, the suction cannula is passed subcutaneously from the suprapubic incision to the same lateral waist incision. The clamp is removed and the tie is passed through the cannula to now exit the suprapubic region (Fig. 32c). Again, the cannula is removed over the tie and clamped. Another pass of the suction cannula is made from the lower umbilical incision toward the suprapubic incision. The tie is passed through the cannula in the same fashion from suprapubic to lower umbilicus and the cannula is removed (Fig. 32D, E).

Attention is then turned to the contralateral side, where the same steps are followed. At this point, two separate ties should be clamped at the upper umbilical incision, with their distal ends clamped at the lower umbilical incision (Fig. 32F).

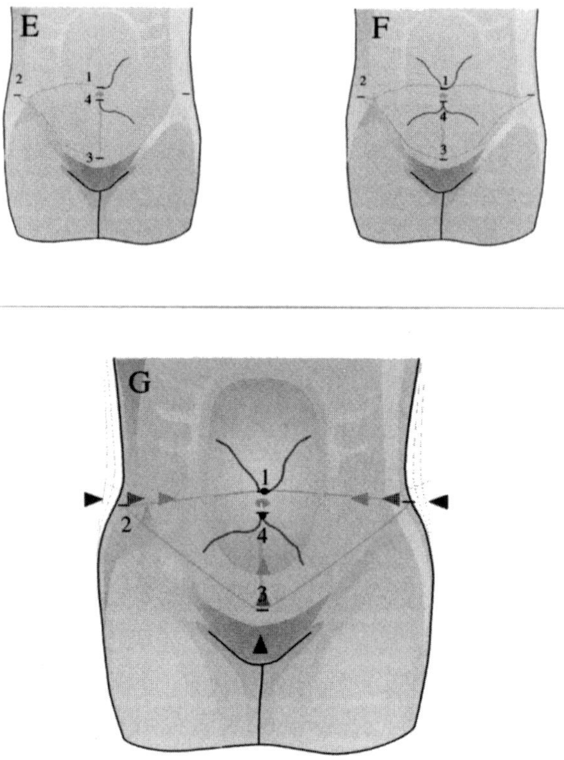

FIGURE 32 Continued

Tension is applied by pulling on both sets of clamps, while at the same time visually inspecting for a "dimpling effect" and the proper waistline tightening. Once we are satisfied with the result, the lower umbilical ties are kept under tension while the upper umbilical ties are secured with eight to 10 knots. The same is then done for the lower umbilical ties (Fig. 32G).

Clinical Cases

Case 24. A 46-year-old male patient with a wide waistline and obese abdomen. The patient wanted abdominoplasty for reduction of the waistline. The patient underwent UAL and SAL of the abdomen flanks with waistline cincture. A total of 4,000 ml was aspirated. The patient is shown 1 month after surgery. The patient is happy that he did not have abdominoplasty (Fig. 33).

Case 25. A 47-year-old male patient underwent UAL of the flanks and SAL of the breast, abdomen, and back, with etching of the abdominal wall and waistline cincture. A total of 3,100 ml was aspirated. The patient is shown 6 months after surgery (Fig. 34).

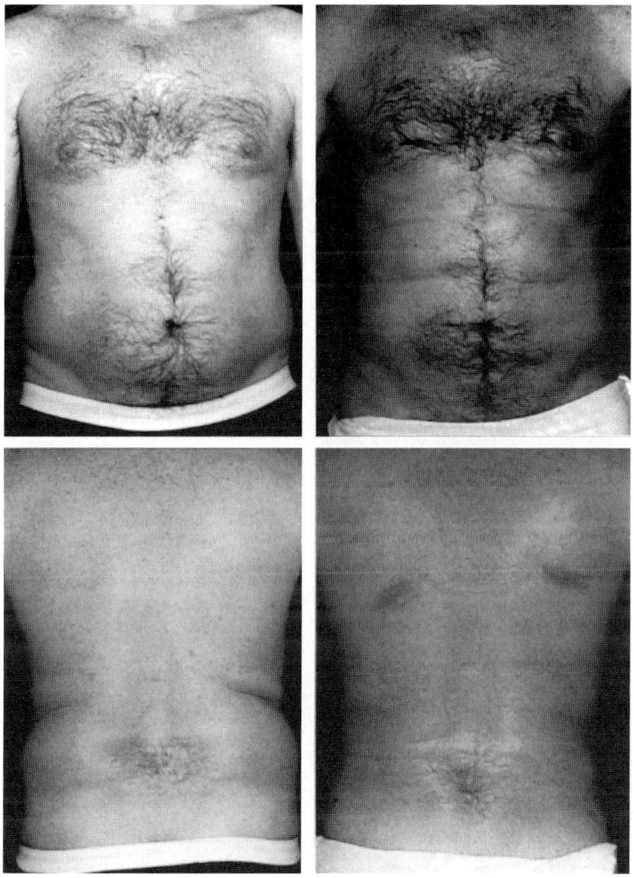

FIGURE 33 See p. 608 for details.

MULTIPLE PROCEDURES

When liposuction is performed in conjunction with other reduction procedures, the suctioning is performed first. Reduction mammoplasty and/or abdominoplasty is then performed. Additional touch-up suctioning or lipograft will be performed last.

Clinical Cases

Case 26. A 59-year-old female s/p abdominoplasty, suction of the abdomen and flanks. She is shown after surgery and 4 years after surgery (Fig. 35).

Case 27. A 37-year-old female had a history of hypothyroidism and right hip pain secondary to hip fracture 17 years earlier, and also complained of back pain. The patient's right femur was shorter than the left. Before surgery, her weight was 220 lbs. The patient underwent abdominoplasty and 1500-ml UAL and SAL of each flank. After surgery, her back and hip pain improved substantially. Her exercise level increased. Her 6-month postsurgical weight was 193 lbs (Fig. 36).

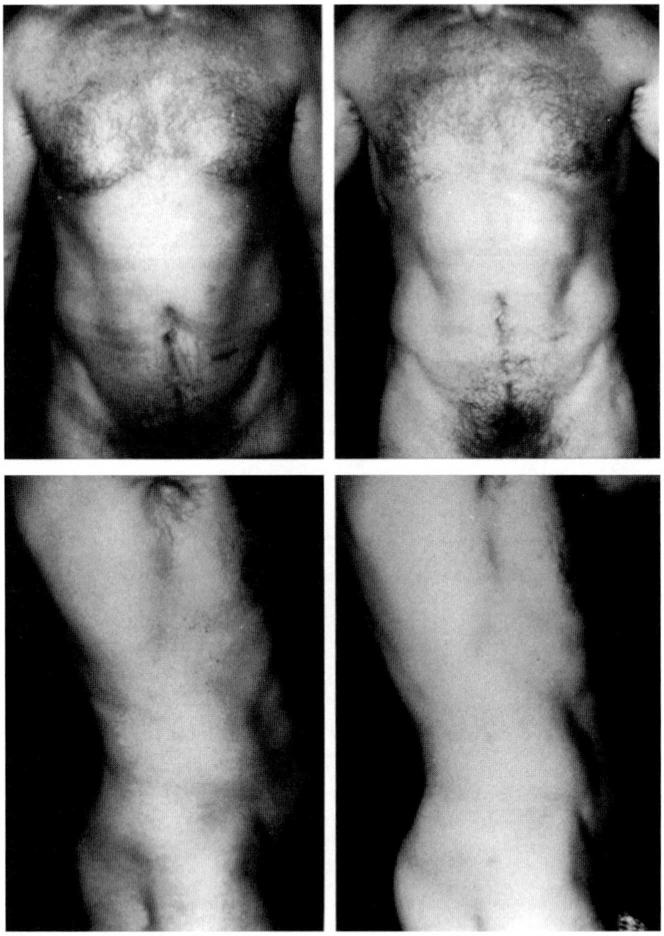

FIGURE 34 **See p. 608 for details.**

Case 28. A 47-year-old male with chronic back pain, skin irritation, and gynecomastia. Presurgical weight was 250 lbs. He underwent 5 minutes of UAL to each breast and chest wall and 950-ml SAL of each breast. The inframammary line was released and extended abdominoplasty was performed. The weight of abdominal specimen was 10 lbs. The patient is shown 1 year after surgery. He no longer complains of back pain. He is able to exercise and his 1-year postsurgical weight is 210 lbs (Fig. 37).

Case 29. A 47-year-old overweight female with breast hypertrophy and back and neck pain. The patient received physical therapy for 1 year with no relief. The patient's presurgical weight was 167 lbs. The patient underwent bilateral breast reduction, abdominoplasty, and 750-ml SAL of each flank. Release of supra flank and back depression with lipograft and suction of elevated folds. After surgery, the patient

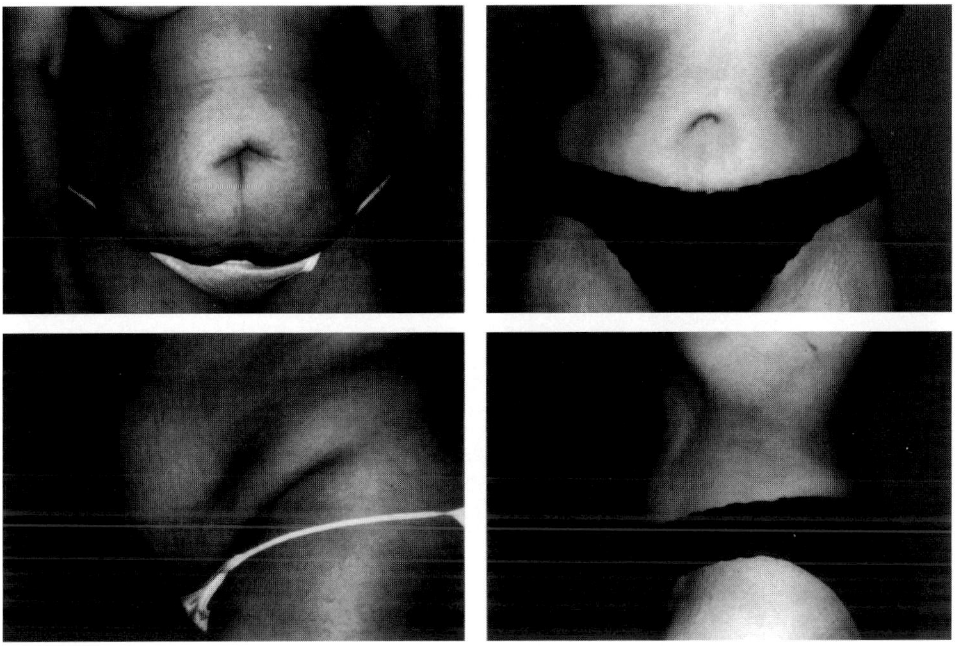

FIGURE 35 **See p. 609 for details.**

reported no neck or back pain. The patient stopped physical therapy. At 1 year, her postsurgical weight was 153 lbs (Fig. 38).

Case 30. A 48-year-old female underwent bilateral breast reduction, suction lipectomy of the torso, and abdominoplasty. The patient is shown 9 months after surgery (Fig. 39).

Case 31. A 40-year-old female with weight gain presented for weight reduction surgery. Her presurgical weight was 289 lbs. The patients underwent bilateral breast reduction with removal of 4 lbs, abdominoplasty, and suction lipectomy of the flanks and back. Six months later, the patient underwent 18-L UAL and SAL of the trunk and flanks with lipograft to the depressed area. The patient received two units of autologous blood transfusion after surgery. The patient's weight decreased to 242 lbs. Her clothing size went from 26 to 18. The fullness in the epigastric area is attributable to intra-abdominal obesity. The patient is shown 1 year after surgery (Fig. 40).

Case 32. A 40-year-old female after a 65-lb weight loss underwent bilateral mastopexy, abdominoplasty, 350-ml SAL of each flank, SAL of each trunk side fold, and 50-ml of lipograft to side depressions and inner thigh lift. The patient also had superficial liposuction of the supraumbilical region in the midline of the abdominal wall. The patient is shown 1 year after surgery (Fig. 41). Despite SAL of the flanks, the patient still has flank fullness that required flank excision of extended abdominoplasty.

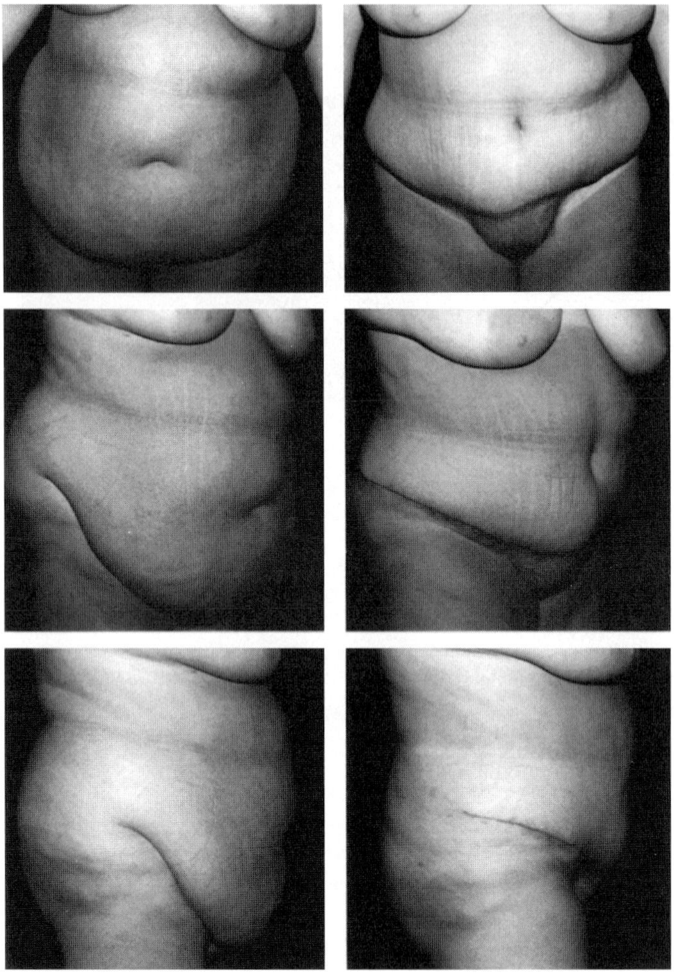

FIGURE 36 See p. 609 for details.

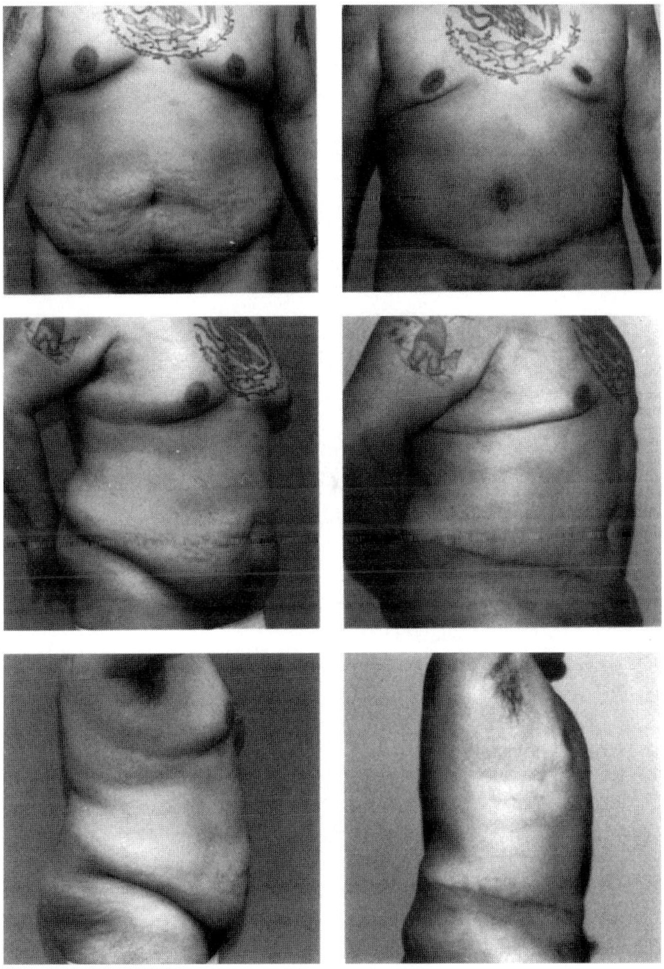

FIGURE 37 **See p. 610 for details.**

FLANKS AND BACK

Evaluation

Liposuctioning of the flanks is usually performed before completing the abdomen or lower extremity. The back usually requires suctioning in obese patients or when there are multiple folds. Also, thick lateral chest and back make the body disproportionate to the arm and the neck. Therefore, all these areas need to be marked for suctioning.

Marking and Surgery

If the patient has mild and anterior flank fat deposits, the access can be obtained in the supine position through an iliac incision. However, if the fat deposit is postero-lateral, we use the lateral decubitus position for suctioning. All supra flank depressions will be accessed through a small incision to release and lipograft. Also, if

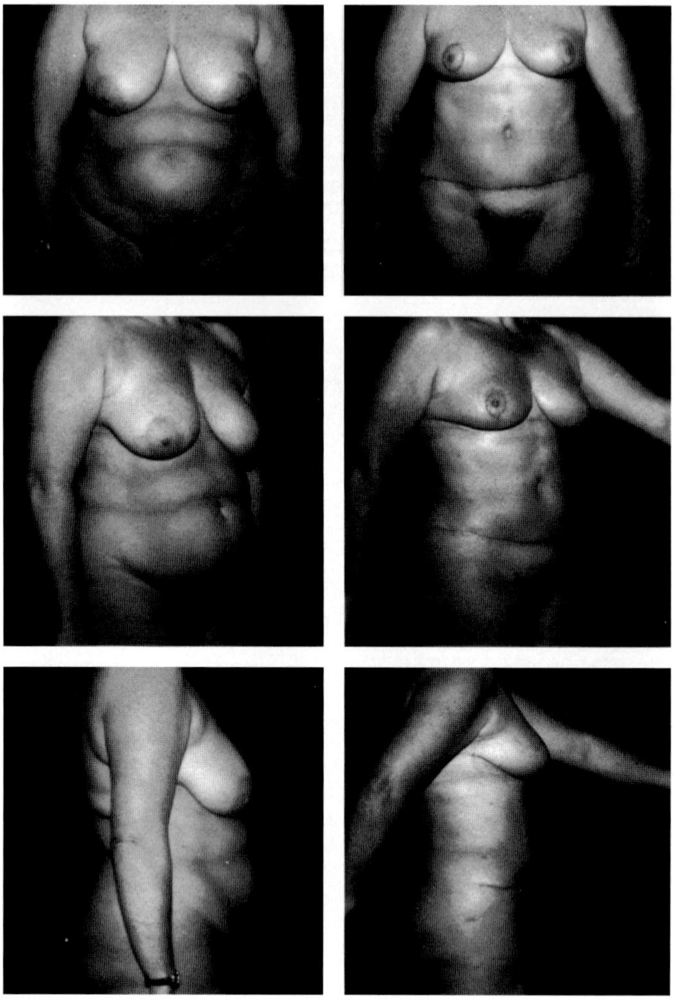

FIGURE 38 See pp. 610–611 for details.

needed, a second incision is made posteriorly for posterior and upper gluteal SAL. The central area of the back over the spine area should be avoided. If the patient has had previous lumbar surgery, that area is also avoided (Fig. 42).

Clinical Cases

Case 33. A 32-year-old female with back truncal obesity with no definition between the trunk and the buttocks. Also, the patient had multiple folds on the back. The patient underwent suction lipectomy of the back as well as release of folds and lipograft. The patient also had extended breast reduction and frontal surgeries. The improvement in the upper-back fold is partially attributable to excision of the fold (Fig. 43).

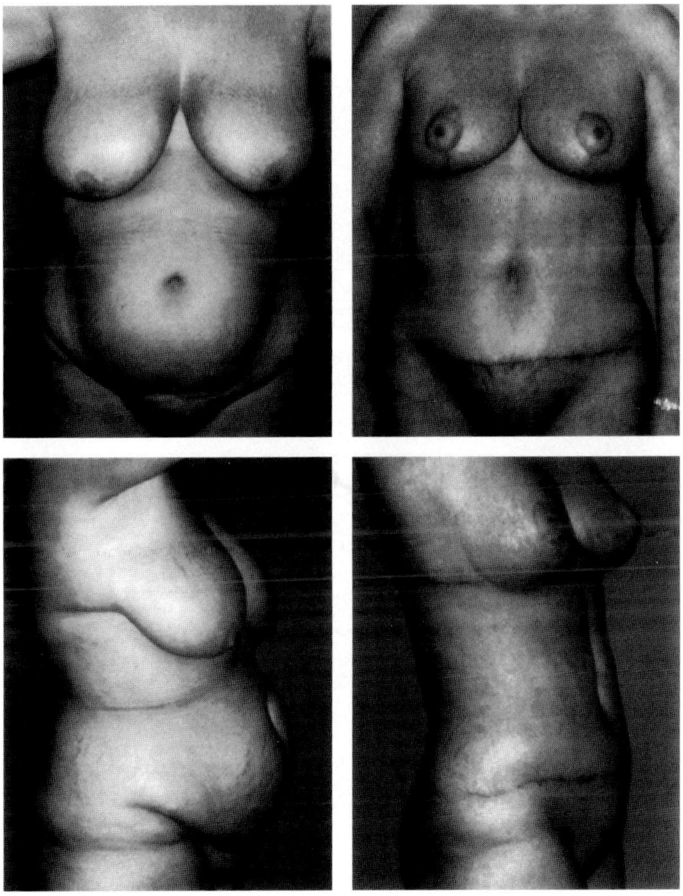

FIGURE 39 See p. 611 for details.

LOWER EXTREMITY

Evaluation

In evaluation of patients for lower extremity suction, flanks need to be studied as part of the lower extremities. The frontal, lateral, and posterior views of the nude, standing patient should be examined [2,38]. The following observations are noted:

1. Flank prominence
2. Trochanteric prominence
3. Squareness or roundness of posterior silhouette
4. Presence of cellulitis
5. Presence of asymmetry
6. Lateral gluteal depression and presence of banana fold
7. Status of skin
8. Asymmetry of gluteal fold

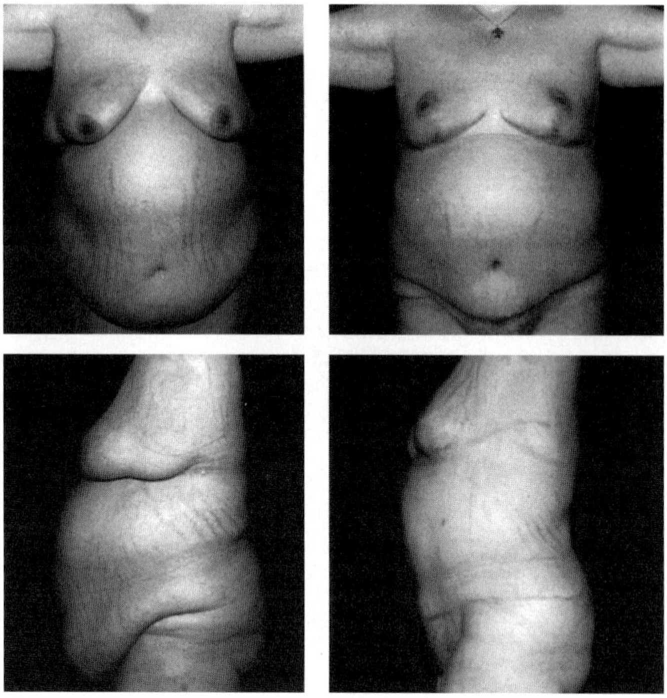

FIGURE 40 **See p. 611 for details.**

Again, the patient's goals from liposuction are determined. Patients with large thighs and a small waist may have difficulty with tight-fitting clothing. Patients more frequently desire improvement in both the belt and thigh areas. Also, the patient needs to contract the gluteal muscle while the trochanteric area and flank are evaluated. This maneuver can shift some of the soft tissue that can present after surgery as swelling or bulges. Patients with very loose and thin skin may have a worsening of their appearance with suctioning. These patients may be better candidates for extended abdominoplasty and inner-thigh lift [38] or lower-body lifting [39,40]. Finally, the fat around the knee and calf is assessed for suctioning to give the patient better definition.

The patient is advised that for 6 to 8 weeks after surgery, tight garments are to be worn and treated areas are to be massaged. If the patient is unable to carry this out, liposuction should not be considered. Also, the patient should be cautioned that there is a chance of irregularities and that further surgery may be required [33].

Marking and Surgery

Our marking for trochanteric liposuction is the same as L. Toledo's [2]. The lateral point of the trochanter is marked. Then, a mark is made at the lateral aspect of the gluteal fold to the trochanter. If there is a banana roll medial to that area, it is marked.

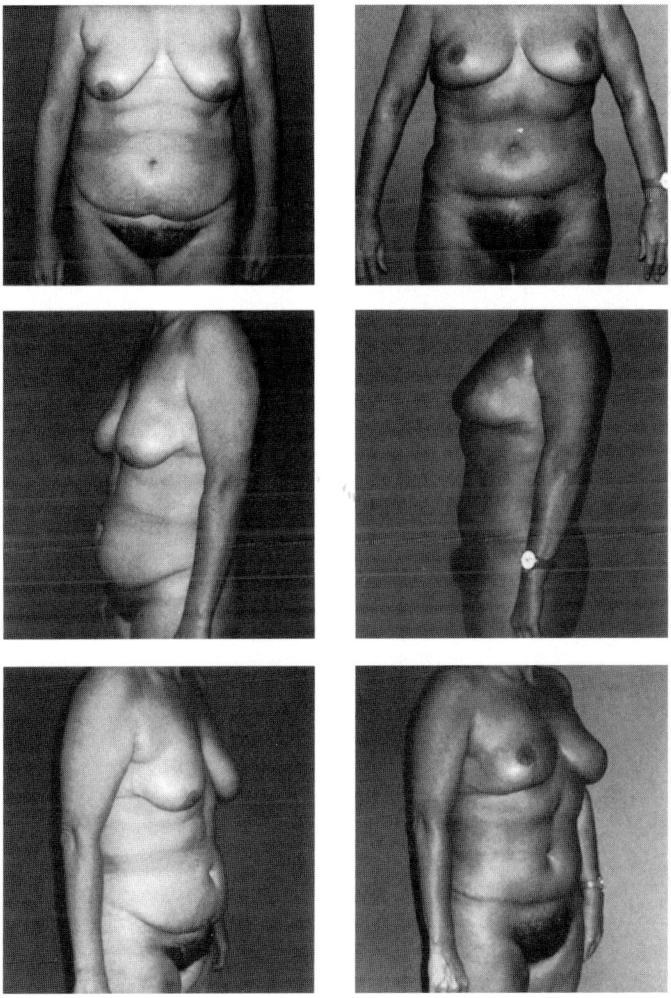

FIGURE 41 See p. 611 for details.

Care is taken when suctioning to avoid the posterior upper-mid thigh because this may lower the gluteal fold. This is very noticeable for patients that wear high-cut bikinis, where the buttock ptosis appears and any asymmetries become noticeable. Depressions from cellulite are marked for release. Superior to the trochanteric area, depressions are marked for fat augmentation.

After marking, the patient is placed in the supine and lateral decubitus position to observe the shift of fat. This is helpful in estimating the amount of fat to be removed. Some heavy patients require reduction of the buttock. Buttocks access can be obtained in the lower lumbar area. Access can be obtained through the flank area

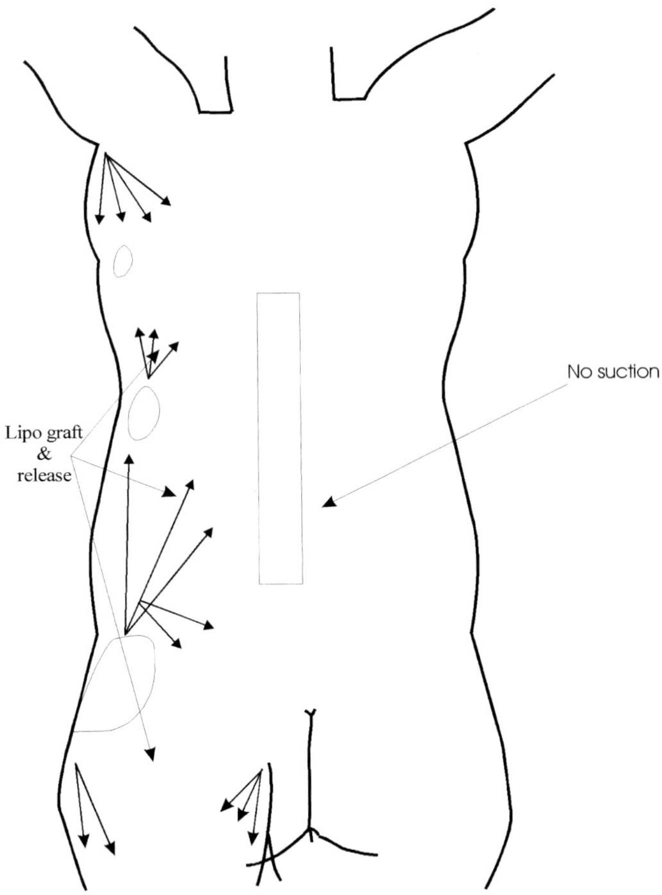

FIGURE 42 Access sites for suction lipectomy of the back and flanks. The areas for suction and release with lipografts are shown.

for lateral and superior gluteal areas. Also, in extremely obese legs, the anterior thigh area may need SAL (Fig. 44).

The portal for suctioning the knee is marked at the popliteal fossa crease anteriorly. Through this incision, areas above and below the knee can be reached. Lateral access is marked lateral to the patella. Occasional access is gained superior to the patella. Also, sometimes through mid-medial thigh access, the knee area can be suctioned. The calf can be accessed proximally from the medial and lateral popliteal fossa area and distally through access at either side of the achilles tendon (Fig. 45).

Clinical Cases

Case 34. A 22-year-old patient had square buttocks and prominent flanks. The patient underwent SAL of the flanks, trochanter, and inner thigh with fat graft to infraflank area. The patient is shown 1 year after surgery. The patient appears taller with thinner thighs (Fig. 46).

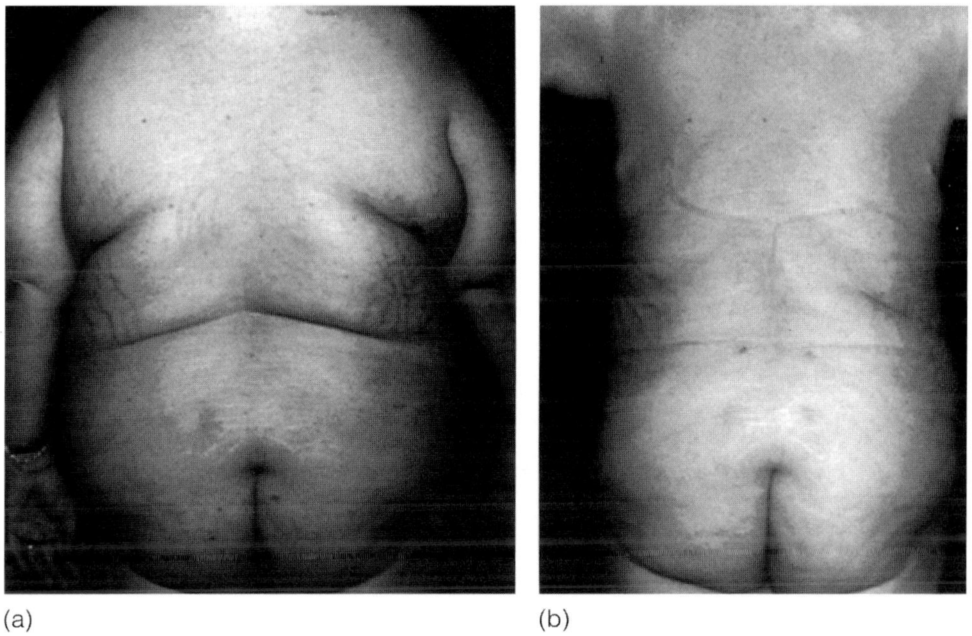

FIGURE 43 (a) Before surgery; (b) after surgery.

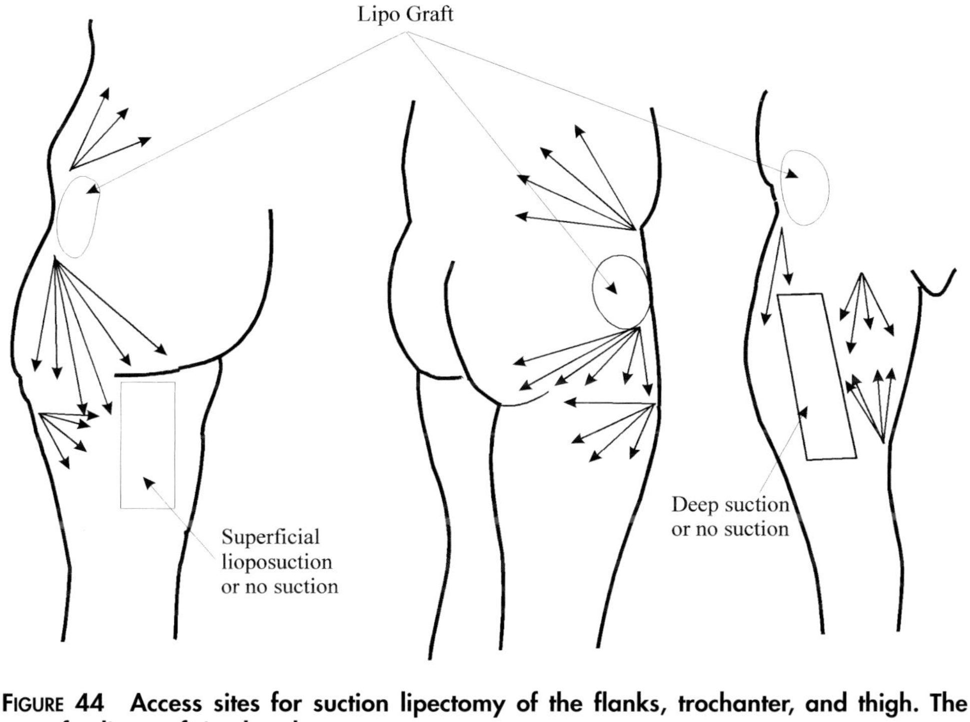

FIGURE 44 Access sites for suction lipectomy of the flanks, trochanter, and thigh. The area for lipograft is also shown.

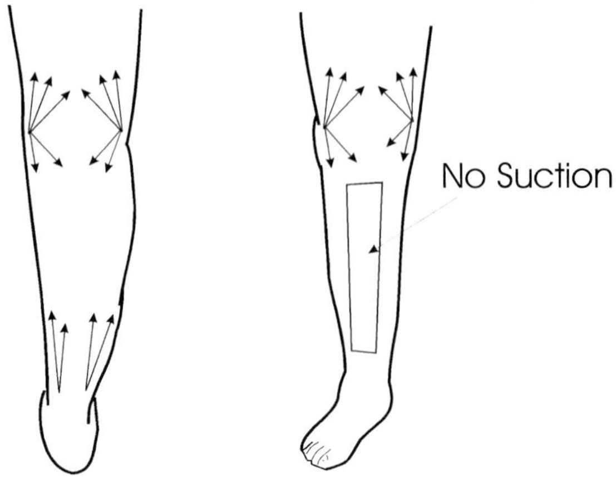

FIGURE 45 Access sites for suction lipectomy of the knee and calf areas.

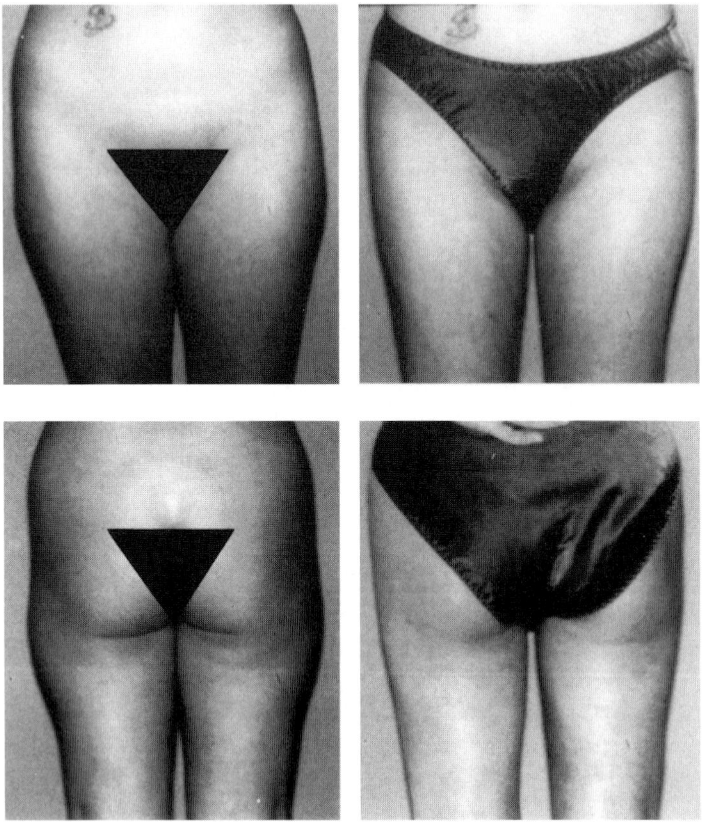

FIGURE 46 See p. 618 for details.

Case 35. A 40-year-old patient underwent SAL of the trochanter, flanks, and inner thigh with lipograft to depressed intraflank area (Fig. 47).

Case 36. A 38-year-old patient underwent approximately 8,000-ml UAL and SAL of the thigh and trochanter. The patient is shown 1 year after surgery and after weight gain (Fig. 48).

Case 37. A 40-year-old patient with a heavy calf underwent two-thirds semicircumferential suctioning of both knees and legs. The patient is shown 18 months after surgery (Fig. 49).

Case 38. A 37-year-old patient underwent semicircumferential suctioning of both knees and legs. The patient is shown 5 months after surgery (Fig. 50).

LIPOSUCTION FOR DIFFERENT PURPOSES

Liposuction can be used to debulk flaps, assist in closure of wounds without undermining, reduce the extent of the scar, or reduce depression of the wound after excisional surgery. In addition, suction lipectomy can be used for salvage cases.

Clinical Case

Case 39. A 42-year-old patient underwent secondary breast reduction with lowering of the nipple and areola by another surgeon. The patient developed partial areola and breast necrosis. The patient developed a flat and deformed asymmetric breast with loss of cleavage. The patient was salvaged after healing with lateral breast, chest wall, and sternal liposuction, plication of the chest skin to the sternum, and bilateral subpectoral augmentation mammoplasty with nipple and areola reconstruction. The patient, who had lost her self-confidence, now feels whole again (Fig. 51).

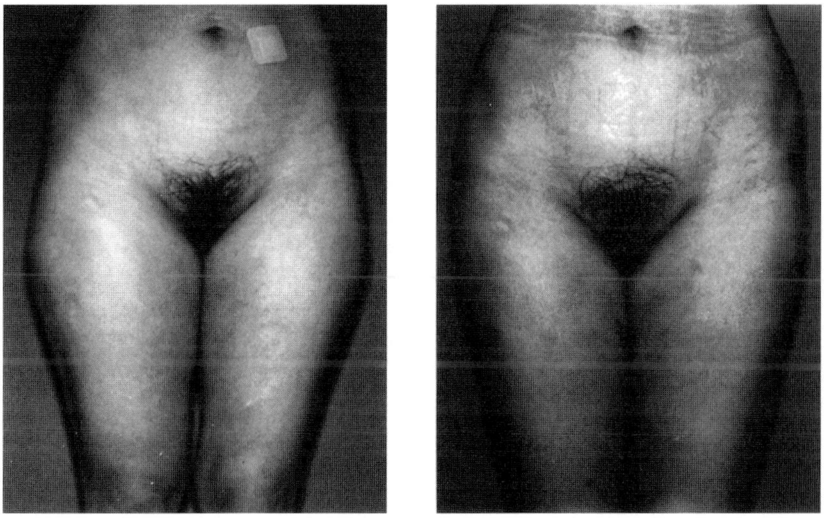

(a) (b)

FIGURE 47 (a) Before surgery; (b) after surgery.

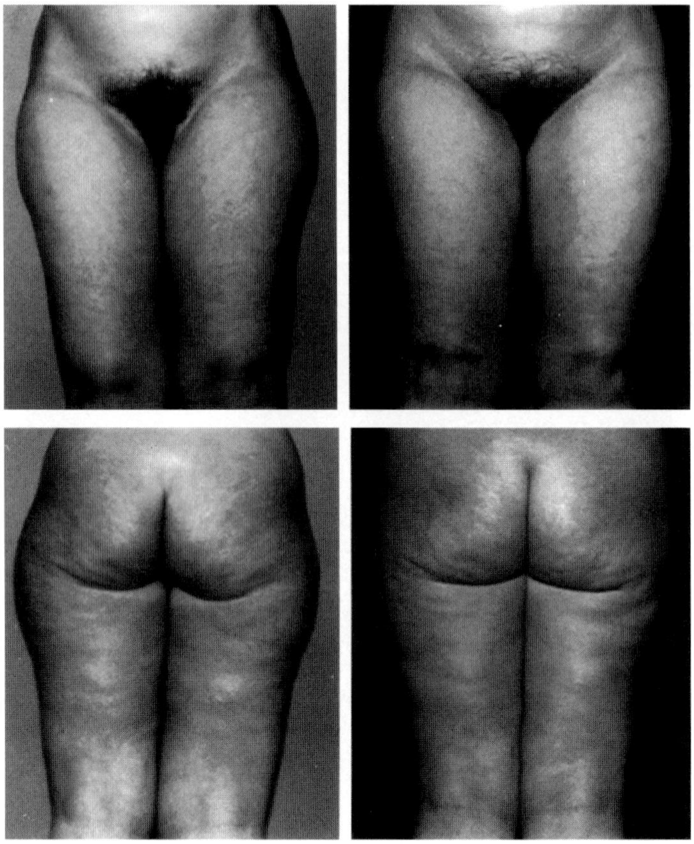

FIGURE 48 See p. 621 for details.

COMPLICATIONS OF SAL AND UAL

The incidence of complications from SAL has been reduced as a result of the improved cannula and suction machine design. However, complications still do occur.

Excessive bleeding after SAL is rarely a problem with the use of tumescent solution [41]. However, there have been reports of complications secondary to tumescent solution injection, such as pulmonary edema [42,43] and acute median nerve compression [44]. Procedural complications, such as fat embolisms [45], toxic shock syndrome [46], and necrotizing fasciitis [47], have been reported. Surgeons performing liposuction should be aware of each of these potential complications and be skilled in their management. Incorrect technique has been associated with cutaneous hyperpigmentation [48], rupture of the pectoralis muscle [49], and even penetration of the abdominal wall resulting in death. We are also aware of four cases of foot drop after liposuction of the lower extremity. Recovery of function occurred in each patient. In our opinion, this is a result of increased pressure on the peroneal nerve during surgery.

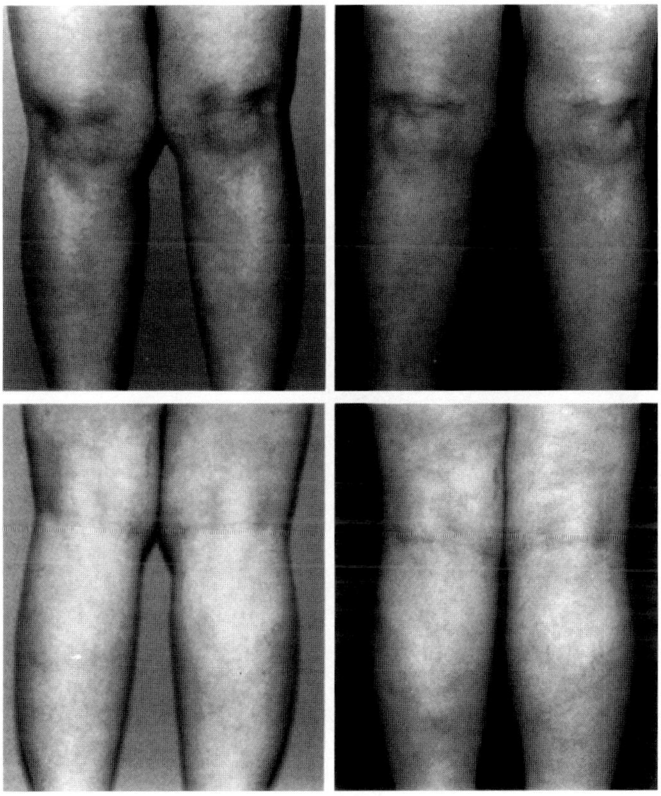

FIGURE 49 See p. 621 for details.

The most common complication associated with liposuction of the neck area is overtreatment that results in a contour deformity (Fig. 52). In addition, thin flaps scar to the platysma, giving an aesthetically displeasing result.

Aesthetically poor results also occur when suctioning of the lower face is not performed or the skin is not adequately undermined. The patient's central part of the neck will look good but laterally there are excess fat and bulges (Fig. 53). The treatment for this problem is facelift or lower-face suction with extensive neck undermining.

In the past, we used expanded poytetrafloroethylene (gortex) suture for plication. Our experience included one patient who rejected the gortex and another patient who had prolonged drainage and cellulitis (Fig. 54). As a result of these complications, we now use absorbable sutures for interlocking plication in the midline and anchoring to the mastoid fascia laterally.

Suction lipectomy of the face in individuals with thin skin can cause contour deformity secondary to hematomas and fat necrosis. Systemic steroid may be helpful, but local steroid injection can also lead to fat necrosis. The treatment for this problem is incision and drainage with scar release, which is necessary to correct the contour deformity. Also, secondary fat injection and secondary facelift with laser treatment may be required (Fig. 55).

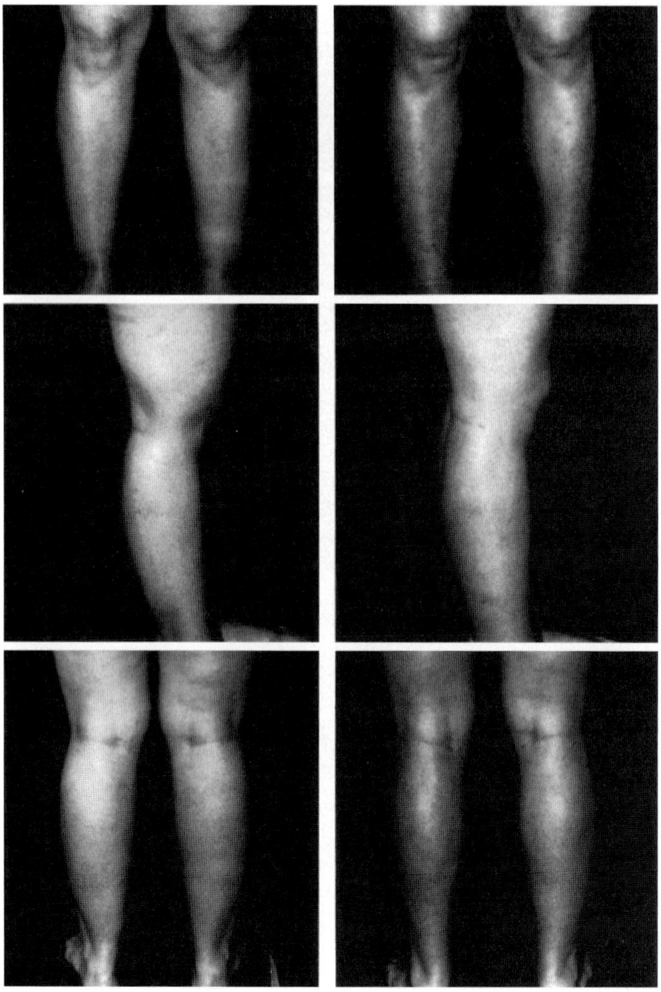

FIGURE 50 See p. 621 for details.

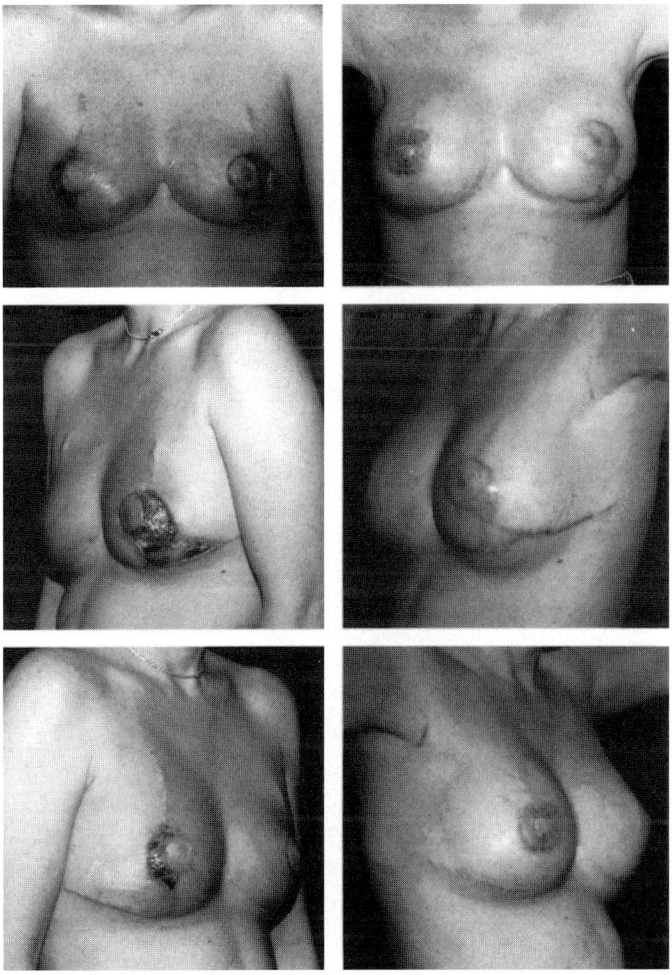

FIGURE 51 Before surgery (left) after partial necrosis of the breast and areola; after surgery (right).

(a)

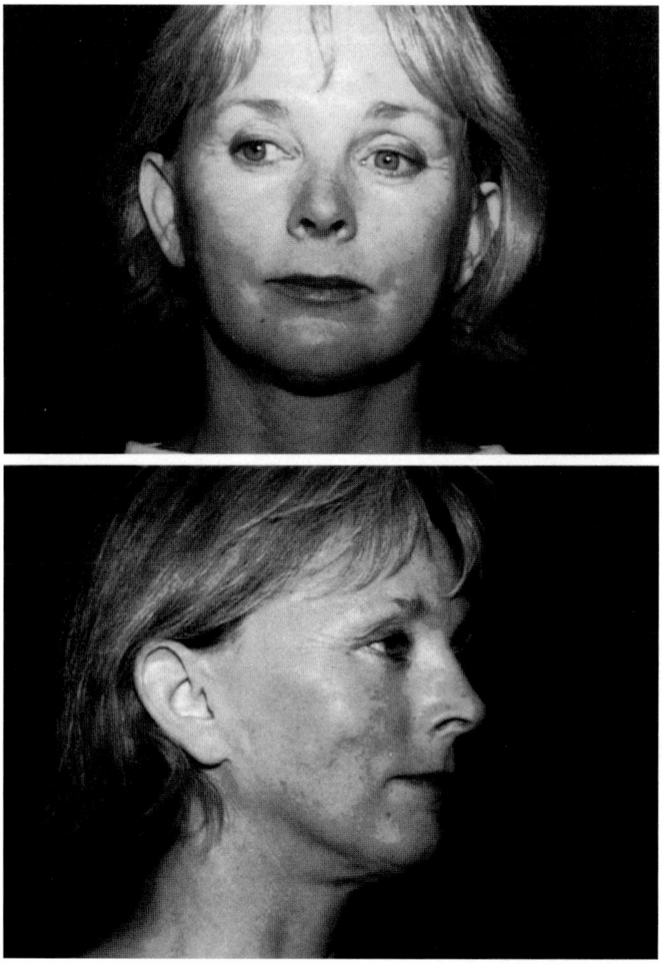

(b)

FIGURE 52 Presurgical correction, (a) and (b) show skin irregularity in the neck secondary to excessive liposuction and facial asymmetry secondary to excess removal of fat from the right side of the face.

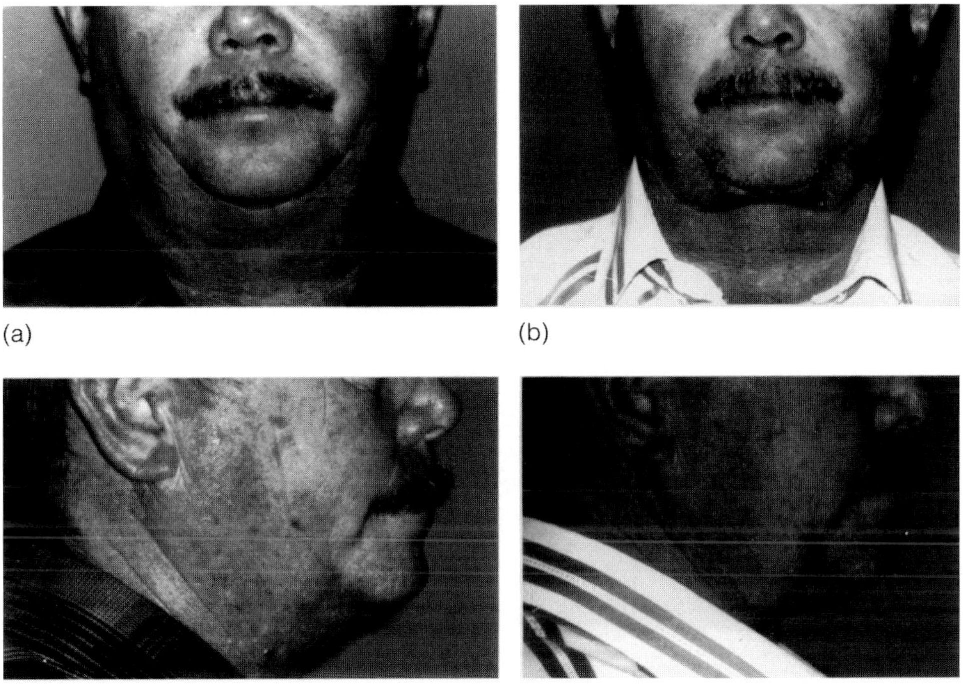

(a) (b)

(c) (d)

FIGURE 53 (a–d) Central removal of fat with platysmal plication. There is excess fat in the lateral neck and face areas. This could be corrected with facelift or combined face and neck SAL and extensive skin undermining.

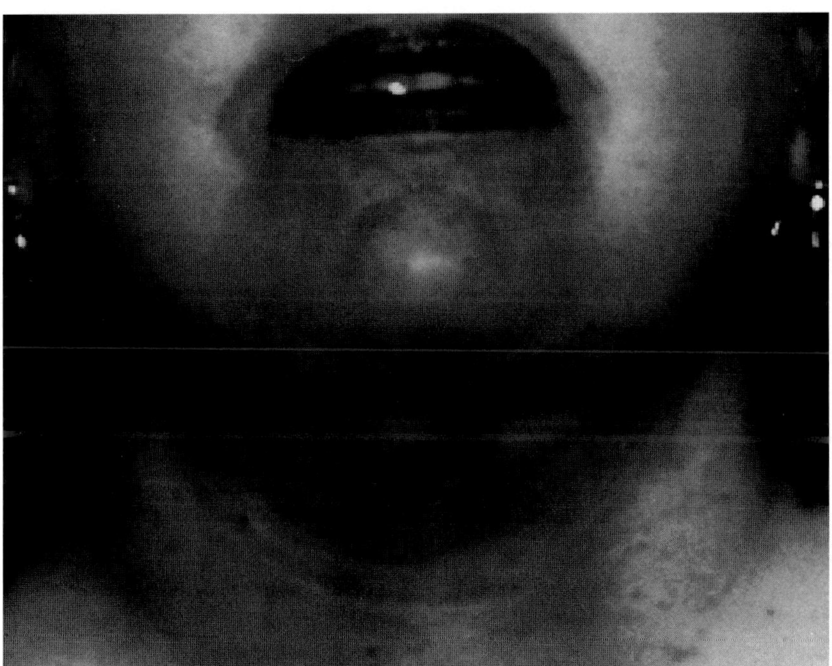

FIGURE 54 Drainage in the mid neck area with sinus tract to the gortex suture for midline interlocking plication.

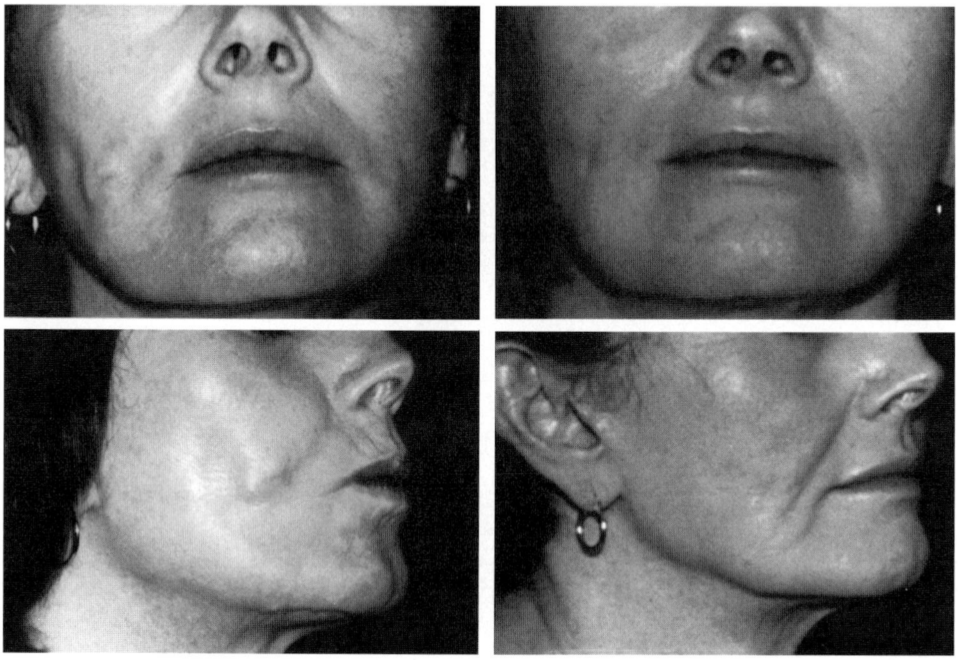

FIGURE 55 Skin irregularity with fat necrosis and scar contraction of the right cheek (left); after surgery (right).

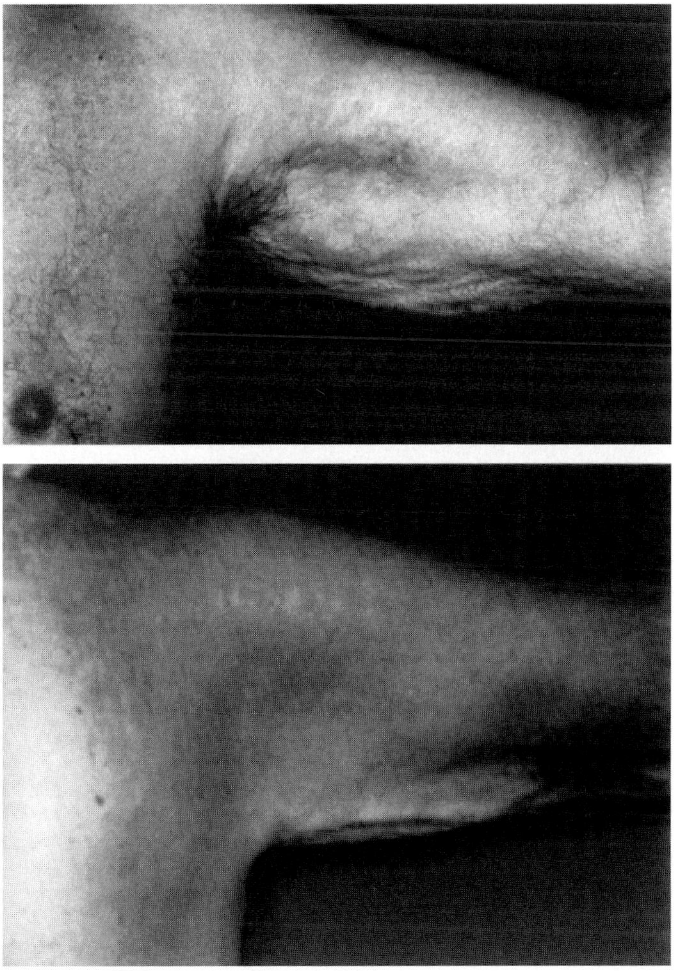

(a)

(b)

FIGURE 56 Medial SAL of the arm in the patient with loose skin caused wrinkles and worsened the skin looseness. (a) shows the frontal view, (b) shows the posterior view after SAL of the arm.

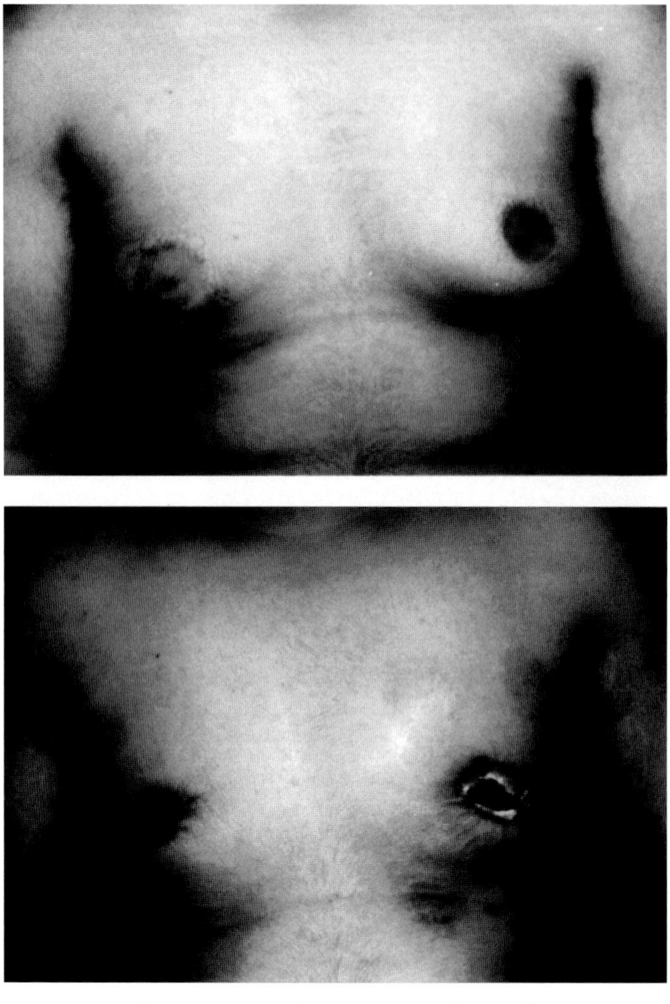

(a)

(b)

FIGURE 57 (a) Before surgery; (b) postsurgical complication. Partial breast necrosis after breast liposuction and areola reduction.

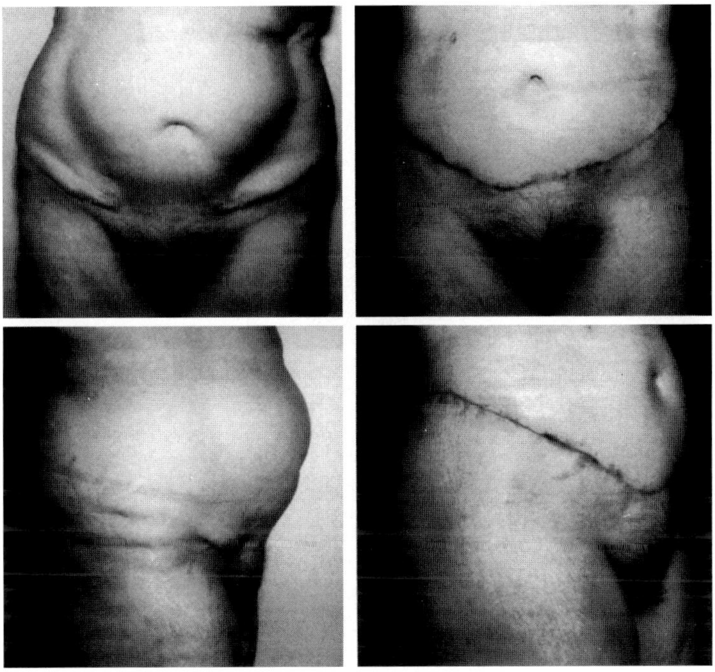

FIGURE 58 Postsurgical mini-abdominoplasty (left); postsurgical revision (right), with SAL and extended abdominoplasty.

Excessive and inappropriate suctioning of the inner arm leads to redundant arm skin, causing "bat wings" to appear worse (Fig. 56). The treatment for this complication is brachioplasty (Figs. 24, 25).

Excessive suctioning of the lateral or central aspect of the breast for gynecomastia in a muscular patient can lead to depression. Patients with third-degree gynecomastia require release of the inframammary line, or wrinkling of the lower breast skin and/or accentuation of inframammary fold will occur. Simultaneous SAL and areola reduction can cause areola necrosis, and should not be performed (Fig. 57).

With the advent of SAL for the abdomen, some clinicians have attempted to use this as the sole treatment and not perform full abdominoplasty. An aesthetically satisfactory result usually does not occur if this is done. These patients commonly require a standard or extended abdominoplasty in conjunction with SAL. It should be noted that mini-abdominoplasty in older patients may cause contour deformities (Fig. 58).

UAL of the abdomen with or without abdominoplasty can cause prolonged seroma with capsular formation, skin discoloration, skin irregularities (Fig. 59), and skin necrosis (Fig. 60).

Suction lipectomy of the abdomen and flanks with narrowing and lowering of the waistline may make the patient with heavy thighs appear shorter (Fig. 61). One

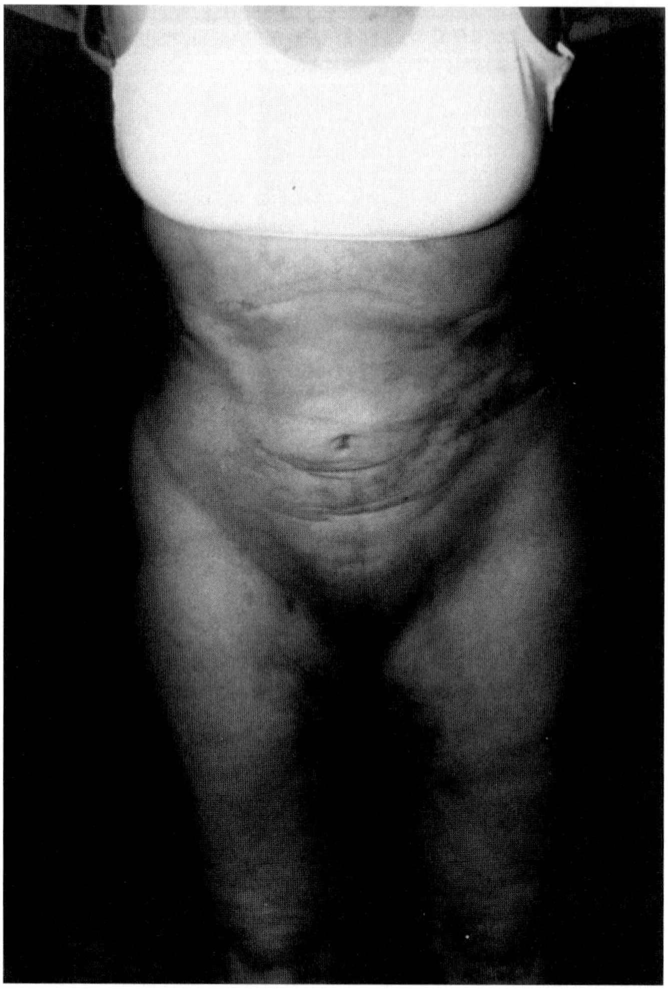

FIGURE 59 Skin wrinkling with discoloration after UAL and SAL of the abdomen.

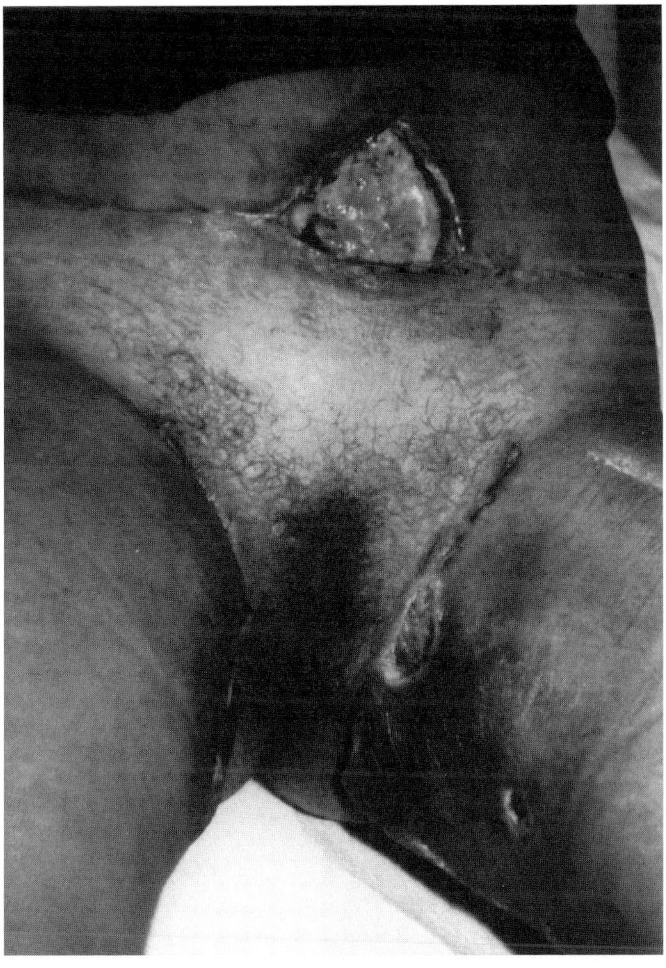

FIGURE 60 Skin necrosis after UAL of the abdomen and inner thigh.

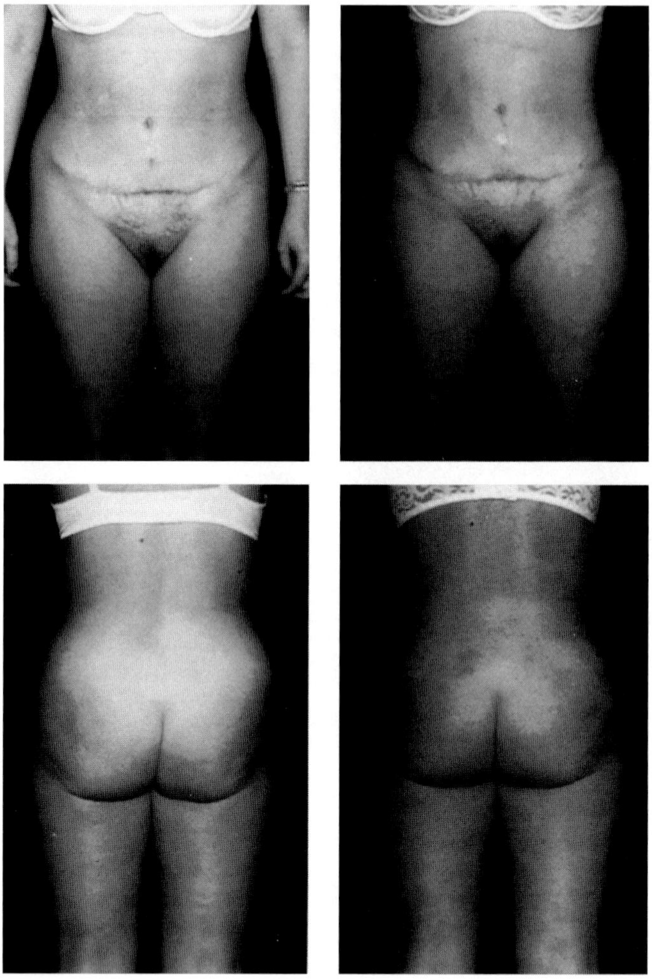

FIGURE 61 Before surgery (left); after surgery (right), presurgical SAL of the thighs, trochanter.

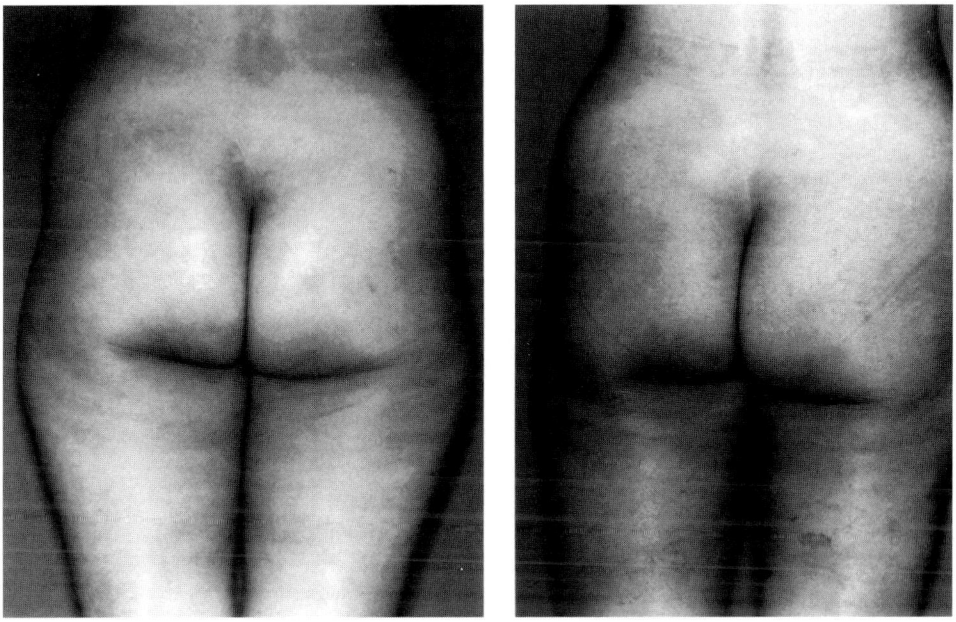

(a) (b)

FIGURE 62 (a) Before surgery; (b) after surgery.

of the treatments for this problem is SAL of the trochanter and thighs to make the lower extremity thinner, appear longer, and more proportionate to the waistline (Figs. 46, 47).

The SAL and UAL of the thigh and buttocks in the patient with loose skin can cause buttocks ptosis, posterior gluteal fold asymmetry, lowering (Fig. 62), and banana fold formation [29]. The best way to avoid this problem is to not disturb the fold and to avoid suctioning of the posterior and superior aspect of the mid thigh. In addition, suction lipectomy of the lower extremity of patients with loose skin improves the form but can increase the skin contour irregularities. Some of these patients' problems can be improved with lower-body lift of a Lockwood type [40] or extended abdominoplasty and inner thigh lift (Fig. 63) [38].

In patients with multiple back folds, SAL alone cannot improve the deformity. A backlift or extended abdominoplasty with fold release and lipograft to depressions are required to improve the lower back (Figs. 63, 64). However, the persistent upper-back folds may need excision. This is performed as an extension of the inframammary line laterally and posteriorly with release, SAL, and lipograft (Fig. 43).

ACKNOWLEDGMENT

We would like to thank Tiffany Sullivan for her editorial assistance.

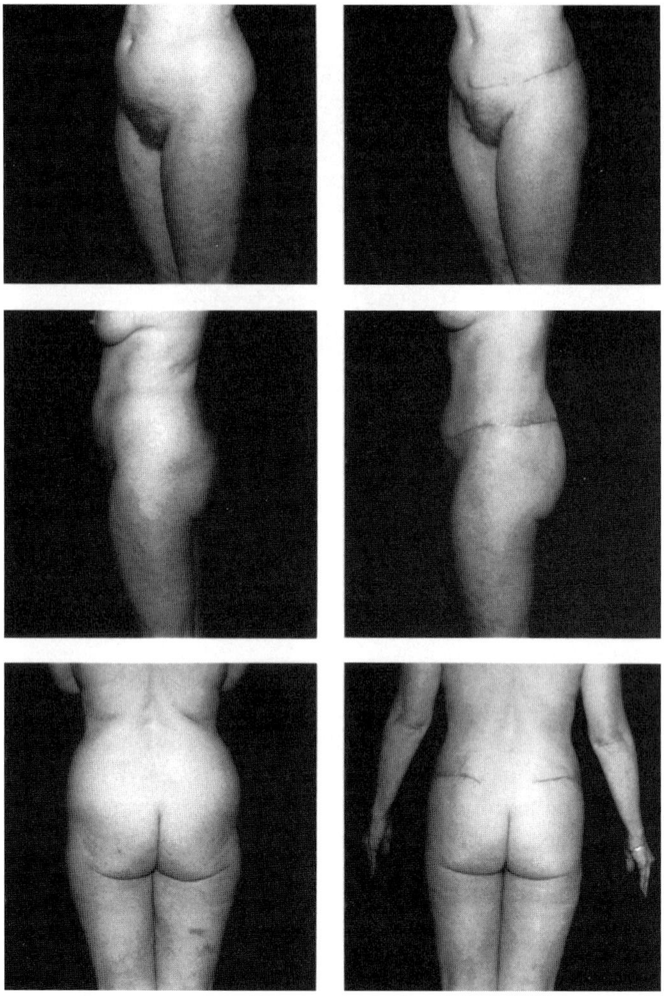

FIGURE 63 See p. 635 for details.

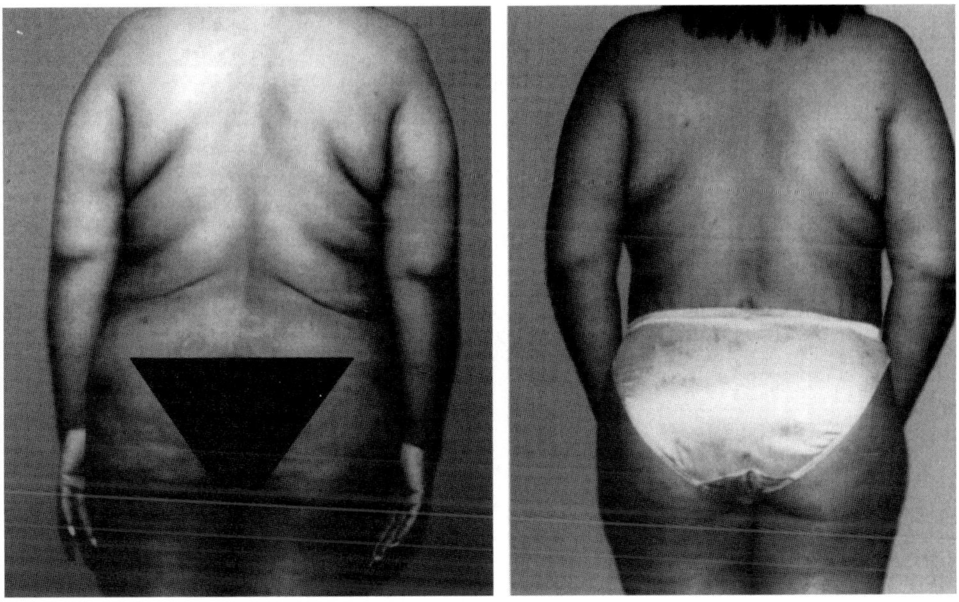

(a) (b)

Figure 64 **(a) Before surgery; (b) after surgery.**

REFERENCES

1. Teimourian B, Rodgers BW. A national survey of complications associated with suction lipectomy: a comparative study. Plast Reconstr Surg 1989; 84:628–663.
2. Gasparotti M, Lewis CM, Toledo LS. Superficial Liposculpture Manual Technique. New York: Springer-Verlag, 1993.
3. Pitanguy I. Trochanteric lipodystrophy. Plast Reconstr Surg 1964; 34:280–283.
4. Hausman G, Campion D, Martin R. Search for the adipocyte precursor cell and factors that promote its differentiation. J Lipid Res 1980; 21:657.
5. Bjorntorp P. The fat cell: a clinical review. In: Bray G, ed. Recent Advances of Obesity Research. London: Newman Publishing, 1978.
6. Toledo LS. Syringe liposculpture: a two year experience. Aesth Plast Surg 1991; 15: 321–326.
7. Illouz YG. Body contouring by lipolysis: a 5 year experience with over 3000 cases. Plast Reconstr Surg 1983; 72:591–597.
8. Narins RS. Liposuction and anesthesia. Dermatol Clin 1990; 8(3):421–424.
9. Klein JA. Tumescent technique for local anesthesia improves safety in large-volume liposuction. Plast Reconstr Surg 1993; 92:1085–1098.
10. Fournier PF, Otteni FM. Lipodissection in body sculpturing: the dry procedure. Plast Reconstr Surg 1983; 72:598.
11. Kesselring UK. Regional fat aspiration for body contouring. Plast Reconstr Surg 1983; 72:610.
12. Grazer FM. Suction-assisted lipectomy, suction lipectomy, lipolysis, and lipexeresis. Plast Reconstr Surg 1983; 72:620.
13. Fischer G. Liposuction 2: evaluation of the patient for liposuction. J Dermatol Surg Oncol 1991; 17:741–743.

14. Hanke CW, Lee MW, Bernstein G. The safety of dermatologic liposuction surgery. Dermatol Clin 1990; 8(3):563–568.
15. Simmon BE, Hoffman S, Kahn S. Classification and surgical correction for gynecomastia. Plast Reconstr Surg 1983; 7:155.
16. Teimourian B. Problems in suction lipectomy. Plastic Surgery Educational Foundation. Boston, 1985.
17. Teimourian B. Discussion: suction lipectomy: a retrospective analysis of 100 patients. Plast Reconstr Surg 1984; 73:795.
18. Gheradini G, Matarasso A, Serure AS, Toledo LS, DiBernardo BE. Standardization in photography for body contour surgery and suction-assisted lipectomy. Plast Reconstr Surg 1997; 100:227–237.
19. Courtiss HE. Suction lipectomy: a retrospective analysis of 100 patients. Plast Reconstr Surg 1984; 73:779.
20. Voukidis TE. Letter to the editor: reply to suction lipectomy. Plast Reconstr Surg 1985; 75:137.
21. Klein JA. Anesthesia for liposuction in dermatologic surgery. J Dermat Surg Oncol 1988; 14:1124.
22. Gilliland MD, Lyos AT. Cast liposuction: an alternative to brachioplasty. Aesth Plast Surg 1997; 21(6):398–402.
23. Pittman GH. Liposuction and Aesthetic Surgery. St. Louis: Quality Medical, 1993.
24. Tebbetts JB. Minimizing complications of ultrasound-assisted lipoplasty: an initial experience with no related complications. Plast Reconstr Surg 1998; 102:1690–1697.
25. Teimourian B. Letter to the editor: ultrasonic-assisted liposuction. Plast Reconstr Surg 1997; 100:1623–1625.
26. Gonzales-Ulloa M. Ptosis of the chin. The witch's chin. Plast Reconstr Surg 1972; 50: 54–57.
27. Teimourian B. Suction Lipectomy and Body Sculpturing. St. Louis: The C.V. Mosby Company, 1987.
28. Adham MN. A new technique for nasal tip cartilage graft in primary rhinoplasty. Plast Reconstr Surg 1996; 97:649–655.
29. Teimourian B, Perlman R. Surgery for gynecomastia. Aesth Plast Surg 1983; 7:155.
30. Matarasso A. Abdominoplasty. Clin Plast Surg 1989; 16:289.
31. Rosenburg GJ. A new cannula for suction removal of parenchymal tissue of gynecomastia. Plast Reconstr Surg 1994; 94:548.
32. Vogt PA, Baroudi R. Brachioplasty and brachial suction-assisted lipectomy. In: Cohen M, ed. Mastery of Plastic and Reconstructive Surgery. 1st ed. Boston: Little, Brown, 1994, pp. 2219–2236.
33. Teimourian B, Malekzadeh S. Rejuvenation of the upper arm. Plast Reconstr Surg 1998; 102:545.
34. Grazer FM. Atlas of Suction Assisted Lipectomy in Body Sculpturing. New York: Churchill Livingstone, 1992.
35. Mentz HA 3rd, Gilliland MD, Patronella CK. Abdominal etching: differential liposuction to detail abdominal musculature. Aesth Plast Surg 1993; 17:287–290.
36. Teimourian B, Adham M, Malekzadeh S. Waistline cincture. Aesth Plast Surg 1998; 18: 458.
37. Illouz YG. Body Sculpturing by Lipoplasty. New York: Churchill Livingstone, 1989.
38. Teimourian B, Adham MN. Anterior periosteal dermal suspension with suction curettage for lateral thigh lipectomy. Aesth Plast Surg 1982; 6:207.
39. Pfulg ME. Complications of suction for lipectomy. Plast Reconstr Surg 1982; 69:562.
40. Lockwood T. Lower body lift with superficial fascial system suspension. Plast Reconstr Surg 1993; 92:1112.

41. Samdal F, Amland PF, Bugge JF. Blood loss during suction-assisted lipectomy with large volumes of dilute adrenaline. Scand J Plast Reconstr Surg and Hand Surg 1995; 29:161.
42. Pitman GH. Tumescent liposuction complicated by pulmonary edema. Plast Reconstr Surg 1997; 100:1363–1364.
43. Gilliland MD, Coates N. Tumescent liposuction complicated by pulmonary edema. Plast Reconstr Surg 1997; 99:215–219.
44. Lombardi AS, Quirke TE, Rauscher G. Acute median nerve compression associated with tumescent fluid administration. Plast Reconstr Surg 1998; 102:235.
45. Fourme T, Vieillar-Baron A, Loubieres Y, Julie C, Page B, Tardin F. Early fat embolism after liposuction. Anesthesiology 1998; 89:782.
46. Rhee CA, Smith RJ, Jackson IT. Toxic shock syndrome associated with suction-assisted lipectomy. Anesth Plast Surg 1994; 18:161.
47. Barillo DJ, Cancio LC, Kim SH, Shirani KZ, Goodwin CW. Fatal and near fatal complications of liposuction. Southern Med J 1998; 91:487.
48. Mateu LP, Hernandez JJ. Cutaneous hyperpigmentation caused by liposuction. Aesth Plast Surg 1997; 21:230.
49. Khan JI, Ho-Asjoe M, Frame JD. Pectoralis major rupture post suction lipectomy for surgical management of gynecomastia. Aesth Plast Surg 1998; 22:16.

27

The Cook Weekend Alternative to the Facelift

William R. Cook, Jr.
Coronado Skin Medical Center, Inc., Coronado, California

INTRODUCTION

In this chapter, I will describe a ten-step, laser-enhanced face and neck procedure which I call the Cook Weekend Alternative to the Facelift™. I have codeveloped this procedure over a period of years with my partner, K. K. Cook. I currently use this procedure on most of my face and neck patients [1,2].

During the Cook Weekend Alternative to the Facelift™ procedure, I perform liposculpture of the lower face, neck and jowls, as well as laser resurfacing of the platysma and underside of the dermis, vaporization of subcutaneous fat, resection of a small ellipse of excess submental skin, separation of the neck septae, and plication of the platysma. If indicated, I may do a chin augmentation as well. Using laser technology, all the surgical procedures can be performed in a properly equipped outpatient surgery room under tumescent local anesthesia at the same time as the liposculpture.

The results of this procedure can be striking—much superior to the results of traditional liposculpture alone. In many cases the results are comparable to the results of traditional surgical rhytidectomy, but without the substantial side effects and extended healing period of rhytidectomy. These superior results are achieved with minimal incisions, rare complications, and a very rapid recovery. Instead of needing weeks to recover from a rhytidectomy, the average patient can undergo this procedure literally "over the weekend," with surgery on Thursday or Friday and a return to normal activities the following week.

This extended procedure creates a more natural-looking cosmetic improvement. Sagging or fatty neck areas are transformed by facial and neck sculpting, tightening of the neck, marked reduction in skin laxity, and reduction of the platysmal bands. Patients with round and heavy-appearing faces gain a thinner-appearing, more attractively sculptured look. The cheekbones are more prominent, the mandible is more sharply defined, and facial features are in better balance.

HISTORICAL OVERVIEW

Tumescent liposculpture of the face, neck, and jowls is a very effective and safe procedure when properly performed [3–5]. It is widely performed and will improve the appearance of many patients. But in some patients, liposculpture alone is not as cosmetically effective as a traditional rhytidectomy procedure [6–8].

For many years I have been looking for ways to improve the cosmetic treatment of the face and neck, while avoiding the extensive surgical intervention that a patient is subjected to with rhytidectomy. I have developed a combined liposculpture and laser surgical procedure that I call the Cook Weekend Alternative to the Facelift™. This procedure was developed using well-tested surgical principles, beginning with liposculpture, cautiously adding incremental improvements, including the surgical laser, and combining the techniques into a method that produces consistently good clinical results.

PRESURGICAL CONSIDERATIONS

Presurgical Evaluation

Indications

Liposculpture may be indicated to correct lipodystrophic changes of the lower face and neck, including "turkey neck" and "double chin." The Cook Weekend Alternative to the Facelift™ is especially useful for patients who display poor cervicomental angles, lax platysma, and moderately lax skin. However, the technique will not help a person whose skin is severely inelastic beyond repair. Some individuals whose facial and/or neck skin shows poor elasticity may be helped by first performing either a chemical peel or laser skin resurfacing. Then they can be re-evaluated as candidates for the Weekend Alternative to the Facelift™.

Cosmetic changes in the face, neck, and jowls can occur at any age but generally become more pronounced with aging. I have performed facial liposculpture on patients of 15 to 75 years of age.

Patients at the younger end of the spectrum generally desire correction of a genetic pattern of fullness of the neck and face and perhaps a recessive chin. The history often reveals that the same appearance was also present in the grandparents and parents. Although this appearance can be present in the teens and 20s, it may become more pronounced with advancing age.

Changes in the appearance of face and neck are as individual as patients themselves, but many patients begin to show significant changes in the appearance of their face and neck around 35 years of age. At that time, the submental fat pad becomes more prominent, the platysma muscle is weaker, and the skin begins to lose its elasticity. By 45 years a frank double chin may be present. The skin loses more of its elasticity, the jowls become thickened and begin to sag, and in many cases the eyelids begin to droop and the skin surface to wrinkle. At 55 years the eyelids may be heavy with many lines, skin folds are deeper, and jowls are sagging more. A "turkey neck" and/or double chin may be present. In many cases there are horizontal platysmal bands forming a ringlike configuration around the neck in several folds.

These effects of time, gravity, heredity, and sun exposure can often be helped by the Weekend Alternative to the Facelift™. In some patients, additional procedures such as blepharoplasty, laser resurfacing of the skin, trichloroacetic acid (TCA) peel, and Cook Total Body Peel of nonfacial areas may also be indicated [2].

Clinical Evaluation

As with any liposculpture procedure, careful consideration must be given to clinical findings, goals, and realistic expectations on both the surgeon's and the patient's part. Patients need to understand that, although significant improvement is seen within days, a patient's appearance will continue to improve for several months after the procedure.

In the initial consultation with a candidate for this procedure, I carefully evaluate the distribution of the patient's facial adipose layer. I consider the general facial characteristics of that individual and also the family history. One must determine whether the cosmetic problem is principally caused by bulging of excessive fat or laxity of the skin and muscles. In particular, the "turkey neck" deformity needs to be evaluated as to the relative contributions of fat content versus lax platysma muscle. The platysma tends to become more redundant and lax with the aging process, and this is often the most significant cause of bands in the submental area. Sagging jowls may be caused by excess fat or a hypertrophic masseter muscle.

If enlarged submandibular glands are present, I point them out to the patient and emphasize that they will still be present after surgery. The position of the larynx and hyoid bone should be considered, as well as the underlying bony structure of the face. I also study the cervicomental angle, to see if the patient's appearance might be improved by inserting a chin implant and suctioning the ptotic chin pad.

In addition to the direct examination, I often find that the clinical evaluation is enhanced by the use of photographs and/or computer imaging. Many investigators have defined various profile lines and proportions [9]. A study of the profile in terms of vertical lines can be especially helpful to the surgeon in assessing the need for possible chin augmentation.

When assessing the patient for a possible chin implant, no hard and fast rules apply. The size and shape of the implant must be carefully chosen. The goal is to achieve a natural appearance with which the patient is comfortable.

Presurgical Work-Up

Before performing the Weekend Alternative to the Facelift™ or any other surgical procedure, I obtain the following laboratory tests: complete blood count (CBC), complete chemistry panel, coagulation profile, hepatitis screen, and urinalysis. The results are evaluated before the scheduled surgery date so that any needed additional studies or corrective action may be undertaken.

At the presurgical visit a medical history is obtained, with an emphasis on allergies and medications. A brief physical examination is performed. A medical clearance is requested from the primary physician. Photographs are taken from several angles, which are useful as references during surgery and also provide a permanent record of the patient's presurgical appearance.

Presurgical Instructions

Patients are instructed not to take aspirin, ibuprofen, or Vitamin E before surgery. They are told not to drink alcoholic beverages for several days before the scheduled date of the procedure. Patients are instructed to shower the night before surgery and the morning of surgery with Hibiclens cleanser, and to eat a light meal the morning of surgery.

I generally place the patient on prophylactic antibiotics, starting the day before surgery and continuing for 7 days. A 2-week course of vitamin K may be helpful as well to reduce postsurgical bruising; if some patients do not tolerate this medication well, they can discontinue it. Vitamin K is not given if the patient has any history of thrombophlebitis or emboli.

Patients must arrange for a responsible adult to drive them to my office on the day of surgery, take them home afterward, and remain with them until the next morning.

Paperwork

See Appendixes 1 and 2.

EQUIPMENT

Anesthesia

The Cook Weekend Alternative to the Facelift(TM) is performed under tumescent local anesthesia. This technique requires an infiltration pump or other device to deliver the tumescent solution from the intravenous bag in which it is mixed to the areas of the body undergoing treatment.

Incision sites are first anesthetized with a small bleb of commercial anesthetic solution containing 2% lidocaine and 1:100,000 epinephrine. The more dilute solution used for tumescent anesthesia is infiltrated through the incisions. Initial infiltration is performed using a spinal needle with the infusion pump at a low setting. The tumescent anesthetic solution is infused all around the incision site in a spokelike radial fashion. Then the main volume of tumescent anesthetic solution is infused using an infiltration cannula until the sites are well tumesced and clinically anesthetic.

Tumescent anesthetic solution should be made up fresh on the day it is used. It is very important to make up this solution under precise controls, so that the proper amount of each ingredient is present. I use a tumescent solution that contains 0.1% lidocaine and 1:1,000,000 epinephrine. This solution is made up as follows: to 1000 ml of normal saline solution in an infusion bag, I add 10 ml of 8.4% sodium bicarbonate, 50 ml of 2% lidocaine, 1 ml of epinephrine 1:1000, and 1 ml of triamcinolone acetonide (Kenalog) in the form of a 10 mg/ml suspension. The epinephrine and Kenalog are added just before the mixture is infused.

Before infusion, I warm the tumescent solution to 39 to 40°C. The average face and neck will require 500 to 800 ml of tumescent anesthetic fluid for this procedure.

Tumescent Liposculpture

Tumescent liposculpture requires a variety of cannulas. I usually prefer Klein and Capistrano spatula-type cannulas for sculpting the neck and face. I may use any of the following cannulas during this procedure: 16-gauge, 14-gauge, and 12-gauge Klein cannulas in the 4 inch and 6 inch lengths, or 16-gauge Capistrano cannulas in the 4 inch and 6 inch lengths.

Like most liposculpture surgeons, I prefer to use a mechanical vacuum pump during liposuction procedures.

Laser Surgery

I use a Coherent UltraPulse 5000 surgical laser during this procedure. I recommend an ultrapulsed laser like this for superior surgical results. Ultrapulsed lasers produce less heat, less coagulation necrosis, less injury to tissues, less bruising, and a greatly shortened recovery time compared with unpulsed surgical lasers or traditional metal scalpels. It is important that the surgeon and all ancillary personnel be properly trained in the surgical use of lasers, because lasers involve important safety issues. These include electrical safety, fire prevention, respiratory precautions, and eye protection for both staff and patient.

Other Surgical Procedures

The Cook Weekend Alternative to the Facelift™ requires the use of a Toledo tissue dissector and a Valley electrosurgical unit with a special suction cautery tip. If chin augmentation is performed, a Rich periosteal elevator will be needed.

Chin Augmentation

I use Silastic silicone-rubber implants, which are commercially available in various sizes and shapes. This material is biocompatible with the existing soft tissue, and it stimulates the development of a fibrous connective tissue capsule that abuts the implant surface. The Silastic implants are very inert and resist changes in local conditions of the tissues.

Ultrasound

In many cases I like to apply external ultrasound to the tumesced areas before commencing liposculpture [10]. When properly used by trained personnel, this presurgical external ultrasound can make liposculpture procedures easier for the surgeon and decrease postsurgical bruising, swelling, and discomfort for the patient. I use a Rich-Mar external ultrasound unit. For face and neck areas I use a 5 cm transducer and a setting of 1 watt/cm^2, continuous wave, at 1 mhz.

THE DAY OF SURGERY

Preparation of the Patient

Before any sedation is given, a final review of the planned procedure, alternatives, and risks is carried out with the patient. A brief presurgical physical examination is performed. The patient's ride home is confirmed to be a responsible adult. The surgical areas are scrubbed with Hibiclens, avoiding the eyelids.

Marking the Surgical Areas

I mark the surgical areas with a gentian violet marking pen with the patient in a sitting position. Markings should include the lower face, jowls, chin, and neck. The markings should show the extent of the planned suctioning, any pre-existing elevations or depressions, the midline of the chin, and underlying bony structures such as the mandible. Incision points should be clearly marked. These include two 1-mm incisions in the submental crease, a pair of infra-auricular incisions, and an incision in the mucosal surface of the lateral aspect of the upper lip.

ANESTHESIA

Freshly made up tumescent solution with a lidocaine concentration of 0.1% is infiltrated through incisions approximately 1 mm in size in the submental and infra-auricular areas. The entire anterior and lateral neck, jowls, and lower one third of the face are infiltrated at this time. The average face and neck will require 500 to 800 ml of fluid to achieve good tumescence for this procedure. If indicated, external ultrasound may be applied after infiltration is complete.

SURGICAL PROCEDURE

The Cook Weekend Alternative to the Facelift™ is a 10-step technique for tumescent cosmetic surgery to the face, neck, and jowls. The steps may be summarized as follows:

1. Tumescent liposculpture to the lower third of the face, the nasolabial mound, the jowls, excess fat in the ptotic chin, and the entire anterior and lateral neck, covering an area from the mandible to the base of the neck and laterally to the anterior border of the sternocleidomastoid muscle; this removes fat and allows redraping of the submental skin
2. Laser resection of excessive submental skin (only a small ellipse of tissue is removed)
3. Complete transsection of septae on the anterior and lateral neck, so that complete redraping occurs
4. Separation of the insertions of the platysma muscle to the horizontal bands of the neck, which reduces and in some cases eliminates horizontal bands of the neck
5. Tumescent liposculpture of the subplatysmal fat pad
6. Laser vaporization of remaining fat globules on the platysma and undersurface of the skin of the neck
7. Laser resurfacing of the fascia of the platysma muscle to produce tightening of the muscle
8. Laser resurfacing of the underside of the dermis to produce tightening of the skin of the neck
9. Insertion of a chin implant, when indicated
10. Plication of the anterior border of the platysma muscle to produce maximal tightening and reduced platysmal bands, followed by closure of the submental incision.

Tumescent Liposculpture of the Lower Face, Jowls, and Neck

I wait approximately 20 minutes after infiltration of the anesthesia to allow good vasoconstriction. I then commence tumescent liposculpture through the submental incision sites. I use two small incisions in the submental fold or the area of the submental incision. (In some patients who are scheduled for a chin implant, the submental incision is placed slightly inferior to the submental fold.) I perform liposculpture in the submental region, crisscrossing the area and forming a honeycomb pattern in the sites of involvement.

After this initial submental suctioning is completed, I use the infra-auricular incision to suction the lower one third of the face, the jowl area, and the adjacent area of the lateral neck. This is performed in the mid or deeper plane to avoid ridging of the cheeks, making precise passes carefully spaced.

The next area of suctioning is through an incision approximately 1 mm in size in the mucosal surface of the lateral aspect of the upper lip. I suction the adjacent jowl area and the mound portion lateral to the nasolabial fold, if indicated. I use small cannulas in this area, so that the incision site will close nicely without suturing and leave no apparent cosmetic defect.

The neck region is now sculpted. During this final sculpting, I thoroughly cover the areas from the mandibular ridge down to the base of the neck, so that all apparent excess fatty tissue is removed.

Resection of Excess Submental Skin

I now outline a 2.5 cm submental ellipse approximately 2 to 3 mm in width. I use the UltraPulse 5000 laser (Coherent Medical Group, Palo Alto, CA) with initial settings of 15 mJ and 4 W to make the initial incision of the narrow skin ellipse. I then use the 7 W setting to excise the elliptical piece of skin.

Transection of Septae of the Neck

A Toledo tissue dissector is inserted into this submental incision and is used to break all visible septae in the entire anterior and lateral neck. The plane of dissection is important, staying relatively superficial. Adequate hemostasis is achieved by using the Valley electrosurgical unit with or without suction cautery.

Separation of the Platysma

I then use the Toledo tissue dissector to separate the insertion of the platysma muscle into the horizontal bands of the neck. Hemostasis is again controlled with a Valley electrosurgical unit equipped with a special suction cautery tip.

Tumescent Liposculpture of the Subplatysmal Fat Pad

I next infiltrate the mid portion of the platysma muscle with a solution of 2% lidocaine and 1:100,000 epinephrine, approximately 1.5 to 2.0 ml injected into the muscle. This provides anesthesia and vasoconstriction for subplatysmal suctioning.

A small incision is made in the midline of the superior aspect of the platysma muscle. The subplatysmal fat pad is carefully visualized through this small opening and is gently aspirated. The fat is this area is very soft, and extreme caution and very slow movements of the cannula are needed, so as not to traumatize any of the adjacent structures. After suctioning I carefully monitor the area for good hemostasis.

After the subplatysmal pad is removed, direct visualization is made of the jowl areas. Any residual globules of fat in this area are carefully removed.

Vaporization of the Remaining Fat

Using the Coherent UltraPulse 5000 laser, I perform spot vaporization of any persistent fat lobules on the platysma and undersurface of the skin.

Resurfacing the Platysma

I then use the UltraPulse 5000 laser in a defocused mode on a 7 W setting to gently resurface approximately 10 to 20% of the anterior surface of the platysma muscle by using a crisscrossing randomized pattern. This tightens the fascial surface of the platysma.

Resurfacing the Dermis

To tighten the skin, I then carefully resurface the undersurface of the dermis in a crisscrossing randomized fashion by using the UltraPulse 5000 laser on a 7 W defocused setting. Care must be taken to keep the laser beam moving continuously. The amount of resurfacing performed on the undersurface of the skin will depend on the skin laxity, the skin thickness, and the amount of tightening desired. Resurfacing should only be performed on 20 to 30% of the skin undersurface, rather than a total or dense pattern as is used with external skin resurfacing procedures.

Chin Implant (Optional)

In patients with slight to moderate microgenia, the mandible may be augmented to maximize the cervicomental angle. I initiate the implant procedure at this time by using the UltraPulse 5000 laser on the 7 W continuous setting to carefully separate the platysma muscle in a horizontal line proceeding down to the periosteum on the mandible, corresponding to the desired position for the implant. The periosteum is then incised with the laser. A Rich periosteal elevator is used to create a pocket subperiosteally along the border of the mandible. The pocket for the implant should be located so that the implant will seat comfortably and squarely over the chin prominence and will not extend higher than the natural labiomental groove.

Once the pocket is freed and hemostasis is achieved, the implant is positioned and is secured to the periosteum with 4-0 clear nylon sutures. The fibers of the platysma muscle are then reapproximated with 4-0 Vicryl suture. This fixes the implant in place and helps to prevent malposition and extrusion.

Plication of the Platysma and Closure

Platysmal tightening is then performed to further improve the cervicomental angle and to reduce neck banding. After liposuction, severing of the septae, and removal of the platysmal insertions into the skin of the neck, the pattern of the particular individual's platysma muscle can clearly be noted. Because of the support given by the platysma and its role in the creation of the cervicomental angle, there is no substitute for a very thorough plication of the medial platysma to create the best results in the neck.

The medial borders of the platysma muscle are carefully sutured together using a plication stitch of 3-0 Vicryl. I prefer a vertical mattress type of suture, which gives better strength to the plicated muscle so that it will heal very firmly.

Below the point of plication, I resect a small wedge of muscle from each of the anterior platysmal borders to break the continuity of the band and allow the creation of a sharp cervicomental angle. This allows the muscle to conform to the cervicomental angle rather than forming a "bowstring" across it.

With good hemostasis achieved in all areas, the submental incision is closed with 4-0 Vicryl in the subcutaneous layer and 5-0 running and interrupted clear Prolene sutures in the skin surface. The remaining incisions in the infra-auricular and lip areas are left open to promote drainage.

Stretch foam tape (3M) is applied to the neck and lower facial areas. The stretch foam tape must be positioned very carefully so as not to induce any folds in the skin. The tape is then covered by elastic neck support with Velcro attachments to hold the tissues in the appropriate position.

POSTSURGICAL CONSIDERATIONS

Immediate Postsurgical Care

On returning home, the patient is advised to rest for the remainder of the day, with the head elevated and ice packs in position over the lower face and neck, 15 minutes "on" and 15 minutes "off" while awake. This will help to reduce tissue swelling and prevent ecchymosis of the areas. Good hydration should be maintained through adequate water intake. The first full postsurgical day is spent in quiet activities, with periodic rest, head elevation, and application of ice packs. After 1 to 2 days, patients return to my office for removal of the tape.

Thereafter patients can return to work and normal activities. However, vigorous exercise or physical exertion should be avoided for approximately 1 week after surgery. Immersion in water, such as in a swimming pool, hot tub, or bath, must be avoided until all the incisions have closed and the sutures are removed. I leave the sutures in place for 21 days to assure good healing of the area and good approximation of the wound.

Patients undergoing this procedure generally experience no to minimal postsurgical ecchymosis and usually no postsurgical discomfort. Occasionally the chin implant site may be tender for 1 to 2 days after surgery. The average patient is usually able to return to work and social activities on the third postsurgical day.

Long-Term Postsurgical Care

This procedure allows significant surgical intervention with very rapid recovery. In many cases, the patient's appearance will continue to improve for 2 to 3 months after surgery.

Complications and Treatment

Some patients will recover more rapidly than others, depending on the amount of skin retraction that must occur. Rarely a small seroma may develop during the postsurgical period. This may easily be drained, and recovery will then proceed uneventfully. Individuals with a history of keloid formation need to be monitored, and treated with intralesional Kenalog as indicated. The usual complications possible in any surgical procedure must be explained to the patient, but are rare occurrences.

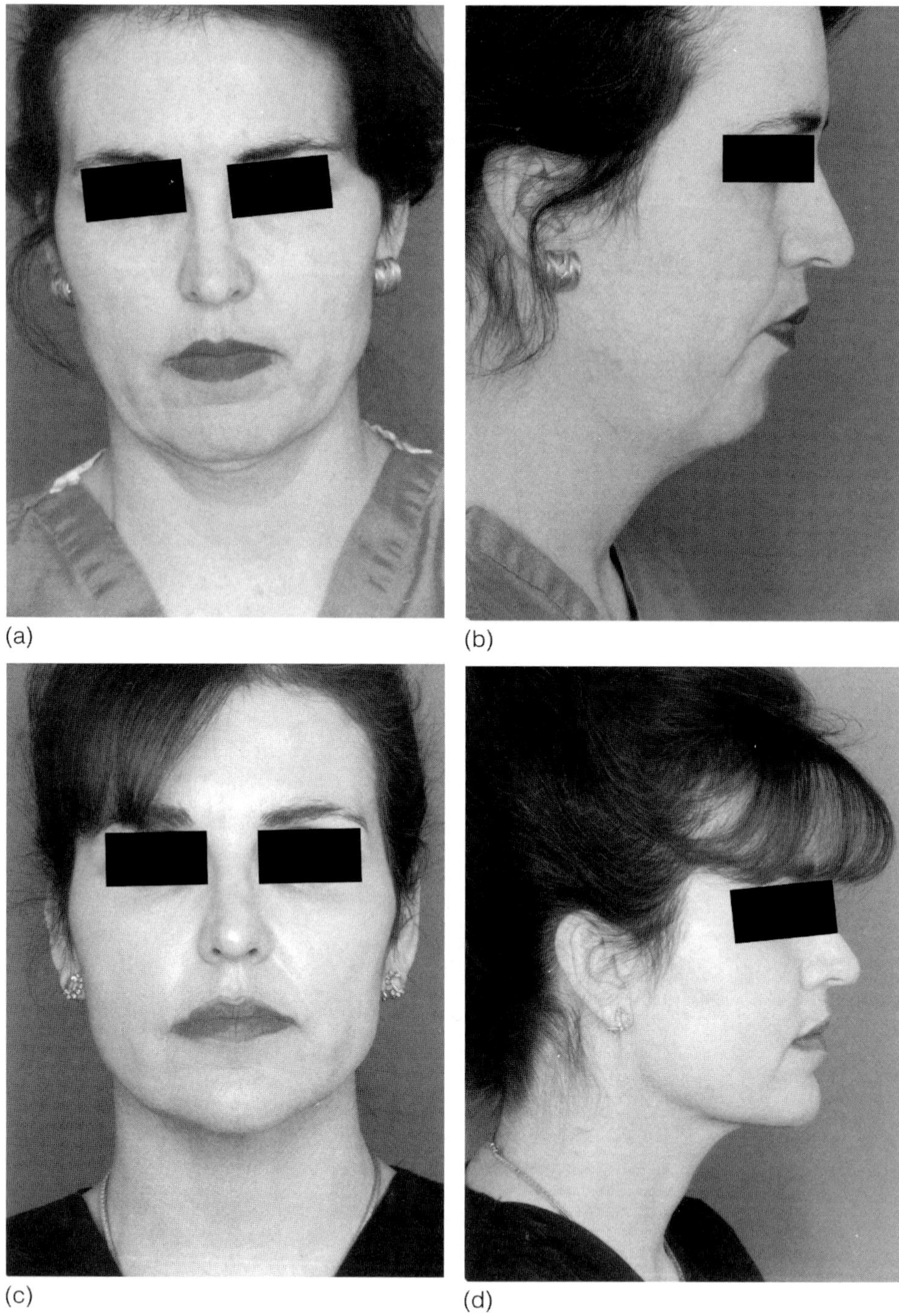

FIGURE 1 Patient (a, b) before and (c, d) after the Cook Weekend Alternative to the Facelift™ with chin implant.

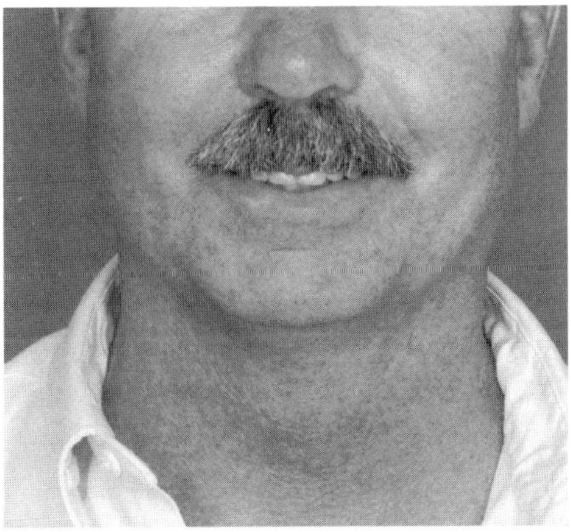

(a)

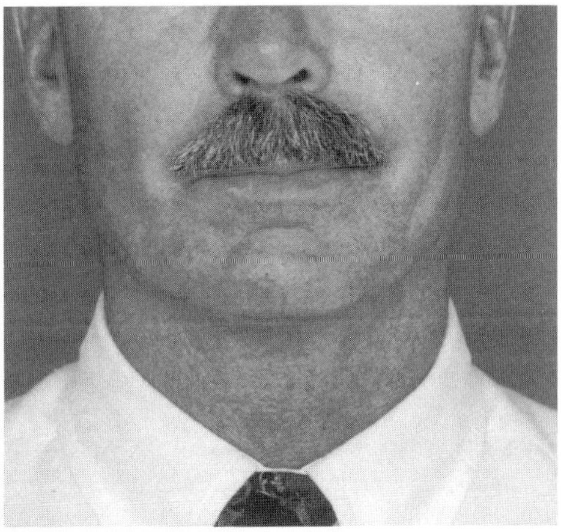

(b)

FIGURE 2 Patient (a) before and (b) after the Cook Weekend Alternative to the Facelift™ with chin implant.

SUMMARY

After this procedure, "turkey neck" deformity, neck banding, and double chins are significantly reduced. Patients with round and heavy-appearing faces gain a slimmer look with more prominent-appearing cheekbones. Patients with receding chins gain a more attractive profile. The cervicomental angle is excellent and the mandible is more sharply defined. Overall the facial features are in better balance (Figs. 1–3).

In summary, the Cook Weekend Alternative to the Facelift™ offers the following advantages over liposculpture alone or traditional rhytidectomy:

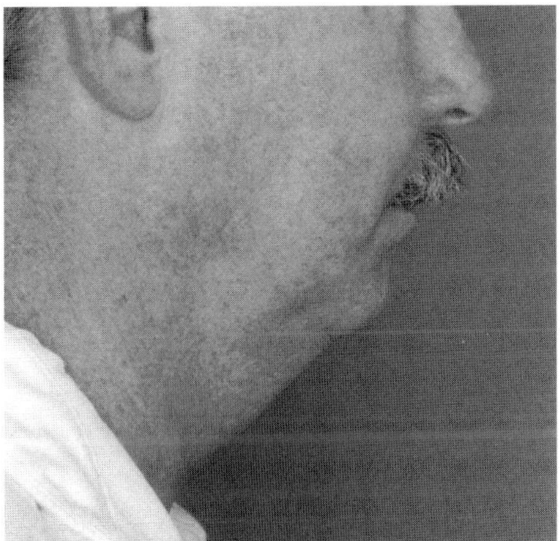

(a)

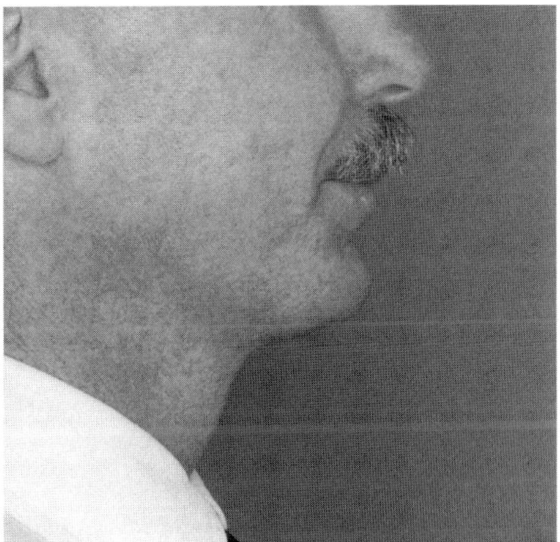

(b)

FIGURE 3 Patient (a) before and (b) after the Cook Weekend Alternative to the Facelift™ with chin implant.

- Excellent cosmetic results
- No need for general anesthesia
- Minimal incisions
- Little or no postsurgical discomfort
- Rapid healing and recovery
- Minimal to no complications

REFERENCES

1. WR Cook Jr. Laser neck and jowl liposculpture including platysma laser resurfacing, dermal laser resurfacing, and vaporization of subcutaneous fat. Dermatol Surg 23:1143–1148, 1997.
2. WR Cook Jr, KK Cook. Manual of Tumescent Liposculpture and Laser Cosmetic Surgery. Philadelphia: Lippincott William & Wilkins, 1999.
3. JA Klein. The tumescent technique for liposuction surgery. Am J Cosmet Surg 4:263–267, 1987.
4. CW Hanke, G Bernstein, S Bullock. Safety of tumescent liposuction in 15,336 patients. J Dermatol Surg Oncol 21:459–462, 1995.
5. W Coleman. Liposuction. In: W Coleman, C Hanke, T Alt, S Asken, eds. Cosmetic Surgery of the Skin. Philadelphia: BC Decker Inc, 1991, pp. 213–238.
6. B Chrisman. Liposuction with facelift surgery. Dermatol Clin 8:501–522, 1990.
7. S Hamra. Composite rhytidectomy. In: T Rees, G LaTrenta, eds. Aesthetic Plastic Surgery. Philadelphia: WB Saunders, 1994:708–721.
8. S Asken. The Face-lift-cervicofacial rhytidectomy. In: W Coleman, C Hanke, T Alt, S Asken, eds. Cosmetic Surgery of the Skin. Philadelphia: BC Decker Inc, 1991, pp. 335–354.
9. LG Farkas, P Sohm, JC Kolar, MJ Katic, IR Munro. Inclinations of the facial profile: art versus reality. Plast Reconstr Surg 75:509–519, 1985.
10. WR Cook Jr. Utilizing external ultrasonic energy to improve the results of tumescent liposculpture. Dermatol Surg 23:1207–1211, 1997.

APPENDIX 1

1. Operative Consent Form

PATIENT'S OPERATIVE CONSENT FOR FACIAL SURGERY
(THE COOK WEEKEND ALTERNATIVE TO THE FACELIFT™)

Patient name: ______________

Patient states: I am aware that the Cook Weekend Alternative to the Facelift™ (including but not limited to liposculpture, platysma muscle revision, laser dermal resurfacing, etc.) is a contouring process. Dr. Cook and assistants have carefully explained to me the nature, goals, limitations, and possible complications of this procedure and alternative forms of treatment. I have had the opportunity to ask questions about the procedure, its limitations, and possible complications.

I clearly understand and accept:

A. The potential benefits of the proposed procedure(s);
B. The possible alternate medical procedure(s);
C. The probability of success;

D. The reasonable anticipated consequences if the procedure(s) are not performed;

E. The possibility that additional services/fees may be required, including, but not limited to, anesthesia, laboratory, medications, and/or surgical facility or hospital use.

2. I realize that the goal of cosmetic surgery is improvement, not perfection. Satisfaction is based on realistic expectations. No one should expect that the procedure will remove all excess skin, all excess fat, or every wrinkle, or smooth and tighten skin perfectly. It does not guarantee the reduction of any measurements or weight.

3. The average time off from work and social activities is usually 2-3 days, but in some patients this may be extended.

4, The final result may not be apparent for 3-6 months postoperatively.

5. Occasionally, to achieve the best possible result, additional procedures may be necessary. There will be a charge for any additional operation performed.

6. Strict adherence to postoperative instructions is necessary in order to achieve the best possible results.

7. The surgical fee is paid for the operation itself and subsequent postoperative visits.

8. I will not drive for 24 hours after the procedure.

9. I give my permission for the administration of anesthesia, as deemed appropriate by the physician.

10. Protective eye covering will be provided to protect my eyes from accidental laser exposure. Accidental exposure to laser is extremely rare but possible.

Although complications following surgery are infrequent, I understand that the following may occur:

1. Bleeding is rare. In rare instances it could require hospitalization and blood transfusion. It is possible that blood clots or fluid may form requiring surgical drainage or medication.
2. Swelling, crusting, skin irregularities, lumpiness, hardness, and dimpling may occur postoperatively. Most of these problems will disappear with time and massage, but they may persist permanently.
3. If loose skin is present in the treated areas, it may or may not shrink to conform to the new contour. In rare cases wrinkling may persist.
4. Infection is rare, but should it occur, treatment with antibiotics and/or surgical drainage may be required.
5. Possible numbness or increased sensitivity of the skin over treated areas may persist for months, and in rare cases may be permanent.
6. Objectionable bruising and scarring are rare but possible, and may result in discoloration or texture changes of the skin. This is usually temporary but may rarely be permanent. To minimize the chances of this, I understand that it is important for me to follow all preoperative and after-care instructions carefully.
7. Dizziness may occur following surgery, particularly upon rising from a lying or sitting position. If dizziness occurs, exercise caution while walking and do not attempt to drive a car.
8. As the dermal resurfacing heals and the skin redrapes itself, in rare instances the skin may appear more wrinkled and the neck may

feel tighter. In almost all cases this resolves, but in rare instances it may persist.

9. Allergic or toxic responses to anesthesia are extremely rare, but possible.

10. In addition to these possible complications, I am aware of the general risks inherent in all surgical procedures and administration of anesthetic.

11. (For chin implant procedures only) Rare but possible complications include: extrusion (pushing out of the implant), malposition (abnormal location of the implant), bone absorption, hypesthesia of the lip (full or partial loss of sensation), and allergies. These complications may require removal of the implant.

Patient signature: ________________ Date

APPENDIX 2

2. Medical History Form

MEDICAL HISTORY

Name of patient: _____________

Name and address of your family doctor: __________________

____

May we contact your doctor in regard to any medical problem which may arise?

Are you considered a healthy person?

Are you now taking ANY drugs or medications? Which ones and how often?

Are you allergic to ANY medications? Which ones?

Have you ever received local anesthesia (Novocaine or Xylocaine) from a dentist or doctor?

Have you ever received general anesthesia?

Have you ever had any bad reaction to either local or general anesthesia? Please describe.

Do you take blood thinners? Which ones?

Do you take vitamins regularly? Which ones?

Do you take aspirin products or anti-inflammatory medicines or headache medicines? Which ones?

List all previous surgeries, peels, and dates:

Have you had:
- malignant hyperthermia
- fever blisters (herpes simplex)
- heart trouble
- blood pressure related problems
- liver problems, gallbladder problems, or yellow jaundice
- kidney disease
- diabetes
- stomach problems, indigestion, or ulcers
- bleeding tendency or excessive bruising
- any part of your body paralyzed or numb
- psychiatric consultation
- epilepsy - convulsions or seizures
- broken bones of the face, neck, jaw or back
- back trouble
- abnormal chest x-rays

abnormal electrocardiogram (ECG)
asthma or other respiratory problems
any medical treatment for nervous condition
excessive scarring or abnormal healing (explain)
tuberculosis
thyroid problems
any other illness. If so, please list:

Do any family members have:

heart trouble
excessive scarring
diabetes
asthma
excessive bruising
bad reaction to anesthesia
tuberculosis
high blood pressure
psychiatric or "nerve" problem
thyroid problems
excessive bleeding tendency
malignant hyperthermia

Do you:

wear contact lenses?
have dentures, false teeth, caps, or bridges?
smoke? how much?
drink alcohol? how much?
have any loose teeth or gum disease?

object to blood transfusions?

think you are pregnant? date of last menstrual period: ________

Have any contagious or infectious conditions? which ones?

28

Abdominal Contouring: Liposuction, Abdominal Rectus Plication, and Crescent Tuck Abdominoplasty to Contour the Abdomen

Edward B. Lack
The Center for Liposculpture and Cosmetic Surgery, Ltd., Des Plaines, Illinois

INTRODUCTION

During the evolution of body contouring, several pioneers in the field of liposuction promoted the concept that liposuction could be refined to an art form called liposculpture. To be sure, skeptics have questioned whether there is a difference between the two techniques, but over the past 5 years demonstrations at meetings of cosmetic surgeons have confirmed that an artistic and holistic approach to contouring produces superior results. The concept of body contouring was discussed by G. Fenno, in 1989–1990, and he conceived its application to abdominal contour reconstruction as a combination of liposuction, rectus muscle plication, and modified abdominoplasty. The geometry of the modified abdominal tuck was altered by B. Risch, who designed a trapezoidal excision to develop the necessary flaps to simultaneously enhance the appearance of the abdomen, waistline, and hips.

J. Klein promoted the conceptualization of liposculpting with the introduction of tumescent anesthesia and microcannulas [1]. Not only does tumescence allow the safe and relatively painless removal of fat, but also the swelling of the adipose unit makes it feasible to sculpt by creating a larger, more penetrable mass within which one can whittle [2]. Likewise, the introduction of microcannulas facilitated creating subtle alterations in the fat mass, which could not be achieved with large instruments. Lastly, reducing the friction of a cannula traversing a distended wet environment allows greater dexterity when sculpting.

The abdomen is one of the classic cosmetic units to consider when appreciating body sculpting—as it integrates with the waist laterally, the chest and rib cage superiorly, and the pelvis inferiorly. Its appearance is defined by its contour as well as by its surroundings. Designers appreciate that an item such as a picture can be made to look larger by placing it within a larger frame or smaller by confining the frame to the borders of the picture. Similarly, the abdomen is defined by its shape and by the presence or absence of protrusion as well as by its frame—the waist, ribs, and pelvis.

Laxity of the rectus muscles and their sheaths secondary to genetic predisposition, the effects of aging, and the effects of pregnancy render some female patients susceptible to visceral abdominal protrusion regardless of the presence of subcutaneous abdominal fat. Similarly, the same causal factors may produce superficial fascial laxity in combination with stretching and redundancy of the abdominal wall skin. These patients require surgical reconstruction of the abdominal wall at the level of the rectus sheath (rectus muscle plication) and at the level of the skin (full or modified abdominoplasty). The text in this chapter will focus on combining modified abdominoplasty and rectus must plication with liposculpting to obtain the best possible abdominal contour for the patient who presents with abdominal subcutaneous fat deposits, diastasis recti, and redundant abdominal skin.

HISTORY OF ABDOMINAL CONTOURING

Before the early 1980s, abdominal contouring referred to panniculectomy for patients with redundant skin and subcutis of the apron of the abdominal wall, or full abdominoplasty with incisions extending from anterior iliac crest to anterior iliac crest [3]. With the increasing popularity of liposuction in the mid 1980s, abdominal liposuction became a contouring technique. After J. Klein introduced tumescent anesthesia in 1986, more profound changes could be effected in abdominal contouring without significant bleeding or general anesthesia. As previously noted, by 1990 G. Fenno popularized the notion of combining liposuction with a modified abdominoplasty, which contoured the abdomen and accentuated the concavity of the waist and the convexity of the hips. Subsequently, A. Matarasso published his findings on abdominoplasty and showed that less than 20% of the patients in his series required a full abdominoplasty [4].

By 1990, articles were written noting morbidity of combined excisional procedures with liposuction—specifically, abdominoplasty and liposuction [5,6]. The abdominal wall obtains its vascular supply from three sources. Superiorly it is fed by the internal mammary arteries; inferiorly it is fed by the deep circumflex iliac arteries; and laterally it is fed by the intercostal perforators. Extensive undermining of the abdominal flap severs the superior and inferior perforator system, and if liposuction is carried out laterally the intercostal system is blocked as well, leading to necrosis of the abdominal wall flap. In addition, previous surgery, such as cholecystectomy, creates scars, which further interrupts blood supply to the cutaneous wall. Cases of hemorrhage, pulmonary embolism, and fat embolisation syndrome have appeared in the literature [7,8] and enthusiasm for combined procedures waned. As modified flap techniques evolved and were combined with rectus plication at or below the umbilicus, combined procedures again became popular [9].

The need for combined procedures was re-examined in the first half of the 1990s. The nature of liposuction with tumescent anesthesia in itself induces skin retraction—probably through principles of tissue-tissue interaction as mediators are released in the absence of contiguity of the skin flap with its underlying fascia. Presumably these mediators induce a reduction in the surface area of the skin until contiguity is re-established. P. Lillis published descriptions of retraction of abdominal apron skin redundancy after aggressive liposuction of the pannus [10]. Similarly, investigators have reported anecdotal evidence of skin retraction enhanced with the use of ultrasonic-assisted liposuction. Yet, regardless of the degree of skin retraction, some female patients desired taut, scaphoid abdomens that could not be achieved by skin retraction alone, and other female patients with inferior abdominal diastasis recti still required plication of the rectus sheath below the umbilicus to reduce abdominal protrusion secondary to pressure from abdominal viscera.

What follows in this chapter is my view of the candidate for combined liposuction of the abdomen with rectus muscle plication and modified abdominoplasty, as well as the procedure itself. In this discussion, no attempt will be made to discuss full abdominoplasty. Thus the ideal patient for this discussion is a postpartem female in her 30s or 40s; who does not anticipate conceiving more children; who does not have excessive abdominal visceral fat deposits; and who presents with subcutaneous fullness accompanied by rectus diastasis and moderate abdominal skin laxity below the umbilicus, with minimal laxity above the umbilicus. The goal is to obtain a flat to slightly scaphoid abdominal contour, which enhances appearance. The design of the flap for the crescent tuck not only minimizes skin flaccidity and flattens the stomach, but also accentuates the flow of the waist as it sweeps over the iliac crests and joins the anterior abdominal wall.

THE PATIENT CANDIDATE

Before initiating a consultation, criteria are established to define as objectively as possible the evaluation of the patient's physiognomy. The patient should be examined in the anterior, posterior, and lateral (profile) positions. In the anterior view an imaginary line may be drawn from the shoulders to the floor (Fig. 1). Ideally, the hips and thighs lie within the boundaries of these lines. There is a convex curvature from the axilla to the waist that accents the lines of the latissimus dorsi and extends to the iliac crest. From the iliac crest a second convex line proceeds to the inferior lateral thigh and then to the lateral knee. Ideally, the abdomen appears to extend from the sternum and rib cage above in a scaphoid or slightly concave fashion to the pubic bone below. As the waist proceeds anteriorly over the hips there is a gentle sweep, that curves into the lower abdomen. In profile, the scaphoid or slightly concave shape of the abdomen is more apparent and blends into the concavity of the waist just above the iliac crest (Fig. 2). In the female, the breasts protrude anteriorly beyond the abdomen and are slightly overbalanced posteriorly by the protrusion of the buttocks. In the male, the chest protrudes anteriorly beyond the abdomen and is balanced by the posterior projection of the buttocks.

Commonly, many female patients present in the anterior view with a bilobed protrusion of the abdomen with the larger protrusion extending from the umbilicus to the pubic bone. The fat pad of the hip extends above the iliac crest, which visually shortens the waist, and redundant rolls of skin and fat often characterize the waist. In the lateral view, the protrusion of the abdomen is excessive and is not balance proportionately by the breasts or the buttocks (Fig. 3). In an anterior view, the male abdomen is often characterized by an upper abdominal protrusion, which extends inferiorly into bulbous protrusions of the lateral waist, known as love handles.

When considering a modified crescent tuck, the patient is examined with respect to skin redundancy and flaccidity. When considering rectus muscle plication, diastasis recti is evaluated by having the patient valsalva in the diver's position while

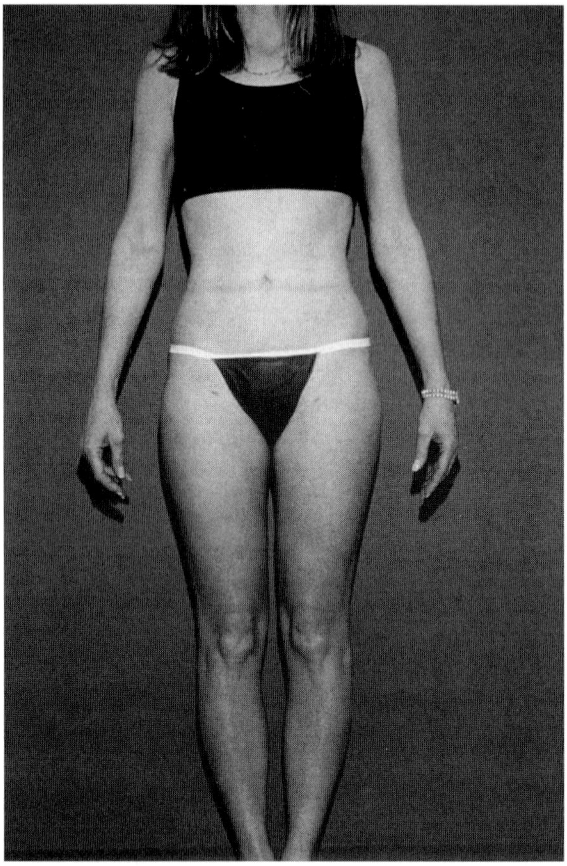

FIGURE 1 In the anterior view ideally the hips and thighs lie within the boundaries of imaginary lines dropped from the shoulders to the floor.

standing, and by palpating the junction of the rectus sheaths in the supine position while elevating the head to a 30° angle. During the physical examination, the presence or absence of hernias is noted—especially umbilical hernias. An umbilical hernia is not a contraindication for the procedure but will need to be avoided and repaired. Patients with significant skin laxity above and below the umbilicus or significant rectus diastasis above the umbilicus are candidates for full abdominoplasty and will not do as well with a modified abdominoplasty. Patients with pathology limited at or below the umbilicus are excellent candidates for this procedure.

THE CONSULTATION

The prospective patient consultation is an opportunity to educate both the physician and the patient. The patient needs factual information with which to decide whether the contemplated procedure is desirable. The physician needs to evaluate the patient as to the advisability of a procedure for this person as well as the psychological make-up of the person who is planning to undergo cosmetic surgery.

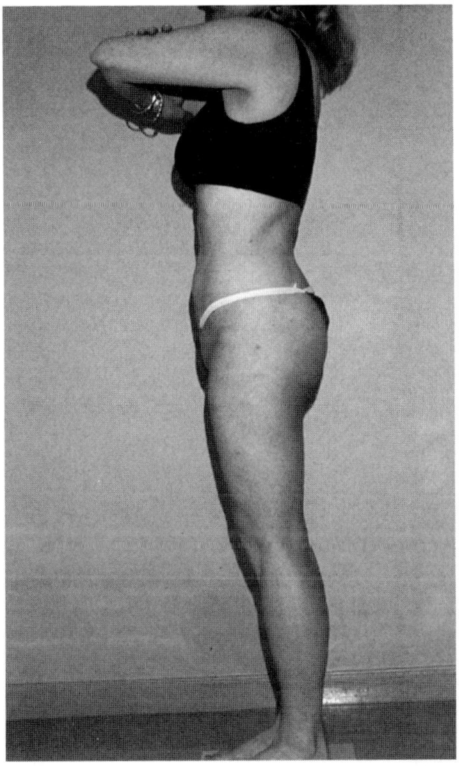

FIGURE 2 In profile, ideally, when an imaginary line is dropped from the shoulder the anterior projection of the female breasts extends beyond the abdomen and is balanced by the posterior projection of the buttocks.

Before the patient's arrival, a packet of information is sent that outlines the procedures and concerns the patient has expressed to the telephone consultant. The packet may contain "before" and "after" pictures of patients who have had the procedure, as well as information pertaining to how some of the procedure is performed, appropriate concerns for postsurgical care, and possible morbid sequelae of the operation. The patient thus arrives at the consultation with some background information regarding the procedure and several questions as to how the procedure applies to him or her.

The patient is ushered into a comfortable consultation room where a nurse consultant or other qualified person greets them to review the procedure and answer preliminary questions. The patient has already filled out a medical history questionnaire. If possible, the patient is shown a video of some of the procedure that is tastefully edited so as to provide an illustration of how the procedure is performed in a manner that is not offensive to lay people.

The patient is then escorted to an examination room where he or she can disrobe and redress in appropriate paper or cloth garments to facilitate a physical examination. When the physician meets the patient, he or she reviews the patient's medical history and engages in a dialogue regarding the patient's wishes and expectations. The patient can then stand for an examination of the torso, and dispropor-

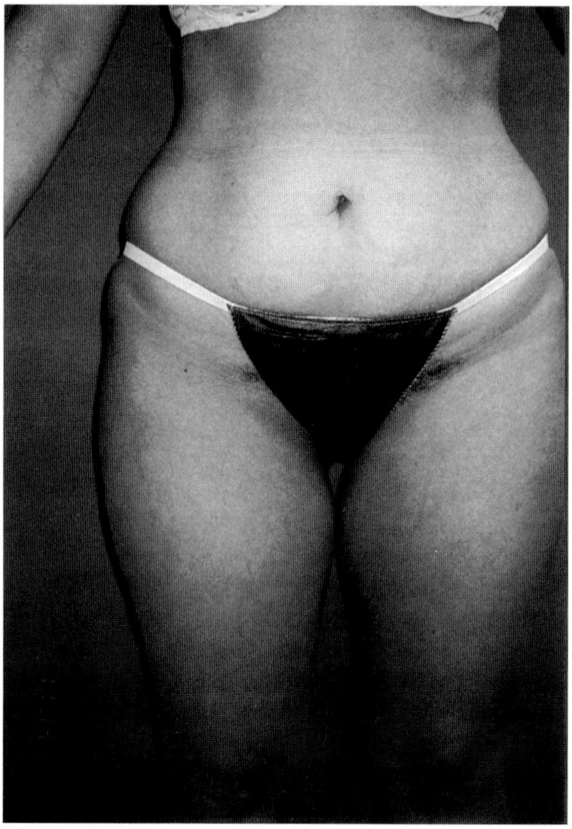

FIGURE 3 Commonly, female patients present with a bilobed protrusion of the abdomen and a superior projection of the fat pads of the hips above the iliac crest.

tionate fat deposits and contours are noted in the anterior, posterior, and lateral positions as described in *The Patient Candidate*. The patient can be checked for inguinal and umbilical hernias at that time and is asked to flex at the waist to check for diastasis recti or ventral hernias. Laxity of the abdominal skin and the presence of a redundant abdominal apron are noted. The patient is then asked to lie in the supine position on the examination table, and with the head flexed at 30° the presence of diastases is again evaluated.

At the conclusion of the evaluation, the patient is placed in a gown or bathrobe and the physician's evaluation is related to the patient's desires and expectations. A comparison of treatment of lax skin with liposculpting alone versus a combined procedure with rectus plication and abdominoplasty is discussed at this time. Ancillary procedures such as liposculpture of the back, waist, and hips can also be discussed.

PRESURGICAL EVALUATION

Two weeks before surgery, the patient returns to the office setting for a physical examination. The timing of this event has several purposes. First, it allows a physical assessment of the patient which, when combined with laboratory tests, and an EKG if the patient is over 40, confirms that the patient is an appropriate candidate for surgery. Second, it allows the patient once more to ask questions and reassess his or her motivation for having cosmetic surgery. Lastly, it is a time to take presurgical photographs, give the patient presurgical and postsurgical instructions, and to review with the patient the expected postsurgical course. At this time, the surgical consent is reviewed and signed by the patient. Medical nurses perform most of these tasks, but the physician should interact with the patient either during this visit or via telephone after the visit is concluded.

During the evaluation for a combined procedure liposculpture of the abdomen and modified crescent tuck abdominoplasty, the patient is checked for diastasis recti once again and the presence or absence of hernias is noted. Blood is drawn for CBC, Chemistry profile, PT, PTT, HIV, and hepatitis screen.

The patient is told to shower with Hibiclens soap the night before and the morning of surgery. Cephalexin (500 mg) is taken at 6:00 p.m. and 10:00 p.m. the night before surgery. Zantac (150 mg) is taken the night before and the morning of surgery. If the patient has a history of anxiety, Xanax (0.25 mg) may be taken the night before and the morning of surgery. The patient is kept NPO for 8 hours before surgery except for the sips of water necessary to take their morning pills.

Postsurgical instructions are described to the patient, and a written copy of the postsurgical plan is given to the patient. They are instructed to expect copious drainage from the 3-mm incision sites used for liposuction. At times the drainage will be considerable, and they are told to place maxipads over or below drainage sites. Specific postsurgical instructions are described later in this chapter (see Postsurgical Care).

SURGICAL INSTRUMENTATION

The combined procedure involves exposing the underside of the abdominal wall, the superficial fascia, and the rectus sheath. Therefore, a fully equipped operatory with monitoring facilities and appropriate staffing is essential for the protection of the patient and the successful completion of the surgery. Instrumentation for tumescent liposuction has been well documented in other publications and will not be expanded on in this chapter except to note the need for infusing equipment and appropriate cannulas, usually 2.5 to 4.0 mm in diameter. Cannulas may vary from 15 to 25 cm in length, and I favor shorter cannulas for better control. Likewise, the aggressiveness of the design of the cannula varies from the standard single hole to the three port mercedes design. The modified abdominoplasty requires a full instrument table appropriate for abdominal surgery. I have found the DeBakey forceps, the Mayo scissors, and the heavy needleholder to be very helpful for developing the abdominal flap, and the maleable retractor and the bear claw retractors very helpful for developing good exposure of the surgical field.

The choice of suture is personal, but I prefer 0 PDS, 2-0 PDS, 2-0 Prolene, 2-0 Ethibond, 4-0 vicryl, and 4-0 nylon.

ANESTHESIA

Tumescent anesthesia is sufficient for liposuction of the superficial fascia of the abdominal wall, and provides hemostasis and an excellent tissue plane for removing fat. It is inadequate, however, for muscle tightening and the necessary patient relaxation to perform the rectus muscle plication. Although IM sedation might be sufficient to perform the procedure, I consider it marginal at best and may introduce an element of risk as titration of anesthesia is not possible.

Therefore, intravenous sedation and general anesthesia are appropriate for this procedure, and in either case require the expertise and administration of a certified registered nurse anesthetist or a board-certified anesthesiologist. In both cases, sedation is titrated and monitored and may involve the use of midazolam, fentanyl, and propofol. General anesthesia uses the same medications along with muscle relaxants and/or halogenated inhalants. Dissociative agents (ie, Ketamine), when combined with tranquilizers, have been used with favorable results in selected patient groups.

TECHNIQUES OF SURGERY

Anatomical Considerations

The abdomen is framed by the rib cage superiorly, the waist and hips laterally, and the pubis inferiorly. Ideally, a concave waist, a bony hip, and a flat pubis frame a scaphoid abdomen. Liposculpting these areas will help to achieve the frame necessary to highlight a flat abdomen. Similarly, as will be reviewed in the discussion of the crescent tuck, the rotation of the flap closure for the abdominoplasty can highlight the concavity of the waist and the prominence of the iliac crest.

The Fascial Layers

The vascular supply is an important consideration whenever combined procedures of liposuction and flaps are discussed. While it is possible to perform the two procedures on different occasions, it is a more difficult undertaking if abdominoplasty is performed months or years after liposuction because of the copious amounts of fibrosis in the superficial fascial layer and its adherence to the rectus sheath. Lysing these fibrous bands produces more bleeding and pain than if fibrosis is not present, as is the case with a combined procedure. Cosmetic results are usually superior with the combined procedure because there is no distortion from previous fibrosis.

By the early 1990s, combined procedures had been performed with full abdominoplasty and liposuction under general anesthesia and reports appeared in the literature of significant blood loss and morbid sequelae, such as fat emboli syndrome and pulmonary emboli syndrome [11]. In addition, flap necrosis was reported because of the disruption of the blood supply to the abdominal wall [12].

In 1990, when G. Fenno and B. Risch conceived of a combined procedure of liposuction with a modified crescent tuck abdominoplasty, they felt that the minimal flap dissection would preclude vascular compromise of the abdominal wall. In reality, it also reduced systemic morbidity to that approximating liposuction of the abdomen alone.

Another major advantage of this combined procedure is that a limited flap dissection enhances the ability to liposculpt the surrounding cosmetic units of the abdomen without fear of compromising the vascular supply of the abdominal wall. Although extensive undermining of the abdominal wall and its surroundings severely compromises this collateral circulatory system, the modified tuck minimizes under-

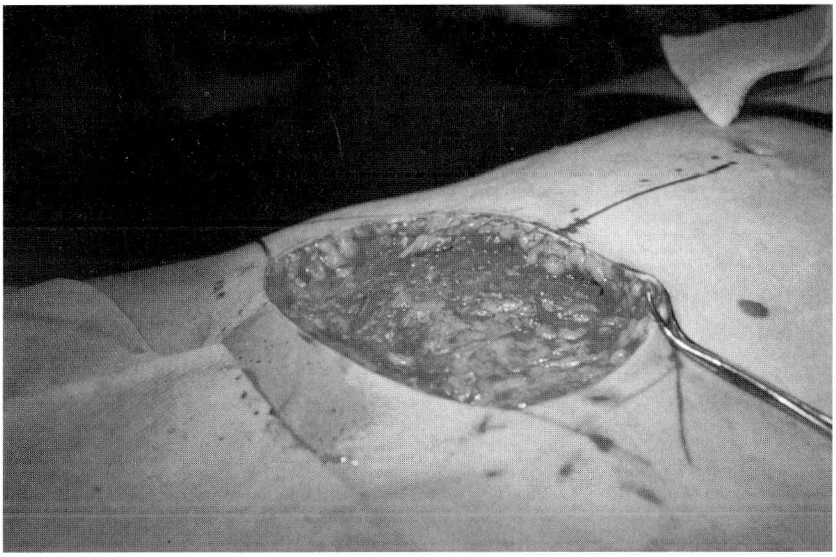

FIGURE 9 Scarpa's fascia lies in tact and glistening above the rectus sheath.

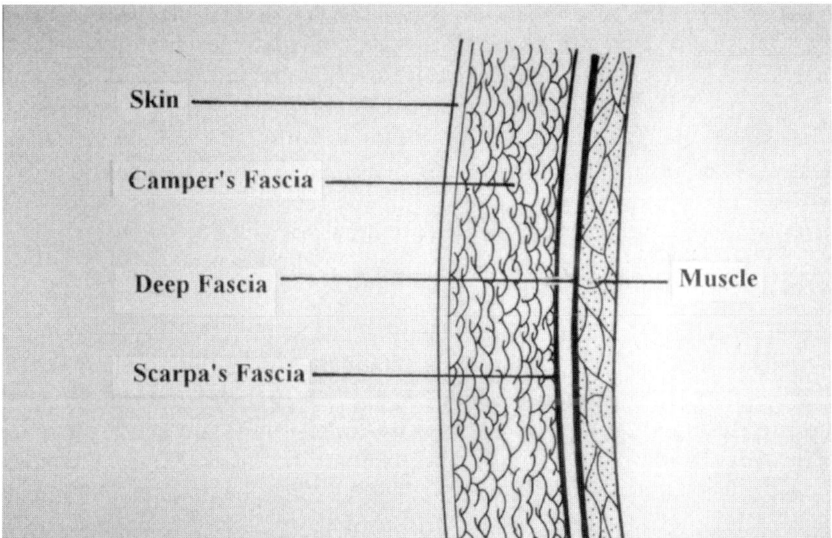

FIGURE 10 Scarpa's fascia is a thin fibrous tissue which is the most inferior layer of the superficial fascia of the abdominal wall and is separated from the rectus sheath by a potential space.

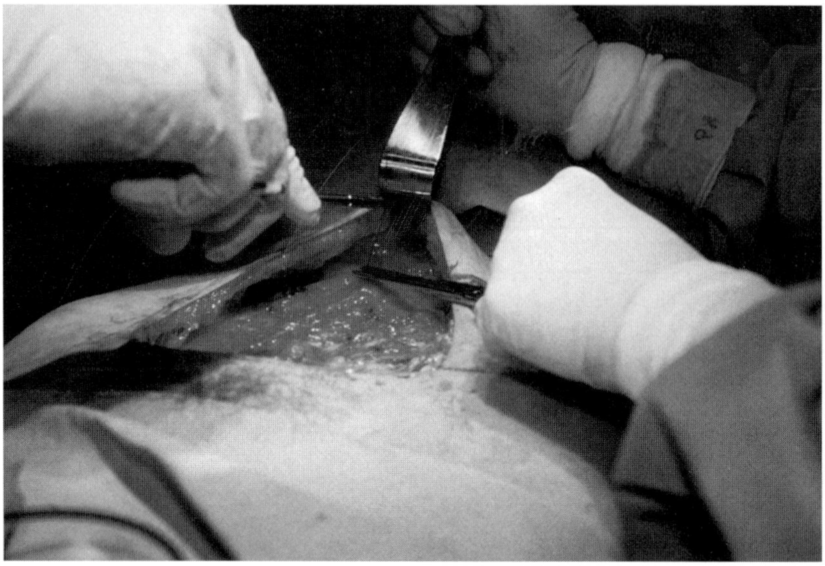

FIGURE 11 Plication of the rectus sheath is performed from the umbilicus to the pubic symphysis.

plication invaginates the rectus sheath upon itself medially. It is important not to disturb the apposition of the fascial layers or the risk of seroma is greatly increased. When Scarpa's fascia and the rectus sheath are in apposition, placing a drain is usually unnecessary. Alternatively, if destruction of Scarpa's fascia has occurred secondary to liposuction, the placement of a drain is advisable.

At the conclusion of muscle sheath plication, the trapezoidal defect is closed (Figs. 12–15). The sides of the trapezoid are rotated medially and inferiorly, and three subcutaneous/dermal tacking sutures are placed in the midline and halfway between the lateral poles and the midline with 2-0 PDS sutures. The subcutaneous/deep dermal border of the rotation flap is then closed with 2-0 PDS sutures. The dermis is closed with interrupted 4-0 vicryl sutures and the wound edges are opposed with running 4-0 nylon sutures.

POSTSURGICAL CARE

At the conclusion of surgery, Polysporin ointment covered with Telfapads are applied to the liposuction incision sites as well as the suprapubic suture line. Reston Foam is applied to the abdominal wall and to contiguous cosmetic units that have been sculpted. Maxipad absorbent dressings are taped inferior to the foam at the pubis to absorb drainage, and absorbent chucks are taped around the torso. A lycra/spandex garment is applied over the thighs and lower half of the abdomen, and an abdominal binder 6 to 9 in is applied to the abdomen. The patient remains in recovery for 1 hour and, after showing an ability to eat crackers, drink fluids, and void, is discharged home in the care of an adult.

The patient has the option of changing the chucks and maxipads in 6 hours, and at 12 hours the chucks are discarded. Because chucks are lined with plastic, they

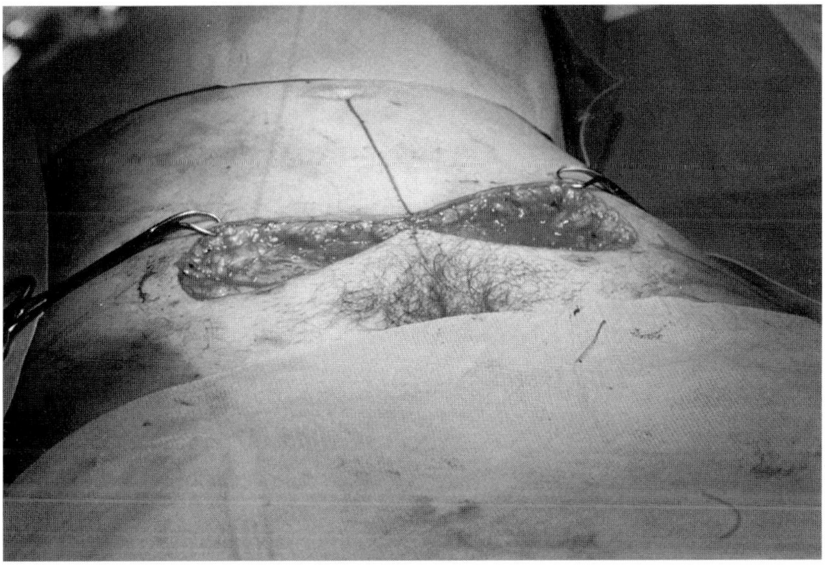

FIGURE 12 A key stitch is placed in the midline with a deep subcutaneous 00-PDS suture.

tend to elevate body temperature and are cumbersome. For the next 48 to 96 hours, maxipads will be used to absorb drainage at the level of the pubis. The patient is instructed to walk 2 miles in a leisurely fashion the first morning after surgery and 4 miles per day thereafter. The patient must avoid lifting more than 10 lbs or engaging in physical exercise other than as prescribed for approximately 12 weeks. At

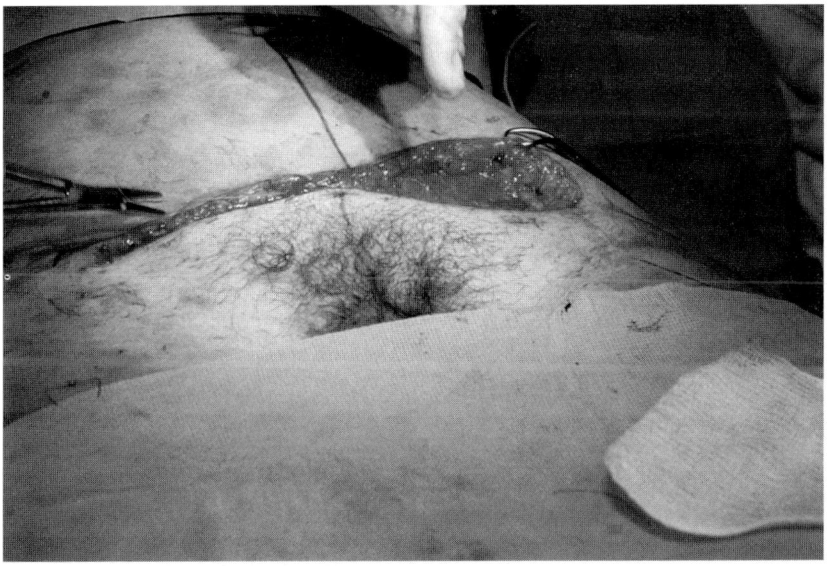

FIGURE 13 The lateral wall of the trapezoid is rotated inferior and lateral and another key suture is placed.

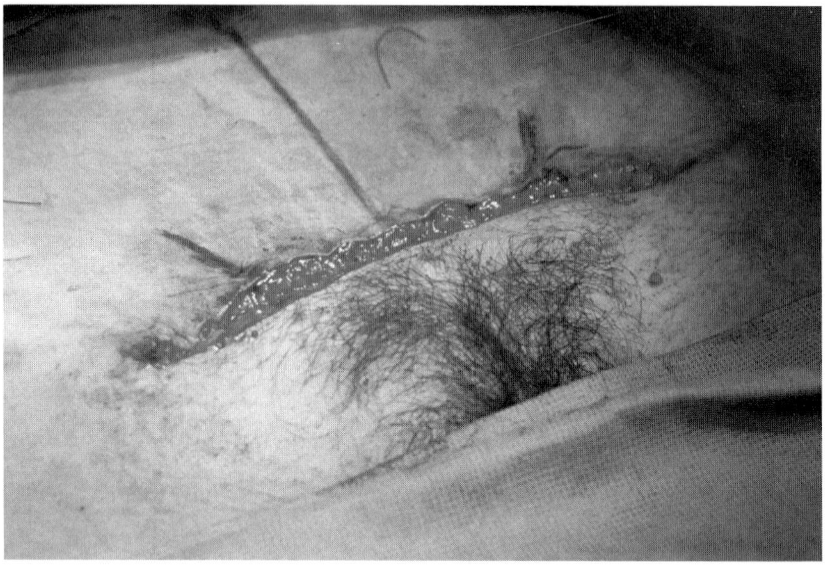

FIGURE 14 The subcutis is closed by the rule of halves.

72 to 96 hours after surgery, the patient returns to the office for removal of the Reston Foam. This is performed with the patient in the recumbent position to avoid an inadvertent vasovagal maneuver. The abdomen is examined for swelling or tenderness and any evidence of a hematoma or seroma. If the latter is noted, it is drained at that time. The patient is then discharged home with a lycra/spandex garment and an abdominal binder that is worn at all times when the patient is ambulating.

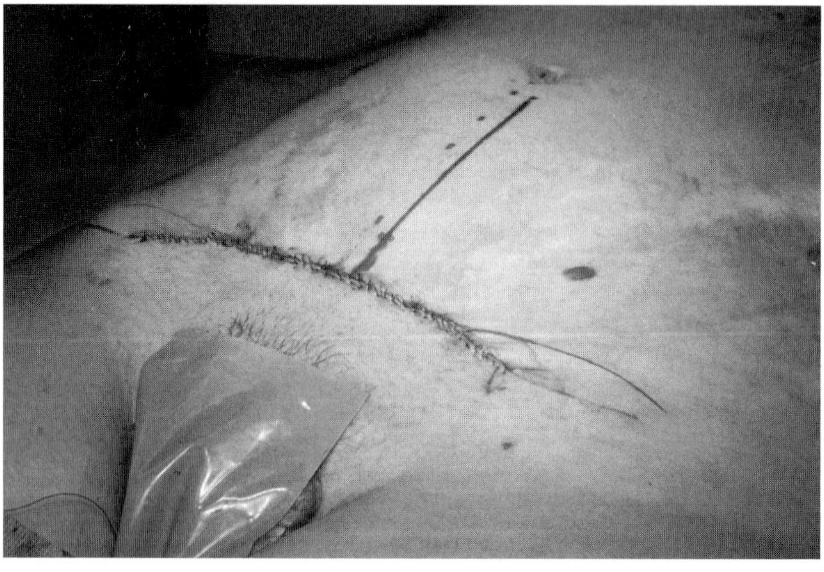

FIGURE 15 The cutis is closed with running 4-0 plain gut suture.

The patient returns to the office 7 days after surgery for examination. If induration is significant, physical therapy in the form of low-amperage electrical stimulation or low-energy pulsed ultrasound massage may be applied to the abdominal wall. These treatments are repeated daily or on alternate days until significant improvement is noted. If evidence of a hematoma or seroma appears, it may be drained with a seroma needle or standard 16-gauge needle between the tenth and fourteenth day. The patient is encouraged to continue walking 4 miles per day for exercise and rehabilitation. Showers are allowed after foam has been removed, but no form of immersion in water, whether bathing, swimming, soaking, or hot tubs, is allowed for 4 weeks.

At the conclusion of 12 weeks after surgery, the patient is allowed to resume normal lifting and normal exercise. Although many patients resume full activities after 8 weeks, I have seen sudden reoccurrence of the diastasis recti after vigorous exercise.

COMPLICATIONS AND TREATMENT

The complications of a combined procedure of liposuction of the abdomen and a modified crescent tuck abdominoplasty are identical to those of liposuction of the abdomen alone with the possible addition of more significant hemorrhage, hematoma, and wound dehiscence. The complications related to both procedures separately or combined include induration, edema, seroma, infection, skin necrosis, bowel perforation, fasciitis, neuropraxia, and contour irregularities. Avoidance of these complications includes the practice of meticulous, sterile technique. In the event of acute hemorrhage or hematoma, the wound must be reopened and the superficial fascial plane explored to determine and ligate the source of bleeding. Infection is usually staphylococcal or streptococcal and is limited to skin wounds, but gram negative sepsis, pseudomonas infection, atypical mycobacterium infections, and toxic shock syndromes have been reported. I am unaware of any reports of acute necrotizing fasciitis. Treatment is based on culture and sensitivity studies, and is initiated with broad-spectrum coverage. In the case of abscess formation, incision and drainage are required. Consultation with general surgery and infectious disease specialists is advisable.

Wound dehiscence may be treated with re-excision and closure if the wound is uncontaminated. If the dehiscence is small, healing by secondary intent may suffice. Skin necrosis may be treated with topical ointment and healing by secondary intent, or, if significant, by debridement or excision and primary closure. Induration and mild fasciitis may be treated with physical therapy modalities of low-amperage electrical stimulation or low-dosage ultrasound massage, as well as pharmacologically with nonsteroidal anti-inflammatory drugs, prednisone, and broad-spectrum antibiotics if there is any evidence of infection. Acute necrotizing fasciitis, although heretofore not reported, must be treated with open fasciotomy and massive appropriate antibiotic therapy in a hospital intensive care facility.

Seromas require repeated drainage and the use of broad-spectrum antibiotic coverage. If left untreated, they may result in pseudobursa formation and require excision.

SUMMARY

Physicians and patients have become more sophisticated in their evaluation of body contour, and procedures to enhance body contour have improved during the past decade. Combined abdominal procedures have become more specific to patient presentation and safer to perform. The combination of liposuction of the abdomen, abdominal rectus plication, and a modified crescent tuck abdominoplasty is a successful approach to patients with abdominal subcutaneous fat deposits accompanied by rectus muscle diastases and cutaneous laxity.

REFERENCES

1. Klein J. The tumescent technique for lipo-suction surgery. Am J Cosmet Surg 1987; 4: 263–267.
2. Klein J. Anesthesia for liposuction in dermatologic surgery. Dermatol Surg 1988; 14: 1124–1132.
3. Mataraso Alan, Mataraso S. When does your liposuction patient require an abdominoplasty? Dermatol Surg 1997; 23:1151–1160.
4. Matarasso A. Abdominoplasty: a system of classification and treatment for combined abdominoplasty and suction-assisted lipectomy. Aesthet Plast Surg 1991; 15:111–121.
5. Dillerud E. Abdominoplasty combined with suction lipoplasty: a study of complications, revisions, and risk factors in 487 cases. Ann Plast Surg 1990; 25:333–338.
6. Hester WE Jr, Baird W, Bostwick J III, Nahai F, Cukic JPA. Abdominoplasty combined with other major surgical procedures: safe or sorry. Plast Reconstr Surg 1989; 83:997.
7. Hester WE Jr, Baird W, Bostwick J III, Nahai F, Cukic JPA. Abdominoplasty combined with other major surgical procedures: safe or sorry. Plast Reconstr Surg 1989; 83:997.
8. Christman KD. Death following suction lipectomy and abdominoplasty. Plast Reconstr Surg 1986; 78:428.
9. Floros C, Davis PKB. Complications and long-term results following abdominoplasty: a retrospective study. Br J Plast Surg 1991; 44:190–194.
10. Lillis P. Liposuction for excessive lower abdominal fat accumulation in females over 60. Cosmet Dermatol 1994; 7:11–14.
11. Voss SC, Sharp HC, Scott JR. Abdominoplasty combined with gynecologic surgical procedures. Obstet Gynecol 1986; 67:181.
12. Ousterhout DK. Combined suction-assisted lipectomy, surgical lipectomy, and surgical abdominoplasty. Ann Plast Surg 1990; 24:126–133.

29

Multivector Face/Neck/Browlift: An Anatomical and Biomechanical Approach

Elliott H. Rose
The Mount Sinai/NYU Medical Center, and The Aesthetic Surgery Center, New York, New York

INTRODUCTION

The prospect of facial rejuvenation surgery can be one of the most exciting, yet intimidating, decisions facing the 40-year-old or older man or woman. With the advance of less invasive incisions, more anatomically directed dissections, and sophisticated ancillary techniques (eg, microliposuction, laser resurfacing, lipoinjection, etc.), results are more predictable and long lasting. State-of-the-art outpatient surgical facilities and "twilight" sedation techniques make the surgery safer, more comfortable for the patient and family, and economically more affordable. Attention to skin care and postsurgical camouflage make-up techniques reintegrate patients to their work and social environments in the time it takes for a moderate length vacation.

The typical facelift patient is in his or her late forties, self-controlled, socially poised, and more oriented towards action and independent [1]. Many emphasize their intense commitment to their jobs and/or social activities where youthful appearance is extremely important. Unlike patients with major congenital or traumatic defects, cosmetic patients are not seeking a removal of a deformity, but rather restoration to the "ideal state" that existed in their youth. The results are generally reviewed as very favorable, because the outcome is a positive enhancement of already existing narcissism and represents an addition to the customary armamentarium of adaptive behavior patterns [2]. In a society where youth and beauty are at a premium, it is not surprising that psychological studies have confirmed that physically attractive people are likely to have better jobs, better marriages, and more fulfilling lives [3].

SURGICAL ANATOMY OF THE FACE RELATED TO THE AGING PROCESS

Upper Face (Forehead, Eyebrows, Nasion)

Biomechanically, forehead tone (and thus eyebrow position) is influenced by the delicate interaction between the three depressors and one elevator muscle bilaterally

(Fig. 1) [4]. The paired frontalis muscules course vertically through the forehead and are contiguous with the galea aponeurotica, the dense muscle/fascial layer of the scalp. Having no bony origin, the frontalis muscle interdigitates inferiorly with the procerus muscle at the nasion, the corrugator supercilli muscles at the medial brow, and fibers of the orbicularis muscles more laterally. With contraction, the frontalis elevates the eyebrow and causes deep transverse wrinkling in the forehead. Frontalis elevation is opposed by the depressor pull of the paired procerus, corrugator, and orbicularis oculi muscles. The fanshaped corrugator muscle arises from the frontal bone near the superomedial orbital rim and inserts into the frontalis muscle and skin in the medial brow [5]. The action of the corrugator muscles is to pull the eyebrows together and produce the vertical wrinkles of the forehead ("frown lines") [6].

The vertically oriented procerus muscles, arising from the nasal bones and inserting into the mid forehead skin between the most medial fibers of the frontalis [5], are responsible for the wrinkles of the glabellar nose. The concentric orbicularis oculi muscles in closing counteract the upper pull of the frontalis muscle. The frontalis and corrugator muscles are innervated by the temporal branch of the facial nerve, which travels within the superficial musculoaponeurotic layer (SMAS) over the zygomatic and temporal areas approximately one fingerbreadth lateral to the

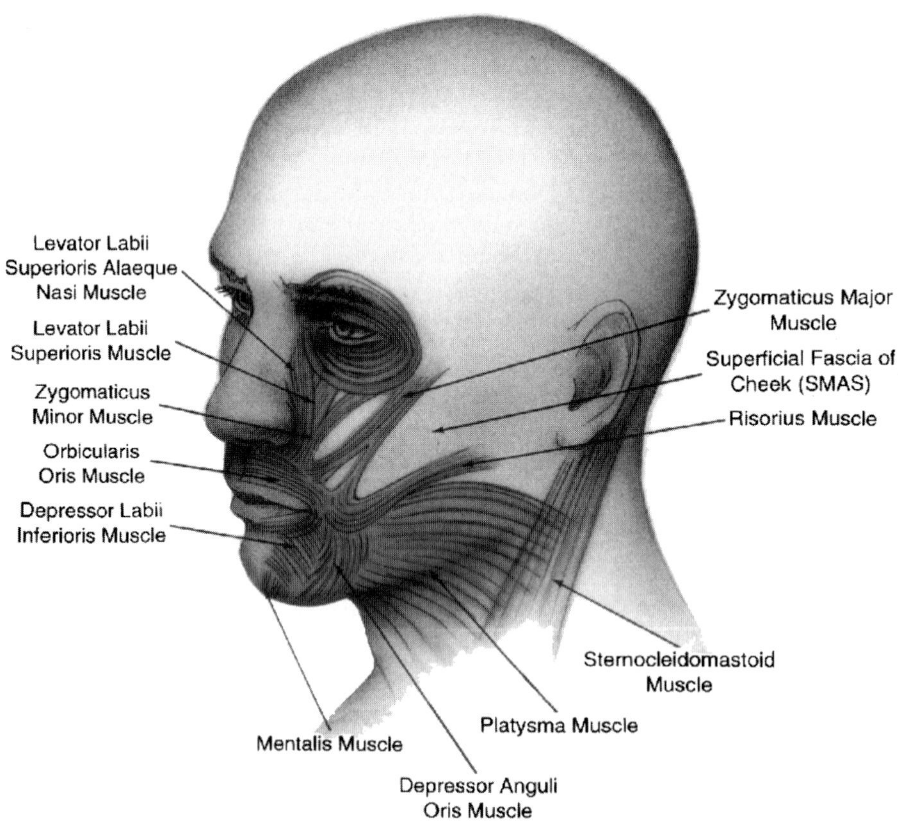

FIGURE 1 Surgical anatomy of the upper face.

orbital rim and enters the undersurface of the frontalis muscle 1.5 cm above the eyebrow [7].

The vascular supply to the mid forehead is via the paramedian supraorbital and supratrochlear arteries, terminal branches of the ophthalmic arteries of the internal carotid system. They, along with the supraorbital and supratrochlear nerves, terminal branches of the ophthalmic division of the trigeminal nerve, exit the supraorbital rim 2.7 cm and 1.7 cm from the midline, respectively [8]. The supraorbital nerve and artery pedicle exits through a small foramen in the supraorbital rim or through a palpable notch in the bone at that time [9]. The supraorbital arterial branches anastomosis laterally with the anterior branch of the superficial temporal artery and the zygomatic orbital arteries [10].

Typical eyebrow configuration is gender related. The ideal female brow is at least 1 cm above the supraorbital rim [11] and is arched at its highest point above the lateral limbus [6]. The male brow, on the other hand, is more horizontal and lies along the supraorbital rim. Numerical guidelines further assist in establishing proper aesthetic brow/forehead/pupil relationships. Ideal distances in females are as follows: brow to hairline 5 to 6 cm; brow to supratarsal crease 1.6 cm; and brow to mid pupil 2.5 cm [12].

With aging, the frontalis muscle loses tone in response to gravity and brow ptosis ensues. Low brow position contributes to "hooding" of the thicker infrabrow skin and the appearance of blepharochalasia. Transverse forehead wrinkling ("furrows") is the sequela of the constant strain of the frontalis muscle to elevate the descended upper eyelid skin for unobstructed and comfortable forward vision [13]. The attenuated frontalis muscle (elevator) alters the biomechanical balance and allows the corrugator and procerus muscles (depressors) to contract unopposed. The net effect is the marked exaggeration of the glabellar "frown lines" between the brows [13] and deepening of the transverse nasion lines.

Mid Face (Figures 2, 3)

The SMAS (originally described by Mitz and Peyronie [14]) invests and interdigitates with the superficial mimetic muscles of facial expression (orbicularis oculi, depressor anguli oris, zygomaticus major and minor, and risorius) (Figs. 2, 3). The muscle contraction is translated to expressive movements through vertical septae extending from the SMAS into the dermis [14]. The fascia, comprised of elastin and collagen fibers with similar viscoelastic properties to dermis [15], is thicker over the parotid gland but thins out anteriorly over the masseter and buccal fat pads [16]. The SMAS is contiguous with the lower margin of the orbicular oculi muscles but becomes wispy within 1 cm of the zygomatic arch [17]. The stout zygomaticus ligaments (Fig. 4)—6 to 8 mm in length, originating from the inferior border of the zygoma behind the insertion of the zygomaticus muscles, and inserting into dermis—serve to anchor the malar soft tissue against gravitational change [18].

The superficial mimetic muscles of the mid face (zygomaticus major and minor, levator labii superioris, levator labii superioris alaque nasi), derived embriologically from sphincter coli muscles, have a direct bony origin, in contrast to the muscles of the lower face and neck, derived from the embrionic primitive platysma which lacks bony insertion [6]. A less rigid line of fibrous septa, the masseteric cutaneous ligaments, interconnect the superficial and deep fascial layers in the mid face at the

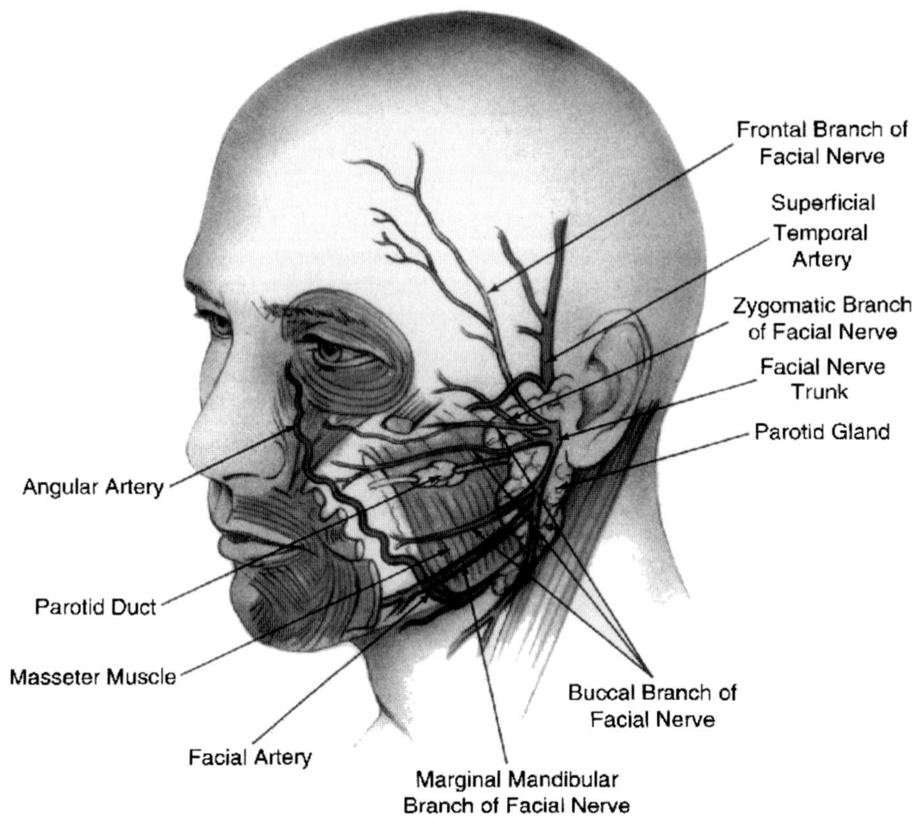

FIGURE 2 Surgical anatomy of the mid and lower face.

anterior margin of the masseter muscle [16]. Weakening of these retaining ligaments allows for anterior-inferior descent of the lipodystrophic fibro-fatty layer overlying the zygomatic prominence (malar fat pad), leaving an infraorbital hollow and deepening of the nasojugal groove.

Anteriorly, the SMAS extends across the cheek to the nasolabial fold where it merges with the superficial orbicularis oris muscles in the upper lip [19]. The nasolabial crease is a distinct fusion separating the cheek from the upper lip at the line where the mimetic muscles and SMAS insert into the orbicularis oris muscles [20]. Medial to the crease there is almost no subcutaneous fat between the dermis and the orbicularis oris sphincter; laterally a generous layer of fat exists between the mimetic muscles and dermis to allow for a smooth gliding plane with animation [21].

During the aging process, the nasolabial crease remains in an anchored position because of the constant pull of the SMAS and mimetic muscles to retain the resting tone and activity of the upper lip [20], whereas the less fixed fibrofatty structures lateral to the crease descend with gravity and aging to overhang the fixed crease, thereby increasing the fullness and depth of the nasolabial fold [22,23]. A popular misconception is that the lateral pull of the SMAS layer of the mid face will flatten the nasolabial fold. In fact, lateral traction in the SMAS actually deepens the crease

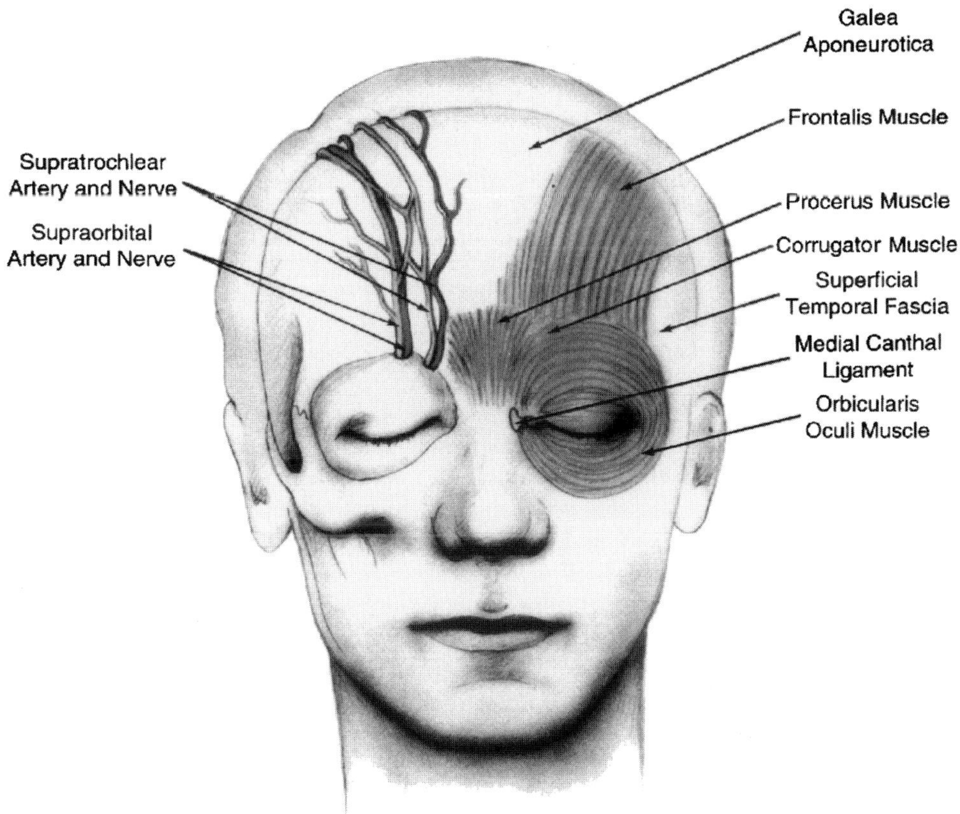

FIGURE 3 Deeper anatomy of the mid and lower face.

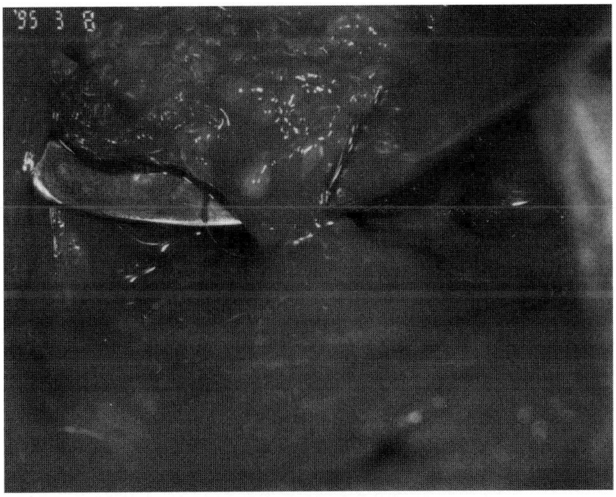

FIGURE 4 Broad, stout zygomaticus ligament.

and accentuates the nasolabial fold. Conversely, in the paralyzed face, when the SMAS and mimetic muscle tone is weakened, the nasolabial fold flattens as the lip elevators elongate and the nasolabial crease descends more medially. Logically, an aesthetically acceptable softening of the nasolabial fold requires release of the tethering of the zygomatic ligaments, resuspension of the superficial fibrofatty layer of the nasolabial fold (malar fat pad) in a vector directed over the malar prominence, and redraping of the cheek skin in a lateral oblique direction.

In the mid face, the buccal branches and zygomatic branches of the facial nerve exit the anterior border of the parotid gland and course over the masseter muscle deep to the SMAS. In this region the facial nerve branches lie beneath the thinned parotidomasseteric fascia as it drapes over the deep buccal fat pad [16]. Peripherally, the buccal and zygomatic branches divide 2.0 cm beyond the anterior edge of the parotid before innervating the mimetic facial muscles [24]. The more superficial muscles (zygomaticus major and minor, levator labii superioris alaque nasi, levator labii superioris) receive their innervation on the deep surfaces whereas the buccinator and levator anguli oris muscles are innervated on their outside surfaces [25]. The larger ramus of the zygomatic branch crosses deep to the zygomaticus major muscle at its lower one third [26].

The facial skin is supplied by a series of paired musculocutaneous perforators arising from the main arterial trunks—the facial, superficial temporal, and ophthalmic arteries [27]. The dermis of the lateral cheek area of the face is supplied predominantly by fasciocutaneous perforating branches of the transverse facial artery passing through the subcutaneous and SMAS layers to branch extensively in the subdermal plexus. Whetzel and Mathes were able to predict with 95% certainty the location of the single perforator in the mid face on a line extending from the external auditory canal to the nasal spine [28]. Inclusion or exclusion of the SMAS layer in the dissection had no effect on the perfusion or viability of the lateral face flap [29]. Preservation of this lone perforator in a deep flap dissection greatly enhances blood flow to an area extending 1 to 2 cm above the zygomatic arch, anteriorly to the lateral canthus, inferiorly to within 2 cm of the mandibular border, and posteriorly to 1 to 2 cm of the tragus [29]. More medially in the cheek, the anterior face is supplied by multiple small perforators of the submental, superior, and inferior labial artery, and the lateral nasal and ophthalmic arteries [27].

Lower Face (Neck, Jawline, and Jowls)

The platysma muscle, a broad, thin quadrangular muscle, originates at the upper chest, clavicle, and shoulders and sweeps obliquely across the anterior lateral neck where it fuses with the SMAS and the perioral mimetic muscles of facial expression (orbicularis oris, depressor anguli oris, depressor labii inferioris, and risorius muscles) (Figs. 2,3) [14]. At the anterior border of the masseter, the platysma is adherent to the deep fascial layer via the masseteric cutaneous ligaments [16]. Unlike the mimetic muscles of the upper face which have their origin from bony attachments, the platysma and mimetic muscles of the lower face lack bony insertions [6] and, with the exception of the dense mandibular ligament at the anterior jaw [16], are entirely suspended by the fibroelastic SMAS fascia. With aging, the platysma and subcutaneous fat respond to gravitational changes and weakening of the masseteric cutaneous ligaments, allowing inferior migration of the cheek soft tissue below the mandibular border [30]. The labiomental crease extending from the lateral lip commissure to the parasymphysis represents the adhesion of the superficial and deep fascia at the point of attachment of the osseocutaneous mandibular ligament [16]. The mid mandibular jowl, therefore, is bordered anteriorly by the tethered mandibular ligament and posteriorly by the anterior masseteric border. "Softening" of the mandibular jowl is achieved by contouring of the fat pad, redirection of the vector of the SMAS/platysmal support along the jawline, and redraping of the cervical skin above the mandibular border.

In the anterior neck, the platysma muscle may fully decussate at the midline above the hyoid or be entirely separated [31]. Because the medial edges of the platysma are firmly attached to the deep cervical fascia, platysmal "bands" represent "lateral pleats" caused by laxity of the muscle [32]. Fat in the submental regions may either be supraplatysmal or in the "subplatysmal space" bounded laterally by the digastrics, deeply by the myelohyoid muscle, and superficially by the platysma muscle [33].

The marginal mandibular branch of the facial nerve leaves the parotid gland 1 cm below the angle of the mandible and courses deep to the platysma along the inferior border of the body of the mandible, but drops 1 cm below 19% of the time [34]. It recrosses the mandibular border anterior to the facial artery to supply the labii inferioris and mentalis muscles on their superficial rather than deep surfaces [35]. Gosain has shown in cadaver dissections that the marginal mandibular nerve consistently passes through the mandibular ligament at the anterior margin of the jaw [36], which perhaps accounts for Barton's report of a 15% incidence of injury in combined deep plane and subcutaneous rhytidectomies [37].

HISTORICAL PERSPECTIVE OF FACELIFT SURGERY

From a historical perspective, facial rejuvenation surgery has evolved from a simple undermining and advancement of facial skin to complex alteration of the deeper supportive structures based on understanding of the three-dimensional anatomical interrelationships and biomechanical principles of stress/relaxation of facial components. The first description of a "surgical lift" is credited to Hollander in 1901 [38]. Lexer in 1910 describes subcutaneous dissection through two "S" temporal and postauricular incisions [39]. Bettman in 1920 published photographs showing temporal and preauricular incisions used in modern facelifts [40]. This technique remained relatively standard until 1974 when Skoog introduced the concept of a deeper dissection beneath the platysma to suspend the "foundation" structures of the lower space [41]. This was followed by Mitz and Peyronie's anatomical dissections and delineation of the SMAS [14]. In 1977, Owsley combined the Skoog technique and Mitz and Peyronie's description of the SMAS to develop an entirely subfascial/subplatysmal suspension of the cheek and neck in continuity [42]. Others followed with large series and modifications of sub-SMAS/platysmal advancement [43–48]. Hamra's "composite" rhytidectomy, introduced in 1992, raised the deep SMAS and skin layers as a single unit to achieve cheek repositioning [49]. Others have worked in multiplanes of dissection, combining deeper and more superficial approaches [50–52].

Long-term efficacy of the extended SMAS suspension when compared with conventional facelift procedures had not been shown [53], although biomechanical studies in cadavers have shown the deep tissue support using the SMAS technique decreases skin closure tension [54]. Arterial perfusion to skin flaps is better preserved in composite dissection than in subcutaneous or biplanar techniques [55].

Despite increasingly aggressive approaches to SMAS or deep plane suspension, it was apparent that SMAS traction alone could not "soften" nasolabial fullness of the mid face. In fact, excessive pull could further deepen the nasolabial groove [56]. Many attempts at "contouring" the nasolabial fold by excision, curettage, or liposuction have been described [57–59], but it was not until the intricate anatomy of the nasolabial fold complex was better delineated [20,60] that more definitive approaches to nasolabial suspension could evolve. With the understanding of the gravitational descent of the fibrofatty layer lateral to the fixed insertion of the SMAS to the orbicularis oris at the nasolabial crease, numerous investigators have described very effective methods of superior "resuspension" of the cheek fat over the malar prominence, thereby "softening" the nasolabial fold [61–64].

In 1986, Psillakis described yet a deeper plane, a subperiosteal facelift approach, for correction of the aging face [65]. By continuing the subgaleal dissection of the temporal area deep to the periosteal plane of the zygomatic arch, the deep fascia of the masseter muscle could be undermined to lift the cheek malar mound in a vertical direction [66]. Adaptation of endoscopic techniques from other surgical subspecialties has furthered the development of the subperiosteal facelift as well as the coronal browlift through shorter, less invasive incisions [67–70].

VIDEO IMAGING

As part of the initial consultation, sophisticated imaging software is used to assist the surgeon in the complex facial analysis and projection of "reasonable outcome" after surgical modification (Fig. 5). Traditionally, the plastic surgeon has used "intangible" adjectives such as "elegant," "refined," or "soften" to depict his or her visual perceptions of the anticipated surgical result to the patient. These descriptions, based on the surgeon's own intuitive creativity and experience, often differ from the patient's "fantasy" of her desired outcome. This "communication gap" is often bridged by the surgeon's representation of other patients "before and after" photographs as proof of his skills and/or the patients' furnishing portfolios of magazine photographs of the "desired look." In either instance, the aspired changes do not specifically "fit" the unique facial architecture or shape of the prospective patient.

In our office, we use Mirror II imaging software (Mirror Imaging Technology, Lynwood, WA) to modify the facial image and develop a surgical protocol that is acceptable to both patient and surgeon. This "communication tool" eliminates "surprises" and gives the patient a feeling of participating in the decision-making process. The surgeon benefits by being able to develop a specific "map" of the multiple surgical procedures that can assist in surgical planning and be referred to at the patient's presurgical visit. Prints, both of the original face and modified image, can be printed on a high-resolution Sony Video Printer to be taken to the surgery room for viewing.

Image modification is accomplished with the use of a Wacon tablet with cordless pen to manipulate the "paint" software. The most commonly used tool is the warp tool, which stretches the skin in a given plane (ie, nasolabial fold and eyelids) or creates new lines of profile (ie, submental lipectomy, malar and chin augmentation,

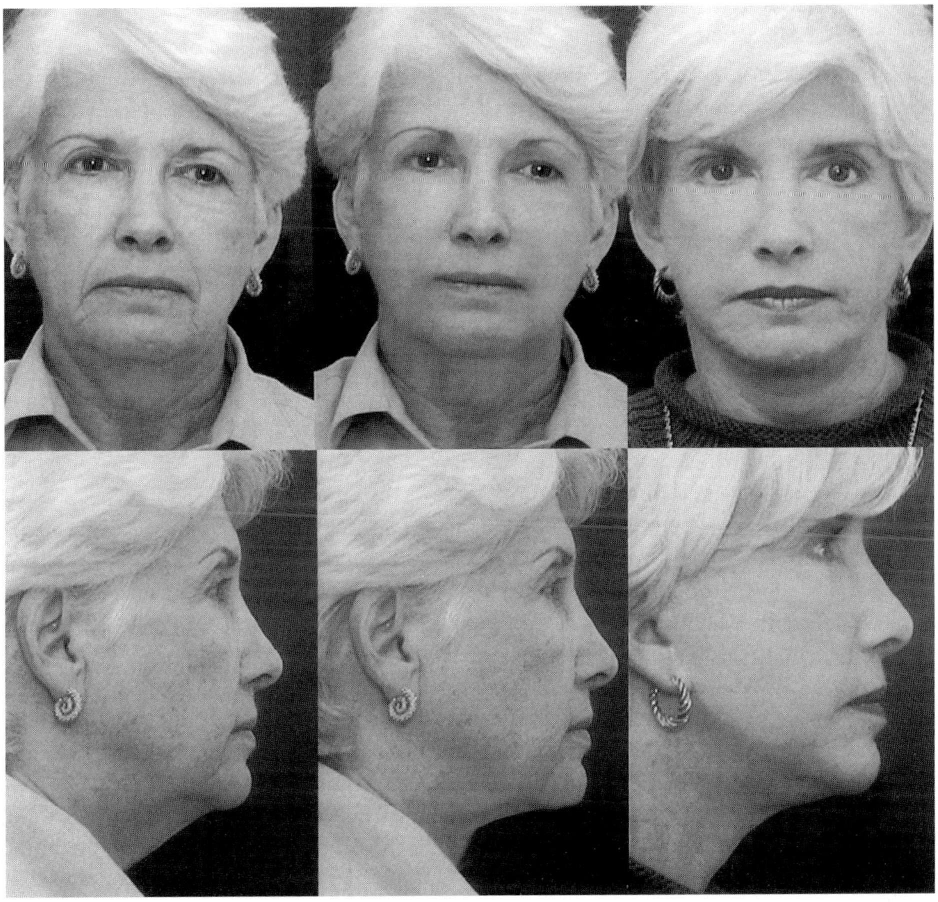

FIGURE 5 Video imaging. Sixty-three-year-old female. (left) Presurgical views. (middle) Computer projection of surgical outcome. (right) Actual postsurgical view after face/neck/browlift and laser resurfacing of perioral and "frown lines."

and neck advancement). The blend tool "airbrushes" out fine wrinkles and eyelid crepiness. The cutout tool elevates fixed structures such as eyebrows, lip vermillion, and so on. The copy tool permits overlay of a facial segment from one image to another, which is particularly useful in facelift comparisons between natural and "pulled" sides.

During the course of the consultation, the patient is apprised that there is no guarantee that the final surgical outcome will match the projected computer image. Most patients are very understanding and appreciate the opportunity to have direct input into the surgical planning. In my experience, the actual surgical outcome is often better than the projected computer image because of the three dimensionality of living tissue compared with the flatness of the video image on the monitor (Fig. 5). Nevertheless, all patients are required to sign an informed consent before medical imaging and photography (Appendix 1).

INITIAL EVALUATION AND MULTIVECTOR ANALYSIS

The patient is examined in the sitting position and facial features evaluated in a systematic cephalad to caudad direction (Fig. 6). The position of the frontal hairline is noted to be high or low—a factor determining prehairline or posthairline placement of the browlift incision. The presence of the transverse brow furrows are noted (? laser resurfacing). Depth of glabellar frown lines and transverse nasion lines are determined passively and with animation to assess the need for corrugator and/or procerus resection. Eyebrow position related to the superior orbital rim and degree of infrabrow upper lid laxity is assessed to determine the need for a mini-browlift. Simple digital vertical elevation of the brow perpendicular to the midpupillary (Vector I) to the desired position can predict changes in upper lid contour and the need for upper lid blepharoplasty. Often, upper lid blepharoplasty is no longer necessary after the brow has been re-elevated to the proper position. Lateral traction is placed in an upward outward direction in the temporal region (Vector II) to position the lateral brow and assess softening of the lateral crow's feet.

The skin texture (thin vs. thick), moisture (dry vs. oily), color (ruddy vs. sallow), and elasticity (mobile vs. fixed) of the mid face are evaluated. Architecture and symmetry of the malar bones are observed. Higher cheekbones will allow for more convexity in redraping the lax soft tissue structures of the mid face. Recessed malar prominences contribute to "flatter" infraorbital rims, nasojugal grooves ("tear troughs"), and excessive pouching of the infraorbital, medial, and lateral fat pads. Downward gravitational descent of the malar fibrofatty layer (see anatomical explanation on p. 682) creates the fullness of the nasolabial fold and the depth of the nasolabial crease. Lateral digital traction in a vector perpendicular to the nasolabial fold (Vector III) will reasonably accurately predict the resuspension of the malar fat pad over the malar bony prominence and degree of flattening of the nasolabial fold. Fine wrinkling along the vermillion border of the upper and lower lips and at the lateral lip commissure and those paralleling the nasolabial crease in the buccal cheek are observed. These latter lines are often softened by the lateral traction of the cheek advancement, whereas the perioral lines are not affected by the facelift procedure and require laser resurfacing (see section on Ancillary Procedures). "Crepiness" of the lower eyelids should be noted both before and after lateral cheek traction. These fine wrinkles are often exaggerated by mid face advancement.

The lower face is evaluated for jawline contour, mid-mandibular jowl laxity and lipodystrophy, and depth of the labiomental crease ("marionnette lines"). Lateral pull directed along the jaw line (Vector IV) predicts the correction of the platysmal laxity and redraping of the cervical skin above the mandibular border (see anatomical explanation on p. 684). Persistent lipodystrophy of the mid-mandibular jowl is an indication for contouring by microliposuction. A ptotic submandibular gland may be palpated as a firm mass along the mid-inferior mandibular border.

In the lower neck, the cervicomental angle, position of the hyoid, vertically oriented submental skin folds, and anatomy of the anterior platysma muscles are assessed. Upward oblique traction in a line from the thyroid cartilage to the earlobe (Vector V) will determine the acuteness of the cervicomandibular angle and degree of softening of the vertical submental folds. A low set hyoid and thickly palpable myelohyoid upper neck muscles predict an obtuse cervicomental angle. Voluntary platysmal animation (clenching the teeth and grimacing) show the degree of decus-

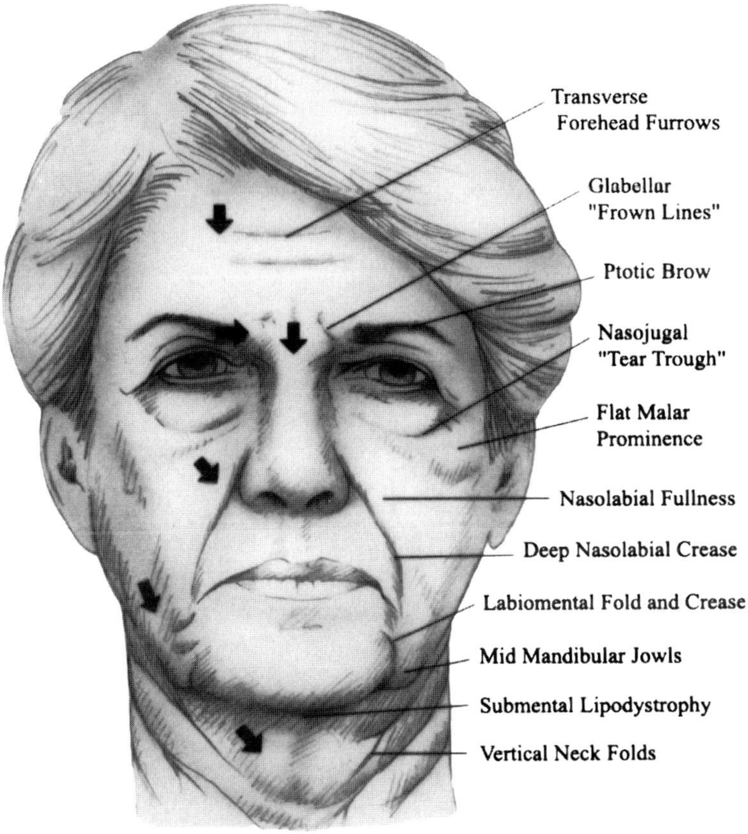

FIGURE 6 Characteristics of the aging face. Arrows represent biomechanical forces of gravity and muscular pull.

sation or dehiscence of the anterior platysma muscle at the midline. Tensely bulging fat in the submental triangle of the neck indicates a deposit of preplatysmal fat.

In addition to the facially focused clinical exam, a comprehensive medical history is obtained from the patient (see Appendix 2). For all patients planning to have surgery, a medical clearance for sedation anesthesia is obtained from the primary care physician. Routine blood work includes CBC, protime, and PTT at a minimum. An EKG is obtained for all patients above 50 years of age or with a history of cardiac abnormalities. An eye clearance is necessary from an ophthalmologist if periocular laser abrasion or eyelid surgery is included with the facelift. Informational brochures and comprehensive instruction sheets describing the surgery, postsurgical care, risks, and potential complications are given to the patient for review at home, and are discussed at the presurgical visit.

PRESURGICAL INSTRUCTIONS/PREPARATION/CONSENT

All patients are seen 10 to 14 days before surgery for a comprehensive presurgical visit. At this time, the video-image and surgical plan is reviewed with the patient.

She or he is given the opportunity to ask questions about the procedure, postsurgical instructions, or risks involved with the surgery. An "informed consent" specifically listing the surgical procedure and date is signed by the patient and witnessed by a staff member (Appendix 3). For premenopausal women, a "pregnancy waver" is signed (Appendix 4). A complete checklist of presurgical administrative details is followed by me during the visit (Appendix 5). Presurgical instructions are as follows:

1. Wash your face thoroughly and shampoo hair with Phisoderm soap the night before your surgery. Remove all makeup.
2. No jewelry should be worn to the outpatient surgical facility.
3. Wear a front-buttoned blouse or shirt. Pullover shirts will be difficult to put on or take off over the facial dressing.
4. Do not eat or drink after midnight the night before surgery.
5. Arrange in advance to have a family member or friend take you home from the surgical facility after your procedure.
6. Please leave all valuables at home with family members.
7. Family or friends should wait in the surgical waiting area. Dr. Rose will discuss the case with them after completion of the surgery.
8. No alcohol 24 hours before surgery.
9. Notify the doctor of any abnormal bleeding tendencies in you or your family.
10. Avoid taking aspirin, vitamin E, or non-asteroidal anti-inflammatory medications at least 10 days before surgery.
11. Notify the doctor if you are taking any of the following medications: Atromid, Butzolidin, Indocin, Thorazine, Tofranil, Elavil, Heparin, Coumadin, and/or Sinequan.
12. Advise the doctor of any significant medical problems that affect your health, eg, high blood pressure, diabetes, angina, heart failure or abnormal rhythm, weak bladder, kidney, respiratory infection, or skin abscesses.
13. Absolutely no smoking 2 weeks before surgery.

THE AMERICAN ASSOCIATION FOR ACCREDITATION OF AMBULATORY SURGERY FACILITIES (AAAASF) CERTIFICATION

Most cases are carried out in our state-of-the-art, office-based outpatient surgical facility (The Aesthetic Surgery Center, Inc., New York, NY). This entity is licensed by New York State as a corporation and has a separate Tax ID number for billing purposes (important for third-party indemnification).

The facility is accredited as Class B facility (intravenous sedation without the use of endotracheal intubation or general anesthesia) by The American Association for Accreditation of Ambulatory Surgery Facilities, Incorporated (AAAASF), a national accreditation program certifying to the medical and lay communities that a surgical facility meets nationally recognized standards. Each facility is meticulously inspected initially and every 3 years afterwards by a certified surgeon inspector. Criteria include physical conformity of the surgery and recovery room; adequacy and maintenance of monitoring equipment; emergency "crash cart" for airway control and updated intravenous medications administration; uniformity and consistency of medical records; program of quarterly quality assessment and peer review; and employee standards and their record verification [71]. Each facility must be directed by a full-time registered nurse. All surgeons must be Board-certified or Board-eligible and hold unrestricted hospital privileges for each and every procedure performed at the AAAASF facility. Additionally, each facility must be current in compliance with the American Disabilities Act (ADA) guidelines; National and Occupational Safety and Health (OSHA) regulations; and National Fire Protection Association (NFPA) standards. Cumulatively, adherence to the strict AAAASF standards of physical and regulatory compliance assure the patient of the highest quality of outpatient care and protection. In fact, pending legislation in the New York State Legislature may soon require all outpatient surgical facilities to be certified by AAAASF or similar accreditation agencies.

INTRAVENOUS "TWILIGHT" SEDATION

Approximately 95% of our facelifts are carried out under intravenous "twilight" sedation in our office base AAAASF-certified ambulatory surgery facility. Older patients (more than 70 years old) or patients with medically labile hypertension, cardiac abnormalities, or insulin-dependent diabetics are treated in the hospital.

All patients selected for intravenous "twilight" sedation are ASA Class I (no organic physiological, biochemical, or psychiatric disturbances) or Class II (mild to moderate systemic disease that is readily correctable) as defined by The American Society of Anesthesiologists [72].

Although there is no legal evidence that the surgeon is more liable when working with a nurse anesthetist than an anesthesiologist [73], I feel more comfortable (and protected) in the presence of a Board-certified anesthesiologist.

Patients are not routinely given oral or intramuscular premedication. An intravenous injection of Midazolam (Versed), a rapid-acting water-soluble benzo diazepine produces immediate sedation and amnesia in titrated doses of 0.02 to 0.03 mg/kg intravenously. Glycopyrolate 0.2 mg intravenously, a quatenary amine compound with no central nervous effect, is given to dry oral and airway secretions. Fentanyl, a short-acting narcotic is infused in 0.25 mg increments until the patient is sleepy but arousable.

The anesthetic agent of choice is Propofol, a short-acting hypnotic of the alkyl phenol class, which is administered with an initial intravenous bolus of 0.05 to 0.1 mg/kg followed by a continuous infusion of 0.01 to 0.02 mg/kg. Its rapid onset (less than 60 sec) and quick awakening (4 to 8 min on reversal) make it an ideal hypnotic for outpatient monitored anesthesia care (MAC) surgery. Nausea and vomiting are infrequent after Propofol induction, but prophylactically Metoclopromide (Reglan) 10 mg, an effective antiemetic, is given a half hour before conclusion of the procedure to decrease gastric emptying and gastric secretions. Ondansetron (Zofran) is given 4 mg intravenously after surgery only if the patient complains of nausea and vomiting before emergence or in patients with a strong history of prior postsurgical nausea and vomiting experience [74].

In the recovery room, all patients are monitored by assessment of vital signs at 15-minute intervals and continuous pulse oximetry. Discharge criteria, according to standard guidelines [75], are as follows:

1. Stable vital signs
2. Protective cough and gag reflex (particularly after intraoral and nasal surgery)
3. Minimal nausea and vomiting
4. Tolerable pain
5. Ambulatory with minimal dizziness

Patients must be accompanied by a family member, friend, or attendant. All patients sign a recognition statement before surgery that someone will be present to escort him or her home. Patients are called the evening or morning after the surgery by the registered nurse to assess postsurgical pain, nausea, status of the dressings, drainage, recalled surgical procedure, and so on.

SURGICAL TECHNIQUE OF MULTIVECTOR FACE/NECK/BROW LIFT

The topographical anatomy of the face and direction of pull is marked with methylene blue (Fig. 7). The course and direction of the zygomaticus major and minor

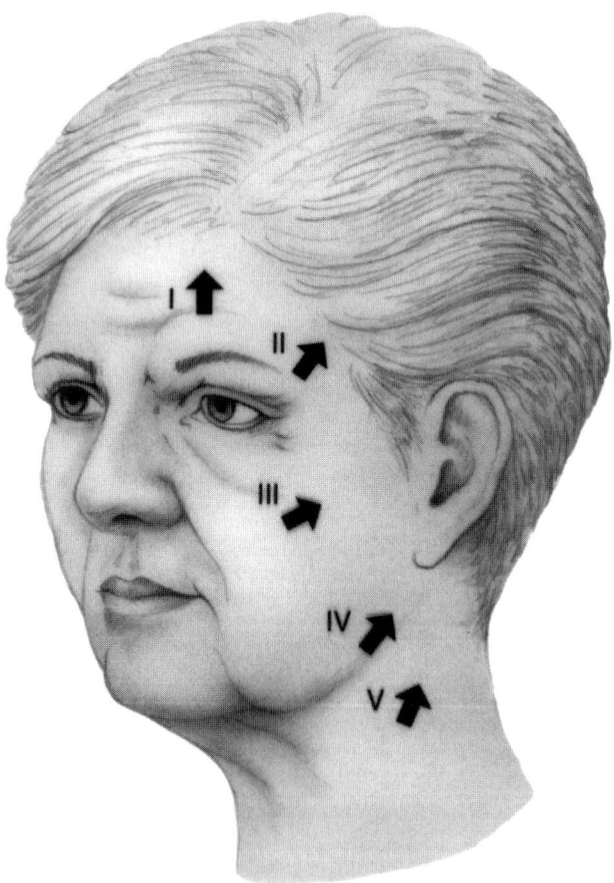

FIGURE 7 Multidirectional forces of pull in multivector face/neck/browlift.

are outlined. The extent of the skin undermining is defined by a "lazy S line" in the medial cheek following lateral orbital rim and extending over the mid-buccal cheek and then dropping obliquely across the mid body of the mandible. Periauricular and scalp/face/neck/brow lift incisions are marked (Fig. 8).

Areas of dissection and incision lines are infiltrated with a mix of 0.25% Marcaine and 0.5% Xylocaine with 1:200,000 Epinephrine using a #25 spinal needle. Local anesthesia is superficially instilled at the desired level of dissection at each facial region. While the local anesthesia is taking effect (10–15 min), the face is prepared and scrubbed with Septisol soap and draped.

Mini-Browlift (Vector I)

The mini-browlift is a quick, minimally invasive, nonendoscopic method of correcting the lax frontalis muscles and overpull of the eyebrow depressors. Elevation and symmetry of the eyebrow position is achieved, often precluding lid resection of the ptotic infrabrow skin (Fig. 9).

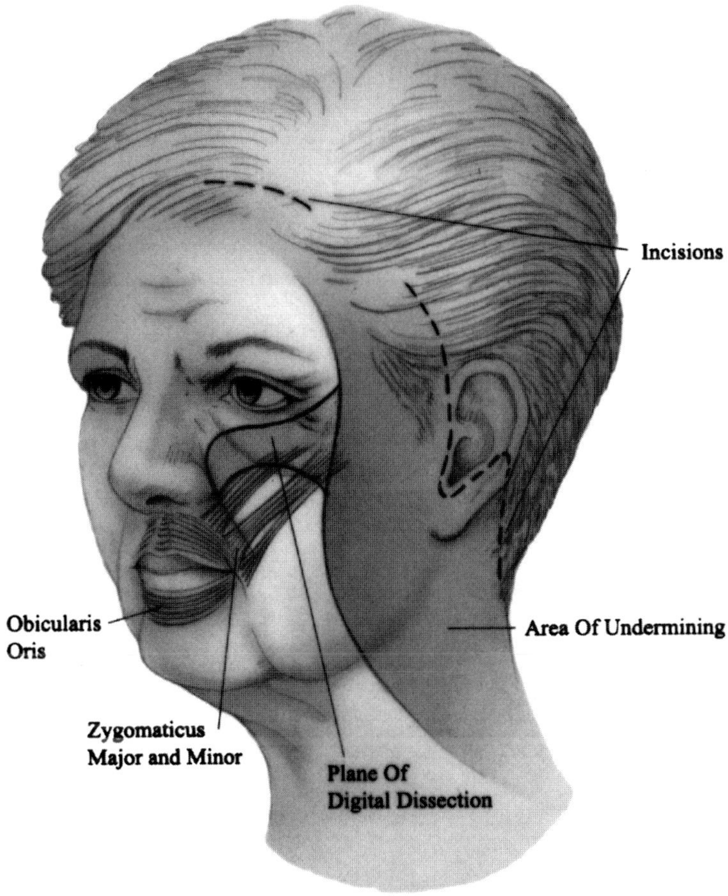

FIGURE 8 Topographical markings and planes of dissection in multivector face/neck/browlift.

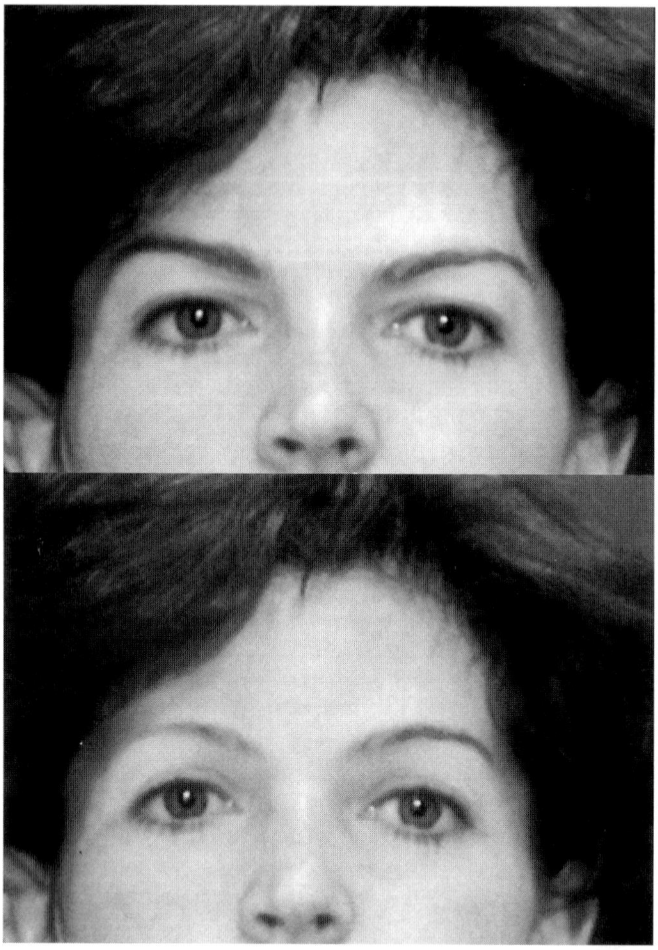

(a)

(b)

FIGURE 9 Thirty-eight-year-old female. (a) Ptotic brows with infrabrow ptosis. (b) After mini-browlift.

A curvilinear 1.25-in incision is outlined in the frontal scalp 1.5-cm posterior to the frontal hairline and centered over the mid-pupillary line (Fig. 10a). In those patients with a high forehead or in males with a receding hairline, the incision is placed in the frontal hairline. The incision is carried deep to the galea until the glistening periosteum of the frontal bone is encountered. With a sweeping motion of the blunt-tip facelift scissors, a plane is created deep to the galea (Fig. 10b). At a point 1 cm superior to the orbital rim, the periosteum is scraped blindly with an elevator to release the deep fibrous attachments of the brow to the supraorbital rim. In the region of the supraorbital nerve and artery (palpable by the supraorbital notch), the dissection is in a vertically oriented direction with the blunt curved-tipped scissors to avoid injury to the nerve and bleeding. The tip of the scissors are also used to strip the corrugator muscle attachments from the dermis beneath the vertical "frown lines" and the procerus muscle attachments from the transverse nasal creases in the midline of the nasion. In the lateral forehead, the periosteum is elevated by a

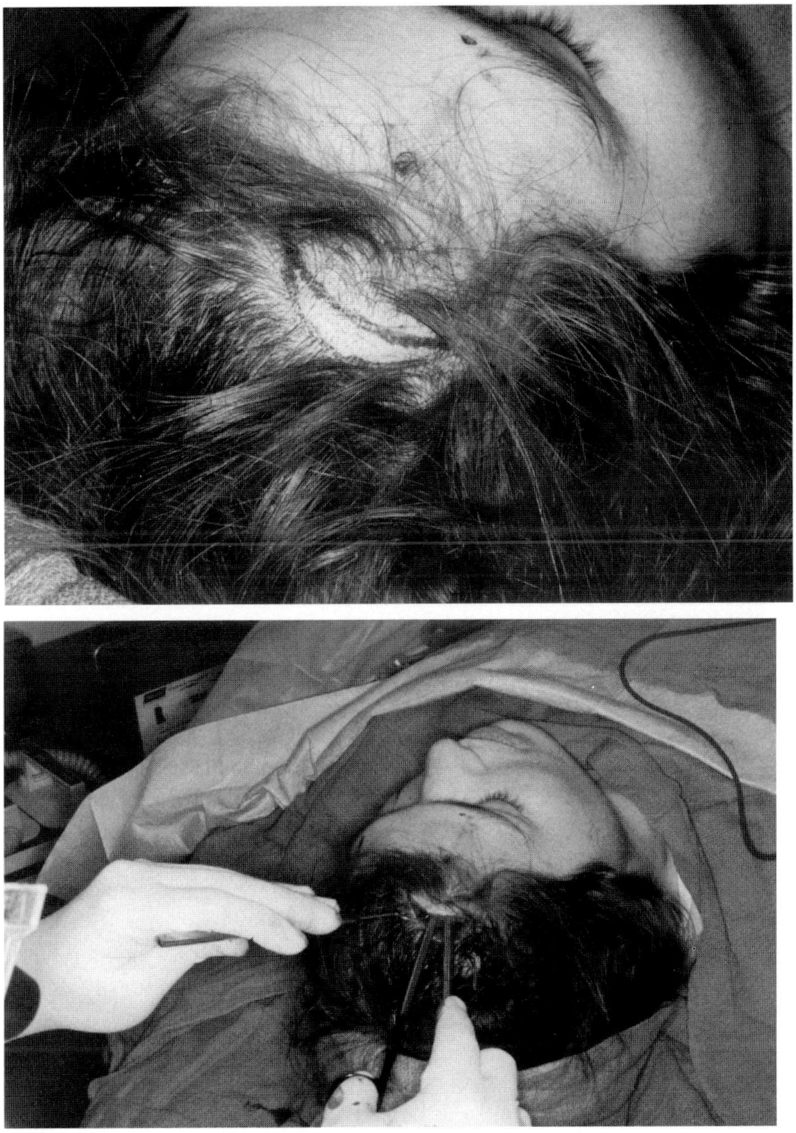

(a)

(b)

FIGURE 10 Mini-browlift technique. (a) Outline of crescent in frontal scalp centered over midpupillary line. (b) Deep dissection beneath galea to release brow attachments.

sweeping motion from the anterior temporal crest (deep to the frontal branch of the facial nerve) to completely mobilize the Hemi-forehead flap. Traction is placed in a vertical direction (Vector I) on the Hemi-forehead flap until the arch of the brow is 0.5 to 1.0 cm, above the supraorbital rim in females and at the level of the supraorbital rim in males. A crescent of frontal scalp skin is excised and the deep galea is plicated to the pericranium with 3-0 PDS suture. The scalp skin is closed subdermally with 4-0 Monocryl and surgical staples for epidermal approximation. Symmetry of brow position is achieved as the Hemi-forehead flap is advanced on the contralateral side.

The Temporal Lift (Vector II)

The pull of the temporal lift is in an upward-outward direction within the temporal region to elevate the lateral brow and reposition the sagging edge of the orbicularis oculi muscle (Fig. 7). Redraping of the temporal skin often softens the radially oriented "crow's feet." The temporal incision is a scythe-shaped incision beginning at the cauda helix and extending 3.5 cm superiorly (Fig. 8). Undermining of the temporal flap is at the level of the superficial temporal fascia deep to the hair follicles. Anterior to the temporal hairline, a transition is made to the subcutaneous plane (superficial to the frontal branch of the facial nerve). In patients with prominent crow's feet, dissection at the subcutaneous plane by transillumination is carried all the way to the lateral orbital rim. Fibers of adherent orbicularis oculi muscle are gently teased digitally and by sharp dissection from the dermis. The fascial temporal flap is rotated and advanced until the lateral brow and lateral canthal eyelid skin is at the desired height. An anchor stitch of 3-0 PDS is placed through the deep temporal fascia at the cauda helix. The temporal flap is trimmed and inset with deep 4-0 PDS sutures and surgical staples.

The Mid-Face Lift (Vector III)

The vector of the mid face is directed perpendicular to the nasolabial fold in an upward oblique line extending from the mid-nasolabial crease to the tragus of the ear (Fig. 7). Advancement of the mid face along this vector line flattens the nasolabial fold and resuspends the descended malar fat pad over the malar bony prominence (Figs. 5, 11, 14). The mid-face incision (contiguous with the temporal incision) begins slightly above the cauda helix and follows the curve of the crus of the helix (Fig. 8). At the anterior ear, I prefer a retrotragal incision carefully following the natural tragal margin with triangular darts into the superior and inferior tragal notches (Fig. 12). Elevation of the lateral cheek flap is performed sharply under direct vision at the depth of the SMAS (but not deep to it). Supra-SMAS undermining of the cheek flap is carried out to the extent of the topographical markings. Fiberoptic illumination assists in hemostasis and division of the masseteric cutaneous ligaments. An attempt is made to preserve the vascular supply of the fasciocutaneous perforators off the transverse facial artery in the mid-cheek region (see anatomical description on p. 684). Under fiberoptic illumination, the inferior lateral fibers of the orbicularis oculi muscle are identified and teased away from the lateral orbital skin. Inferomedial to the orbicularis muscle, the fibers of the zygomaticus major muscle are identified coursing towards the modiolus of the lateral lip commissure. Long tenotomy scissors are used to tease the zygomaticus major fibers from the overlying fibrofatty layer. The tight fibrous zygomaticus ligaments, originating from the inferior border of the zygoma behind the insertion of the zygomaticus major muscle and inserting into the dermis (see p. 681 on surgical anatomy), are sharply divided, thereby freeing the malar soft tissue for advancement. With gentle digital pressure a plane is created superficial and medial to the zygomaticus major muscle beneath the malar fat pad (Fig. 13). The finger is directed obliquely towards the nasal ala and then turned at a right angle inferiorly towards the lateral lip commissure (Fig. 13b). With this

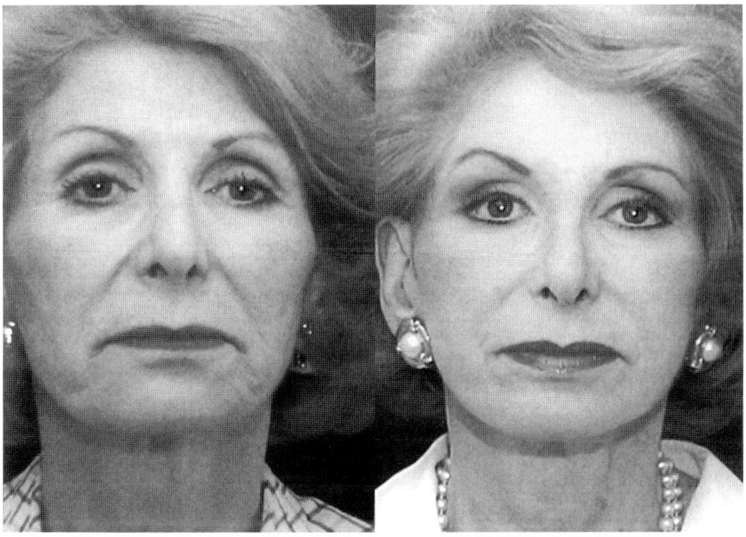

(a) (b)

FIGURE 11 Sixty-one-year-old female. (a) Before surgery. Prominent nasolabial folds and descended malar fat pads. (b) Postsurgical after face/necklift with malar fat pad resuspension.

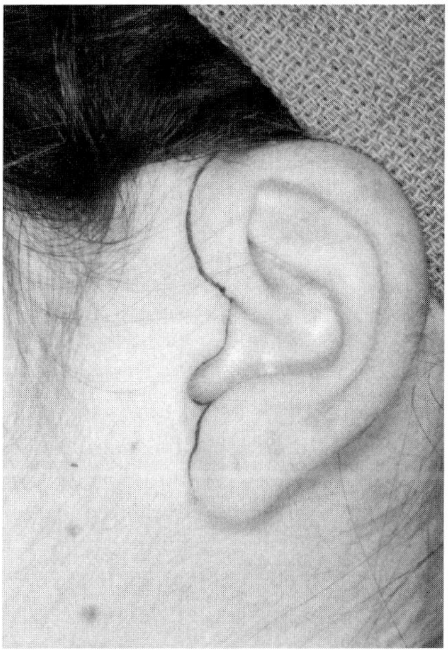

FIGURE 12 Outline of retrotragal incision. Note triangular darts into supra- and infra-tragal notches.

(a)

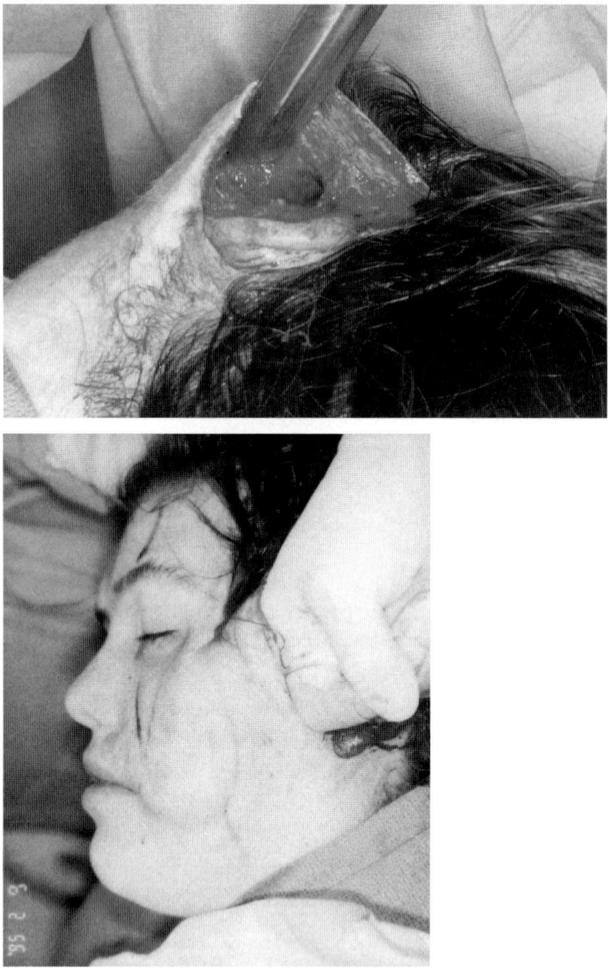

(b)

FIGURE 13 Midface dissection. (a) Tunnel created superomedial to zygomaticus major and minor muscles after release of zygomaticus ligaments. (b) Digital dissection beneath descended malar fat pad (nasolabial fold).

maneuver, the fibrofatty tissue of the nasolabial fold is freed from its deep attachments. Applying traction along Vector III, the nasolabial fold visibly flattens as the malar fat is "resuspended" to its more youthful anatomical position over the convexity of the bony malar prominence (Figs. 5, 11, 14). The skin of the medially based mid-face cheek flap is advanced posterosuperiorly and distributed over the length of the preauricular incision. A 3-0 PDS deep plication stitch is placed at the cauda helix, securing the cuff of superficial temporal fascia to the deep temporal fascia. This deep stitch maintains traction along Vector III and sustains the suspension of the malar fat pad over the malar prominence (I tend to avoid a deep stitch directly anchoring the malar fat pad to the denuded zygoma because of the potential for dimpling of the dermis of the skin). Excessive skin is trimmed along the "natural" border of the tragus. 4-0 nylon stitches are placed in the tips of the darts designed

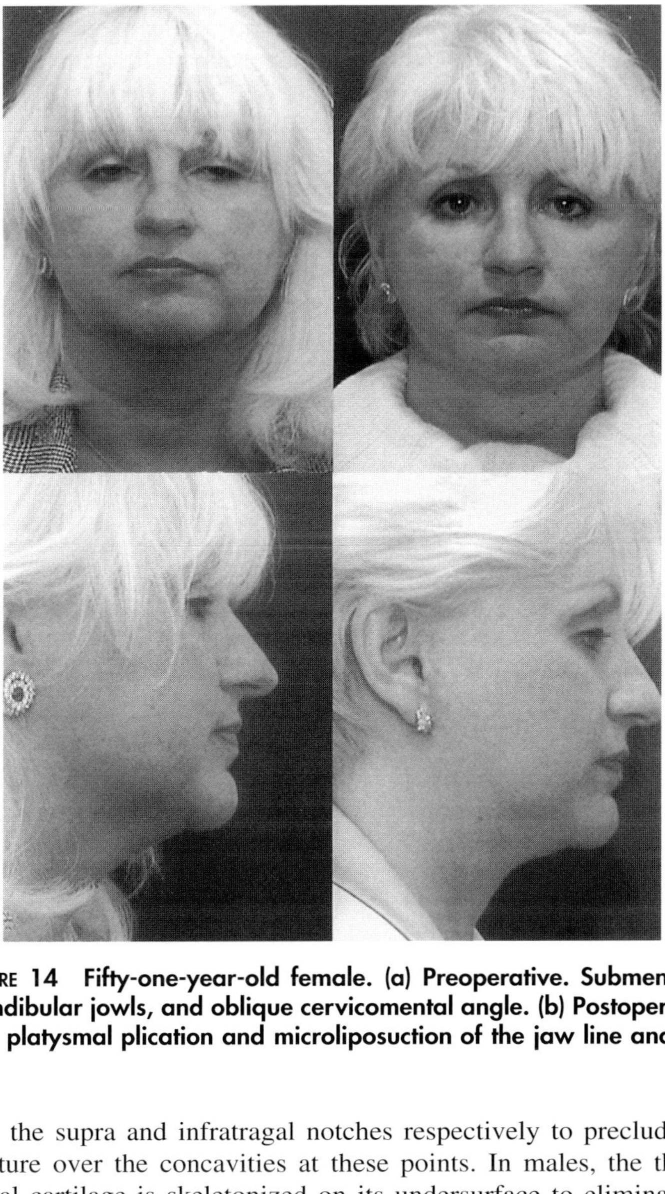

(a) (b)

FIGURE 14 Fifty-one-year-old female. (a) Preoperative. Submental lipodystrophy, mid-mandibular jowls, and oblique cervicomental angle. (b) Postoperative after face/necklift and platysmal plication and microliposuction of the jaw line and submental region.

into the supra and infratragal notches respectively to preclude secondary scar contracture over the concavities at these points. In males, the thin skin overlying the tragal cartilage is skeletonized on its undersurface to eliminate subdermal hair follicles. The skin of the preauricular incision is closed with deep 4-0 Monocryl subdermal stitches and a running interlocking 5-0 nylon cuticular stitch.

The Lower Face and Neck Lift (Vectors VI and V)

Attention to the lower face is directed towards recontouring the jaw line, resuspending the lax platysmal muscle and labiomental folds, eliminating the vertically oriented submental skin and/or platysmal folds, and sharpening the acuteness of the cervicomental angle (Figs. 7, 14).

Before dissection of the neck, the mid-mandibular and submental fat pads and lower face are sculpted by microliposuction through stab incisions in the submental crease and base of the earlobes (see p. 701). The incision (contiguous with the midface incision) begins at the inferior tragal notch, extends around the curve of the ear lobe, and into the retroauricular sulcus (Figs. 8, 15a). The posterior incision is carried near the apex of the mastoid hairline. The entire ear lobe is detached from the underlying areolar tissue (Figure 15c); this maneuver allows for true vector advancement along the jaw line and rotation of the posterior neck flap (Fig. 7). Skin is elevated over the angle and posterior one half of the body and the anterior triangle of the neck by sharp dissection immediately above the platysma muscle fibers. Fibrous attachments over the sternomastoid muscle are divided under direct vision, assisted by fiberoptic illumination. The posterior neck and retroauricular skin is sharply elevated by knife and needle point cautery dissection from the mastoid fascia.

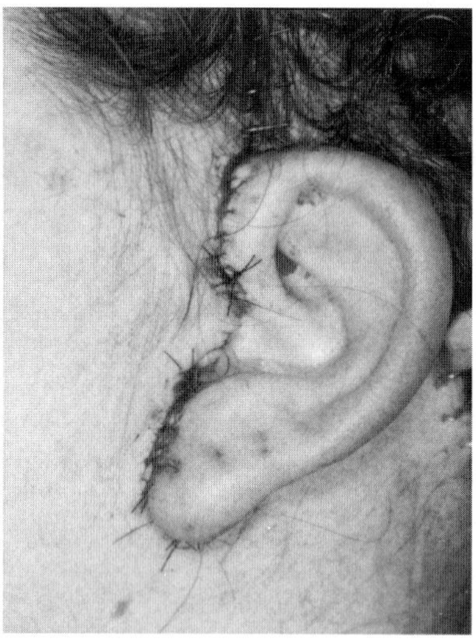

(a)

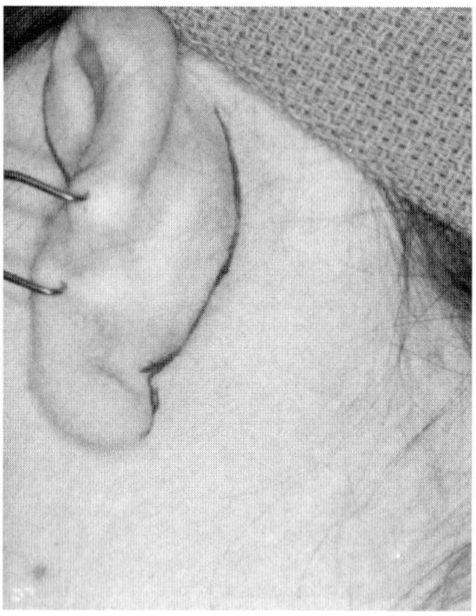

(b)

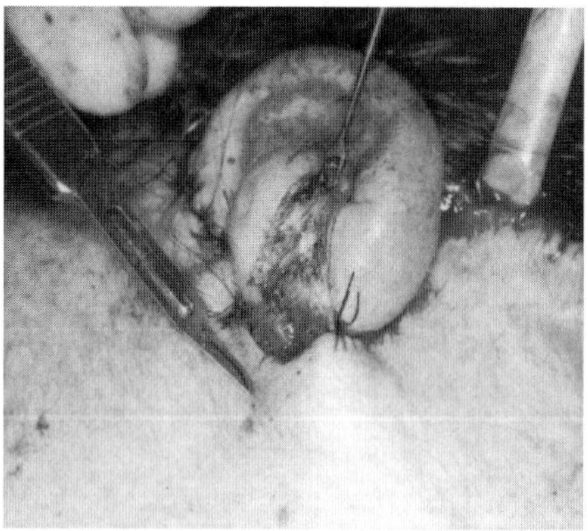

(c)

FIGURE 15 (a) Design of retroauricular incision for necklift. (b) Earlobe reinset anatomically under no tension. (c) Earlobe completely detached to allow for neck advancement and rotation.

Double hooks are placed in the anterior and posterior neck flaps, respectively. While the assistant retracts the anterior flap, the surgeon sharply undermines at the subcutaneous plane under fiberoptic illumination, teasing the fibrous attachments from the posterior edge and muscle mass of the sternocleidomastoid muscle. At the subcutaneous level, the arborizing branches of the greater auricular nerve at a point 6.5 cm below the external auditory canal are protected [76]. With the ear lobe retracted, an inferiorly based 3 × 1.5 cm triangular cuff of preauricular SMAS is elevated from the parotid fascia (Fig. 16a). The contiguous platysma muscle is undermined by blunt dissection over the angle of the mandible and anterior triangle of the neck. The inferiorly based SMAS/platysma flap is rotated 60 to 75° posteriorly to align itself along the axis of the inferior border of the mandible (Vector IV) (Fig. 16b,c). A back cut along the anterior border of the sternomastoid muscle is necessary for adequate rotation. As traction is placed on the platysma along Vector IV (the jaw line), the labiomental fold is seen to flatten and the lateral commissure of the lip is drawn slightly upward and outward. The triangular platysma/SMAS flap is anchored to the mastoid fascia and posterior conchal ear cartilage with 3-0 PDS suture. The preauricular SMAS defect is repaired with buried 4-0 PDS plication sutures. In patients with deep labiomental sulci, a separate stab incision may be necessary in the submental crease to release the fibers of the adherent osteocutaneous mandibular ligament. If prominent anterior platysmal bands are not completely flattened by the posterior platysmal advancement, a separate counterincision is made in the submental crease to plicate the dehisced borders of the paired platysma muscles (approximately 10–20% of patients).

The neck flap is rotated upward and in a counterclockwise direction at a 45° angle. The most cephalad border is plicated to the apex of the retroauricular incision with a surgical staple. The dog ear created is excised in a triangular wedge excision with the hypotenuse following the cervical hairline. The length of the backcut along the hairline is shorted by more anterior rotation of the posterior neck flap. With one jaw of the curved facelift scissors following the convexity of the conchal wall, the excised skin is trimmed to a point anterior to the lobule. A plication stitch of 4-0 nylon is placed through the skin and cartilage of the infratragal notch to anchor the flap. The postauricular incision is closed with a deep 3-0 PDS suture, securing the dermis in the neck flap to the conchal cartilage. Skin is approximated with an interlocking 4-0 nylon cuticular suture. A quarter-inch Penrose drain is placed along the inferior neck gutter and brought out through the apex of the postauricular incision. The ear lobe is then reinserted at the divergence of the anterior and posterior neck flaps. Percutaneous methylene blue marks are traced around the natural curve of the ear lobe. The skin is excised, and the lobe secured, with a deep 4-0 Monocryl and running/interrupted 5-0 nylon sutures. The ear lobe is set at "zero" downward tension, therefore precluding a "pixy ear" deformity (Fig. 15a).

ANCILLARY TECHNIQUES

Microliposuction

The use of microliposuction for facial contouring in the jaw line, submental lipodystrophy, and prominent nasolabial folds has eliminated the need for wide under-

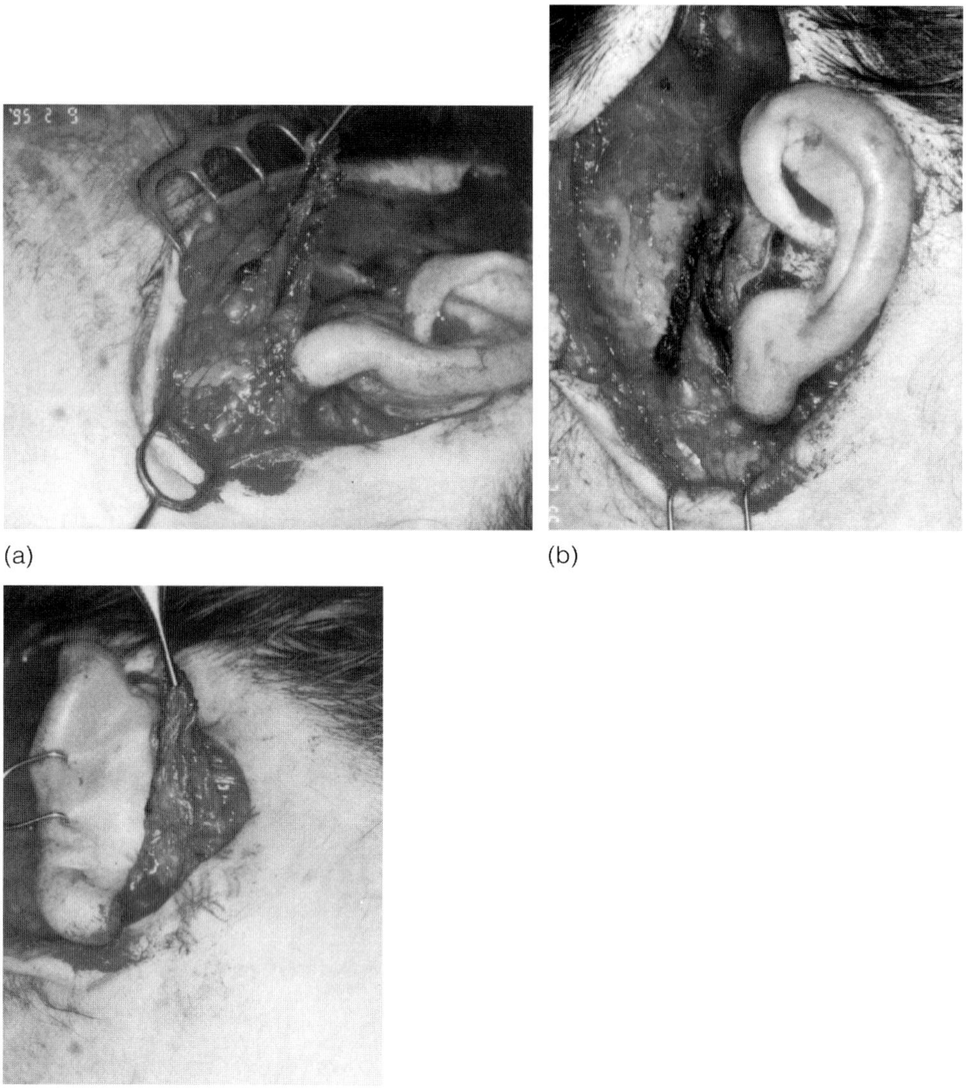

(a) (b) (c)

FIGURE 16 Platysma/SMAS rotation flap. (a) Design of inferiorly based SMAS/Platysma flap. (b) Flap transposed and inset into mastoid fascia. (c) Flap elevated and ready for transfer.

mining to gain exposure of these areas, thereby preserving blood supply and shortening the access incisions (Fig. 14).

In the lower face, small stab incisions are made in the paramedian submental creases 2 to 2.5 cm apart. A tiny 2.4 mm Mercedes tipped cannula is introduced into the subcutaneous layer 3 to 4 mm below the surface. A "crosshatched pattern" is used to aspirate subcutaneous fat from the submental pocket. If a "bulge" persists, deep penetration is made beneath the anterior platysma muscle to reach the subplatysmal fat pocket. The head is turned to each side respectively and fat is aspirated along the jaw line, lower face and the mid-mandibular jowls. Separate counterincisions are made at the base of each ear lobe and the cannula is swept in a radial direction across the lower face and anterior triangle of the neck. The tip of the cannula may be extended as far as the lateral commissure of the lip. With elevation of the neck flap, the "honeycombed" pattern of the fibrous lattice network [77] is easily visualized. Additional fat may be aspirated under direct vision beneath the neck flap using a spatulated cannula.

The nasolabial fold may be approached through stab incisions at the alar base. I, however, am hesitant to remove fat from the nasolabial fold because I prefer to use this fat for resuspension over the malar prominence. Over time, extensive removal of the fat from the nasolabial folds may also lead to a "gaunt" look in the midface as the subcutaneous fatty layer naturally thins with the aging process. In "round" faces, the technique of buccal fat excision through an intraoral approach can flatten the submalar cheek [78].

Autologous Fat Injections

Microlipoinjection is a new method of "filling out" unwanted facial depressions, "frown lines," "laugh lines," or enhancing lip fullness (Fig. 17). In contrast to other materials using animal protein (ie, bovine collagen) or synthetic materials (Gortex), lipoinjections are entirely one's own tissue extracted from excess fat deposits in the hips, thighs, or lower abdominal regions. Tiny stab incisions are made in inconspicuous areas and the fat is aspirated through thin cannulas (2–3 mm) attached to a suction device. The fat is then processed for reinjection by serial emulsification, purification, and centrifugation. The "pure" liquid fat is reinjected into contour defects of the face with a 14 to 16 gauge needle, leaving no marks or surgical incisions. Excess syringes of fat are labeled and frozen at 0°C. These syringes may be thawed at 9 to 12 month intervals over a period of 2 to 3 years to be reinjected into depressed areas.

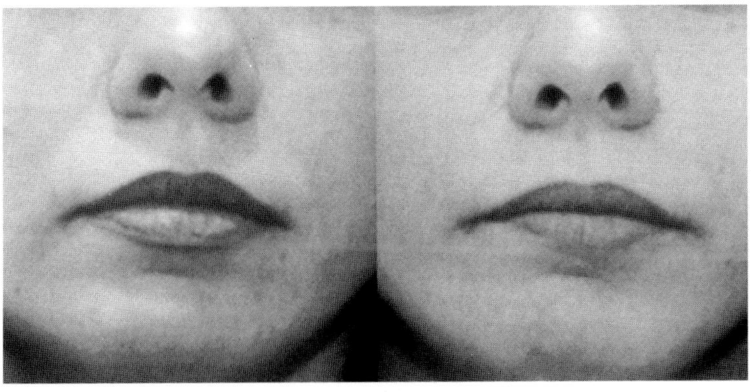

(a) (b)

FIGURE 17 Autologous fat injections. (a) Depressed nasolabial creases in 39-year-old female. (b) After autologous fat injections into "laugh lines."

This technique has been proven to be highly successful in resculpting facial irregularities [79]. Clinical and histological studies have shown the long-term efficacy of free fat transfer [80–82]. Absorption rates are approximately 20 to 30% at 1 year, although this may vary from individual to individual. Generally, depressed areas are slightly "overfilled" at the initial procedure to compensate for this absorption. "Lumpiness" at the injection site is common for 7 to 10 days right after the procedure, but this smoothes out with time and light message to achieve a smooth surface contour.

Alloplastic Chin and Malar Implants

Architecture of the facial framework may not be entirely compensated by redraping the facial soft tissue. These deficiencies, are often visualized on presurgical computer imaging, may be ameliorated by the addition of alloplastic implants in conjunction with the facial surgery (Fig. 18). Silicone implants for bony augmentation have been used since the early 1950s [83], but have the potential drawbacks of: (1) mobility, (2) migration, and (3) autoimmune response. My preferred choice of alloplastic material is porous polyethylene (Porex surgical; College Park, GA). This material has the advantage of being firm but flexible when placed in boiling water. Used in maxillary facial surgery for 3 decades [84], it can be trimmed, shaped to bony contours, and anchored to bone by wire or prolene suture. Placement in chin, infraorbital, or malar regions is easily accomplished through well-concealed intraoral incisions. The porous nature of the material induces soft tissue ingrowth within 1 week and fixation to bone within 3 weeks [85]. Neovascularization of the implant reduces the incidence of infection even when exposed to sinus mucosa [86c].

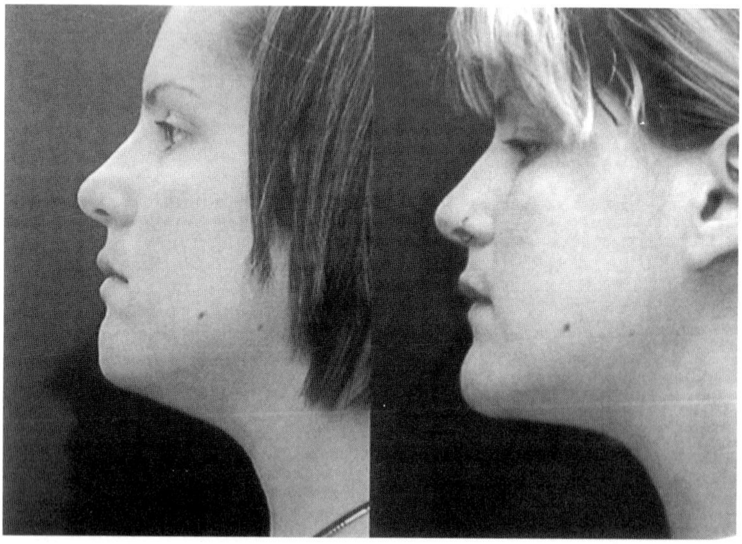

(a) (b)

FIGURE 18 Alloplastic chin implant. (a) Retrusive chin in 26-year-old. (b) After Porex chin implant and microliposuction of neck.

Laser Resurfacing

Fine vertical wrinkles in the upper and lower lip and lateral commissure regions are unaffected by mid and lower face advancement (Fig. 19). These wrinkles, along with the mid-glabellar "frown lines," lateral "crow's feet," and transverse forehead creases may be eliminated or substantially softened by laser resurfacing. Introduced in the mid 1990s, high energy ultrapulsed CO_2 laser systems emit light at 10,600 nm, which is absorbed by water and vaporizes the outer layers of skin into a smooth surface [86b]. Commercially available units achieve depth of 50 to 100 μm per pass [87]. The first pass typically removes the epidermis; the second pass, the mid-papillary dermis; and the third pass deeply into the papillary or into the reticular dermis [88]. Penetration of the dermis stimulates remodeling by formation of new collagen. New collagen formation leads to further "contraction" and "tightening" of the skin up to 90 days after the procedure.

Clinically, the CO_2 is applicable for a variety of surface irregularities including surgical rhytids, solar damage, focal scarring, acne nodules, and pigmentation abnormalities. Patients are advised of prolonged erythema post–laser treatment lasting at least 3 to 6 months. Sun avoidance or sun block with SPF 15 or greater should be worn continuously until the erythema is completely resolved. Postsurgical hyperpigmentation may occur in darker skin or olive-complected patients, and rarely occurs in Fitzpatrick Type I or Type II skin types [88]. In patients predisposed to hyperpigmentation, pre- and postsurgical bleaching agents are a necessary adjunct (hydroquinone 4–6% concentrations).

Dermal Strip Grafts

Excised facelift skin, usually discarded, is an excellent source of "filler material" for deep nasolabial creases to pump up retruded lip elements or to smooth lip ver-

(a)

(b)

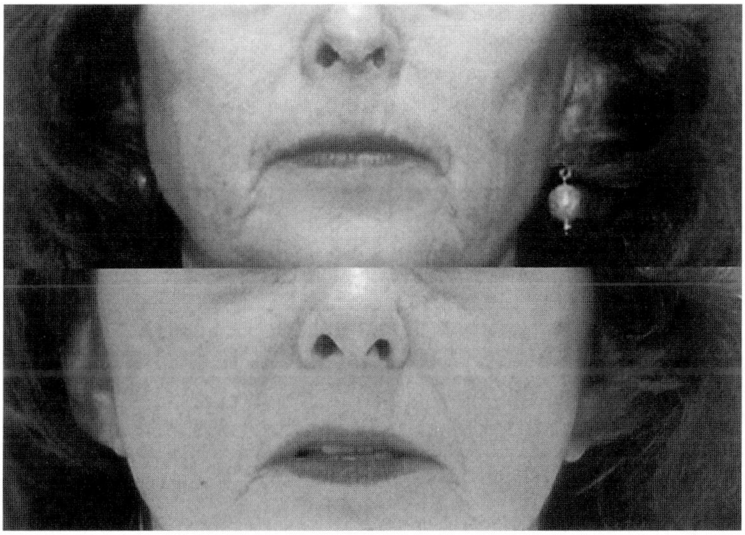

FIGURE 19 Laser resurfacing. (a) Fine perioral vertical wrinkles in a 51-year-old female. (b) After laser resurfacing.

million irregularities. The de-epithelialized dermal fat grafts survive by ingrowth of rich vascular network within the dermis as well as retention of the thin layer of fat cells included beneath the dermis in the graft [89]. Thompson has reported "take" of approximately 90% after free transfer of nonvascularized subcutaneous dermal fat grafts for filling of soft tissue contour defects, as well as hemifacial atrophy [90]. A 20% absorption rate was usually expected at 1 year.

The cuff of preauricular facelift skin is de-epithelialized before trimming (Fig. 20a). For lip augmentation, the excised skin is tailored and "rolled" into a cylindrical configuration secured with a 5-0 Monocryl suture (Fig. 20b). A submucosal pocket is created beneath the vermillion border through stab incisions at the lateral com-

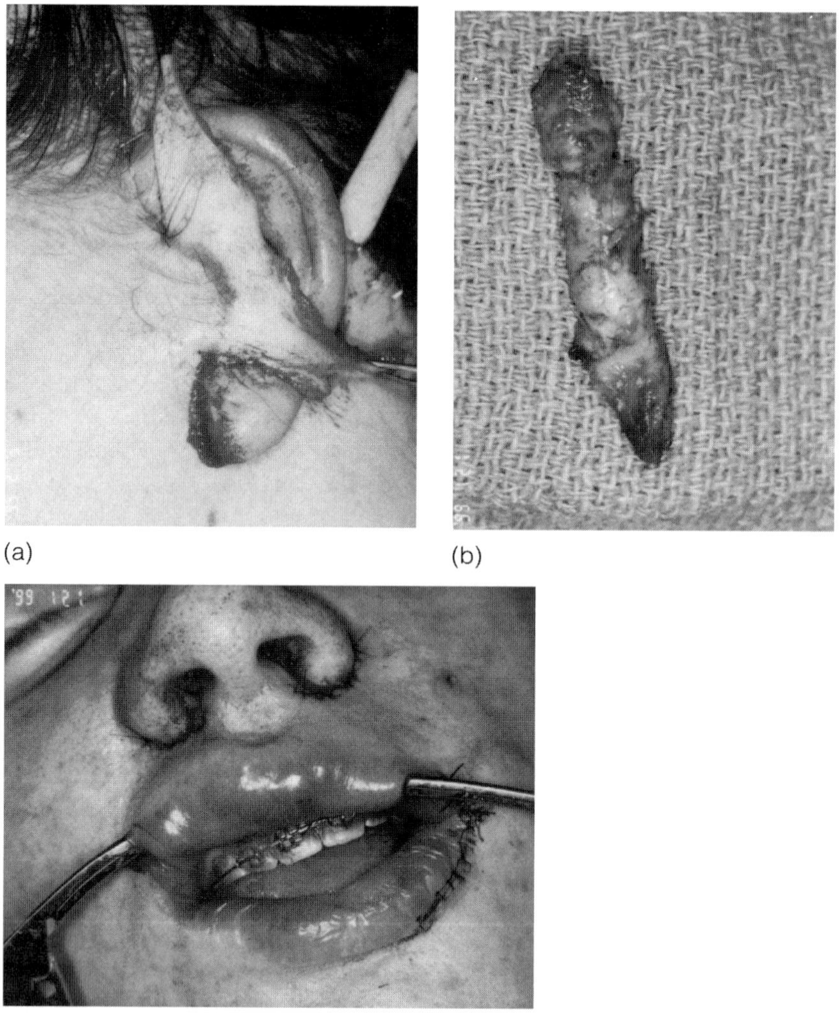

(a) (b) (c)

FIGURE 20 Dermal strip graft. (a) Excess preauricular facelift skin. (b) Skin de-epithelialized and rolled into cylinder. (c) Tendon passer used to pull dermal strip graft through submucosal tunnel.

(a)

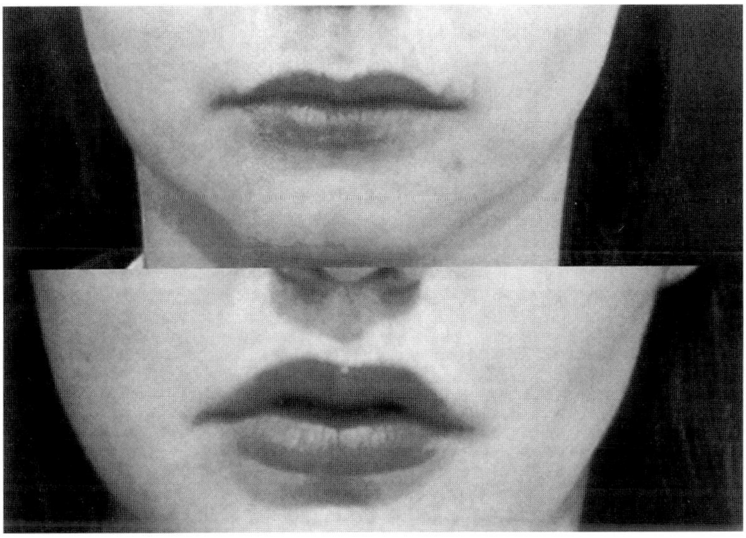

(b)

FIGURE 21 Dermal strip graft. (a) Thin upper lip in 36-year-old woman. (b) One year after dermal strip graft.

missures. The "rolled" dermal fat graft strip is tunneled beneath the vermillion with a curved tendon passer (Fig. 20c). The thicker "roll" in the midportion of the graft allows for greater lip enhancement in the midtubercle region (Fig. 21). Vermillion stab incisions are closed with buried 5-0 Monocryl sutures.

POSTSURGICAL CARE/DRESSINGS

Face/necklift patients receive 1.0 g intravenous Kefzol intrasurgically and are maintained on systemic oral antibiotics for 3 days after surgery (Duricef 500 mg p.o. twice daily). Eight to 12 mg Dexamethasone are administered intrasurgically to preclude swelling. A Medrol Dose Pak is initiated on the first day after surgery. Additionally, SinEcch (Arnica) 500 mg, a homeopathic antiecchymotic, is given three times daily perisurgically for 4 days.

Smoking, alcohol, and aspirin-containing drugs are restricted for 2 weeks after surgery. The head is kept elevated. Ice water compresses are placed frequently over both eyes for comfort and edema reduction. A blenderized or liquid diet is required for the first 2 to 3 days and then advanced to a soft, easy-to-chew food for another week.

The large turban-like dressing is removed at the first office visit, usually on the second day after surgery. This is replaced by a flesh-colored prefit elastic Caromed chin/neck strap. Velcro fasteners allow for easy removal and incorporation of the periauricular gauze dressings beneath the strap. Hair shampoo may be initiated after the head wrap has been removed. Clots are removed with a wide-toothed comb or soft bristle brush. Hair is padded dry and Bacitracin ointment is applied to suture lines.

Drains are removed at the first dressing change. Preauricular sutures are removed at 5 to 7 days. Earlobe and postauricular stitches and scalp staples are left in until the tenth day after surgery.

Ecchymosis and swelling begin to resolve by the tenth to the fourteenth day. Most patients are "very presentable" with the application of a light concealer or cover make-up by the third to fourth week. No bending, straining, lifting, laughing, or excessive facial movement is allowed for 10 days. Strenuous exercise (eg, tennis, swimming, jogging, etc.) are avoided for 4 to 6 weeks, although patients may get back to light treadmill walking within 7 to 10 days.

Complete healing of the surgical scars may take 6 to 12 months longer. Fortunately, most scars are hidden within or behind the ears or in the scalp line and may easily be covered with make-up or hairstyle. A postsurgical regimen of .025% Triamcinolone cream and Neutrogena Healthy Skin (Vitamin A, E, and C cream with sunblock) is applied twice daily to scars after the third week.

SKIN CARE/CORRECTIVE CAMOUFLAGE COSMETICS

All postsurgical skin care and custom make-up application is supervised by our full-time skin care coordinator. At the time of the presurgical visit, a kit of skin care products and a list of instructions are given to the patient for preparation.

The daily skin care regimen is initiated 2 to 3 days after surgery. Gentle lotion and sensitive skin cleansers are applied twice daily to face and neck in an upward circular motion, massaging for a few seconds to loosen surface irregularities. The skin is rinsed with tepid water and washed with a soft facial sponge. After cleansing the skin, an antioxidant toner is applied with a cotton pad, or simply sprayed to freshen the skin. After cleansing and toning, an antioxidant moisturizing cream is gently massaged into the face and neck. In the morning, an SPF 15 or greater sun protective cream with optimal UVA and UVB protection is spread and allowed to penetrate for a few seconds. This is followed with application of custom-prepared flesh-colored concealers beneath the foundation of choice. Lavender or green neutralizer may be used beneath the make-up to color-correct bruising or erythema, respectively. Exfoliatory and antioxidant mask are used on a weekly basis at 4 to 6 weeks. The skin care regimen is supplemented with nightly Renova 0.05% cream and/or 8 to 10% alphahydroxy program for exfoliation or dead surface of skin cells and skin rejuvenation. Heavy sun exposure is avoided for 4 to 6 weeks after surgery.

COMPLICATIONS

On the whole, facial rhytidoplasty is a relatively safe procedure, and complications, even when they occur, cause minimal morbidity and are usually self limiting. Complication rates have been extensively overviewed by several investigators [91–93].

Infection

The incidence of postsurgical infection requiring readmission is very low (0.18%) [94]. The most common organism cultured is Staphylococcus. However, in infections occurring more than 1 week after surgery, gram negative coverage should also be considered [94]. Drainage and/or systemic antibiotic coverage is the treatment of choice. Scars heal by secondary intent and are usually imperceptible after a period of prolonged erythema and scar management.

Hematoma

Hematomas requiring surgical evacuation are less than 2% and all occur within 48 hours [95]. Age, presurgical tests, medical history, gender, periosurgical medication, pre- and postsurgical blood pressure, and treatment of SMAS do not affect the incidence of hematoma formation [95]. The incidence of hematoma was 1.1% with general anesthesia and 0.87% in the intravenous sedation group [95].

Hematoma can be avoided by meticulous hemostasis, a "second look" before closing, and judicious placement of drains. In my experience, the application of bulky gauze dressings supported by microfoam pressure tape (3M Corporation, St. Paul, MN) precludes the development of capillary-related hematoma development and seems to reduce postsurgical swelling.

Postsurgical hematomas are characterized by bluish discoloration of the lips and cheeks, associated with intense pain. Treatment of larger hematomas is by open evaluation, identification and ligation of the bleeding vessel, and drainage. Smaller clot formations, particularly beneath the temporal and mastoid flap, may be "milked out," expressed, and treated with a pressure dressing.

Hypertrophic Scar

The most common sites are in the retroauricular sulcus and near the tragus. These are treated by repeated intralesional injections of Depo-Medrol (diluted with 1% Xylocaine and 0.25% Marcaine solution) using a fine 30-gauge needle. Scar management with Triamcinolone 0.025% and Health Skin (Vitamin A, E, and C cream with sunblock) is continued until erythema subsides. In recalcitrant hypertrophic scars, a combination of laser and dermabrasion is used for flattening of the scars. The dermabrader mechanically lowers the ridges to a flat plane with the skin surface and the laser "feathers" the scar into the surrounding skin.

Impaired Wound Healing

Decreased vascularity may range from superficial blistering to full-thickness skin slough, most commonly at the apex of the posterior neck flap and occasionally at the margin of the preauricular skin flap. Smokers are 12.46 times more likely to experience skin slough than patients who do not smoke [96]. In smokers, I routinely treat the patient perisurgically with a calcium channel blocker (Nifedipine 10 mg p.o. three times daily) 2 days before and 10 days after to vasodilate the peripheral vessels. In smokers, skin flaps are undermined less widely and raised to the deeper plane.

Skin slough is treated as deep second- or third-degree burn by topical application of silver sulfadiazine cream 1% and allowed to heal by re-epithelialization or secondary intent. This method is preferable to excision and skin grafting. Ensuing hypertrophic scars are treated by intralesional cortisone injections and/or laser/dermabrasion resurfacing.

Nerve Palsy

Facial nerve weakness occurs in 1 to 3% of facelifts. The most common nerves injured are the frontalis and marginal mandibular branches of the facial nerve. Although disconcerting to the patient and the surgeon, these palsies are usually transient and will resolve within 3 to 6 months. Prevention of injury to the marginal mandibular and frontalis nerve is by careful dissection superficial to the platysma and superficial temporal fascias, respectively (see operative technique on pp. 696 and 700).

Parotid Cyst

An often misdiagnosed complication after facelift surgery is the parotid pseudocyst. With deeper dissections beneath the SMAS, exposure of the parotid parenchyma is at greater risk. A parotid pseudocyst typically manifests itself as a ballottable mass in the buccal cheek or angle of the mandible at a week or 10 days after surgery. Needle aspiration yields clear fluid. Laboratory assay for amylase is extremely high (500,000 units or greater).

Repeated percutaneous needle aspiration over a 3- to 6-week period may eventually lead to resolution [97], but the danger is further extension by enzymatic erosion, thinning of the skin, and preclusion of sealing of the injured parotid parenchyma. Preferred treatment is the more aggressive approach of insertion of a flat Jackson-Pratt drain attached to a suction reservoir [98]. Resolution of the cyst is usually within 5 to 7 days, after which the drain is removed. Parotid secretions can be further diminished by a pharmacological regimen of an anticholinergic (Probanthine 10 mg t.i.d.).

Hair Loss

Focal alopecia most frequently occurs in the temporal scalp region. This occurs because of inadequate depth of flap elevation with subsequent injury to the deep subcutaneous hair follicles. I personally prefer to elevate the temporal flap under 4½ power magnification with sharp dissection at the level of the superficial temporal fascia to assure that the deep hair follicles are preserved. Transition to the subcutaneous plane at the anterior temporal hairline will avoid injury to the frontal branch of the facial nerve which lies within the superficial temporal fascia. Excessive tension on the temporal flap or posterior neck flap can also decrease vascularity to the sensitive hair follicles, further contributing to focal alopecia.

Early manifestation of hair loss can be treated with follicle stimulants (Rogaine or Propecia). Definitive alopecia may require excision and scalp advancement or micro-minifollicular hair transplant techniques.

Anesthetic Ear

Periauricular numbness is common after facelift procedures but permanent hypesthesia is usually the result of surgical transection of the greater auricular nerve. This nerve is located 6.5 cm inferior to the external auditory canal at the midportion of the sternocleidomastoid muscle [98]. Injury can be avoided during dissection by retracting the anterior cheek flap and the posterior cheek flap simultaneously as the tenacious fibrous bands overlying the sternocleidomastoid muscle are sharply divided under direct vision by transillumination. If the greater auricular nerve is inadvertently injured, it should be repaired immediately by microneural repair with 7-0 nylon sutures.

SUMMARY

A good facelift will last 8 to 12 years. In my experience, younger patients (mid-40s to mid-50s) have a better skin elasticity and therefore not only "set back the clock" further, but tend to age at a slower rate because of the collagen reorientation that occurs at the plane of dissection. This collagen "foundation" anchors the skin envelope and decelerates the soft tissue response to gravity and loss of elasticity. The average length of time between primary and secondary facelift surgery is 8.48 years [99], although maintenance procedures performed every 2 to 3 years (ie, neck tightening, laser, microliposuction) will increase that interval. Secondary facelifts often do not require undermining or deep plane dissection as extensive as the primary procedure.

Facelift patients perceive themselves an average of 9.31 years younger after surgery [99]. Overall satisfaction rate is high and the "positive" surgical experience and renewed self esteem encourages patients to seek further facial rejuvenation surgery [99].

REFERENCES

1. Webb WL, Slaughter R, Meyer E. Mechanisms of psychosocial adjustment patterns in patients seeking face lift operations. Psychosom Med 27:183, 1965.
2. Gifford S. Cosmetic surgery and personality change: a review and some clinical observations. pp. 11–33.
3. Dion K, Berscheid E, Walster E. What is beautiful is good. J Pers Soc Psychol 24:285, 1972.
4. Lemke BN, Stasior OG. The anatomy of eyebrow ptosis. Arch Ophthalmol 100:981, 1982.
5. Krize DM. Transpalpebral approach to the corrugator supercilii and procerus muscles. Plast Reconstr Surg 95:52, 1995.
6. Larrabee WR, Makiekski KH. Surgical Anatomy of the Face. New York: Raven Press, 1993.
7. Pitanguy I, Ramos AS. The frontal branch of the facial nerve. The importance of its variation in face lifting. Plast Reconstr Surg 38:352, 1996.
8. Isse N. Endoscopic facial rejuvenation. Endo forehead, the functional lift. Case reports. Aesth Plast Surg 18:21–29, 1994.
9. Toranto IR. The subperiosteal forehead lift. Clin Plast Surg 477–485, 1992.
10. Whetzel TP, Mathes SJ. Arterial anatomy of the face; an analysis of vascular territories and perforating cutaneous vessels. Plast Reconstr Surg 89:591, 1992.
11. Ellenbogen R. Transcoronal eyebrow lift with concomitant upper blepharoplasty. Plast Reconstr Surg 71:490–499, 1983.
12. McKinney P, Mossie RD, Zukowksi MC. Criteria for the forehead lift. Aesth Plast Surg 15:141, 1991.
13. Flowers RS, Caputy GG, Flowers SS. The biomechanics of brow and frontalis function and its effect on blepharoplasty. Clin Plast Surg 20:255–268, 1993.
14. Mitz V, Peyronie M. The superficial musculoaponeurotic system in the parotid mid cheek area. Plast Reconstr Surg 58:80, 1976.
15. Harshai Y, Bodner SR, Egozy-Golan D, Lindenbaum ES, et al. Mechanical properties and microstructure of the superficial musculoaponeurotic system. Plast Reconstr Surg 98:59, 1996.
16. Stuzin JM, Baker TJ, Gordon HL. The relationship of the superficial and deep fascias; relevance to rhytidectomy and aging. Plast Reconstr Surg 89:441, 1992.
17. Gosain AK, Yousif NS, Madiedo G, Larson DC, Matloub HS, Sanger SR. Surgical anatomy of the SMAS; a reinvestigation. Plast Reconstr Surg 92:1254, 1993.
18. Furnas DW. The retaining ligaments of the cheek. Plast Reconstr Surg 83:11, 1989.

19. Yousif NS, Mendelsohn DC. Anatomy of the midface. Clin Plast Surg 22:227–240, 1995.
20. Yousif NS, Gosain A, Matloub HS, et al. The nasolabial fold: an anastomotic and histological reappraisal. Plast Reconstr Surg 93:60–69, 1994.
21. Barton FE, Gyimesi TM. Anatomy of the nasolabial fold. Plast Reconstr Surg 100:1276, 1997.
22. Yousif NS. Changes of the mid-face with age. Clin Plast Surg 12:213–226, 1995.
23. Gosain AK, Amarante MTS, Hyde JS, Yousif NS. A dynamic analysis of changes in the nasolabial fold using magnetic resonance imaging: implications for facial rejuvenation and facial animation surgery. Plast Reconstr Surg 98:622, 1996.
24. Davis RA, Anson BS, Budinger JM, Kurth LE. Surgical anatomy of the facial nerves and parotid gland based on a study of 350 cervicofacial halves. Surg Gyn Obstetr 1021: 385, 1956.
25. Freilinger G, Grober H, Happak W, Pechmann U. Surgical anatomy of the mimetic muscle system and the facial nerve. Plast Reconstr Surg 80:686, 1987.
26. Gosain AK. Surgical anatomy of the facial nerve. Clin Plast Surg 22:241–251, 1995. Yousif NS, Gosain A, Sanger JR, et al. The nasolabial fold: a photogrammetic analysis. Plast Reconstr Surg 93:70, 1996.
27. Blanco-Davila F, Arrendondola, DeLa Garga O, Montemayor R, et al. Anatomical study of the blood supply to the skin in rhytidectomy. Aesth Plast Surg 19:175–181, 1995.
28. Whetzel TP, Mathes SJ, Arterial anatomy of the face: an analysis of the vascular territories and perforating cutaneous vessels. Plast Reconstr Surg 89:591, 1992.
29. Whetzel TP, Stevenson TR. The contribution of the SMAS to the blood supply in the lateral face lift flap. Plast Reconstr Surg 100:1011–1018, 1997.
30. Stuzin JM, Baker TS, Gordon HL, Baker TM. Extended SMAS dissection—an approach to mid face rejuvenation. Clin Plast Surg 295–311, 1995.
31. Vistnes LM, Souther SM. The platysma muscle: anatomic considerations for aesthetic surgery of the anterior neck. Plast Reconstr Surg 10:441, 1983.
32. McKinney P. The management of platysmal bands. Plast Reconstr Surg 98:999–1000, 1996.
33. Lambros V. Fat contouring in the face and neck. Clin Plast Surg 19:401–414, 1992.
34. Dingman RO, Grabb WC. Surgical anatomy of the facial nerves and parotid gland based upon a study of 350 cervicofacial halves. Surg Gyn Obst 102:385, 1956.
35. Lemmon ML. Color atlas of SMAS rhytidectomy. New York: Thieme Medical Publishers, 1992, pp. 1–11.
36. Gosain AK. Surgical anatomy of the facial nerve. Clin Plast Surg 22:241–251, 1995.
37. Barton FE Jr. Rhytidectomy and the nasolabial fold. Plast Reconstr Surg 90:601, 1992.
38. Hollander E. Cosmetic surgery. In: Joseph M, ed. Hanbuch der Kosmetik. Leipzig, Verlag von Veit, 1912.
39. Lexer E. Zur Gesichtsplastik. Arch Klin Chir 92:749, 1910.
40. Turpin IM. The modern rhytidectomy. Clin Plast Surg 15:383–400, 1992.
41. Skoog T. Plastic Surgery—New Methods. Philadelphia: W.B. Saunders, 1974.
42. Owsley JQ. Platysma-fascial rhytidectomy. Plast Reconstr Surg 60:843, 1977.
43. Connell BF. Contouring the neck in rhytidectomy by lipectomy and a muscle sling. Plast Reconstr Surg 61:376, 1978.
44. Guerrero-Santos J, Espaillat L, Morales F. Muscular lift in cervical rhytidectomy. Plast Reconstr Surg 54:127, 1974.
45. Webster RC, et al. Comparison of SMAS plication with SMAS imbrication in face lifting. Laryngoscope 92:901, 1982.
46. McKinney P, Tresley GE. The "maxi SMAS" management of the platysma bands in rhytidectomy. Ann Plastic Surg 12:260, 1984.

47. Lemmon ML, Hamra ST. Skoog rhytidectomy. A five year experience with 577 patients. Plast Reconstr Surg 65:283, 1980.
48. Peterson R. The role of platysma muscle in cervical lifts. In: Gouliari D, Courtiss EH, eds. Symposium on Surgery of the Aging Face. St. Louis: C.V. Mosby, 1978.
49. Hamra ST. Composite rhytidectomy Plast Reconstr Surg 90:1, 1992.
50. Hamra ST. The triplane face lift dissection. Ann Plastic Surg 12:268, 1984.
51. Kamar FM, Halsey W. The two layer rhytidectomy. Arch Otolaryng 107:450, 1981.
52. Teimourian B, Delia S, Wahrman A. The multiplane face lift. Plast Reconstr Surg 93: 78, 1994.
53. Ivy EJ, Lorenc LP, Aston S. Is there a difference? A prospective study comparing lateral and standard SMAS face lifts with extended SMAS and composite rhytidectomies. Plast Reconstr Surg 98:1135, 1996.
54. Gamble WB, Manson PN, Smith GE, Hamra ST. Comparison of 9 skin-tissue tensions using the composite and the subcutaneous techniques. Ann Plast Surg 35:447–457, 1995.
55. Schuster PH, Gamble WD, Hamra ST, Manson PN. A comparison of flap vascular anatomy in three rhytidectomy techniques. Plast Reconstr Surg 95:683, 1995.
56. Larson DL. An historical glimpse of the evolution of rhytidectomy. Clin Plast Surg 207–212, 1995.
57. Millard DR Jr, Yuan RT, Devine JW Jr. A challenge to the undefeated nasolabial fold. Plast Reconstr Surg 80:37, 1987.
58. Ellenbogen R, et al. Currette fat sculpture in rhytidectomy: improving the nasolabial and labiomandibular folds. Plast Reconstr Surg 88:433, 1991.
59. Teimourian B. Face and neck suction assisted lipectomy associated with rhytidectomy. Plast Reconstr Surg 72:627, 1983.
60. Barton FE Jr. The SMAS and the nasolabial fold. Plast Reconstr Surg 89:1054, 1992.
61. Barton FE Jr. Rhytidectomy and the nasolabial fold. Plast Reconstr Surg 90:601, 1992.
62. Owsley JR. Lifting the malar fat pad for correction of prominent nasolabial folds. Plast Reconstr Surg 91:463, 1993.
63. Furnas DW. Strategies for nasolabial levitation. Clin Plast Surg 22:265–278, 1995.
64. Mendelson DC. Correction of the nasolabial fold. Extended SMAS dissection with periosteal fixation. Plast Reconstr Surg 89:822, 1992.
65. Billarkis JM, Rumsley TO, Camargos, KA. A subperiosteal approach as an improved concept for correction of the aging face. Plast Reconstr Surg 82:383, 1988.
66. Ramirez OM, Maillard GF, Musolas H. The extended subperiosteal face lift: a definitive soft tissue remodeling for facial rejuvenation. Plast Reconstr Surg 88:227, 1991.
67. Vasconez LO, I Askren CC, Gore G. Endoscopic technique in coronal face lifting. PSEF Videotape Library No. 9313, 1993.
68. Ramirez OM. Endoscopic full face lift. Aesth Plast Surg 18:363–371, 1994.
69. Isse NG. Endoscopic facial rejuvenation, endo forehead, the functional lift. Aesth Plast Surg 18:21–29, 1994.
70. Hamas RS. Reducing the subconscious frown by endoscopic resection of the corrugator muscles. Aesth Plast Surg 19:21–25, 1995.
71. Standards and Check List for Accreditation of Ambulatory Surgical Facilities. American Association for Accreditation of Ambulatory Surgery Facilities, Inc., 1997.
72. Dripps R, Eckenhoff J, Uaddam L, eds. Introduction to Anesthesia, 6th ed. Philadelphia: WB Saunders, 1982, pp. 17–18.
73. Rosenbach ML, Cromwell J, Ketler JH, SH, et al. Payment options for non-physician anesthetists under Medicare's prospective payment system. Center for Health Economics Research, 1988.
74. AO Cutrone. Personal communication.
75. Bogetz MS. Recovery and discharge following outpatient surgery. In: University of California San Diego Anesthesia Update, 1991. San Diego, UCSD, 1991, pp. 46–52.

76. McKinney P, Katrana DJ. Prevention of injuries to the greater auricular nerve during rhytidectomy. Plast Reconstr Surg 83:11, 1989.
77. Rose EH, Vistnes CM, Ksander GA. A microarchitectural model of regional variation in hypodermal mobility in porcine and human skin. Ann Plast Surg 1:254, 1978.
78. Matarasso A. Buccal fat pad excision: aesthetic improvement of the mid face. Ann Plast Surg 26:413, 1991.
79. Coleman SR. Facial recontouring with lipostructure. Clin Plast Surg 24:347, 1997.
80. Niechajer I, Sevcuk O. Long term results of fat transplantation: clinical and histological studies. Plast Reconstr Surg 94:496–506, 1994.
81. Moscona R, Ullman Y, Har Shai Y, et al. Free fat injections for correction of hemifacial atrophy. Plast Reconstr Surg 84:501–507, 1989.
82. Wilkinson T. Fat grafting. In: Practical Procedures in Aesthetic Plast Surgery. New York: Springer-Verlag, 1994.
83. Brown JB, Fryer MP, Randall P. Silicones in plastic surgery. Plast Reconstr Surg 12: 374, 1953.
84. Rubin LR. Polyethylene as a bone and cartilage substitute; a 32 year retrospective. In: Rubin LR, ed. Biomaterials in Plastic Surgery. St. Louis: Mosby, 1983, pp. 477–493.
85. Wellisz T, Kanel G, Anooshian RV. Characteristics of the tissue response to MEDPORE porous polyethylene implants in the human facial skeleton. J Long Term Effect Biomed 3:223, 1993.
86a. Dougherty W, Wellisz T. The natural history of alloplastic implants in orbital floor reconstruction. An animal model. J Craniofac Surg 5;26, 1994.
86b. Weinstein C, Roberts TL. Aesthetic skin resurfacing with the high energy ultrapulsed CO_2 laser. Clin Plast Surg 24:379, 1997.
87. Anderson RR. Hair transplantation and skin resurfacing with lasers. Laser physics and scanner technology. Symposium on Skin Resurfacing and Hair Transplantation Using Novel Laser Flash Scanner Techniques, New York, 1995.
88. Lask G. Laser skin resurfacing with the Silk Touch Scanner. Symposium on Skin Resurfacing and Hair Transplantation Using Novel Laser Flash Scanner Techniques, New York, 1995.
89. Stallins SO, Vandenbus K, Storene WS, et al. The reverse dermis graft—a choice not a flap. J Iowa Med Sci 61:606, 1971.
90. Thompson N. The subcutaneous dermis graft. Plast Reconstr Surg 26:1, 1960.
91. Baker TJ, Gordon HL. Complications of rhytidectomy. Plast Reconstr Surg 40:31, 1967.
92. Baker DC. Complications of cervicofacial rhytidectomy. Clin Plast Surg 10:543, 1983.
93. Rees TD, Aston SJ. Complications of rhytidectomy. Clin Plast Surg 5:109, 1978.
94. Le Roy JL, Rees TD, Nolan WB III. Infections requiring hospital readmission following face lift surgery. Incidence, treatment, and sequelae. Plast Reconstr Surg 93:533, 1994.
95. Rees TD, Barone CM, Valauri FA, et al. Hematomas requiring surgical evacuation after face lift surgery. Plast Reconstr Surg 93:1185–1190, 1994.
96. Rees TD, Liverett DM, Guy CL. The effects of cigarette smoking on skin flap survival in the face lift patient. Plast Reconstr Surg 73:911, 1984.
97. Bansberg SF, Krugman ME. Parotid salivary fistula following rhytidectomy. Ann Plast Surg 24:61, 1990.
98. McKinney P, Zuckerbraun BS, Smith JW, et al. Management of parotid leakage following rhytidectomy. Plast Reconstr Surg 98:795, 1996.
99. Guyuron B, Bokhari F, Thomas T. Secondary rhytidectomy. Plast Reconstr Surg 100: 1281, 1997.

APPENDIX 1. INFORMED CONSENT

Patient Computer Imaging

In the course of consultation and discussion of with Dr. Rose, I may have been shown or provided certain brochures, pictures of actual patients or pictures on an electronic computer imaging device. I do understand that those pictures and alteration of these pictures seen are solely for the purpose of illustration, discussion and to provide improved communication with Dr. Rose. I do understand that the outcome of any type of surgical procedure is directly related to my individual characteristics and health. I further understand and acknowledge that because of the obvious significant differences in how living tissues react to surgery my final actual surgical result may be different than the electronic image created. Use of the computer imaging system offers an opportunity for me to discuss my desires and to allow improved communication with the medical staff.

Photography

I have been asked to sign this Consent for Photography. I understand that the photographs are kept strictly confidential. They are primarily used in the preoperative planning and postoperative assessment of the results by Dr. Rose. On occasion there are used for teaching purposes and may be shared with other health care professionals or shown in scientific publications.

I have read and understood all the above and give my permission for photographs. I reserve the right to request return of all photographic material at the conclusion of my treatment.

Patient:______________________________

Surgeon:______________________________

Witness: ______________________________

Date: ________________________________

APPENDIX 2. MEDICAL QUESTIONNAIRE

Today's date______________________________ DOB____

Name:____Age:________Height__________Weight___________

Please provide us with the name of your personal physician: (Internist, Family Physician, Pediatrician, etc.):

Pharmacy Name and Number:____

Do you have any serious or chronic illnesses? Yes______ No_________ If yes, please specify:

____

____

WHAT MEDICATIONS ARE YOU CURRENTLY TAKING?_______________________________________

____

DO YOU HAVE OR HAVE YOU HAD AN ALLERGIC REACTION TO ANY DRUGS OR MEDICATIONS? (IF NO, LEAVE BLANK, IF YES, GIVE DATE OF OCCURRENCE):___________________________

____

DO YOU HAVE OR HAVE YOU HAD? (IF NO LEAVE BLANK, IF YES, GIVE DATE OF OCCURRENCE)

Stroke___________	Shortness of Breath___________	Kidney Disease___________	Hepatitis___________
Cancer___________	Chest Pain___________	Visual Disorders___________	Heart Attack___________
Tuberculosis_______	Migraines___________	Arthritis___________	Ulcers___________
Leukemia_________	Frequent Headaches___________	Dizzy Spells___________	Swelling___________
Bronchitis_________	Colitis___________	Rheumatic Fever___________	Nervous___________
Epilepsy__________	Seizure___________	Goiter___________	Bleeding Tendency______
HIV+___________	Pneumonia___________	Bladder Infection___________	AIDS___________
Diabetes__________	Asthma___________	Heart Problems___________	

High Blood Pressure____

No Yes Do you frequently have bleeding gums?

No Yes Do you have nosebleeds? How Often?____

No Yes Have you ever bled excessively from a tooth extraction?

No Yes Do you bleed excessively from a laceration?

No Yes Do you take aspirin regularly? How Often?____________________________________

(IF YES STOP TAKING THEM UNTIL AFTER YOUR SURGERY)

No Yes Do you take any drugs containing salicytates or anti-inflammatory medications, Bufferin Anacin, Alka Seltzer, Excedrin, Motrin, Advil, Nuprin, Darvon compound, Clinoril, Feldene, etc? Which ones and how often?_______________________________________

____

No Yes Have you taken steroids in the past two years? Why?___________________________

No Yes HAVE YOU EVER CONSULTED A PLASTIC SURGEON? When?______________

No Yes Do you regularly smoke? How much?_______________ For how long?______________

No Yes Do you regularly drink alcohol or beer? How much?_____________________________

No Yes Have you had any psychiatric treatment? Please explain.:_________________________

No Yes Do you have any unsightly scars? Where?___________________________________

WOMEN ONLY:

NUMBER OF PREGNANCIES:_____________MISCARRIAGES_______________CHILDREN_________

No Yes Are you currently taking birth control No Yes Are you pregnant?

APPENDIX 3. INFORMED CONSENT

PATIENT:

I have consulted with Dr. Rose on prior visit(s). I am discussing with Dr. Rose the following surgical procedure(s) .

Face/neck lift; mini-brow lift.

They supplied me with an information sheet and brochure for this particular type of surgery, and I have read them and understood their contents to my satisfaction.

Dr. Rose has reviewed the surgery in understandable detail; the potential outcome, the various risks, and possible complications. Dr. Rose has explained to me all the surgical alternatives and that the decision to have surgery is mine alone.

I understand the importance of following the preoperative and postoperative suggestions and recommendations, and I will return for follow-up visits as requested. Dr. Rose has informed me of the importance of these appointments, and the fact that negligence may seriously jeopardize the final results of the surgery.

I consent to the use of my chart in a periodic peer review, and am assured that confidentiality will be maintained at all times.

I consent to the administration of intravenous sedation, to be administered by

____

At this time, I feel that I am thoroughly familiar with all aspects of the procedure, and understand that Dr. Rose cannot guarantee or warranty results of this procedure. I am satisfied with the explanations which have been given to me, and it is my decision to proceed with surgery on the 16th of December, 1998 to be performed by Dr. Rose and his associates.

________________________	________________________
Surgeon	Patient
________________________	________________________
Witness	Date

APPENDIX 4. PREGNANCY TEST WAIVER

It is recommended that all female patients of child bearing age take a pregnancy test prior to a surgical procedure.

The reason for this precaution is possible damage to any unborn child. If you wish to waive this pregnancy test and assume this risk yourself, releasing The Aesthetic Surgery Center and Dr. Elliott Rose from all responsibility and liability for any complications that may occur, please sign below.

____________________ Patient

____________________ Date

____________________ Surgeon

____________________ Witness

APPENDIX 5. PRESURGICAL VISIT

Date: ____________________

Presurgical testing ____________________

Medical clearance ____________________

Autologous blood ____________________

Prescriptions ____________________

Postsurgical visit ____________________

Postsurgical instruction sheet ____________________

Garments ____________________

Consents ____________________

Deposit ____________________

30

Blepharoplasty

Gregg M. Menaker
Harvard Medical School, Boston, Massachusetts

Ronald L. Moy and Philina Lamb
VA-West Los Angeles Medical Center, University of California at Los Angeles, Los Angeles, California

INTRODUCTION

It has been said that the eyes are the seat of the soul. The eyes are not only responsible for many facial expressions but they are also a major component of facial attractiveness and youthfulness. However, the aging process alters the paraorbital tissues, rendering change to the once-youthful face. In the Caucasian face, there are three changes that occur in the typical aging eye: degeneration, delamination, and displacement [1–6]. Degeneration of the lateral canthus causes a rounding and downward displacement of the eyelids. In addition, skin degeneration, as a result of gravity, oxidation, and ultraviolet (UV) light, leads to elastosis and wrinkling. Delamination of the orbital septum allows the upper lid fat, normally sandwiched between the orbicularis oculi and the levator aponeurosis, to project downward over the eye and obliterate the tarsal crease by separating the levator aponeurosis from the upper eyelid skin. Lastly, protrusion of the orbital fat pads may occur secondary to deterioration of the elastic paraorbital tissues. It is mainly the downward displacement of these fat pads that contributes to the "bags-under-the-eyes" or aged appearance [7].

Blepharoplasty is mainly a cosmetic procedure that is performed to eliminate fatty prominence in the upper and lower eyelids and to reestablish the upper eyelid crease that has been obliterated by tissue ptosis [7]. When lid ptosis interferes with superior and lateral visual fields, blepharoplasty can be a corrective procedure rather than a cosmetic procedure [7,8]. Eyelid deformities that can be managed with blepharoplasty can be classified into six categories: (1) blepharochalasis, (2) dermatochalasis, (3) orbicularis oculi hypertrophy, (4) protrusion of intraorbital fat, (5) a combination of any of these, and (6) hooding of the upper eyelids secondary to ptosis of the eyebrows [1,2,7–9].

Blepharochalasis is defined as atony or relaxation of the upper lid skin, which becomes wrinkled and hangs over the eyes like a curtain. Dermatochalasis primarily involves the upper eyelids and is distinguished from blepharochalasis as being hypertrophy of the upper eyelid skin. The fascial bands that connect the skin to the orbicularis muscle and orbital ostium relax, and the thickened skin hangs down over the eye as a pouch, or pseudoptosis. Hypertrophy of the orbicularis muscle is common in individuals who smile or squint often, or in patients with blepharospasm. This hypertrophy is seen as a horizontal bulging immediately below the lower lid margin. This is in contrast to protrusion of orbital adipose tissue, which is seen more inferior to the lash line. Orbicularis hypertrophy can be treated with an elliptical excision of the muscle without excision of the overlying skin. Protrusion of orbital fat occurs secondary to weakness in the orbital septum and orbicularis muscle. This is a pseudoherniation because there is no disruption of the fascia or musculature. In rare instances, a true herniation can develop with adipose protruding through an actual defect in the orbital septum [9]. Combinations of these conditions can be seen. In fact, it is common for two of these conditions to coexist. Hooding of the upper eyelids secondary to ptosis of the eyebrows is very common. Hooding occurs as a result of the aging process, which leads to gravitational descent of the eyebrows. Differentiation between hooding of the eyelids due to eyebrow ptosis is important to the surgeon in that hooding requires correction of the eyebrows with a browlift procedure and not with a correction of the eyelids via blepharoplasty.

ANATOMY

The upper eyelid, above the superior palpebral fold (or upper eyelid crease), is commonly referred to as the preseptal portion. It is composed of seven major layers: skin, orbicularis muscle, orbital septum, orbital fat, levator aponeurosis, Muller's muscle, and conjunctiva [6,7] (Fig. 1). The skin superficial to the tarsus is very thin, and contains very little dermis. The orbicularis oculi, located directly beneath the

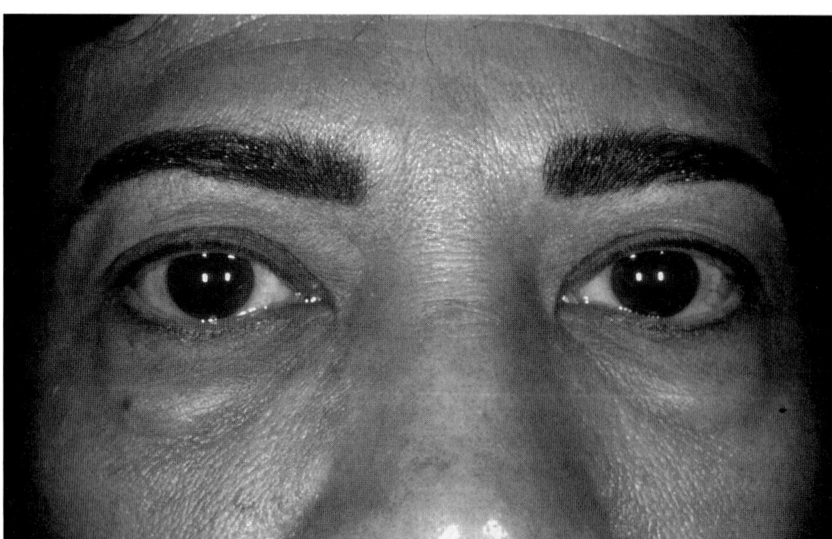

FIGURE 1 The patient complained of bags under her eyes.

skin of the eyelid, functions to close the eyelids. This muscle is further divided into pretarsal, preseptal, and orbital sections. The orbicularis also forms the lateral and medial canthal tendons. The temporal branch of the seventh cranial nerve innervates all three sections of the orbicularis [6,9,10,11].

Deep to the orbicularis muscle is the fibrous orbital septum, originating at the arcus marginalis of the supraorbital rim, and coursing inferiorly to insert on the anterior surface of the levator aponeurosis, 3 to 4 mm superior to the tarsus. It is critical to avoid damage to the levator aponeurosis as this will lead to upper eyelid ptosis. The tarsal plates of the upper and lower lids are composed of dense fibrous connective tissue. The tarsal plates act as support to the eyelids and are attached to the medial and lateral canthal tendons [6,7,9–11].

In the Caucasian eye, the upper eyelid crease is formed by the attachments of the levator aponeurosis fibers to the overlying orbital septum and orbicularis fibers. These attachments follow a crescent pattern: 3 to 5 mm above the lash line, rising to 8 to 14 mm centrally, and descending to 4 to 8 mm laterally. The height and shape of the crease can vary widely, even in the same individual and especially between the sexes. The crease in women is higher at 8 to 10 mm, whereas the crease in men is usually at 6 to 8 mm. In the Asian eye, the attachment of the levator aponeurosis occurs much closer to the ciliary margin, thus giving the appearance of a less-defined or "single" crease. Because of the formation of this lower crease, the preaponeurotic fat is allowed to move more inferiorly, thus contributing to a less prominent upper eyelid fold [6,10,12–15].

The paraorbital adipose tissue plays a prominent role in the aesthetic quality of the eyes (Fig. 2). The fat pads lie deep to the orbital septum, it is believed that this tissue has a strong hereditary predilection [16]. The paraorbital fat is separated

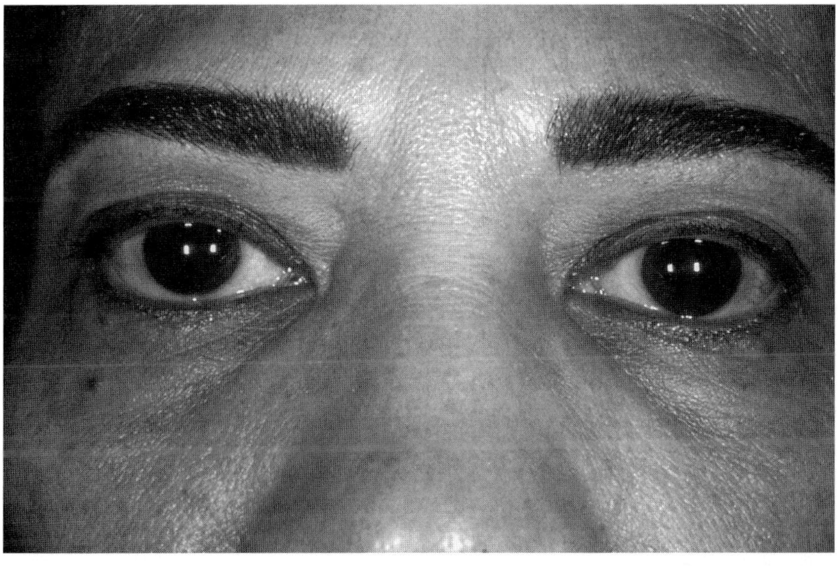

FIGURE 2 Six months after a transconjunctival blepharoplasty with only a small amount of fat removed. There is only moderate improvement. The patient may have had a better result if fat were moved and sutured to the nasal jugular groove.

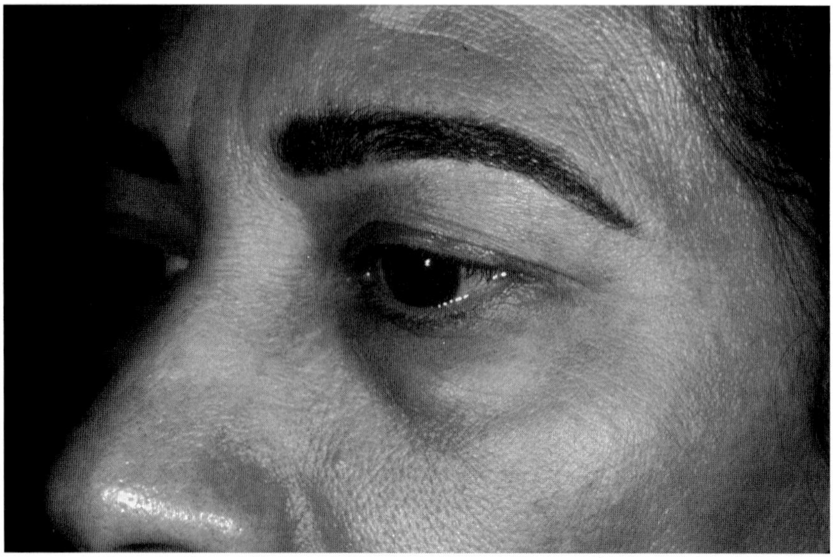

FIGURE 3 Presurgical to transconjunctival blepharoplasty.

into five compartments in each eye: two (medial and lateral) in the upper eyelid and three (lateral, middle, and medial) in the lower eyelid. The compartments are divided by thin fibrous sheaths. In the lower eyelid, the middle and medial compartment are also divided by the inferior oblique muscle, whereas the arcuate expansion of the inferior oblique separates the lateral and middle compartments.

The lacrimal gland is located in the superior temporal quadrant of the orbit and is separated into firm lobules by the lateral horn of the levator aponeurosis (Fig. 3). It differs in its pink coloration from orbital fat, which is yellow, to white in color. Prolapse of the lacrimal gland will be seen as fullness in the lateral area of the upper eyelid and is seen with a greater incidence in females. It has been estimated that 15% of patients undergoing blepharoplasty show displacement of the lacrimal gland. Left uncorrected, this will result is postsurgical fullness in the lateral aspect of the upper lid. However, if misdiagnosed as orbital fat, portions of the lacrimal gland will be mistakenly resected and abnormalities of lacrimal function will result [6,9,10,16].

The lower eyelid is attached to the bony orbit by the medial and lateral canthal tendons. The medial canthal tendon serves as an excellent source of support; the lateral canthal tendon, however, is less supportive and lies 1 to 2 mm superior to the medial canthus (3 mm in Asians). The lower eyelid retractors are composed of the inferior tarsal muscle and the capsulopalpebral fascia; this is analogous to the levator aponeurosis and Mueller's muscle of the upper eyelid. The three fat pads of the lower eyelid are found between the orbital septum and the lower lid retractors. The lateral fat pad is more superior than the middle and medial fat pads; however, the middle fat pad is the most prominent [6,7].

PRESURGICAL EVALUATION

More likely than not, the patient presenting for aesthetic blepharoplasty will be healthy with a relatively straightforward medical history. Because of these factors, the majority of the consultation may be devoted to determining the patient's concerns and expectations of the surgery. In addition, it is important for the surgeon to determine which patients should or should not have surgery and which surgeries or procedures ought to be performed to improve the patient's appearance. This discussion will minimize complications and avoid any patient dissatisfaction after surgery [17–26].

The use of a mirror will assist the patient in showing the surgeon which specific areas of the eyelids he or she would like to have altered. This will also enable the physician to point out the limitations and the specific areas that are not correctable by blepharoplasty. Features such as periorbital rhytides, hyperpigmentation ("dark circles under the eyes"), festoons, or chronic edema will not be repaired or refined with lower lid transconjuctival blepharoplasty. It is paramount that the patient understands what the surgery will accomplish along with limitations, failures, and potential complications. Patients with grandiose and unrealistic expectations are often poor surgical candidates [7,8].

A review of the past medical history and current medications is important to reveal any contraindications or underlying illnesses that may affect the surgery. Taking a detailed ophthalmic history is imperative before performing blepharoplasty. The patient may undergo a full ophthalmic evaluation by an ophthalmologist before surgery. Postsurgical complications are often a result of an exacerbation of an underlying ophthalmic problem. Important medical conditions that may affect the patient's physical ability for surgery are summarized in Table 1. Special attention needs

TABLE 1 Medical History

Personal or familial ocular disease
Glaucoma
Dry eyes
Unilateral blindness
Previous orbital trauma or surgery
Thyroid problems and associated ophthalmic involvement
Exophthalmos
Myxedema
Systemic disease
Recent myocardial infection
Unstable angina pectoris
Congestive heart failure
Uncontrolled hypertension
Diabetes mellitus
Multiple sclerosis
Medications or coagulopathies that increase bleeding
Allergic history that may be exacerbated by or contribute to periorbital edema and blepharochalasis
Dermatological conditions
Rosacea
Seborrhea
Keloids

Source: Refs. 7, 9, 15, 26, 27.

TABLE 2 Physical Examination

Visual acuity with or without glasses or contact lenses.
Thorough evaluation of the tissues from the anterior scalp hairline to the midcheek region.
Observation for thyroid symptoms.
  Exophthalmos
  Myxedema
Eyebrow and eyelid evaluation for ptosis.
Evaluation for atony of the eyelids.
Fat pad estimate
Lacrimal gland evaluation for prolapse.
  Prolapse is seen in the temporal region of the upper lid. Often, this is mistaken for fat and erroneously resected.
Levator excursion with the patient looking up and then down.
  This measurement should be at least 12 cm.
Palpebral fissure width and length
Medial/lateral canthal evaluation for laxity.
Scleral show
Schirmer's test to assess presurgical tear production.
Lower-eyelid "snap back" test to assess laxity of the lower lid.
  The middle of the lower lid is grasped between the index finger and the thumb and pulled forward and upward. The lid is then released and allowed to "snap" back against the globe. An audible sound may confirm that there is little or no loss in elasticity. With laxity, the sound becomes absent and the lid may not return to its original position.
Lower-eyelid pinch test
  The middle of the lower lid is grasped between the index finger and the thumb and pinched together. If there is a distance greater than 6 mm between the globe and the lid edge, the patient may have lower-lid laxity.
Visual field examination
  Important for documentation of presurgical vision.
  Limitation of vision in the upper and outer gaze is an indication for therapeutic blepharoplasty. This is usually secondary to hooding of the lateral half of the upper lid.*
Extraocular movements assessment
  Important for presurgical documentation.
Presurgical determination of planned incision lines.

**Source*: Ref. 8.
Source: Refs. 14, 27.

to be directed towards patients with thyroid disease, bleeding diatheses, and acute angle glaucoma—conditions that may preclude the patient from blepharoplasty. The patient's general health and the use of systemic or topical medications may also affect the ability to undergo blepharoplasty. Important components of the physical examination are summarized in Table 2.

Photographs

Presurgical clinical photography of both eyes is essential in documenting existing eyelid and orbital anatomy. Photographs aid in presurgical planning and intrasurgical decision making [28]. Variables that may lead to photographic distortion, such as head tilt, brow relaxation, visual focal point, the plane of the camera, lighting, and smiling, need to be minimized [29]. The recommended standard presurgical photographic views include: (1) full face in repose and smiling; (2) close-up views of eyelids and periorbital structures in repose and smiling; (3) close-up views of the eyelids and periorbital tissues in upgaze and downgaze; (4) close-up lateral views of eyelids and periorbital tissues; and (5) close-up oblique (45° angle) views of the eyelids. With the patient in upward gaze, the lower lid herniated fat is accentuated, whereas the downward gaze emphasizes upper lid dermatochalasis. The oblique views of the eyelids make evident excessive upper lid temporal skin, lower lid herniated orbital fat, and ptotic eyebrows.

Presurgical Marking

Accurate marking of the eyelids before infiltration with local anesthesia is critical. Incisions are marked with the patient in the upright sitting position with the surgeon facing the patient; this allows the surgeon to optimally assess the effect of gravity on the paraorbital tissues [8,9,30–32]. Once the patient has assumed the supine position, the orbital fat sinks into the orbit and the gravitational effect on the eyebrows disappears [32].

Upper Lid

Marking of the Inferior Incision. The patient is instructed to close the eyes and the surgeon identifies the upper eyelid crease. This will serve as the inferior incision. With a fine-tipped surgical marker, the physician marks the midtarsal point (approximately 10 mm in women and 8 mm in men, with a single dot) usually in the upper lid crease. The medial aspect of the inferior incision is drawn approximately 5 mm above the upper punctum, extending to the lateral canthus, and then sloping slightly upward in one of the lateral canthal eyelid creases, somewhat beyond the lateral canthus (Fig. 4).

Marking of the Superior Incision. The middle upper eyelid crease and the redundant skin superior to it are gently grasped with forceps. The amount of pinched tissue is adequate when all excessive eyelid skin is eliminated, the lashes are minimally everted, and there is minimal elevation of the upper eyelid from the lower eyelid. A mark is made centrally at the edge of the superior forceps blade. This procedure is repeated medially and laterally. The medial and lateral markings are then connected to each other and to the ends of the inferior incision. In general, more skin is excised laterally because of the hooding and extra skin of the lateral upper eyelid (Fig. 5).

Lower Lid

If transconjuctival blepharoplasty is to be performed on the lower eyelid, no marking of the lower eyelid is required, although it is helpful to mark out the areas of protruded adipose tissue.

Instrument Tray

The following should be on the instrument tray:

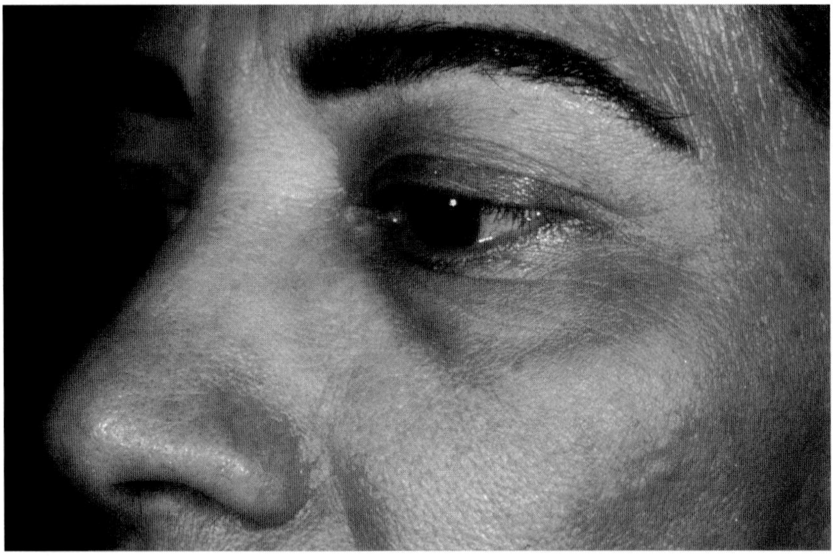

FIGURE 4 Moderate improvement after 10 months.

- Electrocautery machine with bipolar capabilities
- Colorado needle or CO_2 laser in the cutting mode (for transconjunctival blepharoplasty)
- Scleral shields
- Castroviejo caliper
- Bard-Parker scalpel handle and No. 15 blade

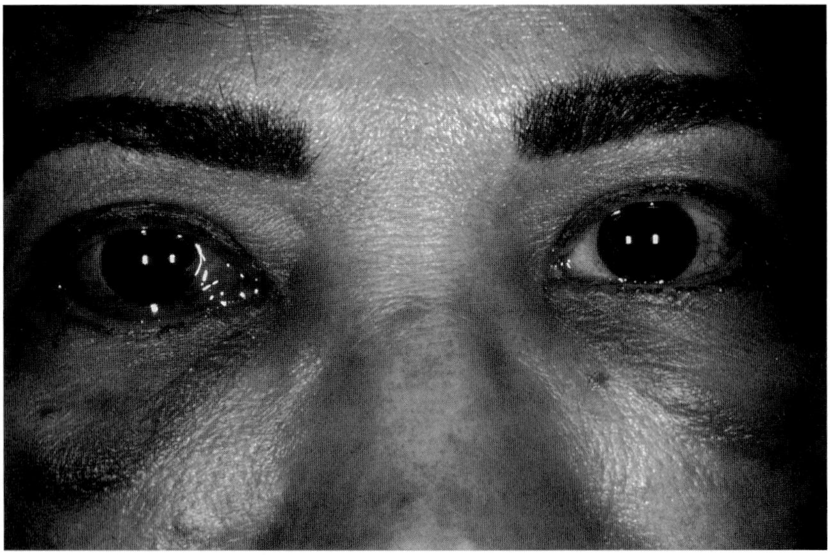

FIGURE 5 Two days after surgery the patient has bruising of sclera.

- Desmarres lid retractor
- Jaeger lid plate
- Adson forceps
- Scissors
- Needle holder
- Nonabsorbable sutures, eg, silk (6-0), nylon (6-0), Prolene (6-0), or absorbable suture such as fast absorbing plain gut (6-0)
- Surgical dressings
- Cotton-tip applicators
- Wound closure tape

ANESTHESIA

Blepharoplasty can be performed under local or general anesthesia [14,30]. Most dermatologists prefer the use of local anesthetics alone or possibly with intravenous sedation. The advantages of local anesthesia include the following: (1) the patient is able to inform the surgeon when there has been excessive pulling on orbital structures or if corneal irritation has occurred, (2) the patient can respond to commands to test extraocular movements, (3) there is less postsurgical nausea and vomiting, thus minimizing the risk of hematoma, and (4) the surgeon is able to assess any changes in visual acuity [9].

Presurgical markings of the lids are made before injection of local anesthesia. Tetracaine 0.5% drops are placed in each eye and the incision sites are infiltrated with lidocaine mixed with 1:100,000 epinephrine. At the surgeon's preference, hyaluronidase (Wydase) may be added to the infiltrative anesthesia to aid in the even distribution of anesthetic and to minimize postinjection tissue distortion [31]. As the eyelid is pulled upward and outward, anesthetic is slowly injected in a temporal to nasal direction with a 0.5 inch 30-gauge needle subcutaneously. This will avoid globe penetration with the needle. A small amount is injected deeper, aiming for the fat compartments. Even if the patient is under intravenous sedation, a local anesthetic with epinephrine is required to facilitate hemostasis [33]. Light pressure is then held for 10 minutes to reduce the amount of bruising that may occur secondary to needle penetration. Twenty minutes are allowed to elapse before the surgery begins. This allows the epinephrine in the local anesthetic to reach its optimal vasoconstrictive effect [9,12,33].

UPPER-LID BLEPHAROPLASTY

Skin excision alone without excision of orbicularis or adipose tissue is sufficient to correct dermatochalasis. However, if the patient has "heavy" eyelids, characterized by protruding fat and orbicularis hypertrophy, the patient will require excision of skin, hypertrophied orbicularis, and protruding orbital fat [6,9,10,12,13,14,25,27] (Figs. 6 and 7).

In women, the main objective in upper lid blepharoplasty is to obtain relatively high symmetric creases (10–12 mm) above the lash line. This is usually accomplished by liberal excision of muscle and fat. In men, however, the goal is to design a lower crease, which maintains the "masculine" look and eliminates the bulky, heavy, and fatigued appearance. Designing the male eyelid with a high crease will

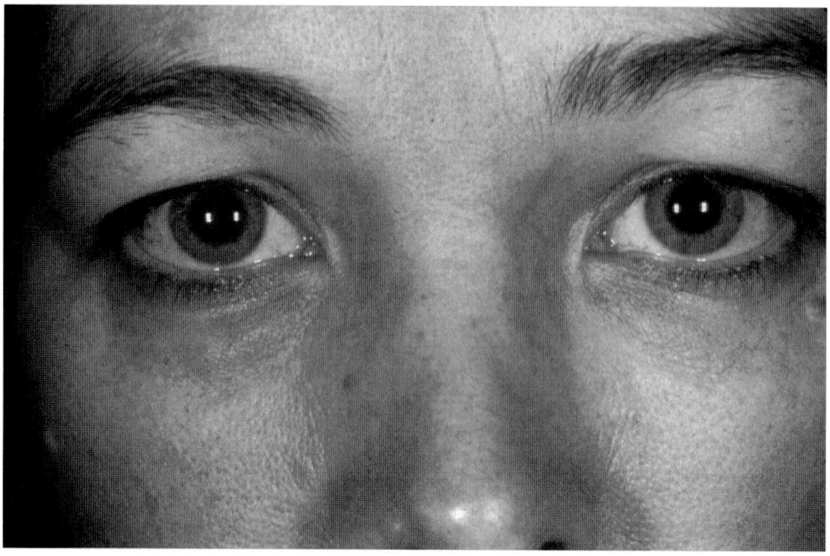

FIGURE 6 The patient complained of heavy eyelids.

lead to feminization. Upper lid blepharoplasty in the male will usually require conservative muscle excision and minimal fat excision [10,12,14,27].

In the Asian eye, the attachment of the levator aponeurosis occurs much closer to the lash line, thus giving the appearance of a less-defined or "single" crease. The superior palpebral fold is present in approximately 50% of Asians [13]. Because of the formation of the lower crease, the preaponeurotic fat is allowed to move more

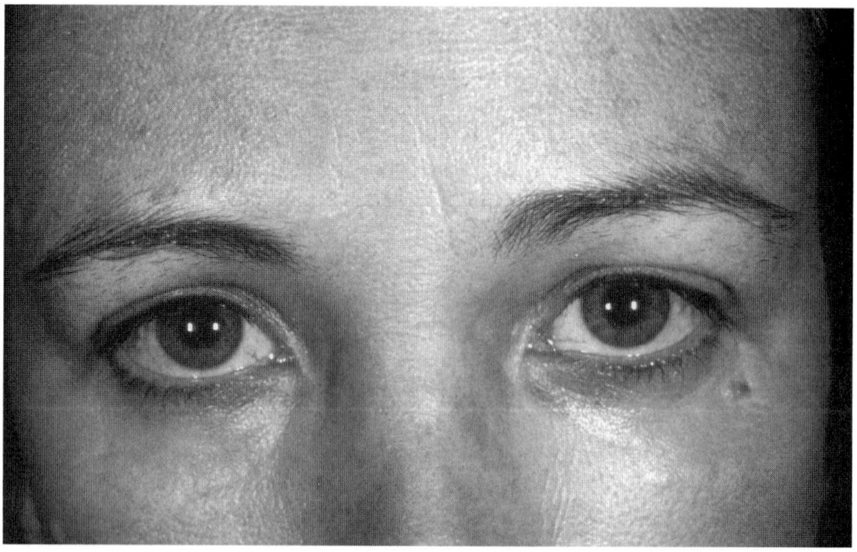

FIGURE 7 Postsurgical upper-lid blepharoplasty shows more of the patient's upper eyelids.

TABLE 3 Complications Specific To Asian Blepharoplasty

Eyelid crease asymmetry
Abnormal contour of the eyelid folds
Formation of a shallow crease
Temporary crease formation

inferiorly and thus contribute to a more prominent upper eyelid fold [6,10,12–14,62]. When performing blepharoplasty in the Asian patient, it is important to ask if the patient desires "westernization" of the eye. If the patient does not want to "westernize" the eye, excision of fat and skin will be sufficient. However, if the western eyelid is to be created, adequate excision of muscle is also necessary to allow for spontaneous supratarsal fixation and crease formation or, for a very sharp crease, fixation with sutures [10,12–14,34] (Table 3).

Surgical Technique

The surgeon sits above the patient, and the surgical assistant is on the patient's left side if the surgeon is right-handed. With marking and anesthesia complete, a No. 15 scalpel blade is used to incise the outlined skin in a nasal-to-temporal direction, first over the inferior margin and then over the superior margin (Fig. 8). Each margin is incised with one smooth motion to avoid any irregularities.

The assistant then applies upward traction on the eyebrow and downward traction on the upper lid margin. As the surgeon grasps the lateral edge of the incised skin with toothed forceps, the underlying orbicularis can be separated and excised from the skin with scissors (Fig. 9). Electrocautery is used to control bleeding.

A thin strip of preseptal orbicularis is removed separately after the skin is excised (Fig. 10). The orbicularis must be grasped in an upward and outward fashion, away from the globe. Careful attention must be given while excising the orbicularis; the dissection must be superficial to avoid cutting into the levator aponeurosis and the retroseptal fat. The orbital septum is then visualized (Fig. 11).

As slight pressure is applied to the globe, the medial region of the orbital septum should be visualized for tenting by the protruding adipose tissue. The orbital septum at this site is grasped with toothed forceps and a small incision is made using scissors (Fig. 12). A slight bulge of fat should be seen through this opening. Pressure is again applied to the globe and fat should protrude more freely. The fat is then grasped with forceps and pulled outward. Gentle pulling on the fat is imperative. The preaponeurotic fat is attached to the posterior fat pad, through which both the ophthalmic and ciliary vessels pass. Excessive tension may inadvertently lead to retrobulbar hemorrhage. The orbital fat is excised with the laser or Colorado needle attached to an electrocautery unit and cauterized. Some [31] believe that clamping causes increased traction on orbital vessels with an increased risk of orbital hemorrhage. The remaining stump of fat is inspected for any bleeding and then allowed to retract into the orbit. The same procedure is applied to the other eyelid. Potential intrasurgical complications are summarized in Table 4.

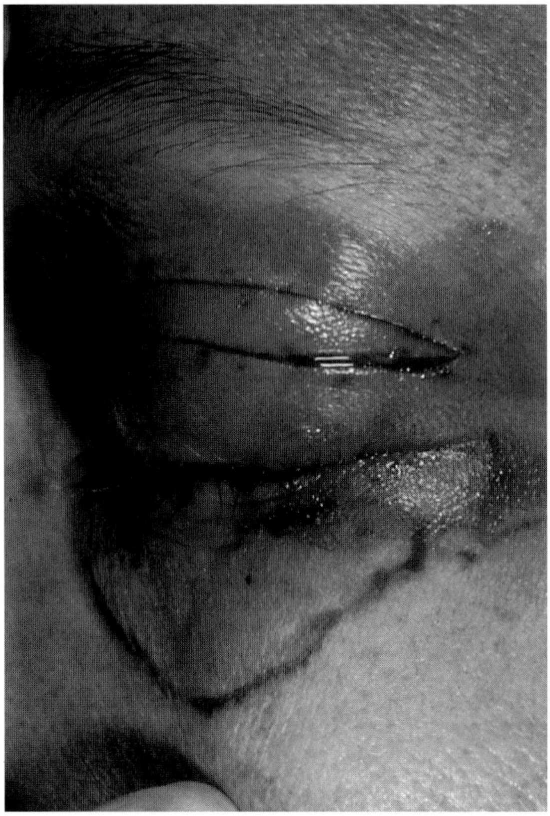

FIGURE 8 Skin incision for upper-lid blepharoplasty.

The skin incisions are closed with continuous intradermal, nonabsorbable sutures, or simple interrupted fast-absorbing sutures (Fig. 13). The wound is then gently cleansed with normal saline and wound closure tape is placed. Potential complications of upper-lid blepharoplasty are summarized in Tables 4 and 5. Complications specific to laser patients are summarized in Table 7.

LOWER-LID BLEPHAROPLASTY

Lower lid blepharoplasty can be approached via the transcutaneous route or the transconjunctival route. Traditional transcutaneous lower blepharoplasty requires dissection through the skin, orbicularis muscle, and anterior orbital septum. The skin-flap approach of transcutaneous blepharoplasty is used when excessive lower-lid skin needs to be resected. The skin-muscle flap (ie, skin-orbicularis flap) is used when there is both herniated orbital fat and excessive skin in the lower eyelid.

Theoretical advantages of transcutaneous blepharoplasty include less chance of globe or corneal injury, less risk to deeper structures of the orbit, and better visualization of anatomy. Despite excellent results, it is well documented that this approach can lead to lower-eyelid retraction at an estimated incidence of 15 to 20% [35–37]. This results in a lateral depression with "rounding" of the lower lid. This

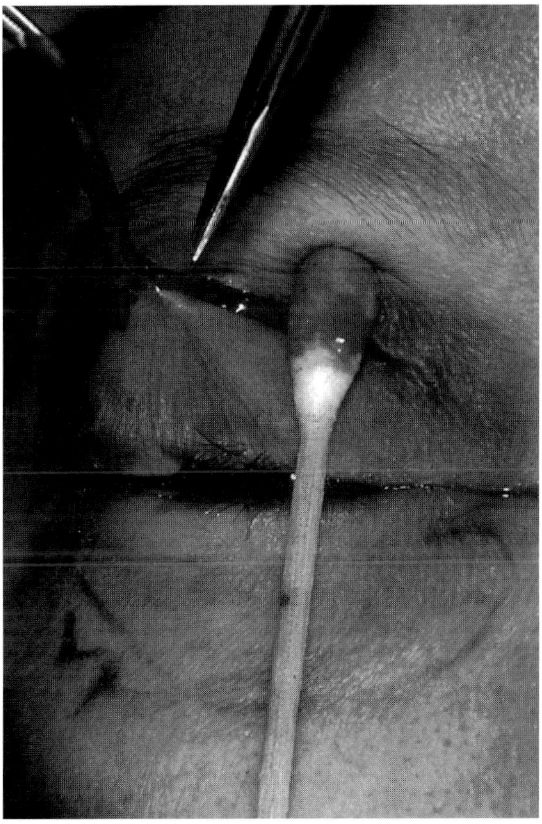

FIGURE 9 Excision of upper-lid skin.

"rounding" can be accentuated by scarring in the lateral canthal region. Severe lower-lid retraction results in scleral show and "dry eye." The most severe consequence of lower-lid retraction is frank ectropion, where dry eye and corneal exposure are most extreme.

In contrast, the transconjunctival approach leaves the skin, orbicularis, and orbital septum intact. This technique is best in patients who show protruding orbital fat but minimal excess skin [35]. However, adjuvant techniques, such as CO_2 laser resurfacing or a pinch technique of skin excision, can supplement blepharoplasty to tighten excess skin. Advantages of the transconjunctival approach include the following: removing excess fat from the lower eyelids without an external scar, less chance of eyelid retraction, and improved patient acceptance [38,39]. Netscher et al. reported no significant statistical difference in appearance or in subjective patient complaints between transconjunctival and transcutaneous groups [38]. Complications of transconjuctival blepharoplasty include the following: increased risk of corneal injury, excessive lower-lid stretch with potential for traction ectropion, symblepharon formation, excessive scarring in the fornix, postsurgical dry-eye symptoms, damage to the inferior oblique muscle, entropion, and, most importantly, underresection of fat [33,38]. Baylis et al. [36] reported that 7.4% of their patients required a second surgery for incomplete removal of fat.

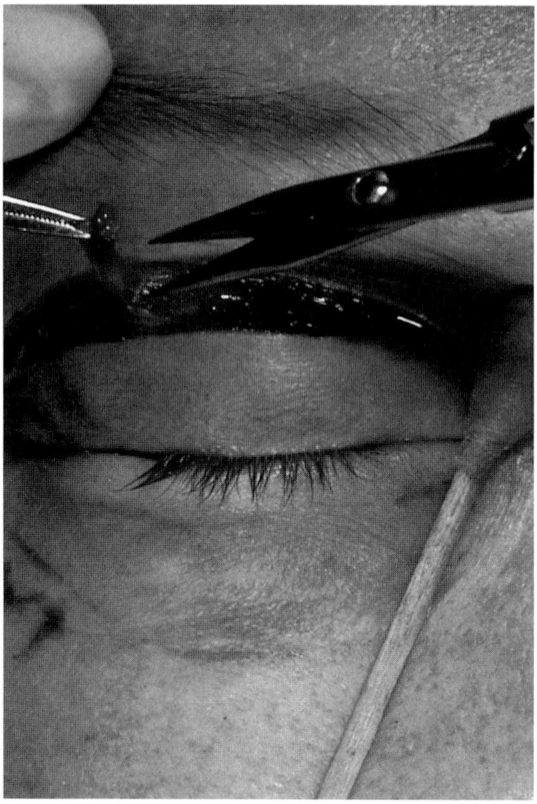

FIGURE 10 Excision of orbicularis oculi strip.

Proper patient selection in lower-lid blepharoplasty is important. Patients with excess lower-lid fat, fine rhytides, and less than 1 mm of forceps-tested redundant skin are better candidates for transconjunctival blepharoplasty. If necessary, this procedure can be immediately followed by laser resurfacing [27,33]. In patients with greater than 2 mm of forceps-tested redundancy and lax lower eyelids, transconjunctival blepharoplasty combined with lateral canthoplasty are often better options [27]. Several investigators stress that apparent skin excess does not exclude a patient from transconjunctival blepharoplasty. This excess is more theoretical than real, and the skin is able to recontour the lower eyelid after fat excision and laser resurfacing [28,40].

Transconjunctival Blepharoplasty Surgical Technique

After appropriate anesthesia has been administered, the assistant retracts the lower lid with a small Desmaires retractor to expose the inferior palpebral conjunctiva. The Jaeger plate is held by the assistant's other hand, angled from above, and placed in the sulcus below the orbital rim and directly against the orbital floor. A slight bulge is created between these two retractors (Fig. 14).

Using electrocautery, an incision is made between the two retractors directed at the infraorbital rim at a 45° angle. The incision should be placed below the inferior

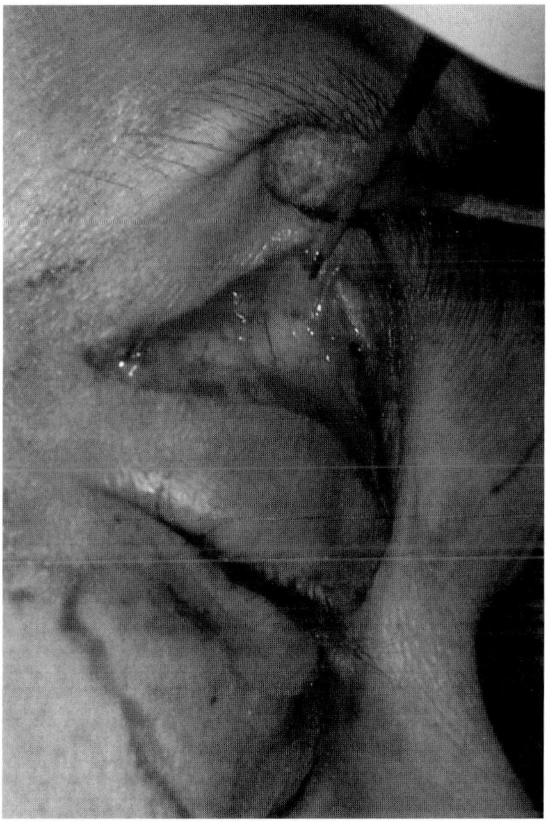

FIGURE 11 Orbital septum exposed.

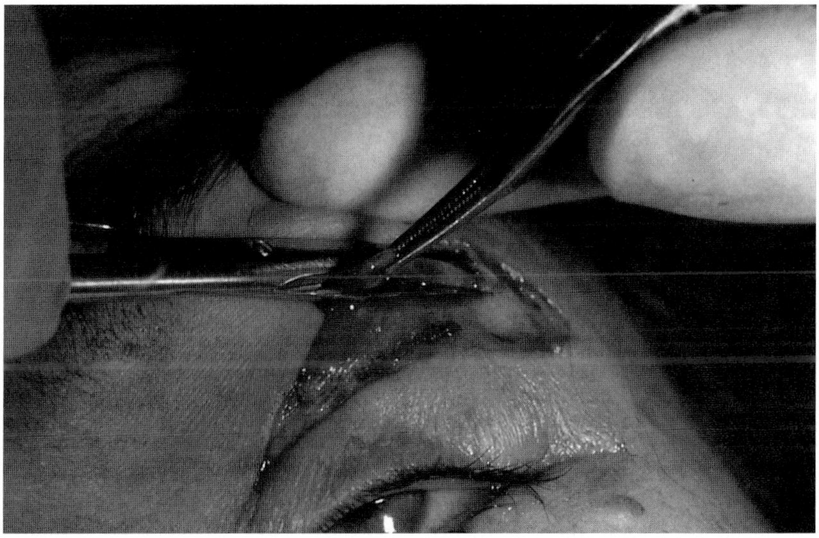

FIGURE 12 Incision of orbital septum exposing the underlying fat.

TABLE 4 Potential Complications Arising Intrasurgically and Postsurgically

Intrasurgically	Bleeding
	Corneal injury/globe penetration
	Anesthetic reaction
	Cardiovascular
	Central nervous system
	Respiratory
	Allergic
	Angle closure glaucoma from epinephrine
	Fire and explosion with oxygen supplementation
Postsurgically (early)	Hematoma
	Vision loss
	Pain
	Infection
	Diplopia
Postsurgically (late)	Diplopia
	Residual skin
	Residual fat
	Excessive fat removal
	Excessive skin removal
	Suture tracks/cysts/granulomas/milia
	Scars (hypertrophic/keloid)
	Diplopia
	Superior oblique injury
	Inferior oblique injury
	Inferior rectus injury
	Lid malposition (ectropion, entropion)
	Dry-eye syndrome (irritation, burning, tearing)
	Pigmentation (hematoma)
	Dehiscence

border of the tarsus, 7 to 8 mm wide, and considerably above the inferior border of the fornix. Often an arcade of vessels is apparent, which is just posterior to the incision. The incision begins centrally and extends medially, directed downward towards the caruncle and away from the lacrimal punctum. Laterally, it approaches the lateral canthus. The incision is made through the conjunctiva and the capsulopalpebral fascia of the lower-eyelid retractors (Fig. 15). The assistant then presses on the Jaeger plate to produce the maximum bulge of orbital fat. The yellow orbital fat will be seen protruding after spreading open the orbital septum with fine scissors (Fig. 16). After teasing the fat away from the lower-lid retractors, the Desmaires retractor and the Jaeger plate can be removed. This will allow the surgeon to visualize the eyelid as it will appear without the fat. To simulate the effects of gravity on the eyelid, the assistant may put gentle pressure on the globe in the upper-lid area.

The key landmarks are the arcuate expansion of the inferior oblique muscle, which separates the middle from the lateral fat compartment, and the inferior oblique muscle, which separates the middle and medial compartments. In order to prevent separation of the lower-lid retractors, and thus postsurgical retractor dysfunction, the

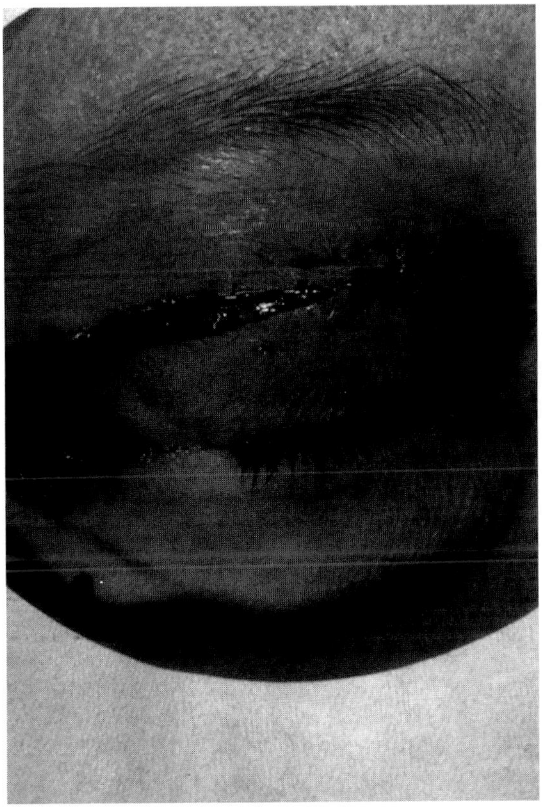

FIGURE 13 **Skin closure with 6-0 fast absorbing gut suture.**

arcuate expansion is left intact and a separate incision is made to isolate the lateral fat pad. After identification of all three fat pads, they are grasped with forceps and dissected with the aid of a cotton-tip applicator. The extruded fat is cauterized or lasered, excised, and coagulated (Fig. 17) [33,39]. The orbital tissues are then restored to their original anatomical positions and the conjunctiva is left unclosed. Some surgeons advocate closing the conjunctiva with one or two sutures for precise

TABLE 5 **Complications Specific to Upper-Eyelid Blepharoplasty**

Ptosis
Inadequate excision of fat and/or skin
High or low lid crease
Asymmetric lid creases
Medial tension lines
Lagophthalmos
Superior sulcus syndrome
Lacrimal gland injury
Diplopia

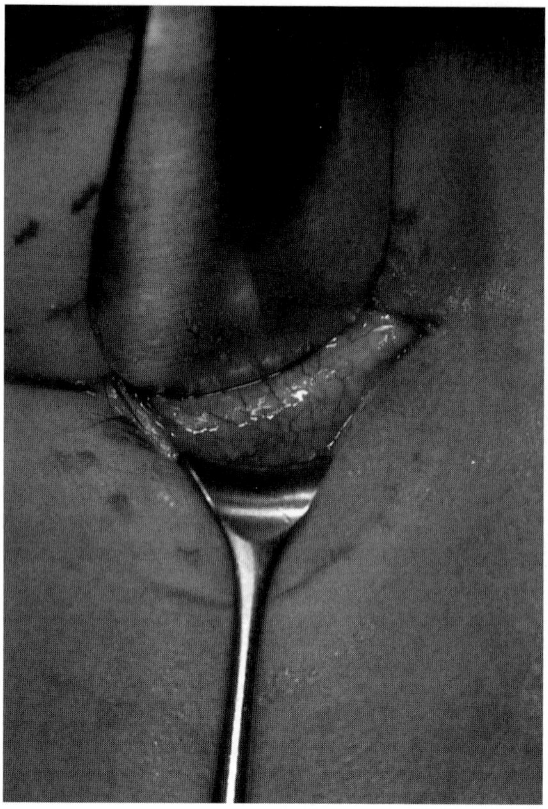

FIGURE 14 Retractors in place for conjunctival incision.

restoration of anatomical position [12,33]. However, suture material can irritate the conjunctiva and, possibly, lead to granuloma formation [35]. Potential intrasurgical complications and complications specific to transconjunctival lower-lid blepharoplasty are summarized in Tables 4 and 6.

Because fine rhytides will not be removed with transconjunctival blepharoplasty alone, laser resurfacing can be performed to eliminate these wrinkles after surgical closure [33,41].

Fat Repositioning in Lower Lid Blepharoplasty

Over the past decade, there has been a paradigm shift in the arena of lower lid blepharoplasty. For many years, the focus of lower lid blepharoplasty has been the removal of excess fat from the lower eyelids. However, it is widely accepted that the appearance of lower eyelid bags is related more to a downward displacement and herniation of fat than to an actual increase in the amount of fat present [42–44]. Furthermore, it is well accepted that excess removal of fat during lower lid blepharoplasty can actually contribute to the overall hollowing of the naso-jugal groove as the patient ages [45]. Because of this, in many instances, fat repositioning during lower lid blepharoplasty is actually preferred over fat excision. Though this approach leads to excellent cosmetic improvement, further studies need to be un-

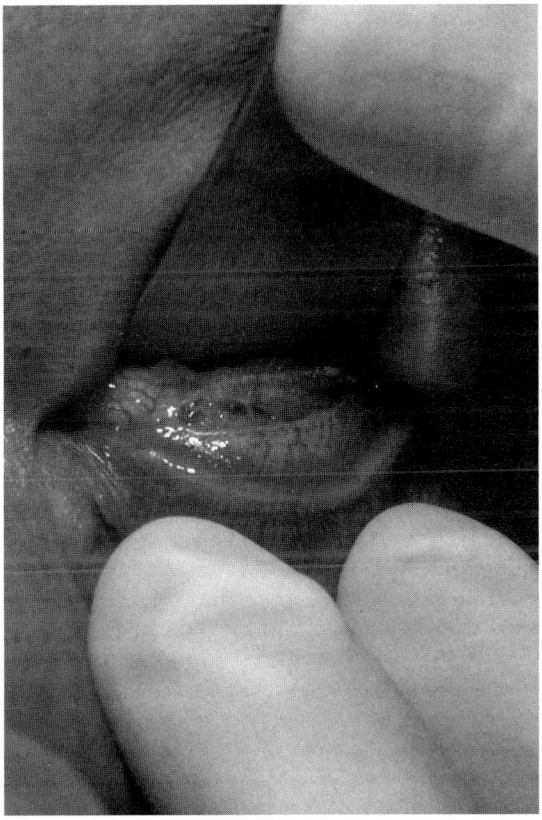

FIGURE 15 Conjunctival incision using electrosection.

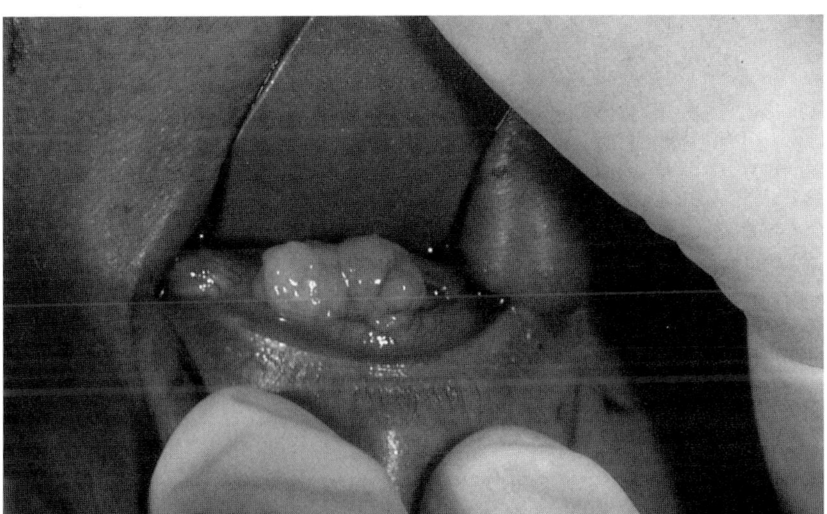

FIGURE 16 Orbital fat protruding through the orbital septum.

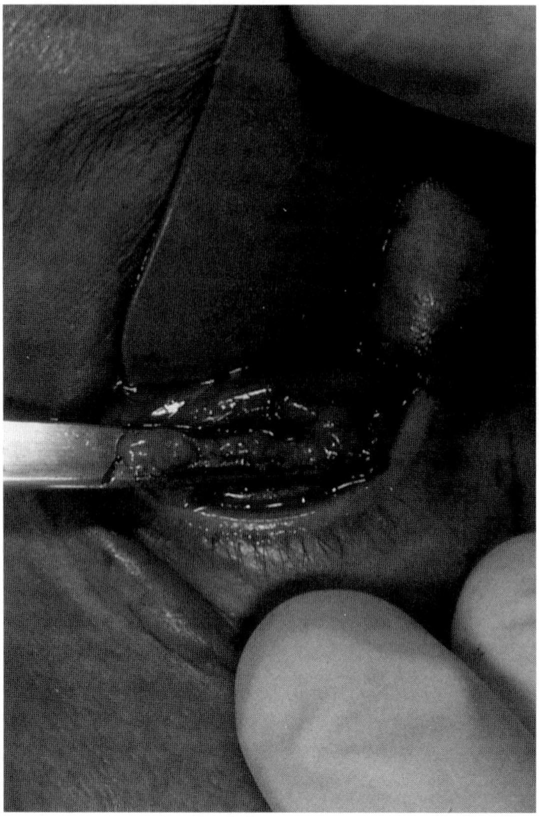

FIGURE 17 Orbital fat is clamped and excised using electrosection.

dertaken to assess the long-term value of this approach. It is not known whether augmentation of the soft tissue overlying the bony orbit will prevent the appearance of aging or if progressive thinning of the tissues overlying the repositioned fat will result in unsightly bulges in the lower lid region.

Either the transcutaneous or the transconjunctival approach may accomplish fat repositioning in lower lid blepharoplasty. Though the transconjunctival approach has the benefit of avoiding a cutaneous incision, the transcutaneous approach offers better exposure of the relevant anatomy [46]. For the transcutaneous approach, after excision of excess lower eyelid skin, a standard skin muscle flap is raised and dissected

TABLE 6 Complications Specific to Lower-Eyelid Blepharoplasty

Ectropion
Eyelid malposition
Lower-eyelid retraction with scleral show
Underexcision/overexcision of skin or adipose tissue
Injury to the inferior oblique muscle

1.5 cm inferior to the bony orbital rim exposing the suborbicularis oculi fat. At this point, the orbital system is incised from the medial to the lateral canthus exposing the intraorbital fat. To assist in mobilizing the intraorbital fat, the arcuate expansion may be divided. The intraorbital fat is then draped over the medial half of the bony orbital rim and sutured with the inferior aspect of the septum to the periosteum using 5-0 absorbable suture. The suborbicularis oculi fat is then carefully mobilized and sutured to the lateral half of the periosteum of the orbital rim. Alternatively, a subperiosteal pocket may be dissected, and the fat pedicles can be placed into the pocket and secured by sutures [47]. The skin muscle flap is then redraped, and the lateral aspect of the orbicularis muscle is sutured to the lateral orbital rim periosteum to support the lower lid.

A transconjunctival approach may be used for fat mobilization as well. Adequate surgical exposure is more challenging using this approach, but it carries the advantages of no cutaneous incisions. A standard transconjunctival incision is made, and dissection through the lower-lid retractors is carried out. Dissection is carried out in the preseptal plane to 1.5 cm inferiorly over the orbital rim just above the periosteum utilizing blunt dissection. At this point, an incision is placed through the orbital septum from the medial to the lateral canthus exposing the intraorbital fat. The fat is repositioned and sutured in the same fashion as the transcutaneous approach. The conjunctival incision may either be sutured with 6-0 fast absorbing gut sutures, or left to heal naturally.

Careful preoperative assessment is essential to determine whether any excess fat should be excised during the fat repositioning procedure. Furthermore, sitting the patient up intraoperatively to insure that the repositioned fat has an even contour can improve the final cosmetic results. Overall, fat repositioning has become a widely used modality in the management of lower eyelid contour deformities.

LASER BLEPHAROPLASTY

The use of laser technology in blepharoplasty was first described in 1984 when the conventional CO_2 laser was used in upper-lid blepharoplasty and transconjunctival lower-lid blepharoplasty [48,49]. David [50], a dermatologist, further described the surgical technique for transconjunctival lower-lid blepharoplasty using the CO_2 laser in 1987. The advantages in using the laser in upper and lower blepharoplasty may include better visualization of anatomy with greater precision in tissue removal, improved hemostasis, decreased surgery time, less postsurgical swelling and ecchymosis (depending on the investigator), and quicker recovery of the patient [26,41,51–63]. Disadvantages of laser blepharoplasty include: expensive cost of laser equipment, technical difficulty, eye and laser safety, and delayed wound healing [26,57,63].

CO_2 Laser

The CO_2 laser can be used for skin resurfacing along with upper and lower blepharoplasty. Ideal patients for concurrent skin resurfacing have fine static rhytides, perioral or periorbital wrinkles, full-face photoaging, or acne scars [56]. The CO_2 laser works by removing 50 to 150 μm of skin in a chain of rapid short pulses [56]. Because the duration of the high power wave is less than the thermal relaxation time of tissue, vaporization occurs with superficial penetration of skin and minimal thermal damage [58].

Controversy has surrounded the benefits of the CO_2 laser in blepharoplasty. Some investigators [53–55] reported slightly to moderately less bruising and swelling on the laser-treated side versus the scalpel-treated side, whereas other investigators [54] could not prove any benefits of laser surgery when compared with the scalpel-treated side. Apfelberg [56] reported average blood loss of 14.8 ml in upper-lid blepharoplasty and complete resolution of bruising and swelling in 10.1 days. No ectropion was observed in his patients and it was rare to observe any lid-position change. Weber [27] observed poor immediate hemostatic capabilities on larger vessels with the CO_2 laser compared with pinpoint electrocoagulation during lower-eyelid fat pad resection.

ND:YAG Laser and KTP Laser

The ND:YAG laser (1064 nm) uses energy, transmitted through fiber optics to scalpels with sharpened quartz tips or special sapphire tips, to simultaneously cut and coagulate small blood vessels to a depth of 6 mm [51,58]. Rapid pulse repetition is effective for surgical cutting and hemostasis of the skin, muscle, and fat. The ND:YAG laser differs from the CO_2 laser in that it readily penetrates through water and is absorbed by hemoglobin and other pigmented tissues. However, this laser causes a zone of thermal injury to surrounding tissue, reported experimentally to be approximately 50 to 200 μm in width; this zone can be resected before closure to decrease wound dehiscence and scar formation [51–53,58]. It has been reported that the zone of thermal damage to surrounding tissue is less with the CO_2 laser [51,58]. However, the YAG laser produces less bleeding and less laser plume than the CO_2 laser [51,58].

The KTP (potassium titanyl phosphate) is a double frequency ND:YAG laser that operates at 532 nm. This energy is also transmitted through fiber optics to scalpels equipped with sharpened quartz tips or special sapphire tips. The energy is able to penetrate tissue 2 to 3 mm in depth and is able to vaporize, cut, and coagulate simultaneously [58,63]. Because of its absorption by red pigment (ie, hemoglobin), this laser is less effective in cutting subcutaneous tissue [58].

Comparisons between the ND:YAG laser and conventional blepharoplasty have been described by several investigators [51–53,59]. The YAG laser did not alter procedural time, and postsurgical pain and discomfort, swelling, and ecchymosis were all decreased in patients treated with the laser. An average of 12.4 days was needed for bruising to completely disappear [51]. When one eye was treated with the YAG laser and the other eye with standard blepharoplasty, the laser-treated side showed disappearance of bruising and swelling 8 to 11 days earlier. Blood loss of less than 3 ml has been reported for all four lids [51,58]. Resumption of normal activities occurred within 7 to 10 days in laser-treated patients compared with 14 to 21 days in standard patients. Laser-treated patients did not require additional hemostasis with electrocautery [51]. However, because of the potential for deeper penetration of tissue, patients may experience more postsurgical swelling [58].

Comparisons between the KTP laser and conventional blepharoplasty have been described by Ginsbach [63]. There were less postsurgical symptoms with the laser and there were no major complications. However, better long-term results with the laser versus conventional techniques were not shown.

Laser Safety

Laser safety is imperative when using the laser in blepharoplasty. Before beginning the surgery, there are four important safety considerations: (1) eye protection, (2) safe laser utilization, (3) plume and smoke evacuation, and (4) the use of oxygen and its potential for fire.

The eye is a delicate structure and is very susceptible to severe damage (ie, corneal burn and ulceration with possible blindness) by laser radiation. Nonreflective metal eye shields covering the cornea and sclera should be used [58]. The use of plastic eye shield is not recommended because the laser energy may penetrate through the plastic [57]. Maximum protection during upper blepharoplasty is obtained with the use of the David-Baker clamp, a sandblasted stainless steel instrument, and during lower blepharoplasty, a Jaeger plate can be used to protect the globe [57]. Before placement of the corneal shields, ophthalmic tetracaine is instilled into each eye, followed by a non–water-absorbable ocular lubricant. The surgeon, when using the CO_2 laser, must wear clear protective eyewear; prescription eyewear and contact lenses are not adequate to protect the eyes. The clear glass windows in the surgery suite need not be covered. However, if the surgeon prefers the ND:YAG or KTP laser, the clear windows of the surgery suite need to be shielded and tinted glasses with protective filtering for the specific wavelength must be used [58]. Ocular damage is preventable in both the patient and the surgeon 100% of the time. In addition, the laser should be in standby position whenever it is not in use; this will prevent misdirected laser beams to the surgical staff [58]. Because plume and smoke generated by the laser have been shown to be potentially harmful, an assistant should hold a suction wand within 1 cm of the laser energy contact with skin [58]. External supplementation with oxygen should be limited to minimize the chance of fire during surgery. One case of intrasurgical fire during laser blepharoplasty has been reported in the literature [64].

Potential complications of laser blepharoplasty are summarized in Table 7.

POSTSURGICAL CARE

Postsurgical care is the same for upper- and lower-eyelid blepharoplasty. No dressings are required after surgery. A simplified postsurgical-care regimen to decrease the amount of manipulation of the wounds is preferred [30].

TABLE 7 Complications Specific to Laser Blepharoplasty

Complication
Perforation of the cornea or globe
Corneal injury (ulceration or burn)
Injury to the levator muscle
Retinal injury
Buttonholing of the skin
Inadequate removal of fat
Loss of lashes
Burn injury
Intrasurgical fire*

**Source*: Ref. 64.

Cold compresses are used as tolerated for the first 48 hours. These applications should be fairly constant for the first few postsurgical hours. After that, the compresses can be applied for 20 minutes, with 15 minute rest periods, until bedtime. Liberal use of eye ointments and drops are encouraged when the patient has a presurgical history of dry-eye symptoms or when dry-eye symptoms develop within the first 24 hours after surgery.

To minimize postsurgical edema, the patient is advised to sleep in a bed with the head elevated 45°. For the first 24 hours, the patient is advised to be in the care of another individual. Assessment of vision, proptosis, and pain should be made regularly. Blepharoplasty is a relatively painless procedure. If the patient complains of excessive pain, loss of vision, or proptosis, the patient must immediately call the surgeon and be taken to the emergency room. The skin sutures can be removed on postsurgical day 4. The incision at the lateral canthal border can then be reinforced with steri-strips for another 3 days.

MANAGEMENT OF COMPLICATIONS OF BLEPHAROPLASTY

Major Complications

Orbital Hemorrhage

The most serious complication of blepharoplasty is retrobulbar hemorrhage, which may result in blindness [9,65]. The incidence of blindness secondary to hemorrhage was estimated to be 0.04% [65]. The incidence is probably less recently because of improved techniques and education of physicians. A retrobulbar hemorrhage results from the dissection of bleeding vessels within the orbital fat into the muscles and the surrounding tissues, thus increasing intraorbital pressure. Increased intraorbital pressure may lead to tamponade of the bleeding artery, possible occlusion of the central retinal artery, and mechanical (or vascular) compromise of the optic nerve. The retina is very sensitive to diminished oxygen delivery and blood flow; 6 minutes of decreased blood flow can result in permanent retinal damage and possibly blindness [9].

Bleeding may occur 20, 60, or up to 150 minutes after the surgery [9]. A retrobulbar hemorrhage should be suspected if there is: (1) acute and severe onset of pain, (2) progressive swelling and ecchymosis of the eyelids, (3) proptosis, (4) raised intraocular pressure (normal less than 20 mmHg), (5) fundoscopic findings of pallor of the optic disk, and (6) rapid onset of blindness.

Immediate action is required once reduced vision is documented secondary to orbital hemorrhage. The incision site is reopened, clots are evacuated, and an attempt should be made to isolate the vessel and cauterize it. If visual acuity does not improve, a lateral canthotomy with or without lysis of the superior and inferior crus of the lateral canthal tendon is required. Decadron (0.3 mg/kg every 6 hours for 24 hours) can be given intravenously to lessen the degree of ischemia. If orbital pressure continues to be elevated, hyperosmotic agents, such as mannitol or acetazolamide, should be given. If blindness persists beyond 10 minutes, an anterior chamber paracentesis needs to be performed by an ophthalmologist. Because of the seriousness of this complication, an ophthalmologist should be consulted immediately once clinical suspicions are confirmed [8,9,65].

Globe Perforation

Globe perforation is a rare albeit serious complication that may occur during administration of local anesthesia or while using the laser [57,65]. The needle can unintentionally pass into the globe or the beam of the laser can inadvertently strike the globe without the awareness of the surgeon. Some patients complain of light flashes or visual changes immediately. However, these changes in vision may not be apparent until much later because of the protective eyeshields and the intravenous sedation. If globe penetration is suspected, an immediate dilated examination with indirect ophthalmoscopy must be performed to determine the point of entry and the appropriate treatment.

Hematoma

Hematoma is seen in approximately 3% of blepharoplasties [9]. As the hematoma resolves, the blood products will break down and hemosiderin will be deposited into the superficial layers of the tissue, leaving a bluish-green hue for 3 to 6 months [8]. The best treatment for this problem is prevention during surgery with meticulous hemostasis and delicate traction on the orbital fat pads. However, if a hematoma is present in the immediate postsurgical period, prompt evacuation is necessary, with mild pressure to the area, and cold compresses to prevent recurrence [8,9]. If a hematoma is present several days after the procedure, the coagulum should be allowed to liquefy and then be aspirated with an 18-gauge needle. In addition, the patient should be instructed to avoid aspirin-containing products or excessive vitamin E supplements 2 weeks before surgery, and excessive straining, bending, vomiting, or alcohol ingestion should be avoided for 48 hours after surgery.

Ectropion

Ectropion refers to drooping of the lower eyelid such that the conjunctiva is no longer in contact with the globe. This is often a result of excessive skin excision or over-aggressive laser resurfacing of the lower-eyelid skin [66].

Keratoconjuctivitis Sicca

Keratoconjuctivitis sicca, or the "dry-eye syndrome," is usually a consequence of aggressive skin removal from the upper or lower lid. More often than not, patients have an underlying or borderline dry-eye syndrome that is exacerbated by overly aggressive skin removal during blepharoplasty. However, it is common for patients who have undergone blepharoplasty to experience some drying and irritation several days to weeks after surgery. This is usually secondary to disturbance of the orbicularis muscle during surgery such that there is incomplete eyelid closure and blinking. These patients can be managed with aggressive topical lubricants until orbicularis muscle tone returns [65].

Ptosis

Ptosis usually occurs as a result of injury to the levator aponeurosis by direct incisional injury, stretching secondary to hematoma, or restriction secondary to inadvertent suturing to the skin incision. Postsurgical management of ptosis depends on the severity. Ptosis less than 2 mm requires strict monitoring of the patient; most cases resolve spontaneously in several days and are most likely, secondary to postsurgical edema. If ptosis persists for greater than 3 months, the patient will likely require surgical correction. Ptosis greater than 2 mm with poor to absent levator function should be treated immediately to prevent late fibrotic changes. This is usually a result of laceration of the levator aponeurosis.

Minor Complications

Edema

Edema in modest degrees is inevitable postsurgically and is not considered a complication unless it is marked. Edema may cause mild diplopia [8,9,65]; however, both will usually clear spontaneously. Edema can be lessened by the use of cold compresses postsurgically and by elevating the head of the bed for 2 weeks.

Incomplete Fat Removal

Incomplete removal of protruding orbital fat in the medial compartment of the upper lid may occur. Ullman et al. [16] further separates the medial fat compartment of the upper eyelid into superior and inferior portions: this was found after several patients returned after blepharoplasty with fullness on the medial side of their upper eyelids. The lateral compartment of the upper eyelid contains two fat pads in about 44% of patients [16].

Incomplete removal of protruding orbital fat in the lower lid often occurs as a consequence of poor technique. Unless the surgeon is specifically looking for the lateral fat pad in lower-lid blepharoplasty, it can easily be missed. This situation occurs because the lateral fat compartment is slightly superior to the middle and medial compartments. This complication is seen 2 to 3 months after lower-lid blepharoplasty as a slight bulge in the lateral aspect of the incision area. This may be mistaken as postsurgical edema; however, this "edema" does not resolve with time. This problem can be corrected by a stab incision through the skin and muscle followed by direct excision of the protuberant periorbital adipose tissue or by correction through the original incision site [9].

Excessive Fat Removal

Excessive removal of orbital adipose tissue leads to a concavity or a "sunken" eye appearance, a complication that can be avoided with adequate surgical planning. It is imperative to resect only fat that freely protrudes into the surgical field. Excessive pressure on orbital contents with excessive dissection of orbital fat can frequently result in this unaesthetic deformity [9].

Infection

Infections occurring after blepharoplasty are rare, although one case of necrotizing fasciitis has been reported [67]. The low incidence of infection can be attributed to the high vascularization of the eyelid skin and the "clean" surgical field of the eye. Antibiotic prophylaxis in clean surgical cases is not indicated because of the potential for the emergence of resistant strains and for the lack of proven efficacy. The overall incidence of infection in clean surgical cases has been estimated to be 2% [67]. In a survey of oculoplastic surgeons, 85% did not use antibiotic prophylaxis in blepharoplasty cases [68]. It has been advocated that there is no need for routine, prophylactic antibiotic use in blepharoplasty [67].

Milia

Milia occur frequently in the upper lid and less frequently in the lower lid after blepharoplasty. This is usually a result of the puncture wound created during suture closure and will resolve spontaneously in several days. If necessary, these areas can be opened up with a sharp needle and their contents expressed. Milia can be prevented by removal of the suture material by postsurgical day 4 [8,9].

Wound Dehiscence

Wound dehiscence may occur for several reasons; however, the most common reason is attributed to the patient who rubs the eyes inadvertently. This can be treated by reinforcing the area with wound closure tape or resuturing of the incision site. If handled appropriately, this should not result in a significant cosmetic deformity [9].

Allergy

Allergic reactions after blepharoplasty are usually a result of either the topical antibiotic ointment or the suture material used. These reactions are associated with the classic symptoms of allergic contact dermatitis: erythema, pruritus, and vesicle formation [8].

REFERENCES

1. Wolfort FG, Gee J, Pan D, Morris D. Nuances of Aesthetic Blepharoplasty. Ann Plast Surg 1997; 38:257–262.
2. Castanares S. Classification of baggy eyelids deformity. Plast Reconstr Surg 1977; 59: 629–637.
3. Gonzalez-Ulloa M. The senile eyelid. Arch Ophthalmol 1967; 78:365–369.
4. Flowers RS. Upper blepharoplasty by eyelid invagination. Clin Plast Surg 1993; 20: 193–199.
5. Flowers RS. Peri-orbital aesthetic surgery for men: eyelids and related structures. Clin Plast Surg 1991; 18:689–698.
6. Shorr N, Enzer YR. Considerations in aesthetic eyelid surgery. J Dermatol Surg Oncol 1992; 18:1081–1095.
7. Collins PS. Blepharoplasty. In: Robinson JK, Arndt KA, Leboit PE, Wintroub BU. Atlas of Cutaneous Surgery. Philadelphia: W.B. Saunders Company, 1996, pp. 301–314.
8. Alt TH. Blepharoplasty. Dermatol Clin 1995; 13(2):389–430.
9. Gross SC, Kanter WR. Pre-operative assessment for eyelid surgery. In: Wolfort FG, Kanter WR, eds. Aesthetic Blepharoplasty. Boston: Little, Brown, and Co. 1995, pp. 53–77.
10. Dailey RA, Wobig JI. Eyelid anatomy. J Dermatol Surg Oncol 1992; 18:1023–1027.
11. Siegel RJ. Essential anatomy for contemporary upper lid blepharoplasty. Clin Plast Surg 1993; 20(2);209–212.
12. Lask GP, Moy RL. Principles and Techniques of Cutaneous Surgery. McGraw Hill, 1996.
13. Fernandez LR. The east asian eyelid open technique. Clin Plast Surg 1993; 20(2):247–253.
14. Bosniak SL. Cosmetic Blepharoplasty. New York: Raven Press, 1990, pp. 25–35.
15. Liv D. Asian Blepharoplasty. In: Bosniak S, ed. Principles and Practice of Ophthalmic Plastic and Reconstructive Surgery, pp. 702–714. Volumes 1 and 2. Philadelphia: W.B. Saunders Company, 1996.

16. Ullman Y, Levi Y, Ben-Izhak O, Har-shai Y, Peled IJ. The surgical anatomy of the fat in the upper eyelid medial compartment. Plast Reconstr Surg 1997; 99:658–661.
17. Jelks GW, Jelks EB. The influence of orbital and eyelid anatomy of palpebral aperture. Clin Plast Surg 1991; 18:183–188.
18. Farkas LG, Kolar JC. Anthropometric guidelines in cranioorbital surgery. Clin Plast Surg 1987; 14:1–12.
19. Bartlett SP, Wornom I, Whitaker LA. Evaluation of facial skeletal aesthetics and surgical planning. Clin Plast Surg 1991; 18:1–11.
20. Tolleth H. Concepts for the plastic surgeon from art and sculpture. Clin Plast Surg 1987; 14:585.
21. Zide BM, Jelks GW. Surgical Anatomy of the Orbit. New York: Raven Press, 1985:21–32; 51–58.
22. Rathbun JE. Eyelid Surg. Boston: Little, Brown, and Company, 1990, pp. 173–199.
23. Putterman AM, ed. Cosmetic Oculoplastic Surgery. 3rd ed. Philadelphia: W.B. Saunders, 1999, pp. 11–22.
24. Moses JL, Tanenbaum M. Blepharoplasty: Cosmetic and functonal. McCord CD Jr, ed., Tanenbaum M. Oculoplastic Surgery. 3rd ed. New York: Raven Press, 1995. pp. 285–318.
25. Rathbun JE. Blepharoplasty and Brow Elevation. In: Waltman SR, Keates RH, eds. Surgery of the eye. New York: Churchill Livingstone Inc. 1987. pp. 483–506.
26. Kikawa DO, Lemke BN. Orbital and eyelid anatomy. In: Dortzbach RK. Ophthalmic Plastic Surgery. Prevention and Management of Complications. New York: Raven Press, 1994, pp. 1–30.
27. Weber PJ. Nuances in ophthalmic plastic surgery. A dermatologic surgeon's perspective. J Dermatol Surg Oncol 1992; 18:1117–1121.
28. Jelks GW, Jelks EB. Preoperative evaluation of the blepharoplasty patient. Bypassing the pitfalls. Clin Plast Surg 1993; 20(2):213–223.
29. Flowers RS, Flowers SS. Diagnosing photographic distortion. Decoding true postoperative contour after eyelid surgery. Clin Plast Surg 1993; 20(2):387–392.
30. Tebbetts JB. Blepharoplasty. A refined technique emphasizing accuracy and control. Clin Plast Surg 1992; 19(2):329–349.
31. Perman KI. Upper eyelid blepharoplasty. J Dermatol Surg Oncol 1992; 18:1096–1099.
32. Flowers RS, Flowers SS. Precision planning in blepharoplasty. The importance of preoperative mapping. Clin Plast Surg 1993; 20(2):303–310.
33. Dodenhoff TG. Transconjunctival blepharoplasty: further applications and adjuncts. Aesth Plast Surg 1995; 19:511–517.
34. Liu D, Hsu WM. Oriental eyelids: anatomic difference and surgical consideration. Ophthalmic Plast Reconstr Surg 1986; 2:59–64.
35. Zarem HA, Resnick JI. Minimizing deformity in lower blepharoplasty. Clin Plast Surg 1993; 20(2):317–321.
36. Baylis HI, Long JA, Groth MJ. Transconjunctival lower eyelid blepharoplasty: technique and complications. Ophthalmology 1990; 96:1027.
37. McGaw BL, Adamson PA. Postblepharoplasty ectropion: prevention and management. Arch Otolaryngol Head Neck Surg 1991; 117:852.
38. Netscher DT, Patrinely JR, Peltier M, Polsen C, Thronby J. Transconjunctival versus transcutaneous lower eyelid blepharoplasty: a prospective study. Plast Reconstr Surg 1995; 96:1053–1060.
39. Asken S. The preseptal and the retroseptal approaches in transconjunctival blepharoplasty. J Dermatol Surg Oncol 1992; 18:1110–1116.
40. Zarem HA, Resnick JI. Minimizing deformity in lower blepharoplasty: the transconjunctival approach. Plast Reconstr Surg 1991; 88:215.

41. Rosenberg GJ, Gregory RO. Lasers in aesthetic surgery. Clin Plast Surg 1996; 23(1): 29–48.
42. Hamra ST. The role of orbital fat preservation in facial aesthetic surgery: a new concept. Clin Plast Surg 1996; 23(1):17–28.
43. Eder H. Importance of fat conservation in lower blepharoplasty. Aesth Plast Surg 1997; 21:168–174.
44. de la Plaza R, Arroyo JM. A new technique for the treatment of palpebral bags. Plast Reconstr Surg 1988; 81(5):677–687.
45. Loeb R. Naso-jugal groove leveling with fat tissue. Clin Plast Surg 1993; 20(2):393–401.
46. Baker SR. Orbital fat preservation in lower-lid blepharoplasty. Arch Facial Plast Surg 1999; 1:33–39.
47. Goldberg RA. Transconjunctival orbital fat repositioning: transposition of orbital fat pedicles into a subperiosteal procket. Plast Reconstr Surg 2000; 105:743–748.
48. Baker SS. Carbon dioxide laser upper lid blepharoplasty. Am J Cosmet Surg 1992; 9: 141.
49. Baker SS, Muenzler WS, Small RG, Leonard JE. Carbon dioxide laser blepharoplasty. Ophthalmology 1984; 91:238–243.
50. David LM, Sanders G. Carbon dioxide laser blepharoplasty: a comparison to cold steel and electrocautery. J Dermatol Surg Oncol 1987; 13:110–114.
51. Apfelberg DB. YAG laser meloplasty and blepharoplasty. Aesth Plast Surg 1995; 19: 231–235.
52. Keller G. KTP frequency doubled YAG laser forehead and facelift. Am J Cosmet Surg 1992; 9:177–180.
53. Beeson WM, Kabaker S, Keller GS. Carbon dioxide laser blepharoplasty: a comparison to electrocautery. Int J Aesth Restor Surg 1994; 2:33–36.
54. Mittelman MD, Apfelberg DB. Carbon dioxide laser blepharoplasty: advantages and disadvantages. Ann Plast Surg 1990; 24:1–6.
55. Morrow DM, Morrow LB. CO_2 laser blepharoplasty. J Dermatol Surg Oncol 1992; 18: 307–313.
56. Apfelberg DB. The ultrapulse carbon dioxide laser with computer pattern generator automatic scanner for facial cosmetic surgery and resurfacing. Ann Plast Surg 1996; 36: 522–529.
57. Biesman BS. Precautions in the use of the laser for blepharoplasty (letter). Plast Reconstr Surg 1997; 99(1):275–277.
58. Bosniak SL, Zilkha MC. Cosmetic blepharoplasty and facial rejuvenation. 2nd edition. Philadelphia: Lippincott-Raven. 1999, pp. 117–126.
59. Putterman AM. Scalpel Nd:YAG laser in oculoplasty surgery. Am J Ophthal 1990; 109: 581–584.
60. David LM. The laser approach to blepharoplasty. J Dermatol Surg Oncol 1988; 1:741–746.
61. Trelles MA, Sanchez J, Sala P, Elspas S. Surgical removal of lower eyelid fat using the carbon dioxide laser. Am J Cosmet Surg 1992; 9:149–152.
62. Spadoni D, Cain CL. Laser blepharoplasty. AORN J 1988; 47:1184–1193.
63. Ginsbach G. Periorbital aesthetic surgery with the KTP laser. Aesth Plast Surg 1995; 19:505–509.
64. Greco RJ, Gonzalez R, Johnson P, Scolieri M, Rekhopf PG, Hecfkler F. Potential dangers of oxygen supplementation during facial surgery. Plast Reconstr Surg 1995; 95:978–984.
65. Popp JC. Complications of blepharoplasty and their management. J Dermatol Surg Oncol 1992; 18:1122–1126.

66. Wule AE. Oculoplastic surgery. An overview. J Dermatol Surg Oncol 1992; 18:1033–1038.
67. Ray AM, Bressler K, Davis RE, Gallo JF, Patete ML. Cervicofacial necrotizing fasciitis. A devastating complication of blepharoplasty. Arch Otalaryngol Head Neck Surg 1997; 123:633–636.
68. Hurley LD, Westfall CT, Shore JW. Prophylactic use of antibiotics in oculoplastic surgery. Int Ophthalmol Clin 1992; 32:165–178.

31

Cosmetic Upper and Lower Eyelid Blepharoplasty: The Ophthalmologist's Perspective

Jean Carruthers and Alastair Carruthers
University of British Columbia, Vancouver, British Columbia, Canada

INTRODUCTION

The teamwork of the surgical ophthalmologist and surgical dermatologist has never been more essential than it is now in the rapidly expanding field of interventional aesthetic facial enhancement. Each discipline approaches the anatomy, physiology, pathology, and treatment of the periocular region from somewhat different points of reference in their residency and fellowship programs and so can teach and help each other. Commonly today, both groups not only treat periocular neoplasia, but also use lasers for treatment of rhytides, pigmented and vascular lesions, and perform surgical browlifts and blepharoplasty. Both groups are very aware of the need for excellent technique so that individuals seeking aesthetic enhancement can achieve their goals without the development of avoidable complications such as blindness, symptomatic keratoconjunctivitis sicca, "round-eye," and frank upper and lower eyelid malposition.

This partnership is also evident in the tools available to each group. Although two dermatologists, R. Fitzpatrick and M. Goldman [1], first described the use of the CO_2 laser for facial resurfacing, an ophthalmologist, Sterling Baker [2], first described the use of the continuous wave laser beam for aesthetic blepharoplasty. Today we use both laser modalities simultaneously to achieve the most polished and refined result for our patients.

THE PRESURGICAL EVALUATION

The pretreatment eye examination is important to define the baseline structure and function of the eyes and their adnexae. Best corrected visual acuity, evaluation of tear film adequacy (ie, the presence of pre-existing keratoconjunctivitis sicca), eyelid excursions (including eyelid closure with the mouth wide open), Bell's phenomenon, levator function, and assessment of horizontal lower eyelid laxity should all be examined and recorded in the chart.

We must also be aware of common coexisting problems such as asymmetric brow height to frank brow ptosis, eyelid ptosis including Horner's Syndrome, lacrimal gland ptosis, frank lower eyelid malposition such as ectropion and entropion, proptosis, upper eyelid retraction, and vertical strabismus.

History of Any Previous Periocular Treatments?

1. BOTOX? Collagen? Hylaform?
2. Ptosis repair?
3. Resurfacing with laser or chemical peel?
4. Blepharoplasty?
5. Artificial tears or punctal occlusion?
6. Orbital decompression (thyroid, tumor)
7. Browlift? Which approach?
8. Glaucoma filtering surgery? NB Stainless steel contact lenses?
9. Contact lenses, PRK, or LASIK? NB Beware the flap when inserting the stainless steel contacts, Baker clamp, Desmarres retractor, or Jaeger plate.

Wy Cosmetic Surgery Now?

1. Personal/social reason for desiring personal facial enhancement at this time? Are expectations realistic? For example, blepharoplasty alone will likely not save your marriage, achieve your promotion, etc.
2. Any previous aesthetic procedures? Perceived results? Satisfaction?
3. Relationship with previous surgeon(s)?
4. Complications?
5. Lawsuits?

Discussion of Personal Desires and Preferences for Surgical Goals

1. Brow height, both medial and lateral (endoscopic browlift, lateral browlift only, including transblepharoplasty brow pexy)
2. Height of superior palpebral furrow (for platform)
3. Angulation of upper lid lashes (supratarsal fixation)
4. Position of medial and lateral extents of upper and infralash incisions
5. Extent of desired fat removal, including superolateral sculpting of Retro Orbicularis Oculi Fat (ROOF), which is the fat immediately behind the orbicularis and anterior to the septum in the upper lid [3].
6. Ancillary safety procedures including Webster suture, Tarsal strip procedure, and Sub Orbicularis Oculi Fat (SOOF) lift. The SOOF is contiguous with the midface malar fat pads [3].

A documented presurgical discussion of the patient's microexpectations as relate to your incision placement is an explanation. A postsurgical discussion of these same topics will be perceived as an excuse and the patient may possibly be unhappy with a result you are proud of.

Presurgical Physical Examination

1. Visual acuity with glasses, contact lenses, or pinhole. This should be recorded separately for each eye and recorded in universal Snellen notation, eg, 20/50, 20/20, etc. for each eye, stating whether recorded at distance or near fixation, with or without optical correction.
2. Periocular anatomy

Document on a line drawing (Fig. 1) the following measurements, as in points 1, 2, 3, 5, and 10:

1. Brow height as relates to the superior bony orbital margin [3]. Eighty percent of middle-aged women have asymmetric brow height—usually no more than 1–2 mm. BOTOX presurgically into the brow depressors on the side of the lower brow allows the surgeon to remove the correct amount of eyelid skin at the time of surgery rather than making the error of removing too much, effectively pulling the lower brow even lower and creating a permanent asymmetric, intense expression [4].
2. Vertical height of palpebral aperture with eyes in primary (ie, straight-ahead) position.
3. Natural and desired height of superior palpebral furrow.
4. R & L Levator excursion with brow immobilized (N = 15 mm)
5. Margin-reflex distance (N = 3–4 mm)
6. Tear film breakup time (N = 10–15 seconds)
7. Schirmer Test (N = 2–3 mm in 30 seconds) [5]
8. Strabismus—an eccentrically positioned globe will alter the eyelid position. Repair before assessment for blepharoplasty.
9. Pre-existing proptosis (Fig. 2) Measure with the Hertel exophthalmometer. Dysthyroid ophthalmopathy is common and should be evaluated by an ophthalmologist before any cosmetic lid surgery is entertained as the patient may need all possible lid skin to protect the globe and can lose vision if the globe is exposed.

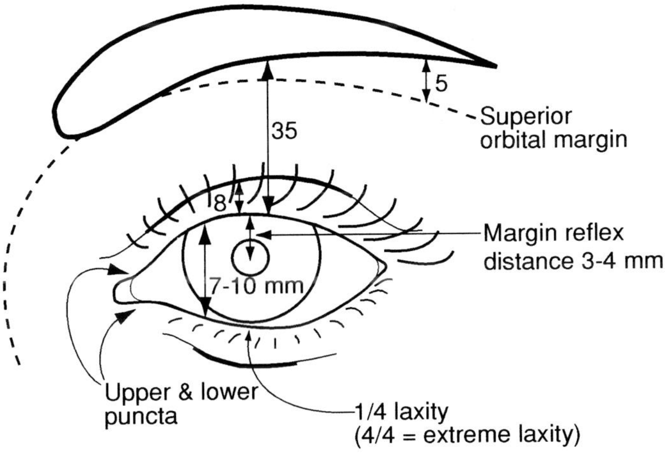

FIGURE 1 Line drawing to summarize important presurgical measurements.

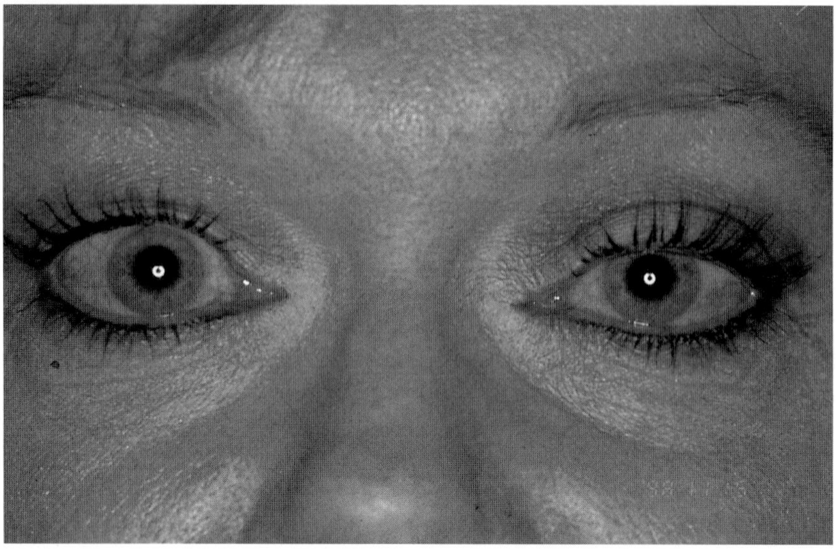

FIGURE 2 Dysthyroid ophthalmopathy. Patient presented wanting surgery on the right upper lid to match it to the left. MRI scan showed enlarged extraocular muscles bilaterally, despite asymmetry of anterior clinical presentation.

10. Lower lid elasticity—snap or pinch test (Fig. 3). The lower lid should briskly flex back to its normal position, and if not, you are warned that a traditional infralash blepharoplasty will give a good chance of post-surgically lower lid malposition.
11. Will the lids close when the mouth is wide open (Fig. 4)? If not, reconsider your surgical approach, particularly if there is coexisting dry eye

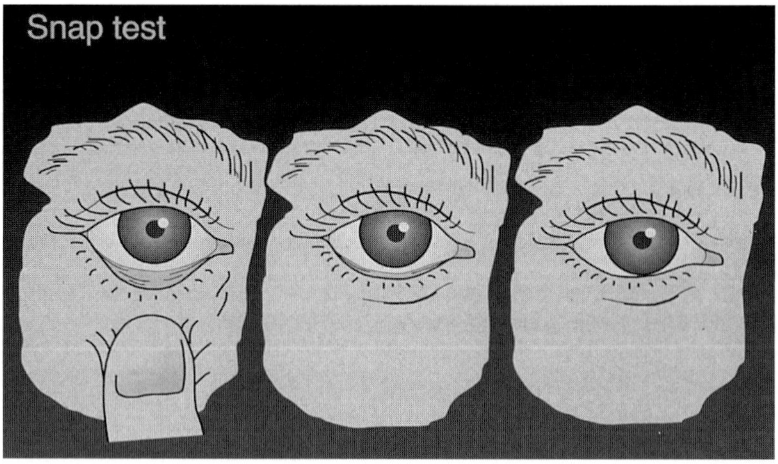

FIGURE 3 Clinical evaluation of lower eyelid laxity—snap test should be performed on every patient. Any loss of elasticity makes the lower lid "float" back to the globe rather than with the normal sharp "snap."

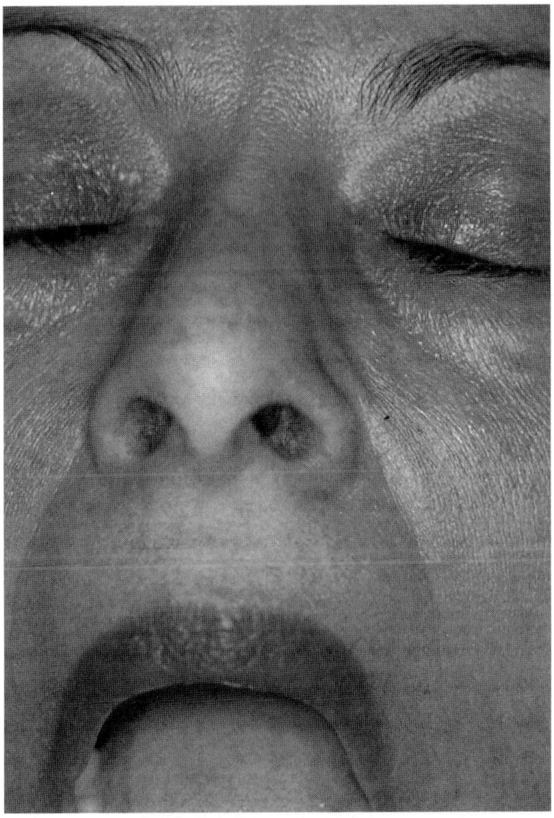

FIGURE 4 Eyelid closure with the mouth open. Some individuals have incomplete lid closure even presurgically, so great caution is needed in further shortening of the anterior lamella.

and poor Bell's phenomenon so the cornea will dessicate postsurgically, causing constant ocular discomfort, blurred vision, and potential corneal ulceration.

Presurgical Photography

Surgery should not commence until the pretreatment photographs are on the chart. Polaroid and 35 mm slides or 4 × 6 color prints are excellent, particularly when taken in a standard format:

1. Full face, eyes straight ahead, in upgaze and with eyes closed and mouth open. Magnification 1:10, F4.
2. Closeup macro with eyes in primary position, and also right and left semiprofile. Magnification 1:3, F8 (Fig. 5)
3. Closeup macro with lids marked and eyes closed to show a/symmetry (Fig. 6).

I use a Lester Dine 35 mm macro camera with electronic ring flash for the 35 mm photos and Lester Dine Professional quality polaroid for the backup photos. We show

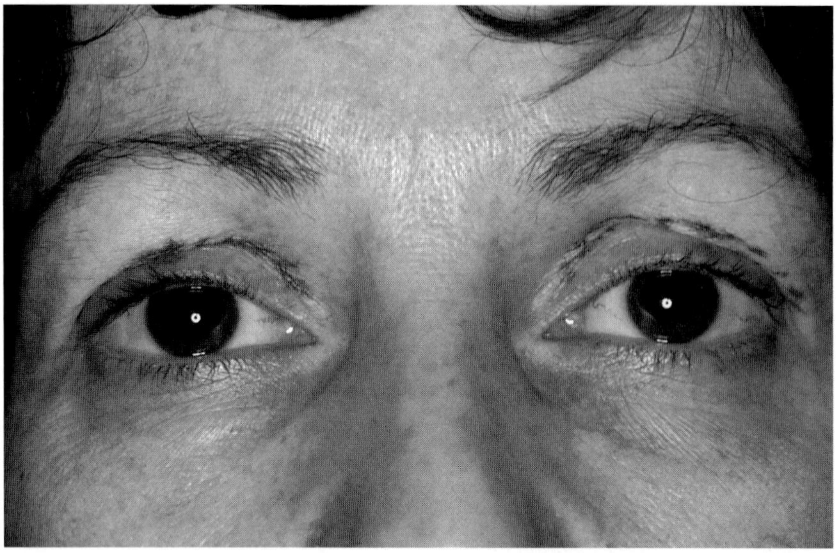

(a)

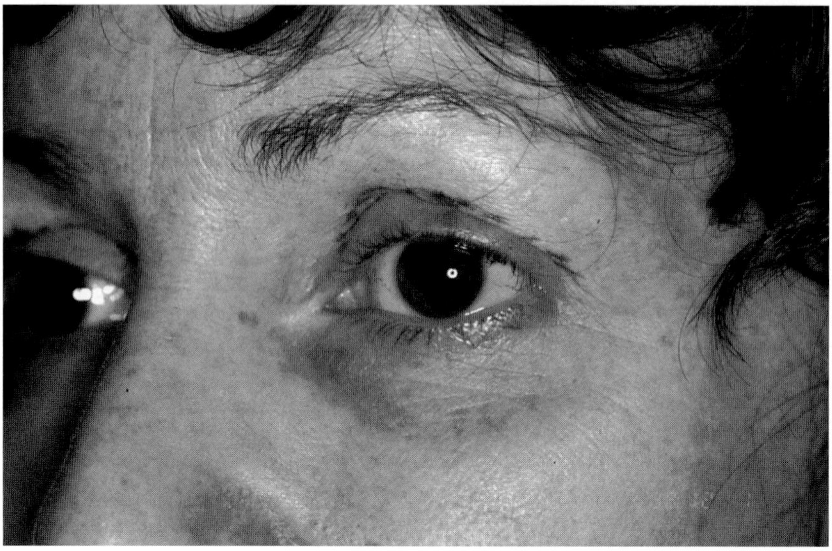

(b)

FIGURE 5 (a, b) Closeup of the eyes in primary position and one semiprofile. Camera set on 1:3 magnification.

all the photos to the patient before surgery because it is the norm for individuals to notice pre-existing asymmetry and details of their periocular anatomy they had never noted before at this time, thus preventing them noting these features after surgery and feeling that the surgery created these "problems." We also explain that asymmetry is normal because of each side of the face developing from a separate embryologic growth process.

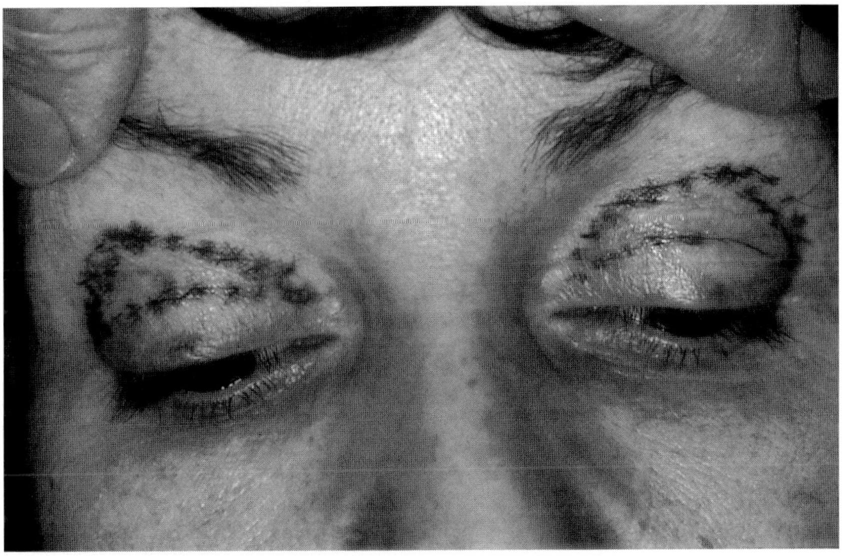

FIGURE 6 Closeup of the lids closed after marking shows relative symmetry.

Instructions

The best surgical technique is no match for the constant oozing of the aspirin-non-steroidal-Vitamin E anticoagulated patient. Some foods also contain salicilates, for example, tomatoes, red pepper, garlic, and onion.

We give the patients a list of foods to avoid starting 2 weeks before sur-

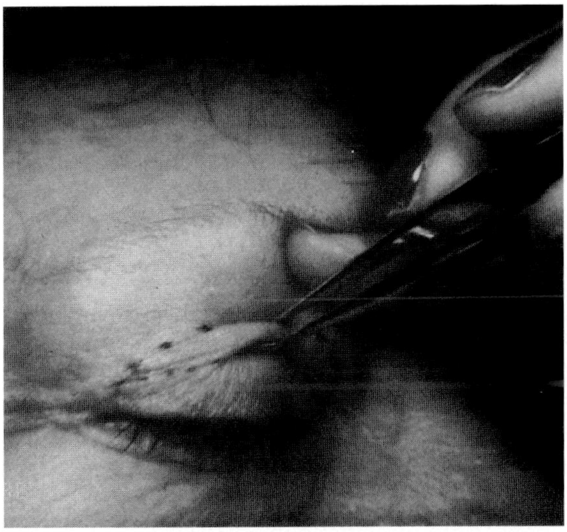

FIGURE 7 Greene forceps are used to evaluate amount of upper or lower eyelid skin that can safely be removed.

gery. They are also informed that their surgery will be cancelled for their own safety if they have inadvertently taken these medications or foods in that time interval. Platelet function must be normal. Individuals on coumadin group anticoagulants bleed normally and surgery can be performed without stopping their medication.

On the day of surgery, we ask individuals to take their oral medications, especially antihypertensives, as usual. We ask them to have water or ginger ale only, and no solid foods. We also like them to arrive 1 to 1½ hours early to avoid delays in traffic. They wear a comfortable track suit and flat shoes, no make-up, jewelry, or perfume (alcohol may be a fire hazard with laser). They bring their own ice packs for the drive home afterwards.

We go over the postsurgical instructions, the consent, and the contact persons and phone numbers one more time and resign the consent. Any photographic views not already in the chart are taken with our polaroid camera.

Consent

Individuals desiring aesthetic enhancement of their lids must thoroughly understand the possible benefits as well as risks of this as with any other surgery. Our consent is appended (see Appendix 1). In addition, the mechanisms causing postsurgical blindness must be discussed presurgically so that the patient properly respects the need for dietary discretion as previously discussed and also the postsurgical care regimen including the need to remain in contact with the surgeon for several days postsurgically. If a patient says they have an engagement requiring travel in the 3 days after surgery, we reschedule their surgery time.

An acute orbital hemorrhage will occlude the flow in the central retinal artery and requires immediate drainage, evacuation of clot, and detailed observation in the following days. The most common time for them to present is intrasurgically, but I have had individuals call at 6 a.m. the next day complaining of reduced vision with bruising and pain, and had them back on the surgery table within the hour. Any cosmetic blepharoplasty surgeon must be familiar with the correct emergency procedures to treat this rare but justifiably feared complication and the properly prepared patient is an enormous help in early diagnosis.

Anesthesia

In the several presurgical visits, we discuss the individual's previous surgical experiences as well as their own perceived anxiety level about the surgery. If the individual is calm and stoical, in good health, with no history of chronic use of central nervous system depressants such as Valium or alcohol and having only a two-lid blepharoplasty, we will use local anesthesia only.

Most individuals desiring a four-lid repair and especially those who require resurfacing are more comfortable with intravenous sedation in addition to local anesthesia. The intravenous route gives superior control and flexibility over depth of analgesia and sedation. We usually use a combination of Propofol, Versed, and a short-acting narcotic such as Sufentanyl. Intramuscular demerol, Versed, and promethazine are other alternatives, but some patients will become relatively apnoeic so they require verbal encouragement throughout the procedure to breathe deeply.

Narcotic and minor tranquilizer antagonists are sometimes helpful to restore normal breathing patterns.

Local anesthesia with Lidocaine 2% with 1/100,000 adrenaline, approximately 1.5 to 2 ml per lid, is injected 20 minutes before the surgical procedure starts. I don't use Wydase because the analgesia wears off too fast. Waiting allows beautiful hemostasis in the surgical field. Using a 30-gauge needle, I inject a bleb of local at the outer superior palpebral furrow of the upper lid and massage it along the furrow medially. I find a good time to inject the medial and central fat pads is after the myocutaneous flap is elevated and this can be performed easily under direct visualization.

In the lower lid I inject similarly in the subcutaneous plane, then place Proparacaine 0.5% eyedrops in the conjunctival sac, evert the lower lid and inject a further 0.5 ml Lidocaine/epinephrine into each of the three fat pads. We always have another syringe of local on the sterile tray in case more is needed intrasurgically.

THE SURGERY

How-to Techniques

Upper Eyelid Blepharoplasty

After detailed discussion with the patient, the fat pads and area of lid skin to be excised are marked with a sterile surgical marking pen. It is important to have the patient in the seated position with the eyes directed in forward gaze. Greene or other forceps are used to check the safe amount of upper lid skin to be removed (see Fig. 7), so that when the skin fold is gently pinched in the forceps, the lids will close with only the tiniest gap of lagophthalmos.

The medial and lateral extent of the blepharoplasty incision are marked after discussion (Fig. 6). The medial extent should not be more medial than the upper punctum; the lateral should not extend more than 2 to 3 mm beyond the lateral bony orbital margin and should be 4 mm above the lateral canthal angle with the eyes in primary position. The vertical extent of the excision is often 10 mm centrally, but the surgeon should measure the amount of skin between the lowest eyebrow cilium and the superior ciliary margin and ensure that at least 23 to 25 mm of skin are present, or difficulty with postsurgical eyelid closure in most individuals can be anticipated.

The orbital septum is opened with the laser, gentle pressure is placed on the globe, and the medial and central fat pads will prolapse into the wound (Fig. 8). The excessive fat can be lasered away in a piecemeal fashion against the sand-blasted Jaeger plate. In most women, the medial fat pad is more prominent than the central in the upper eyelid.

If thinning of ROOF fat is needed, the Desmarres retractor is used to gently elevate the superolateral orbicularis so that the fat can be gently sculpted (Fig. 9). Some individuals have such prominent superolateral bony orbital margins that the bone can also be burred flatter to soften the semiprofile perspective.

If corrugator excision is preferred to BOTOX injections, this too can be accomplished through the blepharoplasty incision [6], as can a temporal browlift to the frontal periosteum [7].

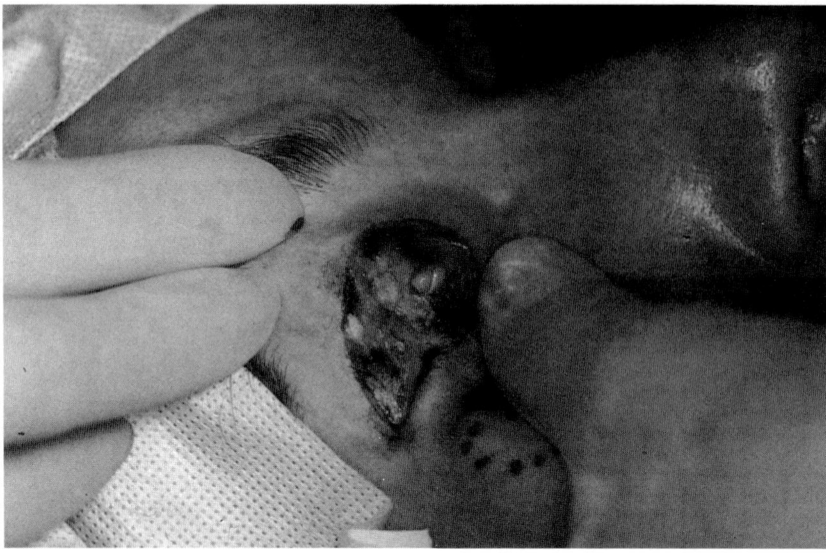

FIGURE 8 Mild pressure safely prolapses the fat forward into the surgical field.

Lower Eyelid Blepharoplasty

Traditional Infralash Blepharoplasty

Infralash blepharoplasty was the standard technique before the advent of the CO_2 laser made fat sculpting from the transconjunctival approach (often combined with simultaneous skin resurfacing) an increasingly popular approach.

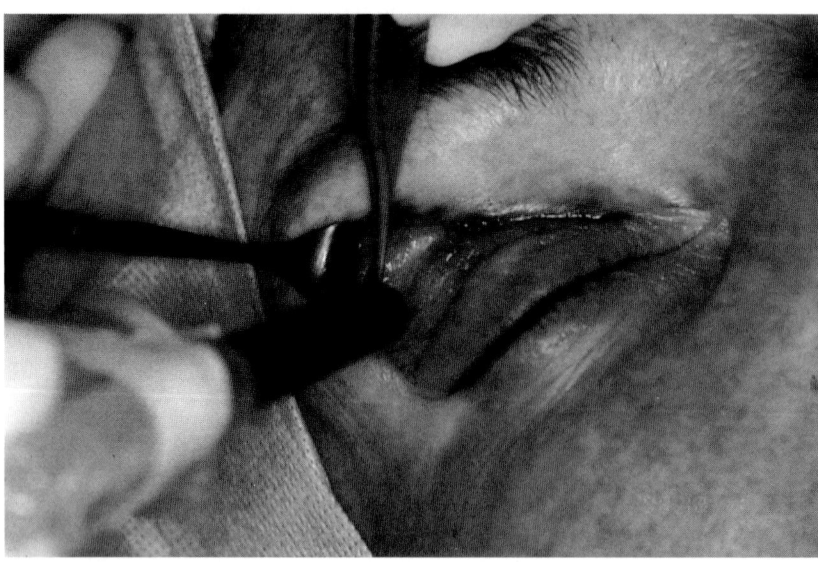

FIGURE 9 Gentle laser sculpting of the ROOF fat exposed by the traction with the Desmarres retractor.

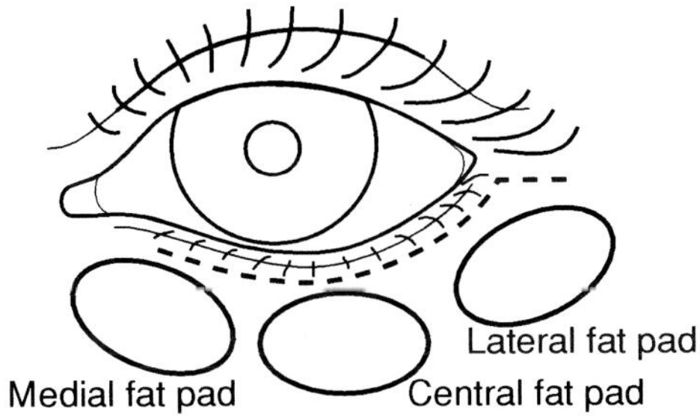

FIGURE 10 Anatomy of the infralash blepharoplasty incision.

Marking the Incision. The incision is marked approximately 1.5 to 2 mm below the ciliary margin starting 1 to 2 mm lateral to the lower punctum and extending to the lateral canthus (Fig. 10). I prefer not to extend the incision line over the lateral orbital margin because it is perennially visible afterwards, but in many individuals a horizontal extension along the lateral canthal tendon allows for redraping in individuals with greater amounts of excess skin.

Local Anesthesia and Globe Protection. Topical proparacaine 0.5% eyedrops are instilled into the conjunctival sac. Paired stainless steel contact lenses are inserted into the conjunctival sacs protecting the globes from laser and operating light (Fig. 11). Lidocaine 2% with 1/100,000 epinephrine is injected subcutaneously along the marked incision line in the immediate subcutaneous plane. The lower lid is gently everted and 0.5 ml of local anesthetic are injected into each of the three lower eyelid fat pads.

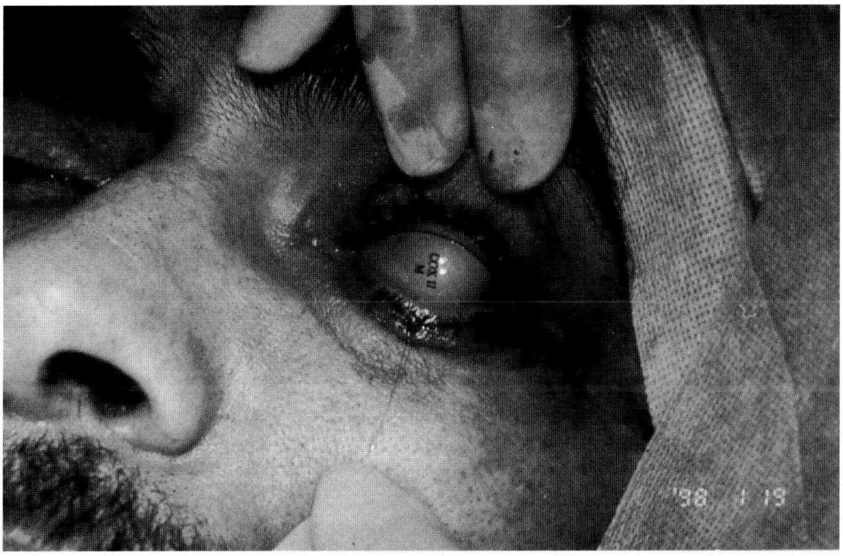

FIGURE 11 Stainless steel high domed sandblasted contact lens inserted into the conjunctival sac.

Incision and Dissection. The CO_2 laser beam is set at 7 W power on continuous wave beam and the incision line is opened. The skin is dissected from the orbicularis muscle with the Westcott scissors until a plane of dissection is established. A 6/0 silk traction suture is placed through the tarsus at mid position on the lid, and the assistant gently provides elevation of the posterior flap. The subcutaneous dissection is usually carried down to the level of the orbital margin and if the dermatochalasis is more marked the dissection can be carried 10 mm below the bony lower orbital margin.

To remove orbital fat, the orbicularis muscle is incised parallel to the orbital margin across the entire horizontal extent of the lower lid by beginning centrally with a gentle tenting of the orbicularis muscle away from the underlying orbital septum. The orbital septum is identified and incised. Gentle pressure on the globe above presents the fat pads. I usually take the lateral fat pad first and work across the central and then to the medial fat pad.

Large veins are often seen in the fat pads, particularly in the medial. Caution with traction is important to avoid tearing vessels posteriorly in the orbit, producing an orbital hemorrhage. The CO_2 laser beam is used to gently abscise the fat in a piecemeal fashion against the sand-blasted Jaeger plate. For larger diameter vessels cautery with the Bovie may be needed pre-emptively before the laser is used.

Webster Suture. Before skin closure, I place a nonabsorbable 4:0 mersilene suture between the lateral canthal tendon and the periosteum of the lateral orbital margin at the level of the lateral orbital tubercle (Webster suture).

Skin Redraping. The skin is then redraped with the patient holding the mouth wide open and the lids closed. I mark the incision line first and usually am very conservative with the amount I exercise because I wish to avoid postsurgical lower eyelid malposition caused by excessive shortening of the anterior lamella. I use interrupted 6/0 plain gut sutures which usually fall out in 4 to 6 days.

Transconjunctival Lower Eyelid Blepharoplasty

The advantage of the transconjunctival approach is its anatomic simplicity, its lack of visible postsurgical scar, and its suitability for individuals with pre-existing, horizontal lower eyelid laxity because it does not violate the orbital septum. It also is perfect for individuals who have little dermatochalasis (baggy skin) but who may desire simultaneous laser resurfacing as well as those who have dysthyroid orbitopathy with lower eyelid retraction.

Marking and Anesthesia. I mark the extent of the lower eyelid fat pads with the patient sitting upright and also leaning forward (Fig. 12).

Topical proparacaine 0.5% eyedrops are instilled into the conjunctival sacs. Lidocaine 2% with 1/100,000 epinephrine (0.5 ml) is injected into each fat pad from the conjunctival surface with the 30 g needle aimed downward to the orbital rim.

If simultaneous lower lid or orbital resurfacing is also to be performed, subcutaneous lidocaine 1.5 to 2 ml is injected into each lower eyelid.

Incision and Dissection. The lower lid is gently everted and the globe is protected with the sandblasted stainless steel Jaeger late. The assistant applies gentle pressure to the globe with the plate so that the fat balloons forward (Fig. 13). The incision is made with the 0.2 mm CO_2 laser beam in continuous wave mode at 7 W.

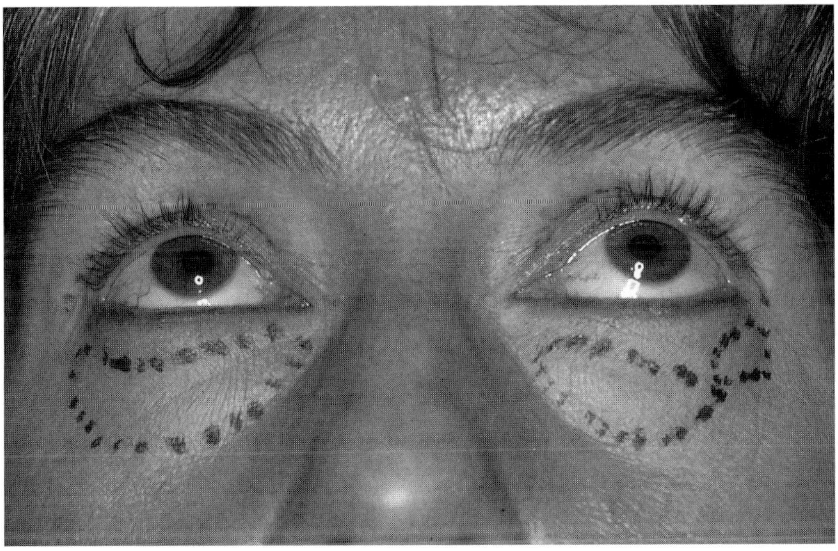

FIGURE 12 Presurgical cutaneous marking of the lower lid fat pads before the injection of local anesthetic which would blur the visible margins.

It is sited 10 mm below the lower lid margin and extends from 1 to 2 mm lateral to the lower punctum to the lateral fornix. I usually angle the incision more posteriorly laterally because otherwise it can be difficult to remove the full amount necessary of the lateral fat pad.

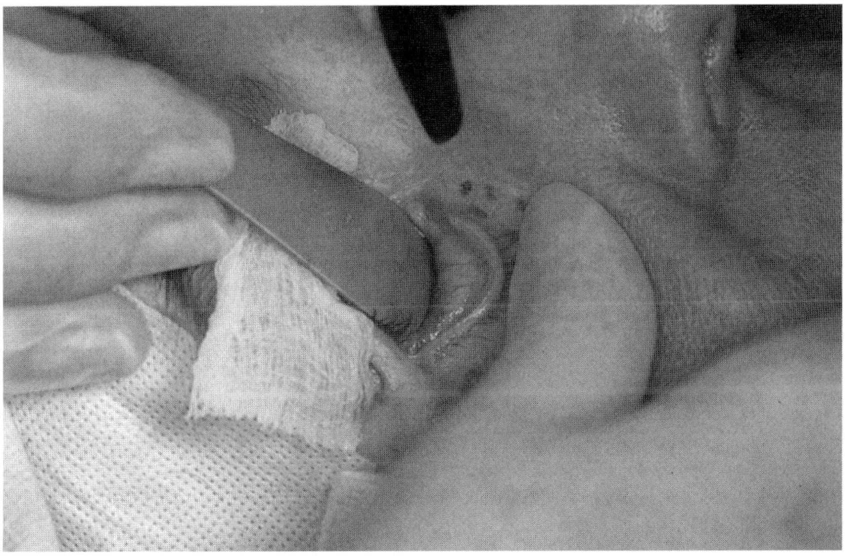

FIGURE 13 Gentle pressure on the globe prolapses the lower lid fat into the surgical field.

As with the external infralash approach, the lateral fat should be removed first because otherwise it tends to fall posteriorly away from the surgical field.

When the surgeon judges that adequate but not excessive fat has been removed and that hemostasis is complete, a fine-toothed forcep is used to gently redrape the lower lid. I do not use any sutures in the conjunctiva or capsulopalpebral fascia and simply insert antibiotic ointment into the conjunctival sac.

IMMEDIATE POSTSURGICAL CARE

Ice, Positioning, and Wound Care

I take a Polaroid photograph of each lid immediately after the surgical drapes are removed. The patient sees the result and then is reminded about the need to apply frequent cold compresses and ice packs in the 48 hours after surgery. We also instruct our patients to sleep sitting up for the first two nights. Although this may seem uncomfortable, the lack of bruising and swelling achieved means that most individuals are ready to reappear in public in 4 to 5 days instead of the traditional 2 to 3 weeks.

All patients use peroxide (10 volume) every 4 hours applied with a cotton swab to remove any drying blood products from external incisions. They also then apply a broad-spectrum antibiotic such as Bactraban or Tobrex 0.3% to the incision line.

Blepharoplasty Plus Resurfacing

I prefer the patients not to use topical antibiotic on newly resurfaced skin. All my resurfacing patients use oral broad spectrum antibiotic such as Biaxin and oral Valtrex.

We ask them to sleep with head elevated and to use regular cold water/ice soaks and topical Vaseline until re-epithelialization has occurred.

Keratoconjunctivitis Sicca

Particularly in traditional infralash blepharoplasty, pre-existing marginally compensated sicca can become an intense short-term problem. Topical lubrication with artificial tears by day and Lacrilube or Tear Gel by night can help mild problems. For the more major problems, Eagle punctal plugs, bandage contact lenses, external moisture chambers, and crazy glue to perform a temporary tarsorrhaphy may also be needed.

COMPLICATIONS AND THEIR TREATMENT

Retrobulbar Hemorrhage

A retrobulbar hemorrhage occurs rarely but is a true ocular emergency (Fig. 15). Delay in recognition and treatment can result in blindness [8,9].

The patient presents with pain, loss of vision, and a hard, purple orbit. On examination, the visual acuity is reduced from the presurgical evaluation, the intraocular pressure is elevated, and there may be a relative afferent pupillary defect. Management begins immediately with reopening of the wounds, evacuation of clot,

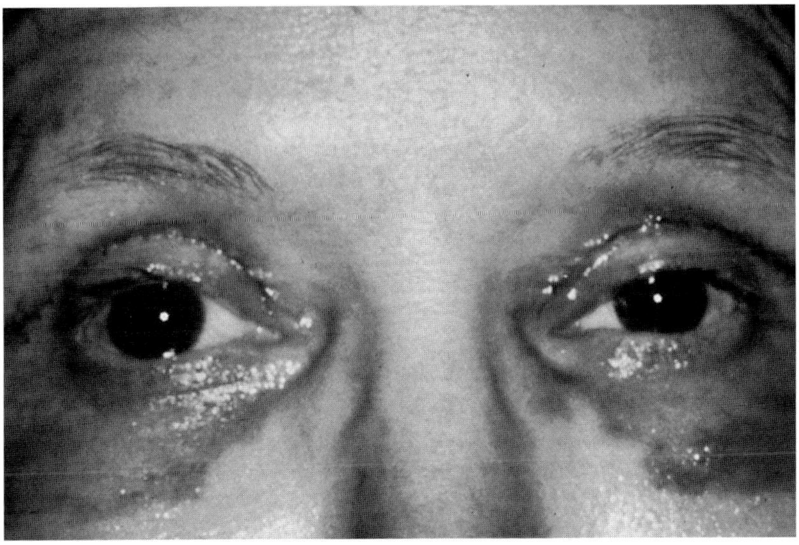

FIGURE 14 Simultaneous laser resurfacing of upper or lower lid or whole facial skin at the same time as surgical blepharoplasty enhances the overall aesthetic result.

and identification of bleeders. If this is not sufficient, the intraorbital pressure can be reduced with a lateral canthotomy and cantholysis of upper and lower lateral canthal tendons. If this is not sufficient, the orbital pressure must be further reduced by intravenous mannitol (1.0–2.0 g/kg) followed by 250 to 500 mg Diamox intramuscularly and followed by 250 mg by mouth every 6 hours.

If the orbital pressure is still not diminished enough to restore circulation to the globe, emergency orbital decompression of the medial wall or floor using a transconjunctival approach is indicated. Most centers have an ophthalmologist whose specialty is orbital surgery and who would have experience in performing emergency orbital decompression procedures.

Hematoma

Individuals who raise their venous pressure after surgery are particularly prone to hematomas. Common examples are smokers who cough, or individuals who take analgesics containing codeine and become nauseated. The surgeon should also ascertain if the patient went back on their aspirin, nonsteroidal antiinflammatory agents or took Vitamin E after surgery. If the hematoma is small, it can be locally drained or else observed. If there is any question of visual change, they must be taken back to the surgery room and treated as for orbital hemorrhage.

Blindness

Blindness is usually attributable to the orbital hemorrhage occluding the blood supply to the optic nerve, retina, and globe [10,11]. Other reported mechanisms include ischemia of the posterior ciliary circulation [12].

Lower Eyelid Malposition

Infralash transcutaneous blepharoplasty commonly results in lower eyelid malposition (40%) (Fig. 16) [13]. This is usually thought to be attributable to incision of the orbital septum (the middle lamella of the lid) with postsurgical scarring and contracture. Individuals who have presurgical increased horizontal lower eyelid laxity (as shown on the presurgical snap test) or who have pre-existing malar hypoplasia are at particular risk.

Careful evaluation of the postsurgical features will show whether the retraction is attributable to excessive skin removal from the anterior lamella or to an inadequately suspended orbicularis oculi muscle. In the former situation, more skin can be provided with a mid-facelift through the previous lower blepharoplasty incision or, if necessary, with a skin graft. In the latter situation, the lateral canthus can be supported with a Webster suture to the lateral orbital periosteum at the level of the lateral canthal tendon, and some may also require a tarsal strip procedure.

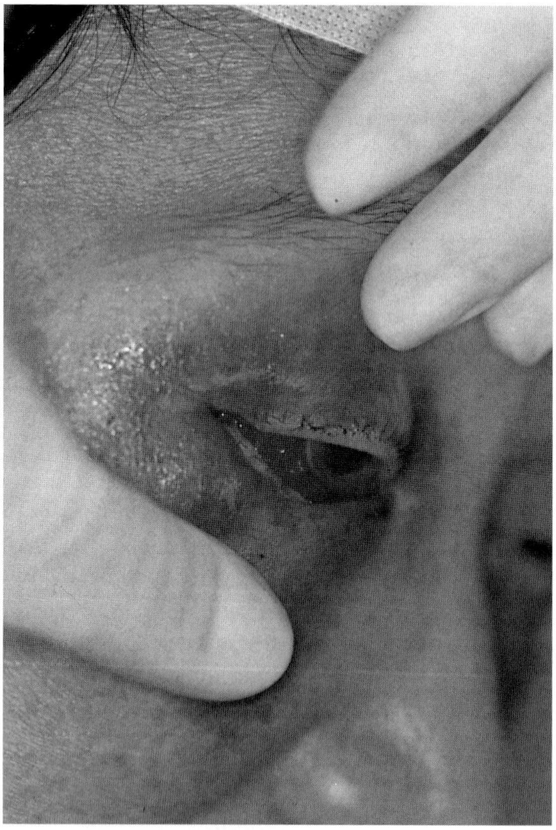

FIGURE 15 Acute retrobulbar hemorrhage presenting 12 hours after uneventful transconjunctival lower lid blepharoplasty.

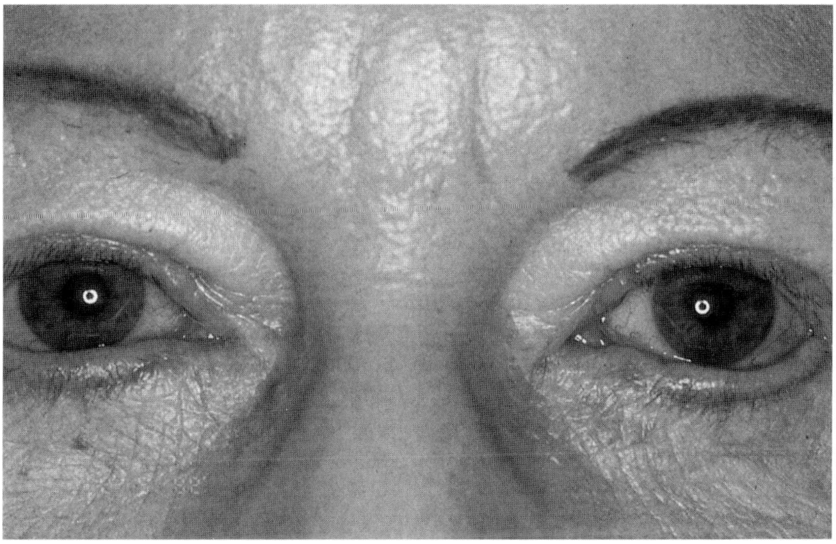

FIGURE 16 Right lower lid malposition and ectropion after bilateral infralash lower lid cosmetic blepharoplasty.

Extraocular Muscle Injury

Superior Oblique

The superior oblique tendon and trochlea are susceptible to injury with overzealous extraction of deeper aspects of the upper medial fat pad. Constant vertical and oblique diplopia particularly bothersome on attempting to read or work can result. The message is to always push orbital fat forward into the wound rather than reach in for it.

Inferior Oblique

The inferior oblique is situated between the medial and central fat pads in the lower lid. Meticulous removal of surrounding fat with direct visualization can avoid scarring and thus constant vertical and oblique diplopia particularly noted on upgaze and gaze to the opposite side.

Surgery for repair of injury to these important extraocular muscles may need to be delayed several months to await spontaneous resolution. In the meantime, the patient may not be legally able to drive or work without wearing a patch or prism to achieve single vision. Working with an ophthalmologist who is experienced in the field of oculomotor dysfunction is essential to the proper resolution of the problem.

Complications Related to Use of the CO_2 Laser for Blepharoplasty

Damage to the globe from either the incisional or resurfacing beams of the laser have been reported [14]. In either instance, the globe was not pre-emptively protected by insertion of a sand-blasted stainless steel contact lens or Jaeger plate (Figs. 11, 13).

SUMMARY

Cosmetic blepharoplasty is one of the most common and most successful surgical procedures in the realm of facial rejuvenation. CO_2 laser–assisted blepharoplasty as first described by Baker [2] has rapidly become one of the most popular approaches, both because of the superior hemostasis and because of the natural adjunctive treatment with CO_2 and Erbium-YAG laser resurfacing [1].

As with any other surgical approach, the surgeon must work with the aesthetically concerned individual to customize the approach to give each patient the best cosmetic result. Whether the surgeon is by primary residency or fellowship training a surgical ophthalmologist or surgical dermatologist, by paying extremely close attention to the underlying anatomic, physiologic, and surgical features, a functional and cosmetic result is the rule rather than the exception.

No matter whether the basic educational background is in ophthalmology or dermatology, each surgeon must be aware of the potential complications and their management in order that the highest standards of safety and excellence are observed for each eyelid and for each individual.

REFERENCES

1. Goldman MP, Fitzpatrick RE. Cutaneous Laser Surgery: The Art and Science of Selective Photothermolysis. St. Louis: Mosby Year-Book, 1994, pp. 198–258.
2. Baker SS. Carbon dioxide laser ptosis surgery combined with blepharoplasty. Dermatol Surg 1995; 21:1065–1070.
3. Lemke BN, Stasior GO. The anatomy of eyebrow ptosis. Arch Ophthalmol 1982; 100: 981–986.
4. Carruthers J, Carruthers A. The adjunctive use of Botulinum-A exotoxin. Dermatologic Surg 1998; 24:1244–1247.
5. Putterman AM. Upper eyelid blepharoplasty. In: Hornblass A, ed. Oculoplastic, Orbital and Reconstructive Surgery, Vol. 1. Baltimore: Williams and Wilkins, 1988, p. 474.
6. Knize DM. Limited-incision forehead lift for eyebrow elevation to enhance upper blepharoplasty. Plast Reconstr Surg 1996; 97(7):1334–1342.
7. Stasior OG, Lemke BN. The posterior eyebrow fixation. Adv Ophthalmol Plast Reconstr Surg 1983; 2:193–197.
8. Smith B, Nesi FA. The Complications of cosmetic blepharoplasty. Ophthalmology 1978; 85:726.
9. Liu D. A Amplified technique of orbital decompression for severe retrobulbar hemorrhage (see comments). Am J Ophthalmol 1993; 116:34–37.
10. De Mere M, Wood T, Austin W. Eye complications with blepharoplasty or other eyelid surgery. A national survey. Plast Reconstr Surg 1974; 53:634–637.
11. Goldberg RA, Marmor MF, Shorr N. Blindness following blepharoplasty. Two case reports and a discussion of management. Ophthalmic Surg 1990; 21:85–89.
12. Hepler RS, Sugimura GI, Straatsma BR. On the occurrence of blindness in association with blepharoplasty. Plast Reconstr Surg 1976; 57:233–235.
13. Hamako C, Baylis HI. Lower eyelid retraction after blepharoplasty. Am J Ophthalmol 1980; 89:517–521.
14. Widder RA, Severin M, Kirkhof B, Krieglstein CK. Corneal injury after carbon-dioxide laser skin resurfacing. Am J Ophthalm 1998; 125(3):392–394.

APPENDIX 1. COSMETIC LASER BLEPHAROPLASTY OPERATIVE CONSENT

I hereby authorize Dr. Jean Carruthers and her associates to perform a ______________________________. I fully understand that this procedure has limited applications. No guarantees or assurances have been given to me by anyone as to the results that may be obtained. Dr. J. Carruthers and assistants have carefully explained to me the nature, goals, limitations, and possible complications of this procedure and have discussed alternative forms of treatment.

By placing my initials next to these items, I clearly understand and accept the following:

INITIAL
HERE

___ 1. The potential benefits of the proposed procedure(s).
___ 2. The possible alternate medical procedure(s).
___ 3. The probability of success.
___ 4. The reasonably anticipated consequences if the procedure is not performed.
___ 5. The possibility of ancillary services/fees including, but not limited to, anesthesia, laboratory, medications, and/or surgical facility use.
___ 6. The goal of laser surgery, as in any cosmetic procedure, is improvement, not perfection. Satisfaction is based on realistic expectation.
___ 7. Although the procedure is intended to improve my appearance, in rare cases it may leave it unchanged or in some cases worsened.
___ 8. The final result may not be apparent for 3 to 12 months after surgery.
___ 9. To achieve the best possible result, additional procedures may be required. There will be a charge for any additional procedure performed.
___ 10. Strict adherence to the postsurgical regimen discussed by Dr. J. Carruthers (ie, medications, creams, postsurgical care instructions and all other regimens discussed) is necessary in order to achieve the best possible results.
___ 11. The surgical fee is paid for the surgery itself and subsequent postsurgical office visits. There is no guarantee that the expected or anticipated results will be achieved.
___ 12. I give my permission for the administration of anesthesia, as deemed appropriate by the physician.
___ 13. Protective eye covering will be provided to protect my eyes from accidental laser exposure, but accidental exposure to laser is possible.

Although complications after these procedures are infrequent, by placing my initials next to the following I understand that they may occur and that other procedures may be needed to correct them:

INITIAL
HERE

___ 1. ORBITAL HEMORRHAGE. Can occur in one out of 2300 cosmetic blepharoplasty cases.
___ 2. BLINDNESS: Can occur in one in 40,000 cosmetic blepharoplasty cases.
___ 3. BRUSING/BLEEDING/SWELLING: In some cases, bruising/bleeding of the treated area may occur. Additionally, there may be some swelling noted.
___ 4. INFECTION: Infection is rare. Should it occur, treatment with antibiotics and/or surgical drainage may be required.
___ 5. SCARRING: Scarring is a rare occurrence, but it is a possibility when the skin's surface is disrupted. To minimize the chances of scarring, it is important that I follow all postsurgical instructions carefully.
___ 6. VISUAL changes, dry eyes, ulcerations, and cysts are rare.
___ 7. ALLERGIES: Allergic or toxic responses to anesthetic are extremely rare, but possible.
___ 8. GENERAL RISKS: In addition to these possible complications, I am aware of the general risks inherent in all surgical procedures and anesthetic administration.

My signature certifies that I have discussed the above material thoroughly with Dr. J. Carruthers and assistants. I understand the goals, limitations, and possible complications of the above procedure(s), and I wish to proceed with them. I authorize and direct Dr. J. Carruthers and/or associates or assistants of his/her choice to perform these procedure(s) on me and/or to perform any other additional therapeutic procedure that his/her judgement may dictate to be advisable, reasonable, or necessary for my well being.

____
PATIENT SIGNATURE DATE

____
PATIENT PRINTED NAME

____
WITNESS DATE

____
PHYSICIAN SIGNATURE DATE

APPENDIX 2. LASER BLEPHAROPLASTY (LID LIFT)

1. WHAT IS BLEPHAROPLASTY?

Blepharoplasty, or lid lift, is a delicate surgical procedure in which the laser beam is used as a means of removing excess skin and/or fat from both upper and lower eyelids. The eyes then have a more open, youthful, and bright appearance.

2. WHAT IS INVOLVED?

Dr. Carruthers uses the Sharplan $C0_2$ laser beam to perform the lid lift surgery. This laser beam is 1/5 mm in diameter and seals tiny blood vessels as it cuts, so that there is very little swelling and bruising. This translates to a shorter recovery time and reduced discomfort for the patient. Most individuals are ready to go back to their normal activities in 5–7 days.

3. WHAT IS THE DIFFERENCE BETWEEN LASER AND TRADITIONAL "COLD-STEEL" SURGERY?

With previous "cold-steel" surgery, eyelids could be bruised-looking for 2 to 3 weeks after blepharoplasty. With the use of the laser beam as the cutting instrument, bruising is dramatically reduced and many individuals are able to be back at work with only slight residual swelling by the end of the first week after surgery.

4. WHAT ARE THE ADVANTAGES?

Usually, the upper lid fold starts to be hidden in the mid-thirties, and this appearance can make one look tired, angry, and frustrated. Lifting the excess skin and fat away gives the sparkle back to the eyes and the expression again. Lid lift surgery is a most effective way to restore an open, relaxed, and youthful appearance.

In the lower lid, the prominent fat pockets can be removed from the inside (transconjunctival blepharoplasty) so that there is no visible scar afterwards. We also resurface lower and upper eyelid skin right after the CO_2 laser incisional surgery, using the Erbium-YAG laser or CO_2 laser because it dramatically changes tired, crepey skin, to a new, youthful, smooth translucent skin. Laser resurfacing is precise and the length of time to recover from the resurfacing parallels the time for recovery from the procedure so it is most efficient to perform both procedures at the same surgical appointment.

5. WHAT IS THE RECOVERY TIME?

We recommend that individuals should take at least 1 week off their regular activities. With make-up, individuals can often go out a day or two earlier.

6. HOW LONG WILL IT LAST?

Blepharoplasty turns back the clock but we must continue with our ongoing skin maintenance program and sunscreen, AHA, and Vitamins A and C therapy. If the lid skin does become crepey again, instead of the blepharoplasty, a resurfacing of the lid skin using the Erbium-YAG laser or CO_2 laser is an effective adjunctive procedure.

7. CAN OTHER PROCEDURES BE COMBINED WITH AN EYELID LIFT?

YES. As previously mentioned, laser resurfacing of the skin around the eyes helps produce a new, smooth, youthful look. Also, BOTOX to the forehead and brow furrows and crow's feet results in a more youthful appearance.

COSMETIC LASER BLEPHAROPLASTY OPERATIVE CONSENT

I hereby authorize Dr. Jean Carruthers and her associates to perform a blepharoplasty on my ______________________________ lids.
I fully understand that this procedure has limited applications. No guarantees or assurances have been given to me by anyone as to the results that may be obtained.
Dr. J. Carruthers and assistants have carefully explained to me the nature, goals, limitations and possible complications of this procedure and have discussed alternative forms of treatment.

By placing my initials next to these items, I clearly understand and accept the following:

INITIAL
HERE

___ 1. The potential benefits of the proposed procedure(s)
___ 2. The possible alternate medical procedure(s)
___ 3. The probability of success
___ 4. The reasonably anticipated consequences if the procedure is not performed
___ 5. The possibility of ancillary services/fees including, but not limited to, anesthesia, laboratory, medications and/or surgical facility use.
___ 6. The goal of laser surgery, as in any cosmetic procedure, is improvement, not perfection. Satisfaction is based on realistic expectation.
___ 7. Although the procedure is intended to improve my appearance, in rare cases it may leave it unchanged or in some cases worsened.
___ 8. The final result may not be apparent for 3 to 12 months postoperatively.
___ 9. To achieve the best possible result, additional procedures may be required. There will be a charge for any additional operation performed.
___ 10. Strict adherence to the postoperative regimen discussed by Dr. J. Carruthers (i.e. medications, creams, postoperative care instructions and all other regimens discussed) is necessary in order to achieve the best possible results.
___ 11. The surgical fee is paid for the operation itself and subsequent postoperative office visits. There is no guarantee that the expected or anticipated results will be achieved.
___ 12. I give my permission for the administration of anesthesia, as deemed appropriate by the physician.
___ 13. Protective eye covering will be provided to protect my eyes from accidental laser exposure, but accidental exposure to laser is possible.

Although complications following these procedures are infrequent, by placing my initials next to the following I understand that they may occur and that other procedures may be needed to correct them:

INITIAL
HERE

___ 1. ORBITAL HEMORRHAGE: Can occur in one out of 2500 cosmetic blepharoplasty cases.
___ 2. BLINDNESS: Can occur in one in 40,000 cosmetic blepharoplasty cases.
___ 3. BRUSING/BLEEDING/SWELLING: In some cases, bruising/bleeding of the treated area may occur. Additionally, there may be some swelling noted.
___ 4. INFECTION: Infection is rare. Should it occur, treatment with antibiotics and/or surgical drainage may be required.
___ 5. SCARRING: Scarring is a rare occurrence, but it is a possibility when the skin's surface is disrupted. To minimize the chances of scarring, it is important that I follow all postoperative instructions carefully.
___ 6. VISUAL changes, dry eyes, ulcerations, and cysts are rare.
___ 7. ALLERGIES: Allergic or toxic responses to anesthetic are extremely rare, but possible.
___ 8. GENERAL RISKS: In addition to these possible complications, I am aware of the general risks inherent in all surgical procedures and anesthetic administration.

My signature certifies that I have discussed the above material thoroughly with Dr. J. Carruthers and assistants. I understand the goals, limitations and possible complications of the above procedure(s), and I wish to proceed with them. I authorize and direct Dr. J. Carruthers and/or associates or assistants of his/her choice, to perform these procedure(s) on me and/or to do any other additional therapeutic procedure that his/her judgement may dictate to be advisable, reasonable or necessary for my well being.

____
PATIENT SIGNATURE DATE

____
PATIENT PRINTED NAME

____
WITNESS DATE

____
PHYSICIAN SIGNATURE DATE

EYELID SURGERY IMMEDIATE AFTERCARE INSTRUCTIONS

1. **DO NOT DRIVE** until the day after surgery. After the first day, you may drive if you are not taking medications which cause drowsiness.

2. **REST IN BED** the day to prevent bruising and swelling.

3. **ELEVATE YOUR HEAD** at all times; and sleep with your head elevated to prevent bruising and swelling.

4. **APPLY COLD PACKS** to your eyes 15 minutes "on" alternating with 15 minutes "off" for the first 8 hours. Bags of frozen peas or soft ice packs are excellent cold packs – buy 4 so you can keep 2 in the freezer while you are using the other 2. You may want to put the cold packs in plastic wrappers to keep your eyes dry. DO NOT put ice cubes directly on skin. Do not push or put any pressure on your eyelids. Just gently lay the cold packs on your face.

5. **CONFINE YOUR ACTIVITIES TO RESTING** and activities which do not elevate your heart rate or blood pressure for 48 hours after surgery to prevent bleeding and bruising. Do not bend over so that your head is lower than your heart. Dr. Carruthers will advise you when you may resume exercise – usually 4 days after surgery.

6. **DO NOT TOUCH OR CLEAN OR RUB YOUR EYELIDS.** If you have had upper eyelid surgery, you will have stiches in place. These will fall out in 3-4 days. Do not pick or pull at the stitches.

7. **YOU MAY HAVE DRAINAGE** from lower eyelids which appears as crusting or reddish fluid along the lower eyelid edge. This is normal and can be cleaned off with a wet Q-tip (water only).

8. **DO NOT WEAR CONTACT LENSES** for at least two weeks after surgery.

9. **PLEASE CALL** the office at anytime if you have questions or problems. The office number is 555-1234, or page one of our nurses:

    Jane Doe 555-2345 OR

    John Doe 555-3456

32

Brow Rejuvenation

Alan Matarasso
Albert Einstein College of Medicine, New York, New York

Ivo Pitanguy and Henrique N. Radwanski
Pontificial Catholic University of Rio de Janeiro and Carlos Chagas Institute of Post-Graduate Medical Studies, Rio de Janeiro, Brazil

Giulio Gherardini
The National Centre for Cosmetic Surgery, Birmingham, United Kingdom

INTRODUCTION

The concept of beauty is related to the search for harmony as a means of achieving intimate well-being. The human body is a fundamental aspect of this harmonizing process. Aging brings changes that are often undesirable, such as skin flaccidity, marked lines of expression, and fat deposits. The face, because of its exposure and expressivity, is frequently the main focus of anxiety in individuals who have attained a certain maturity. Aging in the upper face becomes evident with a descent in the level of the eyebrow and the appearance of wrinkles and furrows, sometimes from an early age. These are a direct consequence of muscle dynamics, responsible for the multitude of expressions so characteristic of man.

Facial rejuvenation surgery is often sought with deeply hidden motivations. Patients should be made aware that the ultimate goal in facial rejuvenation is not to return lost years, but rather to make him or her accept their biological age naturally, permitting for a better adjustment between a period of intense activity and social interaction and a more mature phase of life. On the other hand, a satisfactory result of an aesthetic facial procedure is obtained when signs of a surgery are undetectable and no anatomical landmarks have been altered.

In general, facial aesthetic surgery has witnessed enormous progress since the first descriptions from the beginning of the century, and is sometimes described as a relatively complex procedure. Forehead–brow rhytidoplasty has traditionally been advocated for senile brow ptosis. As the procedure became more widely accepted, it became a routine consideration in facial rejuvenation surgery. Indeed, over time, forehead–brow rhytidoplasty has also withstood the initial criticism that it was of limited longevity, and it is now recognized that, as with all other lifting procedures, this procedure will gradually succumb to time, gravity, and the aging process. Moreover, refinements in techniques have added versatility to the procedure so that a variety of problems encountered in the upper face in addition to brow ptosis can be addressed. Consequently, an eclectic population with a range of deformities benefits from the procedure.

The surgeon must be knowledgeable in details of surgical technique and its variations to attain the best result for each individual case. Facial anatomy should be carefully examined for an individualized diagnosis, and classification of patients and selection of the proper technique are important aspects of successful outcome. Just as well-placed incisions result in imperceptible scars, incisions that are grossly apparent and that cause anatomical distortion are extremely displeasing. In this chapter we describe patient assessment and the surgical approach to rejuvenation of the upper face.

ANATOMY

In the execution of a browlift several anatomical structures are of significant importance. These are the frontalis (FM), corrugator (CM), and procerus (PM) muscles. The supraorbital (SON) and the supratrochlear (STN) sensory nerves, as well as the frontal branch (FB) of the facial nerve, are also encountered. The galeal aponeurosis is a continuous fibromuscular sheet that extends from the occiput to the brow anteriorly. Posteriorly it attaches to the external occipital protuberance, while in its most anterior portion it invests the frontalis muscle. The paired FM is innervated by the frontal branches of the facial nerve. During contraction the FM raises the position of the eyebrows and nasal skin. The CM muscles are a pair of pyramical-shaped muscles located deep to the frontalis and the orbicularis oculi muscles (Fig. 1). They arise from the periosteum of the medial portion of the supercilliary arch and insert into the deep surface of the eyebrow skin. During animation, contraction of the CM causes the development of the vertical and oblique glabellar frown lines. The CM are innervated by the distal portion of the frontal branch of the facial nerve. The PM is a musculofascial slip arising from the fascia of the nasal bones, inserting into the skin of the lower forehead as well as decussating with the caudal portion of the frontalis muscle. During animation it creates the transverse frown lines of the glabella and the suprabrow. The PM is innervated by the superior buccal branch of the facial nerve. The SON and the STN provide sensation to the glabella and the suprabrow area, and are visualized during the dissection of the forehead. Both nerves are the continuation of the trigeminal nerve after it enters the orbit via the superior oblique fissure. There is a constant spatial relationship of the SON and the STN with respect to each other and to the midline. The STN is interposed between the body of the CM.

AESTHETICS AND PATIENT EVALUATION

The "ideal" brow position is a subjective concept. Measurements that provide a guide are useful, but should serve to complement the aesthetic judgment of the surgeon. Brow ptosis is considered to be present if the distance from the mid pupil to the arch of the eyebrow is less than 2.5 cm. Ideal brow to frontal hairline distance is 5 to 6 cm. The patient is considered to have a high forehead if the distance from

TABLE 2 Indications of Brow-Forehead Plasty and Goals of Surgery

Indications	Goals
Primary	
Eyebrow malposition (ptosis)	
a. Senile	Elevate forehead and eyebrows
b. Congenital	Balance, position, symmetry
Secondary	
1. Frown muscle imbalance	Minimize corrugator-procerus activity and central frown folds
2. Forehead rhytids	Decrease frontalis muscle hyperactivity and transverse rhytids
3. Enhancing medial/lateral eyelid incision (aesthetics)	Confine the eyelid incision to within the tarsal crease
4. Lateral brow laxity (temporal lift)	Restore temporal, lateral brow, and canthal regions
5. Abnormal/unattractive expression	Adjust brow position to normalize expression (sad, tired, angry)

retained its contractility, probably account for the beneficial effects of surgery without requiring excess brow-flap elevation or skin excision. These are the theoretical bases for endoscopically assisted forehead–brow rhytidoplasty (Fig. 4b). This recently introduced technique is particularly useful in a variety of "secondary" or "minor" indications for browplasty. Although endoscopically-assisted browplasty has a short follow-up, some indications and contraindications to its use have been identified (Table 2).

Although followup does not exceed 5 to 6 years, good flap stability can be achieved by a variety of fixation methods, including bony cortical tunnels.

The planes of dissection will vary according to the method. In an open procedure our preference is a subgaleal dissection and in a closed procedure we prefer a sub-periosteal approach.

SURGICAL TECHNIQUE

Surgery can be performed in the hospital or office surgicenter on an inpatient basis or in an ambulatory setting. Before surgery, patients are instructed to cleanse their hair, face, and ears with an antimicrobial solution, and on the morning of surgery are given presurgical sedation before entering the surgical center, if desired. Patients undergoing brow surgery do not require a blood transfusion; hematocrit and coagulation profile are the routine laboratory tests required. General anesthesia or local anesthetic infiltration with monitored sedation by an anesthesiologist can be used, and the surgery can be carried out alone or in conjunction with other surgeries. If associated with facialplasty, we prefer to perform brow surgery last. (Only a rhinoplasty would come after forehead surgery.) Positioning the patient for brow surgery is important. The patient's hands should be lightly restrained, the head of the surgery table elevated about 15°. A foam plastic ring under the head and standard antiseptic and head-drape preparation are commonly used.

Open or Coronal Brow Rejuvenation

The procedure begins by parting the hair and marking the lines of incision with Methylene blue or a marking pen along a gull wing type arc, from ear to ear, keeping a distance of approximately 5–7 cm behind the anterior line of hair implantation, and joining the prolongation of the temporal portion of a facelift incision. The midline is carefully scratched with a blade so as to be permanently marked. A solution of 0.25% Xylocaine and epinephrine (1:200.000) is infiltrated, along the coronal incision, the orbital rims, and the root and dorsum of the nose.

An incision is made in the premarked area, and dissection is carried down to the subgaleal plane. The flap is developed by sharp dissection to within 2 to 3 cm of the supraorbital rims and is then completed with blunt (pushing) dissection, and the forehead flap folded forward 180°. If elevation of the brows is necessary or if there is asymmetry, the lateral-brow periosteum is incised and freed from the restraints of the orbital rims in a subperiosteal plane. The midline of the flap to the tip of the nose is then established, and the procerus muscle and the orbicularis oculi are detached with a periosteal elevator. In the patient where the aging process has resulted in a drooping nose, the nasal tip and the membranous septum can be manipulated by dissecting with a long scissors in a subcutaneous plane, starting at the root of the nose and freeing Pitanguy's ligament. There are now three planes of dissection: subcutaneous, subgaleal, and subperiosteal. The supratrochlear nerve branches are located in a deeper plane within the fibers of the corrugator muscle, approximately 8 to 12 mm from the supraorbital branches. The corrugator muscle is widely resected carefully preserving the interposed ST nerves. The glabellar lines are then transferred to the undersurface of the flap with a 25-gauge needle and are skeletonized and undermined to the dermis to assist in relaxing the rhytid.

A small rectangle of frontalis muscle 1 to 2 cm above the orbital rims is then marked between the supraorbital nerves and excised, with care taken to preserve the fat (Fig. 5). Alternatively, the muscle can be cross-hatched to weaken it, or in certain circumstances not treated at all. The flap is then returned to its position. Hemostasis of the edges of the scalp is restricted to the large vessels that run in the deep plane, so as not to damage hair follicles. This along with avoidance of tension and minimal flap ischemia assists in preserving hair follicles. Final sutures will guarantee total hemostasis of the edges of the incision. When the brow lift is associated with a cervicofacial rhytidectomy, no traction is applied to the forehead until the facial and cervical flaps have been appropriately dissected, pulled, and blocked. This "blocking" of the flaps is performed with key stitches in the supra-auricular and retroauricular regions. This assures that when the brow is tractioned, no alterations in facial anatomy will occur. The amount of tension that is applied to the forehead flap and direction of traction is dependent on the degree of eyebrow ptosis, skin laxity, and vertical dimension of the forehead. The forehead is initially pulled straight back with gentle traction, the overlap of the scalp is incised along the midline to the point previously determined, and a temporary suture is placed. The forehead flap is thus divided in two equal halves, and each will be tractioned individually yet with the same tension and in a symmetrical manner.

Final closure of the forehead incision is performed in layers above the temporalis muscle, and the full length of the incision is closed with staples. When the nose has been dissected, adhesive tapes are placed starting from the tip up to the

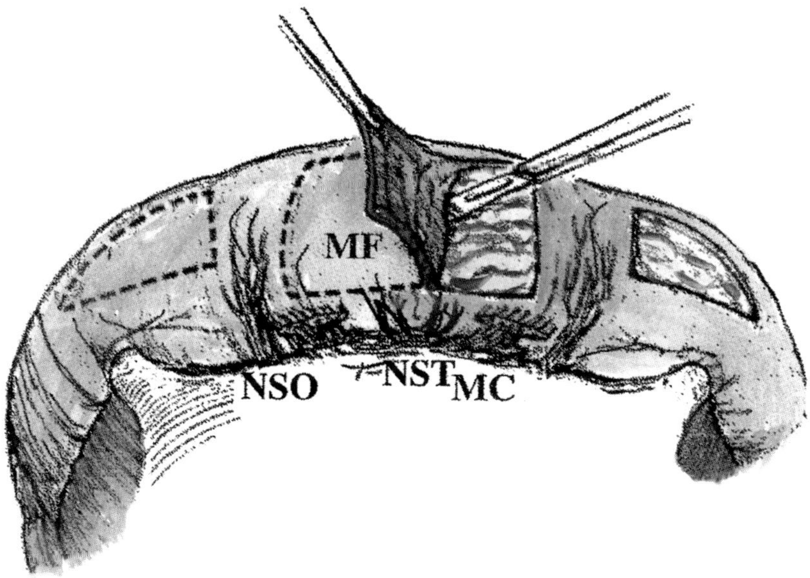

FIGURE 5 Undermining has proceeded to the nasal tip. Cutaneous markings are transferred to the undersurface of the flap for treatment of the muscles of animation. A wedge of frontalis is excised. The glabellar creases are treated. NSO, supraorbital nerve; NST, supratrochlear nerve; MF, frontalis muscle; MC, corrugator muscle.

dorsum so as to fix the undermined skin to the underlying osteocartilaginous skeleton and avoid formation of blood collection at the tip.

At the end of the procedure the hair is carefully washed of all blood with generous amounts of saline. It is helpful to comb the hair neatly before placing final dressings, which consists of wet gauges along the incision line and soft padding. A bandage is wrapped around the head with enough tension to exert a comfortable compression (Pitanguy). Others prefer no dressing (Matarasso).

Endoscopic Brow Rejuvenation

A standard tray of surgical instruments used for the coronal technique and endoscopic instruments are necessary. A number of manufacturers make endoscopic forehead instruments. A 4-mm, guarded, 30° down-angled endoscope (with a focal length of 2.54–7.62 cm), high-resolution video equipment, and xenon light source are used.

With the patient in a sitting position, the locations of the motor and sensory nerves, incisions, and frown lines are marked. The procedure can be performed under local or general anesthesia; the surgical field is infiltrated with a solution of 0.25% Xylocaine and epinephrine (1:200.000) along the coronal incision, the orbital rims, and the root and dorsum of the nose.

The procedure begins with a vertical, 3-cm central incision in the hairline at the level of the midline of the nose and carried down to the level of the galea. Two other lateral incisions are made outside the course of the supraorbital nerves or 4 cm from the midline. The dissection proceeds medially across the superficial temporal crest line. Anteriorly, using facelift scissors a subgaleal plane is dissected to 2 cm above the orbital rims. Posteriorly, undermining is performed until the occipitalis muscle is engaged or to the extent necessary, based on the amount of excess skin that must be redraped. The incisions are then connected. Using standard long scissors, an optical cavity is bluntly developed toward the membranous septum of the nose. The endoscope is introduced into the cavity via the central incision in the scalp and, under direct endoscopic vision (with the overhead lights turned off), sharp periosteal elevators are used to free the lateral periosteum from the orbital rims. Once the plan is established, bimanual sweeps can be used as the periosteum is freed lateral to the supraorbital nerve and around the canthus. In order to maintain proper orientation, palpation with the nondominant hand and redirection of the relationship between the endoscope and the instruments will aid in positioning. The depressor muscles are then thoroughly addressed with the aid of the endoscope. A small, blunt elevator is used to release the restraining fibers of the orbicularis oculi muscle from the root of the nose toward the medial canthus. The procerus muscle is elevated and transected, preserving its substance for bulk. The corrugator muscles are then identified through the endoscope and a 2-0 nylon suture is placed over the corresponding skin surface to provide external retraction. Another retraction suture can be placed over the outline of the supraorbital nerve. After incising the corrugator fascia, the muscle is dissected by vertical spreading and completely excised (avulsed) with the aid of a Takahashi biopsy forceps or grasper; a large vein is often encountered at the medial aspect of the muscle. Individual branches of the supratroclear nerve are located and preserved. When indicated, the frontalis muscle is interrupted by incising it with a slit knife within the limits of the supraorbital nerves or by excising a wedge. The skin is mobilized and redraped cephalically, using the eyebrow–supraorbital rim relationship as a reference. Alternatively, the initial flap dissection can be performed in the subperiosteal plane. In this case, using a large periosteal elevator, the periosteum is elevated from the skin incisions inferiorly to the supraorbital rim, laterally to the temporal fossa remaining superficial to the temporalis muscle fascia, and posteriorly as far as the occiput.

In patients with significant ptosis or poor skin quality, the flap can be fixed by external support (bunching the skin between bolsters, percutaneous screw fixation, or a suture placed between staples), internal suspension (advancing the temporoparietal fascia to the deep temporal fascia, spraying with fibrin glue), or excision techniques (ellipses of skin or *Y* to *V* advancements). In general, we favor external suspension with screw fixation or internal suspension with screw suspension. The former is performed by drilling a hole in the outer cortex (1.5-mm tip), in the most posterior point of the two lateral scalp incisions, and inserting a screw (2 × 2–14 mm). The forehead skin is then pulled posteriorly with a skin hook, and the incision is stapled in the new position under tension, over the screws. Postsurgically the periosteum reattaches rapidly. Therefore, since there are no natural fixed points, the value of fixing the flap is in suitably positioning it and thus avoiding random attachment at an undesirable level; rather than securing it. After closing the wounds, additional compression is placed at the junction of the nasal and frontal bone, where a large dead space is common, and over the temporalis muscle. When the first sutures are removed, the bandage is replaced with a snug headband that is to be worn as much as possible over the next 2 or 3 weeks. Cortical tunnels can also be utilized by placing a suture from the anterior portion of the incision, grasping the fascia and advancing it through the tunnel.

Postsurgical Care

Postsurgically, periorbital and malar ecchymosis and edema are common sequelae and transient paresthesias are reported, although scar complaints, itching, and hair loss are less frequent. A long-acting steroid and broad-spectrum antibiotics are used in the postsurgical period, and a variety of vitamins are prescribed. In the endoscopic brow lift the screws are removed in the office on postsurgical day 9 to 10.

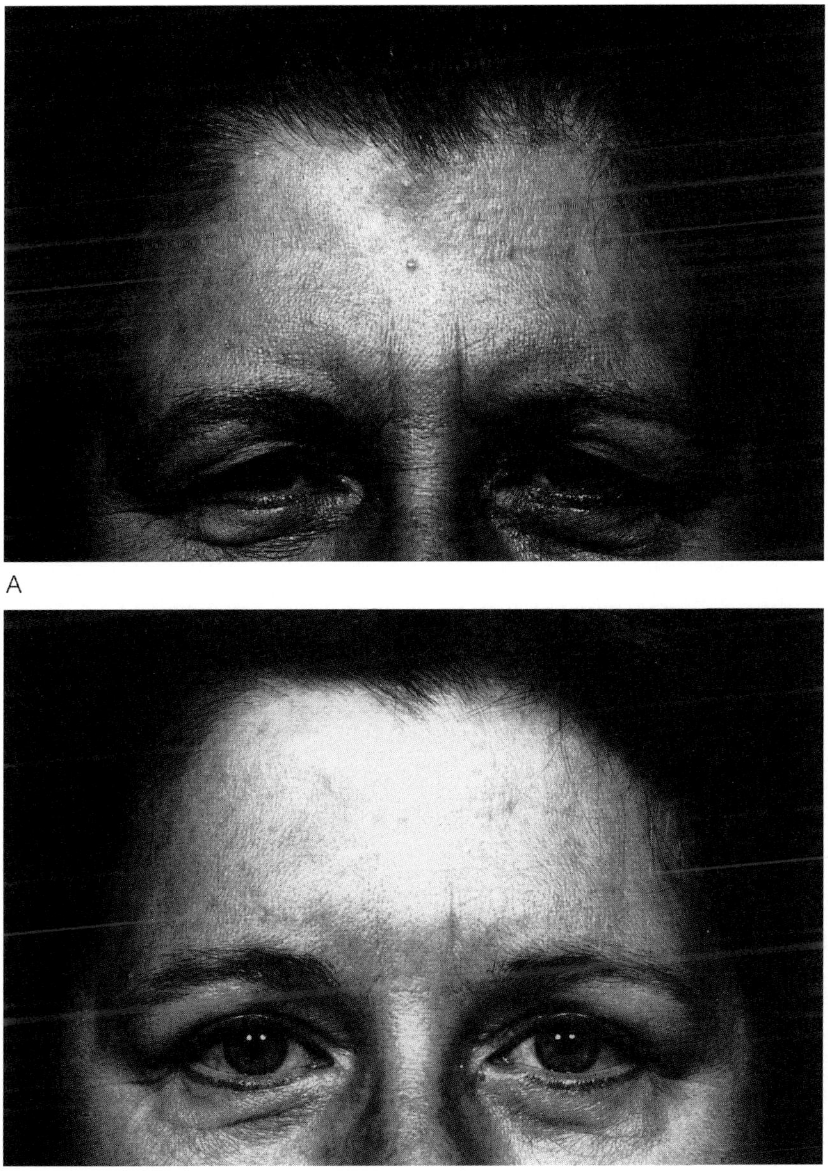

A

B

Clinical Case 1

CLINICAL CASES

Clinical case 1: [A,B] The main complaint of this 53-year-old woman was a strong, heavy, frowning look due to procerus and corrugator dynamics [A]. She had been submitted to a facialplasty 8 years earlier. Her relatively short forehead permitted for a bicoronal approach with traction of the brow, after crossing incisions of the frontalis-procerus corrugator aponeurotic expansion. The patient is seen three years

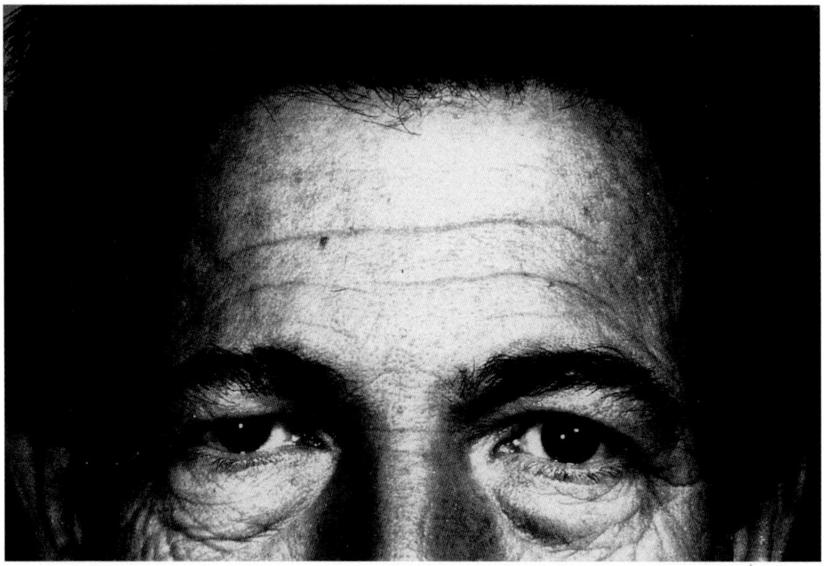

A

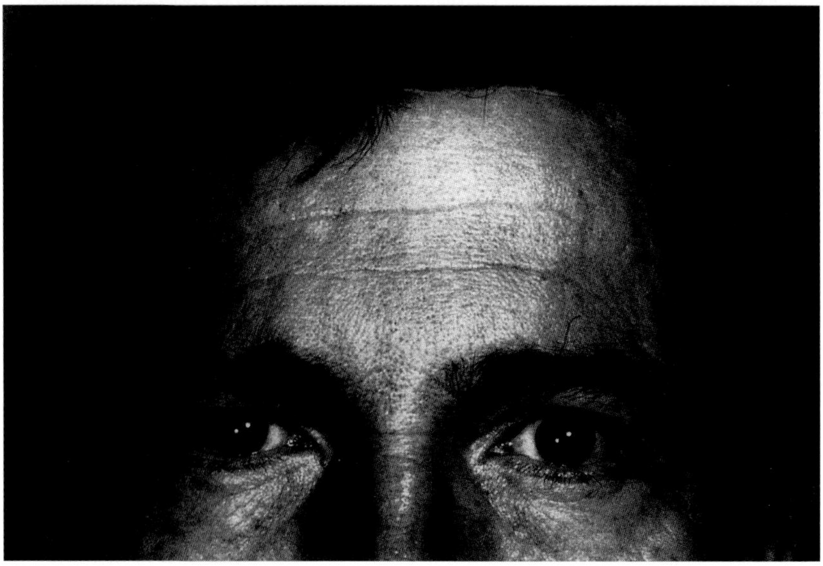

B

CLINICAL CASE 2

post-operatively; she is particularly pleased with what she called a "lighter look" to her brow [B].

Clinical case 2: [A,B] This 51-year-old man requested a younger appearance to his face. [B] Brow lifting, associated with a lower blepharoplasty, was done by the bicoronal prepilose technique. He is seen 1.5 years post-operatively.

SUMMARY

The face, because of its exposure and expressivity, is frequently the main focus of anxiety in individuals who have attained a certain maturity. Aging in the upper face becomes evident with a descent in the level of the eyebrow and the appearance of wrinkles and rhytids. The wide variety of surgical techniques for rejuvenation of the brow, including newer instrumentation and minimal accesses, only serves to indicate that no single procedure offers the ideal solution to every problem encountered in the upper face. Surgical correction of the eyebrows should follow a problem-oriented analysis of the face and each subunit, and the appropriate technique should be chosen accordingly. In this chapter, we described principles of brow-rejuvenation surgery that have provided consistent results over the years. Furthermore, an algorithm has been formulated that integrates the patient's primary complaint with any concomitant procedures being performed (Table 3).

TABLE 3 Forehead and Brow Rejuvenation Algorithm

Indications	Associated procedures		Treatment
1) Forehead rhytids	None	→	Botulinum toxin, +/− laser resurfacing*
2) Glabellar creases/corrugator muscle hypertrophy	a) None	→	Endoscopic corrugator muscle excision or Botulinum toxin, +/− laser resurfacing*
	b) Upper eyelid surgery	→	Corrugator muscle excision through upper lid, +/− laser resurfacing
3) Lateral brow laxity	a) None	→	Limited procedure (i.e., endoscopic temporal lift) Upper lid browpexy
	b) Rhytidectomy	→	Lateral browlift through temporal aspect of facelift incision
4) Brow ptosis	With or without rhytidectomy	→	Coronal browlift Anterior hairline browlift for high (>5–6 cm) forehead Endoscopic browlift

*An array of soft tissue fillers/substitutes (i.e., collagen replacement products, fat injections, liquid injectable silicone) can also be utilized.

BIBLIOGRAPHY

1. Adamson PA, Johnson CM Jr, Anderson JR, Dupin CL. The forehead lift: a review. Arch Otolaryngol 111:325, 1985.
2. Artz JS, Dinner MI, Foglietti MA. Planning the aesthetic foreheadplasty. Ann Plast Surg 25:1, 1990.
3. Bames HO. Frown disfigurement and ptosis of the eyebrows. Plast Reconstr Surg 19: 337, 1957.
4. Bruck JD, Baker TJ, Gordon H. Facial mimics and the coronal brow lift. Aesthetic Plast Surg 11:199, 1987.
5. Castanares S. Forehead wrinkles, glabellar frown and ptosis of the eyebrows. Plast Reconstr Surg 34:406, 1964.
6. Connell BF, Marten TJ. The male foreheadplasty: recognizing and treating aging in the upper face. Clin Plast Surg 18:653, 1991.
7. Guyuron B. Subcutaneous approach to forehead, brow and modified temple incision. Clin Plast Surg 19:461, 1992.
8. Kaye BL. The forehead lift: a useful adjunct to face lift and blepharoplasty. Plast Reconstr Surg 60:161, 1977.
9. MacGregor FC. Social, psychological and cultural dimensions of cosmetic and reconstructive plastic surgery. Aesth Plast Surg 13:1, 1989.
10. Matarasso A. Endoscopically assisted forehead-brow rhytidoplasty: theory and practice. Aesth Plast Surg 19:141, 1995.
11. Peterson RA. The custom face lift: design and maintenance, an opinion. Clin Plast Surg 19:415, 1992.
12. Pitanguy I. Section of the frontalis-procerus-corrugator aponeurosis in the correction of frontal and glabellar wrinkles. Ann Plast Surg 2:422, 1979.
13. Pitanguy I. Indications for and treatment of frontal and glabellar wrinkles in an analysis of 3404 consecutive cases of rhytidectomy. Plast Reconstr Surg 67:157, 1981.
14. Pitanguy I. Aesthetic Plastic Surg of Head and Body. Berlin-Heidelberg: Springer-Verlag, p. 202, 1981.
15. Pitanguy I, Bretano JM, Salgado F, Radwanski HN, Carpeggiani R. Incisions in primary and secondary rhytidoplasties. Rev Bras Cir 85:165, 1995.
16. Rees TD. Aesthetic Plastic Surg. First edition. Philadelphia, W.B. Saunders, Vol. 2, p. 731, 1980.
17. Matarasso A, Hutchinson O. Evaluating rejuvenation of the forehead and brow: an algorithm for selecting the appropriate technique. Plast Reconstr Surg. Sept 2000.
18. Matarasso A. Endoscopic surgical correction fo glabellar creases. Dermatologic Surgery 21:695, 1995. (Cited in Yearbook of Dermatologic Surgery, Mosby-Year Book, Chicago, IL, 1997.)

33

Combination Cosmetic Procedures

William P. Coleman, III
Tulane University School of Medicine, New Orleans, Louisiana

Many patients, often from an early age, anticipate that one day they will have a facelift. Intrinsic to this notion is the concept that one procedure (facelift) will take care of all their cosmetic concerns. Experienced cosmetic surgeons, however, are well aware that each patient presents with a unique set of aesthetic problems. In almost all cases, several separate procedures are required to obtain the best cosmetic result. The latter half of the 20th century has spawned a great number of new surgical techniques for cosmetic rejuvenation. During any aesthetic consultation, the surgeon must carefully educate the potential patient on the options available and the sequence in which they best would be used. The informed patient should recognize that cosmetic surgery is not a one-time event, but rather a process of various interventions to delay or reverse the natural aging process.

STRATEGIES FOR COMBINATION COSMETIC SURGERY

Cosmetic procedures can be used simultaneously (at the same time on the same part of the body), segmentally (at the same time on different parts of the body), or sequentially (at several different surgeries) [1]. The main reason for using procedures at the same time is to allow simultaneous recovery as well as to limit exposure to anesthesia and the general trauma of surgery. However, attempting too much surgery at the same time may expose the patient to more complications. Wound healing is compromised by exceeding the patient's capacity for recovering from multiple injuries. The surgeon must educate the patient and temper enthusiasm for convenience at the expense of safety.

Practical concerns may also dictate whether procedures can be performed at the same time. For instance, the elastic garments required after liposuction of the neck would irritate facial skin healing from a chemical peel or laser resurfacing. The surgeon must consider the details not only of the surgical procedure but the post-surgical plan as well before deciding whether or not to combine two procedures.

Procedures that have specific risks should not be combined with others that have similar risks. For instance, abdominoplasty has a finite risk of thromboembolism. Combining this procedure with vascular surgery, such as sclerotherapy or ambulatory phlebectomy, may not be wise.

Procedures that are difficult to combine during one surgical session can be separated by a few days so that the patient will still have the advantage of simultaneous recovery. For instance, soft-tissue augmentation can be performed several days after laser resurfacing or chemical peeling. In fact, the increased vascularity in the resurfaced skin may enhance the take of a tissue filler.

The variety of options available to the surgeon in combining cosmetic procedures is practically endless. However, before embarking on this course, it is wise to plan the sequence carefully and be sure the patient is well informed and participates in the planning process. Often a sense of partnership emerges between the patient and the surgeon as this process evolves, resulting in a sense of mutual satisfaction.

COMMON COMBINATION COSMETIC SURGICAL PROCEDURES

Combining Resurfacing Techniques

With the advent of laser resurfacing, many surgeons falsely assumed that chemical peeling and dermabrasion would disappear. In fact, in many ways laser resurfacing has only served to enhance the popularity of these other techniques. Laser resurfacing, chemical peeling, and dermabrasion each provide unique advantages and disadvantages for skin resurfacing. Combining these procedures allows the surgeon to maximize the advantages of each one while minimizing their disadvantages. Furthermore, each of these procedures can be used more or less aggressively to allow even more flexibility.

Superficial chemical peeling must typically be used on several occasions to obtain a visible cosmetic result. Recovery from superficial chemical peeling, however, is quite rapid and often requires little down time. When a patient is undergoing a variety of cosmetic procedures, superficial peeling can often be used at the same time as another procedure but on a different part of the body. For instance, a patient who returns two or three times a year for soft-tissue augmentation or BOTOX treatments might have simultaneous superficial peeling of the extremities during each of these visits. This combination of minimal morbidity procedures allows the patient to return to public life rapidly after each treatment while gradually improving in appearance.

Medium-depth chemical peeling, on the other hand, typically requires a week away from work or social activities. This procedure can often be combined with other techniques that require similar down time. Many patients who might benefit from skin resurfacing have significant rhytides of the upper lip and periorbital areas with only medium photodamage of the rest of the face. In these cases, full-face laser resurfacing would unnecessarily expose most of the facial skin to a deep resurfacing procedure with its attendant potential complications, slow recovery, and expense. Instead, medium-depth chemical peeling can be used over most of the face with CO_2 laser resurfacing only of the eyelids and/or lip (Fig. 1).

It is important when combining these two modalities to peel first and use the laser second. If the peeling solution overlaps the lasered skin deeper injury results and scarring is possible. In combination resurfacing cases, although the lasered skin heals more slowly than the peeled skin, there is usually a nice eventual blending that avoids lines of demarcation. It is important to use the laser only in single anatomic units and not overlap onto the cheeks. Alternatively, such patients could be treated

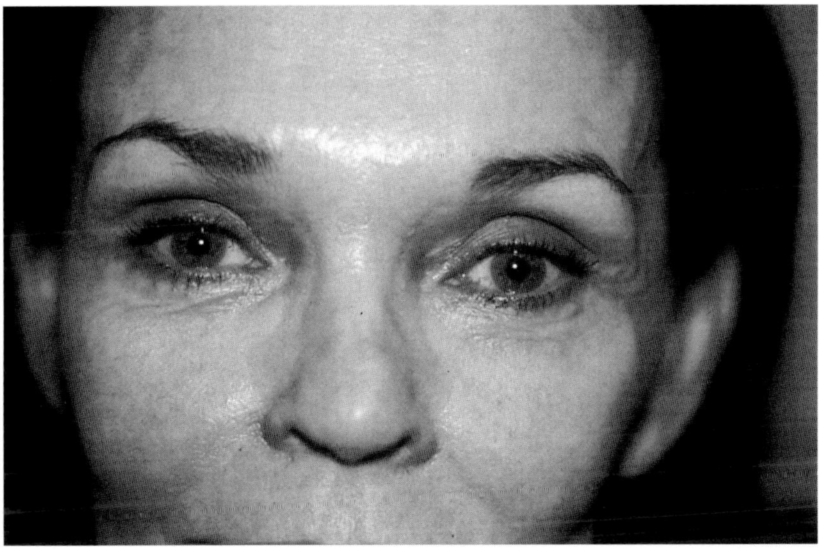

(a)

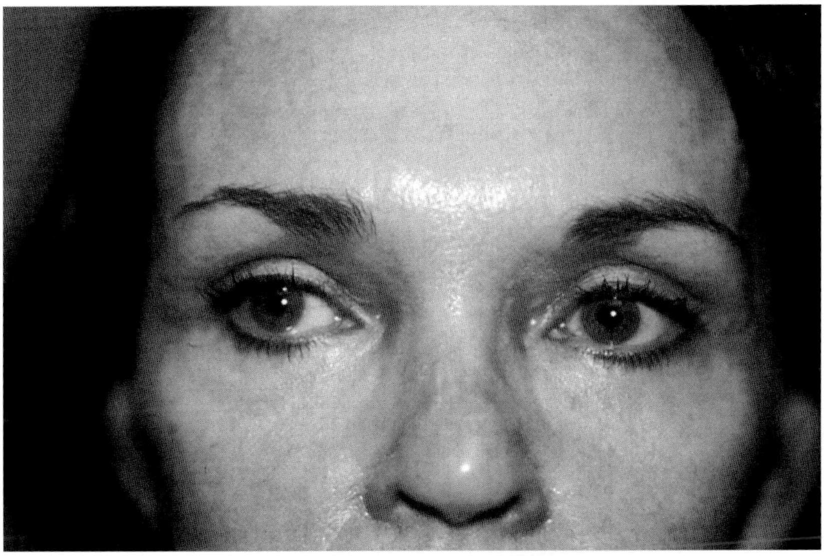

(b)

FIGURE 1 (a) Before and 6 months after laser resurfacing (b) of the lower eyelids with medium-depth chemical peel of the less-damaged rest of the face.

with an Erbium:YAG laser resurfacing over most of the face with CO_2 laser resurfacing of the lips and/or eyelids.

Chemical peeling of a variety of depths can also be used at the same time. Deep chemical peeling using Bakers phenol solution is an excellent approach for upper lip rhytides. Deep peeling can be limited to this area or perhaps also used on the eyelids with medium deep peeling used over the rest of the face. Below the mandible, superficial peeling can be used to avoid a line of demarcation while improving the color of sun-damaged cervical skin.

Wire brush or diamond fraise dermabrasion usually provides excellent improvement of acne scars, traumatic scars, and severe photodamage. It is still unclear whether or not CO_2 laser resurfacing improves acne scars as well as dermabrasion. Many patients present with significant acne scarring of the cheeks and chin with photodamage and aging changes of the rest of the face. In these cases, dermabrasion can be used for the acne-scarred areas, remaining within cosmetic units. The rest of the face can then be treated with medium-depth chemical peeling or CO_2 laser resurfacing (Fig. 2). A common combination in these patients includes dermabrasion of the cheeks and chin, laser resurfacing of the upper lip and eyelids, and chemical peeling of the forehead, brows, nose, and neck. These kinds of combinations allow the surgeon to take advantage of the benefits of each of these procedures while allowing simultaneous healing.

Manual dermabrasion has become increasingly popular in recent years [2]. This more superficial form of dermabrasion can easily be combined with either chemical peeling or laser resurfacing. Manual dermabrasion can be used after TCA peels on areas that require deeper treatment. In patients who desire improvement of the lower eyelids only, manual dermabrasion can be used at the periphery of CO_2-lasered lower lids to feather the resurfacing. (Alternatively, laser resurfacing can be performed at different depths to allow a similar feathering effect.)

Combining Blepharoplasty or Rhytidectomy and Resurfacing

The recent development of deep plane facelifts may allow the skin to retain enough vascularity to endure an additional external insult from resurfacing. However, this is still not a universally held view. In general, facelifting and skin muscle flap blepharoplasty are performed several months apart from resurfacing procedures to avoid complications. Many patients will benefit from this sequential approach because blepharoplasty and facelift do not address the quality of skin, only the quantity.

The recent popularity of transconjunctival blepharoplasty, however, has increased the practice of simultaneous laser resurfacing. CO_2 laser resurfacing can safely be performed immediately after transconjunctival blepharoplasty without increased risks of scarring (see p. 792).

Laser resurfacing can also be combined with traditional facelifting when it is restricted to the areas not undermined. A common combination is resurfacing of the upper lip and lower eyelids performed during the same surgical session as the facelift. The advantage to this is that patients can heal from these two procedures at the same time.

Facelifting or blepharoplasty can be combined with medium-depth chemical peeling of the extremities or trunk. Peeling of this depth in nonfacial areas often requires a week or more of recovery. This can be ideally combined with significant facial surgery to allow simultaneous healing.

Combining Facial Surgery with Body Liposuction

Many patients with limited vacation time may ask to have as much treated as possible at the same time. The main surgical objection to this is the potential risk of increased

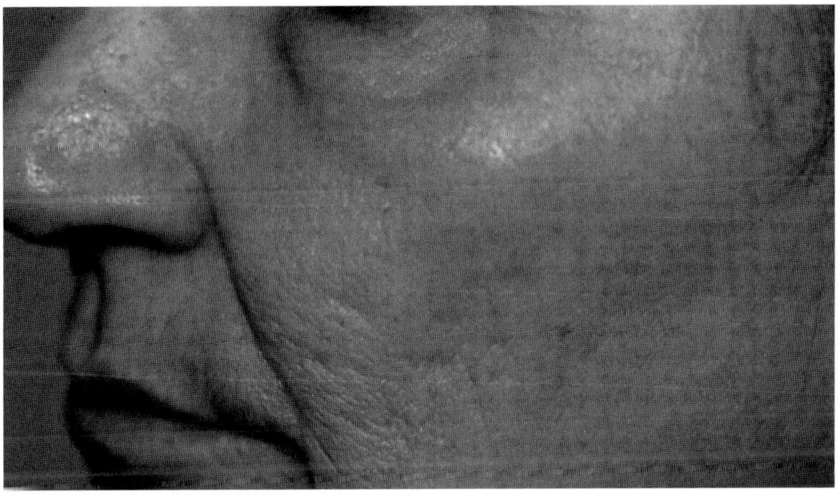

(a)

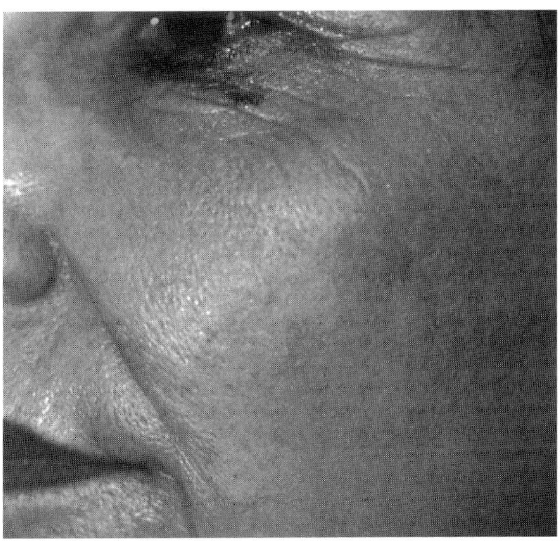

(b)

Figure 2 (a) Before and 1 year after dermabrasion (b) of the cheeks and medium-depth chemical peeling of the rest of the face.

anesthesia time. Also, physician fatigue may reduce the precision of the second procedure. In general, extensive body liposuction should not be combined with face-lifting. However, more limited facial procedures can easily be performed at the same time as body liposuction. In addition, facelifting and minimal liposuction may safely be combined.

Blepharoplasty and liposuction of the neck are a common combination. These procedures can both be performed under local anesthesia and surgical fatigue is usually not an issue. Postsurgically, neck liposuction requires wearing an elastic garment for 3 or more days, whereas blepharoplasty patients are often not ready for public appearance for several days after surgery. This simultaneous recovery is an advantage.

Full-face facial resurfacing may be combined with liposuction of the trunk or extremities. However, this should be reserved for patients with strong constitutions. Although both procedures can be performed under local anesthesia or with mild sedation, the simultaneous recovery may be too much for some individuals. This is especially true with CO_2 laser resurfacing. Medium-depth chemical peeling is well tolerated after surgery and can easily be combined with liposuction elsewhere on the body.

Combining Soft-Tissue Augmentation with Other Cosmetic Procedures

Resurfacing procedures that extend down into the dermis cannot be combined with dermal augmentation simultaneously. However, once the dermis has regenerated, soft-tissue augmentation can be used while the skin is still healing. Subcutaneous augmentation materials, such as fat, can be injected several days after medium-depth chemical peeling or laser resurfacing. The increased vascularity of the healing skin appears to support the viability of the implanted fat (Fig. 3). Because the fat is injected subcutaneously and not into the dermis, this technique can be used as soon as swelling has subsided and the contours can be determined.

BOTOX deinervation is quite useful immediately before skin resurfacing. Paralyzing the active facial muscles before resurfacing allows the skin to heal with minimal movement. Thus, the impressions in the skin formed by muscle activity are diminished and do not return as rapidly [3].

Soft-tissue augmentation of the lower face is often combined simultaneously with BOTOX treatment of the upper face. Dermal augmentation of the periorbital rhytides has diminished in popularity since the introduction of BOTOX. Softform, GoreTex, Zyderm Collagen, Fat Transplantation, Dermolagen, etc., can be used in the nasolabial furrows and/or chin areas whereas BOTOX is injected into the forehead, medial brows, and canthal regions. Because both of these procedures require minimal recovery, they are ideally suited for a combination approach. Patients who are on a monthly program of superficial facial chemical peels can also undergo these procedures at the same time.

Soft-tissue augmentation is also commonly performed simultaneously with body liposuction. When fat transplantation and/or lipocytic dermal augmentation are used, the fat can be extracted by syringe before beginning machine liposuction and then reinjected during the same surgical session. Typically, additional fat is also extracted for freezing and subsequent injection. Physicians who use fat transplantation often extract fat to be saved for possible later injection during most liposuction procedures. Because the fat can be stored quite safely for at least 6 months, the patient can decide whether or not to use the banked fat at any time during this period.

Soft-tissue augmentation is also commonly used simultaneously with treatment of benign skin lesions. Laser techniques for vascular or pigmented lesions can easily be combined with soft-tissue augmentation of other areas. Soft-tissue augmentation is also commonly combined with excision of dermal or subcutaneous lesions, cryosurgery, and electrosurgery.

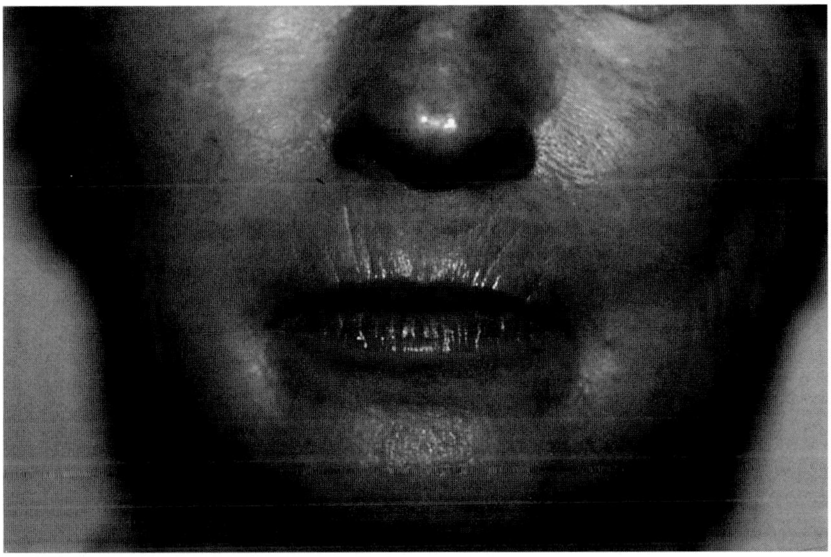

(a)

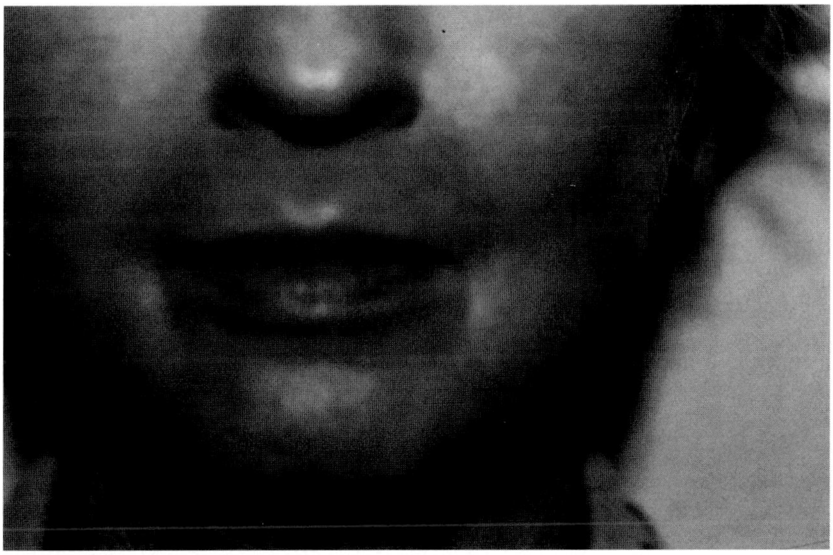

(b)

FIGURE 3 (a) Before and 6 months after laser resurfacing (b) with fat transplantation of the cheeks performed 1 week after laser.

Combining Hair Transplantation with Other Procedures

Cosmetic procedures that do not involve the scalp can conveniently be combined with hair transplantation. This allows the patient the convenience of simultaneous recovery from two or more procedures. Because most hair transplantation is performed under local anesthesia, there is no risk of adding additional minor procedures.

Blepharoplasty and hair transplantation are a useful combination of procedures. Many men over 40 years of age can benefit from blepharoplasty as well as hair restoration. Many blepharoplasty patients can return to public life within 5 to 7 days. When performed simultaneously with hair transplantation, they can hide from the public for this short time and obtain two cosmetic improvements with one recovery.

Although liposuction of the neck is often indicated in many men who present for hair transplantation, the surgeon must be sure that the postsurgical elastic dressings required for cervical liposuction do not impede the healing from the hair transplantation procedure. Although full scalp dressings are often used after hair transplantation, the neck elastic garment may shift and potentially loosen grafts after surgery. Liposuction of the body can easily be combined with hair transplantation. Neither procedure causes a great deal of postsurgical discomfort and the combination is tolerable. However, when local anesthesia is used, the surgeon must be sure that the safe levels of plasma lidocaine are not exceeded. When liposuction is performed using the tumescent technique, lidocaine, which is lipophyllic, does not cause significant elevations in plasma levels even when doses of up to 55 mg/kg are used [4].

However, lidocaine physiology has not been well studied for facial and scalp work. Generally, tumescent anesthesia used for hair transplantation does not exceed 7 mg/kg [5]. This is the original published safe dose for more concentrated lidocaine infiltration. However, the surgeon must be keenly aware of the potential for lidocaine toxicity when extensive liposuction and hair transplantation are combined.

Hair transplantation is also commonly combined with removal of benign skin lesions, superficial chemical peeling of nonfacial skin, soft-tissue augmentation and other minor procedures. Male patients are notoriously eager to minimize visits to the physician's office and appreciate a combined recovery from multiple procedures when it is feasible and safe.

Intrinsically Combined Procedures

The number of surgical procedures that combine a variety of techniques on the same anatomical area is increasing. The notion of conservatively using a variety of techniques at the same time instead of aggressively using one to accomplish the same task is attractive. However, the surgeon must be certain that the combination is not used in such a way as to cause overlapping complications.

Cook's combined neck approach uses liposuction, platysma muscle repair, augmentation with a chin implant, and subdermal laser resurfacing all performed at the same time [6]. This combination of a variety of techniques allows the surgeon to overcome the disadvantages of one of these used alone. For instance, liposuction of the neck in many individuals may not achieve sufficient skin tightening to allow complete redraping. The addition of the chin implant to provide superior tension as well as laser resurfacing for skin tightening makes this combined procedure more effective than liposuction alone. However, when using this technique the surgeon must be certain not to be too aggressive with any of the components. This could lead to too much tightening resulting in scarring or dehiscence of the submental incision.

The combination of transconjunctival blepharoplasty and CO_2 laser resurfacing has become quite popular in recent years. There is apparently no significant risk of scarring from combining these approaches because the skin is not undermined. The combined effect of subcutaneous fat removal with skin resurfacing allows improvement of both the contour of the eyelids as well as the skin appearance. Using either one of the procedures alone does not accomplish the same degree of improvement. This is a particularly satisfying approach for surgeons who have performed blepharoplasty without resurfacing for many years but have been unable to satisfy patient complaints of failing to remove fine rhytides.

Primum Non Nocere

The first job of the physician is to do no harm. Although it is often convenient for the patient and the physician to combine multiple procedures, safety must be the primary guiding principle. When convenience and safety conflict then convenience must be sacrificed. There are countless possible combinations of cosmetic surgical procedures. Certainly, this number will grow as new techniques appear on the horizon. Undoubtedly, the simultaneous use of multiple procedures on the same anatomical area will also increase.

However, there will also likely remain many patients who are happy to correct one problem at a time. This allows them the benefit of judging the effects of one change on their appearance and self image before proceeding to another surgery. Many patients have one major flaw that is quite distressing to them. Once this flaw is corrected they are quite happy with the remainder of their appearance even though they may have significant aesthetic problems elsewhere. Surgeons must keep in mind that the decision for cosmetic surgery is a partnership and not allow enthusiasm or confidence in skill to override the wishes of the patient. True satisfaction and happiness from a cosmetic surgical practice is dependent on happy patients. What makes each person happy is quite different from what makes another happy. The best surgeons offer their patients a variety of possible approaches for improving their appearance and use these in a skillful and thoughtful manner.

REFERENCES

1. Coleman WP III, Narins RS. Combining surgical methods for skin resurfacing. Sem Cut Med Surg 15:194–199, 1996.
2. Harris DR, Noodleman FR. Combining manual dermabrasion with low strength trichloroacetic acid to improve actinically injured skin. J Dermatol Surg Oncol 20:436–442, 1994.
3. Carruthers J, Carruthers A. Combining botulinum toxin injection and laser resurfacing for facial rhytides. In: Coleman WP, Lawrence N, eds. Skin Resurfacing. Baltimore: Williams and Wilkins, 1998, pp. 235–243.
4. Ostad A, Kageyama N, Moy RL. Tumescent anesthesia with a lidocaine dose of 55 mg/kg is safe for liposuction. Dermatol Surg 22:921–927, 1996.
5. Coleman WP III, Klein JA. The use of the tumescent technique for hair transplantation, dermabrasion, and soft-tissue surgery. J Dermatol Surg Oncol 18:130–135, 1992.
6. Cook WR. Laser neck and jowl liposculpture including platysma laser resurfacing, dermal laser resurfacing, and vaporization of subcutaneous fat. Dermatol Surg 23:1143–1148, 1997.

34

Hair Transplantation with Alopecia Reduction

Walter P. Unger
University of Toronto, Toronto, Ontario, Canada

Paul C. Cotterill
Private Practice, Toronto, Ontario, Canada

The field of hair transplantation and alopecia reduction (AR) has changed substantially over the last decade. Numerous new instruments, techniques, and objectives are now routinely being used, providing for an increased number of patient and physician options. This chapter will deal briefly with many alternatives; however, our specific approach will be described in more detail. The reader is advised to refer to one of the major hair transplantation textbooks for a more in-depth description of alternative approaches [1,2].

HAIR TRANSPLANTATION

History

Modern-day hair transplantation and its popularization began with Norman Orentreich, a New York dermatologist, who in 1959 published a paper describing the use of small autografts that were used to study various types of alopecias. Among his findings was a phenomenon that he termed "donor dominance" in male pattern baldness (MPB). Specifically, he found that if a small graft was taken from the hair-bearing rim of a patient with MPB and transplanted into the alopecic area, after an initial effluvium the hair would grow back and persist in its new site [3]. (The first publication on successful hair transplantation dates back to an 1822 doctoral thesis by a German physician named Dieffenbach [4]. He in turn credited his teacher, Carl Unger, with the concept.) From 1959 until the 1980s, round "standard" grafts, 4 to 5 mm in diameter, were used almost exclusively to treat alopecic areas of the scalp. In the early 1980s Nordstrom and Marritt introduced 1 to 2 hair "micrografts" to refine the front hairline [5,6] and Bradshaw began dividing 4-mm punch grafts into smaller "quarter" and "half" grafts containing 2 to 4 follicles that were transplanted into scalpel blade incisions—the first "slit" grafts [7]. The main advantages of the smaller grafts was the minimization of the short-term "plugginess," which was inherent in the use of the standard sized grafts, and a correspondingly more natural appearance with fewer sessions and/or lower hair density objectives.

The most common reason for performing hair transplantation is for the surgical correction of MPB in men. However, hair transplantation can also be beneficial for women with female pattern alopecia [8,9]; eyebrow, eyelash [10], and mustache transplantation [11]; and cicatricial alopecia secondary to trauma, rhytidectomy, inactive dermatoses, and burns [12].

Presurgical Consultation/Consideration

The initial interview between the patient and physician for assessment of hair restoration should never be hurried. It is important to weigh carefully the patient's objectives against the present as well as future donor/recipient area ratio and to establish realistic goals that are acceptable to him/her. For treatment of MPB an educated estimate of its eventual severity must be made (Fig. 1). It should be based on the patient's age, family history, and presenting physical findings. It is generally inadvisable to treat a patient under 25 years of age because the younger the individual the more difficult it is to predict future hair loss. However, the degree of psychological distress caused by MPB may in some instances make treatment as early as the late teens advisable [13].

One of the most common reasons for a poor result in hair transplantation is improper long-term planning. Certain principles should be followed when dealing with the younger patient: (1) assume the worst reasonable scenario (most patients will not develop Type VI or VII MPB before their eighties, so all patients should not be treated as if they will); (2) always plan to leave some permanent donor hair in reserve for future use; (3) limit the size of the recipient area to be transplanted to the anterior one third or two thirds of the scalp unless AR is used or will be used in the future (do not put grafts into areas you plan to excise later); (4) limit yourself to micrografts and minigrafts in order to produce natural-looking results while conserving donor tissue, because these types of grafts also minimize any damage to existing hair in the recipient region (Fig. 2); and (5) transplant areas that are still hair-bearing but can be reasonably anticipated to lose hair in the future. Thus one avoids a seemingly never-ending chasing of an enlarging bald area (Fig. 3).

Hair texture, frizz, curl, color, and skin type must also be considered. Generally, the finer the texture the less contrast there is between graft hair and the surrounding scalp or residual thinning hair. Thus, fine hair is advantageous for the treatment of "early" MPB if density objectives are relatively low. A more feathered and natural-looking result can also be achieved with the use of fine-haired micrografts in the hairline zone. (The finest hair can often be found in the temporal and inferior occipital areas). At the other end of the spectrum of hair type, kinky Negroid-type hair or frizzy hair can give the appearance of more density and allows for the use of fewer grafts and/or sessions to achieve the appearance of good density. Curly hair always produces a denser-looking result when compared with the same number of straight hairs in a given area. The less contrast between hair color and skin color the better. For example, lighter colored hair produces a denser appearance than dark

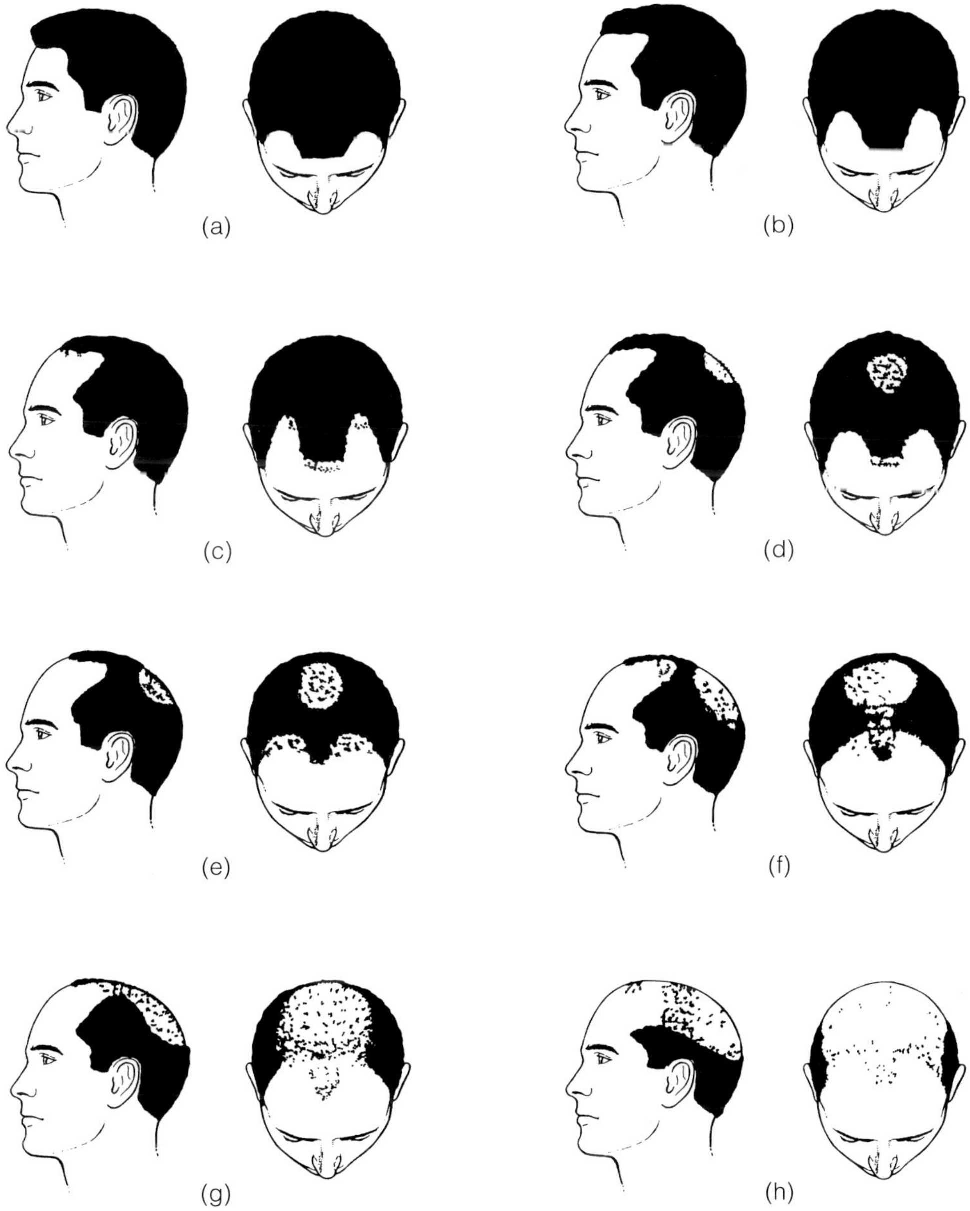

FIGURE 1A Norwood Classification of Male Pattern Baldness.

colored hair against light-colored scalp. The best colors for Caucasians, in decreasing order of preference, are white, "salt and pepper," blond, light brown or red, and darker brown to black.

Various techniques are available to assess donor-hair density, and the number of grafts that can be produced from donor strips. Table 1 is a sample outline of the

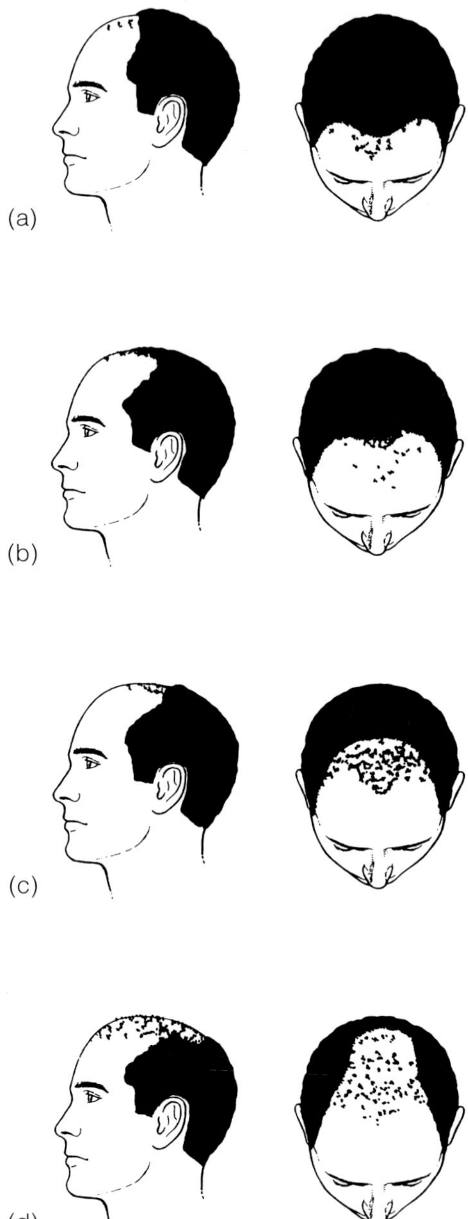

FIGURE 1B Norwood Classification for Type A variant Male Pattern Baldness.

length of the donor strip required for different numbers of mini/micrografts [14], assuming the use of a triple bladed knife with 2 mm spacers and average hair density. Grafts with more and/or denser hair are best used 2 to 3 cm posterior to the most anterior hairs in the hairline zone. Those with finer and/or fewer hairs are used in creating the hairline zone, the whorl of the vertex, and the part side of the area of MPB.

(a)

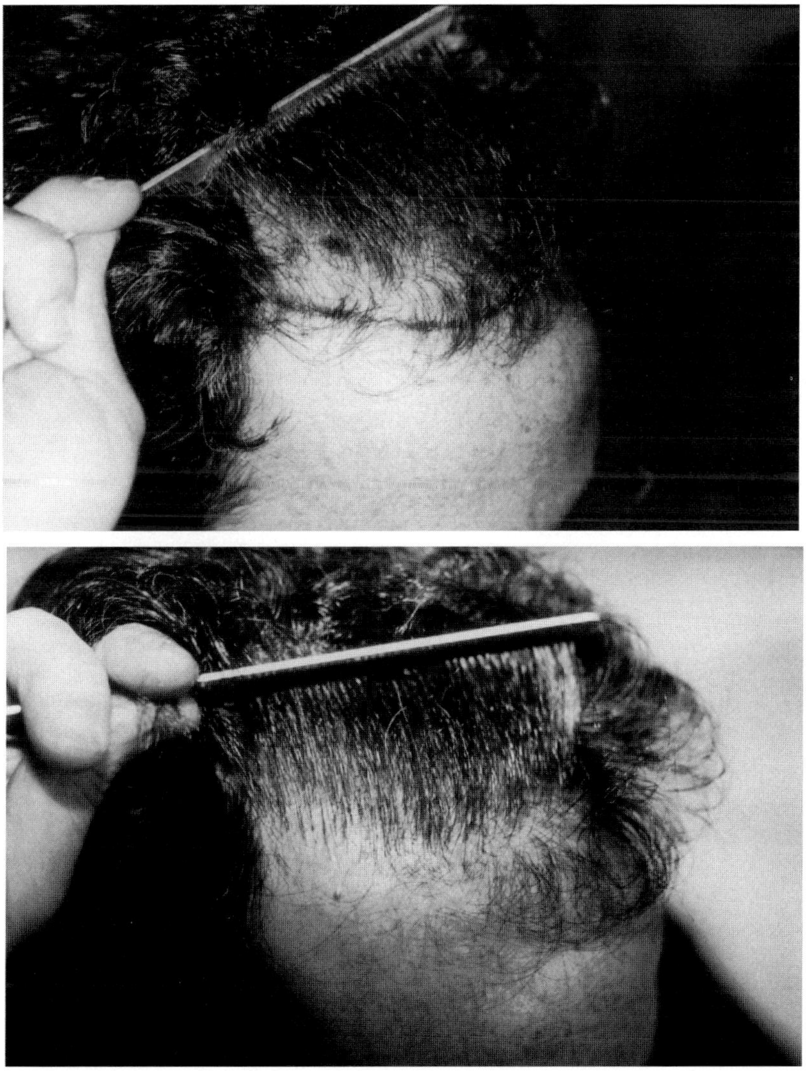

(b)

FIGURE 2 (a) Patient D.S. before treatment. The patient only wanted one surgery of subtle thickening and to conserve existing hair. (b) One year after a single session of 203 micrografts, 163 "Beaver" grafts, and 222 small slit grafts.

Hairline Design

It is a good idea to use a black grease pencil to draw a suggested hairline on the patient during the first consultation. This ensures that the patient has a clear understanding of what you are recommending. A hairline that is designed poorly (eg, too low, too high, or too rounded in the frontotemporal recessions) is one of the most common causes of a poor cosmetic result in hair transplantation. The physician and patient must keep in mind that the chosen hairline must be suitable for the present,

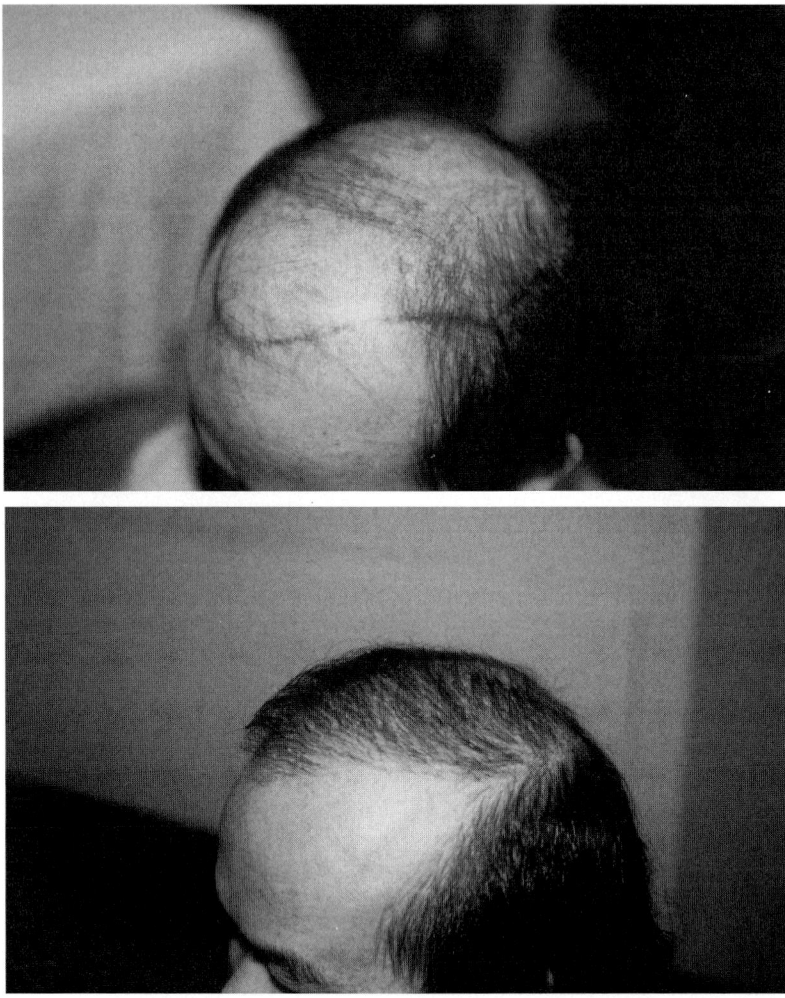

(a)

(b)

FIGURE 3 (a) Patient before first session. Patient wanted a light coverage of hair and only one session. Notice black grease pencil line denoting hairline extending into lateral ledge of existing hair-bearing area. Patient has less than ideal hair characteristics, ie, black, straight, sparse, coarse hair with extensive thinning. (b) One year after one session of 210 micrografts and 400 "Beaver" grafts. The result is a thin, feathered appearance that has extended into the lateral ledge in order to anticipate future thinning. The patient has the option of further sessions for added density.

but that it will also be the hairline when he is in his sixties, seventies, eighties, and beyond.

The midline anterior-most point of the hairline generally begins 8 to 11 cm above the midglabellar line at approximately the place where the forehead goes into transition from being more or less vertical to sloping gradually posteriorly [14]. The anterior/superior most temporal points are then chosen based on the prognosis for

TABLE 1 Example of Requirements of Donor Strip Length and Spacing

Desired number of grafts	Required length of 4-mm wide strip			
	Single	1.00 mm	1.25 mm	1.5 mm
50	1.25 cm	2 cm	3 cm	4 cm
100	2.50 cm	4 cm	6 cm	8 cm
150	3.75 cm	6 cm	9 cm	12 cm
200	5 cm	8 cm	12 cm	16 cm

Strip taken with triple bladed knife, and 2 mm spacers.
These measurements are for patients with average donor density (18–22 hairs in a 4 mm circle).
Adjustment Factor: Reduce 10% of total length if hair density is >22. Increase 10% if hair density is <18.
Source: Ref. 21.

their ultimate location when MPB is fully developed (Fig. 4). The specific location of points A, B, and C are modified depending on the patient's individual facial features, age, hair characteristics, and goals [14]. The hairline when viewed laterally should run more or less horizontally from the anterior midline point. By accentuating a bell shape to the hairline or using an AR to raise the anterior/superior most temporal points [14], the midline point may be moved superiorly in order to decrease the length of the area of MPB to be treated without losing the horizontal orientation of the hairline.

As noted earlier, when constructing the hairline zone the surgeon is attempting to create a subtle irregular-shaped zone that begins with relatively sparse hair that gradually becomes denser and coarser as one moves more posteriorly. This is done by using the finest textured one-hair grafts most anteriorly followed by one to two hair grafts posterior to them and then grafts with gradually denser and coarser hair as one moves still further posteriorly (Fig. 5). Rose has described four components of natural hairlines that warrant attention and with which we agree: (1) an undulating line, (2) an uneven dispersion of hair, (3) variable hair density at different points along the hairline, and (4) random hairs anterior to the main body of the hairline zone [15].

Despite attempting to treat future areas of alopecia, perfect prognostication in all patients is an impossibility. Thus the development of alopecic alleys between the superior margin of the tempoparietal hair and the most medial grafts can occur as the MPB progresses with age. There are a variety of options available to deal with this eventuality:

1. Place micro- and minigrafts into the lateral borders of the recipient area (Fig. 5). If it extends beyond your prognosis it will simply look like a large isolated frontal forelock (IFF) [16].
2. Design an IFF (Fig. 6) whose purpose is to break up the expansive bald area between the left and right temporoparietal areas, but intentionally leaves the alopecic alleys untransplanted.
3. Include AR in the treatment plan to excise thinning alleys.

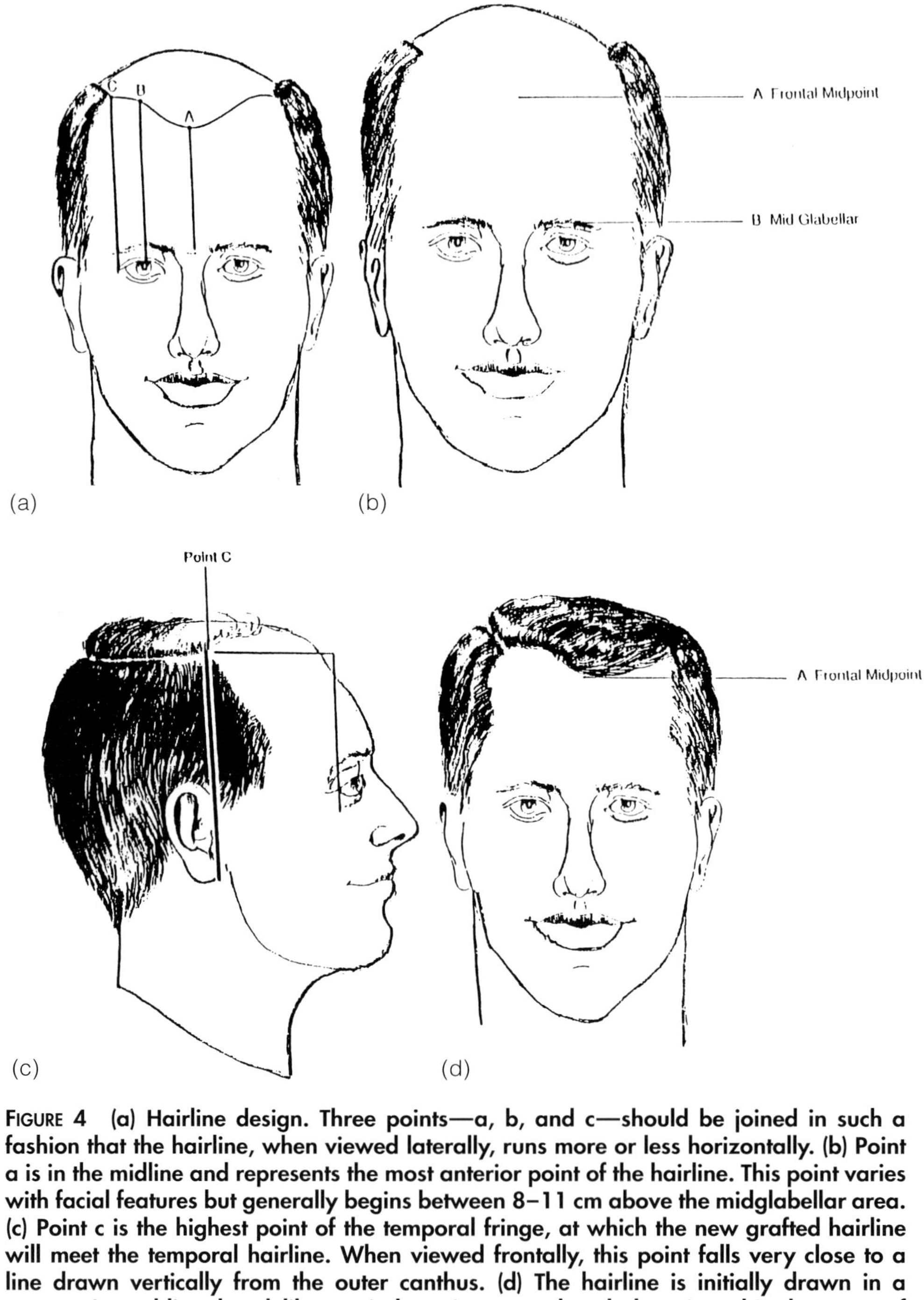

FIGURE 4 (a) Hairline design. Three points—a, b, and c—should be joined in such a fashion that the hairline, when viewed laterally, runs more or less horizontally. (b) Point a is in the midline and represents the most anterior point of the hairline. This point varies with facial features but generally begins between 8–11 cm above the midglabellar area. (c) Point c is the highest point of the temporal fringe, at which the new grafted hairline will meet the temporal hairline. When viewed frontally, this point falls very close to a line drawn vertically from the outer canthus. (d) The hairline is initially drawn in a symmetric oval line, but deliberate indentations are placed along it and in the areas of the temporal recess [21].

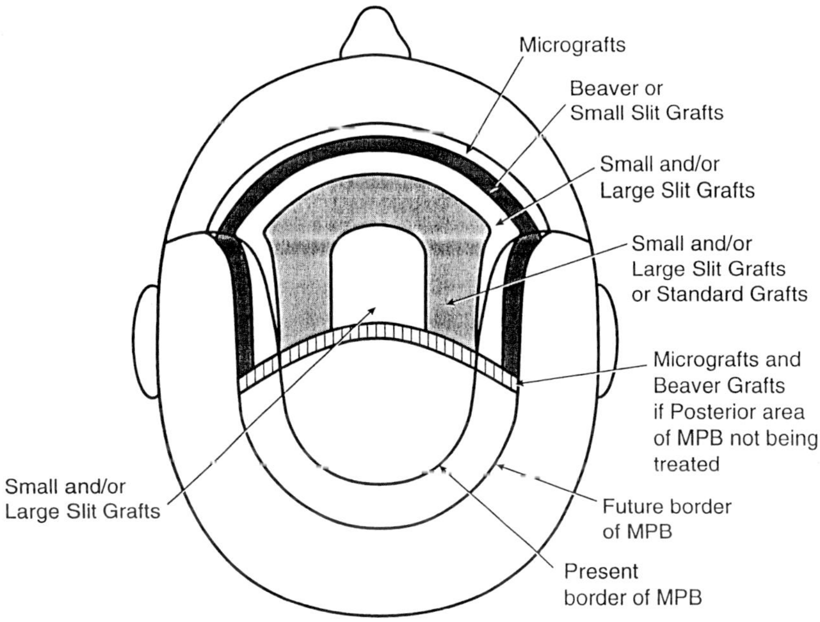

FIGURE 5 General distribution of various graft types. An attempt is made to recreate a natural-appearing hairline by using small 1–2 hair grafts most anteriorly blending in to somewhat larger grafts as one moves more posteriorly. Note also that 2–4 hair minigrafts are used at lateral and posterior borders. If MPB later progresses beyond your original prognosis, a natural-looking large isolated frontal forelock will have been created.

Although some practitioners have recommended an IFF for virtually all patients [17], we feel it is an appropriate pattern only for older patients with limited objectives or very young patients in whom there is a reasonable likelihood of the development of Type VI or VII MPB. The appearance of only a frontal forelock is less than most young men want or can reasonably hope to accomplish. Studies by Unger et al. have shown that 13% of men by age 80 will develop Class VI MPB and only 11% Class VII MPB [18]. Thus more than 75% of men will develop Type V or less MPB. Furthermore, most Type VI patients can be converted with AR to Class IV or Class V. Additionally, Unger has shown that there is nearly always enough donor hair available to produce at least six sizable sessions of minigrafts and micrografts [18]. As such, many young men do not need to be limited to an IFF. Shiell and Stough have reported on a variation of the IFF that they have named a "cadre de cheveux" [19] in which the forelock pattern is extended more posteriorly to involve the mid-scalp area as well.

Another method aimed at framing of the face but without attempting to produce a frontal tuft is to create a "bridge" of micrografts and minigrafts [20] that spans the area between the left and right temporoparietal fringes. This can allow the patient to cautiously proceed with transplants without creating the need for further sessions, but leaves the option open for additional grafting anterior or posterior to the "bridge over troubled waters" if he so desires. The appearance is that of the "comb-over"

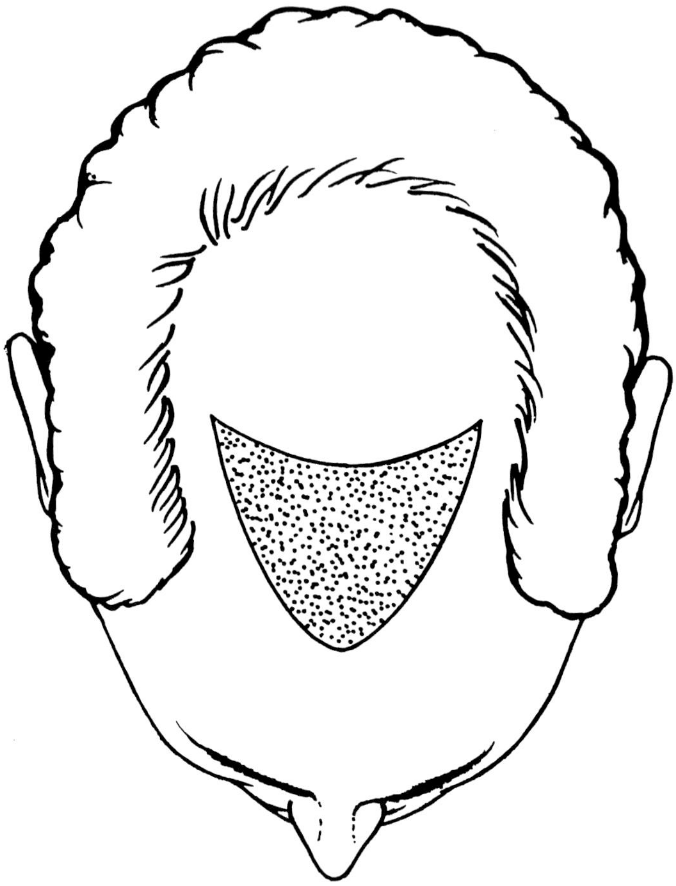

FIGURE 6 (a) Design of an isolated frontal forelock. Micrografts are generally placed at the periphery of the forelock with grafts of gradually increasing size as one moves progressively towards the central area. (b) Ultimate isolated frontal forelock with black grease pencil mark drawn on to show zones of differing sizes of grafts to be used. Note: No attempt is made to join the lateral fringe with the forelock [20].

technique that some patients use in combination with hair spray, but without its obvious and disturbing cosmetic subterfuge.

AR will be more fully dealt with in the second half of this chapter; however its role in long-term planning will be discussed at this point. In brief:

1. AR is advisable for patients who want maximum coverage. Generally speaking, it is wise to not attempt to transplant both frontal and vertex areas on any patient under the age of 40 years without planning to possibly use AR at some point—or without carrying out AR before transplanting of the vertex area [21].
2. AR is extremely useful in the treatment of any previously transplanted individual who has subsequently developed cosmetically unacceptable alopecic areas but lacks sufficient remaining donor areas to adequately transplant them.

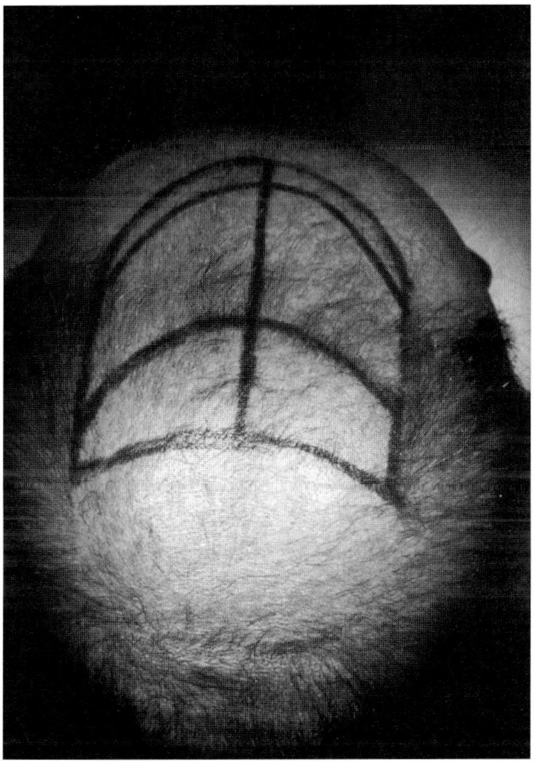

FIGURE 6 Continued.

3. It is always important to choose an AR pattern that will not leave a scar in an area that you are not planning to transplant in the future.

As implied above, AR may be performed before transplanting or between sessions. It is advisable to leave 3 to 6 weeks between AR and hair transplantation to allow adequate blood supply to return to the alopecic area, to enable the donor region to regain some of its laxity, and to allow grafts to be placed successfully into an AR scar.

When planning AR for MPB, it is wise not to aim to excise all the alopecic area because an abnormal hair direction at the midline (sometimes referred to as "parting of the Red Sea") will always occur. This cosmetic defect is difficult to transplant or correct. If a large area of alopecia can be decreased in width to approximately 5 to 6 cm then any remaining area can be treated with grafts that can be oriented to produce a more natural hair direction. The exception to this rule is aggressive scalp extension (Frechet), used to achieve rapid elimination of alopecic areas. Scalp extension intentionally leaves a slot defect that is corrected with the Frechet 3-Flap Slot Correction procedure [22]. Too many ARs can also negatively impact the hair density of prospective donor areas. However, with two or three modified major ARs [23] or their equivalent, there is rarely a significant reduction in hair density of the donor rim.

Graft Selection and Graft Numbers

Table 2 summarizes and defines the types of grafts currently being used in hair transplanting. All grafts are obtained by carefully sectioning various widths of excised strips of donor tissue.

As indicated, a micrograft always contains a single follicular unit. Each "follicular unit" typically contains one to two hairs but some have three, four, or even five hairs. In addition, the follicular units are sometimes grouped into "families" of two or more follicular units in close proximity to each other [24]. Transplanting only single follicular units is currently referred to as "follicular transplantation." The use of families of units has also been referred to as follicular transplantation, but these grafts contain the same number of hairs as the smaller types of minigrafts. The difference between follicular family grafts and minigrafts is that in the former there is less hairless tissue between the follicular units and therefore they can be placed into smaller recipient sites, which in turn can be placed closer together to produce greater density.

Micrografts and minigrafts are used to achieve the least amount of noticeable plugginess during the course of treatment and will generally produce less density per session. They are therefore ideal for the hairline zone and center of the whorl of the vertex, or to produce light, even coverage of a larger recipient area in a single session. Even the most experienced practitioners of follicular transplantation can produce only 126 hairs per cm^2 in four sessions [25], whereas the use of standard grafts can produce 207 hairs per cm^2 [26]. The reason for this is that no human has thus far successfully transplanted follicular units as close together as they occur in nature. On the other hand, a density of 80–100 hairs per cm^2 is adequate to produce cosmetically satisfactory results for a substantial majority of patients.

The use of a zone of standard round grafts is most suitable in the following circumstances: (1) patients who want maximum density and have good *long-term* donor/recipient area ratios; (2) patients with good hair characteristics, such as fine texture and/or light coloring; (3) those with some hair still present in the recipient region; (4) individuals who are aware and accept that they may need up to four

TABLE 2 Graft Terminology

	Number of hairs	Type of recipient site	Number of follicular units	Tissue removed
Micrograft (always a single follicular unit)	1–3	puncture hole	1	No
Large micrograft	2–3	small blade slit	2	No
Minigraft "small"	3–4	hole or slot	2–3	Yes
"large"	5–6	hole or slot	2–4	Yes
Slit graft "small"	3–4	blade slit	2–3	No
"large"	5–6	blade slit	2–4	No
Standard graft	8–30	3.0 + mm hole	6–22	Yes

sessions in the long run to fill in any circular alopecic spaces between the standard grafts that may result with ongoing hair loss, and (5) in combination with other graft types to repair cosmetically unsatisfactory older transplants in which standard grafts had been used. Because standard grafts are used in only 5 to 10% of our patients (excepting those seen for correcting unsatisfactory transplants), it will not be dealt with in great detail in this chapter. The reader is directed to current texts on hair transplantation for a more in-depth description [27]. It is important to note, however, that when they are used in patients with no preceding transplantation they are used only in a four to six graft wide band between zones of micro/minigrafting anterior, posterior, and lateral to them (Figs. 5, 7, 8).

Follicular transplanting or a combination of micrografts and minigrafts should be used if a male patient wants maximum undetectability after each session and is prepared for light to moderate hair density. With young patients, one can never be sure of the total extent of future hair loss. Aiming for less density in the recipient region requires the use of less donor tissue and allows conservation of the donor area for the future. Additionally, with slit grafts and micrografts, or follicular units, one can take advantage of any existing hair in the recipient region because none of it is removed during the creation of the recipient sites. This maximizes postsurgical camouflage as well as initial hair density. Finally, micrografts and minigrafts are ideal for recreating the whorl of the crown. Because there is no overlapping hair in the center of the whorl of the vertex, it is important to keep plugginess to a minimum. In our experience, the use of a combination of micrografts and minigrafts will produce more density per session than one consisting of micrografts or follicular units alone. If the size of minigrafts used is appropriate, it will not appear to be any pluggier than if only micrografts had been used, except perhaps on very close inspection.

As noted above, slit grafting and micrografting are advantageous when transplanted into areas containing hair because none of that hair is removed during the course of treatment. This approach is also especially appropriate for the female patient with female pattern thinning [8]. Because the pattern of thinning in women is more of a general diffuse thinning, without total hair loss, slit grafts, and micrografts augment density without disturbing existing hair, and can therefore produce quite thick-looking results (Fig. 9). In areas of female scalp hair loss, where there is generalized thinning with scattered small, totally alopecic spots, one uses a combination of micrografts, slit grafts, and small round grafts (where these spots have been punched out).

If micro- and minigrafts are used exclusively in the first one or two treatments, in order to take advantage of pre-existing hair, as the patient goes on to more complete loss of pre-existing hair, small circular minigrafts or "slot" grafts [created with special "slot punches" (Redfield Slot Punch, Montvale, NJ)] can be used in between the previously transplanted slit grafts (in areas that are now devoid of hair) in order to increase hair density. Bald skin, or potentially bald skin, is removed with the use of round grafts or slot grafts, but is not eliminated with the use of slit grafts and micrografting. One can therefore achieve greater density with the use of round grafts and slot grafts than with slit grafts and micrografts given the same amount of donor tissue. Slit grafts unfortunately can also produce a phenomenon referred to as "compression" or dense lines of hair that are as unsightly as "plugs"—especially if the hair is dark colored and/or coarse. This is because no tissue is being removed and

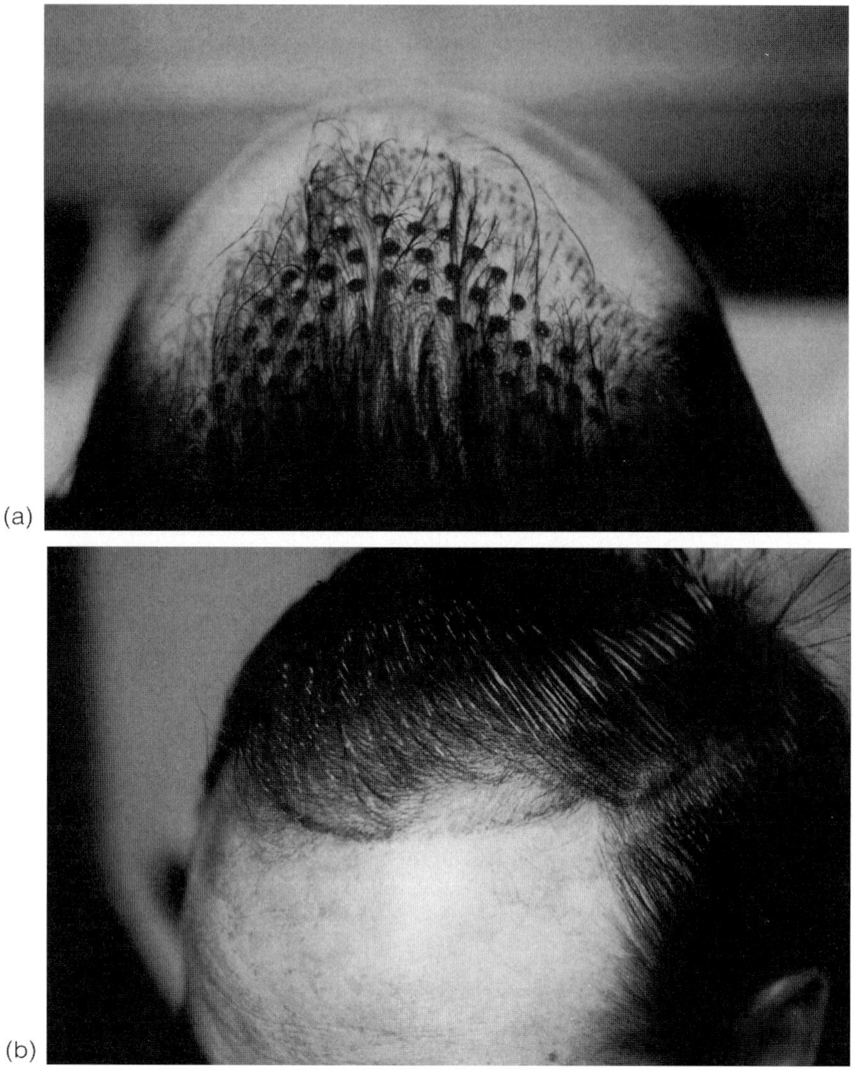

FIGURE 7 (a) First session of transplantation using a combination of grafts. (48 micrografts, 108 large slit grafts, and 68 standard round grafts). (b) Patient shown in (a) before transplantation. (c) Seven months after first transplantation session with the hair combed back for critical evaluation. Using a combination of grafts plugginess is avoided as small micro/minigrafts are placed most anteriorly. However, there is the added benefit of increased density afforded by the standard round grafts [21].

a graft is simply wedged into the recipient site. In patients with dark and/or coarse hair, using slit grafts with no more than three or four hairs eliminates this possibility because there are simply too few hairs per graft to create noticeable compression. The decision to use slits or small circular minigrafts and/or standard grafts behind an anterior zone of micrografts should be based on the patient's expectations, age,

(c) 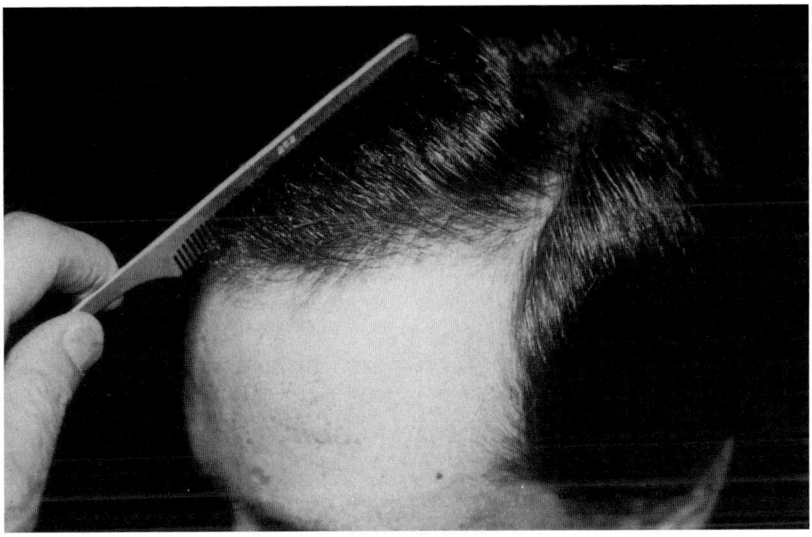

FIGURE 7 Continued.

hair type, and scalp color. There is a tendency for some physicians to use one graft type for all patients; however, we suggest treating each patient on an individual basis using a variety of grafts to be used for specific and different purposes [28].

The decision as to how many grafts to transplant in a single session is one that varies from patient to patient and from surgeon to surgeon. Several factors should be considered when making this choice: the size of the area of alopecia to be treated, the characteristics and density of the hair in the donor region, expectations and goals of the patient and surgeon, experience and skill of the surgeon and assistants, and, finally, the type of graft to be employed. It is appropriate to indicate to the patient not only the number of grafts that will be transplanted but also the number of hairs that will be moved within those grafts from the donor to recipient area. To a patient, 2,000 grafts sounds better than 600 grafts; however, if all 2,000 grafts are single-hair micrografts and the 600-graft session used various sizes of grafts, which yielded a total of 2,000 hairs, then the number of hairs being transferred would be the same. However, in the first instance one session of 2,000 micrografts would nearly always produce a thinner look spread over a larger area than that produced by a comparable number of hairs transferred in the form of micrografts, minigrafts, and possibly standard grafts (Table 3).

Megasessions are defined here as any session of more than 1000 grafts, and larger megasessions may involve 2,500 or more grafts. "Dense packing" of these grafts less than 1 mm apart has been used in some instances in order to accomplish in one session what might be achieved in two to three sessions or with a combination of micrografts and minigrafts. There are several potential problems with larger megasessions combined with dense packing. These include the need for eight to 12 rotating assistants, increased procedure time (8–12 h), patient and surgeon fatigue, possible medical compromise of the patient, and only 65% or even less hair survival attributable to excessive graft handling and/or vascular compromise of the recipient

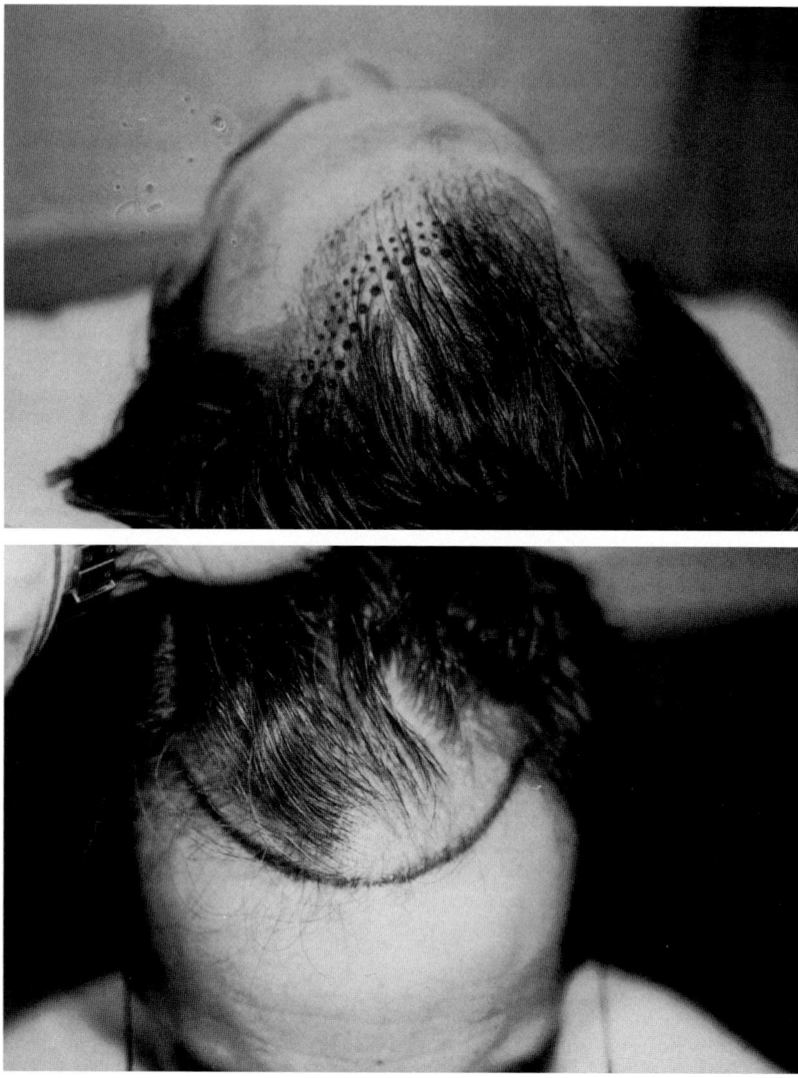

(a)

(b)

FIGURE 8 (a) Example of the use of a combination of many graft types. (b) Before transplantation. Same patient as shown in (a). (c) One year after first session. (60 micrografts, 162 large slit grafts, 100 2-mm grafts, 22 standard round grafts.) (d) Photograph taken at same time as (c) but with hair combed back for critical evaluation. Minimal plugginess is evident with the benefit of added density afforded by circular grafts. (e) After three sessions with hair parted through middle [21].

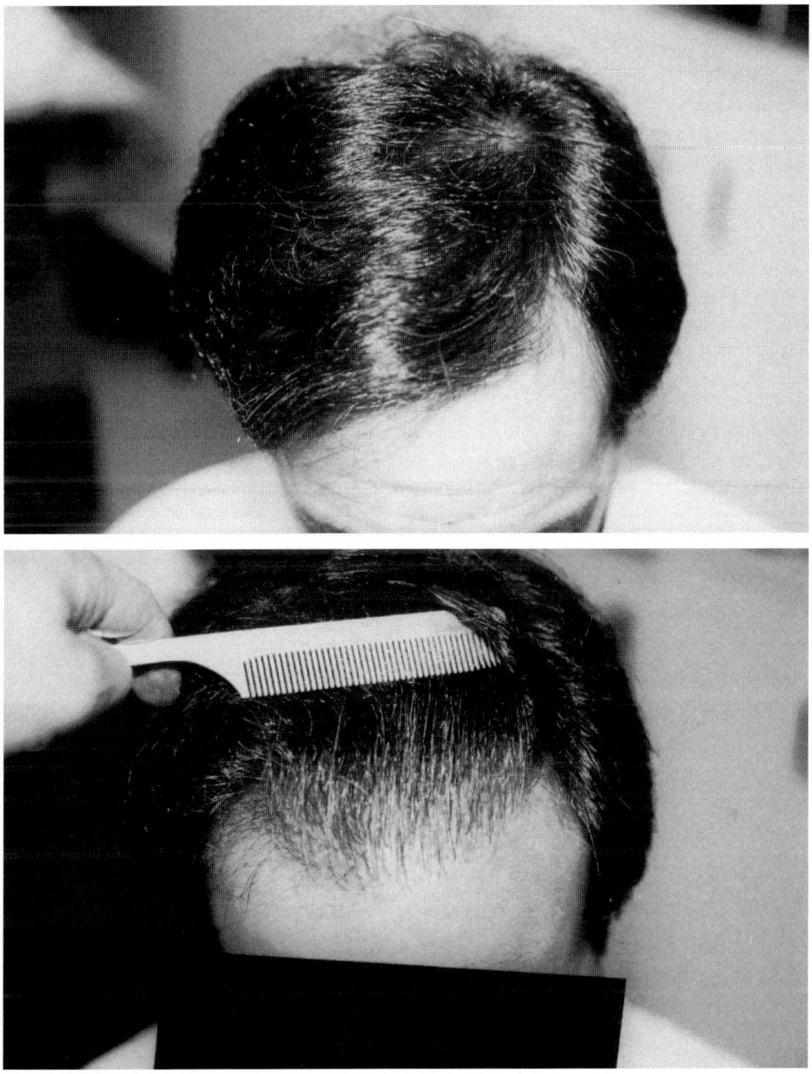

(c)

(d)

FIGURE 8 Continued.

area secondary to so many incisions so close together [29,30]. Because of these drawbacks, after an initial spurt of popularity, the use of sessions of 1500 or more grafts per session has dropped precipitously and is now being routinely performed by only a handful of surgeons. It would be wise for novice hair transplant surgeons to begin with a more modest number of micro/minigrafts (350–500) and then as the level of skill of the physician and staff increases larger and/or more complex sessions can be performed.

(e) 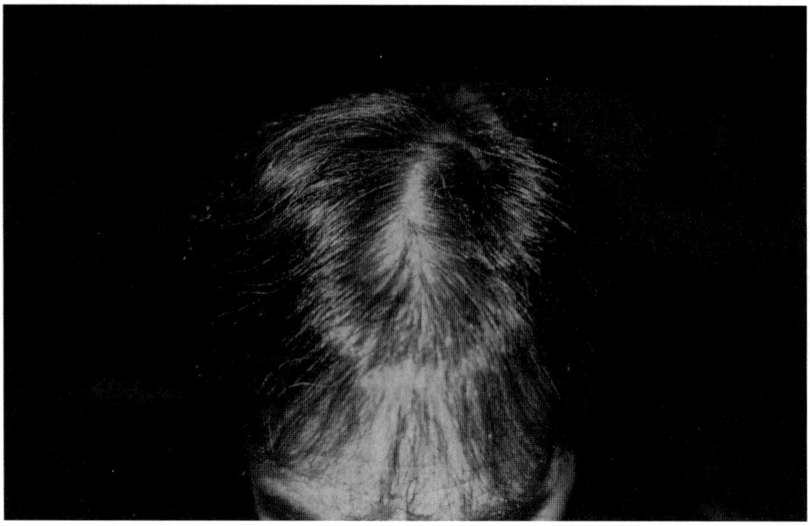

FIGURE 8 Continued.

Presurgical Instructions

In the appendix, the reader will find consent forms, pre- and postsurgical instructions, and the equipment suggested for a hair transplant procedure. Patients are requested to avoid Acetasalicylic acid and Vitamin E capsules for 3 weeks before surgery. Topical Minoxidil, and any other oral medications that might result in excessive bleeding, are also discontinued 1 to 7 days before surgery. Synkovite (Vitamin K) 5 mg daily can be used 1 week before surgery if it is suspected that the patient may have more than average bleeding. Other medications that should be avoided are Monoamine oxidase inhibitors, beta blockers, and anticoagulants [31]. All presurgical instructions are sent out 10 weeks before surgery, with laboratory requisitions for a CBC and screening for Hepatitis B, C, and HIV. If there is a history of keloid formation, then the procedure should be delayed until such a time as a test graft has been performed without subsequent keloidal healing [32].

The patient is sent a prescription for Cefadroxil (Duricef) 500 mg. One gram is taken 2 hours presurgically and 6 hours later unless there is an intolerance or allergy to Penicillin or Cefadroxil. Otherwise, Erythromycin or Trimethoprin-Sulfanethoxazole (Septra DS) can be used instead [31]. Patients are instructed to wash the scalp with a Chlorhexidine Gluconate soap wash (Hibitane) the night before and the morning of surgery.

When the patients arrive on the day of the procedure they sign procedure and photograph consent forms (see Appendix). They are then given Diazepam (Valium) 20 mg orally 30 minutes before surgery to minimize susceptibility to lidocaine toxicity as well as anxiety. For patients that want to be asleep for the initial injections of the donor/recipient area, an anesthetist can be present to deliver twilight intravenous sedation with the use of Propofol (Diprovan), Versed, and/or Fentanyl. Oral Meperidine Hydrochloride (Demerol) 50 mg, or Oxycodone (Percocet) may be given with the Diazepam for patients with low pain thresholds or more than average ner-

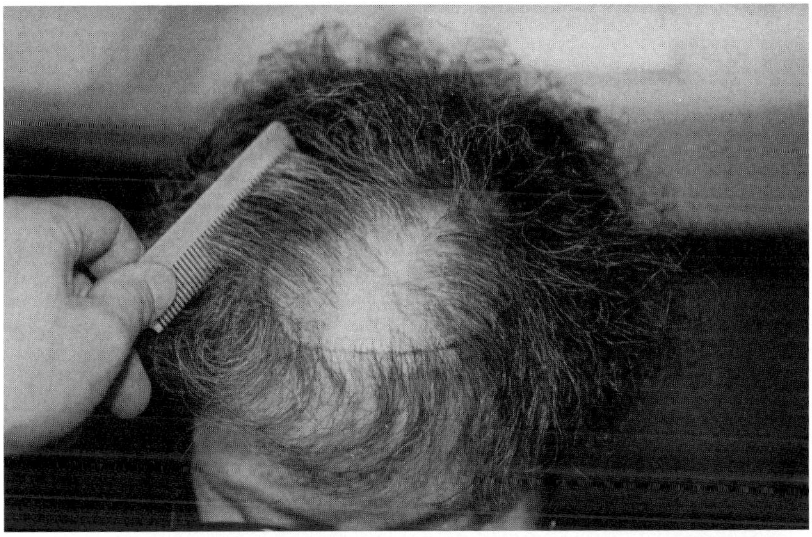

(a)

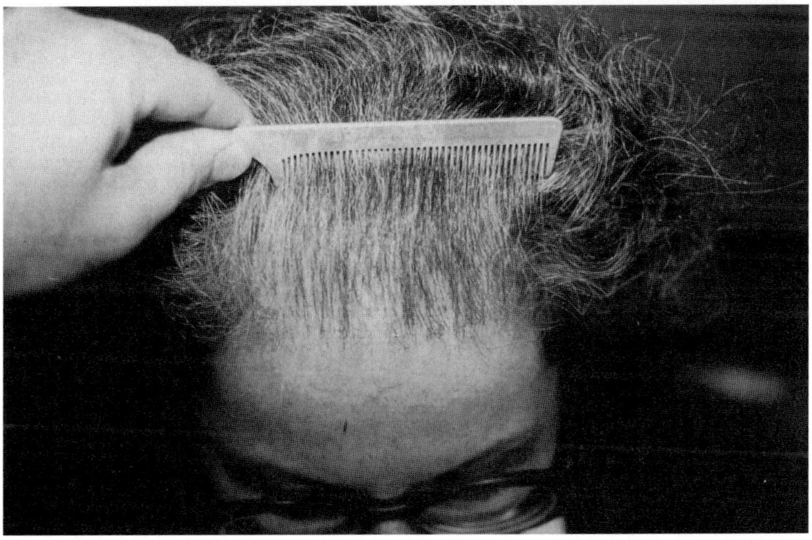

(b)

FIGURE 9 (a) Before first session showing area to be treated indicated with black grease pencil. Typical female pattern thinning with maintenance of the front hairline with generalized thinning posteriorly. (b) 10 months after first session using a combination of 206 slit grafts and 60 micrografts. With the use of slits none of the pre-existing hair was sacrificed. (c) Photograph taken at same time frame as (b) with hair parted through transplant for critical evaluation.

(c)

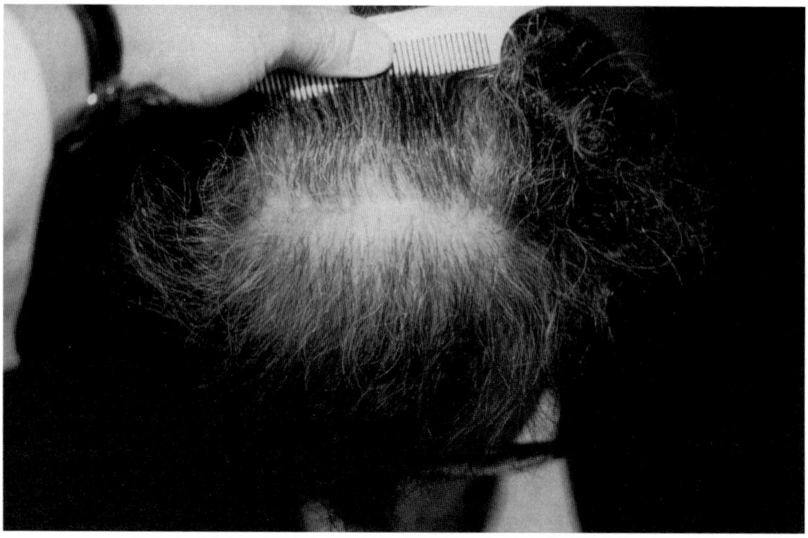

FIGURE 9 Continued.

TABLE 3 Number of Hairs Transplanted per Transplant Session Based on Number of Hairs per Graft

Type of session	Number of each graft type	Number of hairs transplanted	Number of grafts transplanted
All micrografts (Average of 2.3 hair each)	1000 2000 3000	2300 4600 6900	1000 2000 3000
All micrograft and small (3–4 hair) minigrafts	200 micro = 460 hairs 400 small minigrafts 200 × 3 hairs = 600 hairs 200 × 4 hairs = 800 hairs	1860	600
All micrografts, small and large (5–6 hair) minigrafts	200 micro = 460 hairs 200 small minigrafts 100 × 3 hairs = 300 hairs 100 × 4 hairs = 400 hairs 200 large minigrafts 100 × 5 = 500 hairs 100 × 6 = 600 hairs	2260	600
Mixed micrograft, Beaver, Small Minigraft, Standard graft (Average hair count in three of author's recent patients was 23 hairs per 3.5 mm^2 graft)	200 micro = 460 hairs 150 Beaver 75 × 2 hairs = 150 hairs 75 × 3 = 225 hairs 200 Small Minigrafts 100 × 3 hairs = 300 hairs 100 × 4 hairs = 400 hairs 60 × 3.5 mm^2 = 1380 hairs	2910 (equivalent to 1265 micrografts)	610

vousness. Intramuscular Methylprednisolone acetate (Depomedrol) 40 mg/ml is administered in a 2 ml dose just before beginning surgery to minimize postsurgical edema unless there is a contraindication.

Anesthesia

Our method of choice is to use a tumescent anesthetic solution for the donor area. The tumescent anesthetic solution is prepared as follows: add 5.0 ml of 2% lidocaine without epinephrine and 0.4 ml of 1/1000 epinephrine to a 100 ml intravenous (IV) bag of saline. This can also be used in the vertex recipient area; however, it is not used in the anterior recipient area because of a tendency for more postsurgical facial edema. Tumescent anesthesia has the following advantages: (1) reduced lidocaine toxicity, (2) decreased bleeding, (3) increased tissue turgor, resulting in donor area strip removal with minimal damage to hair follicles, and (4) tumescence of the vertex recipient area allows sites that are a given distance apart to move closer together once the tumescence has dissipated, resulting in greater hair density.

Field blocks are produced in the donor and recipient areas by using buffered 1% lidocaine with 1:100,000 epinephrine for the former and 2% lidocaine with 1:100,000 epinephrine for the latter. This allows for the creation of field blocks with minimal pain and no pain superior to them. Buffering of the lidocaine is accomplished by adding sodium bicarbonate to produce mixtures containing 5.2 meq/ml of sodium bicarbonate [33].

The donor area field block is initiated by using a 30-gauge needle to produce four or five wheals approximately 3 cm apart along a line 2 to 3 cm inferior to the proposed donor area. Sixty to 90 seconds later, the field block is completed by injecting through the already anesthetized sites. Once the field block is in place, 50 to 100 ml of the tumescent solution is infiltrated superior to it, using an 18-gauge 3.5 inch spinal needle. The needle is introduced at approximately the midpoint of the donor area and advanced to just beyond the limits of the donor area in one direction. It is then slowly withdrawn concomitant with infiltration of the solution. This is then repeated in the opposite direction through the same entry point. The result should be a very turgid donor region. An automated Klein pump can be used to inject the solution to minimize hand strain [33]. Just before collecting the donor strips, an additional 30 to 40 ml of the tumescent solution may be administered into the intended donor site to maximize tissue turgor. Five ml of 2% lidocaine with 1/100.000 epinephrine should be available for the reinforcement of occasional "hot spots" that need additional anesthesia, but this is rarely needed. Some physicians will add a field block of Bupivicane (Marcaine) 0.05% to the donor area just before the patient leaving the office at the end of the procedure.

Once the donor area has been collected and sutured, a field block is produced in the recipient area. (Some physicians advocate the use of supraorbital nerve blocks before this field block in order to minimize discomfort and give more profound anesthesia [34]). The recipient area field block is placed approximately 2 cm anterior and lateral to the recipient area borders. This is followed by 8 to 10 ml of unbuffered 2% lidocaine with 1/100,000 epinephrine to produce a second field block immediately superior and medial to the first one. Although buffering of the anesthetic solution produces less pain on injections, buffering also causes more bleeding by accelerating the denaturing of epinephrine in the solution. Therefore, an unbuffered

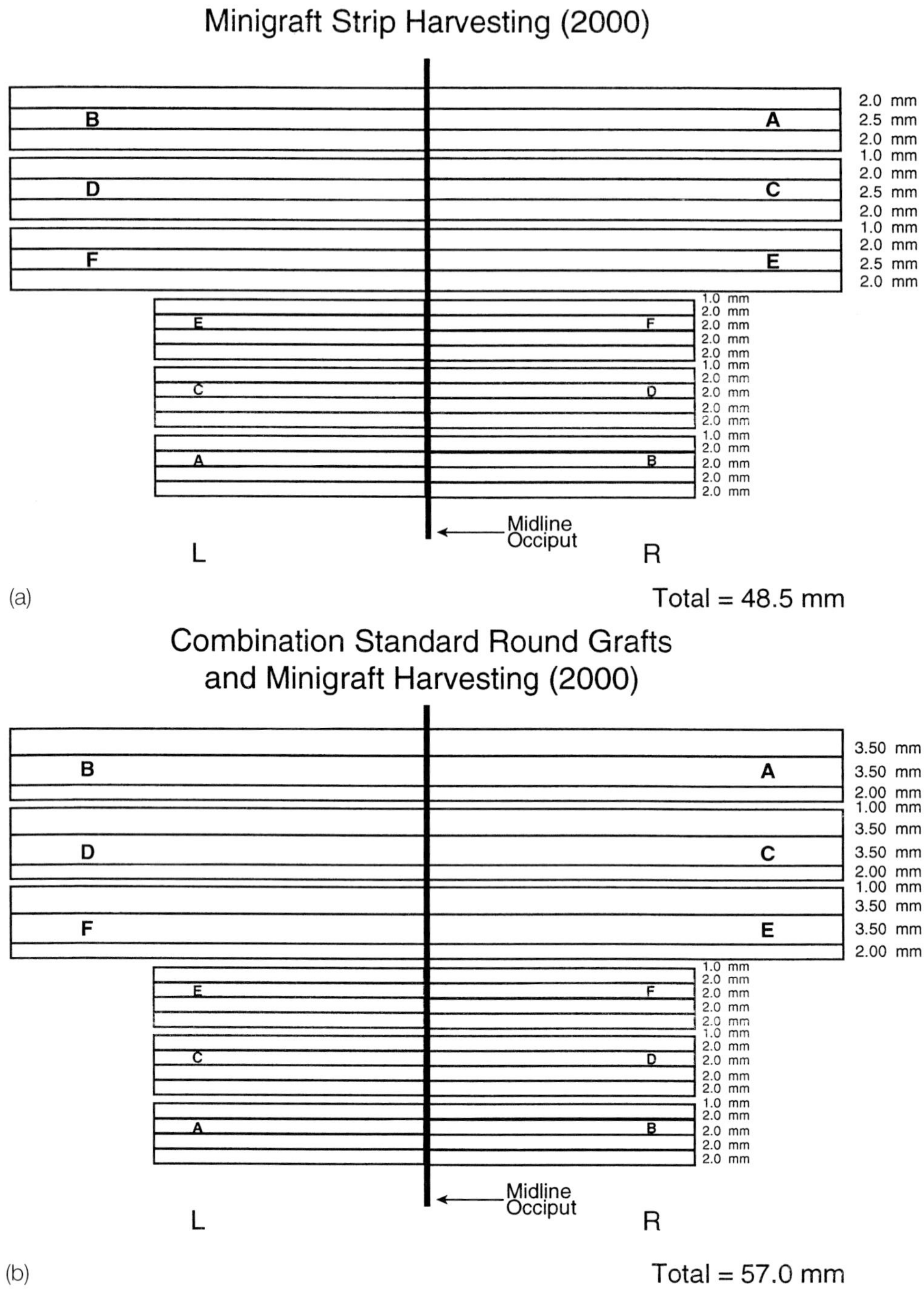

FIGURE 10 **(a) Example of total strip collecting technique by using six donor zones (A, B, C, D, E, and F for sessions 1,2,3,4,5,6). The width of strips taken is shown on the right side of drawing. A 1-mm space has been left between donor sites from different sessions to represent a scar line. A total of 48.5 mm donor tissue would be used for six sessions to yield approximately 300 micrografts and 450–500 or more minigrafts per session. For each session, an inferior donor zone is used to obtain micrografts for finer**

field block superior to the first is used in any area where incisions will be made. Ten ml of 1/50,000 epinephrine should be infiltrated very superficially in small amounts in multiple spots into the rest of the recipient area to minimize bleeding during surgery.

The physician should know the toxicity levels of all drugs used, be certified in advanced cardiac life support, and be prepared to deal with emergencies. Oxygen and a full crash cart set-up should be available.

Surgical Technique

Excision of Donor Area

We usually use two donor zones, one in the left or right inferior occipital area in areas that we feel will permanently maintain good hair density, and another contralateral zone more superiorly that extends from the midline into the parietal area and as far anteriorly as a line drawn perpendicularly from the tragus (Fig. 10). The inferior occipital zone contains hair that is generally finer textured and somewhat sparser than the more superior donor zone. It is used for reconstituting a feathered hairline zone or central vertex. The superior donor zone contains hair that is coarser and somewhat denser and can be used posterior to the hairline zone and/or for a major part of the vertex area. Because it extends into the temporal area, it also contains hair that will usually grey earlier than occipital area hair. This hair when used in the frontal recipient area will grey at the same rate as hair in the temporal area. As the patient ages, the color of temporal and frontal hair will match each other better. If the patient has similar texture and density of donor hair throughout the donor region, then a single long narrow rectangular donor zone extending from just superior to the left ear to just superior to the right ear can be used instead of the collecting pattern described above. The hair is clipped in the donor zone to approximately 2 mm in length and is then rubbed with alcohol, followed by the application of a povidone-iodine (Betadine) solution. Chlorhexidine (Hibaclens) can be used instead of povidone-iodine if the patient is allergic to the latter. Unger has described a "safe" donor area for 80% of patients under the age of 80 years (Fig. 11) [35]. In the occipital regions, the area was found to be 70 mm high, in the parietal region approximately 80 mm high, and in the temporal region approximately 50 mm high.

The patient lies on his stomach with his face in a prone pillow. A multibladed scalpel (Universal handle, straight; Robbins Instruments, Chatham, NJ) with four or

---

hair to be used at the hairline and center of the whorl of the vertex, as well as a superior and contralateral donor zone to obtain coarser, denser hair. (b) Typical widths of strips excised for standard round grafts, minigrafts, and micrografts. A total of 57.0 mm donor tissue is needed to yield six sessions of grafts consisting of approximately 300–350 or more minigrafts, 300 micrografts, and 50–60 standard round grafts per session. The standard round grafts would be obtained from the more superior donor zone. The 2-mm strips in each of the superior donor rows are used to produce micrografts and additional minigrafts. The 1-mm spaces shown between adjacent sessions represents scar tissue. Any scar is re-excised during each subsequent harvesting so that at most only two continuous scars should be left in the donor zone regardless of the number of sessions [21].

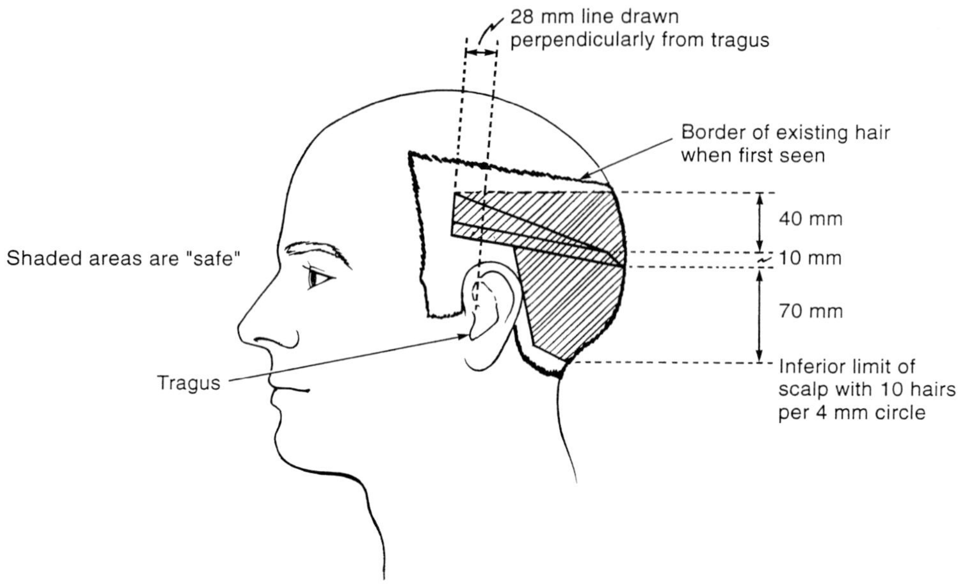

FIGURE 11 Unger's safe donor zone for 80% of patients under the age of 80 years as determined from studies of 328 men aged 65 years or older [35].

five #11 Persona Plus blades is typically used to incise the donor tissue. Some physicians prefer to excise an ellipse instead of multiple strips. We generally use two bladed multibladed handles or an ellipse only when re-excising areas where there is a combination of scar and hair. In such instances, hair direction is often distorted by adjacent scar, and the fewer blade incisions the less likely follicles in the tissue will be inadvertently injured. Although proponents of routine elliptical excisions cite the production of more grafts from the same amount of donor tissue, this may occur with some physicians and not others [36]. Spacers used with the multiblade handles vary from 1 mm to 3 mm depending on hair density and the size of graft required.

The blades are inserted into the midsubcutaneous level of the scalp at the midline. The angle of insertion must be kept parallel to the existing angle of hair at that site in order to avoid transecting follicles. The blade is drawn smoothly across the full length of the donor zone in a continuous motion. It is suggested that novice surgeons stop every 1 inch or so to check that the blade is being held at the correct angle. A #15 scalpel blade is then used to produce triangular tapering of both ends of the wound. One end of the donor tissue is lifted with small-tooth forceps, and either small curved scissors or a #15 blade scalpel can be used to separate the tissue from its underlying bed. A hyfrecator set at 80 and unipolar delivery is used to cauterize vessels that are bleeding excessively. Some physicians advocate the use of an infrared coagulator instead of a hyfrecator. We have not found infrared coagulators satisfactory. Plumes produced from electrocautery of blood vessels can contain benzines, aldohydes, hydrocarbons, carcinogenic carbonized particles, virus, and bacteria. A smoke evacuator system to vacuum the plume is required. The excised strips are then immediately placed in a petri dish containing normal saline to keep the strips moist. The grafts can be kept cool by placing the petri dish on ice and ensuring that the grafts are not left under any hot overhead lights for any prolonged period of time.

Undermining of the wound edges before suturing the defect is not usually necessary, but should be carried out if any significant tension is anticipated without it. Keep in mind that undermining can result in more vessel transection requiring in turn more cauterization, which often results in more postsurgical pain. If a large amount of tumescent fluid has been used, then one can apply modified towel clamps to the skin edges for a short period of time to allow fluid to dissipate and to allow for some additional laxity to return. 2-0 Monocryl violet monofilament on a tapered CT needle is used to close the wound with a continuous running suture. Some physicians advocate the use of staples instead of suturing. In our experience there is less postsurgical discomfort and better hemostatis with the use of sutures. Sutures or staples are removed in 7 to 14 days.

Scars from previous surgery are excised as part of subsequent harvesting in the same area. This "total excision technique" results in no more than two donor area scars no matter how many surgeries have been carried out. The usual width of spacers are shown in Figure 10. When removing donor strips for micrografts and minigrafts, the strip widths can be increased slightly if the donor hair density is lower than average or decreased slightly if it is higher than average. If standard round grafts are required, a triple strip can be removed from the donor area with two 3.5 to 3.75 mm wide spacers and one that is 2.0 mm (Fig. 10). The wider strips can then be sectioned into pieces to produce roughly square grafts of 3.5 to 3.75 mm. These are placed into round holes made with 3.25 to 3.5 mm trephines.

The technique of strip collecting as is shown in Figure 10, allows for six sessions to be carried out in a donor zone that is substantially smaller than 70 mm high and will fall well within the "safe" donor zone area described earlier. Each session will yield 300 or more micrografts and either 450 to 500 or more minigrafts, or 300 to 350 or more minigrafts and 50 to 60 standard round grafts.

The Recipient Area

The "hairline zone" is approximately 2.5 cm wide. Its anterior border consists of 1 to 3 hair micrografts that are inserted into recipient sites prepared with a #16- to #18-gauge needle, a Nokor needle (Bekton Dickinson and Company, Rutherford, NJ), a Lightning knife with an SP90 mini-blade (A–Z Surgical), or a 1.8 minde-knife (A–Z Surgical). Typically, 300 to 350 micrografts are placed approximately 1 mm apart from each other in an irregular fashion as described in the section on planning. Dilators are not used in our office but may be used if your technicians are not expert at atraumatic insertion of such small grafts. The hairline zone is completed with 2 to 3 and then 3 to 4 hair slit grafts posterior to the micrografts. The recipient sites for these grafts are usually prepared with either a Beaver mini-ES blade, or a 2.5 to 3.0 minde-knife for the 2 to 3 hair grafts, and a #15 blade scalpel for the 3 to 4 hair grafts. Great care is taken to exactly follow the angle and direction of the original or previously transplanted hairs so as to not damage them, and to create the most natural flow of hair for that individual. Additional micrografts are usually sprinkled between these small slit sites. Small slit grafts are used to complete the recipient area posterior to the hairline zone during the first session, but in the second or later sessions, if hair texture and color are suitable, large slit grafts or small or large round minigrafts may also be used between the previously transplanted grafts in order to produce more density. Sites for all slit grafts are arranged in a very organized fashion, approximately 3 mm apart from each other (in order to produce the most even coverage of the area after each session), but either 1 mm anterior or posterior to their neighboring slits in order to create the impression of irregularity and naturalness. The author refers to this type of graft dispersion as an "organized disorganization" (Fig. 12). We currenty routinely use approximately 300 micrografts and between 400 and 500 minigrafts per surgery. Typically, 3 to 3½ sessions are required to produce good density in the anterior third to one half of an area of MPB. Sessions are typically 5 to 6 months or longer apart, though they may be as close as 6 weeks apart. The longer intervals are advantageous in that they provide additional hair for postsurgical camouflage and allow for adjustments in graft type and dispersion in response to what is seen growing from previous sessions. In "early" MPB, only one or two sessions 6 months or more apart are performed. The balance of the 3 to 3½ sessions are carried out in pace with the rate of further hair loss. When only micrografts or micrografts and small minigrafts are used, a single transplant procedure can usually stand well on its own without looking clumpy or unnatural. Some patients may be satisfied with one such session in an originally alopecic recipient site if the goal is relatively low density (Fig. 3).

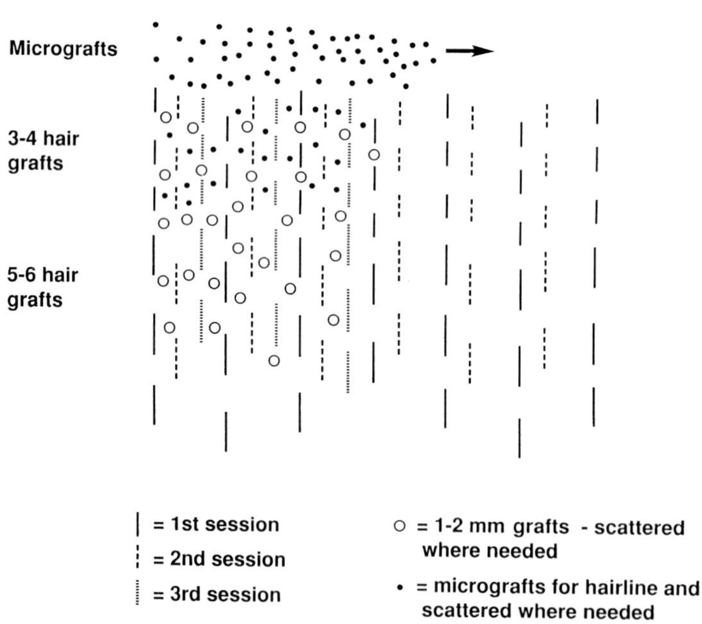

FIGURE 12 Schematic diagram showing creation of a feathered hairline. Organized disorganization is obtained by using micrografts most anteriorly blending in to slightly larger grafts more posteriorly. Grafts should be placed approximately 3 mm apart from each other in the same line as well as being 1 mm anterior posterior to their neighbors. The second and third session are dispersed as shown in a similarly organized fashion. Micrografts are scattered between the slit grafts. As shown, 1–2 mm round grafts may also be used after the first session to give added density where needed [20].

A "U"-shaped pattern of grafting is used in the first session. Subsequent sessions consist of somewhat narrower "U"-shaped patterns combined with grafting of areas not treated in the first session. If the treatment plan includes the use of AR between or after hair transplant sessions, an area should be left in the midline between the "arms" of the transplanted "U" (Fig. 13). It is uncommon to use more than three sessions in a totally alopecic frontal third to half of a typical area of MPB. If treatment of the crown is not part of the objective or AR is not contemplated, then one can treat the entire area of the peninsula between the arms of the "U" after the first session (Fig. 13). In such patients, a posterior "hairline" is created in a concave fashion, so as to leave a more or less natural-looking round alopecic crown. This posterior hairline is created with grafts similar to those described previously for the anterior hairline.

Treatment of women with female pattern androgenetic alopecia (FPAA) differs somewhat from that of their male counterparts. Women with FPAA usually maintain reasonable hair density in the frontal hairline zone and have generalized thinning more posteriorly. As noted earlier, slit grafts are the grafts of choice in most cases, as one does not want to remove any hair in the recipient area, even temporarily. Small circular grafts are used only in areas devoid of hair. Cotterill has reported that 70% of women seen in consultation with androgenetic alopecia are satisfactory candidates for hair transplantation; however, it is important to choose your patients carefully and screen for unrealistic expectations [9]. Women in particular should be warned about the possibility of telogen effluvium affecting existing hair. Topical Minoxidil 3% applied twice daily for 6 weeks after surgery is very helpful in min-

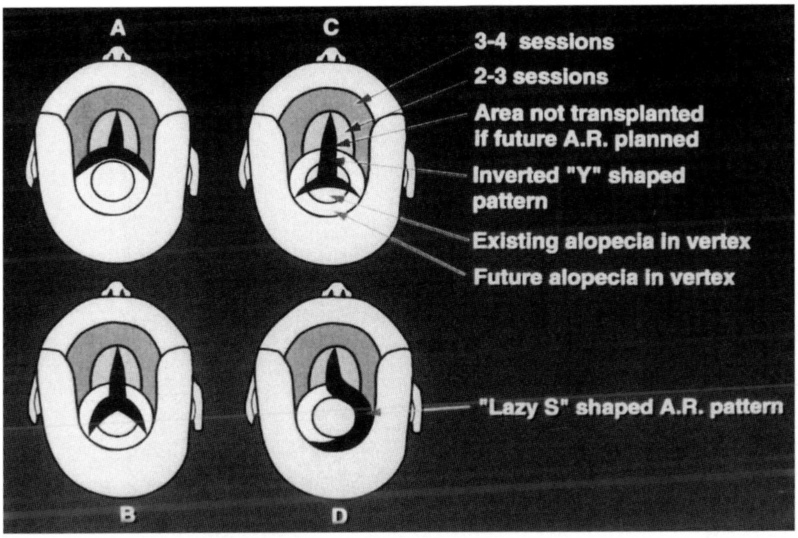

FIGURE 13 Schematic drawing to show general planning of transplanting (hair) density and incorporation of AR into planning. The first and second sessions to the front half of the scalp are made so as to form a "U" pattern. The center of the "U" is left untreated in order to incorporate scalp reduction. If scalp reduction will not be used, then the center of the "U" can be treated during the second and third session [21]. (From Reference #21.)

imizing its occurrence. Typical feminine hairlines also lack the frontotemporal recessions seen in males with MPB (Fig. 9). Areas of hair loss and scarring secondary to facial cosmetic surgery is the second most common reason for transplantation in females (Fig. 14).

The use of lasers for making recipient site holes or slits has been used since 1992 [37]. The Coherent Ultrapulse laser (Coherent Medical, Palo Alto, CA) and the Sharplan/Silktouch laser (Sharplan Laser Inc., Allendale, NJ) create recipient sites

(a)

(b)

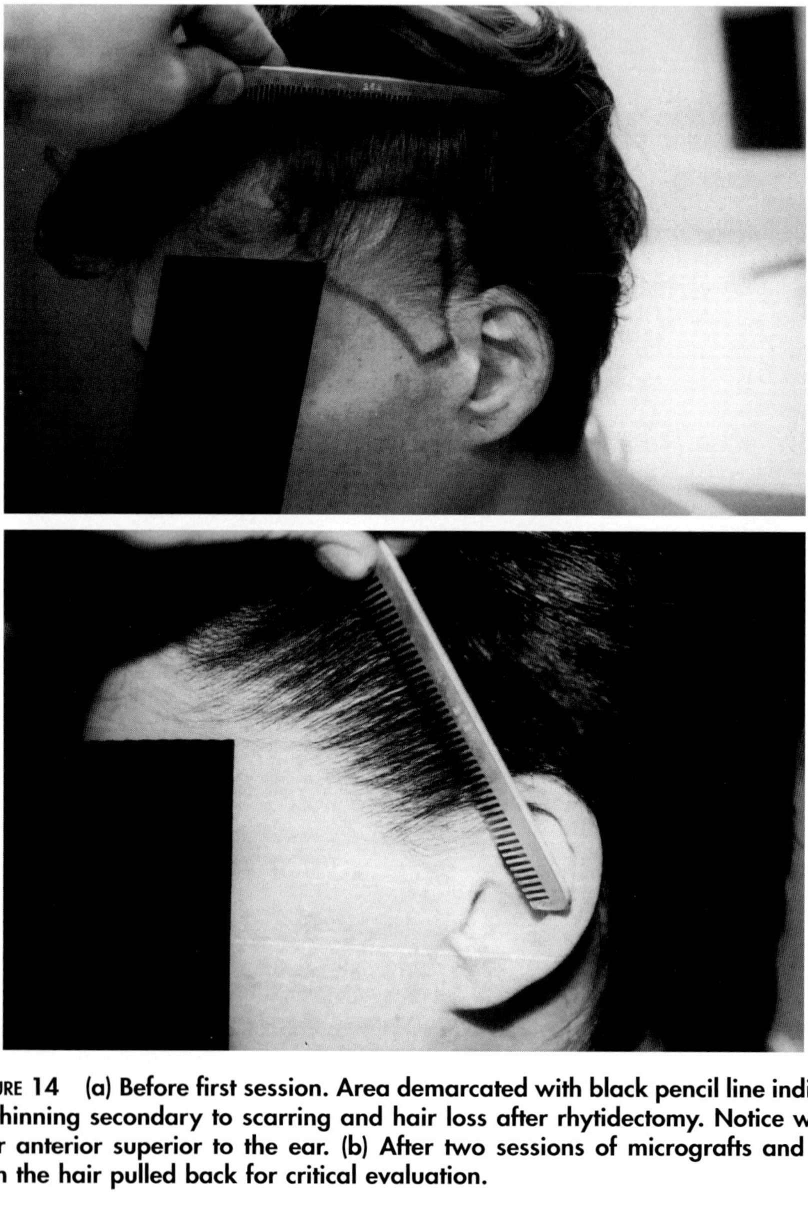

FIGURE 14 (a) Before first session. Area demarcated with black pencil line indicates area of thinning secondary to scarring and hair loss after rhytidectomy. Notice white linear scar anterior superior to the ear. (b) After two sessions of micrografts and minigrafts with the hair pulled back for critical evaluation.

by vaporizing tissue and offer the advantages of no compressions of slit grafts and more control of bleeding. Lasers that are used to produce round holes do not result in superior cosmetic results but can significantly decrease surgery time as the result of less bleeding and eliminating the need to remove tissue from the hole. Disadvantages of using a laser include increased postsurgical crusting in the recipient area and a delay of 2 to 6 weeks longer than that seen with conventional transplanting before hair growth begins. The exact parameters that should be used in laser hair transplantation have not yet been established and good hair survival rates are inconsistent. At the present time the high cost of these lasers also make their purchase difficult to justify unless other uses for the laser—such as resurfacing—exist in the physician's office.

Graft Preparation and Insertion

Once the donor strip has been collected it is placed in a petri dish containing a 4 × 4 inch gauze soaked in normal saline. Cooling of the saline to 4°C has been advocated as means of improving hair survival, but scientific studies to support this contention have never been carried out. If the donor tissue is a large ellipse, it is first sectioned into narrow slices much as one slices bread. These slices are then further divided into smaller grafts. If the donor tissue consists of multiple strips, they are first carefully separated from each other and then subdivided into the desired number and type of grafts. Small jeweller forceps and Persona Super Stainless Shaper blades, double edged Personna shaving blades, or #11 scalpel blades, are used in our office for all sectioning. Small spicules of hair without matrices are removed using jewellers forceps. Great care is taken when sectioning the strip to keep the scalpel blade parallel to the angle of the follicle and to avoid transection. Various aids can be used to better visualize the hair follicles. These include backlighting, magnification loops, and stereoscopic microscopes (38–40). With proper magnification, individual hair follicles and follicular units can be seen so that trauma to the grafts can be minimized. It is imperative that the strips and grafts be kept constantly moist. Dehydration is more likely to damage hair follicles than inadvertent injury to them during sectioning or insertion [41].

When placing the prepared grafts into petri dishes, it is helpful to segregate them into groups according to number of hairs per graft, hair color, and texture. The grafts should be gently eased into the recipient sites using small serrated forceps, or straight or curved jewellers forceps. Care must be taken not to grasp the grafts at the bulb and to approach the recipient site at an angle and direction that will minimize trauma to the grafts during insertion. Some surgeons advocate the use of dilators placed into the sites for at least five minutes before placement of grafts, but we virtually never use dilators. It is better to leave a graft protruding slightly above the level of surrounding skin than below it, as inclusion cysts or "dimpling" can occur.

Postsurgical Care

Bandaging

A small overnight dressing that does not cover the ears is usually used to keep the grafts in place and to prevent them from being accidentally dislodged out of position during the first postsurgical night [42]. The bandage also helps to absorb small amounts of serosanguinous fluid that might develop. Baciquent ointment is applied to both donor and recipient areas followed by Telfa sheets on the recipient area only. Four by four inch gauze squares are placed on top of the Telfa and directly over the donor area. Cotton batting is then placed behind the front of the ears to minimize pressure on them. Make sure that the ears are lying flat against the head rather than being accidentally bent forward during application of the bandage. Two Kerlix bandages should be used to hold everything in place. Generally, two assistants are needed to do this. While the first Kerlix is encircling the head, the second is passed from front to back and back to front. Each passing and circling Kerlix bandage anchors in place the one being passed back and forth. The bandage is removed the next day. Patients may leave the office without a bandage if there is no bleeding during the first two postsurgical hours and the recipient area is in the frontal half of the area of MPB. As implied, a bandage is always used if the posterior half of the area of MPB is the recipient area.

A hairdryer set on cool is used to dry any minor exudation around the grafts in order to accelerate clotting and create a firmer adhesion between them and their recipient sites. Whether or not a bandage is applied, the patient should return the next day to confirm proper placement of the grafts as well as to clean the scalp of any blood clots that may have developed overnight. Hydrogen peroxide–soaked gauze and cotton-tipped swab sticks are used for the latter. The hair is then carefully washed, blown dry, and styled.

The First 24 Hours

Intramuscular ketorolac tromethamine (Toradol) 30 to 60 mg is very effective in eliminating postsurgical pain for 4 to 6 hours in virtually all patients. It is used for all individuals without a prior history of asthma or gastrointestinal ulcers. In addition, when the patients leave the office on the day of surgery, they are given a supply of Acetaminophen tablets with 30 mg Codeine (Tylenol 3), Oxycodone (Percocet), and Meperedine Hydrochloride (Demerol) 50 mg to be used as required. Most commonly, Tylenol 3 is all that is needed.

Patients are telephoned that evening to ensure they are using the medication correctly and do not have any unanswered questions. An anti-inflammatory injection, as mentioned earlier in this chapter, will have been given just before the procedure to minimize edema. However, patients should have been forewarned about the possibility of postsurgical swelling, which typically begins 2 to 3 days after surgery and is usually gone within 7 to 10 days. In approximately one of every 50 patients there can be significant swelling and ecchymoses around the eyes.

Long-Term Postsurgical Course

Patients are instructed to bathe twice a day, soaking the back of the scalp in order to soften and loosen the crusts. After 15 minutes, they gently shampoo both the recipient and donor areas. Sutures are removed 7 to 10 days after surgery. By 10 days to 2 weeks, all the crusting on top of the recipient grafts should have fallen off.

The transplanted grafts will shed their hair in 2 to 6 weeks, although some may retain a few hairs that will continue to grow without effluvium. New hair growth usually begins 10 to 20 weeks after surgery, but can occur somewhat earlier in micrografts and minigrafts than in standard round grafts. In order to accelerate regrowth of dormant hair, patients can be given a 3% solution of Minoxidil to be used twice daily for 5 to 6 weeks after surgery. This solution also minimizes the possibility of temporary loss of hairs adjacent to the recipient sites.

Patients are told that hair growth begins at approximately 3 months, and by 6 months from the day of surgery they will have a fairly good idea of how much hair they are going to have. However, the full cosmetic benefit isn't achieved until 9 to 12 months after surgery, by which time hair length and caliber are well developed.

Postsurgical hypoesthesia of the scalp usually occurs and lasts for 3 to 6 months, although it can persist for as long as 18 months. In approximately 1% of cases, there is a permanent decreased sensitivity in one or more small areas of the scalp. Patients are instructed to return for re-evaluation 6 to 9 months after surgery.

Complications and Their Treatment

Complications after hair transplantation can be divided into medical/surgical complications and cosmetic/aesthetic complications.

Medical/Surgical.

1. Postsurgical infection in the recipient area occurs in fewer than 0.1% of patients. It usually begins as papules or papulo pustules. In the donor area, infection occurs around sutures. Swabs of any exudate should be taken for culture and sensitivity and patients should be placed on an appropriate systemic antibiotic. Patients are also instructed to apply hot saline compresses to the area three times a day, followed by a topical antibiotic ointment.

2. "Cobblestoning" occurs when grafts remain elevated above the surrounding skin. It is more common with the use of larger grafts, such as standard grafts, but even when the latter are used it is quite unusual. Such grafts can be easily flattened with light electrodesication.

3. Depressed grafts may also occur. They should be excised and replaced with grafts placed flat with the surrounding skin.

4. Inclusion or epidermal cysts occur when small grafts have inadvertently been placed on top of one another at the time of their insertion (piggy-backing), or when a small graft has fallen beneath the surrounding skin, which subsequently heals over it. They should be incised with a #11 or #15 blade and their contents expressed. A small curved forceps with teeth is used for extracting any material from within these epidermal cysts that is not easily ejected. These can include whole minigrafts, balls of hair, or small pieces of buried epidermis.

5. Bleeding can occur intrasurgically or postsurgically in either the donor or recipient area. This can be controlled with direct pressure, electrocautery, or ligation.

6. Excessive scarring can occur in the donor area and is usually either hypertrophic or keloidal. In these patients, there is usually a family history of poor scar formation. Hypertrophic scarring can be revised in subsequent sessions with or without concomitant intralesional infiltration of triamcinolone acetonide to minimize inflammation. Keloids are best treated only with intralesional corticosteroids every 1 to 3 weeks [43]. A "test" graft is recommended 8 weeks or more before surgery in any instance where there is family or personal history of keloid formation. "Hyperfibrotic" healing in the recipient area is a rare complication that is probably secondary to spicules of hair that have accidentally been transplanted [44].

7. Arteriovenous (AV) fistulae occur in approximately 1 in 5,000 surgeries, thought they may be more common than previously reported as a result of many

more recipient graft sites that are made to accommodate minigrafts and micrografts. AV fistulae present as pulsating nodules in either the recipient or donor area. They are caused by the accidental joining of a small severed venule and severed arteriole. AV fistulae will resolve spontaneously in 3 to 6 months. However, if there is a cosmetic concern or worry that the patient might inadvertently puncture the lesion, it can be eliminated by tying off the afferent and efferent vessels.

Other less common medical/surgical complications that are usually self-limiting and mild include telogen effluvium of pre-existing hair, chronic folliculitis, and temporary curly/wiry hair. Wound dehiscence after removal of donor area sutures is a rare complication, and osteomyelitis has been reported in the literature as a complication of hair transplanting only once [45].

Cosmetic/Aesthetic. Poor planning is one of the most common reasons for a cosmetically unsatisfactory result in hair restoration surgery. This can be as a result of improper choice of hairline; improper graft selection; improper graft position, angling, or direction; insufficient donor hair; or improper prognostication of future hair loss [46]. Physicians must also be wary of unrealistic expectations. If a patient has inappropriate expectations, the patient may never be happy, regardless of otherwise excellent results.

ALOPECIA REDUCTION

History

AR has been used for over 20 years to excise areas of bald scalp in order to conserve grafts and allow for coverage of a larger proportion of the originally larger area of MPB with hair transplantation. Blanchard and Blanchard in 1977 published the first description of AR techniques [47], followed by Unger and Unger in 1978 [48]. Since that time there has been a continuous evolution and improvement of methods of removing alopecic areas. Recent significant refinements include Frechet Scalp Extension [49] and Triple Flap Procedure [50], the Brandy Scalp Lift [51], the Unger Prolonged Acute Tissue Expansion (PATE) technique [52], and the Nordstrom suture in conjunction with scalp reduction [53].

Despite the foregoing, over the last 10 years there has been a decrease in the number of AR actually performed. The reasons cited for this are as follows:

1. The concern of "stretchback," which is associated with the rewidening of the hairless zone after scalp reduction. Studies have shown that stretchback is dependent to a large degree on the tension on closure. Understandably greater tension applied at closure results in greater stretchback.
2. The "parting of the Red Sea" effect, with disoriented hair direction.
3. Unsightly noticeable scars.
4. Decreased donor hair density.
5. With the success of micro- and minigrafting techniques, a larger area of the scalp can be given a light natural-looking coverage before the limited number of grafts is exhausted.

AR still remains one of the most efficient techniques of conserving donor tissue in order to achieve greater scalp coverage, as long as the surgeon plans properly and performs the technique in a safe manner with minimal tension on closure.

Unger has listed four types of patients who will benefit significantly from AR [54]:

1. Patients whose goal is complete and maximum coverage. In this group of well-motivated patients, the more aggressive procedures can be used (scalplifting, Frechet scalp extender with three flap slot correction, or Prolonged Acute Tissue Expansion (PATE).

2. Patients with MPB who have had prior grafting, but an extension of alopecia beyond the originally estimated borders resulting in a halo of lost alopecia around the transplanted area.

3. Patients with Type IV to VII MPB who desire maximum coverage.

4. Patients with cicatricial alopecia secondary to trauma, burns and medical conditions such as localized morphea, nevus sebaceous of jadassohn, pseudopelade, cutis congenita, or traction alopecia.

The midline ellipse is the most commonly performed of all the various patterns of AR. The main problems, however, are the production of a slot defect when hair-bearing skin is brought together from either side and a visible midline scar. Figure 15 gives examples of other AR patterns (midline excision, Mercedes, or "Y," Paramedian, Lazy "S," "J," and "U" shape pattern). Marzola introduced the lateral scalplift, which is based on the paramedian scalp reduction incision [55]. Unger has modified the paramedian excision into a "lazy S" pattern, which enables one to excise more alopecic areas by increasing the total length of the AR and avoids a slot defect in persisting occipital hair.

Brandy devised the bilateral occipitoparietal flap, which entails undermining under the donor fringe around the rim of the ear and donor area to the hairline of the nape of the neck with sectioning of both occipital and post-auricular neurovascular bundles. By pre-ligating occipital arteries, extending the plane of dissection below the nuchal ridge and operating on the patient in the prone position, Brandy has lowered the rate of necrosis. The bitemporal flap and the modified bitemporal flap were designed to close the central defect with more anterior movement of tissue. All of these Brandy procedures are relatively aggressive maneuvers that substantially reduce the alopecic area at the cost of somewhat more frequent complications. We do not use them (Fig. 16).

In 1992, Patrick Frechet developed the "scalp extender." An extender is composed of a thin sheet of silicone with two rows of titanium hooks on either end. The sheet is inserted into the subgaleal space after stretching it to approximately double its original length. The hooks are used to attach the stretched sheet into the undersurface of the galea of the fringe hair, on either side of the excision site. The device has a strong elastic memory and will gradually return to its original size stretching the rim hair in the process. Typically, an AR is carried out, the extender is put in place, and the wound is then sutured closed in two layers. Approximately 4 weeks later, the patient returns for a second AR and then either a second extender is inserted or a traditional AR is performed. Frechet has shown that approximately twice the area of alopecia can be removed with the second AR as is eliminated with the first one. Another advantage is that a second AR can be carried out as soon as 30 days after the first instead of after the usual 2 to 3 month interval.

Complications have included increased postsurgical discomfort, an infection rate of approximately 0.5%, and rare seromas. A slot defect can result if the entire area of alopecia is excised. This can be avoided by not removing the entire area of

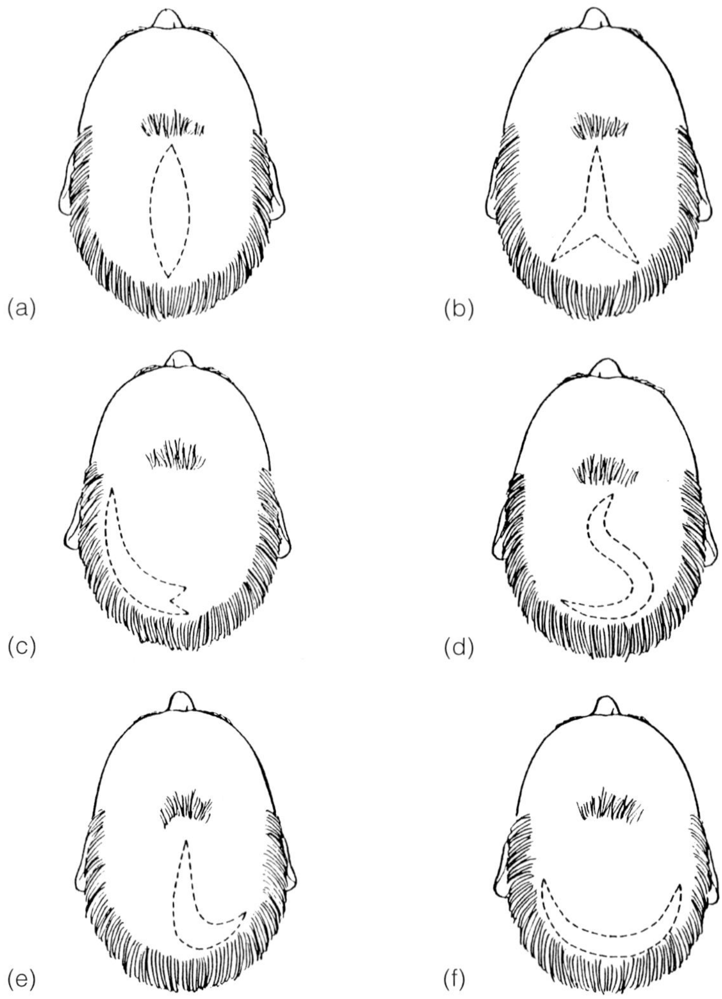

FIGURE 15 Examples of scalp reduction patterns. a, Midline excision; b, Mercedes or "Y" pattern excision; c, paramediam excision; d, lazy "S" excision; e, "J" pattern excision; f, "U" pattern excision.

MPB. However, Frechet prefers total elimination of alopecia with the creation of a slot, which he then corrects with the Frechet three-flap corrective procedure (Fig. 17).

Scalp Expansion

The use of expanders to increase the removal of tissue was first described by Radovan [56]. Its use in conjunction with AR has been available for the last decade. Anderson has described soft-tissue expansion before bilateral advancement transposition and triple advancement transposition flaps with remarkable results [57]. The downside, however, is that cosmetically this procedure is unacceptable for the ma-

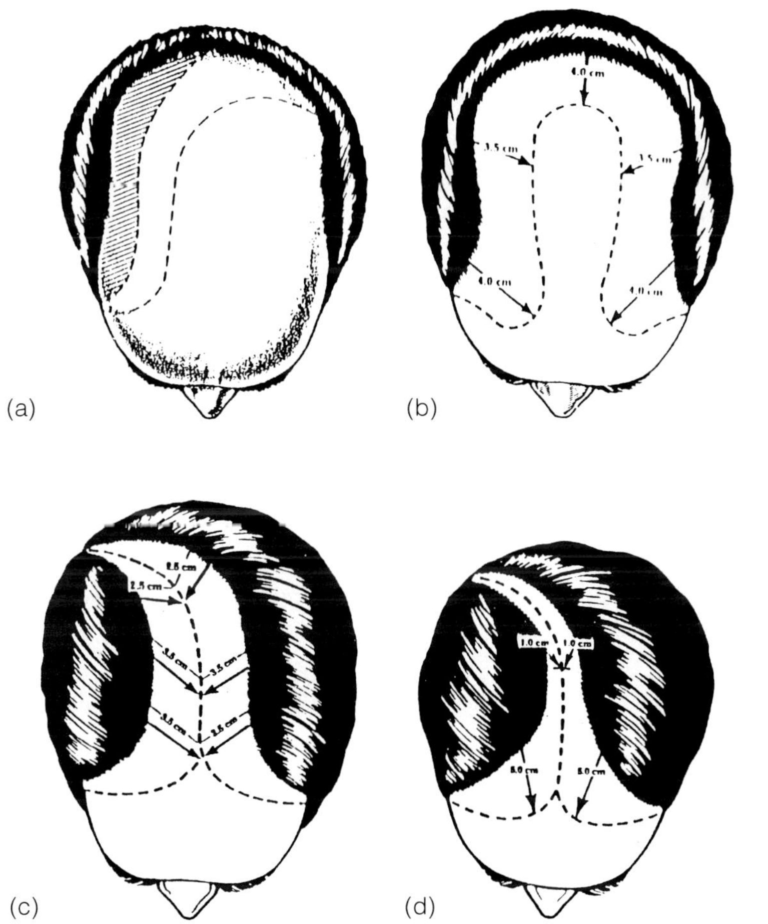

FIGURE 16 a, The Marzola Lateral Lift compared with a paramediam scalp reduction (shaded); b, the Bilateral Occipital Parietal Flap; c, the Bitemporal Flap; d, the Modified Bitemporal Flap.

jority of patients with MPB because of the hydrocephalus-like appearance of the inflated expander at the end of the inflation period.

The most recent innovation to AR has been the development of the PATE technique by Unger [58]. During the course of a modified major scalp reduction, tissue expanders are inserted under the hair-bearing scalp and slowly inflated and deflated through 18 to 20 cycles over a period of 2 to 3 hours while the patient remains in the surgery room under local anesthesia. The AR is then carried out and generally results in the removal of up to 100% more tissue removal than can be expected with traditional AR. It also avoids the cosmetic disadvantages of chronic tissue expansion.

Scalp reduction can be performed before hair transplantation, between transplantation sessions, or after transplantation has been completed. Generally, hair transplantation and scalp reduction are performed separately and approximately 6 weeks or longer apart. Occasionally, however, hair transplantation may be performed after

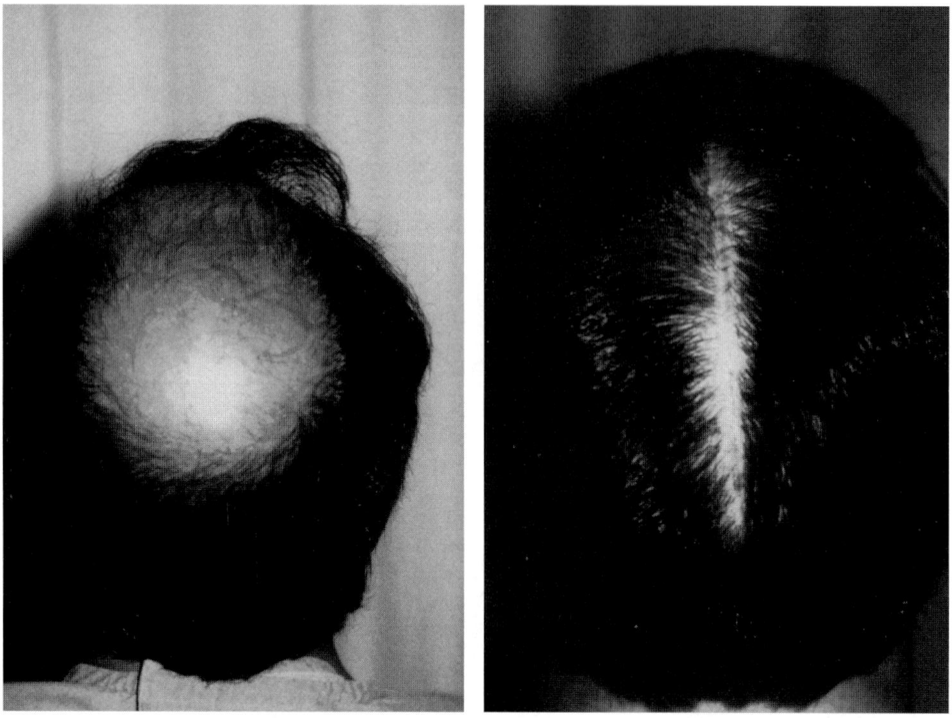

(a) (b)

FIGURE 17 (a) Before alopecia reduction. (b) After removal of extender and completion of reductions. A slot formation has resulted. (c) After slot correction. (Courtesy of P. Frechet).

a limited scalp reduction as long as the reduction has been performed in an area sufficiently distant from the area of transplantation and the grafts do not approach the AR incision.

A presurgical assessment should include blood work for prothombin time, partial thromboplastin, complete blood count, HIV, and Hepatitis B and C. Patients are asked to avoid Acetasalicylic Acid and Vitamin E for 3 weeks before surgery, and topical Minoxidil as well as other medications which might result in increased bleeding for 1 to 7 days before surgery. Patients wash their hair with Hibiclens or Phisohex the morning of the procedure and take 1 g Cefadroxil (Duricef) 2 hours before, and 1 g 6 hours after surgery. Photographs should be taken for postsurgical comparison. It is suggested for the purposes of assessing how much scalp has been removed at the time of the procedure and for later follow-up assessment that pinpoint tattoos be placed bilaterally at the lateral fringes of the hair-bearing regions with the distance between tattoos measured. This also clarifies the benefits of scalp reduction to the patient.

Patterns

The sagital midline ellipse has been the most popular pattern of AR because of its simplicity and safety. However, as has been previously discussed, this leaves a mid-

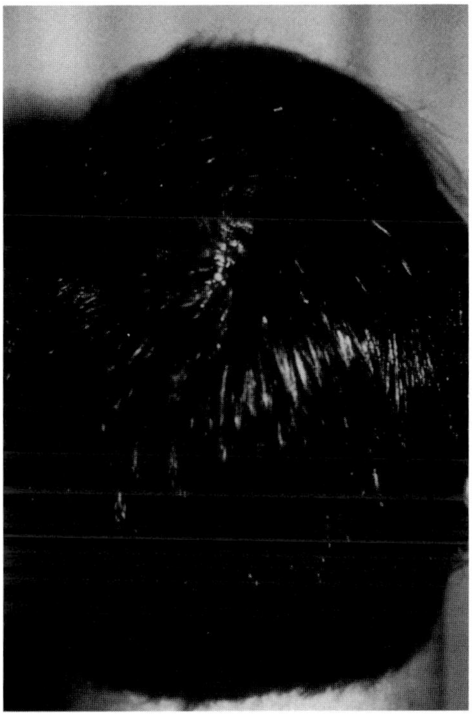

(c)

FIGURE 17 Continued.

line scar until such time as transplantation has been completed. The "Y"-shaped pattern, or Mercedes Benz pattern, allows for greater tissue excision at the posterior aspects with some lifting of the posterior hairline. The goal is not total scalp coverage with hair transplants but the appearance of a smaller bald spot in the crown with no visible scar through it. Grafts are ultimately placed up to and into the "Y"-shaped scar. The lazy "S"-shaped pattern is used when the intention is total scalp coverage with transplants. The reduction is typically placed on the nonpart side and extends into the occipital region. With the "S" as well as the "J"- and "C"-shaped configurations, most of the stretching occurs in hair-bearing tissue rather than in the alopecic areas. The resultant scar is also easier to hide because of its proximity to hair-bearing tissue.

A "U"-shaped pattern that places the open end of the "U" anteriorly with the "U" following the hairline around the crown has the benefit of removing larger areas of alopecic skin than those allowed by other standard AR patterns, but interrupts the blood supply to the remaining alopecic area from three directions with possibly negative consequences to safety and future of graft survival.

Surgical Procedure

Diazepam 15 mg is given orally 30 minutes before surgery. Meperidine (Demerol) 50 mg intramuscularly is optional. The area to be excised is marked with a series of dots using a marker such as the Micropoint Supermarker. The patient is placed in a prone position which gives excellent exposure to the posterior scalp. A field block is created by injecting a circle of anesthetic around the circumference of the head inferior to the expected extent of undermining using a 25-gauge 3-inch spinal needle and 2% lidocaine with 1/100,000 epinephrine. Local anesthetic is also injected along the outline of the proposed AR in order to minimize bleeding. For most patterns, the surgical technique is similar to that used for the elliptical pattern, which is described below. One side of the pattern is incised down to and through the galea aponeurotica. The scalpel blade should be angled to avoid severing adjacent hair follicles. It is recommended that if previous hair transplantation has been performed in the area that a 2 mm margin of safety be left. Surgical skin hooks are used to handle the skin edges and curved mayo scissors are used to undermine under the galea as widely as possible. Unless there has been donor harvesting in the area, undermining in the subgaleal plane is usually relatively bloodless and quite easy. Hemostasis is obtained using electrocautery. The amount of redundant scalp tissue that can be safely excised is determined by draping the tissue to be excised over the incision and the resultant blood stain on the underlying flap is used to mark the extent of scalp to be removed. One can make a series of perpendicular incisions through the top flap stopping at the point where the tissues will meet. By joining the perpendicular cuts the redundant tissue can be removed.

AR are always closed in two layers. The galea aponeurotica is sutured using absorbable sutures such as 2-0 Dexon or Vicryl placed approximately 1.5 mm apart. The skin edges are then approximated with a running 4-0 chromic catgut suture or alternatively using surgical staples. The technique used for the Mercedes pattern is similar to that used for the ellipse, but is dealt with as three separate ellipses [58].

An antibiotic ointment with a nonstick adhesive pad is placed over the wound. Three or four layers of gauze are then applied and held in place with a piece of 6-inch stockinet modified to form a cap. The patient is instructed to remove the dressing himself the next morning, and to return 1 week after surgery for suture/staple removal.

Postsurgical Course and Complications

The patient should be forewarned of postsurgical swelling in the area and to expect some pain the night of the procedure. AR is generally very safe and is associated only rarely with complications. These include postsurgical bleeding, hematoma, seroma, infection, minor skin necrosis, and wound dehiscence. Postsurgical bleeding is extremely rare because the wound is closed under tension and a turban-like bandage is applied. If a hematoma results, it is best to open the wound and evacuate the hematoma. Infections that occur are usually related to a foreign body reaction such as from a suture or from a tissue extender. With any signs of infection a culture should be obtained and the foreign material removed if possible. Scar formation from an AR depends to a large degree on the skill of the surgeon. The vast majority of patients heal with a very fine scar line. However, occasionally with thick scalps the scar may be slightly depressed. Such a scar can be re-excised at a later time with or without another AR. Small noticeable scars are not ultimately significant because the intent should always be to cover them with hair from subsequent transplanting.

REFERENCES

1. Unger W. Hair Transplantation. 3rd ed. New York: Marcel Dekker, 1995.
2. Stough DB, Haber RS. Hair Replacement. New York: McGraw-Hill, 1995.
3. Orentreich N. Autografts in Alopecias and other selected dermatological conditions. Ann NY Acad Sci 1959; 83:463.
4. Dieffenbach JF. Nonnulla de Regeneratione et Transplantatione. Dissertation Inauguralis, 1822.
5. Marritt E. Transplantation of single hairs from the scalp as eyelashes. J Dermatol Surg Oncol 1980; 6:271–273.
6. Nordstrom REA. Micrografts for improvement of the frontal hairline after transplantation. Aesth Plast Surg 1981; 5:97–101.
7. Bradshaw W. Quarter grafts: a technique for minigrafts. In: Unger WP, Nordstrom REA, eds. Hair Transplantation, 2nd ed. New York: Marcel Dekker, 1998, pp. 333–351.
8. Cotterill PC. Hair transplantation in females. In: Unger WP, ed. Hair Transplantation. New York: Marcel Dekker, 1995, pp. 287–292.
9. Cotterill PC. Application and approach to hair transplantation in females. Am J Cosm Surg 1997; 14:137–141.
10. Gandelman M. Eyebrow and eyelash transplantation. In: Unger WP, ed. Hair Transplantation. New York: Marcel Dekker, 1995, pp. 294–311.
11. Unger WP. Mustache transplants. In: Unger WP, ed. Hair Transplantation. New York: Marcel Dekker, 1995, pp. 311–312.
12. Nordstrom REA. Hair transplantation under split thickness skin grafts of the scalp, very thin recipient skin and areas of alopecia secondary to radiation. In: Unger WP, ed. Hair Transplantation. New York: Marcel Dekker, 1995, pp. 312–318.
13. Weidig JC. An approach to the younger patient. In: Stough DB, Haber RS, eds. Hair Replacement. New York: McGraw-Hill, 1995, pp. 62–67.
14. Unger WP, Knudsen R. General principles of recipient site organization and planning. In: Unger WP, ed. Hair Transplantation. New York: Marcel Dekker, 1995, pp. 105–158.
15. Rose P. It's not just a line, the subtleties of the hairline area. Sixth Annual meeting of the International Society of Hair Restoration Surgery, Washington, DC, September 16–20, 1998.
16. Beehner M. The frontal forelock. Hair Transplant Forum 1995; 5:1–5.
17. Marritt E, Dzubow LM. Reassessment of male pattern baldness: a reevaluation of the treatment. In: Stough DB, Haber RS, eds. Hair Replacement. New York: McGraw-Hill, 1995, pp. 30–41.
18. Unger WP. The donor site. In: Unger WP, ed. Hair Transplantation. New York: Marcel Dekker, 1995, pp. 183–187.
19. Shiell R, Stough DB, Cadre de Cheveaux. Am J Cosm Surg 1995; 12:317–319.
20. Unger WP. What's new in hair replacement surgery? Dermatol Clin 1996; 14(4):783–802.
21. Unger WP, Stough DB, Jimenez FJ, Avram M, Fitzpatrick RE. Alopecia reduction. In: Ratz JL, ed. Textbook of Dermatologic Surgery. Philadelphia: Lippincott-Raven, 1998, pp. 499–530.
22. Frechet P. Scalp extension. In: Unger WP, ed. Hair Transplantation. New York: Marcel Dekker, 1995, pp. 625–642.
23. Unger MG. The modified major scalp reduction. J Dermatol Surg Oncol 1988; 14(1): 80–84.
24. Limmer BL. Elliptical donor stereoscopically assisted micrografting as an approach to further refinement in hair transplantation. J Dermatol Surg Oncol 1994; 20:787–793.
25. Marritt E. The death of the density debate. Dermatol Surg 1999; 25(8):654–660.
26. Unger WP. Graft types. Hair Transplant Forum 1998; 8(3):14–16.

27. Unger WP. Recipient area. In: Unger WP, ed. Hair Transplantation. New York: Marcel Dekker, 1995, pp. 215–321.
28. Unger WP. Different grafts for different purposes. Am J Cosm Surg 1997; 14(2):177–183.
29. Cole J. Graft Dissection: Loopes vs. Microscopes, Annual Meeting of the International Society of Hair Restoration Surgery, Oct. 23, 1999.
30. Pomerantz M. More problems with megasessions. Hair Transplant Forum 1995; 5:4–5.
31. Unger WP. Pre-operative instructions. In: Unger WP, ed. Hair Transplantation. New York: Marcel Dekker, 1995, pp. 159–164.
32. Unger WP. Keloids and hypertrophic scars. In: Unger WP, ed. Hair Transplantation. New York: Marcel Dekker, 1995, pp. 367–368.
33. Unger WP. Anesthesia. In: Unger WP, ed. Hair Transplantation. New York: Marcel Dekker, 1995, pp. 165–181.
34. Haber RS, Khan S, Stough DB. Nerveblock anesthesia of the scalp. In: Stough DB, Haber RS, eds. Hair Replacement. New York: McGraw-Hill, 1995, pp. 89–93.
35. Unger WP, Solish B, Giguerre D. Delineating the "safe" donor area for hair transplanting. Am J Cosmet Surg 1994; 11:239–243.
36. Beehner M. Two research studies on follicular unit growth. Sixth Annual meeting International Society of Hair Restoration Surgery, Washington, DC, September 16–20, 1998.
37. Unger WP, David L. Laser hair transplanting. J Dermatol Surg Oncol 1994; 20:515–521.
38. Rose P. Presentation on backlighting. American Hair Restoration Society meeting, Orlando, January 1996.
39. Greco J. Transilluminated graft preparation: the Ergonomic Way. Hair Transplant Forum 1997: 7(3):31.
40. Limmer B. Bob Limmer does it all one hair at a time! Hair Transplant Forum 1991; 2: 8–9.
41. Cooley JE. Follicle trauma in hair transplantation: prevalence and prevention. Fifth Annual meeting of the International Society of Hair Restoration Surgery, Barcelona, October 15–19, 1997.
42. Unger WP. Bandaging. In: Unger WP, ed. Hair Transplantation. New York: Marcel Dekker, 1995, pp. 349–352.
43. Brown M, Johnson T, Swansen N. Extensive keloids following hair transplantation. J Dermatol Surg Oncol 1990; 16:867–869.
44. Unger M. Hyperfibrotic transplants. Hair Transplant Forum 1993; 3(4):8–9.
45. Jones W. Osteomyelitis of the skull following scalp reduction and hair plug transplantation. Ann Plast Surg 1980; 5:480–482.
46. Unger WP. Correction of poor transplanting. In: Unger WP, ed. Hair Transplantation. New York: Marcel Dekker, 1995, pp. 375–388.
47. Blanchard G, Blanchard B. Obliteration of alopecia by hair-lifting: a new concept and technique. J Natl Med Assoc 1977; 69:639–641.
48. Unger M, Unger WP. Management of alopecia of the scalp by a combination of excisions and transplantations. J Dermatol Surg Oncol 1978; 4:670–672.
49. Frechet P. Du Nouveau as la chirurgie de la calvitie. Panorama Med 1992; 3685:7.
50. Frechet P. Occipito-frontal transposition flap combined with scalp extension for extensive baldness. Int J Cosm Surg 1998; 6(1):50–56.
51. Brandy DA. The bilateral occipito-parietal flap. J Dermatol Surg Oncol 1986; 12:1062–1066.
52. Unger M. Prolonged acute tissue expansion (PATE). Ann J Cosm Surg 1995; 12:231–240.

53. Nordstrom REA. The "Nordstrom Suture" for scalp reduction. Fifth Annual meeting for the International Society of Hair Restoration Surgery, Barcelona, October 15–19, 1997.
54. Unger M. Alopecia reductions. In: Unger WP, ed. Hair Transplantation. New York: Marcel Dekker, 1995, pp. 509–624.
55. Marzola M. An alternative hair replacement method. In: Norwood OT, ed. Springfield: Charles C Thomas, 1984, pp. 315–324.
56. Radovan C. Adjacent slot development using expandable silastic implants. American Society of Plastic and Reconstructive Surgery Forum, Boston, September 30, 1976.
57. Anderson R. New expanded scalp flap techniques for elimination of male pattern baldness. In: Unger WP, ed. Hair Transplantation. New York: Marcel Dekker, 1995, pp. 673–691.
58. Unger M. Prolonged acute tissue expansion (PATE). Am J Cosm Surg, 1995; 12:231–240.

Appendices 1–3 follow

APPENDIX 1. PRESURGICAL INSTRUCTIONS

for

____

Date/Time of Surgery: ____

IMPORTANT: YOU MUST STRICTLY FOLLOW THESE INSTRUCTIONS TO AVOID COMPLICATIONS (ie, excess bleeding and/or longer healing process) AND ENSURE THE BEST POSSIBLE RESULTS

THREE (3) WEEKS BEFORE SURGERY:

* ELIMINATE intake of Vitamin E capsules or vitamin pills containing Vitamin E
* Notify office re: any medications you will be taking at time of surgery. It may have to be discontinued or substituted with an alternate drug
* If you live out of town, make arrangements to stay overnight, as traffic and/or weather could delay your arrival at our office. If you arrive late, your appointment may have to be postponed. The day after surgery do not book flights until after 12:00 noon. If you want to be seen very early the day after surgery please arrange this with the booking secretary 1–3 weeks before your appointment.

ONE (1) WEEK BEFORE SURGERY:

* STOP use of Minoxidil (Rogaine)
* DO NOT take any ASPIRIN (ASA) or any drugs containing Aspirin—see enclosed sheet (eg, some cold remedies). Note: You may use Tylenol
* DO NOT drink any alcohol (wine, beer, liquors)
* DO NOT use marijuana or any nonapproved drugs

DAY BEFORE SURGERY:

* PLEASE drink 1 quart (1/2 litre) of fluids the day before surgery

NIGHT BEFORE SURGERY: ____________________________

* WASH hair well with any of the recommended shampoos listed on page 3
* Get a full night's sleep

DAY OF SURGERY: ____________________________

* PLEASE DO NOT be late for your appointment. Allow for unusual traffic delays.
* Take first dosage of antibiotics two hours before scheduled time of surgery—unless otherwise directed.
* **A.M. Surgery:** Shampoo hair well with Hibitane Skin Cleanser 4% and rinse well. Make sure you eat a good breakfast unless you have arranged for intravenous sedation with the anesthetist. If you will be having intravenous

1st Day to 4th Day After Surgery:

* Take antibiotics as directed and sleeping pills as needed. You may use Extra Strength Tylenol and/or Tylenol #3 for any discomfort you may have for the first few days after surgery.

1st Day to 7th Day After Surgery: SWELLING:

* Most people will experience some degree of swelling, the first session usually being the worst. To help prevent swelling, do the following:

  1) You will be given 2 reusable ice packs on bandage removal day. Apply ice packs or a bag of frozen peas as frequently as possible around the forehead and temples for 1–5 days after the procedure. DO NOT PLACE COLD PACKS DIRECTLY ON RECIPIENT SITES OR DONOR AREA. If swelling should occur, continue applying ice packs until the swelling subsides.

  2) Sleep with your head elevated at a 45 degree angle for 1–5 nights after the surgery, by using 3–4 pillows or a reclining chair; if you do experience swelling, keep sleeping with your head elevated until the swelling subsides.

  3) You may have been given an injection to help prevent the postsurgical swelling. If so, you do still need to follow the previous suggestions [in 1) and 2) above].

NOTE: If swelling should nevertheless occur we are sorry if this inconveniences or embarrasses you. Unfortunately if you call the office there is no further treatment or medication available—nature must take its course. It will gradually subside on its own over a 3–7 day period.

2nd Day to 21st Day After Surgery: SHAMPOOING

* Beginning on the 2nd day after surgery and until your stitches are removed from the donor area, you should wash your hair twice a day in the following manner:

  1) Fill bathtub with warm water; lay back in the water until the water covers the donor areas (ie, the stitched areas from where the grafts were taken).

  2) Soak the donor areas for 10 minutes in order to help soften the healing crusts.

  3) After soaking for 10 minutes, gently massage the donor areas for 10 more minutes under the water to help loosen and dissolve the crusts.

  4) Gently shampoo your whole head (donor and recipient areas). Do not be afraid to get a good lather in the recipient areas. Bring a cup into the bath

and with clean warm tap water rinse off the shampoo. If you wish, you may shampoo your hair in the shower; however, DO NOT allow the water to beat directly on the newly transplanted grafts until day 7. Use a weak stream of water and/or use your hand to deflect the direct flow of the shower water.

* After your stitches have been removed you must WASH YOUR HAIR DAILY until all the crusts have fallen off. We recommend the shampoos listed on the following pages. Use daily until all crusts have fallen off from both the donor and recipient areas. The following products are particularly good at removing the antibiotic ointment from your hair. Crabtree & Evelyn Jojoba Foaming Bath Gel, Gillette Foamy Shaving Cream, or Aveda "Hair Detoxifier" shampoo. Lather up and rinse off these products before you shampoo with whatever shampoo is being used.

NOTE: If the crusts from the stitched donor areas do not come off early in the healing process, the tissue underneath will not heal properly and you may end up with a wider scar in the donor area than is usual. The problem is avoidable with proper soaking and massaging as described above.

7th Day to 10th Day After Surgery: SUTURE REMOVAL

* You have been given an appointment approximately 7–10 days after surgery to have the sutures removed. You may want to take 1–2 Extra Strength Tylenol 1 hour before you come to the office for the removal of your sutures to alleviate any slight discomfort that you may experience.

1st Day to 21st Day After Surgery: DISLODGING GRAFTS

* If a plug/graft is accidentaly knocked or combed out, place it in a solution of salt water (1 tsp. of salt to a glass of water) and CALL DR. UNGER OR DR. COTTERILL IMMEDIATELY

1st Day to 21st Day After Surgery: HEALING AND CRUSTS

* Leave the transplanted recipient area open to the air as much as possible; avoid the use of hats and hairpieces unless absolutely necessary. You may gradually expose the transplanted recipient area to the sun but AVOID SUNBURN. When going outdoors use an SPF of 15 or higher.

* A few days after surgery, crusts will begin to form at the transplanted recipient sites. These crusts are part of the normal healing process; DO NOT PICK AT OR OTHERWISE TRY TO REMOVE THE CRUSTS. They will begin to fall off on their own between 1–3 weeks after surgery. If all of the crusts have not fallen off after 3 weeks, please call Dr. Unger/Cotterill's office.

* To encourage the crusts to fall off, we highly recommend that you apply K-Y Jelly (water based) to the crusts starting the night before you are permitted

to shampoo to help soften the crusts. You may want to place a towel on your pillow to protect it from the ointments. Apply a coating on all of the recipient grafts (you may also apply them to the donor areas). Make certain that you shampoo all the K-Y Jelly with each shampoo. Continue to reapply until all of the crusts have fallen off. Vitamin E oil or Bacitracin ointment may also be used. They soften the crusts better than K-Y Jelly but they are more oily and are more difficult to shampoo out.

* If your scalp becomes itchy, a cream may be prescribed by Dr. Unger or Dr. Cotterill if you call the office.

6 Weeks to 4 Months After Surgery: TRANSPLANTED HAIR REGROWTH

* DO NOT expect any hair growth for 3 months. This is perfectly normal. (Some patients experience hair growth starting as soon as 6 weeks after surgery but this is unusual). By 3 months all grafts will have started to grow. However, because hair grows 1/2″ per month your transplanted hair will not be very visible until 6 months after surgery at which point it will be at least 1 1/2″ long. The full cosmetic benefit is not reached until 9 months after surgery.

ADDITIONAL INFORMATION

* **INFECTION:** Infection is rare. However, to help prevent infection, avoid exposure to dirt in the air, at work or at play, for 2 weeks after the surgery. If you experience any redness, swelling, tenderness or "pus pimples," please contact Dr. Unger/Cotterill's office immediately.

* **NUMBNESS:** Many fine nerve endings are cut during each procedure resulting in decreased sensitivity in the donor or recipient area, or both. This decreased sensitivity is nearly always temporary and will resolve on its own in 6 to 18 months.

* **EXERCISE:** For the first 7 days after surgery, you should refrain from exercise, sports activities, and strenuous work. Maximum weightlifting or any kind of heavy lifting must be avoided for 14 days after surgery. You may swim in a clean lake or a clean non-public pool beginning on the 3rd day after surgery. Wait 2 weeks before swimming in a public pool or lake of uncertain cleanliness.

  If you do begin exercising after 7 days or otherwise engage in activities that cause you to perspire, please wash your hair as soon as possible after the activity. Bacteria can grow quickly in any moist warm area and may cause infection in an area that is not completely healed.

* **VITAMINS:** There *may* be some benefit to taking vitamin supplements after surgery. You may take Vitamin E, 800 I.U., per day beginning 24 hours after surgery and continuing for at least 14 days. You may also take Vitamin C, 2000 mg (2 gms), per day immediately after surgery and

continuing for at least 14 days. Swiss herbal One-A-Day Vitamin Mineral supplement (and certain other multivitamin/mineral supplements) may also be taken beginning 24 hours after surgery.

* **MINOXIDIL: (Rogaine) (Apogain)** Sometimes using Minoxidil twice a day for the first 5–6 weeks will result in fewer hairs temporarily falling out of the grafts and/or will stimulate hair in the grafts to begin to regrow a little faster. It is not necessary to use Minoxidil, but if you would like to try it, please ask for a prescription and use the following procedures.

  1) Wash hands thoroughly before each application.

  2) Beginning on the day your bandage is removed, apply Minoxidil twice daily as directed, for 6 weeks, morning and evening (at least 1/2 hour before going to sleep), preferably after you have washed your hair, but before you apply K-Y Jelly or any other medication.

  3) If you intend to have another transplant 6 weeks later. STOP using Minoxidil 1 week before the scheduled date of your next surgery.

* **HAIR PRODUCTS:** Recommended shampoos and conditioners. These can be found in drug stores, Beauty supply shops, and Health food shops):

  —Ionil (without tar), Redken, Nexxus, Neutrogena

  Hair conditioners may be used with every 2nd washing. Light hair spray, gels, and mousses may be used when you begin shampooing your hair, but preferably as little as possible for the first week and must be washed off daily. Recommended hair spray is a non–alcohol-based one.

  Hair coloring and perms should be avoided until all of the crusts have fallen off; generally by 1–2 weeks.

* **CAMOUFLAGE:** You may have an important meeting or function that you must attend after your surgery and would like to be able to use a cover-up to camouflage the recipient areas for a few hours. Two suggestions: 1) Lancome "Maquicontrole," an oil-free water-based make-up (available at large department stores), 2) any other water-based make-up you can obtain more easily, or 3) Institute For Advanced Skin Care, 66 Avenue Road (416)962-0001. They offer a waterproof camouflage make-up (24 skin shades available) with flat opaque tones that can conceal discolorations and smooth uneven skin surfaces.

  Whichever cover-up method you use, you must do so only for the limited time that it is absolute necessary. Shampoo the cover-up off as soon as possible afterwards.

APPENDIX 3. *AS YOU HEAL . . .*

Family & Friends *Support from family and friends is very helpful, but because they may not understand what constitutes a normal postsurgical course, their comments may unintentionally create emotional turmoil for you. We will tell you honestly how you are doing and what we expect your results to be.*

Depression *Some patients experience a brief period of "let-down" or depression the first few days after their hair transplantation. This is in some part due to the Valium and Demerol given presurgically, as well as the pain medication and sleeping pills taken during the postsurgical night. Some may subconsciously have expected to feel and look better "instantly," even though they rationally understand that this will not be the case. Patients sometimes question their decision to have surgery during the first few days after surgery. As the healing occurs, these thoughts usually disappear quickly. If you feel depressed, understanding that this is a "natural" phase of the healing process may help you.*

HEALING *FOLLOWING INSTRUCTIONS:*
Another major factor in the course of healing is whether you follow the instructions given by the doctor verbally and in this pamphlet. Such guidelines are designed to promote the healing process and to prevent the occurrence of anything that may interfere with recovery. It is imperative that you recognize that you are a partner in this process and have a responsibility to follow instructions carefully. Our instructions, based on broad experience, are designed to give you the best opportunity for healing without delay or surprise.

APPENDIX 4. CONSENT FOR USE OF PHOTOGRAPHS

1. **NAME OF PATIENT** ____

2. In the interest of medical science, ________________________________
(Doctor's Name)

   is hereby authorized to take and exhibit

   ____________ with the face exposed

   ____________ with the face completely blocked out

   photographs of the above patient before, during and after treatment.

3. The present consent is given on condition that the said photographs shall be used for scientific purposes only, including publication in scientific and professional publications, and exhibitions to scientific and medical audiences.

4. I hereby expressly waive any and all claims which I might at any time have, or pretend to have, against said Doctor, in any matter whatsoever relating to the said photographs as stipulated in paragraph 3.

DATED THIS ______ DAY OF ______, 19______

______________________ ______________________

Witness Signature

APPENDIX 5. CONSENT TO OPERATION AND/OR DIAGNOSTIC PROCEDURE

I, ______________________ do hereby authorize Dr. __________ to perform the ________________ procedure on me. I have read and understand the procedure and possible complications as set out in the information sheets provided at my interview with Dr. ____________. I have also had the opportunity to ask whatever questions I wished before undergoing the procedure. Should I for any reason and at any time decide to sue Dr. ____________ or any member or members of his staff, I hereby agree that I will contact a lawyer for this purpose only after first consulting with another qualified expert in hair transplanting, and agree to settlement of any legal action by arbitration. I wish to modify my consent in the following manner:

____

____

____

I also understand that I must not operate any motorized vehicle for **8 hours following surgery.** I hereby release (doctor) from any and all actions los or injury sustained by me as a consequence of my operation of any motorized vehicle.

Dated is __________ day of ____________________, 19______.

____

WITNESS PATIENT, PARENT OR GUARDIAN

35

Earlobe Repair, Scar Revision, Actinic Cheilitis, and Other Lip Lesions

Nancy Marchell
Laguna Hills Dermatology, Inc., Laguna Hills, California

Yardy Tse
University of California at San Diego, San Diego, California

This chapter will address general dermatologic surgical procedures that are commonly performed in the office: scar revision, repair of torn earlobes, and treatment of actinic cheilitis and other lip lesions. The revision of existing scars is a frequently requested procedure. Seemingly straightforward, the techniques of scar revision have many nuances that must be considered before initiating any procedure. Similarly, the repair of torn earlobes has become increasingly popular for both male and female patients. Many techniques exist for this procedure; we describe a very straightforward, simple approach. With the advent of laser resurfacing, the treatment of actinic cheilitis has also become fairly straightforward and simple.

SCAR REVISION

Scar revision is an attempt to improve a scar's appearance by changing the direction of the scar, narrowing or repositioning the scar, or eliminating or minimizing the size of the scar via surgical or nonsurgical means. Scars can be categorized by their location, origin, size, shape, contour, function, or color. Some areas of the body are more susceptible to hypertrophic or thickened scarring. These areas include the upper back, shoulders, chest, mandible, and nasal dorsum. Because of constant movement in these areas, the scar may spread in size over time.

The chance of developing a hypertrophic or thickened scar is inversely related to the extent of injury that parallels the relaxed skin tension lines (RSTLs) (1). Relaxed skin tension lines are the natural tissue planes that display the least amount of tension. Ideally, scar placement should fall within the RSTLs that correspond to natural wrinkle lines and run perpendicular to underlying muscle movement. Scars that occur without regard to the RSTL such as acne scars, trauma, ulcers, or burns, often result in disfigurement.

Atrophic scars are somewhat concave in appearance with overlying thinned epidermis. These scars usually result from tissue loss after healing by secondary intention, heavy intralesional steroid use, or from a resolving underlying lesion. Scars that are stretched from high movement areas may also have atrophic features. Also, loss of subcutaneous tissues can result in a depressed scar with atrophy (2).

Several nonsurgical methods are available for scar revision. These include silicone gel sheeting (3–7); soft-tissue augmentation (2) with collagen; Autologen™; Dermologen™; Fibral™; autologous fat and silicone; pulsed dye laser treatment (3,8); treatment using other lasers, including the argon, copper, Nd:YAG, and Helium:neon lasers; cryosurgery (9); irradiation; compression (10); and intralesional therapy, including corticosteroids, 5-fluorouracil (5-FU) (11), interferons (12), prostaglandins (8), and topical tretinoin (13,14).

Surgical options for scar revision include extramarginal excision, intramarginal excision, W-plasty, Z-plasty, V-Y advancement flap, dermabrasion, and laser resurfacing with the CO_2 or erbium:YAG lasers.

History

Scar revision dates back to 1500 BC, where in the Egyptian Papyrus Ebers, use of abrasive pastes of pumice and alabaster particles in honey and milk is described to smooth skin defects. In the late 19th century, the great European dermatologist Unna applied compounds of pumice to facial skin to improve its cosmetic appearance. By 1905, motor-driven dermabrasion was developed by Kromayer to plane facial scars (15). He used cylindrical knives, then later dental burrs and rasps to treat tattoos, nevi, warts, and scars. Considered the father of modern dermabrasion, Kromayer also used CO_2 snow and ether spray both to achieve rigidity of the skin as well as anesthesia.

In 1948, McEvitt described the use of sandpaper abrasion for the treatment of acne scars (16). Kurtin, in the early 1950s, developed motor-driven wire brushes and used ethyl chloride as a skin refrigerant (17). His technique was used in the treatment of acne scars and trauma scars, as well as tattoos, fine wrinkles, keratoses, and keloids.

Dermabrasion had traditionally been performed on scars that were present for 6 months or longer after the original surgery or injury. Vukas, in 1974, stated that aesthetic results were better when the scar was older (18); however, only marginal improvement resulted when dermabrasion was performed after this time interval. Other techniques, such as Z-plasty, W-plasty, and geometric broken line closures, increased in popularity at this time. By changing a straight line into a broken line, the scar was made less apparent to the eye.

Only 20 years ago, in 1979, was the suggestion of earlier surgical intervention made. Burk stated in his text on dermabrasion that scars may be dermabraded 6 to 8 weeks after their formation (15). Collins and Farber reported that dermabrasion on nasal scars 2 to 6 weeks after suture removal increased the cosmetic outcome (19). Yarborough found that facial scars planed with a wire brush 4 to 8 weeks after injury healed without residual scarring compared with older scars (20). Scars abraded during this time period were found to have an increase in collagen bundle density and size with a tendency toward unidirectional orientation of fibers parallel to the epidermal surface (21). Revision of scars with significant dermal components is usually delayed for 6 to 9 months after surgery in order to allow for scar maturation (5).

Presurgical Considerations

When attempting a surgical scar revision, the following factors must be considered (2): (1) a wound needs to have clean viable edges for optimal healing, (2) the edges should oppose with little or no tension, (3) the best orientation must be selected, and (4) the least reactive suture material must be selected.

Extramarginal excision, intramarginal excision, W-plasty, and Z-plasty require precise excision and suturing technique. Other surgical options for selected scars include spot dermabrasion and laser resurfacing.

SURGICAL EXCISION OF SCARS

Presurgical Instructions

Before attempting any type of scar revision, the patient should understand that all forms of scar revision involve exchanging one type of scar for another more cosmetically acceptable scar. Complete eradication of a scar so as to render the treatment or traumatized area "brand new" is often impossible. Thus, complete informed consent and realistic expectations on the part of the patient are of utmost importance.

Patients are instructed to avoid aspirin and ibuprofen products 10 days before and 2 days after surgery in order to minimize bleeding. Similarly, alcoholic beverages should also be avoided 3 days before surgery and 2 days after surgery.

The surgical site is prepared and draped in a sterile fashion, and local anesthesia with 1% lidocaine with epinephrine is administered.

Paperwork

Consent forms for all surgical procedures described in this chapter are essentially the same. The consent form for the surgery must be reviewed with the patient and signed by both the patient as well as the physician. A witness, usually one of the medical staff, also signs the consent. Risks of complications from the procedure and postsurgical risks must be discussed. These include bleeding, infection, necrosis, dehiscence, hypertrophic scarring, and postinflammatory hyper- and hypopigmentation.

Equipment

The basic instruments used in most scar revisions include the following:

1. A fresh sharp blade (Bard-Parker #15 or Persona Plus #15). Multiple lesions may require replacement blades. A #11 scalpel blade will be helpful for precise cutting of angles in a W-plasty.
2. An absorbable suture, such as polyglactin 910 (Vicryl) or similar suture.
3. Nonabsorbable suture such as Prolene or similar suture.
4. Two single prong skin hooks.
5. Electrocautery (Bovie instrument) for hemostasis.
6. 1% Xylocaine with 1:100,000 epinephrine (maximum 70 mg/kg based on the patient's weight). 2% lidocaine is used for nerve blocks (without epinephrine if used on fingers or toes).
7. Needle holder.
8. Marking pen.

Day of Surgery

On the day of surgery, the patient is escorted into the surgical room and the consent form is discussed and signed. Presurgical photographs are taken. For surgical scar revision, the scar is marked with a narrow clear margin of approximately 1 mm. For an intramarginal excision, 2 to 3 mm of surrounding scar tissue is left.

Anesthesia

Local anesthesia using 1% lidocaine is usually effective for scar revision, earlobe repair, and vermilionectomy for actinic cheilitis. Local anesthesia containing epinephrine becomes effective immediately after injection. For maximum vasoconstrictive effect and good hemostasis from the epinephrine, a waiting period of at least 7 minutes should be expected before excision. Blanching of the site is an indication that the vasoconstrictive properties of epinephrine have taken effect. Local anesthesia as a field or nerve block with or without topical EMLA (eutectic mixture of lidocaine and prilocaine) can also be used. For larger areas of scar revision, such as extensive burn contractures, systemic anesthesia (IV sedation or general anesthesia) may be necessary.

Technique

An extramarginal scar excision involves complete removal of scar tissue as an elliptical or fusiform excision. In an intramarginal excision, the purpose is to decrease the bulk of the scar and flatten its contour. Intramarginal scar excision involves excising the scar while leaving a small margin of scar tissue. It has been reported that excision of a hypertrophic scar within the margins of the scar followed by reapproximation produces a better cosmetic result with less subsequent hypertrophy than excision of the scar in its entirety. Studies on hypertrophic burn scars and perioral scars confirmed this finding. There has yet to be any data to explain why a scar within a scar heals better.

A W-plasty is merely a zig-zag configured scar revision to break up a scar visually and to reorient it so that it lies within RSTLs with no increase in length. A Z-plasty, however, is the transposition of two triangular flaps of tissue, resulting in a theoretical gain in length or relaxation of the scar. It can also help to reorient the scar to lie within RSTLs. A V-Y advancement flap is used to revise a moderately sized scar that may be curvilinear or have trap door deformities. A "V"-shaped excision is transformed into a "Y" by advancing the lateral tissue.

The scar excision should be made in natural skin lines (RSTLs) or be altered to fall within these lines. For scars less than 2 cm, elliptical or fusiform excision is best. Larger scars may require a series of excisions at 6 to 8 week intervals, which will result in a single linear scar. If a sunken scar exists, the excision should be made divergent in depth to the deep portion of the scar to help re-establish the loss of tissue that caused the depression. Undermining of the surrounding tissue should be made at the level of the subcutaneous tissue laterally for minimal tension at the wound edges. Little to no undermining of the surrounding tissues is needed for an intramarginal excision. Wound closure with deep dermal absorbable suture is placed in an inverted (knot down) fashion as an interrupted simple suture. This can then be followed by a series of simple interrupted sutures or by a continuous subcuticular stitch using an absorbable or nonabsorbable suture placed from one end of the wound to the other at the level of the deep dermis and epidermis. This will result in a fine linear scar with no punctate or cross tie scarring (Figs. 1, 2). Acne scars can be excised via punch excisions (Fig. 3).

For W-plasty, wounds are closed with a few horizontal mattress sutures followed by simple interrupted sutures at the tips of the triangular flaps. For longer scars, a running subcuticular stitch placed between the triangle tip and base can also be used.

In a W-plasty, complete excision of scar tissue occurs via a series of interlocking triangles or "Ws." The triangles are cut with 60° tips so that they will fit together like a "lock and key" (templates are available) (Fig. 4). Depending on the scar, the

(a)

(b)

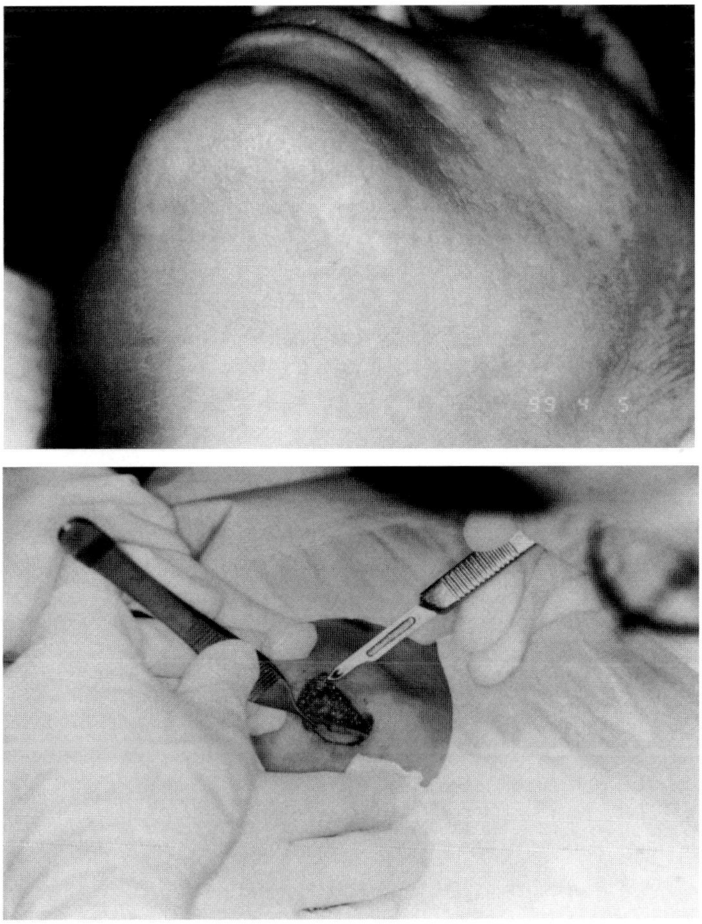

FIGURE 1 (a) Presurgical photograph of submental scar. (b) Scar is outlined and is excised with a #15 blade. (c) Immediately postsurgical scar revision.

(c) 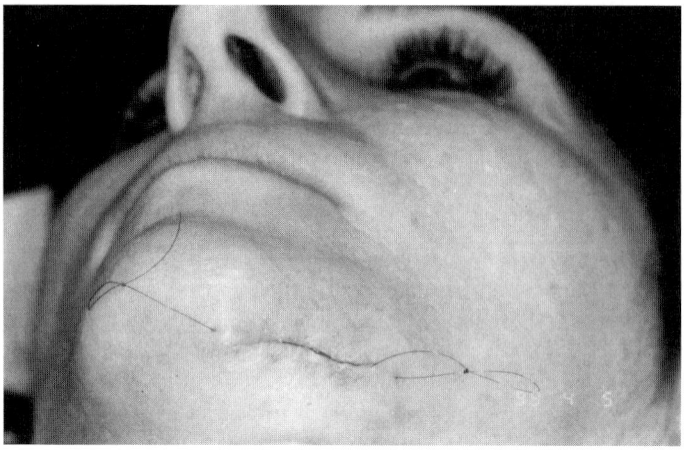

FIGURE 1 Continued.

length, direction, and size of the triangles will vary. For facial scars, triangles should be no larger than 8 mm.

In a Z-plasty, after excision of the main portion of the scar, triangular flaps of 60° are cut to the same length as the central portion. The surrounding tissue is undermined into two triangles, which are then transposed (Fig. 5). This transposition transfers wound tension from the central axis of the scar by lengthening it and shifting tension toward the lateral axis of the scar. The lateral limbs may need to be lengthened 3 to 6 mm more than the length of the central limb in scars with high contraction. The final scar will be approximately three times longer. Multiple Z-plasties can be performed in series on a single scar to produce less tissue contraction.

(a) 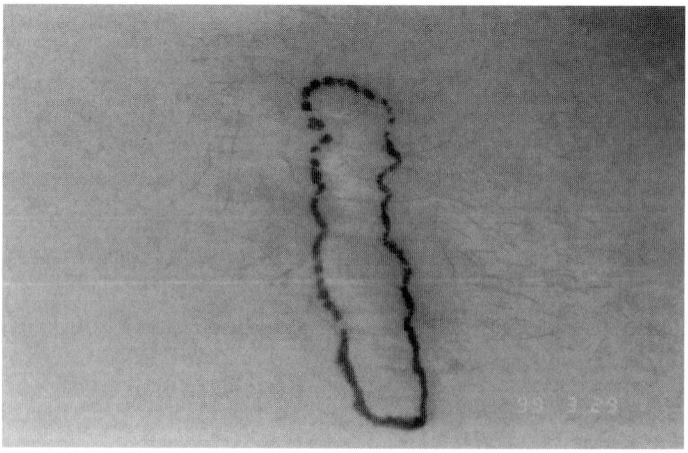

FIGURE 2 (a) Presurgical photograph of spread scar on sacral area. (b) Surgical excision of scar with #15 blade. (c) Immediately postsurgical scar revision.

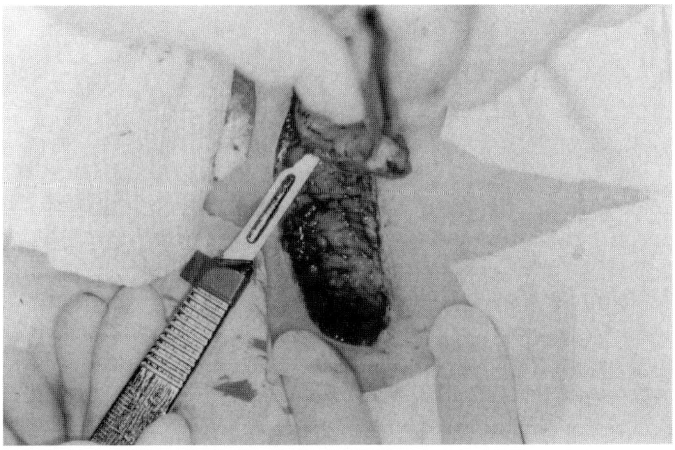

(b)

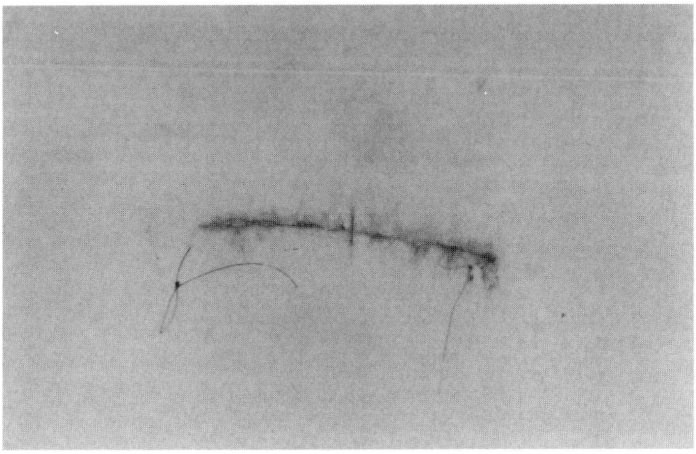

(c)

FIGURE 2 Continued.

To minimize necrosis at the tip of the triangular flaps, a fine nonabsorbable suture should be placed in a horizontal mattress involving only a portion of the dermis in the tip of the triangles.

In a V-Y advancement flap, a "V"-shaped incision is made into the skin surrounding the scar. The skin on either side of the "V" is undermined, advanced, and closed as a "Y" (Fig. 6). Undermining the "V" itself is not necessary because most of the tissue gain is from undermining the lateral tissue.

Postsurgical Care

Antibiotic ointment and a pressure dressing are applied. This pressure dressing should remain in place for 24 to 48 hours after surgery in order to help provide hemostasis. The patient is instructed in daily cleansing and application of antibiotic ointment. To maximize the cosmetic outcome, physical activity, which could cause tension to the

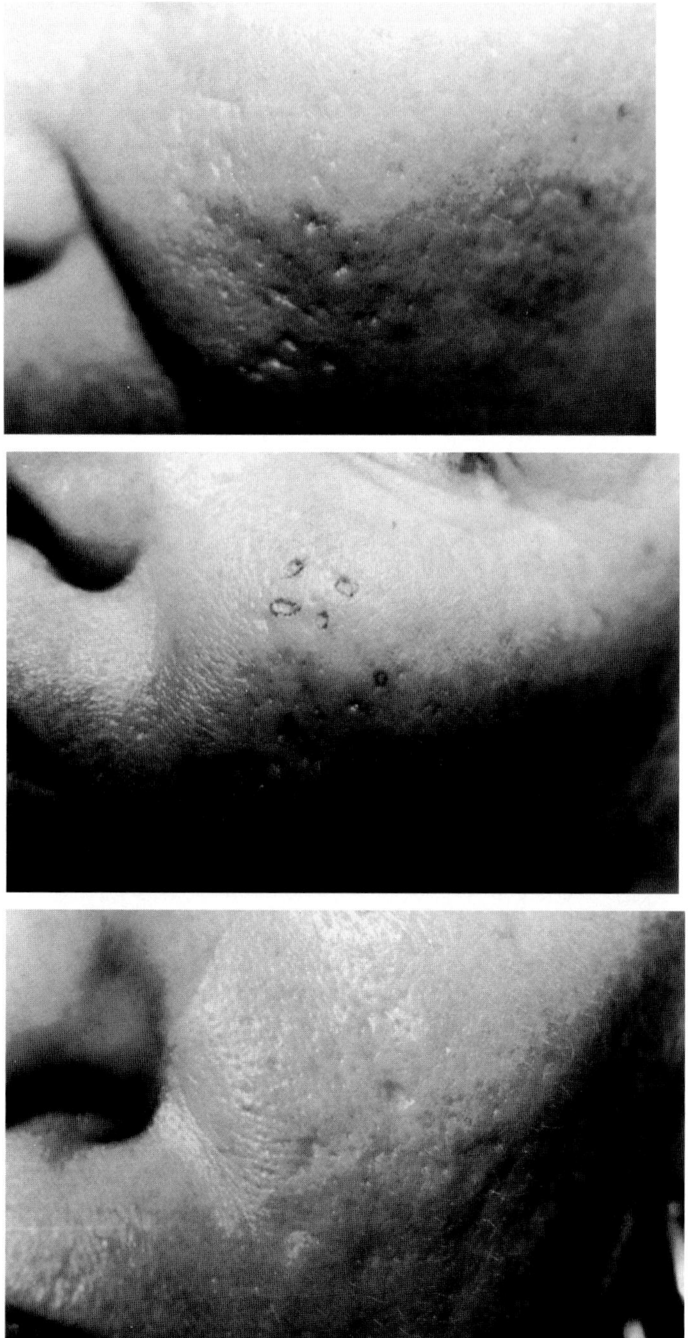

(a) (b) (c)

FIGURE 3 (a) Presurgical photograph of acne scars on left cheek. (b) Individual scars are outlined for multiple punch excisions. (c) Four years after punch excisions of acne scars.

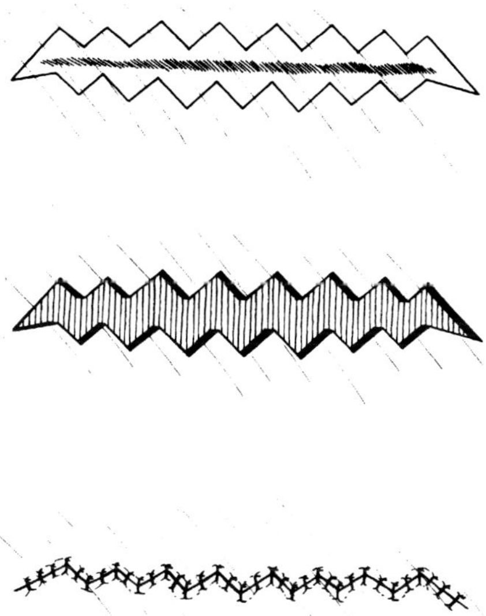

FIGURE 4 W-plasty with interlocking triangles forming a zigzag line. Note that half of the lines are oriented in the RSTLs.

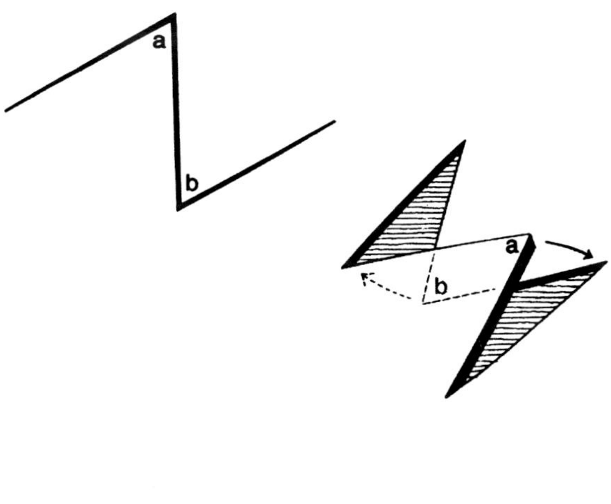

FIGURE 5 Z-plasty with 60-degree transposing flaps a and b. A net gain in length in the vertical direction along the line from a to b has been achieved.

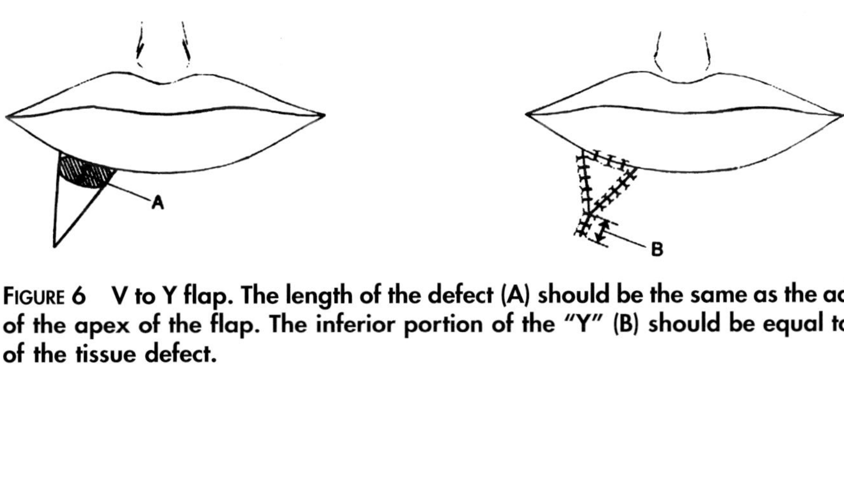

FIGURE 6 V to Y flap. The length of the defect (A) should be the same as the advancement of the apex of the flap. The inferior portion of the "Y" (B) should be equal to the height of the tissue defect.

wound, should be avoided. Swimming in the ocean and tub baths increase the risk of wound infections and should also be avoided before suture removal. Acetaminophen can be taken for pain management, and the use of ice packs are encouraged to decrease swelling.

DERMABRASION

Presurgical Considerations

Early intervention with dermabrasion (approximately 1–3 months after injury) creates optimal results. Any patient who has taken isotretinoin within 1 year has a higher risk of adverse scarring. Thus, dermabrasion should be delayed in these patients.

Presurgical Instructions

Antiviral medication should be initiated several days before the dermabrasion if the treatment area is on the face. Depending on the size of the area to be dermabraded, some physicians will initiate treatment with topical retinoic acid or 4% hydroquinone approximately 1 month before the procedure. This is believed to enhance re-epithelialization and decrease the incidence of hyperpigmentation, respectively.

Equipment

Fraises are available in a variety of shapes and coarseness. Diamond fraises with a motor-driven engine are very effective. A coarse diamond fraise followed by a delicate pea or bullet-shaped fraise can be used for scar revision. Wire brushes, sterile drywall sanding mesh, and aluminum-carbide crystals can also be used.

Technique

The scar is planed, then blended at the edges into the surrounding normal tissue. This may result in a larger defect and patients should be warned of this. At the appearance of pinpoint bleeding, the papillary dermis is reached. When small yellow areas representing sebaceous globules can be seen, the reticular dermis has been reached and dermabrasion should cease. Areas such as the mandible that overlie bony prominences are at high risk for hypertrophic scarring and caution should be taken.

Postsurgical Care

Gauze saturated in ice water should be applied to stop the bleeding. Antibiotic ointment and a bio-occlusive dressing is then applied. The patient is instructed on wound care with an antibiotic ointment. The patient is advised to avoid sun exposure for the next 3 months.

LASER RESURFACING

Presurgical Considerations

Laser resurfacing with the CO_2 or erbium:YAG lasers can provide ablation of thin layers of scar tissue with minimal thermal damage and bleeding. A recent article by

Alster et al. (22) describes the use of concomitant high-energy, pulsed CO_2, and pulsed dye lasers for results superior to CO_2 laser vaporization alone in hypertrophic scar revision. Like dermabrasion, early intervention of a scar revision provides optimal results (1–3 months after injury). Patients need to wait at least 1 year if they are taking isotretinoin.

Presurgical Instructions

As in dermabrasion, preprocedure treatment with antiviral medication should be initiated if the face is to be treated. Patients should be advised that prolonged erythema (up to 6 months) may result. Pigment alteration (particularly hyperpigmentation in skin types III–V) may occur.

Equipment

Many CO_2 lasers can be used for resurfacing. With short tissue exposure times of less than 1 msec, the thermal damage zone is only about 50 microns to 100 microns. CO_2 lasers such as the Sharplan SilkTouch/Feathertouch (Sharplan Lasers, Inc., Allendale, NJ) use a rapidly scanning CO_2 beam to reduce tissue exposure. The Coherent UltraPulse (Coherent Medical Group, Santa Clara, CA) produces high peak power pulses of very short duration. The use of computerized scanners allows for easier delivery and consistency. The erbium:YAG lasers ablate more superficially than CO_2 laser with shorter pulses and more precise ablation. Using erbium:YAG lasers appears to decrease postprocedure erythema, but intra- and postsurgical bleeding may be more significant.

Technique

The surgical area should be prepared with nonflammable agents. Wet towels should be used on the surgical field and eye protection worn by the patient and staff. Moistened gauze may be used to cover the periorbital region if the treatment area is on the face. A single pass of nonoverlapping pulses is first made to the entire scar. The debris is wiped with saline-soaked gauze after each pass with the CO_2 laser. A greater number of passes with the erbium:YAG laser will be required to achieve an endpoint that is similar to that of a few passes of the CO_2 laser. Feathering of the edges of the scar into surrounding tissue with additional passes is performed as in dermabrasion. The resulting scar will appear flatter and somewhat larger but will continue to improve with healing.

Postsurgical Care

Bio-occlusive dressings can be applied along with antibiotic ointment or petrolatum twice a day. Strict sun avoidance should be emphasized for at least 2 to 3 months postsurgically or until postsurgical erythema has subsided.

Surgical Complications and Treatment

No matter how skilled the surgeon or how compliant the patient, adverse results following surgery can always occur. These risks should be discussed in the informed consent.

Bleeding is the most common complication in postsurgical excision. Many patients taking aspirin products or nonsteroidal anti-inflammatory drugs (NSAIDs) should be instructed to stop these products at least 10 days before surgery and for 2 days after surgery. Acetaminophen can be used for pain management. For those patients taking Coumadin, the primary-care physician or cardiologist should be consulted regarding discontinuation of this medication 2 days before surgery and 1 day after surgery. The patient should also avoid alcohol 48 hours after surgery to prevent bleeding and limit physical activity postsurgically.

Most postsurgical bleeding usually occurs within the first 6 hours after surgery. This may result in a hematoma with swelling and discomfort. Hematomas can be aspirated or evacuated by removing the sutures and draining the hematoma. If active bleeding is present, electrocautery or tying off the vessel with an absorbable suture should be performed. A drain may be placed in the incision line and antibiotic therapy should be initiated to decrease the risk of infection. The drain should be removed in 24 hours. Most bleeding can be controlled with adequate pressure (15–20 min) and the patient should be instructed to apply pressure initially if bleeding occurs after surgery.

The risk of infection is infrequent but must be treated early if suspected to prevent prolonged healing time and a poor cosmetic result. Signs of infection can be subtle, such as moderate erythema and swelling, or appear more obvious as purulent abscess formation. Most wound infections occur 4 to 8 days after surgery and can be controlled with oral antibiotics. For dermabrasion and laser resurfacing patients, acetic acid soaks are recommended after surgery on an hourly basis for the first 2 to 3 days to minimize the risk of infection.

If purulent drainage is noted, a Gram stain and culture and sensitivity should be performed. The majority of infections are attributable to Staphylococcus aureus and can be treated with a penicillinase-resistant penicillin (dicloxacillin) or erythromycin. A broad-spectrum cephalosporin will cover some Gram-negative organisms as well. Ciprofloxacin can be used to treat pseudomonas infections.

Wound necrosis results from tissue ischemia secondary to circulatory compromise. The most common cause of tissue ischemia and necrosis is excessive tension on the wound edges. Proper use of subcutaneous sutures will help reduce wound tension before the placement of epidermal sutures. Smokers are at higher risk for tissue ischemia and necrosis, especially if skin grafts or flaps have been performed. The patient should be advised to stop smoking 2 to 3 days before surgery and at least 5 to 7 days after surgery.

Dehiscence, or wound separation, is usually secondary to infection or bleeding, which causes increased swelling and tension on the wound. Trauma to the wound or excessive activity can also cause wound dehiscence. Also, failure to use subcutaneous sutures in high-tension areas may contribute to dehiscence. The addition of Steri-Strips™ at the time of suture removal may provide support to the wound edges and decrease the chance of dehiscence. A wound that opens cleanly from trauma in the first 24 hours can be resutured. Dehiscense secondary to infection should usually heal by secondary intention.

Topical antibiotics are a common cause of contact dermatitis in the postsurgical period, with the most common sensitizing agent being neomycin. The use of petrolatum or other similar ointments may be less irritating for patients with sensitive skin. Treatment of postsurgical contact dermatitis consists of discontinuing the responsible agent and using a mid-strength topical steroid for several days.

Hypertrophic scarring is rare but can occur after dermabrasion or laser resurfacing. This occurs most commonly on the upper lip, mandible, malar regions, periorbital regions, and neck. Higher laser energy settings and greater numbers of passes may contribute to the development of this complication. Wound infections in the postsurgical period also increase the risk of scarring after laser resurfacing. Treatment includes potent topical steroids, injections of intralesional corticosteroids with or without 5-FU, silicone gel sheeting, or pulsed dye laser.

Summary

There are many techniques for scar revision. The choice of technique should be customized to the individual patient. Ultimately, the result should be a scar that is more cosmetically appealing and perhaps with improved functional capability. The surgeon needs to discuss with the patient the options available as well as the risks and complications for each procedure.

EARLOBE REPAIR

Cleft earlobes may be congenital in origin or a result of traumatic injury. Traumatic clefts are often caused by a sudden pull on an earring, wearing heavy earrings, wearing multiple earrings, which weakens the tissue of the earlobes, or from pressure necrosis caused by clip-on earrings. In recent years, there has been an increase in ear piercing attributable to a trend in young men wearing an earring in one and sometimes both ears, and women wearing multiple earrings in each ear. As a result, there has been an increasing incidence of cleft or split earlobe deformities necessitating repair.

History

The surgical technique to repair split earlobes has been recorded since ancient India (23). Correction is usually obtained by excising the cleft margins and suturing the new edges with or without a Z-plasty and with or without preserving the pierced hole. Over the years, many techniques for earlobe repair have been described and all are subject to criticism. (24).

Presurgical Considerations and Instructions

The patient should be instructed to avoid aspirin and Ibuprofen products 10 days before and 2 days after surgery. The patient should also refrain from alcoholic beverages 3 days before and 2 days after surgery.

Equipment

1. A fresh, sharp #15 blade
2. An absorbable 5.0 suture, such as polyglactin 910 (Vicryl) or similar suture
3. Nonabsorbable 6.0 suture such as Prolene or similar suture
4. Two single prong skin hooks

5. Electrocautery (Bovie instrument for hemostasis)
6. 1% Xylocaine with 1:100,000 epinephrine (maximum 70 mg/kg based on the patient's weight)
7. Needle holder
8. Marking pens

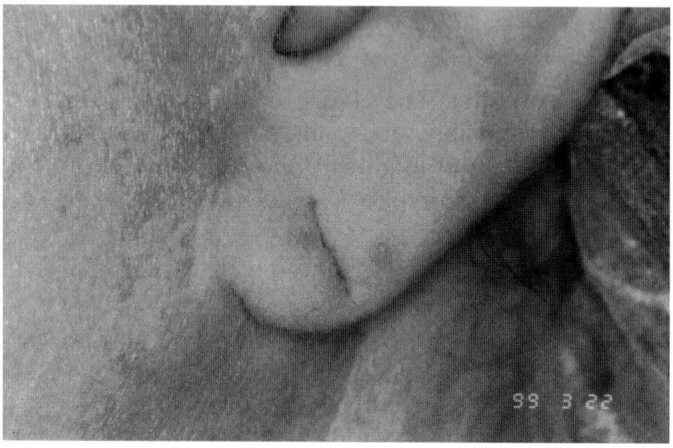

(a)

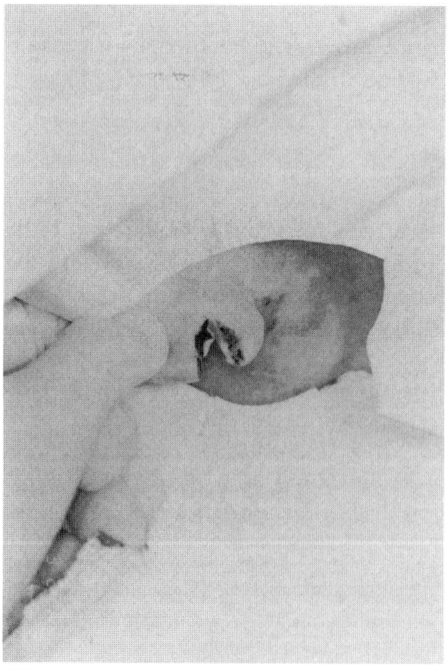

(b)

FIGURE 7 **(a) Presurgical photograph of torn earlobe. (b) Scar has been excised and the skin edges freshened using a #15 blade. (c) Immediately postsurgical earlobe repair.**

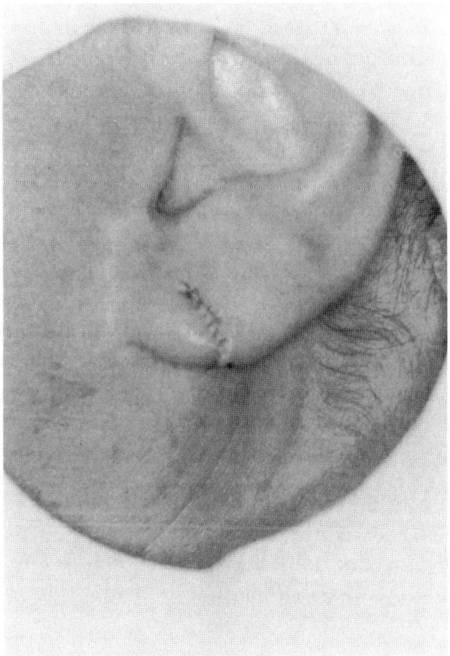

(c)

FIGURE 7 Continued.

Technique

The earlobe is prepared and draped in a sterile fashion (Fig. 7a). The lobule is infiltrated with 1% lidocaine with epinephrine (1:100,000). A 1 to 2 mm margin around the cleft is marked. If the cleft is incomplete, the marking should extend down to the inferior border of the earlobe. A #15 blade is used to excise the cleft tissue through and through down to the inferior border of the lobe including the skin bridge if the cleft is incomplete. Straight edges are freshened and cut to a point just above the superior aspect of the cleft (Fig. 7b). Avoid cross-hatching of the inverted "V" excision. Subcutaneous sutures are placed using 5-0 Vicryl suture. The skin edges are everted and approximated with multiple 6-0 prolene interrupted simple sutures (Fig. 7c). If the cleft is not too large, a 2 to 4 mm punch excision of the existing cleft can be performed and closed with simple sutures (25).

Postsurgical Care

Antibiotic ointment and bandage are applied. The patient is instructed in daily cleansing and application of antibiotic ointment. The patient should avoid swimming in the ocean before suture removal. Acetaminophen can be taken for pain management. Ice packs can be used to decrease swelling.

The sutures are removed in 1 week. The wound is then reinforced with Steri-Strips. The patient is advised against sun exposure for the next 3 months. It has been recommended that the earlobe not be repierced sooner than 4 to 6 weeks after repair to allow the earlobe tissue to soften and assume its final shape (24,26). The patient can wear clip-on earrings if comfortable, but should avoid wearing heavy earrings.

When the ears are repierced after reconstruction, the lobe is smooth and the scar is imperceptible. Piercing can be performed just below the apex of the scar, in the scar, or to either side of the incision.

Summary

The dermatologic surgeon must frequently address the aesthetic repair of cleft earlobes. Many techniques have been described, some preserving the pierced hole. Our procedure is much technically simpler than many others and provides the ability to pierce a new hole in any location on the repaired lobe.

TREATMENT OF ACTINIC CHEILITIS AND OTHER LIP LESIONS

Actinic cheilitis is a superficial keratotic lesion of the lip which, like actinic keratosis, is a precursor to the development of squamous cell carcinoma. It is also known as cheilitis exfoliativa, solar cheilosis, and actinic keratosis of the lip (27). Clinically, patients experience dryness and scaling with intermittent bleeding and occasional erosions of the lip. Patients with Fitzpatrick skin types I and II are prone to this condition, along with those who are habitually exposed to sunlight (28–30). The location of actinic cheilitis is usually the lower lip because this structure usually protrudes, thus receiving more direct rays from the sun. Like actinic keratosis, ultraviolet light is the primary causative factor for the development of squamous cell carcinoma (27). However, less than 3% of cutaneous squamous cell carcinoma metastasize, whereas approximately 10% of those originating in the lip metastasize (31).

There are many other lip lesions presenting as "cheilitis" or an inflammatory process affecting the vermilion of the lips. Because of constant exposure to the environment, the lips can develop an allergic or irritant contact cheilitis from toothpastes, sunscreens, cane reed in instruments, foods, and flavorings (32). Photosensitive cheilitis can also occur or worsen by dryness, windburn, and sunburn. Clinically, scaling, edema, and erythema are noted on the lips or may extend beyond it. Both upper and lower lips are typically involved. A patch test should be performed to identify the offending agent, and treatment consists of 1% hydrocortisone ointment (27).

Angular cheilitis or perleche is an inflammatory process occurring at the oral commissures and frequently seen in HIV-infected patients (33). The clinical features are erythema, atrophy, scaling, edema, fissuring, ulceration, and maceration, and are commonly seen in the elderly. Some possible causes are trapping of saliva at the oral commissures, riboflavin deficiency, candidiasis, streptococcus or staphlococcus infections, and atopic or seborrheic dermatitis. Allergic perleche can be seen in nickle- or rubber-sensitive individuals as well as nail polish–sensitive individuals. Diagnosis is confirmed by potassium hydroxide (KOH) preparation and careful history and examination. Therapy of angular cheilitis involves elimination of the predisposing factor. Nystatin and iodochlorhydroxyquin in a hydrocortisone or fluorinated corticosteroid ointment can be effective (27,31).

Glandular cheilitis is an uncommon disorder with enlargement and secondary changes of heterotopic salivary glands of the lip. Clinically, the lower lip is enlarged and everted with crusting and scaling. Saliva can be expressed from numerous tiny orifices in the lip. Actinic exposure, emotional instability, atopy, and familial macrocheilia have been listed as recurring factors. There has also been associations with squamous cell carcinomas (31,34).

Exfoliative cheilitis is a chronic superficial inflammatory disorder of the vermilion border with persistent scaling. Most patients are young women; a familial incidence has been suggested. History of atopy or emotional disturbance can often be elicited. Treatment consists of reassurance, sedatives, and low-potency topical steroids (35,36).

Factitious cheilitis consists of dryness, scaling, or cracking of the lips from biting or continuous licking of the lips (37). Patients with this condition often also have personality disorders (35,38). The presence of irregular hemorrhagic or keratotic crusting of the lip may suggest a factitious origin and a psychiatric evaluation should be ordered (27,31).

Granulomatous cheilitis is characterized by progressive enlargement of one or both lips because of lymphatic obstruction by granulomatous infiltration (39). When associated with scrotal tongue and facial nerve palsy, it is termed Melkersson-Rosenthal syndrome (40). Other areas of the face may become swollen to the extent of interfering with eating and speaking, and other cranial nerves can be involved (41). Treatment has not been very successful, ranging from intralesional and systemic steroids to surgery (39,41).

Plasma cell cheilitis, the counterpart of Zoons' balanoposthitis, appears as circumscribed plaques of erythema usually on the lower lip of elderly people. Skin biopsy reveals abundant plasma cells in the dermis. Treatment consists of topical fluorinated steroid or intralesional injections of steroid. Griseofulvin has also been used (27).

Various other causes of cheilitis include cheilitis of mongolism secondary to trauma or low-grade infection (42), candidal cheilitis involving the entire lower lip (43), hereditary polymorphous light eruption, which can be treated with topical sunblocks (44), actinic prurigo of the lower lip associated with conjunctivitis, alopecia of the eyebrows and pterygium (45), and a wide range of systemic medications including isotretinoin, anticholinergics, antihistamines, anticonvulsants, antidepressants, antineoplastics, antipsychotics, narcotics, and diuretics (46).

History

The treatment of actinic cheilitis involves the successful removal of the premalignant epithelium and replacing it with healthy tissue. Actinic cheilitis has been treated in the past with vermilionectomy ("lip shave") or with topical fluorouracil. Vermilionectomy has been effective and the treatment of choice; however, several complications have been known to occur. In a 1-year follow-up study on patients treated with vermilionectomy, 25% experienced paresthesias, 7.7% complained of pruritus of the lip, 15.4% experienced labial scar tension during oral movements, 7.6% had persistent and painful discomfort from tension on the labial scar, and 72% of patients complained of a prickling sensation in the upper lip from hairs outside the lower lip surgical scar (47).

Fluorouracil is often used for precancerous skin lesions with good results (48). By inhibiting the enzyme thymidylate synthetase, it acts as an antimetabolite in the biosynthesis of deoxyribonucleic acid (49,50). After topical fluorouracil application, there is a greater inhibition of thymidylate synthetase in actinic keratosis than in normal skin (51). For patients with actinic cheilitis, 5% fluorouracil solution applied topically three times a day for 9 to 15 days is effective with complete healing 2 to 3 weeks after treatment. The major side effect is lip discomfort for several weeks. One study showed a 17% recurrence rate at 22 months follow-up (52). Other chemoexfoliants used to induce re-epithelialization include topical tretinoin (53) and tricholoroacetic acid (54).

A very effective treatment for actinic cheilitis is CO_2 laser ablation, considered by many as the treatment of choice (55). No recurrence occurred in one study at 34 months follow-up (56). In addition, no patient complained of pain after the procedure or any postsurgical paresthesia. Also, there was no occurrence of significant scarring, and preservation of normal lip contour was seen in all the patients.

Presurgical Considerations and Instructions

Options for treatment of biopsy-proven actinic cheilitis must be discussed with the patient. If the patient is not a good surgical candidate, topical fluorouracil may be the best alternative. The patient needs to be warned of the discomfort fluorouracil produces and told to continue using the medication as instructed despite its irritating effects. If surgical vermilionectomy is performed, the patient needs to be informed of the surgical scar and risk of paresthesia, pruritus and scar tightening, as well as surgical risks of bleeding and infection. For patients undergoing CO_2 laser vermilionectomy, risks of bleeding, infection, and scarring need to be discussed. Patients are instructed to avoid aspirin and ibuprofen products 10 days before and 2 days after surgery. Alcoholic beverages should also be avoided 3 days before surgery and 2 days after surgery. For patients undergoing CO_2 laser vermilionectomy, treatment with an antiviral agent and antibacterial agent should be initiated on the day of the procedure.

Equipment

For Surgical Vermilionectomy

1. A fresh, sharp blade (Bard-Parker #15 or Persona Plus #15)
2. An Iris scissor or comparable sharp-tip scissor
3. Nonabsorbable suture such as 5-0 Prolene or similar suture
4. Two single prong skin hooks
5. Electrocautery (Bovie instrument) for hemostasis
6. 1% Xylocaine with 1:100,000 epinephrine (maximum 70 mg/kg based on the patient's weight); 2% lidocaine is used for nerve blocks
7. Needle holder
8. Marking pen or gentian violet

CO_2 Laser Vermilionectomy

Both superpulse and ultrapulsed CO_2 lasers can be used. The superpulsed CO_2 laser has been shown to cause less thermal damage compared with the continuous wave CO_2 laser (57). Fitzpatrick compared continuous wave and superpulsed lasers in treating actinic cheilitis and found less scarring and faster healing with the superpulsed CO_2. The superpulsed CO_2 laser wounds healed by 3 weeks and resulted in a 15% excessive scarring rate, compared with 4 weeks and 47% scarring rate with the continuous wave CO_2 laser (58). However, use of the ultrapulsed CO_2 laser resulted in a 40% reduction in healing time (59).

Scalpel Technique

The simple vermilionectomy begins by marking the extent of the resection with gentian violet. The vermilion border is excised from its anterior edge to the labial mucosa with the use of a scalpel and scissors. The underlying orbicularis oris muscle is left intact. The closure is performed by advancing the labial mucosa to the skin and then approximating the tissue edges with interrupted sutures.

(a) (b)
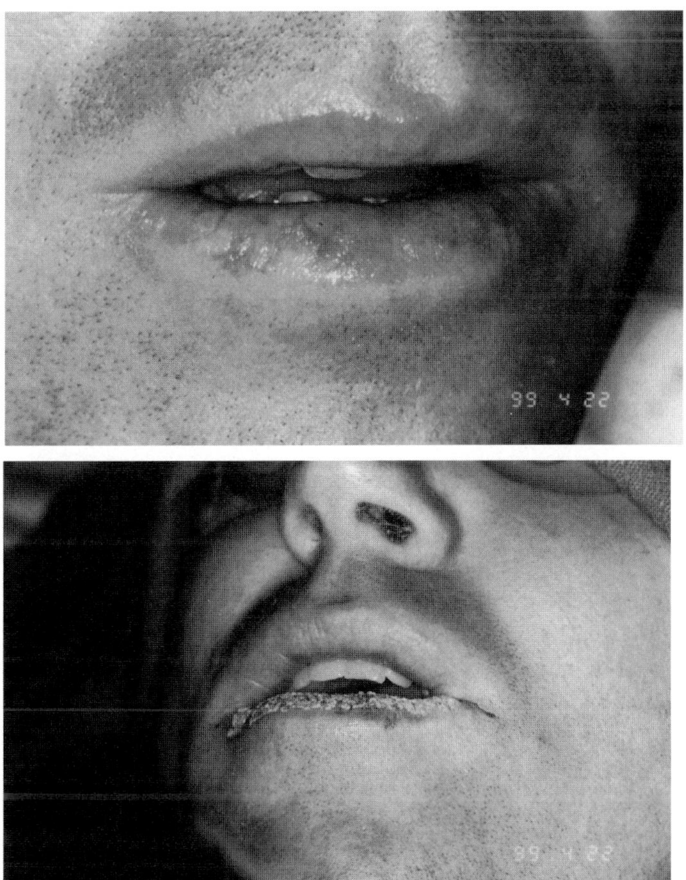

FIGURE 8 (a) Presurgical photograph of actinic cheilitis. (b) One pass of $UPCO_2$ laser performed on the lower lip. (c) One pass of erbium:YAG laser performed after two passes of $UPCO_2$ laser on the lower lip. (d) Immediately after $UPCO_2$ and erbium:YAG lasers for treatment of actinic cheilitis.

(c)

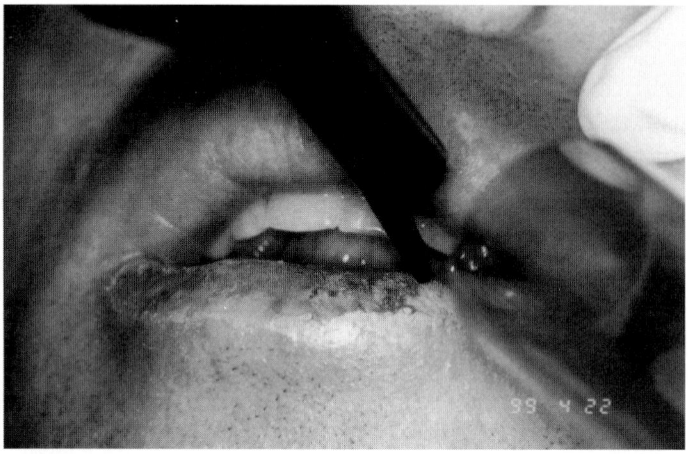

(d)

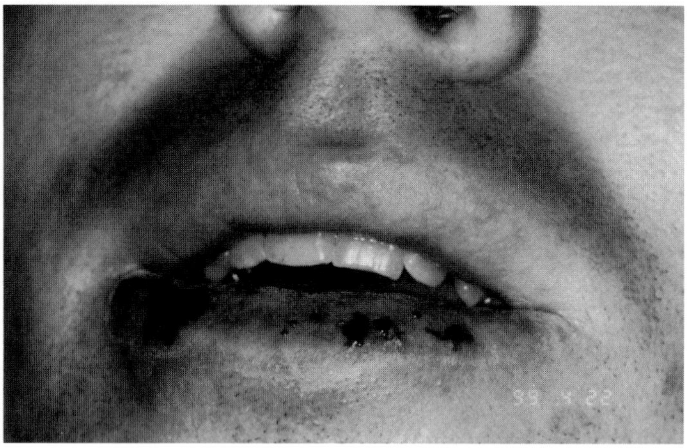

FIGURE 8 Continued.

Laser Technique

The surgical area should be prepared with nonflammable agents. Wet towels should be used on the surgical field and eye protection worn by the patient. Moistened gauze may be used to cover the periorbital region (Fig. 8a). Using the UltraPulse™ CO_2 laser set at 300 mJ and 100 W of power, the lower lip lesion is ablated with non-overlapping pulses and wiped with saline-soaked gauze after each pass (Fig. 8b). Two passes with the $UPCO_2$ laser are usually sufficient. The erbium:YAG laser is then used at 1.7 J/pulse, 10 Hz, with a 4-mm spot size (Fig. 8c). Pinpoint bleeding is present after 300+ pulses with the erbium laser (Fig. 8d).

Postsurgical Care

For surgical vermilionectomy, antibiotic ointment and bandages are applied. The patient is instructed in daily cleansing and application of antibiotic ointment. Acetaminophen and ice packs can be administered for pain and swelling. The sutures are removed in 1 week. The wound is then reinforced with Steri-Strips™. The patient is advised against direct sun exposure to this area for the next 3 months.

For laser vermilionectomy, a bio-occlusive dressing can be applied along with antibiotic ointment or petrolatum twice a day. Frequent soaking with an acetic acid solution (1 teaspoon vinegar to 1 cup tap water) four times a day is advised for the first few days. Strict sun avoidance should also be advised for at least 2 to 3 months after surgery.

For long-term postsurgical instructions, the patient should be advised against lengthy exposure to direct sunlight. A chemical or physical sunscreen may be necessary on a daily and even hourly basis for those with outdoor occupations. Payne (60) evaluated actinic blocking agents and found that those containing para-aminobenzoic acid or its esters resulted in superior protection on the skin and lip.

Summary

Actinic cheilitis needs to be differentiated from other lip lesions. However, once the diagnosis is made, treatment should be initiated as soon as possible because of its potential to progress to squamous cell carcinoma. Patients can be treated successfully with topical fluorouracil and vermilionectomy. However, CO_2 laser ablation with the UltraPulse™ laser is a simple, effective procedure with fewer side effects, less recurrence, faster healing, and excellent results. After treatment, the patient must be advised of the importance of sun restriction and the use of sunscreen on the lips to prevent further actinic damage to this area.

REFERENCES

1. Raju DR, Shaw TE. Results of simple scar excision and layered repair with elevation in facial scars. Surg Gynecol Obstet 1979; 148:699–702.
2. McGillis ST, Lucas AR. Scar revision. Derm Clin 1998; 16(1):165–180.
3. Alster TS, Williams CM. Treatment of keloid sternotomy scars with 585 nm flashlamp-pumped pulsed-dye laser. Lancet 1995; 345:1198–2000.
4. Dockery GL, Nilson RZ. Treatment of hypertrophic and keloid scars with silastic gel sheeting. J Foot Ankle Surg 1994; 33(2):110–119.
5. Kaplan B, Potter T, Moy RL. Scar revision. Dermatol Surg 1977; 23:435–442.
6. Lee SM, Ngim CK, Chan YY, et al. A comparison of silk and epiderm in scar management. Burns 1996; 22(6):483–487.
7. Williams C. Cica-care adhesive gel sheet. Br J Nursing 1996; 5(14):875–876.
8. Gingi H, Ono I, Tateshita T, et al. Clinical effectiveness of an ointment containing prostaglandin E1 for the treatment of burn wounds. Burns 1996; 22:399–405.
9. Ernst K, Hundaker M. Results of cryosurgery in 394 patients with hypertrophic scars and keloids (abstract). Hautartz 1995; 46:462–466.
10. Ng CL, Lee ST, Wong KL. Pressure garments in the prevention and treatment of keloids. Ann Acad Med Singapore 1983; 12:430–435.
11. Fitzpatrick RE. Treatment of inflamed hypertrophic scars using intralesional 5-FU. Dermatol Surg 1999; 25:224–232.
12. Larrabee WF, East CA, Jaffe HS, et al. Intralesional interferon gamma treatment for keloids and hypertrophic scars. Arch Otolaryngol Head Neck Surg 1990; 116:1159–1162.

13. Haas A, Arndt KA. Selected therapeutic applications of topical tretinoin. J Am Acad Dermatol 1986; 15:870–877.
14. Janssen de Limpens AM. The local treatment of hypertrophic scars and keloids with topical retinoic acid. Br J Dermatol 1980; 103:319–323.
15. Burks J. Dermabrasion and chemical peeling in the treatment of certain cosmetic defects and diseases of the skin. Springfield: Charles C. Thomas, 1979.
16. McEvitt WG. Acne pits. J Mich Med Soc 1948; 47:1234–1244.
17. Kurtin A. Corrective surgical planing of the skin. Arch Dermatol 1953; (Suppl 68):389–397.
18. Vukas A. Smallpox-induced scars: treatment by dermabrasion. Postsurgical dermabrasion of the nose. J Dermatol Surg Oncol 1974; 10:476–477.
19. Collins PS, Farber GA. Post-surgical dermabrasion of the nose. J Dermatol Surg Oncol 1984; 10:476–477.
20. Yarborough JM. Ablation of facial scars by programmed dermabrasion. J Dermatol Surg 1995; 21:503–508.
21. Harmon CB, Zelickson BD, Roenigk RK, et al. Dermabrasive scar revision. Dermatol Surg 1995; 21:503–508.
22. Alster TS, Lewis AB, Rosebach A. Laser scar revision: comparison of CO_2 laser vaporization with and without simultaneous pulsed dye laser treatment. Dermatol Surg 1998; 24(12):1299–1302.
23. Majno G. The healing hand. Cambridge: Harvard University Press, 1975, pp. 285–291.
24. Blanco-Davila F, Vasconez HC. The cleft earlobe: a review of methods of treatment. Ann Plast Surg 1994; 33:677–680.
25. Tan EC. Punch technique: an alternative approach to the repair of pierced earlobe deformities. J Dermatol Surg Oncol 1989; 15:270–272.
26. Apesos J, Kane M. Treatment of traumatic earlobe clefts. Aesth Plast Surg 1993; 17: 253–255.
27. Picascia DD, Robinson JK. Actinic cheilitis: a review of the etiology, differential diagnosis, and treatment. J Am Acad Dermatol 1987; 17:255–264.
28. Ayres S. Chronic actinic cheilitis. JAMA 1923; 81:1183–1186.
29. Katzenellenbogen I, Sandbank M. Cheilitis. In: Andrade R, Gumport SL, Popkin GL, Rees TD, eds. Cancer of the skin. Philadelphia: WB Saunders, 1976, pp. 607–634.
30. Van Zile WN. Early carcinoma of the lip: diagnosis and treatment. J Oral Surg 1965; 23:50–59.
31. Rogers RS, Bekic M. Diseases of the lips. Semin Cutaneous Med Surg 1977; 16(4): 328–336.
32. Fisher AA. Contact dermatitis and cheilitis. In: Contact Dermatitis. Philadelphia: Lea & Febiger, 1986; pp. 791–795.
33. Samaranayake LP. Oral mycosis in HIV infection. Oral Surg 1992; 73:171–180.
34. Yacobi R, Brown DA. Cheilitis glandularis: a pediatric case report. J Am Dental Assoc 1989; 228:317–318.
35. Crotty CP, Dicken CH. Factitious lip crusting. Arch Dermatol 1981; 117:338–340.
36. Reade PC, Sim R. Exfoliative cheilitis: a factitious disorder. J Oral Maxillofac Surg 1986; 15:313–317.
37. Perry HO, Lovestedt SA. Disorders of the mouth. In: Conn HF, ed. Current Therapy. Philadelphia: WB Saunders, 1969, pp. 616–623.
38. Thomas JR III, Greene SL, Dicken CH. Factitious cheilitis. J Am Acad Dermatol 1983; 8:368–372.
39. Krutchkoff D, James R. Cheilitis granulomatosa. Arch Dermatol 1978; 114:1203–1206.
40. White JR, Souteyrand P, MacDonald DM. Granulomatous cheilitis. Clin Exp Dermatol 1981; 6:391–397.

41. Rook A. The lips. In: Rook A, Wilkinson DS, Ebling FJG, eds. Textbook of Dermatology. 3rd ed. Oxford: Blackwell, 1979, pp. 1903–1908.
42. Butterworth T, Leoni EP, Beerman H, Wood GW, Strean LP. Cheilitis of mongolism. J Invest Dermatol 1960; 35:347–352.
43. Jansen GT, Dillaha CJ, Honeycutt WM. Candida cheilitis. Arch Dermatol 1963; 88:141–145.
44. Birt AR, Hogg GR. The actinic cheilitis of hereditary polymorphous light eruption. Arch Dermatol 1979; 115:699–702.
45. Mounsdon T, Kratochvil F, Auclair P, et al. Oral Surg Oral Med Oral Pathol 1988; 65: 327–332.
46. Zugarman C. The lips: anatomy and differential diagnosis. Cutis 1986; 38:116–120.
47. Sanchez-Conejo-Mir J, Perez Bernal AM, Moreno-Gimenez JC, Camacho-Martinez F. Follow-up of vermilionectomies: evaluation of the technique. J Dermatol Surg Oncol 1986; 12:180–184.
48. Ott F, Beer HE, Storck H. The local treatment of precancerous skin conditions with 5-fluorouracil ointment. Dermatologica 1970; 14:109–113.
49. Chabner BA, Myers CE, Coleman CN, Johns OG. The clinical pharmacology of autineoplastic agents. N Engl J Med 1975; 292:1107–1113.
50. Eaglstein WH, Weinstein GD, Frost P. Fluorouracil mechanism of action in human skin and actinic keratoses I. Effect on DNA synthesis in vivo. Arch Dermatol 1970; 101: 132–139.
51. Pindberg JJ. Pathology of oral leukoplakia. Am J Dermatopathol 1980; 2:277–278.
52. Epstein E. Treatment of lip keratoses (actinic cheilitis) with topical fluorouracil. Arch Dermatol 1977; 113:906–908.
53. Kligman A. Topical tretinoin: indications, safety and effectiveness. Cutis 1987; 39:486–488.
54. Stanley RJ, Roenigk RK. Actinic cheilitis: treatment with the carbon dioxide laser. Mayo Clinic Proc 1988; 63:230–235.
55. Goldman MP, Fitzpatrick RE. Skin resurfacing with carbon dioxide and erbium lasers. Cutaneous Laser Surgery, 2nd ed. New York: Mosby-Yearbook, Inc., St. Louis, MO, 1999, p. 382.
56. David LM. Laser vermilion ablation for actinic cheilitis. J Dermatol Surg Oncol 1984; 11:605–608.
57. Fitzpatrick RE, Ruiz-Esparza J, Goldman MP. The depth of thermal necrosis using the CO_2 laser: a comparison of the superpulsed mode and conventional mode. J Dermatol Surg Oncol 1991; 17:340–344.
58. Fitzpatrick RE, Goldman MP, Ruiz-Esparza J. Clinical advantages of the CO_2 laser superpulsed mode. J Dermatol Surg Oncol 1994; 20:449–456.
59. Fitzpatrick RE. Treatment of chronic actinic cheilitis: vaporization vermillionectomy with the UltraPulse CO_2 laser. Update Dermatol Laser Surg 1992; 3:1.
60. Payne TE. An evaluation of actinic blocking agents for the protection of lip mucosa. J Am Dent Assoc 1976; 92:409–411.

APPENDIX

DERMATOLOGY ASSOCIATES / COSMETIC LASER ASSOCIATES

PERMISSION FOR SURGICAL CARE

(LASER, COSMETIC & GENERAL SURGERY AND BIOPSIES)

*PATIENT NAME*________________ *ATTENDING PHYSICIAN*________________

PROCEDURE(S)	RECOMMENDED LASER(S)
1.	1.
2.	2.

- While surgery is effective in most cases, no guarantee can be made that a specific patient will benefit from the procedure. Additionally, the nature of surgery may require a patient to return for numerous visits in order to either achieve the desired results or to determine that surgery may not be completely effective at treating the particular condition. Therefore, this Permission For Surgical Care form will continue in effect for any and all subsequent visits with respect to the above outlined procedure(s) and laser(s).
- The objective of cosmetic surgery is individualized improvement, not perfection. In many cases, the final result may not be apparent until six (6) months after performance of the procedure. Cosmetic surgery should be considered only for individualized aesthetic improvement, not for unrelated issues that include, but are not limited to, social acceptance, psychological balance, weight reduction or an increase in physical capabilities/agility.
- I hereby authorize and direct the above named physician, with associates or assistants of his/her choice, to perform the above listed procedure(s). I further authorize the physician(s) to do any other procedure that in their judgment they may dictate to be necessary or advisable should unforeseen circumstances arise during the operation.
- I have been given an opportunity to ask any and all questions concerning the procedure(s) and the legal consequences of this form, and have received satisfactory answers. ________**Initials**
- With the understanding that care will be taken not to reveal my name, I consent to the taking of photographs/videos before, during and after the medical procedure(s). These photographs/videos will be the property of Dermatology Associates of San Diego County, Inc. (DA) and/or its assigns and may be used for medical, scientific, teaching, publication or promotional purposes. ________**Initials**

EACH OF THE FOLLOWING ITEMS HAS BEEN DISCUSSED FULLY WITH ME:

1. Potential benefits of the proposed procedure(s)
2. Possible alternative procedure(s)
3. Reasonable expectations & outcomes of the procedure(s)
4. Reasonably anticipated consequences if the procedure is not performed
5. Possible complications/risks involved with the proposed procedure(s) and subsequent healing period (including but not limited to infection, scarring, recurrence of lesion, bleeding & local nerve damage)
6. Possibility of fees for services including but not limited to, anesthesia, laboratory and/or facility use
7. Possibility of a "touch-up" or follow-up procedure for which I may be charged an additional fee
8. Administration of anesthesia (if applicable)

I AM AWARE OF THE FOLLOWING POSSIBLE EXPERIENCE(S)/RISK(S) WITH LASER SURGERY:

1. **DISCOMFORT** - Some discomfort may be experienced during laser treatment. I give permission for the administration of anesthesia as deemed appropriate by the Physician.
2. **WOUND HEALING** - Laser surgery may result in swelling, weeping, crusting or flaking of the treated area which may require one to three weeks to heal. Once the surface has healed it may be pink and sensitive to the sun for an additional two to four weeks or possibly longer.
3. **BRUISING/SWELLING/INFECTION** - With some lasers, bruising of the treated area may occur. Additionally, there may be some swelling noted, especially when the nose and cheeks have been treated. Infection is a possibility any time a procedure is performed on the skin.
4. **PIGMENT CHANGES** (Skin Color) - During the healing process there is a possibility of the treatment area becoming either lighter or darker in color than the surrounding skin. This is usually temporary, but on some occasions may be permanent.
5. **SCARRING** - Scarring is a relatively rare occurrence but is a possibility when the skin's surface is disrupted. To minimize the chances of scarring, it is important to follow all post-operative instructions carefully.
6. **PERSISTENCE OF LESION** - Some growths, birthmarks, and tattoos may respond only partially or not at all to Laser Surgery. If this situation arises, there may be other treatment alternatives available.
7. **EYE EXPOSURE** - Protective eyewear will be provided and must be kept in place at all times during the treatment in order to protect the eyes from accidental laser exposure.

PATIENTS OWN WORDS: WHAT SPECIFICALLY ARE THEY HAVING DONE TODAY	

BY MY SIGNATURE BELOW, I CERTIFY THAT I HAVE READ AND FULLY UNDERSTAND THE CONTENTS OF THIS PERMISSION FOR SURGICAL CARE FORM AND THAT THE DISCLOSURES REFERRED TO HEREIN WERE MADE TO ME.

Signature ________ ***Print Name*** ________ ***Date*** ________

Witness/DA Representative Signature ________ ***Print Name, Title*** ________ ***Date*** ________

PATHOLOGY CHARGE ACKNOWLEDGEMENT

Print Patient Name ________ **Date** ________

Your physician will be performing a biopsy/excision that requires a pathology reading. Routinely, pathology requires 7-10 days for processing. If you have not heard from us in 2 weeks please call our pathology coordinator (760-944-5888). In some cases , a second opinion reading is necessary to confirm a diagnosis. These slides are sent to an independent pathology lab and read by another physician. As a courtesy, this lab has consented to bill all contracted and non-contracted insurance carriers. However, in some cases you may receive a bill for all or part of this service This is to notify you of this possibility.

I have read the above and understand that I may be financially responsible for this charge and agree to pay for these services.

OWNERSHIP DISCLOSURE: Your physician has an ownership in the pathology lab *Susan P. Detwiler M.D. Inc. and or Laser & Skin Surgery Center of La Jolla.* If such an interest is of concern to you, or you choose to use a different facility please discuss it with your physician and he or she will address your questions.

Patient Signature ________ **Date** ________ **Witness** ________

36

Ancillary Aesthetic Dermatologic Treatments and Procedures

Zoe Diana Draelos
Wake Forest University School of Medicine, Winston-Salem, North Carolina

INTRODUCTION

The skin is the only organ of the body that allows direct observation and easy access. This allows dermatology to be a specialty that describes disease appearance with tremendous accuracy and provides efficient treatment through the application of medication to the exact injury site, as well as allowing the easy development of numerous quasimedical procedures. Some of the aesthetic procedures may offer dermatologic benefit, whereas others are of value strictly for their sensory properties. This chapter discusses some of the ancillary aesthetic dermatologic treatments and procedures, including topical body contouring for cellulite, electrolysis for hair removal, and paramedical facials in a postsurgical setting. The chapter closes with a discussion on postsurgical skin care.

CELLULITE TREATMENT AND TOPICAL BODY CONTOURING

The term cellulite refers to the uneven, lumpy appearance of the skin on the thighs, buttocks, and breasts of postpubertal women. It varies in degree from mild to severe and is not necessarily related to obesity, but worsening occurs with increasing body fat [1]. Cellulite is a common condition, affecting at least 85% of postpubertal women, that is extremely difficult to treat. Liposuction, at first glance, might seem to be a good treatment, because the removal of excess fat might decrease the rumpled skin appearance. However, liposuction actually increases the magnitude of the surface irregularities. This has led to the development of a variety of paramedical treatments designed to improve the appearance of cellulite.

Causal Origins

Before a discussion of therapy, however, it is important to review the pertinent medical facts known about cellulite to evaluate treatment efficacy. It is currently thought that cellulite represents an inflammatory process. Much of this new data are as a result of ultrasound evaluation of the upper thighs [2].

Cellulite may be characterized as a process that progresses slowly over a lifetime. The initial changes leading to cellulite formation may be deterioration of the dermal vasculature, particularly loss of the capillary networks, and the presence of inflammatory cells [3]. As a result, excess fluid is retained with the dermal and subcutaneous tissues. This loss of the capillary network is thought to be caused by engorged fat cells deposited in response to estrogen production. These fat cells ultimately inhibit venous return. Furthermore, the septae between the fat collections may also contribute to adipolysis and mild dermal atrophy [4].

After the capillary networks have been damaged, vascular changes may begin to occur within the dermis, resulting in decreased protein synthesis and an inability to repair tissue damage [5]. There may be the activation of proteinases, such as collagenase and elastase. Ultrasound imaging of skin affected by cellulite reveals thinning of the dermis with subcutaneous fat pushing upward, which translates into the rumpled skin known as cellulite.

Thus, cellulite may be attributable to a variety of factors: hormonally mediated fat deposition, fat lobule compression of capillary vasculature, decreased venous return, formation of clumped fat lobules, deposition of protein substances around clumped fat lobules, activation of proteinases, presence of septae around fat deposits, and inflammatory processes. In short, the exact causal origin is unknown.

Topical Treatment

Topical creams for the treatment of cellulite abound. Most contain some form of methylxanthine. Naturally occurring xanthines include caffeine, while aminophylline and theophylline represent substances traditionally available by prescription. All of these substances inhibit phosphodiesterase and provide beta-adrenergic stimulation. Beta-adrenergic receptors stimulate the hydrolysis of fat stored as triglycerides. Thus, xanthines promote lipolysis by inhibiting phosphodiesterase, which transforms cAMP (adenosine-monophosphate) into AMP, leading to the conversion of triglycerides into free fatty acids and glycerol [6]. It is felt that the topical application of these substances may cause the breakdown and removal of fat stores, ultimately improving the appearance of cellulite.

Whereas the idea is of merit theoretically, the benefit of thigh creams is difficult to assess. Any change in thigh diameter attributable to the use of xanthines would occur slowly, over months, rather than days or weeks. Of course, continued application of the xanthines would be necessary to maintain any effect [7]. However, it is unlikely that the xanthines ever reach the lipocytes in sufficient quantity to induce a biological effect without causing toxicity.

Mechanical Treatments

Most other treatments aimed at cellulite improvement rely on mechanistic means of manipulating the skin to produce a temporary reduction in thigh diameter and the rumpled appearance of the skin. Because decreased circulation and lymphatic return may contribute to cellulite, it is not unreasonable to consider manipulation as a possible treatment.

The original mechanical treatment intended to improve the appearance of cellulite was lymphatic drainage. This involves vigorous rubbing of the skin of the upper thighs and is similar to a manual form of the Jobst pump, commonly used by dermatologists. Vigorous lymphatic massage in the direction of blood flow is designed to encourage removal of extravascular fluid and can reduce thigh diameter in individuals with decreased venous return. Cellulite is not removed with this technique; however, the dimpled skin appearance may be improved as tissue edema is reduced.

A mechanized form of skin kneading is known as endermologie (LPG, Fort Lauderdale, FL.). This technique, based on the use of a patented machine developed about a decade ago in France, involves rubbing the skin with an electrically powered, hand-held box containing two rollers. The skin is sucked between the rollers and kneaded. A technician moves the machine over the hips, stomach, legs, and buttocks, which are covered with a nylon stocking to decrease friction. Initially 15 treatments are administered, followed by monthly maintenance.

A variety of rubbing patterns are used to stroke and pull the skin. Winding movements are used to improve "painful" cellulite, whereas kneading movements are used on areas with intense cellulite, such as the buttocks and upper thighs. Sanding, bouncing, pulling, and figure-eight movements are also combined during the treatment session.

No papers regarding this technique are published in the English literature, but casual correspondence written by French physicians and provided by the company claims efficacy attributable to improving circulation, reducing tissue congestion, and enhancing the removal of waste products [8]. Sometimes skin kneading is used in combination with lymphatic massage because some feel the kneading softens the cellulite which then responds to manual manipulation. Company literature is careful to state that mechanized skin kneading does not remove the cellulite, but rather reduces its appearance [9].

Conclusion

The only permanent method of reducing the appearance of cellulite is to lose weight or exercise to increase muscle bulk. Weight loss reduces the size of the adipocytes, thus decreasing the herniation of the subcutaneous tissue into the dermis. Exercise can aid in weight loss and increase muscle tone, providing support for the overlying subcutaneous tissue. In some individuals, neither of these measures can totally eliminate the appearance of cellulite. At present, it can be safely stated that there are no topical medications or manipulative processes to which advanced cellulite visibly responds in a treatment period of less than 2 months.

ELECTROLYSIS

Unwanted hair removal is a common problem for which patients seek the assistance of a dermatologist. Although there are a number of laser-assisted permanent hair removal techniques that must be performed under the supervision of a physician, electrolysis is unique in that it is a permanent removal technique requiring no medical supervision or training.

Electrolysis involves the insertion of a needle into the follicular ostia down to the follicular germinative cells. The dermal papillae must be destroyed to permanently prevent hair growth. There are several important considerations in determining the effectiveness of electrolysis, summarized in Table 1.

TABLE 1 Important Considerations for Effective Electrolysis

Hairs must be visible for removal by electrolysis.
Anagen hairs can be treated whereas telogen hairs cannot.
Water is necessary for transmitting electrical energy between the needle and dermal papillae. The lower part of the hair follicle is moister than the more superficial follicle, thus the electrolysis needle must be inserted to the depth of the hair follicle.
Larger-diameter hairs require deeper needle insertion for adequate destruction.
Damage to the dermal papillae depends both on the intensity and the duration of the current administered. High-intensity energy may be used for a short duration or lower-intensity energy may be used for a longer duration. Pain increases with higher-intensity energy.
Coarse hairs require longer treatment duration than fine hairs.
Curly, wavy, or kinky hair is more difficult to treat because of problems with accurate needle placement.

Source: Refs. 11 and 14.

Electrolysis Techniques

Electrolysis is actually performed using a variety of techniques known as electrolysis, thermolysis, and the blend [10]. The full name for the technique called electrolysis is "galvanic electrolysis," which uses direct current (DC). The current is passed through a stainless steel needle into the sodium chloride and water in the tissue surrounding the hair follicle. The DC current causes ionization of the salt (NaCl) and water (H_2O) into free sodium ($Na+$), chloride ($Cl-$), hydrogen ($H+$), and hydroxide ($OH-$) ions. These free ions then recombine into sodium hydroxide (NaOH), known as lye, and hydrogen gas (H_2). The caustic sodium hydroxide destroys the hair follicle while the hydrogen gas escapes into the atmosphere. The amount of sodium hydroxide produced is greater at the base of the hair follicle because of increased moisture content, and is minimal at the skin surface. Galvanic electrolysis is the most effective method of producing permanent hair removal, but is tedious and slow.

Thermolysis, also known as short-wave radio frequency diathermy, differs from galvanic electrolysis in that alternating high frequency current (AC) is passed down the needle. This current causes vibration of the water molecules around the hair follicle and produces heat. The needle begins to heat at the tip first and then toward the skin surface. This means that the heat remains longer around the hair follicle than at the skin surface, minimizing discomfort and cutaneous damage. If too much AC current is administered, steam is produced, which exits through the follicular ostia resulting in a burn and possible scarring. Thermolysis is much faster than galvanic electrolysis, but is not as effective. Additionally, thermolysis does not work well on distorted or curved hair follicles.

The blend is a combination of both galvanic electrolysis and thermolysis [11]. Both direct and high-frequency alternating current are passed down the needle at the same time to produce both sodium hydroxide and heat. The hot lye is extremely effective in destroying the dermal papillae, allowing superior results with less re-growth. Furthermore, the tissue damage induced by the thermolysis allows the lye to spread through the hair follicle more rapidly. The blend requires only one fourth the time of galvanic electrolysis alone [12].

Electrolysis Needle Selection

Needle selection is important to the success of any of the forms of electrolysis previously discussed. Needles are available in a variety of shapes: straight, tapered, bulbous, and insulated [13]. Most electrologists prefer to use a straight needle with a gently rounded tip (Fig. 1). Tapered needles (narrower at the tip than the base) are sometimes selected for the removal of deep terminal hairs. Electrolysis of these hairs requires more energy, which can be delivered at the tip without exposing the more superficial tissues to excessive damage.

A variety of needle sizes are also available, because the needle diameter should match the diameter of the hair shaft to be treated. Smaller needles generally get hotter than larger needles, resulting in greater pain. Patient pain can be reduced by selecting the largest needle possible.

Electrolysis Needle Insertion Technique

The needle must be properly inserted into the follicular ostia to insure destruction of the hair follicle without cutaneous scarring. The most popular technique for needle insertion is known as the forehand technique. The needle holder is held much like a pencil between the thumb and forefinger. The removal forceps are then placed between the needle holder and thumb of the same hand. This allows the free hand

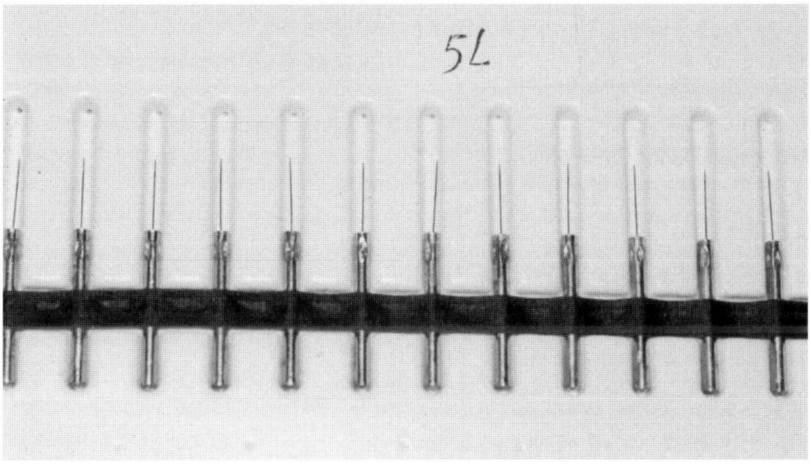

FIGURE 1 Standard electrolysis needles are disposable and made of stainless steel in a variety of diameters. The diameter of the needle selected depends on the thickness of the hair to be removed.

to be used for stretching the skin. Skin stretching is important to open the follicular ostia for needle insertion.

The needle is always inserted parallel to the hair shaft opposite to the direction of hair growth. Hairs may exit the skin at angles varying between 10 and 90°. The needle must be inserted at the same angle as hair growth. If the hair is long and lays on the skin surface, it should be clipped to gain a better appreciation of its exit angle. The needle should also always be inserted below the hair shaft. These steps are necessary to destroy the follicle without scarring the surrounding skin.

It is important that needle insertion occur to the proper depth. In general, coarse hairs have deeper follicles than fine hairs. A slight dimpling of the overlying skin and resistance means that the bottom of the follicle has been reached and the needle should be withdrawn slightly until the dimpling disappears. A proper needle insertion should be painless and bloodless for the patient.

Once the hair has been treated, the needle should be withdrawn at exactly the same angle as it was inserted. The forceps held between the thumb and needle holder are now positioned 90° to the hair shaft for epilation. The hair should be grasped firmly and gently slid out of the follicle if the treatment has been properly performed. Resistance in removing the hair means that the hair has been epilated and not treated with electrolysis; thus, regrowth may occur.

Methods of Minimizing Scarring

Electrolysis must be properly performed to minimize scarring. Table 2 summarizes the pointers that must be followed for successful electrolysis [14]. Care must also be taken to perform the procedure under sanitary conditions to prevent the spread of bacterial and viral infection [15].

Summary

Electrolysis remains a popular method of hair removal for all body sites in men and women. Although it may not be completely permanent, it is safe in the hands of an experienced, well-trained technician.

TABLE 2 Scar Prevention with Electrolysis

The treated hair should be pulled effortlessly from the follicular ostia.
The needle size should be the same as the hair diameter.
The skin should be dry.
The skin should not be blanched after treatment.
The current should only flow when the needle has been completely inserted in the follicular ostia to the level of the follicle.
The needle should only be removed when the current has stopped.
The same follicular ostia should not be re-entered or treated twice.

PARAMEDICAL SKIN TREATMENTS: FACIALS

There are a variety of paramedical skin treatments that may be used in a dermatologic setting. Sometimes these procedures are offered by estheticians as an adjunct to more traditional cosmetic surgery. Facials, or the application of substances to the face, are the most popular of these paramedical treatments. The medical value of the facial is somewhat controversial; nevertheless, the procedure is worthy of brief mention. Facials, also known as masks, may be divided into several types: wax-based masks, vinyl-based masks, hydrocolloid masks, and earth-based masks [16].

Wax-Based Masks

Wax-based masks are popular among women for their warm, esthetically pleasing feel. They are composed of beeswax or, more commonly, paraffin wax to which petroleum jelly and cetyl or stearyl alcohols have been added to provide a soft, pliable material for facial application with a soft brush. The wax is heated and sometimes applied directly to the face or at other times applied over a thin gauze cloth draped over the face. Gauze is used to enable the esthetician to remove the wax in one piece.

Wax-based masks are sometimes used in the postsurgical setting to soothe irritated skin and temporarily impede transepidermal water loss, thereby hydrating the skin of the face. The ability of the wax to improve the appearance of scar tissue is controversial.

Vinyl-Based Masks

Vinyl-based masks are commonly used at home because they are easily applied and removed. They are based on film-forming substances, such as polyvinyl alcohol or vinyl acetate, and are squeezed premixed from a tube or pouch for facial application. The mast is generally left in contact with the skin for 10 to 30 minutes to allow a thin vinyl film to form. Removal consists of peeling the vinyl from the skin.

The evaporation of the vehicle from the wet mask may cause stinging and burning on freshly denuded skin, making this mask a poor choice in the immediate postsurgical period.

Hydrocolloid Masks

Hydrocolloid masks are used both in professional salons and at home. Hydrocolloids are large molecular weight substances, such as oatmeal, that interfere with transepidermal water loss. Botanical anti-inflammatory agents, such as the chamomile derivative bisabolol, are sometimes added for their ability to soothe irritation and decrease erythema.

Earth-Based Masks

Earth-based masks, also known as paste masks or mud packs, are formulated of absorbent clays such as bentonite, kaolin, or china clay. The clays produce an astringent effect on the skin, making this mask most useful in oily complected acne patients. This mask is seldom used in the postsurgical period.

Summary

Face masks are a popular method of cosmetically enhancing the skin among men and women. They can be applied at home, in full-service salons, in aestheticians' offices, or in spas. The dermatologist must evaluate the value of face masks for his or her postsurgical patient in light of possible aesthetic and therapeutic benefits. Paramedical facials may or may not be part of postsurgical skin care, the next topic to be addressed.

POSTSURGICAL SKIN CARE

Postsurgical skin care is aimed at maximizing healing while minimizing scarring. Skin care products that provide cleansing, moisturizing, and sun protection are required.

Cleansers

Cleansers in the postsurgical period must be nonirritating, yet prevent infection. Immediately after surgery, lukewarm water may be the only cleanser required. As serum crusting begins, however, a synthetic detergent cleanser, such as Oil of Olay bar (Procter & Gamble), Ivory Moisture Care bar (Procter & Gamble), or Dove bar (Unilever), can produce gentle cleansing without overdrying the skin. Synthetic detergent soaps, also known as syndets, are generally labeled as "beauty bars." The actual value of an antibacterial soap, containing triclosan or triclocarban, is minimal in the setting of uncomplicated wound healing.

Lipid-free cleansing lotions (Cetaphil, Galderma; Aquanil, Person & Covey), used with or without water, can also gently clean a wound. They do not possess good antibacterial properties, however. In surgical sites where bacterial contamination may be a problem, deodorant soaps containing triclosan (Dial, Dial Corporation) may be appropriate. There are some beauty bar soaps available that also contain an antibacterial (Lever 2000, Unilever) that may meet the needs of some patients.

Moisturizers

Moisturizers are important in the postsurgical patient with large areas of denuded epidermis, because the barrier to transepidermal water loss is absent. This allows water evaporation from the skin, resulting in tightness and pruritus. Furthermore, desiccation impedes wound healing, which proceeds most rapidly in a moist environment.

Immediately after surgery, pure white petroleum jelly may be the best moisturizer. It is an excellent occlusive, thus reducing transepidermal water loss by more than 90%. It is used as a negative control for dermatologic patch testing, thus its irritation and sensitization potentials are low. Furthermore, it is extremely economical. Drawbacks to petroleum jelly are its greasy appearance, odor, and ability to stain natural fiber fabrics; however, it is the only substance shown to reside in the interstices between the corneocytes.

Once re-epithelialization has begun, oil-in-water formulations may be substituted that are more cosmetically elegant. Creams should be selected over lotions because they have a greater moisturizing ability and are less likely to contain irritating vehicles. Products should be chosen for their paucity of ingredients. Therefore, creams with fragrances, herbal or biological additives, and specialty ingredients should be avoided until complete healing has occurred.

Sunscreens

Sun exposure in the surgical site should be avoided immediately after surgery because the skin has lost its ability to adequately protect against photodamage. Once re-epithelialization has occurred sun exposure should be avoided, but many patients will need to continue their daily activities which may include casual sun exposure. All chemical sunscreening agents (PABA esters, cinnamate derivatives, benzophenones, etc.) are potential causes of both irritant and allergic contact dermatitis.

The physician may wish to avoid possible problems by recommending a physical sunblock, containing physical sunscreening agents such as micronized titanium dioxide or zinc oxide. However, the zinc oxide or titanium dioxide particles can become imbedded in a re-epithelializing wound. These products should not be used until re-epithelialization is complete or sutures have been removed.

Summary

Postsurgical skin care products must be chosen with common sense. Simple products with few ingredients seem to perform best while the skin is healing. It should be remembered that most skin care formulations are designed for application on intact skin. This is not the case immediately after surgery. Complex cosmeceutical formulations combining numerous ingredients of dubious benefit only create diagnostic problems for the dermatologist.

CONCLUSION

This chapter has discussed ancillary dermatologic treatments. Although cellulite treatment, hair removal, and skin care fall outside the realm of some dermatology practices, a basic understanding is useful in providing total patient care.

REFERENCES

1. Curri SB, Bombardelli E. Local lipodystrophy and districtual microcirculation: proposed etiology and therapeutic management. Cosmet Toilet 1994; 109:51–65.
2. Salter DC, Hanley M, Tynan A, McCook JP. In-vivo high definition ultrasound studies of subdermal fat lobules associated with cellulite. J Invest Dermatol 1990; 29:272–274.
3. Zalla MJ, Winkelmann RK, Gluck OS. Involutional lipoatrophy: macrophage-related involution of fat lobules. Dermatology 1995; 191:359–364.
4. Draelos ZD, Marenus KD. Cellulite. Dermatol Surg 1997; 23:1177–1181.
5. Curri SB. Cellulite and fatty tissue microcirculation. Cosmet Toilet 1993; 108:51–58.
6. Di Salvo RM. Controlling the appearance of cellulite. Cosmet Toilet 1995; 110:50–59.
7. Jackson EM. Substantiating the efficacy of thigh creams. Cosmet Dermatol 1995; 8: 31–41.
8. Vergereau R. Use of mechanical skin fold rolling in cosmetic medicine. J Cosmet Med Dermatol Surg 1995; 85:49–53.
9. Marchand JP, Privat Y. A new instrumental method for the treatment of cellulite. Medecine au Feminin 1991; 39:25–34.

10. Fino G. Modern Electrology. New York: Milady Publishing Corp., 1987, pp. 35–69.
11. Hinkel AR, Lind RW. Electrolysis, Thermolysis and the Blend. California: Arroway Publishers, 1968.
12. Wagner RF, Tomich JM, Grande DJ. Electrolysis and thermolysis for permanent hair removal. JAAD 1985; 12:441.
13. Gior F. Modern Electrology. New York, Milady Publishing Corporation, 1987, pp. 32–33.
14. Richards RN, Meharg GE. Cosmetic and Medical Electrolysis and Temporary Hair Removal. Ontario, Medric Ltd., 1991.
15. Petrozzi JW. Verrucae planae spread by electrolysis. Cutis 1980, 26:85.
16. Gerson J. Milady's Standard Textbook for Professional Estheticians, 7th ed. New York: Milady Publishing Company, 1992.

37

Laser Hair Removal

Wendy W. Lou
Laser and Skin Surgery Center of New York, New York, New York

Arielle N. B. Kauvar
Laser and Skin Surgery Center of New York, and New York University Medical Center, New York, New York

INTRODUCTION

Hair removal is a recent, novel application of cutaneous laser therapy. A variety of laser or light source systems are now available (Table 1) that can selectively heat and disrupt hair follicles without damaging the skin. Compared with conventional therapies, such as waxing, shaving, depilatories, and tweezing, long-term hair loss can be achieved over large body surface areas safely and efficiently. In addition to a decrease in actual hair counts, hair that does regrow is often thinner and lighter in color. This chapter reviews the basic principles of laser hair removal systems as well as their clinical use.

HAIR ANATOMY AND PHYSIOLOGY

The fundamentals of hair anatomy and physiology are essential to an understanding of the physics of laser hair removal. The hair follicle is a large structure that traverses the epidermis and superficial and deep dermis, with an average diameter of 100 to 300 microns. Hair follicles are comprised of three anatomically distinct units: the infundibulum, the isthmus, and the hair bulb. The infundibulum encompasses the region from the follicular orifice at the surface of the epidermis to the entrance of the sebaceous duct. The region of the follicle extending from the opening of the sebaceous duct down to the insertion of the arrector pili muscle is termed the isthmus. The hair bulb encompasses the region of the follicle extending from the insertion of the arrector pili muscle to the base of the follicle. The matrix cells that produce the hair shaft are contained within the bulb, and surrounding the bulb is the dermal papilla. Viewed in cross section from outside inward, layers of the hair follicle include the outer root sheath, inner root sheath, cuticle, cortex, and medulla.

Hair follicles cycle through three phases of growth: anagen, catagen, and telogen. Anagen is the active growth phase and may last up to 3 years. Hair growth is governed by the duration of this phase, which varies depending on anatomic site, and may last up to 2 to 8 years on the scalp and 1 to 6 months on other parts of

Table 1 Lasers and Light Sources for Hair Removal

Device	Name/ Manufacturer	Wavelength (nm)	Pulse Width	Spot Size (mm)	Maximum Fluence	Pulse Rate	Other
Long-pulse alexandrite	Photogenica LPIR (Cynosure)	755	5, 10, 20 msec	7 10 6 × 10	40 J/cm^2 25 J/cm^2 30 J/cm^2	1 Hz or Single	Cooling tip (optional)
	Gentle LASE (Candela)	755	3 msec	8 10 12	100 J/cm^2 60 J/cm^2 45 J/cm^2	1 Hz	Cryogen spray cooling
	EpiTouch (Sharplan)	755	2 msec	5 7	50 J/cm^2 25 J/cm^2	5 Hz or single	
Diode	Featherlite (LaserLite)	805 ± 25	100 msec	2 2 × 4	60 W	5 Hz	
	Lightsheer (Coherent)	800	5–30 msec	9 × 9	40 J/cm^2	0.5 Hz	Chill tip
Normal mode, long-pulse ruby	EpiLaser (Palomar)	694	3 msec	7, 10	40 J/cm^2	0.5 Hz	EpiWand cooling handpiece
	Chromos 694 (MehlBiophile)	694.3	850 μsec	7	20 J/cm^2	1 Hz	
QS-Nd:YAG with carbon-based suspension	SoftLight (Thermolase)	1064	17 nsec	7	2.5 J/cm^2 (2–3 J/cm^2)	1, 2, 5, 10 Hz	
Intense pulsed light source	EpiLight (Energy Systems Corp)	590–1200	2.7–7 msec	8 × 35 10 × 45	30–65 J/cm^2	2–5 pulse seq.	

the body [1–3]. The majority of hair follicles (80–85%) are in anagen. whereas the remaining follicles are either in the catagen phase (2%) or the telogen phase (10–15%). After the active growth phase of anagen, the follicle moves into catagen, a transitional phase of regression that lasts approximately 3 months.

PHYSICS OF LASER HAIR REMOVAL

The theoretical basis for laser hair removal lies in the concepts of selective photothermolysis [4]. This theory predicts that laser-induced thermal injury can be restricted to tissue structure if the wavelength of light is preferentially absorbed by the target, the laser exposure is shorter than or equal to its thermal relaxation time, and sufficient fluence (energy density) is delivered. Hair follicles are a natural target for laser therapy because they are superficial skin structures and contain melanin, a logical natural chromophore. Within hair follicles, melanin is present in the shaft, hair bulb, and follicular epithelium. Red and infrared wavelengths up to approximately 1000 nm provide the best wavelengths for the desired combination of selective absorption by melanin and deep penetration into the dermis. The 694 nm normal mode ruby laser was the first laser shown to destroy hair follicles by means of selective photothermolysis. Several other lasers and light sources have subsequently been developed for this purpose, including the long-pulsed alexandrite laser (755 nm), the diode laser (800 nm), an intense pulsed-light source (590–1200 nm), and a system that uses a topical carbon suspension in conjunction with a Q-switched Nd:YAG laser (1064 nm).

In addition to wavelength, the other major consideration in developing a hair removal laser is pulse duration. Selective damage to isolated follicular pigmented cells in animals resulting in leukotrichia has been shown after Q-switched ruby laser exposures [5]. Kauvar [6] found long-term reduction (up to 2 years) in human hair counts after three treatments with the Q-switched ruby laser (694 nm, 28 ns; 6.5 mm spot, 6 J/cm^2) where the entire area was treated with double pulsing. Histologically, disruption of the matrix cells was observed in biopsies taken immediately after laser irradiation. The submicrosecond pulses of Q-switched lasers, however, provide insufficient heat transfer to other non-pigmented follicular cells, and are therefore not ideal for follicular destruction. The thermal relaxation time of hair follicles with average diameters of 200 to 300 microns is estimated to be 40 to 100 msec. The optimal pulse duration for a hair removal laser is therefore shorter than 40 to 100 msec, and longer than the approximately 3 msec thermal relation time of the epidermis in order to limit epidermal injury. These exposure times allow the extraction of heat during the laser pulse by conduction from the epidermis while maintaining thermal confinement in the hair follicles. Although significant growth delays can be induced in hairless follicles (epilated sites), presumably because of ample melanin in the follicular epithelium and papillae, the presence of a pigmented hair shaft within the follicle serves as a better chromophore and enhances selective photothermolysis of hair follicles [7].

Because the epidermis contains melanin, epidermal injury by laser light is possible, particularly in individuals with darker skin pigmentation. For this reason, a variety of skin cooling methods are being used, in the form of cooling gels, cryogen sprays, or contact cooling devices, that extract heat from the epidermis during laser pulsing.

The timing of laser hair removal treatment may be critical because the induction of hair loss is dependent on targeting follicular stem cells. Traditionally, hair stem cells were thought to reside in the matrix area of the hair bulb. Recent studies in mice suggest that follicular stem cells are located in a region of the outer root sheath near the attachment of the arrector pili muscle, which has been termed "the bulge" [8,9]. Based on these findings, a new model for the hair growth cycle has been proposed. In this model, the dermal papilla comes in contact with the bulge cells during late telogen, stimulating the bulge cells to proliferate and form an active new hair matrix. The bulge cells grow downward together with the dermal papillae, forming hair matrix cells during the early anagen phase. During anagen, the matrix cells proliferate for a period of time, thereby determining the length of the hair. During catagen, the hair matrix cells regress and the dermal papillae retracts through an area near the bulge, where it remains during telogen.

If the bulge hypothesis is true, important targets for hair follicle destruction by laser are either the bulge, the dermal papilla, or both. The stage of the hair cycle might influence susceptibility of the hair to destruction by laser because of the depth of the dermal papillae varies with the stage of the hair cycle. Papillae are located most superficially in the skin and near the bulge during telogen. During anagen, the papillae are deeper in the dermis, and are therefore more difficult to target by laser light. Susceptibility of the hair follicle to injury may also depend on the activity of the follicular stem cells. For example, bulge cells rapidly proliferate during late telogen, but are inactive throughout the rest of the hair cycle.

The mechanism of laser hair removal using millisecond domain laser or light source pulses is photothermal injury of follicular stem cells. Biopsy specimens taken immediately after exposure with a normal mode ruby laser show thermal coagulation and asymmetric focal ruptures of the follicular epithelium [7]. Hair loss, or hair growth delays, may also be induced via a laser technique that produces a photomechanical rather than a photothermal effect. Irradiation of shaved skin with Q-switched ruby or Q-switched Nd:YAG lasers can produce hair growth delays [6,10]. Another type of hair removal system uses an exogenous chromophore in the form of microparticulate carbon that is propelled down the hair shafts. This method provides a strong follicular chromophore, regardless of the concentration of melanin in the hair shaft, rendering the ability to treat hairs of all colors.

LASERS AND LIGHT SOURCES FOR HAIR REMOVAL

Long-Pulse Ruby Laser

To date, long-pulse ruby laser is the most studied laser system for hair removal (Fig. 1). Several long-pulsed ruby lasers are available with pulse durations ranging from 0.9 to 3 msec and fluences of 10 to 40 J/cm^2. The 694 wavelength of the ruby laser is well absorbed by melanin and penetrates skin to the depth of the hair follicle. With pulse durations in the near millisecond range and sufficient fluence, these lasers satisfy the requirements for selective photothermolysis.

Grossman et al. [7] reported results of the first pilot study evaluating the long-pulse ruby laser (694 nm, 270 μsec, 6 mm spot, 30–60 J/cm^2 Epilaser, Palomar Medical Products) with a cooling handpiece in 13 subjects with fair skin and dark hair. Transient hair loss or hair growth delay lasting 3 to 6 months was shown in all

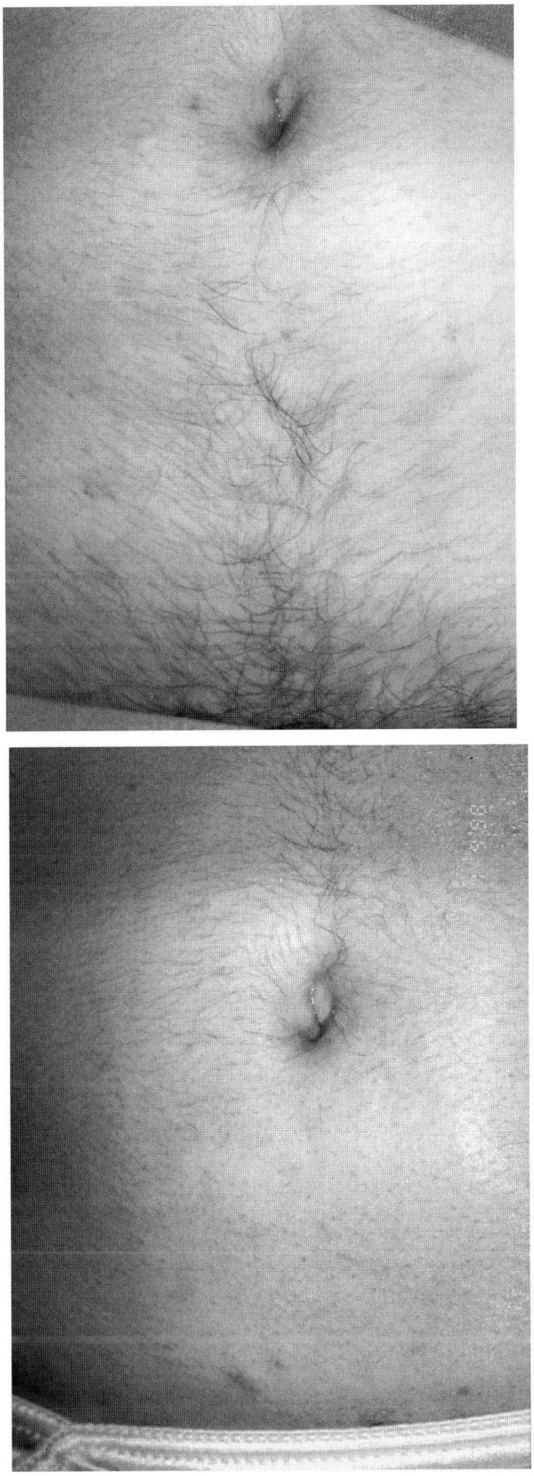

(a)

(b)

FIGURE 1 **The lower abdomen of a fair-skinned, dark-haired patient was treated with the EpiLaser (694 nm, 3 msec) three times with a 7 mm spot at a fluence of 40 J/cm^2. (a) baseline, (b) three months after the last treatment.**

subjects after a single treatment, compared with wax-epilated or shaved control areas. Four subjects showed less than 50% regrowth at 6 months and hair count reduction at 12 months, suggesting a potential for permanent hair removal. In this study, the degree of hair loss was fluence-dependent. Histological evaluation immediately after treatment showed pigmentation of the hair shaft and thermal injury to the follicular epithelium.

A follow-up report [11] of these 13 individuals indicated that permanent, non-scarring alopecia can be induced by a single, high-fluence ruby laser treatment. Significant hair loss (less than 50% regrowth of terminal hairs) was still present in four participants 2 years after one laser exposure. Histologically, there was a reduction in large terminal hairs and a reciprocal increase in miniaturized, vellus-like hair follicles in these subjects. Hair counts in these individuals at 6 months, 1 year, and 2 years were relatively unchanged, suggesting that 6-month follow-up may be sufficient to assess final outcome after laser hair removal.

Lask et al. [12] found 40 to 80% regrowth of arm hair 12 weeks after a single treatment with a different ruby laser (694 nm, 800 μsec, 4–5 mm spot, 10–40 J/cm^2; EpiTouch, Sharplan Laser). Studies [13] on the influence of spot size and skin temperature indicate increased efficacy with the 10 mm compared with the 7 mm spot size, and a decrease in epidermal side effects with skin cooling. Excellent clinical outcomes with minimal adverse effects were found in several other studies evaluating the long-pulse ruby laser for hair removal.

Long-Pulse Alexandrite Laser

The 755 nm long-pulse alexandrite laser has a similar mechanism of action to that of the ruby laser. Several different alexandrite laser systems are now available. The wavelength of 755 nm is well absorbed by follicular melanin, and penetrates even deeper into the dermis. Because this wavelength is less well absorbed by epidermal melanin, it may prove safer in darker skin types. The millisecond duration pulses provide effective heating of hair follicles.

A study of 126 patients receiving up to five treatments with a long-pulse alexandrite (EpiTouch, Sharplan) found 90% hair loss 3 months after the final treatment [14]. Woo et al. [15] treated 392 patients with skin types I to V with a long-pulse alexandrite laser (755 nm, 5–20 msec pulses, 7–10 mm spot, 5–40 J/cm^2; Cynosure), and found a 44% reduction of brown hairs and 50% reduction of black hairs 1 month after treatment. Thirty-five to 40% hair reduction persisted for at least 6 months. The incidence of erosion was 5% in all patients and 8% in patients with skin types IV and V, but no persistent scarring or dyschromia was observed. Similar to the ruby lasers, the 10 mm spot size appears to be more effective than the 7 mm spot size, and higher fluences correlate with increased hair reduction [16]. Higher fluences were associated with an increased risk of blistering and pain, particularly in patients with skin phototypes IV or greater. In a controlled comparison of the long-pulse alexandrite and long-pulse ruby lasers, Nanni and Alster [17] found comparable efficacy and incidence of side effects.

Diode Laser

Similar to the ruby and alexandrite lasers, the 800 nm wavelength of the diode laser provides excellent skin penetration and selectivity for follicular melanin (Fig. 2). In

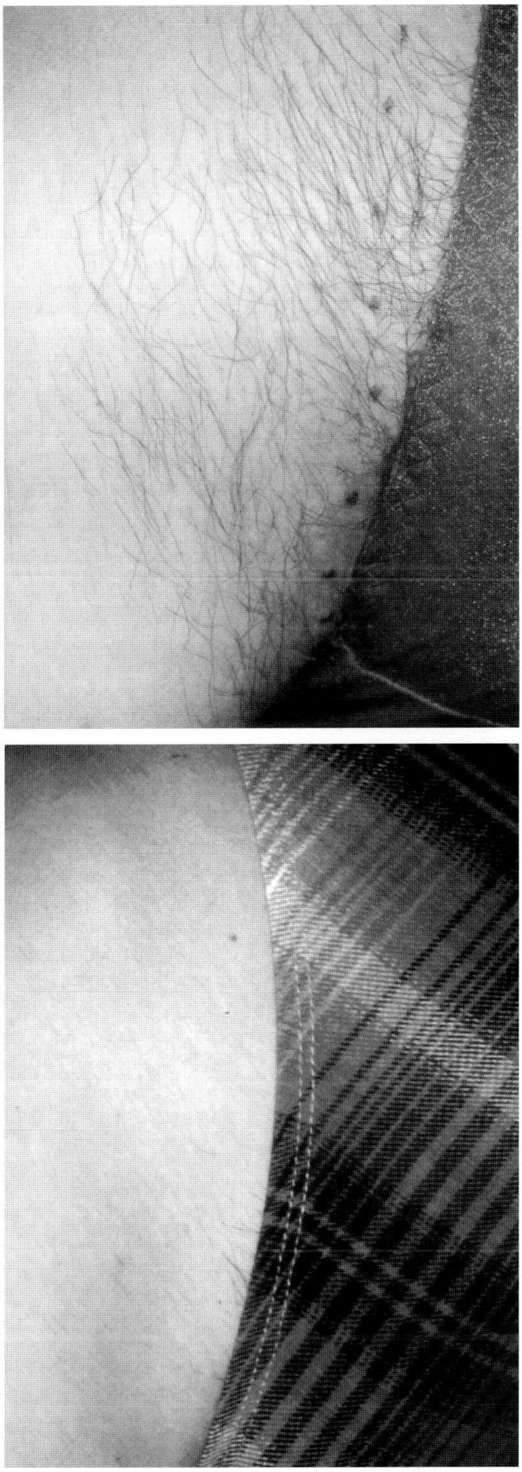

(a) (b)

FIGURE 2 The inguinal region was treated in a 40-year-old female with the LightSheer Diode (800 nm) three times at 39 J/cm^2 with a pulse width of 20 msec and 9 × 9 mm spot. (a) baseline, (b) three months after the last treatment.

a recent study [18] of the diode laser (LightSheer, Coherent), 58 subjects with skin phototypes II and III were treated (5–20 msec, fluence 10–40 J/cm^2) once or twice at 1 month intervals using single or triple pulsing. Approximately 90% of dark-haired subjects and 30% of blonde-haired subjects exhibited hair growth delays. The degree of observed hair loss was fluence-dependent. Statistically significant reductions in hair diameters and lightening of hair color were observed. Triple pulsing did not provide increased efficacy, but doubled the incidence of pigmentary change.

Filtered Flashlamp

The filtered flashlamp (EpiLight, ESC Medical Systems) is a nonlaser device that produces intense noncoherent light of a spectrum ranging from 540 to 1200 nm. A series of cut-off filters are used to adjust the spectrum of light for treatment of various hair/skin color combinations. During treatment, a cooling gel is applied to the skin to minimize epidermal heating and optimize light penetration into the dermis. Gold et al. [19] found a 60% reduction in hair counts 12 weeks after a single treatment with various cut-off filters (34–55 J/cm^2, 2–5 pulses, 1.5–3.5 msec, 20–50 msec delays). Longer delays and multiple pulse modes were used with higher fluences. Adverse effects included post-treatment erythema (7%), hyperpigmentation (3%), and blistering (11%). Similar results were found by other investigators [20,21].

Carbon-Nd:YAG Laser Treatment

The SoftLight system (Thermolase Corporation) uses carbon as an exogenous chromophore that is introduced into the hair follicles in the form of a skin lotion, followed by irradiation with a Q-switched Nd:YAG laser. Carbon particles within the follicle generate photoaucostic waves on absorption of laser light, inducing photomechanical disruption of the follicle. In the original treatment protocol, the carbon suspension was applied to wax-epilated skin. Presently, the hair is shaved 24 hours before treatment, and the carbon suspension is propelled down the hair follicles using the Q-switched Nd:YAG laser at low fluence.

Because follicular melanin is not used as the laser chromophore, light (blonde, red) hair can be treated with the SoftLight system. Another advantage of this system is that absorption at 1064 nm by epidermal melanin is poor, and treatment can be safely performed in individuals with darker skin types. Early studies of the SoftLight system show growth delays up to 3 months after a single treatment [22]. Permanent hair loss has not been shown even after multiple treatment sessions. The nanosecond domain pulses of the Q-switched Nd:YAG produce reversible photomechanical disruption of the follicle, but are incapable of achieving photothermal destruction of follicular epithelium which requires pulse durations in the millisecond range.

Nanni and Alster [23] compared effects of (1) laser treatment alone, (2) waxing alone, (3) waxing plus laser treatment, and (4) waxing plus carbon plus laser treatment. Hair regrowth was observed at 1 month in the wax-epilated control, and in all laser-treated sites at 6 months, regardless of pretreatment with either waxing or carbon solution. This data suggest that the SoftLight method produces a growth delay but no long-term hair loss after a single treatment.

TABLE 2 Directed Patient History and Physical Examination

Patient History	Skin Examination
Metabolic	Hair color
Endocrine	Skin type
Neoplastic	Nevi
Infectious	Tattoos
Medications	Permanent make-up
Skin disease (eg, psoriasis, vitiligo)	Scars, keloids
Scars, keloids	Skin disease (eg, psoriasis, vitiligo)
Isotretinoin use	Skin infection
Local radiation	

PRESURGICAL CONSIDERATIONS

A directed patient history and physical examination should be obtained before treatment (Table 2). When hirsutism appears to relate to an endocrinopathy, metabolic disorder, or medication (Table 3), patients should be referred to the appropriate medical specialist for evaluation. Laser hair removal may prove less effective in these individuals unless the underlying medical problem is treated concurrently.

Active infectons (eg, herpes, cellulitus) are treated before initiating laser therapy, and caution should be exercised when treating immunocompromised patients because of the increased risk of infection. Patients with a history of herpes simplex are treated with antiviral prophylaxis when hair is being treated in a susceptible skin region. Laser hair removal treatment should be avoided in patients undergoing isotretinoin (Accutane) therapy, and careful considerations should be given to treatment of individuals with a history of hypertrophic or keloidal scarring. When treating an individual with a history of koebnerizing skin disease (eg, psoriasis, lichen planus, vitiligo), test treatments should be performed. Treatment of suntanned individuals should be postponed until the tan fades because of the increased risks of blistering and pigmentary alteration.

In general, with the exception of the SoftLight technique, the best candidates for treatment are fair-skinned, dark-haired patients. Individuals with skin phototypes

TABLE 3 Medications Causing Hair Growth

Medications Causing Hair Growth	
Acetazolamide	Minoxidil
Corticosteroids	Oxadiazolopyrimidine
Danazol	Penicillamine
Diazoxide	Phenytoin sodium
Fenoterol	PUVA (Psoralen and ultraviolet A phototherapy)
Hexachlorobenzene	Sodium tetradecyl sulfate
Inteferon	Streptomycin

IV or higher have an increased risk for pigmentary alteration, particularly with the shorter wavelength lasers which are absorbed more strongly by epidermal melanin.

Tattoos or nevi present in the treatment area may be lightened or removed by the lasers and light sources used to treat hair. If a Q-switched laser is being used, patients should be forewarned that tattoo inks and permanent make-ups comprising iron oxide or titanium dioxide pigment may blacken immediately on laser exposure. Patients taking systemic gold therapy are also at risk for immediate skin darkening after Q-switched laser treatment.

TREATMENT GUIDELINES

During treatment, the patient and all personnel in the room must wear wavelength-specific glasses. All hairs in the treatment area are shaved or clipped before laser or light-source treatment. Anesthesia is not routinely needed, but the application of a topical anesthetic cream such as EMLA™ or ELA-Max™ before treatment of sensitive areas, such as the bikini line, axilla, and face, is often helpful.

Individual pulses are applied with minimal (0–10%) overlap, and treatments are performed at the highest fluences tolerated. Perifollicular erythema, edema, and disappearance of the surface hair are the desired endpoints (Fig. 3). Blister formation signifies epidermal damage, and indicates that treatment fluences must be reduced.

Laser pulses are delivered perpendicularly to the skin surface, and the skin is stretched to ensure maximum contact or delivery of laser light. Some of the laser systems, such as the Epilaser (Palomar) and LightSheer (Coherent), contain water-cooled sapphire lenses that permit the safe delivery of higher fluences by cooling the epidermis. Compression of the skin by the laser handpiece is required for optimal skin cooling. Forceful compression also eliminates dermal blood and reduces the distance that light must traverse between the surface and the hair papillae.

Various skin-cooling methods are used by other laser systems. A dynamic cooling device that provides millisecond duration cryogen spurts before each laser pulse is used with an alexandrite (GentleLASE, Candela). With the EpiTouch (Sharplan) and EpiLight (Energy Systems Corp.), a cooling gel is applied to the skin during treatment.

For the SoftLight process, a micronized carbon suspension is applied to the skin surface before laser treatment. One pass of the Q-switched Nd:YAG laser is performed at a low fluence (1 J/cm^2) to propel the carbon into the follicles. A second pass is performed by using higher (2–3 J/cm^2) fluences to disrupt the hair follicles.

POSTSURGICAL CARE

Hydrogel dressings (eg, Spenco™ 2nd Skin or Vigilon™) are applied immediately after treatment to reduce discomfort. Patients are instructed to apply antibiotic ointment (bacitracin or polysporin) twice daily if crusting is present. Sun protection with the use of sunscreens is required for a period of 1 month after treatment.

Complications

Adverse effects fromr laser hair removal are rare. After treatment, patients may develop mild erythema and crusting lasting up to 3 to 4 days. The main concern with

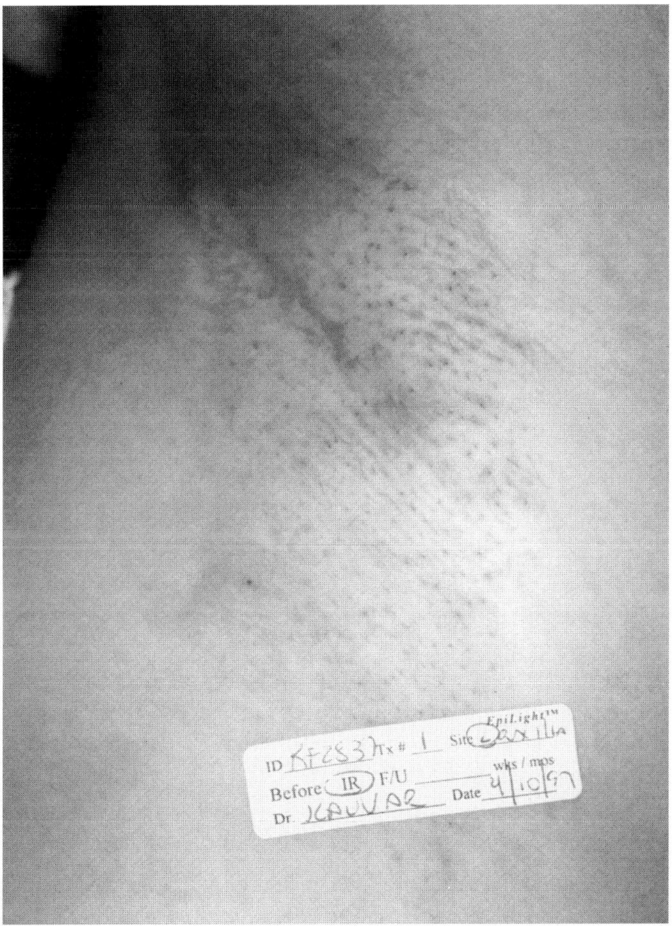

FIGURE 3 Perifollicular erythema and edema immediately after laser treatment with the Epilight.

these lasers is choosing the patient with the appropriate hair and skin-color combination. For the long-pulsed lasers and light sources, fair-skinned, dark-haired individuals show the best response. Fluences must be lowered in individuals with darker skin phototypes and should be adjusted based on the immediate clinical response. With the exception of the 1064 nm Q-switched Nd:YAG laser, the safety of these devices has not been established in skin phototypes V and VI. Skin whitening or blistering implies too high a fluence.

Excessive heating of the epidermis may lead to transient hyperpigmentation and, in rare cases, hypopigmentation. Because erosions are not routinely produced, skin infection is rare. Topical antibiotic ointment should be applied if crusting is present. Scarring is an unexpected outcome but may potentially result from infection, the use of excessive fluence, or multiple pulsing.

SUMMARY

Long-term hair removal is now possible using a variety of pulsed lasers and light sources that selectively damage hair follicles without adversely affecting the skin. Patient acceptance of these procedures is high because large areas can be safely and conveniently treated. Although significant reductions in hair number have been shown for up to 2 years after one laser treatment, the degree of hair loss and duration of benefit varies by the individual patient, treatment area, and laser used. With the present whirlwind pace of laser research and development, it is anticipated that, in the not-too-distant future, parameters will be standardized, results will be more consistent, and patients of all skin and hair types will be successfully treated.

REFERENCES

1. Saitoh M, Uzuka M, Sakamoto M. Human hair cycle. J Invest Dermatol 1970; 54:65.
2. Kligman AM. The human hair cycle. J Invest Dermatol 1959; 33:307.
3. Sactoh M, Uzuka M, Sakamato M, et al. Rate of hair growth. In: Montagna W, Poston RL, eds. Advances in Biology of the Skin. Vol. IX. Hair Growth. Oxford: Pergamon, 1969, p. 183.
4. Anderson RR, Parrish JA. Selective photothermolysis: precise microsurgery by selective absorption of pulsed radiation. Science 1983; 220:524–527.
5. Dover JS, Margolis RJ, Polla LL, et al. Pigmented guinea pig skin irradiated with Q-switched ruby laser pulses: morpholic and histologic findings. Arch Dermatol 1989; 125: 43–49.
6. Kauvar ANB. Hair removal with Q-switched lasers. Presented at the American Society for Dermatologic Surgery, May 1996.
7. Grossman MC, Dierickx C, Farinalli W, Flotte T, Anderson RR. Damage to hair follicles by normal-mode ruby laser pulses. J Am Acad Dermatol 1996; 35:889–894.
8. Cotsarelis G, Sun TT, Lavker RM. Label-retaining cells reside in the bulge area of the pilosebaceous unit: implications for follicular stem cells, hair cycle, and skin carcinogenesis. Cell 1990; 61:1329–1337.
9. Sun T, Cotsarelis G, Lavker RM. Hair follicular stem cells: the bulge-activation hypothesis. J Invest Dermatol 1991; 96:775–785.
10. Kilmer SL, Chotzen VA. Q-switched Nd:YAG hair removal without adjuvant topical preparation. Laser Surg Med 1997; (Suppl. 9):31.
11. Dierickx CC, Melanie MC, Farinelli WA, Anderson RR. Permanent hair removal by normal-mode ruby laser. Arch Dermatol 1998; 134:837–842.
12. Lask G, Elman M, Slatkine M, Waldman A, Rosenberg Z. Laser-assisted hair removal by selective photothermolysis. Dermatol Surg 1997; 23:737–739.
13. Duque V, Dierickx CC, Lin D, Farinelli WA, Anderson RR. Long pulsed ruby laser for hair removal: comparison between different spot sizes, temperatures and interval between first and second treatment. Lasers Surg Med 1998; S10:39, abstr. 187.
14. Finkel B, Eliezri YD, Waldman A, Slatkine M. Pulsed alexandrite lasers technology for non-invasive hair removal. J Clin Laser Med Surg 1997; 15:225–229.
15. Woo TY, Molnar G. Laser assisted hair removal using the Cynosure long pulsed alexandrite laser. Lasers Surg Med 1998; S10:39, abstr. 186.
16. Narurkar V, Miller HM, Seltzer R. The safety and efficacy of the long pulsed alexandrite laser for hair removal in various skin types. Lasers Surg Med 1998; S10:39, abstr. 189.
17. Nanni CA, Alster TA. Complicatons of laser assisted hair removal using the Q-switched Nd:YAG, long-pulsed ruby, and long-pulsed alexandrite lasers. Lasers Surg Med 1998; (Suppl 10):67.

18. Dierickx CC, Grossman MC, Farinelli WA, Manuskiatti W, Duque V, Lin D, Anderson RR. Hair removal by a pulsed infrared laser system. Lasers Surg Med 1998; S10:42, abstr. 198.
19. Gold MH, Bell MW, Foster TD, Street S. Long-term epilation using the EpiLight broad band, intense pulsed light hair removal system. 1997; 23:909–913.
20. Weiss RA, Weiss MA, Marwaha S, Harrington AC. Hair removal with a noncoherent filtered flashlamp pulsed light source. American Society of Laser Medicine and Surgery 1998 Annual Meeting.
21. Smith SR, Tse Y, Adsit SK, Goldman MP, Fitzpatrick RE. Long-term results of hair photoepilation. American Society of Laser Medicine and Surgery 1998 Annual Meeting.
22. Goldberg DJ, Littler CM, Wheeland RG. Topical suspension-assisted Q-switched Nd: YAG laser hair removal. Dermatol Surg 1997; 23:741–745.
23. Nanni CA, Alster TS. Optimizing treatment parameters for hair removal using a topical carbon-based solution and 1064-nm Q-switched Neodymium:YAG laser energy. 1997; 133:1546–1549.

APPENDIX 1. INFORMED CONSENT

I ______________ (patient's name) voluntarily request Dr. ________________ as my physician to use a laser or light source to treat my skin for the purposes of hair removal or reduction. I understand that this is an elective procedure.

I understand that no warranty or guarantee has been made to me as to result or cure. I also understand that multiple treatment sessions are probably necessary. I realize that hair removal by this method may not be permanent, that all of my hair may regrow completely, and that the regrown hair may be lighter and/or thinner.

I understand that this hair removal/reduction procedure is associated with risks including but not limited to the development of pigmentary changes, blisters, scabs, erosions, ulcers, bruising, infection, scarring, and persistent redness. Some potential side effects may require additional treatments. These treatments may include topical regimens such as antibiotic ointments and bleaching agents, or oral antibiotics.

Because of the nature of the lasers and light sources that will be used, I will be required to wear proper eye protection during treatment in order to prevent inadvertent injury to my eyes.

I acknowledge that I have disclosed to my physician all of my medical, surgical, and drug history, as such information may be critical to my medical/surgical treatment.

I hereby state that I have received and understand the pre-operative and post-operative instructions given to me.

I certify that my physician has discussed this procedure with me and that I have been given an opportunity to ask questions about my condition, treatment procedure, risks and hazards involved, and I believe that I have sufficient information to give this informed consent.

I agree to follow the instructions given to me by my physician to the best of my ability, and will notify my physician of any problems following my surgery.

______________________________ (Patient/Guardian name)

______________________________ (Patient/Guardian signature)

______________________________ (Date)

I, hereby certify that I have explained the nature, purpose, benefits and risks of the proposed treatment as well as alternative therapies. I have offered to answer any questions and have fully answered all such questions. I believe that the patient/relative/guardian fully understands what I have explained.

______________________________ (Physician Signature)

______________________________ (Date)

APPENDIX 2. PATIENT INFORMATION SHEET

Hair removal by lasers or light sources is a noninvasive procedure which uses an intense beam of light to heat and disrupt the hair follicles. Unlike electrolysis which treats one hair follicle at a time, large areas can be treated in one session. After treatment, a decreased number of hair will be present in most patients, and some of the hairs may be lighter and thinner. Multiple treatments are usually necessary to achieve long-term hair removal/reduction. These sessions are usually scheduled 4–6 weeks apart.

There is minimal discomfort associated with these procedures consisting of warmth or a pricking sensation. Your physician may recommend a topical anesthetic for more sensitive areas such as the face, bikini area, or areas with thick, dark hair.

EMLA™ cream is the topical anesthetic most frequently used. It is applied in a thick layer to the treatment site with plastic wrap covering for 1–2 hours and removed immediately before treatment.

Following treatment, the area will be red and may be swollen for up to 3 days.

Your physician can discuss in detail the various types of lasers or light sources, and may suggest to treat a test area to assess your response and side effects.

Preprocedure Instructions

- Do not tan for at least one month before, during, and for one month after the treatment series.
- Do not bleach hair in the treatment area for one month before treatment, unless you and your physician have decided to use the carbon suspension assisted Nd:YAG laser system.
- Do not use topical treatment or irritants such as harsh scrubs or topical exfoliants unless specified by your doctor.
- Inform your doctor of any changes in your medical condition or medications.

Postprocedure Instructions

- If crusting is present, a thin layer of antibiotic ointment (bacitracin or polysporin) should be applied twice daily. The treatment areas may be washed with mild soap.
- Do not apply chemical treatments, exfoliants, or bleach to the treated area for one week after the procedure.
- Avoid tanning or sun exposure for one month after treatment. A sunscreen with good UVA and UVB protection and SPF >15 should be worn.
- If there is any evidence of blistering, bleeding, oozing, pain or swelling which persists beyond 3 days, or signs of infection (e.g., pus, drainage, fever), please inform your doctor immediately.
- You may see extrusion of damaged hair follicles during the first week after treatment. This is different from active hair growth.

38

Office Photography in Cosmetic Surgery

David J. Narins
New York University School of Medicine, New York, New York

According to Slue, "[a] medical photograph is a photograph that accurately maximizes clinical information and minimizes irrelevant data" [1]. The professional should strive to take a medical photograph, not a snapshot.

A medical photograph must be both of high technical quality and reproducible. Good photographic records are a necessity in cosmetic surgery. They are helpful in planning the procedure and for patient education, and indispensable in documenting the results of surgery. To evaluate the results of surgery, standardization of photographic technique is necessary. The camera, lens, exposure, lighting, film, patient position, reproduction ratio and background should be constants so that the changes between presurgical and postsurgical photographs can be attributable only to the surgery.

With basic equipment and a modicum of foresight, even a person with limited photographic knowledge can take high-quality, reproducible medical photographs in an office setting. It is especially imperative to take the care necessary to ensure good presurgical photographs because there is only one opportunity to take them.

CAMERA

A 35-mm single lens reflex (SLR) camera is ideal for medical photography (Figs. 1, 2). It can produce very high quality photographs with readily available slide film, or color or black-and-white print film. It is light enough to be easily portable in a medical office. Interchangeable lenses are available so that the best lens for a particular view can be chosen and lenses changed for various clinical situations. The what-you-see-is-what-you-get, through-the-lens (TTL) viewfinder enables the photographer to compose the photographs accurately. A camera that imprints the date on the film is preferable for pre- and postsurgical photography in order to clearly document when a photograph was taken. This feature is built into some cameras; others require an accessory known as a "data back."

A Polaroid camera is also recommended. Use of presurgical Polaroid photographs provides a measure of insurance against having a roll of film lost and thus being left without any presurgical photographs at all. Instant photographs can aid in presurgical planning. Also, instant photographs taken after a patient has been marked

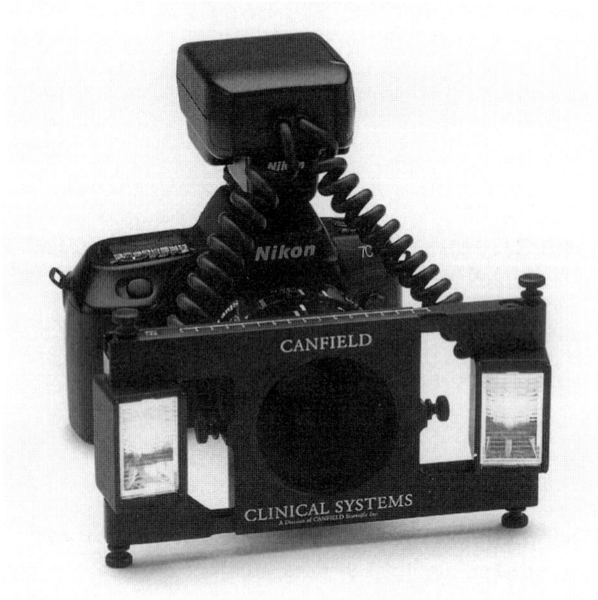

FIGURE 1 Canfield Clinical Systems: 35 mm Nikon N70 camera, 60 mm Slue macro lens, CCS twin flash.

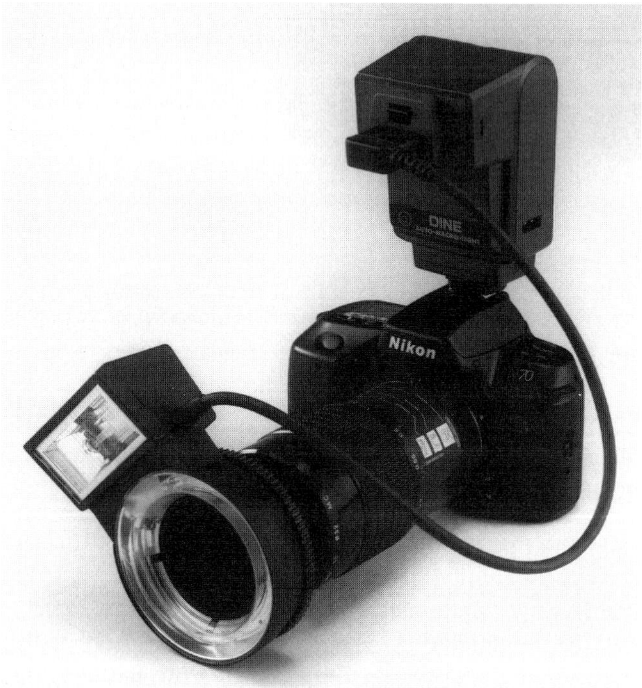

FIGURE 2 Lester Dine 35 mm Nikon N70 camera, 105 mm macro lens, ring/point flash.

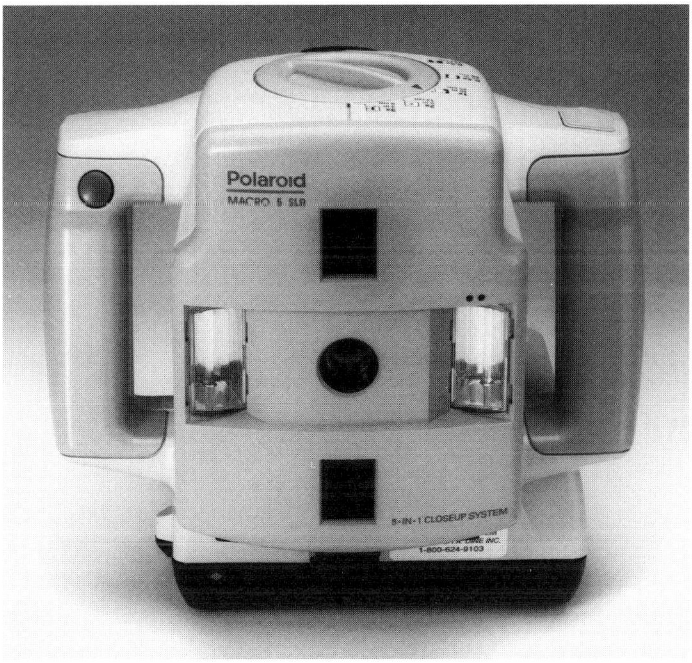

FIGURE 3 Polaroid macro 5 SLR instant camera.

for surgery will often show an asymmetry that might not be appreciated with the naked eye. Either a standard Polaroid camera with a close-focusing feature or the Polaroid Macro 5 SLR model (Fig. 3), which has five predetermined magnification ratios, a grid screen viewfinder for exact alignment, and focuses using converging light beams, may be used. The Macro 5 camera is ideally suited for taking high quality instant photographs using Spectra film.

LENS

A medium-range telephoto lens (90–105 mm) is ideal for most cosmetic surgical procedures. These lenses have minimal distortion and a flat field, which is best for portraits or showing smaller surgical areas. A wider-angle lens will distort the face on close-ups. A 60 mm lens must be used to show larger areas, such as pre- and postliposuction knee-to-shoulder views, because one would have to stand 15 to 20 ft from the patient to include this area with a 105 mm lens. A lens should be selected with a focal length appropriate for the areas to be photographed. It should have macrophotography (close-focusing) capability so that small areas can be photographed without distortion-producing accessory lenses. Macro lenses have adjustments on the focusing ring for the reproduction ratio and the distance to the subject.

EXPOSURE

The exposure is dependent on the film speed (ASA), the lens aperture (f-stop), and the length of time the film is exposed to light. Most modern 35 mm TTL-metered

TABLE 1 Camera Settings—60 mm Lens (ASA 100 Film)*

Subject	Reproduction ratio	Distance from lens (in)	Aperture
Full Body	1:16	72	f4
Full Face	1:10	25	f8
Half Face	1:6	15	f11
Close-up	1:4	10	f16

*Take your own bracketed test photographs to determine settings for your camera and lighting.

cameras can control the exposure automatically during flash photography. Some cameras can be set to full automatic mode and will then control both the lens aperture (f-stop) and the exposure time, but the photographer who enables this mode will be unable to control the depth of field, which is critical in medical photography. In medical photography, a sharp image is crucial because details must be clearly visible. The term "depth of field" refers to the amount of the image which will be in sharp focus. The greater the depth of field, the more of the photograph will be in sharp focus. The smaller the lens aperture (ie, the larger the f-stop number), the greater the depth of field so that more of the picture will be in sharp focus. The choice of lens aperture, therefore, will determine the depth of field. The smallest aperture possible with the available light should be used, because this will produce the sharpest picture. It is an advantage for the photographer to be able to choose the aperture manually. A TTL-metered flash automatically adjusts the length of time during which the film is exposed to light.

To determine the proper exposure, a test roll of film is taken. A limited number of views are usually sufficient to document a given procedure, and one must determine only three or four camera settings to take all the photographs necessary. The camera is set at aperture priority. In this mode, the aperture (lens opening) is selected by the photographer and the camera automatically determines how long the shutter will remain open. For a test roll, one must take several photographs of each view at different apertures, recording the camera to patient distance (and consequent reproduction ratio) and the lens aperture (f-stop) for each exposure. Tables 1 and 2 show

TABLE 2 Camera Settings—105 mm Lens (ADA 100 Film)*

Subject	Reproduction ratio	Distance from lens (in)	Aperture
Full Face	1:10	36	f5.6
Half Face	1:6	24	f8
Close-up	1:4	16	f11

*Take your own bracketed test photographs to determine settings for your camera and lighting.

suggested f-stops for each of the four most common distances (reproduction ratios). Use these as starting-off points and take photographs 1 and 2 f-stops higher and 1 and 2 f-stops lower with your chosen camera and lighting set-up. (If using slide film, bracket the exposure by $\frac{1}{2}$ and 1 f-stop). From the five exposures for each distance, select from the properly exposed photographs the one that was taken with the smallest aperture. It is advisable to record the settings that correspond to the selected photographs to make a camera setting table of your own for your camera and lighting set-up.

LIGHTING

Electronic strobe lights with automatic TTL exposure control are recommended. In the ideal lighting set-up, the main lights are positioned at a 45° angle from the subject and background lights positioned to eliminate shadows behind the patient that would make the patient difficult to distinguish from the background shadow (Fig. 4). Slave flash units, which are triggered by the light from a flash on the camera (thus elim-

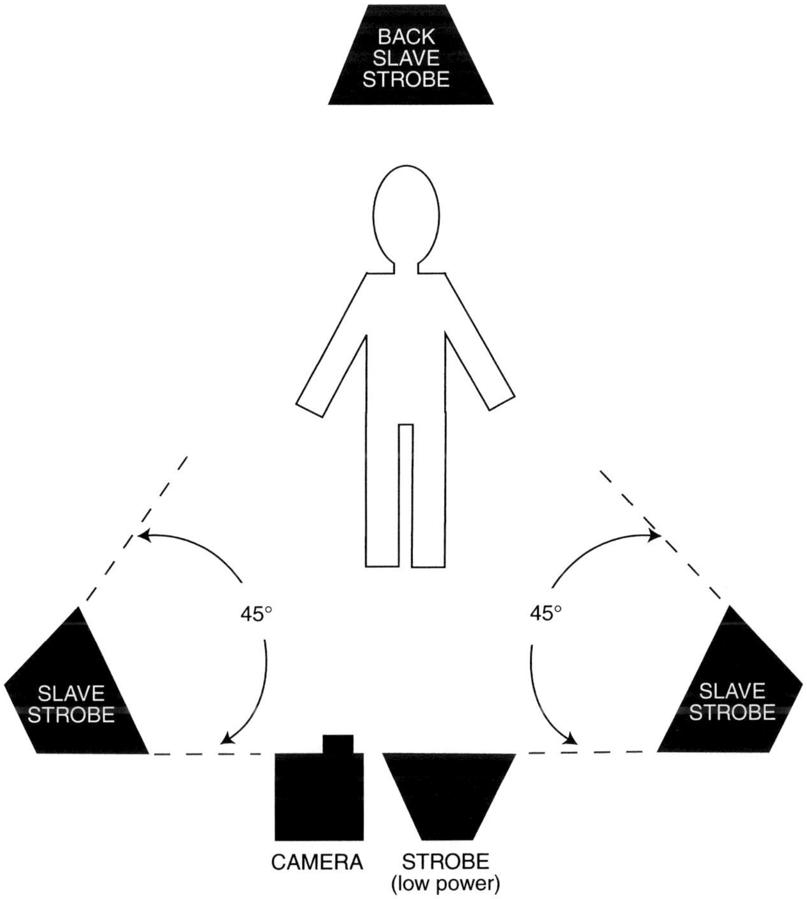

FIGURE 4 Photographic suite set-up.

inating the need for interconnecting wires), can be used. The light intensity of the slave flash units is adjustable. Determine by trial and error how much light each slave unit should give; this setting can then be used for all future photographs. Such a set-up will result in the most evenly lit, shadow-free photographs possible. However, the fact that both the main lights and the background lights are placed on stands at various positions relative to the patient makes it necessary either to have a dedicated photographic space or to spend a moderate amount of time setting up the room before taking pictures of each patient.

A simpler set-up, using a single strobe flash unit on the camera and one background light located directly behind the patient, can also result in photographs of excellent quality and requires far less extra work (Fig. 5). Either a ring flash or a unit that places the flash at the plane of the front of the lens should be used (Figs. 1, 2) If the flash is mounted on top of the camera, it will not illuminate the area being photographed when extreme close-ups are taken (ie, where the camera is very close to the subject). The slave background flash should be set between one-fourth and one-half power so that the background will not be overlit and will appear sky-blue rather than an overexposed white, or produce a halo effect around the subject. Setting the strobe at too weak a setting will result in shadows from the primary flash.

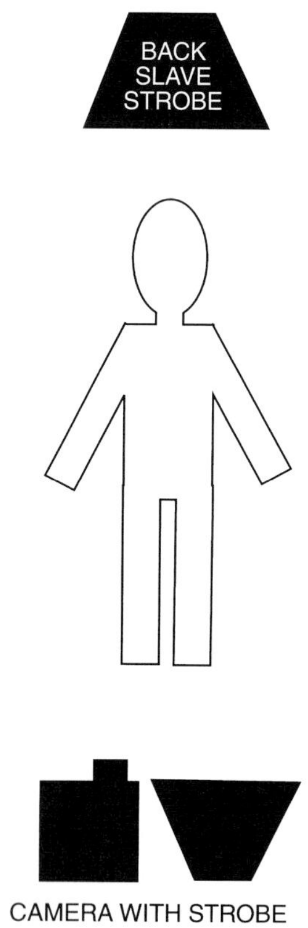

FIGURE 5 Simplified photographic suite set-up.

FILM

The "speed" of a film is a measure of its sensitivity to light. It is measured by an ISO (formerly ASA or DIN) number. Slow film (ie, film with a low ISO number) is less grainy than fast film and shows details better. Because patients are not moving and good lighting is obtained with electronic flash, slow (ISO 64 or 100) film can and should be used. Daylight color film is used with strobe flash units to give proper color balance. Daylight film comes in two types: color negative film for prints and color reversal film for slides. The most vivid and accurate color rendition is obtained with slide film because this is a one-step process. With print film, the print is made from a negative, thus involving a second step which can result in less vivid colors and possible inconsistency from roll to roll. For most medical purposes, either will be acceptable. The choice of slides or prints will depend on the use to be made of the images. Slides are preferable for lectures; prints are easier to use for viewing in the office and for showing patients the results of surgery without having to set up a projector or viewer. Prints can be made from slides more easily than can slides from prints. Kodak, Fuji, Agfa, and Ilford all make good quality film. They reproduce skin tones differently, so you should decide which is most pleasing to you and stick with one brand. Always try to use the same developing laboratory to eliminate the variables inherent in differing processing techniques.

STANDARDIZATION OF VIEWS

Pre- and postsurgical views must be identical so that the photographs will allow for an accurate comparison and contrast. Therefore, the photographer must standardize the views to be taken. Each photograph should be taken at a predetermined distance from the patient with the same camera settings, so the exposure and image size will always be identical. This can be accomplished by having the patient sit in a fixed position and by either marking the floor to indicate the distance for each view or, in the alternative, setting the distance on the macro lens and moving towards the patient until the image is in focus. The latter technique is called "body focusing."

For each procedure, there are certain views that best show the area being worked on. Frontal, oblique, lateral, and posterior views may be taken. A list should be created of the views and magnifications to be taken for any given procedure. Go through the list routinely during each photography session, taking all required photographs at each photography session. In this way, you will have comparison photographs at each stage of the procedure; before surgery, after surgery, and long-term. It is better to take too many photographs than too few. Unnecessary photographs can always be discarded, but one cannot go back in time to retake a photograph he forgot to take. Remember to be especially thorough when taking presurgical photographs, because these can never be retaken.

BACKGROUND

The background is a very important part of a medical photograph. A homogeneous background, free from distracting elements, is essential so that one can focus on the information being presented without being distracted by extraneous details. The color is also important. Sky blue is complementary to skin tones both in color and in black-and-white photography, giving good definition of the clinical area. A satisfactory background can be easily placed in any office. A wall or door can be painted with sky-blue matte paint, or background paper or felt material can be purchased in 4-ft wide strips at photographic supply shops and hung from a wall. Several rooms can be prepared for photography so that patients will not have to be moved to a dedicated photographic area for their photographs and the backgrounds in all photographs documenting the clinical progress will be identical.

RECORD KEEPING

It is necessary to keep systematic records of photographs as they are taken and to be able to file them so they can be easily retrieved. A photographic logbook should be kept with the camera. Each roll should be numbered and there should be a line for each exposure on the roll. You should record the date, patient's name, procedure, and any other relevant notes for each photograph you take. To avoid losing a roll of film during developing, you should take a photograph of your name, address, and telephone number as the first exposure on the roll. In this way, if the film is mishandled at the laboratory, there will be some identification on the roll of film that would enable the photographs to be returned to you. In addition to keeping the logbook, another aid in identifying and filing photographs is to take the first exposure of each series of photographs of a patient of a card with the date, patient's name, and procedure (Fig. 6). Each photograph appearing on the roll until the photograph of the next name card will belong to that patient; this will make filing of the photographs easier.

ARCHIVING

Slides or prints can be stored either in the patient's chart or in a separate file. In either case, you should have a system that enables you to retrieve them easily. You should be able to reference them by patient's name and by procedure so you will be able to get the picture you are looking for with a minimum amount of difficulty. As with all medical records, photographs must be stored in a secure place after office hours.

•Name: ....
•Date: ....
•Notes:

Take a photograph of a card with this information before taking a series of photographs of a patient. All photographs until the next identification photograph will belong to that patient and can easily be identified and filed.

FIGURE 6 Archiving tip.

OTHER CAMERA SYSTEMS

If you do not presently own a suitable camera or are planning to upgrade your system, you might consider the APS system. These cameras are almost identical in feel and use to a 35 mm SLR camera, but use a smaller, 24 mm film cassette. This cassette has practically foolproof drop-in loading which eliminates incorrect loading and unexposed rolls of film. Film can be easily changed in mid-roll if you have a need to switch from color print film to black and white for a particular situation. (There is, as yet, no slide film available in this format, which is a drawback.) A picture quality information exchange (PQIE) feature stores exposure information on a magnetic layer on the film. This information can be used by the photofinisher to improve the quality of each print by making automatic frame by frame adjustments during printing. It also imprints the exposure factors (ISO, f-stop, and shutter speed) on the back of each print so you can change camera settings for future photographs if your results are not satisfactory. The cassette system is also ideal for archiving. Each cassette is numbered and this number is imprinted on the back of each print along with the date, frame number, and exposure factors. An "index print," showing a thumbnail print of each frame and the range of dates of exposure for the roll, allows you to quickly review the contents of each roll. Because the film is returned rerolled into the cassette, it can be filed safety for quick retrieval if copies of a print or a slide have to be made. The index print, film cassette, and information on the back of each print share the same ID number to avoid confusion and help locate the proper negative quickly. The negatives are not handled and are thus less likely to become damaged or lost. The cassettes can also be scanned into a computer for incorporation into a presentation, letter, or e-mail (Fig. 7). Thirty-five mm slides, negatives, or prints can also be scanned into a computer with the appropriate scanner.

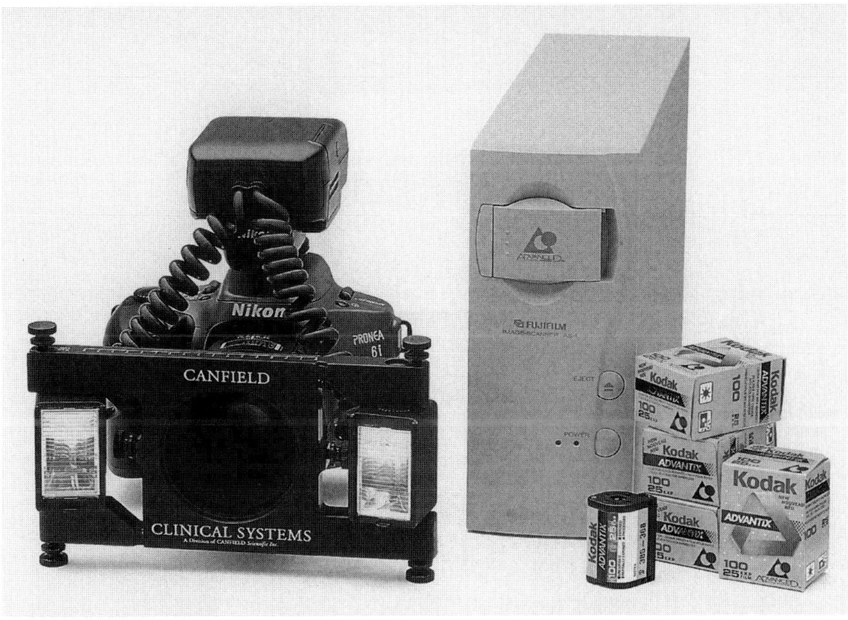

FIGURE 7 APS camera with film cassette scanner.

DIGITAL PHOTOGRAPHY

Digital photography will probably be the standard within several years. Digital cameras record images electronically and these images can be downloaded from the camera to a computer, where they can be stored. Computers are ideal for storing, manipulating, and retrieving photographic images. Images taken with a digital camera are available immediately without the need for processing. With the power of computers and larger, less expensive storage media, large numbers of photographs can be stored in a small space and instantly cross-referenced and retrieved by searching for any information you have included with the image (name, date, condition, surgical procedure, etc., or any combination of criteria). Stored digital images are archival (they will not fade or degrade with time). Color printers can produce laboratory-quality prints and the images can be included in the patient's chart or letters, e-mailed, or incorporated into slides for presentations. Digital images can either be taken with a digital camera (Fig. 8) and downloaded to a computer, or scanned into the computer from 35 mm negatives, slides, or prints.

An electronic image is composed of many small dots called pixels (picture elements). In color digital photography, every pixel contains a red, blue, and green dot, each of which is energized at different intensities to produce different colors. The number of pixels in the width and the number of pixels in the height express the resolution of a digital image (eg, 768 × 504). The larger these numbers, the better the resolution. Pixels are made up of one or more bits (binary digits). Twenty-four bits per pixel are required to get adequate color images. Higher-resolution pictures require more memory for storage, so that fewer can be stored on the media in the camera and will take more time to download to the computer.

Although many medical photographers are currently using digital photography, there are several limitations that make wider acceptance unlikely at this time. To begin with, computers intimidate many people and others feel that they are unreliable as a sole source of storing important patient information. At present, the equipment

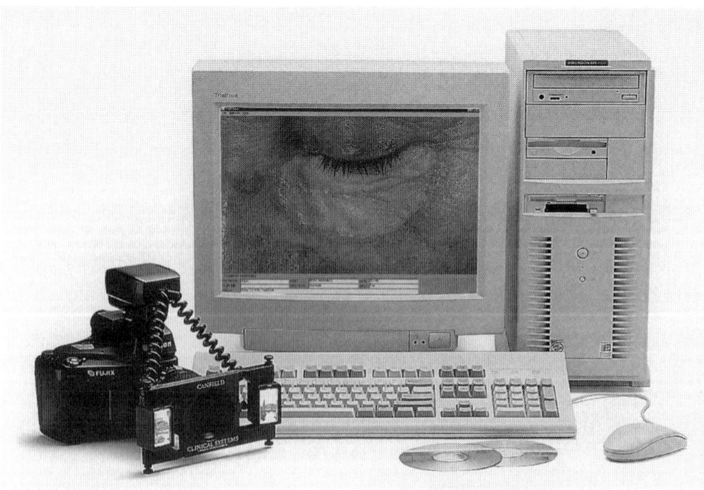

FIGURE 8 **Digital camera with computer.**

is still costly when compared with a 35 mm camera and the resolution (degree of sharpness) of even the best digital cameras is not as good as that of 35 mm film. Chemistry still has the edge over electronics. Top-quality photographic film can have 80 million pixels/in^2 whereas the best digital cameras only have 2.1 million pixels/in^2. Conventional photographs are sharper and reproduce colors more accurately. The storage media in present cameras suffice for only a small number of high-resolution images, and attaching the camera directly to the computer can be unwieldy. An additional limitation is that it is time consuming to download high-resolution images from the camera to the computer.

However, the ability of computers to organize and provide almost instant access to photographic records will make digital photography the standard of the future. The cost of equipment is rapidly decreasing and the resolution of each new generation of cameras has improved. Storage capacity and ease and speed of inputting the images into the computer will improve, as will computer reliability. As with any computer information, backing up all photographs is essential. One day, digital cameras will probably have the same impact on office photography that word processors have had on writing.

One controversial aspect of digital photography is the ease with which the images can be manipulated. It can be difficult to determine if a digitally created image has been electronically altered. Even relatively unsophisticated computer programs can edit images.

This ability to manipulate images is purposely used in "morphing" programs, where the image can be changed to show a patient what can be expected after surgery by showing a digitally created postsurgical view. Whether this is a good idea is debatable. Some say it is an educational tool and gives a patient a better understanding of what can and cannot be accomplished with surgery, whereas others say it can give a false expectation of postsurgical appearance and can be construed as an implied warranty.

CONSENT AND LIABILITY ISSUES

As with all medical procedures, one must obtain consent to take photographs as well as a patient release to use them (see Appendix). This is important if the photographs are intended to be used in publications or lectures and critical if they will be shown to other patients, used in advertising, or placed on a web site for your practice. One should be careful never to show a photograph in which the patient is identifiable without specific consent for that use. Blacking out the eyes or part of the face is not adequate for disguising a patient's identity.

The legal parameters regarding electronic transmittal of patient information are just being developed. Patient's photographs and all clinical information sent by e-mail should be encrypted.

Taking a Photograph

1. Position the patient in front of the blue background
2. Set up the slave background flash
3. Set the camera for manual focus
4. Set the camera for aperture priority

5. Use a TTL-metered flash
6. Set the distance (reproduction ratio) on the macro lens
7. Move in until the image is in focus
8. Take the photograph

Sources of Photographic Equipment

Representative Camera System

Nikon Cameras
Body: N70 or N600
Lens: 60 mm f2.8 AF Micro Nikor
105 mm f2.8 AF Micro Nikor
Flash: TTL Macro Speedlight SB-21 A/B
Slave Flash Controller: SU-4 Wireless Remote Flash Controller
Slave Flash: SB-23 Speedlight

(Note: Canon, Pentax, and Minolta all make excellent camera systems for medical use.)

Slave Flash System

Wein Slave
Procycler Battery Pack
Armatar 100 Flash
VP 1 (Variable Knob) Strobe
Tripod
Armato's Photography
1-718-628-6800

Specialists in Medical Photography, 35 mm, Polaroid, and Digital Systems

Canfield Scientific
253 Passaic Avenue
Fairfield, NJ 07004
Tel: 973-276-0300
Tel: 800-815-4330
Fax: 973-276-0333
e-mail: info@canfieldsci.com
Web Site: http://www.canfieldsci.com

Lester A. Dine, Inc.
351 Hiatt Drive
Palm Beach Gardens, FL 33418
Tel: 561-624-9100
Tel: 800-624-9103
Fax: 561-624-9103
e-mail: dinecorp@emi.net
Web Site: http://www.dinecorp.com

Specialists in Digital Photography and Morphing Hardware and Software

Mirror Software Corporation
12530 128th Lane NE
Kirkland, WA 98034
Tel: 425-823-4111
Tel: 800-841-5678
Fax: 425-823-4113
e-mail: techsupport@mirrorsoftware.com
Web Site: http://www.mirrorsoftware.com

APPENDIX. PERMISSION FOR TAKING AND PUBLISHING PHOTOGRAPHS AND/OR VIDEOTAPES

Patient:________________________

1. I hereby consent that photographs and/or videotapes may be taken of me or the named patient by Dr. __________ in connection with the medical care and treatment which I/the patient am/is receiving from Dr.__________.

2. Such photographs, videotapes, movies, histories, and/or audio recordings may be published, shown, exhibited, or otherwise used by Dr. ___________ for any purpose of medical education, knowledge, or research which Dr. __________may deem proper (including media publicity or other commercial trade purposes).

3. I understand that neither I/the patient nor members of my/the patient's family will be identified by name in connection with any public use of this material, and all care will be used to prevent such identification.

4. I grant this consent as a voluntary contribution and I waive any and all rights I may have to royalties or other compensation in connection with any such use.

Date _____________ Patient/Guardian Signature________________

Witness _____________ Relationship, if not patient __________________

Interpreter (if required)______________________

*The signature of the patient must be obtained unless the patient is an emancipated minor under the age of 18 or is otherwise incompetent to sign.
NOTE: THIS DOCUMENT MUST BE MADE PART OF THE PATIENT'S MEDICAL RECORD.

39

Handling the Dissatisfied or Difficult Patient

Timothy Corcoran Flynn and Mark A. Chastain
Tulane University School of Medicine, New Orleans, Louisiana

Every dermatologist knows difficult patients. The patient with multiple complaints, and who wishes everything treated immediately on the initial visit, is legendary. The loquacious or chatty patient can frustrate the practitioner almost as much as the nebulous patient who is unable to give a simple answer to a straightforward question. Patients who constantly demand special treatment or unusual appointment times can be difficult. Most every dermatologic surgeon knows a bargain-hunting patient who wants treatment at no cost. But some cosmetic patients are extremely difficult, easily dissatisfied, and are best avoided. Minimizing the risk of dissatisfaction and developing a sense for patients who may be difficult will help the dermatologic surgeon maintain a smooth and rewarding practice.

FIRST STEPS TOWARD MINIMIZING DISSATISFACTION

The risk of dissatisfaction in the cosmetic dermatology patient can be minimized with the correct approach during the initial evaluation [1]. The consultative visit allows the physician to take a medical history and obtain a physical examination [2]. It serves to educate the patient regarding the proposed procedure and allows the dermatologic surgeon to identify patients whose personality characteristics, medical and psychological health, and presenting complaint make them good surgical candidates [3].

During the consultation, the physician should be careful not to downplay the extent or risks of the procedure, nor the patient's responsibilities after surgery [4,5]. The surgeon should not exaggerate the improvements that can be expected after the operation [6]. Mindful that the primary goal is to improve the patient's well being, cosmetic dermatologists must be honest in their portrayal of the procedure [7]. The dermatologic surgeon should not be an overly aggressive "salesperson" because the patient who encounters an unpleasant outcome frequently becomes dissatisfied [5,6].

During the initial encounter, good communication establishes rapport and builds trust and respect between the patient and physician. The physician should be seated across from the patient, at eye level, maintaining frequent eye contact. Open-ended questions should be asked, with the first word being "how," "what," or "why" [3,8]. "How can I help you?" is a good initial question. Listen carefully to the patient and respond affirmatively rather than defensively. The use of small pauses, after a patient finishes speaking and before responding, helps to impart a feeling of concern and understanding. The physician should freely thank patients for expressing their feelings and sharing thoughts. Questions asked by the patient are also encouraged and should be answered in a thorough, straightforward, and unhurried manner.

Some factors that can help to build confidence are external. For example, adequate parking, well-equipped restrooms, and an attractive interior design are a favorable reflection on the physician. Being well-groomed, well-dressed, and having a pleasant demeanor are helpful. Any factors that could create doubt or second guesses in a cosmetic patient undermine the patient's confidence in the physician. Good personnel in the office are important in ensuring patient satisfaction and can even play an important role in the physician-patient rapport [9,10]. Many patients may find a surgical assistant or staff member easier to talk with and may form a special bond with them [5].

When nearing the end of the presurgical consultation, it is helpful to ask another open-ended question, such as, "Is there anything else that you feel you should tell me?" [8]. This gives the patient a final opportunity to discuss an important issue that may have been overlooked. Another good technique in this situation is to ask the patient, "Do you have any other questions?," allowing plenty of time for reflection. Occasionally, a second presurgical visit is necessary to confirm the patient's suitability for the procedure and to address any of the patient's last-minute concerns or questions.

THE IDEAL PATIENT

Understanding the ideal cosmetic patient may help the dermatologist recognize the signs that suggest that a particular patient is either a good or bad candidate. Ideal patients seek cosmetic surgery on their own volition and without external pressures. They present to the physician with a specific, well-defined problem to obtain the doctor's opinion. Receptive to the best options available, they are capable of weighing the risks and benefits of the procedure. The ideal patient has realistic expectations and seeks improvement of his or her condition, rather than absolute perfection [7,8]. Ideal patients do not endanger their own financial security in order to have the procedure.

According to Napoleon [11], the ideal cosmetic patient is older than 55 years of age and has concerns limited to one area. Ideal patients are self-motivated, confident, and, despite their interest in cosmetic surgery, do not consider themselves to be unattractive. They are intelligent, knowledgeable, and informed about the procedure [8].

PROBLEM PATIENTS

Although patients present to the cosmetic surgeon from a variety of economic, social, and ethnic backgrounds, the factors associated with a problem patient are common to many groups of people. High-risk patients often have warning signs, or "red flags," signifying that they are a bad surgical candidate. When concern arises about a patient, caution should be exercised and careful consideration given as to whether or not to proceed.

The patient who undergoes a cosmetic procedure with unrealistic expectations is almost invariably dissatisfied after surgery. A patient's presurgical expectation of the postsurgical result is the most reliable predictor of the degree of subsequent satisfaction [7]. For example, a 55-year-old patient may be dissatisfied after laser resurfacing if she were expecting to look 30 years younger. Because patients with such extreme expectations are not content with an excellent aesthetic result, they are poor candidates. Unfortunately, these patients are often adept at concealing their unrealistic goals, which makes identifying them a challenge. During the initial consultation, the physician must listen carefully to patients in order to carefully gauge their perceived notions of the expected result [12]. If a mutual understanding of the risks and reasonable cosmetic benefits cannot be reached, the procedure should be avoided [13].

Some patients presenting for a cosmetic procedure have unrealistic expectations related to an ulterior motivation [7]. These patients are motivated because they expect that cosmetic surgery will solve their personal problems [4]. For example, asking the patient, "What do you hope to achieve from this laser surgery?" is answered by a realistic patient with "Improvement in my sunspots." An unrealistic patient with ulterior motives may respond "for my husband to stop having an affair." Similarly, patients expecting a new job or a more successful acting career as a consequence of surgery are at high risk of becoming difficult or dissatisfied [3]. The dermatologic surgeon should also be wary of the patient who has recently undergone an extreme life stress event [7]. It must be realized that patients with a good surgical outcome may become disappointed, dissatisfied, or difficult unless their underlying motives are commensurate with the surgical goals. Once again, if the physician and patient cannot mutually agree on what is expected as the final result, then avoidance of the surgery is best.

Patients with deficient communication skills can be problem patients after surgery and are thus undesirable candidates. Beware of patients who do not seem to "hear" what they are being told [14]. Some patients have difficulty processing and understanding the physician because they are poor listeners. Without being condescending, the surgeon or a staff assistant should ask the patient detailed questions to assess his or her level of comprehension regarding the cosmetic procedure. A second presurgical visit may be necessary to ensure that both the patient and surgeon are well informed and in mutual agreement regarding all aspects of the procedure. Avoid patients who do not fully understand the procedure, including the risk of potential complications and reasonable outcomes.

Be wary of patients who are extremely vain and obsessively concerned with their appearance. Many of these patients have a dysmorphic body image, which is identified by their preoccupation with a real or imagined defect [15]. They constantly fuss and worry about minor blemishes. They frequently request mirrors during examination to view, point out, and obsess about their problems. These patients typically desire a cosmetic procedure in order to correct a minuscule problem that they perceive to be disfiguring. Sometimes, these patients are psychologically disabled by their concern over "non-problems." These excessively vain patients often have narcissistic personality traits and cannot seem to separate themselves from their external image. An unwillingness to accept unavoidable scars is a characteristic feature and is a reliable warning of postsurgical difficulties [4]. These people are at a high risk for dissatisfaction and require expertise [8].

The physician should be wary of the surgical addict [16–19], or "cosmetic junkie." Often because of their insatiable appetite for perfection, these patients undergo many cosmetic procedures and are repeatedly lured by the "new and exciting result." Occasionally, patients will have the same procedure multiple times or a reversal of a previous procedure. Many "cosmetic junkies" are unhappy people who seek affection and acceptance from others in an attempt to attain happiness [16]. They may use surgery to correct psychological distress [17]. When surgical intervention inevitably fails to deliver complete happiness, the surgical addict may continue to search for perfection through subsequent procedures, often from multiple physicians.

Character traits that may signal a future problem patient include being manipulative, pushy, indecisive, impulsive, untruthful, hysterical, and overly anxious or fearful [8,10,20,21]. Patients with excessively emotional or inappropriate responses to routine questioning are also prone to cause difficulties. The patient whose self-esteem is dependent on others may become troublesome [4]. Patients with multiple complaints or a single, poorly defined complaint frequently have little insight into their condition and can be difficult to manage [22].

THE COSMETIC PATIENT WITH A PSYCHIATRIC CONDITION

Some patients who seek cosmetic procedures may have an underlying psychiatric or emotional disorder [11,20,23,24]. Because these patients are frequently dissatisfied with their postsurgical results, they should be approached cautiously and carefully evaluated. The patient's mental health, medication use, and past hospitalizations are important aspects of the history. If necessary, consultation should occur with a psychiatrist regarding the current status of the patient's condition and the appropriateness of the cosmetic procedure [24]. It is important not to refuse a procedure in patients who have completely recovered from emotional distress in the past. Patients who have succeeded in overcoming a difficult situation may warrant an isolated cosmetic procedure now that their life has "turned around." Three types of patients with diagnosable personality disorders bear concern: the borderline personality disorder, the narcissistic personality disorder, and the obsessive-compulsive patient [8,11,20,21,25].

Narcissistic patients often speak in a grandiose manner and are generally searching for an unattainable, ideal result with cosmetic procedures. These patients are overconcerned with fashion and appearance. They think of themselves as "absolutely wonderful" and "very beautiful." Interestingly, these patients often felt highly attractive as children. They tend to be arrogant, loud, assertive, demanding, and pushy. As cosmetic surgery patients, narcissistic people can be troublesome to manage because they are so frequently unhappy with the result. Regardless how favorable the outcome, it seems never to approach their ideal goal of perfection.

Patients with a borderline personality disorder also require special consideration because of the many difficulties associated with their management [11,19]. The cosmetic surgeon is often envisioned as either "all good" or "all bad" by the borderline patient. These patients initially idolize the cosmetic surgeon, but this worship is often fragile and short-lived. The adoring patient can rapidly become filled with animosity and hatred. From the patient's perspective, the surgeon is transformed, as some have said, "from Saint to Satan" [11]. Borderline patients often suffer from a dysmorphic body image, thereby interfering with their ability to accurately assess the need for a cosmetic procedure or to evaluate a surgical outcome. These individuals have a forward, inappropriate demeanor and usually request an entire "make-over" and want "everything done." Unfortunately, their erratic emotions, judgement biases, and obtrusive personality frequently lead to management difficulties. It is not uncommon for borderline patients to pursue a malpractice claim [11].

Beware of patients who suffer from an obsessive-compulsive disorder as these patients may present problems [15]. Obsessive-compulsive patients are meticulous and perfectionistic. They are rigid, focused, and mentally perseverate on their particular concern. They can devote extreme attention to tiny details at the expense of the overall picture. Compulsive patients may engage in uncontrollable and repetitive behaviors, such as picking at sutures or manipulating scars. The compulsive patient's life can be severely restricted because of overwhelming behaviors and rituals. When these patients undergo a cosmetic procedure, they can contribute to an unfavorable result.

Other psychiatric conditions are associated with management difficulties [20]. Patients with a mood disorder, labile affect, or dependent or histrionic personality disorders are predisposed to cause various difficulties in management [11]. Neurotic patients who experience excessive anxiety, distress, and somatic symptoms are usually risky candidates. Psychotic patients who are confused, out of touch with reality, or afflicted with thought disturbances also make undesirable candidates. Individuals with paranoid schizophrenia or other psychosis may become violent, and there have even been cases in which patients have murdered their surgeons [8,26].

PREVENTING DISSATISFACTION THROUGH PROPER PATIENT SELECTION

The cosmetic dermatologist can easily recognize candidates who exhibit multiple warning signs as well as recognize ideal cosmetic dermatologic patients. However, many candidates rest somewhere in between. Because the physician should attempt to avoid problem patients, it is important to perform a complete assessment both objectively and subjectively. Some patients create a sense of concern or a "bad feeling" in the physician during the pretreatment consultation. Surgeons should respect their own "gut feeling" as an intangible, but important, warning signal of potential difficulties with these surgical candidates. The office staff can also provide input to help identify potentially difficult patients [9,10].

The physician should decline to treat any patient considered to be a poor candidate, whether based on objective facts, subjective impression, or simple intuition. Any patient who is identified as a poor candidate should be treated compassionately as they are further evaluated. The surgeon must delicately refuse the request for treatment without implying in any way that the patient is to blame. For example, "I don't think I can help you achieve the result you are looking for," is far less confrontational than "I know you won't be happy no matter how good it looks." Young dermatologic surgeons who are eager to gain surgical experience may sometimes be reluctant to decline a request for surgery even by an undesirable candidate. In this situation, the dermatologic surgeon must resist the temptation to proceed in order to avoid adverse consequences early in their career [7].

PREVENTING DISSATISFACTION THROUGH COMMUNICATION AND RAPPORT

Many factors contribute to a good physician-patient rapport and therefore play a role in preventing difficult or dissatisfied patients [14]. Good communication between the dermatologic surgeon and patient is essential. In a study of communication behaviors in physicians, those primary care physicians without a history of malpractice claims spent more time during patient visits than physicians with malpractice claims [27]. They made more statements to inform patients as to their progress and what to expect during each visit. These physicians used more facilitative comments towards their patients, such as asking their opinions, verifying their understanding, and encouraging them to talk. The no-claim physicians also laughed and used humor more often. Although this study found significant differences in the communication behaviors between primary care physicians with malpractice claims and those without, this distinction was not identified in surgeons. The surgeons participating in this study practiced either orthopedic or general surgery, and it is unlikely that this finding would hold for dermatologic surgeons.

In nearly every field of medicine, the relationship between patient and physician is the single most important factor leading to malpractice claims [28,29]. This association is particularly true for cosmetic surgery. In general, the likelihood of a lawsuit against a cosmetic surgeon is related much more to patient rapport than to the surgeon's clinical and technical capabilities. Regardless of how difficult the patient is after surgery, the surgeon must never abandon a patient until the problems resolve or until management is undertaken by another physician. If the surgeon notices a deteriorating relationship with a cosmetic patient at any time during the course of management, attempts should be made to re-establish or strengthen the bond.

The strong rapport developed before surgery guards against dissatisfaction and must be maintained throughout the patient's entire surgical course. Maintaining open lines of communication facilitates the detection of signs or symptoms of a difficult or dissatisfied patient [4]. This approach mandates that the physician and staff be available to provide reassurance and address any patient concerns. Support after a procedure is important. A telephone call to the patient at home after the treatment is meaningful and seems to strengthen the bond [30]. Regular follow-up appointments after the treatment are also necessary to maintain a good relationship with the patient and to give the impression of "working together" during the recovery.

APPROACHING THE DISSATISFIED PATIENT

Encountering a dissatisfied patient can often create bad feelings in the cosmetic surgeon [31]. In general, cosmetic surgeons crave excellence, strive for perfection, and frequently resist change [29]. They often remember the dissatisfied patient rather than the satisfied patient because of the intense feelings of distress that both surgeon and patient endure. Because of their wish to be viewed favorably by patients, cosmetic surgeons may be unable to adequately cope with postsurgical difficulties and dissatisfaction [29]. The dissatisfied patient can cause the surgeon to question his or her own competence, talents, and motivations, and can lead to a sense of rejection. The surgeon may become defensive, often manifested by anger and frustration. All of these feelings pose a psychological threat that may interfere with the surgeon's ability to handle the patient's problems. Identifying or recognizing these feelings helps the surgeon retain the confidence necessary to approach the dissatisfied patient in a relaxed and level-headed manner.

The physician must be very attentive to the patient who is experiencing problems after a cosmetic procedure. Most often, patients who are dissatisfied with a procedure express their unhappiness in an emotional manner, outwardly expressing anger, disappointment, and frustration. Dissatisfied patients sometimes appear confused, having trouble finding words to express their dissatisfaction. They may express dissatisfaction in a passive way, such as being tardy for follow-up appointments. Other patients may fail to return for post-treatment visits, which should prompt the office to contact the patient by telephone. It is important that the physician recognize signs of a dissatisfied patient so that they can be identified early and managed appropriately.

Whether the patient is dissatisfied with a favorable or unfavorable result, the same initial approach is taken. The patient must be shown concern, compassion, and support [31]. The physician's disposition should be caring and sensitive while in control of his or her own emotions. Dissatisfied or difficult patients should have undivided attention, and should be encouraged to openly express their own feelings without time constraints. "Tell me exactly what's bothering you," and "How does this make you feel?" are helpful phrases to use. Allowing patients to express themselves and to share their innermost feelings can often provide a therapeutic benefit. Listening is essential. The physician must listen carefully to understand exactly what the patient is trying to express, without arguing or interrupting the patient and without attempting defense. Occasionally clarifying or briefly summarizing the patient's comments emphasizes his or her role as an active listener. The physician should not initially engage in complicated and detailed medical explanations.

Reassurance after a procedure is helpful. Guilt is one of the many emotions expressed in unhappy patients, and reassurance helps to control it [8,22]. Patients are usually quick to second-guess their earlier decision to have the procedure. These patients should be comforted and reassured that their decision was reasonable and was not misguided by their own misconceptions. The physician should tell the patient that "things are going to improve." Patients gain comfort in knowing that if an unfavorable result occurs, it can be improved or corrected in the future.

Some patients suffer from anxiety or depression during their postsurgical course [3]. If these problems are suspected, the physician should express great concern and should reassure the patient that "I want to help you through this." It is not sufficient to proclaim "You need to see a psychiatrist." Some of these patients may benefit from therapeutic counseling or pharmacological intervention. In the cases where assistance becomes necessary, the physician should carefully obtain the patient's approval for being referred to a trusted psychiatrist. Patients with a suspected narcotics addiction should be referred to a health professional trained in the management of this condition. These patients usually complain of excessive pain during the immediate postsurgical period and prolonged discomfort beyond the typical recovery phase. Remember that extreme pain is not only a manifestation of narcotics abuse, but can also signal a pathophysiological problem directly related to surgery.

All dermatologic surgeons encounter individuals who are dissatisfied with their surgical results. Some patients may be dissatisfied with technically satisfactory and cosmetically favorable results [4]. Others may be dissatisfied with an outcome that is truly suboptimal [32,33]. An occasional patient may be satisfied with the surgical outcome while the dermatologic surgeon is not, and in these cases, it is important that the surgeon not project dissatisfaction on a satisfied patient because mutual unhappiness and more management problems are likely to develop [31]. Specific scenarios of dissatisfied patients bear comment, as discussed by Adamson and Kraus [22].

MANAGEMENT OF THE PATIENT DISSATISFIED WITH A FAVORABLE RESULT

Patients who are unhappy with a favorable outcome are frequently encountered and can be extremely problematic. These patients may have an impaired ability to exchange thoughts and ideas in a straightforward, reasonable manner. Unrealistic expectations are the major problem in patients dissatisfied with a favorable result. In most instances, these unrealistic goals were present but not recognized by the surgeon before surgery, only to be discovered during a follow-up visit. It is counterproductive to chastise the patient for "expecting perfection" or for "being ridiculous." Initially, the physician should reassure the patient that he or she is devoted and willing to help with improvements, regardless how minor. Fortunately, the unrealistic expectations often are short-lived. Most patients, who are unhappy with a surgical outcome because their expectations were unrealistic, do not remain chronically dissatisfied [34].

The physician may consider some assistance, which may help these patients feel better [35]. Would a green base cosmetic hide the postlaser resurfacing erythema? Would massage help a tiny hematoma? Would a hair-styling tip help conceal a normal scar? These interventions may yield a small degree of objective improvement yet make a large impact on the patient.

MANAGEMENT OF THE PATIENT WITH AN UNFAVORABLE RESULT

Studies have shown that cosmetic patients are often inattentive when told about possible complications during their surgical evaluation [36]. A true complication is often surprising and difficult to accept for both patient and surgeon, and it must be remembered that suboptimal results and unexpected complications happen to even the most experienced dermatologic surgeons [32].

When initially faced with a disappointing outcome, it is sometimes helpful for the surgeon to spend a few minutes alone in their private office in order to reflect on the situation [14]. This can help the surgeon regain the composure necessary to approach the patient with a poor result. Because physicians typically celebrate successes and deny failures, the urge to avoid the situation can be overwhelming. However, the surgeon who chooses to deny or avoid the issues rather than confront them is likely to encounter a larger problem in the future. The surgeon must learn to accept the poor outcome and approach the patient in a straightforward, conscientious manner.

The patient with a suboptimal result should be assessed for confounding or causative factors that may have contributed to the poor result. Is there a problem with the procedure, the instrumentation, or the medications used? For example, a patient developed a facial ulcer after a minor surgery. The postsurgical interview revealed that she had cared for the wound with hydrogen peroxide as requested. Thinking that "more was better," her husband had obtained from his engineering laboratory a 30% solution that she used on her surgical site. These confounding factors should be clearly documented in the medical record and supplemented with photographs.

Even if there is substantial evidence that the patient's actions contributed to the poor result, the patient should never be directly blamed. It is reasonable to tell the patient that the adverse outcome is unusual, but exclaiming that "Your flap failed because you smoked" undermines the efforts to work together towards a more favorable end result. Accusations put the patient in a defensive position and contribute to their dissatisfaction. On the contrary, a statement of "I know you are not happy with the result and, frankly, neither am I" is usually perceived by the patient as honest and understanding. Acknowledgement of the complication helps rebuild and strengthen rapport.

As previously mentioned, patients should be encouraged to express their feelings openly while the physician listens carefully and provides support and reassurance. The physician should assure the patient that he or she understands the problem, knows how to handle it, and is committed to help resolve it. Patients with complications or an unfavorable outcome should return for frequent follow-up appointments. It is helpful for physicians to show their dedication and commitment to these patients by reminding them of their after-hours availability. These patients appreciate being provided with appropriate telephone numbers, even a home telephone number in case the need arises. Staff and family members should be informed of these "special" patients so that any calls from them are routed directly to the physician. One should never avoid these patients.

If the poor result is a well-known risk of that specific procedure, e.g., a sclerotherapy-induced ulceration, then the presurgical consent will have addressed the risk. Often, the patient does not remember having been informed of the risk. After the patient begins to comprehend and accept what happened, it is helpful to remind him or her that the mutual decision to have the procedure was made with the awareness of the potential complication.

During the long-term management of these patients, the physician should focus on improving the patient's concerns rather than dwelling on specific aspects of the unfavorable result. Asking the patient "How can I help?" or "What do you think needs to be done?" are effective ways to make the patient feel involved in the decisions regarding future therapy. "Let's work together to try and improve the situation" is a wonderful phrase that also acknowledges the patient's participation.

The surgeon should determine if the adverse outcome needs further surgical or medical intervention. For example, offering to dermabrade or laserabrade a scar may be a simple, 5-minute procedure that is an extra step towards achieving the desired result. Would an intralesional injection of corticosteroid improve the patient's concern over a mildly hypertrophic scar? Can a Z-plasty be performed on a contracted scar to change its orientation and improve the appearance? Is a second procedure appropriate?

When the patient returns for the second procedure, it should be approached with the same enthusiasm and interest that was initially present. The surgeon should carefully explain to the patient what to expect and should view the challenge as an opportunity, rather than a "waste of time" or "nuisance." It must be emphasized that the purpose of the second procedure is to achieve "improvement," rather than "correction."

Patients with a suboptimal result may request a second opinion, and the dermatologic surgeon should feel comfortable with this desire. The surgeon's willingness to cooperate with the patient and with other physicians in a collective effort helps to reinforce the patient's faith that the surgeon is truly committed to improving the outcome. The dermatologic surgeon can assist the patient in obtaining an independent consultation with one or more other physicians. In some cases, it may even be necessary to refer some of these patients to a national or international expert in the field. Although the dermatologic surgeon may suggest a specific colleague, the choice of physician should be made by the patient. Attempting to discourage a second opinion or insisting that these patients see only a specific colleague may destroy their trust in the surgeon. The surgeon should tell these patients that he or she will gladly send copies of their medical record, photographs, as well as a cover letter explaining their problems to the consultants. Open and free communication among the patient, original surgeon, and the patient's chosen consultant is essential.

In a patient with a poor outcome or severe complication, it is appropriate to address the issue of risk management. Larger institutions usually have a risk-management department that can assist the dermatologic surgeon in reducing the likelihood or lessening the impact of medicolegal action. Physicians practicing in a smaller environment may wish to notify their attorney. Of course, the surgeon should never be untruthful, blame someone for the bad outcome, or alter the medical record. Suggestions for minimizing the risk of lawsuits are described in the literature [37].

MANAGEMENT OF THE PATIENT WITH DISSATISFACTION FROM A PRIOR SURGERY

Expertise is required with the patient who is dissatisfied with a previous procedure or a previous surgeon [3,14]. These patients must be approached in a careful, cautious manner because they are susceptible to becoming dissatisfied again. As with the initial evaluation of all cosmetic patients, the dermatologic surgeon must take his or her own detailed history, particularly in regards to the prior operation. The consultant surgeon should also determine whether the patient was sent by the original surgeon or the patient presented without referral. The dermatologic surgeon should listen closely to the patient in order to understand the events that led to problems. Gaining insight into these issues from the patient's perspective is helpful in establishing a good rapport and in preventing future problems.

Some patients who are dissatisfied with a prior procedure may have a truly suboptimal result. Other patients may be dissatisfied because of a particular aspect of the experience, even though the final outcome was perfectly acceptable. Some patients simply want reassurance that their previous outcome was good. Regardless how good or bad the prior result, the dermatologic surgeon should never make disparaging comments or give negative feedback about the earlier procedure [14]. Inappropriate comments, such as "Who did that to you?" or "Why did you have that done?" reinforces the patient's anger and disappointment. In contrast, an energetic defense of the prior surgeon or procedure increases the patient's frustration and undermines the attempt to establish good rapport. It can be helpful to make a comment that does not pass judgement in favor or against the prior surgeon or procedure, such as "I'm sure your doctor wanted the very best for you."

The management of these patients is delicate. If the patient's prior outcome is truly favorable, he or she may gain comfort in hearing this from an unbiased physician. The second opinion may clear the air and enable these patients to return to their original physician for further monitoring. In patients with a truly suboptimal result, plans for intervention often depend on the circumstances of the original referral as well as the feelings of both the patient and consultant. Patients who present for a second opinion without being referred may expect the consultant to assume control of their care, and the dermatologic surgeon can either agree to do so or recommend that they return to their original physician. A patient should never be forced to return to the original physician. When the patient is referred by the original physician to a consultant for evaluation, the two physicians should come to an agreement on the patient's management and follow-up. It is important to allow time to pass and to see the patient again for follow-up before a decision is made whether or not to perform an additional surgery. This allows sufficient time for adequate communication with the previous physician who can add relevant historical information towards a better understanding of the situation.

If a decision is made to pursue further intervention, the patient must understand the nature and extent of the procedure as well as the expected goals. Beginning with, "let me explain how I may help you," tells the patient that the physician is interested in improving the situation. Both patient and physician should approach the procedure with a common understanding and focus on the future, rather than dwell on the past [14].

CONCLUSION

In the field of cosmetic dermatology, there is a plethora of "problem patients" who are difficult to manage. The ideal patient presents with a single problem and is satisfied with improvement after a cosmetic procedure. A proper initial encounter can protect against difficult and dissatisfied patients. The dermatologic surgeon must evaluate each patient methodically in order to assess his or her likelihood of becoming difficult or dissatisfied. This assessment is determined by both subjective and objective information in relation to various medical, psychological, aesthetic, and personal factors. Patients having certain character or personality weaknesses may be prone to postsurgical difficulties or dissatisfaction. People with a psychiatric condition, particularly those with narcissism, borderline personality disorder, or obsessive-compulsive disorder, must be handled carefully in order to avoid future problems. Psychotic or neurotic disorders may be found in cosmetic patients and warrant special concern.

Unfortunately, some patients do become difficult or dissatisfied despite all efforts towards prevention. They may be dissatisfied from technically satisfactory procedures with favorable outcomes or they may have an unfavorable result. Regardless of the underlying events that led to dissatisfaction or management difficulties, these patients should be approached in a purposeful, deliberate, and careful manner. Proper management is important in order to resolve difficulties, improve patient satisfaction, and avoid legal claims. The dermatologic surgeon who evaluates, treats, and manages patients by adhering to the principles outlined in this chapter will reduce their burden of difficult patients and have a smooth practice of cosmetic dermatology.

REFERENCES

1. Flynn TC, Narins RS. Preoperative evaluation of the liposuction patient. Dermatol Clin 1999; 17:729–734.
2. Findley C, Kaye BL. Care of the office surgery patient. Clin Plast Surg 1983; 10:333–356.
3. Baker TJ. Patient selection and psychological evaluation. Clin Plast Surg 1978; 5:3–14.
4. Macgregor FC. Patient dissatisfaction with results of technically satisfactory surgery. Aesth Plast Surg 1981; 5:27–32.
5. Katez P. The dissatisfied patient. Plast Surg Nurs 1991; 11:13–16.
6. Caputy GG, Flowers RS. Computer imaging: true or false. Hawaii Med J 1993; 52:349–351.
7. Vuyk HD, Zijlker TD. Psychosocial aspects of patient counseling and selection: a surgeon's perspective. Fac Plast Surg 1995; 11:55–60.
8. Wright MR. How to recognize and control the problem patient. J Dermatol Surg Oncol 1984; 10:389–395.
9. Hockenberger SJ. The nurse's role and responsibilities regarding patient satisfaction. Plast Surg Nurs 1995; 15:187, 189.
10. Dugas B. Dealing with the dissatisfied patient. Plast Surg Nurs 1983; 3:33–35.
11. Napoleon A. The presentation of personalities in plastic surgery. Ann Plast Surg 1993; 31:193–208.
12. Lewis CM. Dissatisfaction among women with "thunder thighs" undergoing closed aspirative lipoplasty. Aesth Plast Surg 1987; 11:187–191.
13. Popp JC. Complications of blepharoplasty and their management. J Dermatol Surg Oncol 1992; 18:1122–1126.
14. Wright MR. Management of patient dissatisfaction with results of cosmetic procedures. Arch Otolaryngol 1980; 106:466–471.
15. Sarwar D. The "obsessive" cosmetic surgery patient: a consideration of body image dissatisfaction and body dysmorphic disorder. Plast Surg Nurs 1997; 17:193–197, 209.
16. Wright MR. Surgical addiction. A complication of modern surgery. Arch Otolaryngol Head Neck Surg 1986; 112:870–872.
17. Menninger KA. Polysurgery and polysurgical addiction. Psychanal Q 1934; 3:173–199.
18. Knorr NJ, Edgerton MT, Hoopes JE. The "insatiable" cosmetic surgery patient. Plast Reconstr Surg 1967; 40:285–289.
19. Groenman NH, Sauer HC. Personality characteristics of the cosmetic surgical insatiable patient. Psychother Psychosom 1983; 40:241–245.
20. Wright MR, Wright WK. A psychological study of patients undergoing cosmetic surgery. Arch Otolaryngol 1975; 101:145–151.
21. Lewis CM, Lavell S, Simpson MF. Patient selection and patient satisfaction. Clin Plast Surg 1983; 10:321–332.
22. Adamson PA, Kraus WM. Management of patient dissatisfaction with cosmetic surgery. Fac Plast Surg 1995; 11:99–104.
23. Jacobson WE, Edgerton MT, Meyer E. Psychiatric evaluation of male patients seeking cosmetic surgery. Plast Reconstr Surg 1960; 20:356.
24. Edgerton MT, Jacobson WE, Meyer E. Surgical-psychiatric study of patients seeking plastic (cosmetic) surgery: ninety-eight consecutive patients with minimal deformity. Br J Plast Surg 1961; 13:136–145.
25. Napoleon A, Lewis CM. Psychological considerations in lipoplasty: the problematic or "special care" patient. Ann Plast Surg 1989; 23:430–432.

26. Hinderer UT. Dr. Vazquez Anon's last lesson. Aesth Plast Surg 1978; 2:375–382.
27. Levinson W, Roter DL, Mullooly JP, Dull VT, Frankel RM. Physician-patient communication: the relationship with malpractice claims among primary care physicians and surgeons. J Am Med Assoc 1997; 277:553–559.
28. Macgregor FC. Cosmetic surgery: a sociological analysis of litigation and a surgical specialty. Aesth Plast Surg 1984; 8:219–224.
29. Wright MR. Self-perception of the elective surgeon and some patient perception correlates. Arch Otolaryngol 1980; 106:460–465.
30. Fallo PC. Developing a program to monitor patient satisfaction and outcome in the ambulatory surgery setting. J Post Anesth Nurs 1991; 6:176–180.
31. Goin JM, Goin MK. Changing the Body: Psychological Effects of Plastic Surgery, Baltimore: Williams and Wilkins, 1981.
32. Leist FD, Masson JK, Erich JB. A review of 324 rhytidectomies, emphasizing complications and patient dissatisfaction. Plast Reconstr Surg 1977; 59:525–529.
33. Scheflan M, Maillard GF, de St Cyr BC, Ramirez OM. Subperiosteal facelifting: complications and the dissatisfied patient. Aesth Plast Surg 1996; 20:33–36.
34. Goldwyn RM, ed. The Unfavorable Result in Plastic Surgery: Avoidance and Treatment. 2nd ed. Boston: Little, Brown and Co, 1984.
35. Hoefflin SM. Surgical pearls in the management of the aging face from A to Z. Dermatol Clin 1997; 15:679–685.
36. Goin MK, Burgoyne RW, Goin JM. Face-lift operation: the patient's secret motivations and reactions to "informed consent." Plast Reconstr Surg 1976; 58:273–279.
37. Gorney M. Malpractice. In: Courtiss EH, ed. Aesthetic Surgery: Trouble, How to Avoid it and How to Treat it. St. Louis: Mosby, 1978, pp 1–13.

40

Facial Implants

Tracy M. Pfeifer
Manhattan Eye, Ear and Throat Hospital, New York, New York

INTRODUCTION

In cosmetic applications, silicone and polyethylene facial implants are used to augment the bony elements of the face and thereby improve facial balance and proportion. In some instances, these facial implants are used to create soft-tissue fill and thereby enhance the appearance of the soft tissues of the face. Noninjectable soft-tissue fillers such as expanded polytetrafluoroethylene (ePTFE) and AlloDerm® are also used to augment soft-tissue fullness of the face as well as reduce the appearance of skin creases. In older patients, these techniques can be used in conjunction with rhytidectomy to improve aesthetic results. In younger patients, augmentation procedures alone can improve facial balance and rejuvenate the early signs of facial aging. This chapter will focus on the use of noninjectable implants to improve facial proportions, balance, and soft-tissue fullness.

FACIAL AESTHETICS

In order to use facial implants effectively, the surgeon must understand the relationships between the bony prominences of the face, the principles of ideal facial proportion, and the effects of aging on the soft tissues of the face. Although some surgeons rely completely on artistic sense, a deliberate and thorough analysis of a patient's facial proportions helps identify areas of facial imbalance. There are many methods by which facial harmony and balance can be assessed. Artists of the Renaissance developed rules of facial proportion, which we use today to define "classic" proportions [1,2]. Farkas et al. significantly contributed to our understanding of attractiveness when he performed anthropometric studies of North American Caucasians to identify norms of facial proportion associated with attractiveness [3–7]. Several additional standards help the surgeon identify facial imbalance and disproportion, which detract from attractiveness. The reader is cautioned that these proportions and facial relationships are just guidelines and it is possible for faces with regions of disproportion to have an overall aesthetically pleasing appearance. Therefore, the scientific analysis must be combined with the artistic sensibility of the cosmetic surgeon to produce an aesthetic result.

Vertical Proportions of the Face

According to the classic principles, the full face is divided into the upper face, middle face, and lower face. In the vertical dimension, each unit occupies approximately one third of the total facial height (Fig. 1). Although not a classic proportion, lower facial height is divided into subunits with the following relationships: the vertical height from the subnasale to the upper lip stomion is one third the lower facial height, and the upper lip stomion to menton is two thirds the lower facial height (Fig. 1).

Another useful analysis principle derived from the Ancient Greeks is the golden proportion (8). This is a mathematical proportion, 1.0 to 1.618, or its reciprocal, 1.0 to 0.618. When applied to human faces, features that are "golden" are aesthetically pleasing. In a well-balanced face, the upper lip:lower lip ratio is in golden proportion, 1:1.618. The ratio of the height of the philtrum to the combined height of the upper and lower lip is golden, 1:1.618. These relationships are helpful when planning lip augmentation.

Transverse Proportions of the Face

Classic proportions tell us the widest portion of the face is located at the level of the malar midface and the width of the face at this level is four times the width of

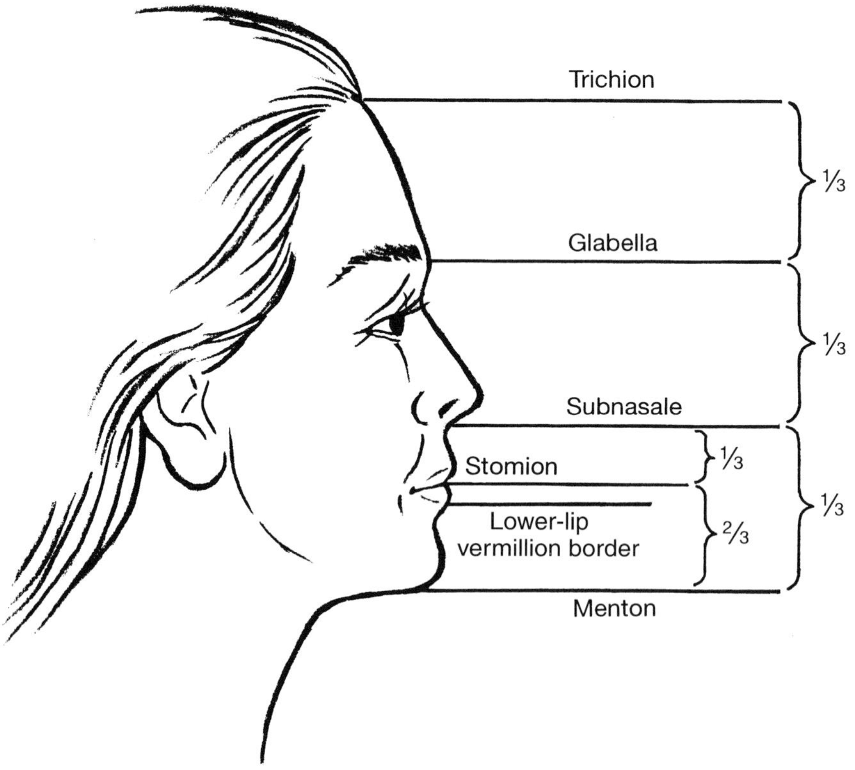

FIGURE 1 Vertical heights of the face and lower facial height relationships. (Courtesy of P. LoBianco.)

the alar base. Anthropometric studies reveal that attractive faces often have bitemporal and bigonial distances that are equal and the malar midface width is 10% wider than the bitemporal distance [6].

Facial Profile Relationships

There are many methods available to evaluate chin point position [9–11]. A simple method to evaluate chin point position using soft-tissue landmarks is often used [12]. A line is dropped perpendicular to the lower lip vermilion border. The soft-tissue chin point position is compared with this line. In women, the soft-tissue chain point should be just posterior to this line; in men, the soft-tissue chin point should be at this line. On profile examination, the lower lip should lie slightly posterior to the upper lip.

HISTORY OF FACIAL AUGMENTATION

Augmentation of the facial skeleton was first performed by Aufricht using autologous tissue to augment the deficient chin [13]. Many of the advances in the field are attributable to plastic surgeons with extensive experience in craniofacial surgery. A background in craniofacial or maxillofacial surgery is often necessary in order to treat some of the complications of alloplastic augmentation of the facial skeleton. Hinderer [14] was the first to describe the use of silicone rubber implants to augment the zygomatic complex. Expanded polytetrafluoroethylene was first used as a vascular conduit in 1971 and in facial reconstructive surgery in 1983 [15]. Lassus reported the use of ePTFE for facial wrinkles in 1991 [16]. AlloDerm® was first used in 1992 for burn patients. In 1995 surgeons began using AlloDerm® for reconstructive plastic surgery applications.

PRESURGICAL PLANNING

When using implants to augment facial proportions, presurgical planning is exceedingly important. Facial implants change the contour, projection, and balance of the bony facial skeleton. The patient's facial proportions and imbalances must be carefully analyzed. Presurgical photographs are essential and should include A-P, lateral, and oblique views. In some cases a cephalogram is helpful.

In addition to the presurgical physical examination and technical planning, the psychological impact of the procedure on the patient must be considered. Experienced cosmetic surgeons are well aware of this impact. The patient undergoing soft-tissue rejuvenation sees a familiar, restored image in the mirror after surgery. After malar or chin augmentation, the patient sees a different, altered face in the mirror. To the observer, the change may be aesthetically pleasing. To the patient, the image is unfamiliar and sometimes impossible to integrate into their self-image. For this reason it is imperative that the patient and the surgeon have excellent communication before surgery. The surgeon must understand the result desired by the patient. The patient is encouraged to bring in photographs depicting the desired result. Computer imaging techniques and drawings can help the surgeon and the patient define the desired change.

Communication with the patient as well as an understanding of the psychological impact of implant augmentation allows the surgeon to understand and meet the patient's expectations. The surgeon performing cosmetic facial surgery is encouraged to familiarize himself/herself with the psychosocial impact and motivations of patients seeking facial aesthetic surgery [16]. Finally, the cosmetic surgeon is advised to carefully study the indications for alloplastic cheek and chin augmentation, identify dental occlusal abnormalities, recognize the limitations of alloplastic augmentation procedures, and thereby identify patients whose needs are best served by osseous facial contouring techniques. These patients should be referred to a plastic surgeon or oral-maxillofacial surgeon.

Patients who request restoration or improvement of soft-tissue fullness usually adapt easily to the fuller contour. Thus, patients of all ages who seek improvement of lip fullness, and softening of nasolabial folds and marionette and glabellar lines readily incorporate the fuller contour into their self-image. In these situations, communication as to the extent of fullness desired and the likelihood of the procedure meeting the patient's desires is most important. The surgeon is cautioned to describe as accurately as possible the degree of fullness that can be achieved by the various techniques. These patients benefit from a thorough discussion of the types of soft-tissue fillers that are available, the longevity of the material, the risks associated with use of each material, the frequency of treatments required to maintain the result, and the various costs.

INFORMED CONSENT

As with any surgical procedure, informed consent must be obtained for patients undergoing facial implant surgery. The patient is informed of the risks, complications, limitations, and alternatives to the proposed procedure. The risks of the procedure and possible complications vary according to the site and the type of implant used. Malar augmentation can be complicated by implant malposition, hematoma, infection, and nerve injury. In addition, chin augmentation, particularly with an implant positioned subperiosteally, can result in bone erosion and soft-tissue abnormalities. The capsule that forms around silicone chin implants can cause soft-tissue distortion on implant removal. In some cases, osseous genioplasty is recommended to prevent this distortion [17].

The use of ePTFE for reduction of the nasolabial fold depth carries a risk of infection and can result in an unnatural appearance [18]. In addition, ePTFE used for reduction of facial skin creases carries the risk of hypersensitivity reaction, inflammation, extrusion, hematoma, induration, and seroma formation.

AlloDerm® implants carry a theoretical risk of virus transmission, although the donors are screened for Hepatitis B and C, HIV, and syphilis. To date there has been no documented case of HIV transmission in patients who received AlloDerm®. The durability of the cosmetic result when AlloDerm® is used to reduce the appearance of creases has not been documented.

Finally, the informed consent should include a clear demonstration of the proposed surgical incision placement and the attendant scars. Patients should be made aware of the possibility of either under- or overcorrection.

TYPES OF IMPLANTS

Silicone

Smooth silicone implants are ideal for augmentation and contouring of the malar-midface and chin areas. Compared with porous implants, silicone implants do not permit tissue ingrowth and, thus, can be easily removed/exchanged. Furthermore, silicone implants can sometimes be salvaged in the advent of infection, whereas porous implants almost always must be removed [19]. When implanted, a fibrous capsule forms around the silicone implant. In general, the capsule, which forms around malar implants, does not cause a problem. Capsular contracture with soft-tissue distortion has been noted after removal of an alloplastic chin implant.

Polyethylene

High-density polyethylene (MEDPOR® implants (POREX Surgical Inc., College Park, GA) have a porous texture, which reduces the tendency for slippage of the implant. These implants are available for use in malar and chin augmentation. The pore structure of the implant allows vascularization and tissue ingrowth [20]. There is some evidence that the bone resorption, which can occur under silicone implants, does not occur with MEDPOR® [21].

Expanded Polytetrafluoroethylene

Expanded polytetrafluoroethylene (ePTFE) is a fibrillated porous tetrafluoroethylene that is inert and biocompatible. In addition, the material will not dissolve or be resorbed. Currently, it is used in aesthetic surgery as a subdermal soft-tissue filler to correct deep facial creases in the nasolabial, marionette, and glabellar areas [22]. It can also be used in lip, malar, and chin augmentation. Limited tissue in-growth occurs so that the implant is stabilized but can easily be removed. The product is available through two manufacturers. GORE Subcutaneous Augmentation Material (GORE SAM; W. L. Gore and Associates, Flagstaff, AZ) is produced in two compositions [23]. One type is reinforced with fluorinated ethylene propylene and is available in sheets and three-dimensional (3-D) shapes used in malar and chin augmentation. A nonreinforced composition is available in sheets and 3-D strands. SoftForm® (Collagen Corporation, Palo Alto, CA) is a single tubule of ePTFE in a preassembled closed trocar delivery system. It is postulated that the lumen of an ePTFE tubule allows tissue ingrowth sufficient to stabilize the implant in mobile areas and may result in lower rates of implant extrusion compared with ePTFE strands. In one animal study, there was a significantly lower extrusion rate of tubed ePTFE (0.83%) compared with an extrusion rate of 4.4% for ePTFE strips [24].

AlloDerm®

AlloDerm® (LifeCell Corp., The Woodlands, TX) acellular dermal graft has recently been used by cosmetic surgeons for augmentation of the lips and correction of deep nasolabial folds and marionette lines. AlloDerm® is collected from human donors and the dermal cells are removed. After implantation, the patient's cells repopulate the collagen framework. The material is nonimmunogenic and feels natural as a result of integration into the host's tissues.

MALAR AUGMENTATION

Presurgical Considerations

After analysis of the overall facial balance, the surgeon must assess the specific areas of the midface and malar regions. Both Binder [25] and Terino [26] have presented useful analysis principles. Terino [27] describes five zones (Fig. 2). Zone 1 includes the malar bone lateral to the infraorbital foramen and the first third of the zygomatic arch. An implant positioned in this zone will increase the anterior-posterior dimension of the malar eminence. Zone 2 is the middle third of the zygomatic arch. Augmentation in this area will result in an increased width across the malar midface. Zone 3 is the paranasal area and is infrequently augmented. Zone 4 overlies the posterior third of the zygomatic arch. This area is avoided in augmentation because dissection in this area risks injury to the zygomatic and temporal branches of the facial nerve. Zone 5 is the submalar triangle defined by the following boundaries: posteriorly, the tendinous origins of the masseter muscle; medially, the lateral border of the nasolabial mound; and superiorly, the inferior margin of the malar eminence. In patients with decreased soft-tissue fullness of the midface, augmentation in the submalar area provides volume that restores a fuller youthful contour (Fig. 3). Augmentation of the submalar area in conjunction with rhytidectomy can be very useful in older patients with minimal soft-tissue fullness of the face who request rhytidectomy and in whom

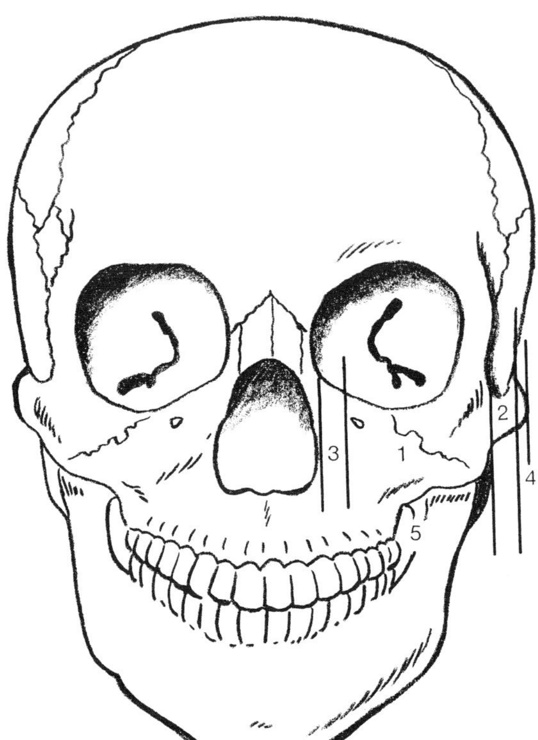

FIGURE 2 Zones of the bony skeleton as described by Terino. (Courtesy of P. LoBianco.)

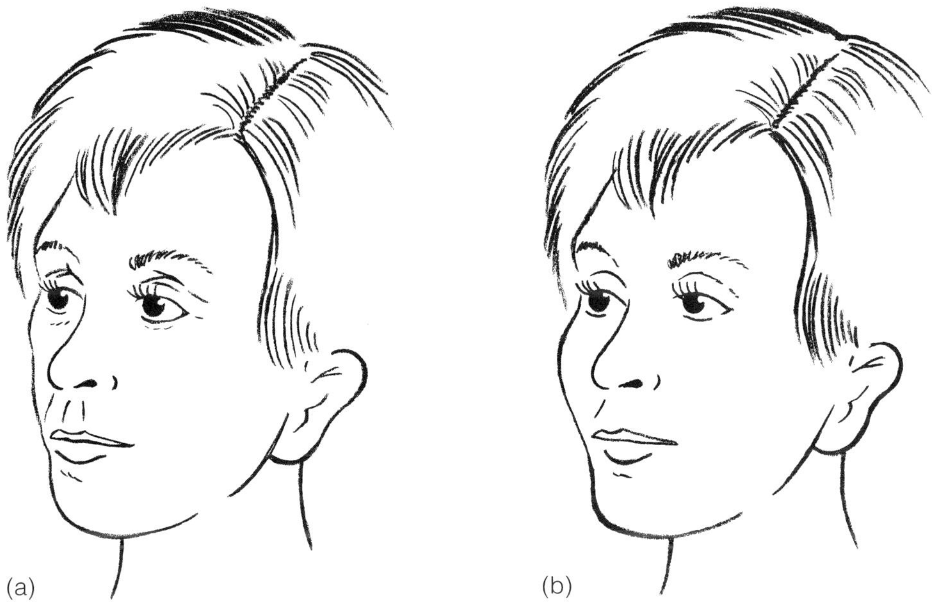

FIGURE 3 Schematic drawing of (a) presurgical appearance and (b) postsurgical appearance after facelift and submalar augmentation. (Courtesy of P. LoBianco.)

the results of rhytidectomy alone can be unsatisfying [28]. Careful analysis of each of these "zones" allows the surgeon to identify the areas requiring augmentation and aids in selection of the appropriately sized implant.

Surgical Procedure

The surgical procedure for augmentation of the midface can be performed under local or general anesthesia. Before surgery, the desired implant position is traced on the skin overlying the area to be augmented. Intravenous antibiotics are administered before the start of the procedure. The approach is usually intraoral, although experienced surgeons may elect a subciliary, coronal, or a preauricular rhytidectomy approach. A small incision is made in a vertical-oblique direction above the canine. A subperiosteal pocket corresponding to the surgical skin marking is created over the maxilla, malar eminence, and zygomatic arch with care taken not to injure the infraorbital nerve. Precise dissection of the pocket is important to maintain the implant in correct position. After placement of the implant, its position in relation to the surgical markings is confirmed. The mucosal incision is closed with several interrupted chromic sutures. The reader is referred to detailed descriptions of this surgical approach [27].

CHIN AUGMENTATION

Presurgical Considerations

In patients requesting chin augmentation, several factors must be considered. First, the need for concomitant or subsequent rhinoplasty is analyzed. Generally, the chin should be addressed first as alloplastic genioplasty may affect the extent of rhinoplasty necessary. Second, the dental occlusion should be assessed. If malocclusion exists, referral to a craniofacial or maxillofacial surgeon is recommended. Third, lower facial height is assessed for vertical deficiencies. Alloplastic implants augment sagittal deficiencies of the chin but do not effectively augment vertical deficiencies of the chin. In patients with vertical deficiencies of the lower face osseous, genioplasty with interposition graft should be considered. Fourth, the amount of advancement of the soft-tissue chin point desired is determined. In general, an 8-mm chin implant will advance the soft-tissue chin point no more than 4 to 5 mm [2]. Patients who require more than a 5 mm increase in the A-P dimension should be considered for osseous genioplasty as implants larger than 8 mm in the anterior-posterior dimension are associated with an increased risk of symptomatic bone erosion [2].

Surgical Procedure

Chin augmentation with alloplastic implants is usually performed using local anesthesia and intravenous sedation. Presurgically, the midline of the chin is marked. One percent lidocaine with epinephrine 1/100,000 is used for local anesthesia and to perform a mental nerve block. Intravenous antibiotics are administered before surgery. Using the submental approach, a 2 to 3 cm incision is made in the submental crease. Next, the platysmal muscle is separated along the muscle fiber axis and a subperiosteal pocket is created. The mental nerves, exiting their foramen halfway down the mandible below the second premolar, are best protected by careful dissection. Ideally, the nerves are never visualized. After placement of the appropriately sized implant, the platysmal muscle is reapproximated. The incision is closed with dermal and skin sutures.

An intraoral approach may also be used. After infiltration of local anesthesia, a 1 to 2 cm transverse incision is made in the gingivolabial mucosa. The mentalis muscles are divided through their median raphe. A subperiosteal pocket is created with care taken to hug the inferior border of the mandible. In this way, injury to the mental nerve is avoided. The implant is positioned. The muscle is closed with absorbable suture and the mucosal incision is closed with interrupted chromic sutures.

LIP AUGMENTATION

Presurgical Considerations

Lip augmentation can be accomplished using either ePTFE or AlloDerm®. Although not discussed here, autologous fat or fascia, collagen, and Dermalogen may also be used. The patient is advised as to the degree of correction that may be achieved by the implant. In general, patients can expect a 50 to 70% correction of the furrow.

The choice of implant is based on patient preference, although AlloDerm® should not be used in patients with connective-tissue disorders. ePTFE has the advantage of permanence compared with fat, collagen, or Dermalogen. Some surgeons prefer the Gore-Tex® multistrand implant for lip augmentation because they believe it is less palpable. Other surgeons prefer the SoftForm® ePTFE facial implant because they believe the prepackaged trocar delivery system allows easier and more accurate implant placement.

AlloDerm®, although not permanent, may provide a more durable result compared with autologous fat, collagen, or Dermalogen. Because AlloDerm® is made from human tissue, it has none of the disadvantages associated with synthetic materials. Compared with synthetic implants, most surgeons believe it is nonpalpable and feels natural.

Surgical Procedure

The techniques for placement of these implant materials are fairly straightforward. Patients with a history of herpes labialis should be considered for treatment with antiviral medication before and after surgery because the procedure may cause a herpes flare-up. The augmentation area is marked before surgery with the patient in the sitting position. The procedure is performed using local anesthesia with or without intravenous sedation. One percent lidocaine with epinephrine 1/100,000 is used to perform a nerve block as well as anesthetize the skin incision sites and subcutaneous tunnel. Prophylactic intravenous antibiotics are administered before surgery. When using AlloDerm®, the implant is cut to the appropriate length, with care taken to taper the ends. Two small incisions are made inside the vermilion border just above the corners of the mouth. A subdermal pocket is created with curved dissecting scissors just inside the white roll. A tendon retriever is passed through the subdermal tunnel and the implant is pulled through. The incisions are closed with absorbable sutures.

Gore-Tex® can be placed using the technique described for AlloDerm®. SoftForm® implant is placed using the closed trocar delivery system. In this technique, the access incisions are made along the vermilion border near the commissure. The cannula is removed while the trocar is stabilized, leaving the trocar with the implant in place. The trocar is then removed and the skin is redraped over the implant. Finally, the implant is trimmed, beveling the ends to reduce visibility.

NASOLABIAL FOLDS, MARIONETTE LINES, AND GLABELLAR CREASES

Presurgical Considerations

The nasolabial folds can be softened by placing a ePTFE or AlloDerm® implant in the subdermal position medial to the crease. The procedure is performed under local anesthesia with or without intravenous sedation. Before surgery the nasolabial fold and/or marionette line is marked with the patient in the sitting position. Small skin incisions are made with a No. 11 blade 3 to 5 mm superior and inferior to the planned placement of the implant. In this way, the implant material is not directly underlying the skin incisions. Access incisions in the facial skin are small and will heal with an inconspicuous scar. The subdermal pocket is created medial to the nasolabial fold from the alar crease to the end of the fold. The AlloDerm® implant is positioned with the aid of a tendon retriever.

SoftForm® facial implants are placed using the prepackaged trocar delivery system described above. The Gore-Tex® ePTFE implant can be placed with the aid of a tendon retriever or by using a closed technique [29]. In the closed technique, stab incisions are made in the skin and a trocar is passed in the subcutaneous plane. The inner trocar is removed and the implant is pulled through with the aid of a suture. After trimming the implant to the appropriate length, the skin incisions are closed with fine, nonabsorbable suture. It is not necessary to secure the implant position with a stitch. The skin incisions are closed with fine nylon sutures. Marionette creases are treated in a similar manner with access incisions placed as necessary. Similar techniques are used for glabellar creases. However, whereas the implant is placed medial to the crease for nasolabial and marionette creases, the implant is placed directly under the crease in the treatment of glabellar creases.

Postsurgical Instructions

All patients are advised to take oral antibiotics for 3 to 5 days after facial implant surgery. Analgesics are taken as needed for discomfort. A soft diet is also recommended for several days. Ice compresses may be used for the first 24 to 48 hours in order to reduce swelling. Patients are advised to avoid excessive talking, smiling, and vigorous mouth movements for several days. The skin incisions are gently cleansed with mild soap and water or half-strength peroxide daily. Antibiotic ointment may be applied and makeup is not permitted until skin incisions are completely healed.

Patients are instructed to notify the office for increasing discomfort, persistent redness, persistent inflammation, or implant visibility. Signs of extrusion in patients with ePTFE implants include pustules at either incision site or persistent drainage.

COMPLICATIONS

Silicone Implants

Complications of alloplastic midface augmentation include the following: implant asymmetries (20%), malposition (5–20%), hematoma/seroma/infection (0.5–15%), extrusion (0.1–20%), temporary nerve dysfunction (10%), permanent sensory nerve dysfunction (0.1–9%), and permanent motor nerve dysfunction (0.5–1%) [19,27]. In experienced hands, the overall complication rate is lower, although asymmetry is still a significant complication [27].

Complications of alloplastic chin augmentation include the following: extrusion, infection, dehiscience, displacement, capsular contracture, lip retraction, paresthesia, and hematoma. In addition, bone resorption under premandibular silicone implants occurs in virtually all patients [30,31]. Because bone resorption occurs to some degree under all silicone chin implants, it is an expected outcome and no longer considered a complication. However, if the implant is positioned too close to the tooth roots, bone erosion could jeopardize the tooth. Implant extrusion after alloplastic chin augmentation is unusual. It is more common after placement via an intraoral incision. Infection is also unusual. One series reported an infection rate of 5% [32]. Lower lip retraction and resultant lower incisor show is most likely related to detachment of the mentalis muscle. This is less often seen after placement via a submental incision.

Careful presurgical assessment and precise surgical execution of the procedure can prevent asymmetries and implant malposition. If an implant requires repositioning, pull-through bolster sutures can be used to maintain the correct position. Hematoma can be avoided by meticulous hemostasis. Hemostasis and appropriate antibiotic prophylaxis can reduce the incidence of infection. Adequate soft-tissue coverage and preventing infection help prevent extrusion.

In the event of extrusion of a silicone chin implant, soft-tissue distortion may occur because of capsular contracture after removal of the implant. After extrusion, the soft tissues should be allowed adequate time to heal and for scar tissue to soften, often several months. Secondary alloplastic augmentation is an option but osseous augmentation techniques may be indicated [32–34].

Polyethylene Implants

Complications of polyethylene implants include infection, exposure, and migration. In one series, an infection rate of 1.5% was noted [35]. Successful treatment of infected implants necessitated implant removal. Several series show low complication rates with polyethylene implants, with no incidence of bone resorption, implant migration, or implant exposure [35–37]. Capsular contracture is less likely with polyethylene chin implants when compared with silicone implants [38].

Expanded Polytetrafluoroethylene

Several studies document an overall complication rate of about 2% for ePTFE implants used in facial surgery [38–40]. With respect to ePTFE, implants in nasolabial and glabellar folds, and lip augmentation, one study revealed no complications after 15 months [41]. Another study of 115 ePTFE implants followed for 2.5 to 4.5 years showed no incidence of implant extrusion or infection; the investigator reported one case of seroma around an upper lip implant and two patients who required further augmentation of nasolabial folds [41].

There are several reports of implant exposure when using ePTFE facial implants [41,42]. Most investigators believe infection and exposure are related to superficial placement of the ends of the ePTFE implant. The ends of the implant must be buried well below the dermis, preferably 2 to 3 mm away from the skin access incisions. Severe inflammatory reaction after ePTFE implant for lip augmentation has also been reported [43].

AlloDerm®

Complications with AlloDerm® are related to infection and graft extrusion. Volume diminution, an expected occurrence rather than a complication, can be up to 50% [51]. Other investigators report 20% volume loss, which stabilizes at 6 weeks [45]. Graft infection occurred in one of 12 patients in one series [45]. However, this was attributed to suturing the graft at the mucosal incision to prevent migration. The graft was trimmed and the infection resolved with oral antibiotics. With respect to graft infection and extrusion, one series of 50 patients reported no complications of graft extrusion or infection [44]. A second series of 85 procedures reported one partial extrusion of the implant, managed conservatively, and implant infection requiring implant removal [46].

SUMMARY

Facial implants can augment the bony prominences of the face and thereby improve facial proportion and balance. Additionally, these materials can act as soft-tissue fillers and restore volume to the aging face. The key to the successful use of facial implants is a thorough understanding of facial proportion, effective communication with the patient regarding the desired change, as well as a realistic assessment of the change the implant can effect. Careful presurgical assessment and meticulous surgical technique help the cosmetic surgeon avoid the problems associated with implant surgery.

REFERENCES

1. Durer A. Della simmetria dei corpi humani. Presso 1, Nicoline, Venetia, 1591.
2. LaTrenta GS. Facial contouring. In: Rees TD, LaTrenta GS, eds. Aesthetic Plastic Surgery. Vol II. 2d ed. Philadelphia: W.B. Saunders, 1994, pp 784–889.
3. Farkas LG. Anthropometry of the Head and Face in Medicine. New York: Elsevier North Holland, 1981.
4. Farkas LG, Munro IR, Kolar JC. Anthropometric Facial Proportions in Medicine. Springfield, IL: Charles C. Thomas, 1987.
5. Farkas LG, Kolar JC. Anthropometrics and art in the aesthetics of women's faces. Clin Plast Surg 1987; 14(4):599–616.
6. Farkas LG, Sohm P, Kolar JC, Katic MJ, Munro IR. Inclination of the facial profile: art versus reality. Plast Reconstr Surg 1985; 75(4):509–519.
7. Farkas LG, Hreczko TA, Kolar JC, Munro IR. Vertical and horizontal proportions of the face in young adult North American Caucasians: revision of neoclassical canons. Plast Reconstr Surg 1985; 75(3):328–338.
8. Ricketts RM. The science and art of aesthetic recontouring of the face. In: Ousterhout DK, ed. Aesthetic Contouring of the Craniofacial Skeleton. Boston: Little, Brown and Company, 1991; pp 71–88.
9. Ricketts RM. Divine proportion in facial esthetics. Clin Plast Surg 1982; 9(4):401–422.
10. Ricketts RM. Esthetics, environment, and the law of lip relation. Am J Orthod 1968; 54(4):272–289.
11. Burstone CJ. Lip posture and its significance in treatment planning. Am J Orthod 1967; 53:262.
12. Sykes JM, Frodel JL. Mentoplasty. In: Cummings CW, Fredrickson JM, Harker LA, Krause CJ, Richardson MA, Schuller DE, eds. Otolaryngology—Head and Neck Surgery. 3d ed. St. Louis: Mosby, 1999, pp 737–753.
13. Aufricht G. Combined nasal plastic and chin plastic; correction of microgenia by osteocartilaginous transplant from large hump nose. Am J Surg 1934; 25:292.
14. Hinderer U. Malar implants for improvement of facial appearance. Plast Reconstr Surg 1975; 56(2):157–165.
15. Neel HB. Implants of Gore-Tex. Arch Otolaryngol Head Neck Surg 1983; 109(7):427–433.
16. Pertschuk M. Psychosocial considerations interface surgery. Clin Plast Surg 1991; 18(1): 11–18.
17. Cohen SR, Mardach OL, Kawamoto HK Jr. Chin disfigurement following removal of alloplastic chin implants. Plast Reconstr Surg 1991; 88(1):62–66.
18. Robertson KM, Dyer WK II. Expanded polytetrafluoroethylene (Gore-Tex) augmentation of deep nasolabial creases. Arch Otolaryngol Head Neck Surg 1999; 125(4):456–461.
19. Terino EO. Chin and malar augmentation. In: Peck GC, ed. Complications and Problems in Aesthetic Plastic Surgery. New York: Gower Medical Publishers, 1992, pp 6.1–6.31
20. Golshani S, Zhou ZY, Gade P. Applications of MEDPOR porous polyethylene in facial bone augmentation. Am J Cosmet Surg 1994; 11:105–109.

of movements that will be compatible with an optimal occlusal restoration and the most aesthetic facial form.

Computer programs have also been developed so that the cephalogram can be digitized. A digital photograph may then be overlayed on the digitized cephalogram and manipulated to simulate the anticipated surgical movements. This has the advantage of providing the patient with a suggestion of the expected postsurgical appearance. However, this technological advance carries with it the potential liabilities associated with varying from patient expectations. The software contains a disclaimer that the simulation is an aid for patient education rather than a guarantee of the surgical result. However, this fact must be reinforced by the surgeon, because computer manipulations, while somewhat unnatural, may often be compelling.

My personal belief is that the clinical examination by a skilled observer is the best way to assess the face. The computer image does not show the patient in full face, the position in which the patient sees himself or herself in the mirror. Nor does the computer show the patient in function. Computerized movements of highlights and shadows of the presurgical patient are merely displaced according to the proposed movements; they do not adapt to the changes in soft-tissue support and muscle function. It is therefore the intuitive appreciation of these factors that allows the surgeon to evaluate the face and convey the information to the patient. Even the cephalometric radiograph, which has been the hallmark for orthodontic and orthognathic diagnosis and planning, must be set aside if its values are in conflict with the clinical intuition of the surgeon. Occasionally, disastrous facial aesthetic results, albeit with excellent occlusions, occur when one goes solely by the numbers.

When we are concerned with restructuring the underlying skeleton rather than with the rejuvenation of the surface of the face, I believe it is more helpful and more diagnostic to consider facial volumes rather than numeric angles and linear measurements. Volume assessment directs one's attention not only to size and position of the parts, but to those highlights and shadows which, if distorted, will convey a heaviness or imbalance, but if appropriate will provide a grace and elegance. Misplaced volume, or the lack of volume, will cause a relative distortion of adjacent parts and may result in a misdiagnosis of the problem by doctor as well as patient.

The early history of orthognathic maxillofacial surgery was devoted to the surgical correction of the prominent mandible. This is easily understood given the experience of the oral and maxillofacial surgeon in treating traumatic injury to the jaws, the profound effect that mandibular discontinuity and displacement have on the dental occlusion, and the relative anatomical simplicity of the mandible compared with that of the maxilla.

The prognathic mandible is attributable to excessive growth of either the mandibular ramus or body, resulting in an exaggeration in the forward projection of the chin. The mandibular dental arch is similarly carried forward creating the Class III occlusion, or underbite. Facial proportions are distorted because of the size and position of the lower third. The face assumes an "aggressive disposition" with the jutting chin and the protruding lower lip. The oblique mandibular angles and the forward displacement of the mandibular breadth further accentuate the distortion (Figs. 1a, 1b).

The earliest efforts to correct mandibular prognathism used a Gigli saw to effect a subcondylar osteotomy. This was accomplished under local anesthesia with the patient seated upright in a dental chair. Relapse was high and this technique was

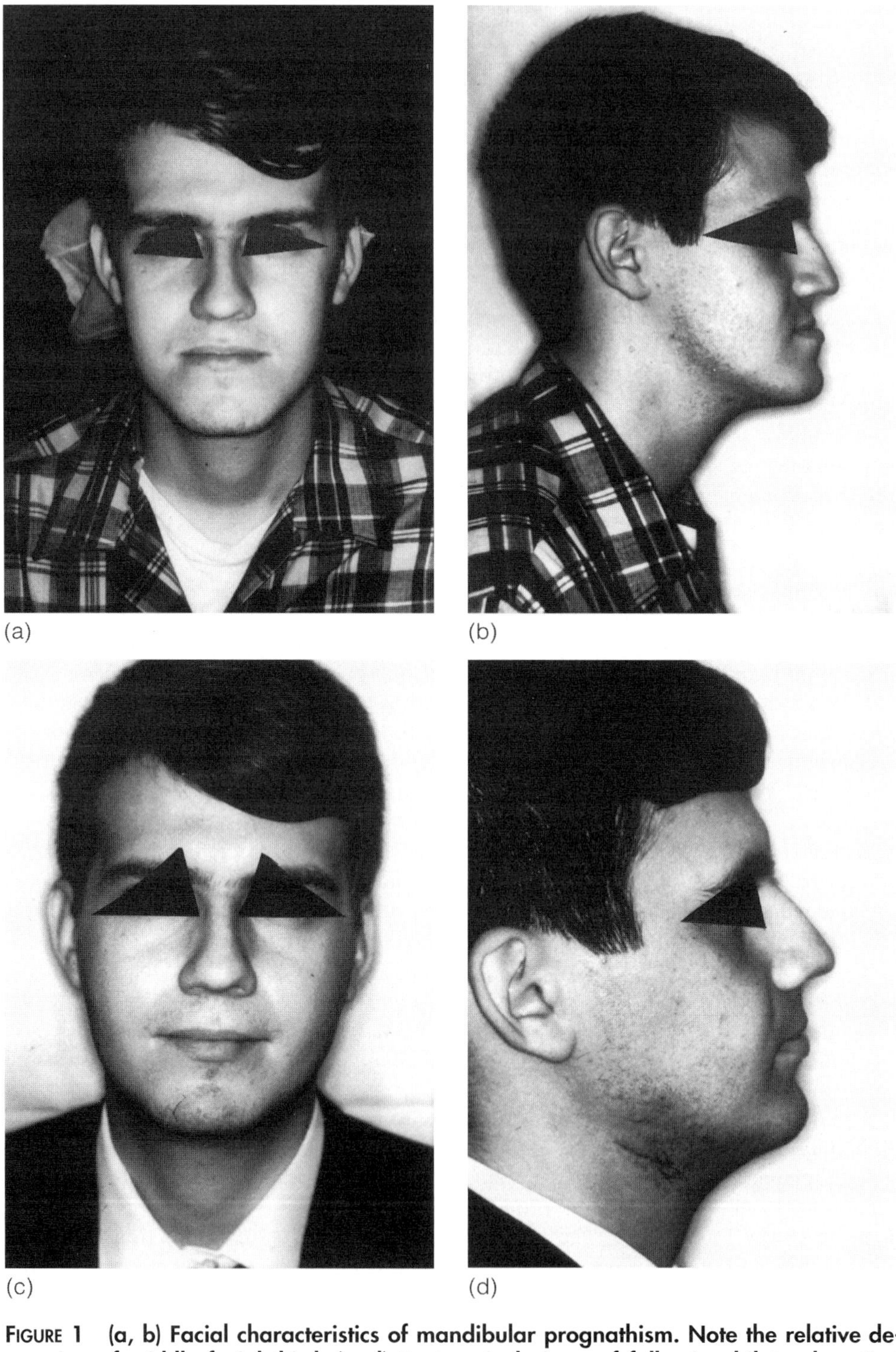

(a) (b) (c) (d)

FIGURE 1 (a, b) Facial characteristics of mandibular prognathism. Note the relative depression of middle facial third. (c, d) Postsurgical views of following bilateral vertical oblique osteotomies of the mandibular rami. The submandibular scar will become barely perceptible. This procedure is now performed intraorally.

understandably abandoned. A procedure designed by Dingman was used to treat excessive growth of the mandibular body. This procedure involved removal of a tooth bilaterally and the excision of measured segments of bone above and below the mandibular canal. It was performed in either one or two stages from an entirely intraoral approach or one that involved both intraoral and external incisions. Again, relapse was a concern as was paresthesia of the inferior alveolar nerve. By the 1960s, numerous osteotomies of the mandibular ramus were described to correct the prognathic jaw as well as other distortions of the mandible such as open bites [4,5] and vertical discrepancies. Some required interpositional bone grafts, whereas others incorporated ingenious bony cuts to maintain bone contact. Much was written about decortication of the segments to facilitate osseous union and minimize the potential for relapse.

The vertical oblique osteotomy of the mandibular rami [6,7] soon became the favored procedure for the surgical correction of mandibular prognathism. Performed bilaterally, it requires an osteotomy from the sigmoid notch to a point near the angle of the mandible. The position of the bony cut is planned on the presurgical cephalometric and panoramic radiographs so that it will pass posterior to the lingula, the entrance of the inferior alveolar nerves and vessels on the medial aspect of the ramus. Identification of this important landmark is also accomplished at the time of surgery by recognition of the antilingula, which is directly visible on the lateral cortex. After the osteotomies have been completed, the distal, tooth-bearing segment is moved to a position predetermined by the occlusion. The bony segments are allowed to overlap with the proximal segment laterally. No bony decortication is necessary. The condylar segments are allowed to remain passively in the glenoid fossae. This procedure was originally performed via Risdon incisions. With the development of the oscillating saws and an armamentarium to perform this procedure intraorally, all external scars are avoided. Surgery is performed efficiently and risk to the inferior alveolar nerve is minimal. Intermaxillary fixation is applied and the jaws remain immobilized for 6 weeks. During this period the patient must remain on a liquid diet. The period of hospitalization, which at one time extended for many days, is now reduced to a single day and, occasionally, the overnight stay is entirely eliminated. Postsurgical swelling can be well controlled with medication; pain is minimal.

Unfortunately, this procedure is primarily directed to the treatment of mandibular displacement, which is correctable with a nonrotational posterior repositioning of the jaw. Bony contact of the segments is a factor of the length of the osteotomies and the amount of overlap. The flare of the ramus as well as its height may require osteotomies which are more angulated and may minimize bony contact. Movements of great dimension may require the removal of the coronoid processes. This lack of versatility and the absolute requirement for intermaxillary fixation has encouraged the use of the sagittal ramusotomy when movements of greater complexity are required and when immobilization of the jaws is unsatisfactory. This procedure will be described in the discussion of the surgical correction of mandibular retrognathia.

Once the prognathic mandible has been corrected, facial form comes into balance (Figs. 1c, 1d). The face softens as the relative proportions of all facial structures change. Cheekbones, nose, eyes, and dentition assume new relationships. It is for this reason that rhinoplasty and orthodontics, except such orthodontic care that is directed toward preparing the dentition for surgery, should be deferred until the dimensions of the reconstructed face can be appreciated.

The experience gained from the correction of mandibular prognathism was then applied to the underdeveloped jaw. The lack of lower-third volume in this facial deformity elicits an entirely new spectrum of facial change (Fig 2). Weakness rather than strength is projected. The face tends to taper into the neck. Structures in the middle third appear larger. The nose seems heavier. The cheek bones, paradoxically, are more prominent, but less defined. Lack of dental support of the lower lip; and eversion of that lip by the maxillary incisors deepens the mentolabial fold and accentuates the Class II malocclusion. As with the Class III malocclusion, the functional efficiency of mastication is compromised. However, with mandibular retrognathia, the tendency to protrude the mandible to incise, as well as the often-noticed habit of forward posturing of the jaw for aesthetic improvement, will not uncommonly result in inflammation of the temporomandibular joints and spasm of the masticatory muscles. Such patients may initially present for the remedy of their pain, with the concern for aesthetic improvement being secondary.

Historically, the external approach to the mandibular rami was initially used for correction of mandibular retrognathia. A vertical oblique osteotomy was effected and the distal segment was advanced. The bony gap, which resulted from the distraction of the parts, was filled with a bone graft collected from the hip (8). Variations on this theme, the inverted L osteotomy and the C osteotomy, were used to maximize the stability of movements in various directions, but the external scar and requirement for a bone graft were unavoidable.

The popularization of the bilateral sagittal osteotomy by Obwegesser [9] revolutionized mandibular orthognathic surgery. This procedure sections the rami so as maximize bone to bone contact. Its versatility allows for the correction of retrognathia, asymmetries, some open-bite deformities and rotational movements, as well as mandibular prognathism. The external scar is eliminated, as is the need for a bone graft. This intraoral osteotomy requires exposure of the medial aspect of the mandibular rami. The entrance of the neurovascular bundle into its foramen is visualized, and these structures are retracted and protected as cuts through the medial cortex and anterior border of the ramus and the buccal cortex of the mandibular body are made with the reciprocating saw and connected. The osteotomy is then completed with appropriate osteotomes. The lateral, condylar segment is noted to move freely and remain passive as the distal segment, which carries the neurovascular structures, is repositioned. A singular advantage of this procedure is the ability to fixate the segments internally with plates and screws and thus to avoid the need for intermaxillary immobilization. The internal fixation hardware is made of pure titanium and is well tolerated by the body. Occasionally a screw may loosen and elicit an inflammatory response. Such events require the removal of the loose hardware. Otherwise the fixation remains in situ. Bioresorbable hardware, which has been recently introduced, stabilizes the parts for healing and is then hydrolyzed and eliminated.

Asymmetry of mandibular growth and development evokes one of the most noticeable distortions of facial aesthetics and is easily appreciated by even the most unsophisticated observer. No doubt every face has a normal variation in symmetry. However, when the normal range is exceeded, facial aesthetics are significantly compromised. Mandibular asymmetry is usually the result of a unilateral restriction of growth that is shown by the antegonial notching of the inferior border of the mandible on radiographic examination. Sometimes a traumatic event or infection can be documented; more often there is no obvious cause. As a result, the affected side is

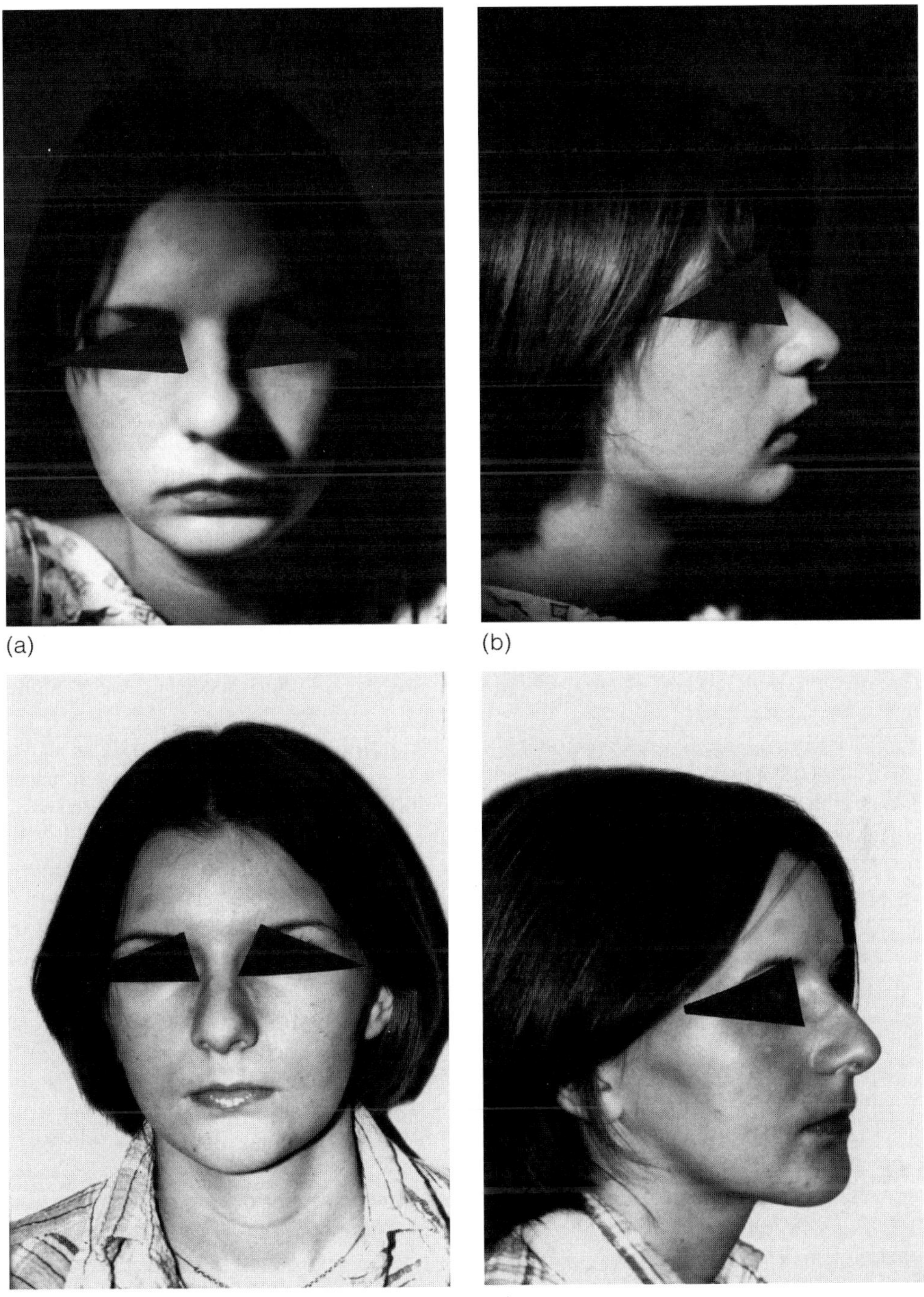

(a) (b) (c) (d)

FIGURE 2 (a, b) Facial characteristics of mandibular retrognathia. (c, d) Postsurgical views following mandibular adancement via sagittal ramusotomies. Note how the facial thirds come into relative balance and nose and cheekbones are enhanced.

foreshortened both in its vertical height and forward projection. The normal growth of the contralateral side results in a deviation of the chin across the facial midline. The "normal" side appears flat and elongated. The dental malocclusion will mirror the skeletal aberration with a unilateral crossbite on the restricted side and a buccal overbite on the other. The dental midlines will not correspond and the chin midline will be displaced even further.

Rarely, unilateral condylar hyperplasia will be the cause of the deformity. However, the radiographic appearance of this disorder is significantly different. Appropriate isotopic scans will reveal the site of persistent growth and condylectomy is in order.

Correction of the mandibular asymmetry in its simplist presentation involves the rotation of the mandible around a vertical axis by elongating the restricted side and shortening the contralateral side. Therefore, those techniques previously described for the correction of both mandibular prognathism and retrognathia will be applied—vertical osteotomy on the elongated side and sagittal osteotomy on the other. As an alternative, the versatile sagittal osteotomy may be used to effect both movements. As a result, the dental midlines will align and the chin will also be more centrally positioned. Occasionally a genioplasty will be required to achieve optimal facial symmetry.

Severe mandibular growth asymmetry, which incorporates a vertical growth component, will result in a compensatory distortion of maxillary position as well. The dental significance of this deformity involves a cant of the occlusal plane. Unless this plane is leveled, the facial asymmetry will persist. For those cants that exceed the corrective measures of the orthodontist, surgery of the maxilla as well as the mandible is required.

Maxillary surgery evolved in a fashion similar to that of the mandible in so far as it was based on a wealth of experience in the treatment of facial trauma. Predictable fracture lines in the LeFort I, II, and III injuries are reproduced, electively, so that the maxilla may be mobilized and repositioned at the appropriate level. The research of Bell, et al. [10,11] provided the scientific justification of this procedure by showing that it could be performed without jeopardizing the vascular supply.

As with the mandible, the initial impetus for maxillary surgery was directed to the correction of skeletal malocclusions—primarily maxillary retrognathia and open-bite deformities. Maxillary deformities are often more subtle than those of the mandible in that the maxilla is a bone fixed in position. Therefore, the effects of functional movements tend not to exaggerate the deformity and, in fact, changes in mandibular position may obscure the characteristics of abnormal midface growth. Vertical maxillary overgrowth may also depress the mandible. The volume excess of the lower third by the downward rotation of the mandible may distract the observer from the primary problem.

The compromise of facial aesthetics attributable to the deficient growth of the maxilla is similar to that associated with mandibular prognathism. However, a skilled observer will be able to recognize the distinct differences between the two. The clinical diagnosis of this deformity is easily confirmed on the cephalometric radiograph. However, perhaps the most revealing technique to determine which jaw is to be treated is the placement of a volume of gauze, consistent with the magnitude of the anticipated movement, under the upper lip. The change in facial appearance is often dramatic, revealing a desirable facial balance or an excessive fullness. In the former instance, the patient will be able to visualize the benefits of surgery; in the latter, mandibular surgery may be elected even if this is contrary to the measurements of the cephalometric analyses.

In the patient with classical maxillary retrognathia, there will be a flattening of the canine fossae, lack of support of the upper lip, and a relative prominence of the lower lip. A lack of support of the nasal tip and a narrowing of the ala breadth as well as a reversal of the arc of the nasolabial fold is also evident (Fig. 3). The Class III malocclusion may be identical to that of a person with mandibular prognathism. Therefore, it is critical that the correct diagnosis be made because the aesthetic results of maxillary surgery versus that of the mandible are drastically different.

Surgical correction of most maxillary deformities require mobilization of the maxilla at the LeFort I level—the level of the floor of the nose and maxillary sinuses. From an intraoral approach, a horizontal osteotomy is performed, above the level of the apices of the maxillary teeth, and through the lateral wall of the maxilla and lateral antral walls. The nasal septum and vomer are also separated from the maxilla. When the attachments of the pterygoid plates are finally separated from the maxillary tuberosities, the maxilla is down-fractured. The maxilla is then repositioned as planned. It may be moved horizontally, vertically, or laterally. If there is pre-existing vertical excess, a segment of bone is removed; if vertically deficient, an interpositional graft is placed. If presurgical planning with the orthodontist requires that the maxilla be segmentalized, this is performed from above so that smaller segments may be precisely repositioned to assist in the dental alignment. The orthodontist will prepare the dentition by providing adequate interradicular space so that the potential for injury to the tooth roots is minimized. It may also be necessary to have the orthodontist alter dental inclinations and occlusal planes before surgery so that the segments, when mobilized, will fit properly. Because this may often worsen the malocclusion before surgery, the patient must be advised of the rationale for such treatment. Internal wire fixation and intermaxillary immobilization were classically used to maintain the improved jaw relationships. Now fixation of the parts is accomplished with internal plating techniques [12] and the mandible is allowed to move freely.

Surgical correction of vertical maxillary excess has the potential to correct not only aesthetic imbalance, but associated functional and physiological sequellae as well. Excessive downward growth of the maxilla will displace the maxillary teeth, and often the gingiva, beyond the confines of the upper lip. The cosmetic compromise is further exaggerated with smiling. The unsightly display of gingiva, which may become red and swollen from the inflammatory changes associated with dessication, the dimpling of the tensed mentalis muscle, which is overworked to achieve lip competence, and the distortion of the upper lip are all correctable with the vertical repositioning of the maxilla. When asymmetric vertical growth occurs, usually in the posterior maxillary segments, the mandible will be prematurely contacted as it rotates to close. Occlusion may be limited to the molars and an anterior open bite may be extreme (Fig. 4). Functional masticatory efficiency will be compromised and abnormal swallowing patterns will evolve as the movements of the tongue, cheeks, and lips will attempt to close occlusal gaps.

One of the most fascinating distortions of facial balance is the Long Face Syndrome [13,14]. This syndrome exhibits features of all the growth deformities of the jaws and, therefore, requires use of all of the various surgical procedures to

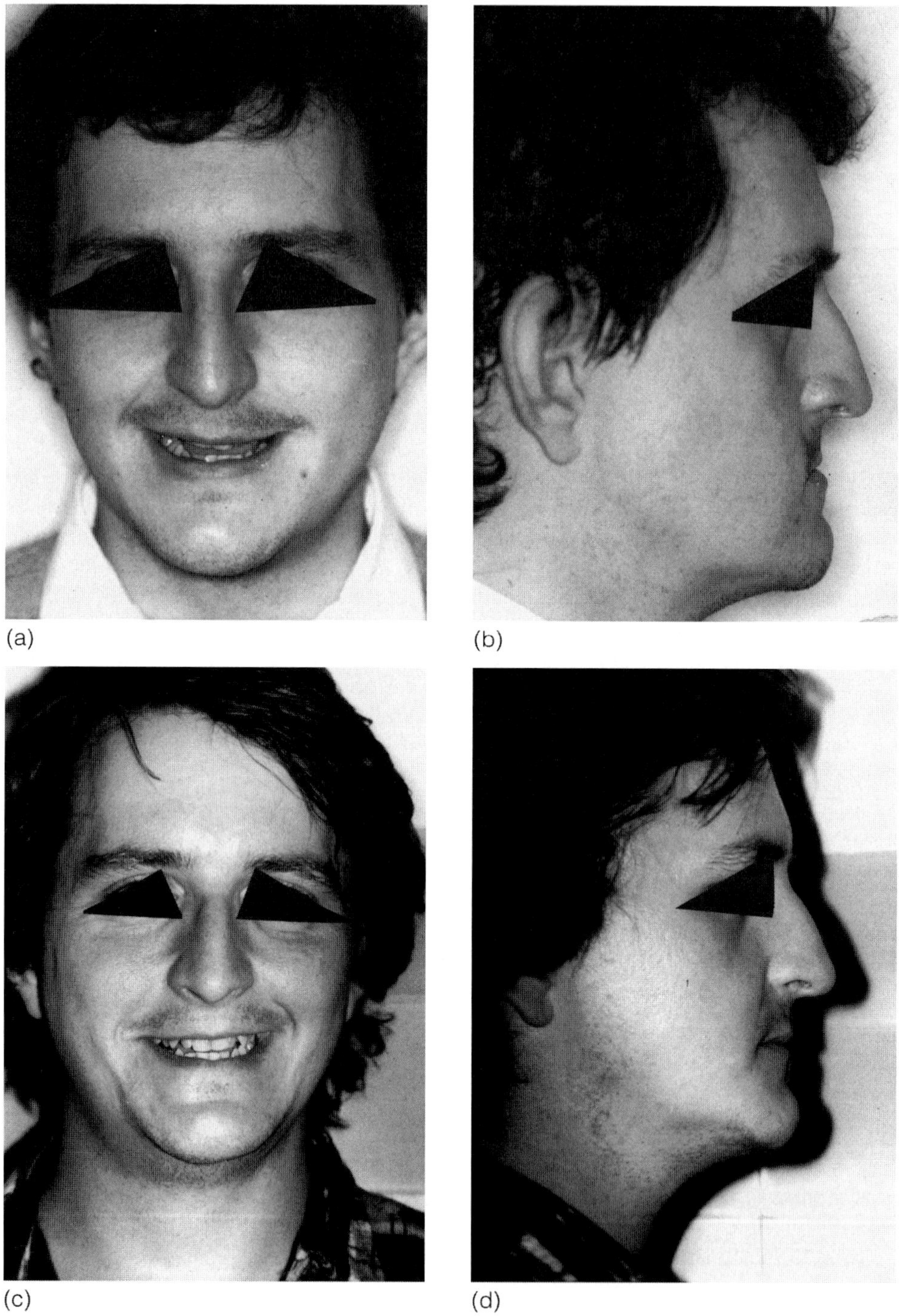

FIGURE 3 (a, b) Facial characteristics of maxillary retrognathia. Note the relative prognathism of the lower jaws, and the lack of upper lip and nasal support. (c, d) Postsurgical views following maxillary advancement at the LeFort I level. The strength of the mandible has been preserved, the nasal tip is well supported, and the nasolabial fold is appropriately directed.

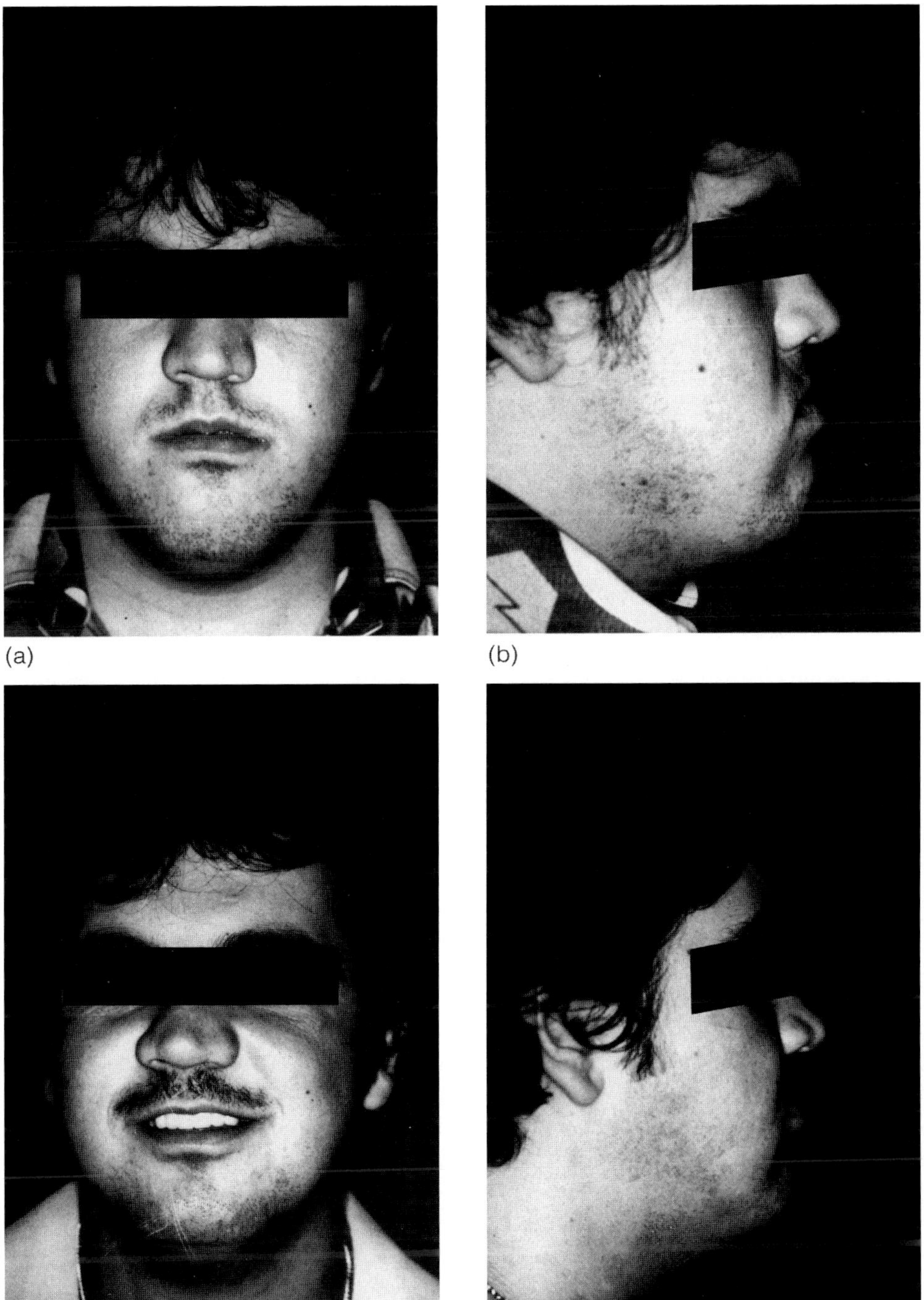

(a) (b) (c) (d)

FIGURE 4 (a, b) Facial characteristics of vertical maxillary excess associated with a severe anterior open bite deformity. (c, d) Postsurgical views following LeFort I ostectomy and mandibular ramusotomies.

correct it. Envision a typical Modigliani portrait and imagine a face made of rubber that is stretched vertically. All the midline structures will become long and narrow. The nose appears elongated, but its most striking feature is the lack of alar breadth. The canine fossae are flat. Maxillary teeth project beyond the upper lip and enclose a high vaulted palate and constricted dental arch. The mandibular arch tends to be narrow as well and sits above an elongated chin that has been flattened by the function of a mentalis musculature that strains to achieve lip competence (Fig. 5a). In profile, the nose has a prominent dorsal hump. The vertical growth excess of the maxilla rotates the mandible downward and backward simulating a retrognathia. Often a true retrognathia exists, further complicating the facial picture as well as the severity of the malocclusion (Fig. 5b).

The Long Face Syndrome has many variations, but all start with a vertical growth excess of the maxilla. Such variations include asymmetries, open bites, and prognathisms (which may be obscured by the backward rotation of the mandible). Precise assessment of the various movements and rotations is critical in the planning for surgery. Articulated study casts, analyses of patient, cephalometric radiographs and photographs, cephalometric and model "operations," and the fabrication of interoperative stents all assist in the work-up and performance of the surgery.

The surgery most frequently requires repositioning of both jaws. The maxilla is elevated and the mandible is usually advanced. As the parts are placed in their proper spatial relationships, the vertical excess is eliminated [15]. The canine fossae are enhanced and, as the support of the nasal floor is reconstituted, the nasal tip is elevated and the dorsal hump becomes less prominent. Teeth and gums relate better to the upper lip and the lips close more easily because of the shortening of the height of the maxilla and the advancement of the mandible, which brings the lower lip into play. Advancement of the mandibular angles provides greater volume to the lower facial third as does the rotational movement of the mandible to a higher spatial plane. Optimal aesthetic change is accomplished with a horizontal ostectomy and advancement of the anterior inferior border of the mandible [16]. This last movement not only provides optimal projection and definition of the chin, but removes the elongated segment and allows for more efficient function of the mentalis musculature (Figs. 5c, 6). In contrast to the mandible, in which the primary concern for undesirable sequellae of long duration is related to the alterations of sensation, that of the maxilla is related to aesthetics. Elevation of the maxilla may cause significant flaring of the nasal alae. This potential must be assessed in the presurgical examination of the nose. If there is concern about the postsurgical width of the nose, this must be expressed to the patient. An alternative treatment plan may be proposed. More commonly, a nasal cinch suture will be used [17]. All maxillary movements have the potential to affect the position as well as the volume of the upper lip [18]. The potential for volume loss and thinning of the lip may be minimized with variations of the V-Y closure [19].

Occasionally, sensory changes of the infraorbital nerves are noted after maxillary surgery. These changes are usually attributable to the effects of soft-tissue retraction and are relatively transient. Deviation of the nasal septum may occur if there is inadequate clearance in the midline or overimpaction of the maxilla. The presence of a pre-existing deviation of the septum must be assessed before surgery to avoid postsurgical confusion regarding this finding.

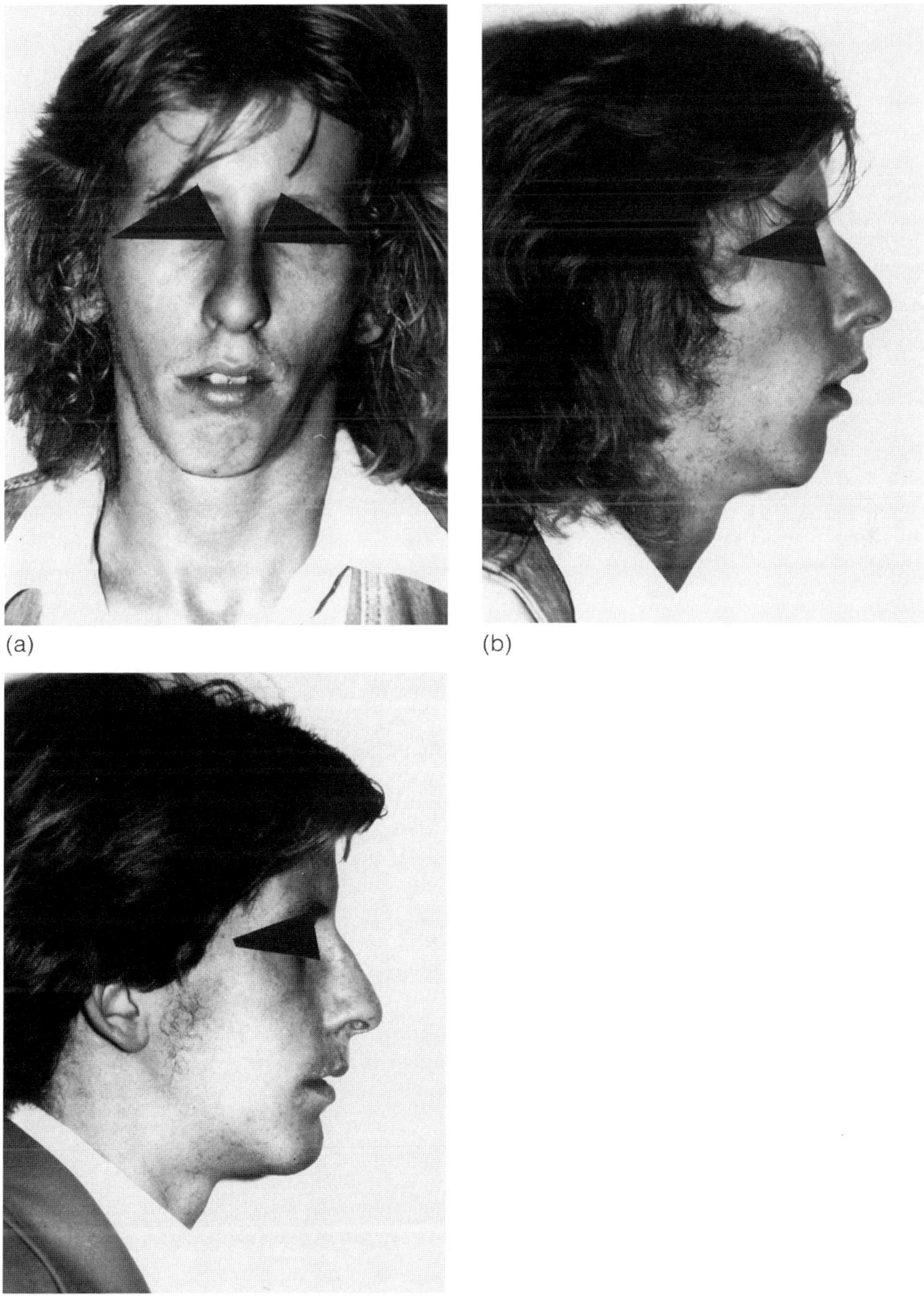

(a) (b) (c)

FIGURE 5 (a, b) Facial characteristics of the Long Face Syndrome. (c) Postsurgical view following LeFort I ostectomy, with midpalatal osteotomy to elevate and expand the maxilla, bilateral sagittal ramusotomies to advance the mandible, and anterior mandibular ostectomy and advancement to achieve optimal chin contour and position.

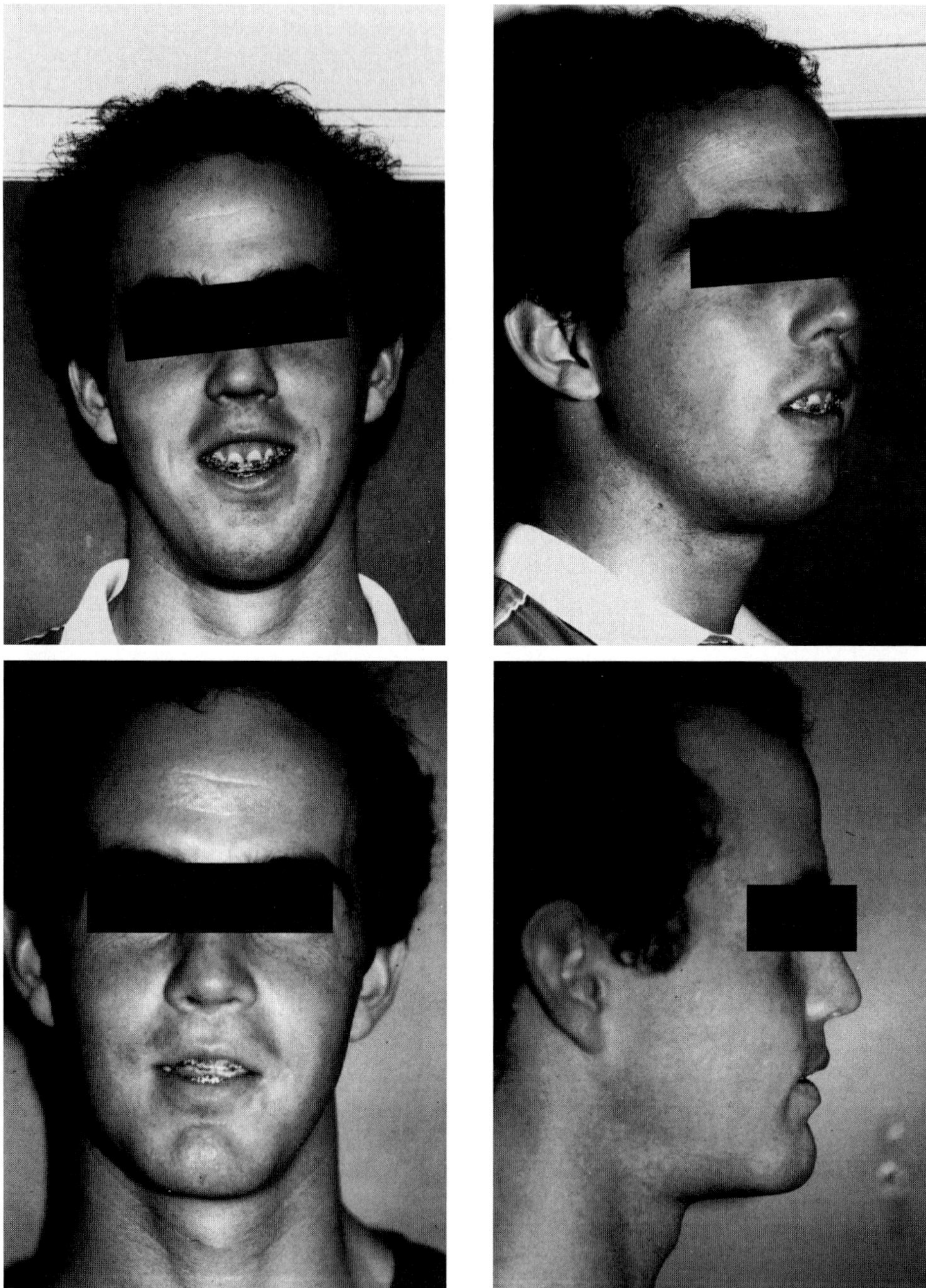

FIGURE 6 Pre- and postsurgical view of Long Face Syndrome and surgical correction.

The Short Face Syndrome is attributable to a deficiency in maxillary vertical growth. It is usually not associated with a particular malocclusion. In fact, one of the hallmarks of the clinical presentation is that it appears to be associated with no malocclusion at all. The patient shows little and often no display of the maxillary dentition similar to that of the edentulous patient or the patient with an inadequate projection of a maxillary denture. Thus the face appears considerably older than the patients chronological years. The mandible tends to close beyond the normal occlusal plane. This work excess will often result in a hypertrophy of the masseter muscles, further exaggerating the characteristic square gonial angles and flat mandibular plane. The aesthetic change from the down-grafting of the maxilla and reangulating the mandibular body rejuvenate the entire face.

Genioplasty is often incorporated in the treatment planning for many of the facial growth deformities. The beneficial effects of a well-defined and well-positioned chin will greatly enhance the aesthetics of many of the aforementioned procedures. However, it may also be performed alone with dramatic results (Fig. 7) [20]. The chin, indeed, is one of the most aesthetically significant landmarks of the facial architecture. As a fixed prominence on the only moving facial bone, its form and functional attachments may significantly complement the facial appearance or greatly detract from its beauty. Often the chin is the primary reason for an unattractive face. It is unrelated to dental occlusion. Its only functional implications are associated with the working of the mentalis muscle and the position of the lower lip. This portion of the mandible can be separated from the mandibular body from an intraoral approach without an external scar. A reciprocating saw is used to effect the osteotomy. According to presurgical planning, the segment can be repositioned backward, forward, up [21], down, and sideways, depending on the deformity that exists and the result desired. The free segment is secured with interosseous wires or appropriate plates [22]. Care must be taken to maintain some of the attachment of the mentalis muscle. If the muscle is completely stripped, the ptotic, "witches chin," may result. In this instance the muscle must be reattached to the bone and periosteum to avoid the aesthetic compromise of this deformity.

The chin can be made stronger or softer without the implantation of foreign materials. Problems associated with the displacement, infection, and exfoliation of various implant materials are thus avoided (Fig. 8). In the presence of labial incompetence, with tensing of the mentalis muscle, the implant will predictably cause bone resorption and is contraindicated [23]. In 6 weeks the osteotomized chin is again continuous with the mandible.

All of the aforementioned surgical procedures are performed under general anesthesia with nasoendotracheal intubation. Most require the facilities of a hospital surgery room and postsurgical care unit. Patients are admitted on the day of surgery. The consent form has already been reviewed, signed, and witnessed (Appendix 1). As with most other surgical procedures, the patient has arrived NPO and has eliminated all medications that may cause persistent bleeding. The fact that most patients who have orthognathic surgical procedures are young and healthy minimizes the presurgical testing requirements. However, consultation with the anesthesiologist regarding the nature of the surgery, the possibility of intermaxillary fixation, and the choice of medications that will minimize the potential for nausea and vomiting should not be neglected. Some procedures take several hours to complete. Hypoten-

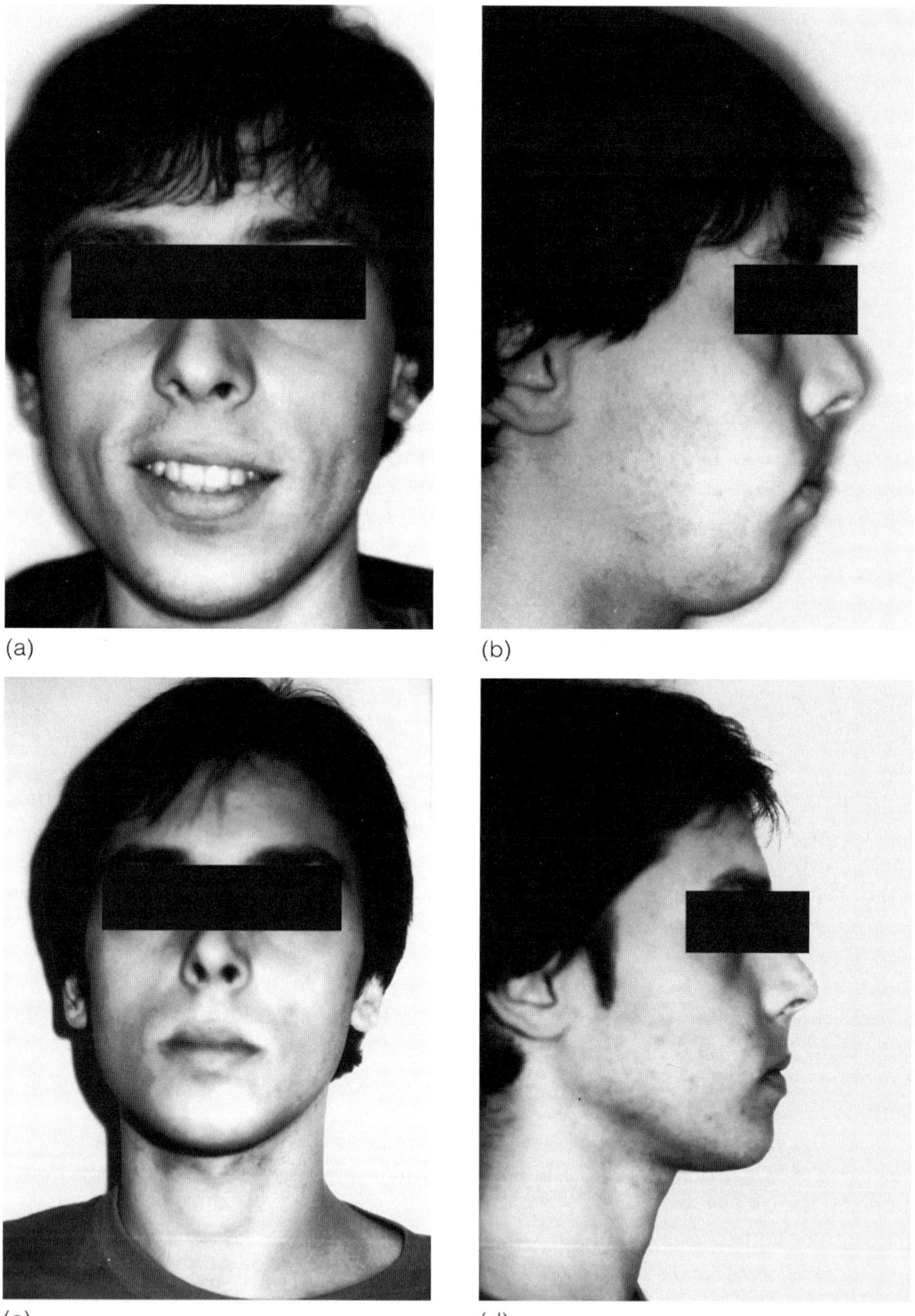

FIGURE 7 (a, b) Facial characteritics of retrogenia and labial incompetence. Chin is retruded and elongated. Patient's complaint was related to fullness of maxilla. (c, d) Postsurgical views following anterior horizontal mandibular ostectomy and advancement of anterior border. Note how maxillary fullness disappears.

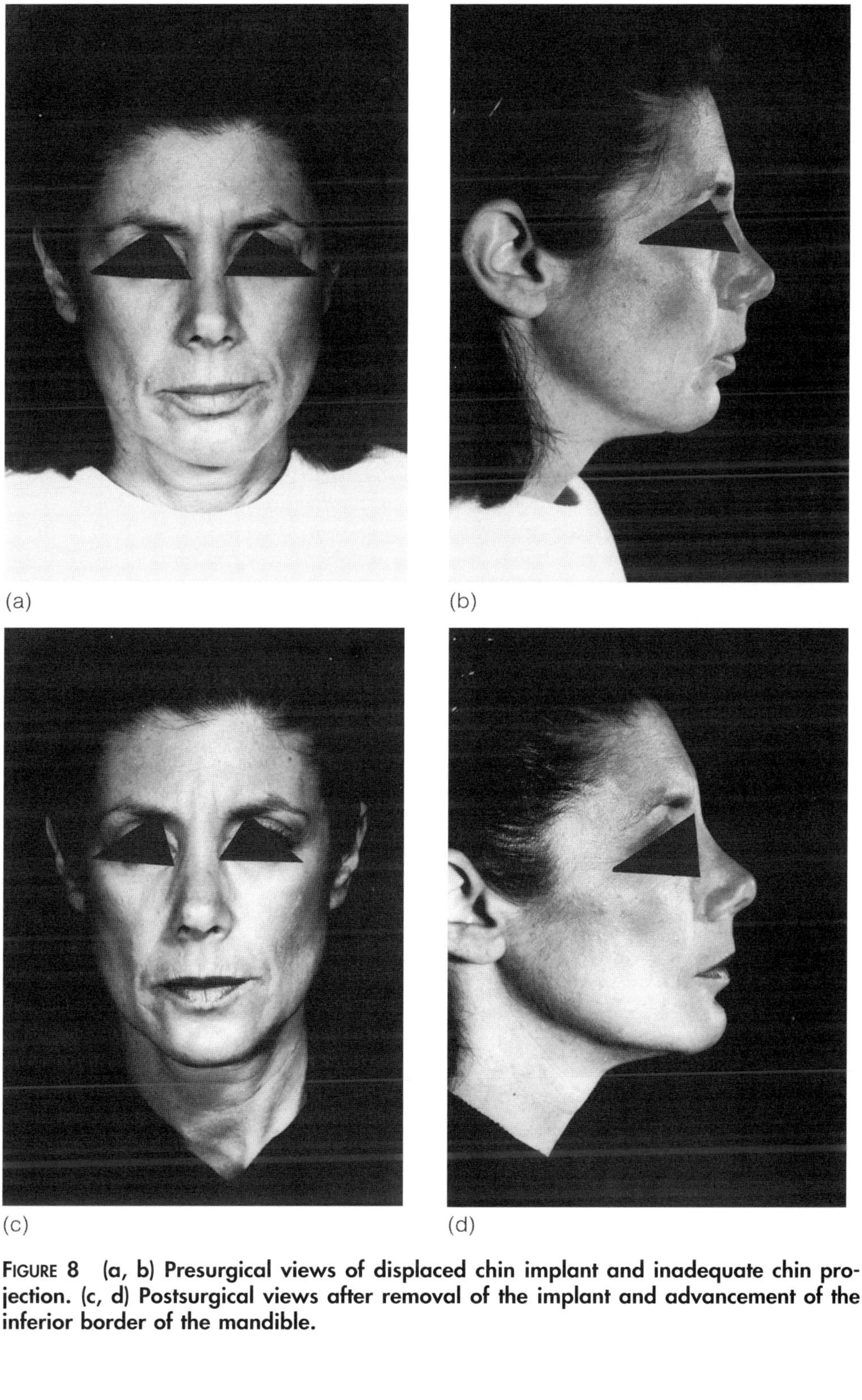

FIGURE 8 (a, b) Presurgical views of displaced chin implant and inadequate chin projection. (c, d) Postsurgical views after removal of the implant and advancement of the inferior border of the mandible.

sive anesthesia, as well as careful dissection, will usually eliminate the need for transfusion.

Postsurgical pain is well controlled with mild narcotic analgesics. Non-narcotic medications are most often quite adequate. Swelling is well controlled with intrasurgical steroids and a repository dose administered on the first postsurgical day. A wire cutter is kept at the bedside of patients in intermaxillary fixation. Cephalometric and panoramic radiographs are taken on the first postsurgical day.

Most patients are discharged from the hospital with prescriptions for an antibiotic, usually a penicillin or cephalosporin. Patients who are allergic to the penicillins receive a prescription for clindamycin. Liquid Tylenol is most often adequate for discomfort. A nasal decongestant is helpful for patients who have had maxillary surgery. Postsurgical nausea and vomiting are of great concern for those patients in intermaxillary fixation. The fact is that the incidence of this problem is relatively uncommon. However, it is most important that the postsurgical diet and medications be reviewed and that the patient be shown exactly where the intermaxillary wire is located. A wire cutter is provided for the patient and is kept handy at all times. Although the patient is on a liquid diet, all foods that may cause nausea are eliminated. Alcohol is forbidden. A liquid antiemetic medication is recommended.

Postdischarge instructions are directed toward taking the prescribed medications, fluids and diet, physical activity, and oral hygiene. Antibiotics are usually continued through the first week. The need to take adequate fluids in excess of the liquid diet is stressed, especially for those patients in intermaxillary fixation. Small fluid volumes, taken many times during the day, are more easily accomplished and tolerated than following the conventional regimen of meals. Patients who have internal rigid fixation and have the ability to open their mandible must also adhere to a diet prepared in a blender. Various dietary and vitamin supplements, which may be purchased over the counter are also advised.

Physical activity is modified to the extent that the patient has had a major surgical procedure, a general anesthetic, a significant change in diet, and, possibly, intermaxillary wiring. This issue is discussed at the office visits, which are scheduled during the 6 weeks of osseous healing. Immaculate attention to oral hygiene is imperative. Surgical arch bars and orthodontic appliances tend to accumulate debris that will irritate the gingiva. Inflamed gums will bleed, hypertrophy, and become sore. Antiseptic rinses are occasionally prescribed.

The past three decades have seen an evolution in the scope of oral and maxillofacial surgery. Skeletal malocclusions and the associated distortions of the facial appearance are now correctable with surgical procedures that are safe, predictable, without any external incisions, and often without intermaxillary fixation. Undesirable sequellae are few and the benefits that accrue from the restoration of the occlusion are great, not the least of which is significant enhancement of facial aesthetics. At present, the potential of distraction osteosysthesis is being investigated.

REFERENCES

1. Tucker MR, et al. Evaluation of treatment of patients with dentofacial deformities: a multidisciplinary approach. NC Dent Rev 3:13, 1985.
2. Steiner CC. Cephalometrics in clinical practice. Angle Orthodontics 28:8, 1959.
3. Burstone CJ, et al. Cephalometrics for orthognathic surgery. J Oral Surg 36:269, 1978.

4. Shira RB. Surgical correction of openbite deformities by oblique sliding osteotomy. J Oral Surg 19:275, 1961.
5. Dattilo DJ, Braun TW, Sotereanos GG. The inverted L osteotomy for treatment of skeletal open bite deformities. J Oral Maxillofac Surg 43:440, 1985.
6. Caldwell JB, Letterman GS. Vertical osteotomy in mandibular rami for correction of prognathism. J Oral Surg 12:185, 1954.
7. Herbert JM, Kent KM, Hinds ED. Correction of prognathism by intraoral vertical subcondylar osteotomy. J Oral Surg 28:651, 1970.
8. Robinson M. Micrognathism corrected by vertical osteotomy of ascending ramus and iliac bone graft: new technique. Oral Surg 10:125, 1957.
9. Obwegeser HL. The indications for surgical correction of mandibular deformity by the sagittal splitting technique. Br J Oral Surg 1:157, 1964.
10. Bell WH. Revascularization and bone healing after anterior maxillary osteotomy. J Oral Surg 27:249, 1969.
11. Bell WH, Fonseca RJ, Kennedy JW, Levy BM. Bone healing and revascularization after total maxillary osteotomy. J Oral Surg 33:253, 1977.
12. Persson G, Hellem S, Nord PG. Bone-plates for stabilizing LeFort I osteotomies. J Maxillofac Surg 14:69, 1986.
13. Bell WH, McBride KL. Correction of the long face syndrome by LeFort I osteotomy. Oral Surg Oral Path Oral Med 44:493, 1977.
14. Wolford LM, Hilliard FW. The surgical orthodontic correction of vertical dentofacial deformities. J Oral Surg 39:883, 1981.
15. Phillips C, Devereau JP, Tullock JF, Tucker MT. Full-face soft tissue response to surgical maxillary intrusion. Int J Adult Orthod Orthognathic Surg 1:299, 1986.
16. Scheidman GB, Legan HG, Bell WH. Soft tissue changes with combined mandibular setback and advancement genioplasty. J Oral Surg 39:505, 1981.
17. Collins PC, Epker BN. The alar cinch. Technique for prevention of alar base flaring secondary to maxillary surgery. Oral Surg Oral Med Oral Path 53:549, 1982.
18. Schendel SA, Williamson LW. Muscle reorientation following superior repositioning of the maxilla. J Oral Maxillofac Surg 41:235, 1983.
19. Hackney FL, Nishioka GJ, Van Sickels JE. Frontal soft tissue morphology with double V-Y closure following LeFort I osteotomy. J Oral Maxillofac Surg 46:850, 1988.
20. Davis HW, Davis CL, Daly BW. Long term bony and soft tissue stability following advancement genioplasty. J Oral Maxillofac Surg 46:731, 1988.
21. Precious DS, Delaire J. Correction of anterior mandibular vertical excess: the functional genioplasty. Oral Surg Oral Med Oral Path 59:229, 1985.
22. Davis W. A simple method to gain symmetry of the intraoral genioplasty. J Oral Maxillofac Surg 46:710, 1988.
23. Matarasso A, Elias AC, Elias RL. Labial incompetence: a marker for progressive bone resorption in silastic chin augmentation. J Plast Reconstr Surg 98:1007, 1996.

APPENDIX 1

CONSENT FOR ORTHOGNATHIC SURGERY

Please initial each paragraph after reading. If you have any questions, please ask your doctor BEFORE initialing.

Orthognathic surgery is being planned for you, and it is important that you understand the benefits and risks of such surgery. This is NOT minor surgery and you have the right to be fully informed about your condition and the recommended treatment plan. The disclosures in this consent are not meant to alarm you, but rather to provide information you need in order to give or withhold your consent to the planned surgery.

____
Patient's Name Date

_____1. I hereby authorize Dr. ________ and staff to treat the condition described as: ________
____
____
____

_____2. The surgical procedure planned to treat the above condition has been explained to me, and I understand the nature of the treatment to be: ______________________
____
____
____

_____3. I have been informed of possible alternative forms of treatment (if any), including: ___
____
____
____

_____4. My doctor has explained to me that there are certain potential risks and side effects of my surgery, some of which may be serious. They include, but are not limited to:

_____A. Facial and jaw swelling after surgery, usually lasting several days.

_____B. Bleeding, both during and after surgery, which may sometimes be severe enough to require blood transfusion. I have been advised of the opportunity for blood donation before surgery so that my own blood may be given back to me (autotransfusion) if necessary.

_____C. Allergic reaction to any of the medications given during or after surgery.

_____D. Delayed healing of the bony segments; rarely requiring a second surgery and/or bone graft to repair.

_____E. Relapse: the tendency for the repositioned bone segments to return to their original position, which may require additional treatment, including surgery and/or bone grafting.

_____F. Bruising and discoloration of the skin around the jaws, eyes and nose.

_____G. Diminished sense of smell (if upper jaw surgery is done).

_____H. A change in cosmetic appearance. Although this is primarily a procedure to restore jaw function, I am aware of some expected change in my appearance. I understand that some other cosmetic changes may result that cannot be exactly predicted.

_____I. Loss of feeling, pain or a tingling numbness in my chin, lips, tongue, gums, or teeth which occurs in a significant number of patients. These symptoms may last for several days, weeks or months. I have been told that there is some chance that it may be permanent.

_____J. Possible decreased function of muscles of facial expression.

_____K. Scarring from external skin incisions if certain rigid fixation methods are used.

_____L. Possible need for additional procedures to remove fixation devices, pins, screws, plates or splints.

_____M. In certain cases where bone cuts may be made in the marrow space between teeth, there is the possibility of devitalization of those teeth which may require later root canal procedures, and may result in the loss of those teeth.

_____N. In upper jaw surgery, the sinus will be affected for several weeks, and there may be a need for further sinus surgery to remedy any lingering problems.

_____O. Post-operative infection which may cause loss of adjacent bone and/or teeth and which may require additional treatment for a prolonged period of time.

_____P. Change in position of the jaw joints (TMJ) which may cause post-operative discomfort, bite change and chewing difficulties. If TMJ symptoms existed before surgery, there may be no improvement and even some worsening of these symptoms after surgery.

_____Q. Stretching of the corners of the mouth with resulting discomfort and slow healing.

_____R. Inflammation of veins (phlebitis) that are used for IV fluids and medications, sometimes resulting in pain, swelling, discoloration and restriction of arm or hand movement for some time after surgery.

_____5. General anesthesia will be used for this surgery and I have been told of the risks, including bronchitis, pneumonia, hoarseness or voice changes, cardiac irregularities, heart attack or death. I am aware of the importance of not having anything by mouth (including clear liquids unless specifically authorized by my doctor or anesthesiologist) after midnight on the day before surgery. I UNDERSTAND THAT IT IS VITAL THAT I HAVE NOTHING TO EAT OR DRINK FOR EIGHT (8) HOURS PRIOR TO MY ANESTHETIC. **TO DO OTHERWISE MAY BE LIFE-THREATENING!**

_____6. I realize the importance of providing true and accurate information about my health, especially concerning possible pregnancy, allergies, medications and history of drug or alcohol use. If I misinform my doctor I understand the consequences may be life-threatening or otherwise adversely affect the results of my surgery.

_____7. If my teeth are wired together after this surgery, I understand there are certain associated risks and complications: oral hygiene will be diminished, there may be resulting gum disease, my teeth will feel slightly loose for some time after the wiring, and there is always some concern about airway obstruction. I agree to carry wire cutters with me at all times when my jaws are wired and to avoid the use of alcohol and other activities that may cause airway problems.

CONSENT

By signing this consent form, I acknowledge that I have read it completely and understand the procedure to be performed, the risks, and the alternatives to surgery. I have had all my questions answered to my satisfaction. I was under no pressure to sign this form and have made a voluntary choice to proceed with surgery. I am fully aware that no guarantee or warranty can be made regarding the results of treatment

____

Patient's (or Legal Guardian's) Signature Date

____

Doctor's Signature Date

____

Witness' Signature Date

Index

AAAASF certification, 690–691
AAAHC. *See* Accreditation Association for Ambulatory Health Care
Abdomen
  liposuction, 600–604
  tumescent liposuction, 559–561
Abdominal contouring
  anatomical considerations, 668
  anesthesia, 667–668
  complications, 677
  consultation, 664–666
  fascial layers, 668–669
  historical development, 662–663
  liposuction, 669
  modified crescent abdominal tuck, 669–670
  patient selection, 663–664
  postsurgical care, 674–677
  presurgical evaluation, 666–667
  rectus plication, 669
  surgery, 668–674
  surgical instrumentation, 667
  technique, 670–674
Accreditation Association for Ambulatory Health Care (AAAHC)
  adjunct standards, 4
[Accreditation Association for Ambulatory Health Care]
  advantages and disadvantages, 4
  office surgical facilities, 2–5
  organizations accredited, 3
  purpose, 3
  sponsoring organizations, 3
  standards, 4
Accutane, 168
  dermabrasion, 180
Acetaminophen, flaps and grafts and, 405
Acne, 89–90
Acne cyst, corticosteroid and, 32
Acne scars. *See also* Collagen
  carbon dioxide laser resurfacing, 112
  dermabrasion, 180
  erbium skin remodeling, 135–137, 150
  fat transplantation, 254
  laser resurfacing, 168
  presurgical photograph, 854
Acquired melanocytic nevi, 371–372
  cause, 372
  treatment, 372–374
    excision, 372
    partial removal, 372, 374
  types, 372

Actinic cheilitis, 862–867
  carbon dioxide laser vermilionectomy, 864–865
  equipment, 864
  historical development of, 863–864
  laser technique, 866
  postsurgical care, 866–867
  presurgical instructions, 864
  presurgical photograph, 865–866
  scalpel technique, 865–866
Actinic keratoses
  dermabrasion, 181
  medicum chemical peel, 51, 52–54
Actinic poikiloderma and, PDL, 471
Acute median nerve compression, 622
Acyclovir, 65
  dermabrasion, 188
  laser resurfacing, 171
Adenoma, dermabrasion and, 183
Adiposis dolorosa, 367
Administration and staffing, 5–9
  employee rights, 7
  job descriptions, 6
  mission statement, 5
  order of authority, 6
  orientation, 7
  personnel files, 6–7
  personnel manual, 6
  professional development, 8
  quality improvement, 8–9
  risk management, 8–9
  salary and benefits, 7
Advancement flaps, 383, 384
After-care instructions in TCA, 78
Aging
  eyebrows, 679–681, 774
  forehead, 679–681
  frontalis muscle, 681
  nasion, 679–681
  surgical anatomy
    face, 679–681
    lower face, 684–685
    mid face, 681–684
Aging face
  aesthetic analysis, 17–26
  anatomic basis, 17–18
  atrophic changes, 221–222
  cartilage and bone changes, 25–26
  characteristics, 689
  combination therapies, 26
  elasticity loss, 25
  musculature changes, 24
[Aging face]
  photoaging, 18–20
  pigmentary system, 20–22
  subcutaneous fat loss, 22–24
  surgical anatomy, 679–684
Alabaster look, 39
Alabaster skin, 82
Alcohol, 14
Alexandrite lasers, 498–499
Algorithm
  brow rejuvenation, 783
  forehead rejuvenation, 783
Allergic reaction, causes of, 423
Allergy
  in blepharoplasty, 745
  local anesthetics in skin testing, 426
AlloDerm, 269, 282–284, 318
  informed consent, 288
AlloDerm facial implants, 929
  complications, 935
  virus transmission, 928
Allogeneic human collagen, 279–284
Alloplastic chin implants, 704
Alloplastic molar implants, 704
Alopecia, 801
Alopecia reduction, 826–833
  complications, 832
  historical development, 826–828
  marking, 832
  patterns, 830–831
  postsurgical course, 832
  surgical procedure, 831–832
Alpha-hydroxy acids, 28
Ambulatory phlebectomy (AP), 525–529
  anatomical locations, 526
  complications, 529
  dressings, 529
  hooks, 526
  instrumentation, 526–527
  sedation, 527
  supplies, 527
Ambulatory surgery centers, surgical suite design in, 1–2
American Association for Accreditation of Ambulatory Surgery Facilities (AAAASF) certification, 690–691
American Society of Anesthesiologists Physical Status Classification, 425
Amide anesthetics, 415–417
Anaphylactic reaction, causes of, 423
Anesthesia. *See also* Sedation
  abdominal contouring, 667–668

[Anesthesia]
blepharoplasty, 439–440, 727
cervicofacial rhytidectomies, 440
Cook Weekend Alternative to the Facelift, 644, 646
cosmetic blepharoplasty, 756–757
epidermal cyst, 356
erbium skin remodeling, 145
facelifts, 440
facial resurfacing, 439
flaps and grafts, 391–394
hair transplantation, 815–817
infralash blepharoplasty, 759
laser resurfacing, 169
liposuction, 573–635
scars surgical excision, 850
transconjunctival lower-lid blepharoplasty, 760
tumescent, 244–245, 547–549
historical development, 662
modified Klein solution, 225
tumescent liposuction, 547–549
Anesthetic ear, in facelift, 710
Anesthetic patches, 420
Anesthetics
amide, 415–417
ester, 413–415
injectable, 412
local. *See* Local anesthetics
topical, 417–419
Angiofibromas
argon lasers, 459
PDLs, 463
Angiokeratomas
argon lasers, 459
copper lasers, 461
Angiolipomas, 367
Angle, Edward, 939
Angular cheilitis, 862
Ankles, tumescent liposuction of, 565
Ankle telangiectasias, laser therapy, 532
Antibiotics
erbium skin remodeling, 152
laser resurfacing, 171
Antiviral medications, erbium skin remodeling and, 152
Anxiety, dissatisfied patient and, 917
Anxiolytics, 427–428
blepharoplasty, 439–440
AP. *See* Ambulatory phlebectomy
Apraclonidine, 339
APS system, 905
Argon lasers, 457–459, 470
Argon-pumped tunable dye lasers, 459–460, 467, 574
vs. PDLs, facial telangiectasias, 466
Arms
liposuction, 590–600
tumescent liposuction, 556
Arrector pili muscle, 881
Arrhythmias, deep peel and, 91
Artecoll, 321
Arteplast, 321–322
Arteriovenous fistulae, hair transplantation and, 825–826
Asian blepharoplasty, 728–729
complications, 728–729
Asian eye, levator apneurosis and, 728–729
Aspiration pump, in tumescent liposuction, 550
Atrophic scars, 847
carbon dioxide laser resurfacing, 111
Atrophy, deep peel and, 90–91
Autografts, disadvantages of, 316
Autologen, 269, 276–279, 318
Autologous collagen. *See* Fat transplantation
Autologous fat injections, facelift and, 703–704
Autologous human collagen, 272–284
Axillary hyperhidrosis, BTX-A and, 348, 350

Back, liposuction of, 613–614
Back tables, 14
Bacterial infection and scarring, 157
Baker-Gordon phenol, deep chemical peels and, 52–53, 58–63
Baker's formula phenol occluded with tape, deep chemical peels and, 57–58
Baldness, male pattern, 795–800
Banana fold formation, 635
Banana roll, tumescent liposuction and, 562
Bandages in hair transplantation, 823–824
Bat wings, 590, 631
Becker's nevi, flashlamp-pumped pulsed dye lasers and, 493
Beckman Laser Institute multicenter trial, 174
Benefits, 7
Benign symmetric lipomatosis, 366
Benign tumors, dermabrasion of, 183
Benzalkonium chloride, 13
Benzodiazepines, 427–428
ambulatory phlebectomy, 527
facelift surgery, 691
tumescent lidocaine, 452

Beta-blockers, epinephrine, 453
Betamethasone, in structural lipoaugmentation, 233–234
Bilateral advancement flaps, 383, 384
Bilateral occipitoparietal flap, 827, 829
Bilobed flaps, 386
Bilobed transposition flaps, 392
Biocell Ultravate, 322
Bionet 2nd skin, erbium skin remodeling and, 152
Bioplastique, 322
Biopsy punch method, incision and drainage, 356–357
Birthmarks, erbium skin remodeling and, 140
Bitemporal flap, 829
Bleach-eze, 82
Bleaching formula for darker skin, 82
Bleaching preparations in erbium skin remodeling, 153–154
Bleeding. *See* Hemorrhage
Blending resurfacing procedures in medicum chemical peel, 51–53, 57
Blepharochalasis, 681, 719–720
Blepharoplasty, 719–745, 749–766
  anesthesia, 439–440, 727, 756–757
  Asian, 728–729
  complications, 742–745, 762–765
  and hair transplantation, 792
  informed consent, 756
    cosmetic laser, 769
  infralash. *See* Infralash blepharoplasty
  instruments, 725–727
  keratoconjunctivitis sicca, 762
  laser. *See* Laser blepharoplasty
  lower eyelid, transconjunctival, 760–762
  marking, 725
  measurements, 751
  medical history, 723, 750
  patient instructions, 755–756, 770
  photography, 724–725, 753
  physical examination, 724, 751
  postsurgical care, 742–743, 762
  presurgical evaluation, 722–727, 749–757
  and resurfacing, 762, 788
  surgical technique, 757–762
  transconjunctival, 731–736
    and carbon dioxide resurfacing, 792–793
    lower eyelid, 760–762
    presurgical, 722
  transcutaneous, 730
[Blepharoplasty]
  upper eyelid, 727–730
    complications, 735
    surgical technique, 729–730, 757
Blindness, blepharoplasty and, 763
Blocks, 429–435
Blue-black tattoos, Q-switched Nd:YAG lasers and, 503–504, 507
Blunt infiltrators, 232
Body liposuction and facial surgery, 788–790
Body peel. *See also* Peel, Total Body
  informed consent, 77
Body warts, copper vapor lasers and, 476
Bone, aging face and, 25–26
Bony skeleton, zones, 930
Borderline personality disorder, in dissatisfied patient, 914–915
Botox, 201, 313, 319
  deinervation before skin resurfacing, 790
  dynamic rhytides, 314–315
  new, 335
Botulinum A exotoxin (BTX-A), 333–350
  adjunctive use, 347–348
  commercially available, 354–355
  complications, 335
  dilution, 335
  dose, 336
  electromyography-guided injection, 340
  paralysis, 354
  problems, 336–337, 341–342
  side effect, 350
  storage, 335
  technique, 336
  toxicology, 333–334
Bovine collagen implants
  adverse treatment responses, 203–205
  correction maintenance, 202–203
  historical development, 267–268, 315, 320
  hypersensitivity, 268
  implantation techniques, 197–198
  indications for, 203
  lip augmentation, 205–207
  patient screening, 197–198
  skin testing, 197–198
Bradycardia, clonidine and, 454–455
Bra fat, tumescent liposuction of, 557
Brandy scalp lift, 826
Breast liposuction
  female, 587–590
  male, 584–587
Brow asymmetry, BTX-A and, 343

Brow depressors, BTX-A and, 341–342
Brow ptosis, 340
Brow rejuvenation, 771–783
  aesthetics, 772–777
  algorithm, 783
  anatomy, 772
  clinical cases, 782–783
  coronal, 777–778
  goals, 777
  incisions, 776
  indications, 777
  measurements, 724
  open, 777–778
  patient evaluation, 772–777
  postsurgical care, 781
  surgical technique, 777–782
BTS-A. *See* Botulinum A exotoxin
Buffalo hump, tumescent liposuction for, 558
Bulge hypothesis, 884
Bupivacaine, 415–417
  tumescent lidocaine, 452
Buttocks ptosis, 635
Butyrophenones, epinephrine, 454

Cafe-au-lait
  flashlamp-pumped pulsed dye lasers, 493
  Q-switched ruby lasers, 497
Calves, tumescent liposuction of, 565
Cameras, 897–899, 905
  setting, 900
Camouflage cosmetics after facelift, 708
Cannulas
  Coleman injection, 245
  extracting, 246
  Klein infiltrating, 245
  liposuction, 577–578, 580
  Luer Lok extraction, 226
  tumescent liposuction, 550
Capsulopalpebral fascia, 722
Carbon dioxide laser resurfacing, 99–115
  complications, 110–114
  contraindications, 102
  with erbium skin remodeling, 151
  history, 99–100
  informed consent, 119
  intraoperative considerations, 105, 107
  laser protocol, 105–108
  log, 122
  patient education, 102–104
  patient selection, 100–103
  postoperative instruction sheet, 120
  postoperative management, 109–110
[Carbon dioxide laser resurfacing]
  preoperative checklist, 121
  preoperative skin preparation, 104–105
  and transconjunctival blepharoplasty, 792–793
  treatment technique, 108
Carbon dioxide lasers
  advantages, 170
  blepharoplasty, 739–740, 765
    controversy, 740
  vs. erbium:YAG lasers, 123–124
  histological effects, 165
  modifications, 164
  physical properties, 12
  risks, 167
  scars, 470
  solar lentignes, 500
  vaporization of myxoid cysts, 364–365
  vermilionectomy of actinic cheilitis, 864–865
  warts, 475–476
Carbon-Nd:YAG for hair removal, 888
Cardiac arrhythmias, deep peel and, 91
Cartilage, aging face, 25–26
Cefadroxil, in liposuction, 577
Ceilings, 10
Cellulite, 871–873
  cause, 871–872
  mechanical treatment, 872–873
  topical treatment, 872
Centrifuge, 228
Cephalexin, in liposuction, 580
Cephalogram, digitized, 940–941
Cephalosporin, in erbium skin remodeling, 152
Cervicofacial rhytidectomies, anesthesia in, 440
Cheeks
  erbium skin remodeling, 150
  fat transplantation, 251–253
  senile lipoatrophy, 252
Cheilitis
  actinic. *See* Actinic cheilitis
  angular, 862
  exfoliative, 863
  factitious, 863
  glandular, 862–863
  granulomatous, 863
  plasma cell, 863
Chemical peels
  complications, 79–98
    acne, 89–90

[Chemical peels]
atrophy, 90–91
cardiac arrhythmias, 91
cold sensitivity, 90
concurrent disease exacerbation, 92
deep peels, 90–92
infection, 87, 89
inherent procedural errors, 92–93
laryngeal edema, 92
milia, 89
persistent erythema, 87–88
pigmentary changes, 80–83
poor physician/patient relationship, 90
pruritus, 87–88
scarring, 83–87
textural changes, 87–89
deep. *See* Deep chemical peels
informed consent, 97
vs. laser resurfacing, 163–164
medium. *See* Medium chemical peels
patient instructions, 96
superficial. *See* Superficial chemical peels
Cherry angiomas
argon lasers, 459
copper lasers, 461
PDLs, 463, 469
Chest, total body peel of, 69–78
Chin augmentation, 931–932
complications, 934
Cook Weekend Alternative to the Facelift, 645
displaced, 955
facelift, 704
presurgical considerations, 932–933
surgical procedure, 933
Chloasmal pigmentation, in erbium skin remodeling, 137
Chlorhexidine, 14
Chloroprocaine, 415
Chronic folliculitis, hair transplantation and, 826
Cleansers, in postsurgical skin care, 878
Clonidine
anxiolysis, 454
bradycardia, 454–455
hypotension, 454–455
sedation, 454
tumescent lidocaine, 455
Cobblestoning, in hair transplantation, 825
Cocaine, 413
epinephrine, 454
Coherent Ultrapulse laser, 164
Cold sensitivity, 90
Cold urticaria, 90
Coleman injection cannula, 245
Collagen, 193–208
historical development, 193
Collagen implants, bovine. *See* Bovine collagen implants
Combes' formula, 29
Combination cosmetic procedures, 785–793
blepharoplasty and resurfacing, 788
combining resurfacing techniques, 785–788
do no harm, 793
facial surgery and body liposuction, 788–790
hair transplantation, 791–792
intrinsically combined, 792–793
soft-tissue augmentation, 790
strategies, 785–786
Comissures, oral, fat transplantation and, 251
Communication, dissatisfied patient and, 913
Concurrent disease exacerbation, deep peel and, 92
Congenital nevi, Q-switched ruby lasers for, 497, 499
Consent. *See also* Informed consent
for photography in hair transplantation, 845–846
Consultation
erbium skin remodeling, 127–135
superficial chemical peels, 29–31
Consultation record
zyderm, 220
zyplast collagen, 220
Contact dermatitis
laser resurfacing, 857–858
scarring, 157–158
Continuous wave lasers, 457
vs. pulsed lasers, for pigmented lesions, 491
Contour deformity, 623
Cook's combined approach, 792
Copper bromide lasers, 457, 460–461, 467–469
Copper vapor lasers, 457, 460–461, 467
vs. PDLs, in facial telangiectasias, 466–467
warts, 476
Coronal brow rejuvenation, 777–778
Corrugator muscle, 772

Corticosteroid, for acne cyst, 32
"Cosmetic junkie," as dissatisfied patient, 914
Cosmetic laser blepharoplasty, informed consent for, 353, 767, 769
Cosmetic procedures, combination. *See* Combination cosmetic procedures
Cosmetics, as camouflage, 708
Crash carts, 15
Crow's feet, BTX-A for, 344–345
Cyst-Abscess, 205
Cysts
  biopsy punch method, 356–357
  dissection technique, 357–366
    complications, 360–361
    electrosurgical technique, 359–360
    excisional removal, 358–359
    medium to large sized, 357–358

Danna method of cyst removal, 359–360
Depressor Anguli Oris, BTX-A and, 345–347
Darker skin, bleaching formula for, 82
Deep chemical peels, 52–59, 787–788
Baker-Gordon phenol, 52–53, 58–63
Baker's formula phenol unoccluded, 57–58
  complications, 64–66, 90–92
  indications, 38–42
  patient selection, 38–42
  persistent erythema, 64–66
  re-epithelialization, 64
  risk factors, 57
  sedation, 52–53, 58–59
  TCA, 52–53
  technique, 59–64
  wound healing, 64–66
Delayed wound healing, 84–85
Dental malocclusion, 940
Dependent personality, in dissatisfied patient, 915
Depressed grafts in hair transplantation, 825
Depression, in dissatisfied patient, 917
Depressor Anugli Oris (DAO), BTX-A and, 345–347
Dercum's disease, 367
Dermabrasion, 179–189, 856
  vs. acid peels, 189
  vs. carbon dioxide laser, 189
  complications, 188–189
  diamond fraise, 788
  equipment, 856
  historical development, 179
[Dermabrasion]
  indications, 179–184
  vs. laser resurfacing, 163–164
  manual, 788
  patient instructions, 96
  patient selection, 179–184
  post-operative management, 188
  postsurgical care, 856
  pre-operative management, 188
  presurgical considerations, 856
  presurgical instructions, 856
  skin chilling, 183–184
  technique, 184–187, 856
  wire brush, 788
Dermal chloasma, 140
Dermal defects, fat transplantation for, 256
Dermal grafting, 319
Dermalive, 322
Dermalogen, 269, 279–282, 319
Dermal strip grafts in facelift, 705–707
Dermatitis
  carbon dioxide laser resurfacing, 112
  contact
    laser resurfacing, 857–858
    scarring, 157–158
Dermoid cysts, 361–362
Diamond fraise dermabrasion, 788
Diazepam
  alopecia reduction, 831
  liposuction, 577, 580
  tumescent lidocaine, 452
  tumescent liposuction, 547
Difficult patient. *See* Dissatisfied patient
Diffuse congenital lipomatosis, 367
Digital myxoid cysts, 363–365
Digital photography, 906–907
  specialists, 909
Digital photoplethysmography of varicose veins, 514, 516, 517–518
Digitized cephalogram, 940–941
Dimpling effect, 608
Dingman procedure, 943
Diode lasers, 462
  hair removal, 886–888
  varicose veins, 534
Displaced chin implant, 955
Dissatisfied patient, 911–922
  character traits, 914
  communication, 913
  cosmetic junkie, 914
  dysmorphic body image, 913
  favorable result, 918

[Dissatisfied patient]
  minimizing, 911–912
  patient selection, 915–918
  prior surgery, 920–921
  with psychiatric condition, 914–915
  surgical addict, 914
  unfavorable result, 918–920
  unrealistic expectations, 913
Distant flaps, 383
Do no harm, 793
Donor strip in hair transplantation, 801
Doppler ultrasound of varicose veins, 513–514, 516–517
Double chin, 642
Drapes, in erbium skin remodeling, 144
Dual luerlock device, 246
Dynamic cooling, 174
Dynamic rhytides, Botox and, 314–315
Dynamic wrinkles, 314
Dysmorphic body image, of dissatisfied patient, 913
Dysport, 335
  storage, 335
Dysthyroid ophthalmopathy, 752

Ear, nerves in, 432
Earlobe, torn, presurgical photograph of, 860–861
Earlobe repair, 859–862
  historical development, 859
  postsurgical care, 861–862
  presurgical instructions, 859
  technique, 861
Earmuffs, erbium skin remodeling and, 144
Earth-based masks, 877
Ecchymosis, structural lipoaugmentation, 234
Ectropion
  in blepharoplasty, 743
  scarring, 158
Edema
  in blepharoplasty, 744
  laryngeal, in deep peel, 92
  laser hair removal, 891
  pulmonary, 622
Elasticity in the aging face, 25
Elective maxillofacial reconstruction, 939
Electrolysis, 873–876
  galvanic, 874
  needle insertion technique, 875–876
  needle selection, 875
  scarring, 876
  techniques, 874–875
Electrosurgical equipment, 14
Elevation test, 775
Emergency power, 10–11
EMLA, 419–421
  contraindications, 418
  depth, 418
  dosage in children, 418
EMLA cream
  erbium skin remodeling, 145
  laser resurfacing, 169
Employees
  orientation, 7
  professional development, 8
  rights, 7
  salary and benefits, 7
Endermologie, cellulite and, 873
Endoscopic brow rejuvenation, 775, 778–781
Epidermal cysts, 355–356
  anesthesia, 356
  hair transplantation, 825
  presurgical consultation, 355–356
  skin preparation, 356
Epidermal melasma, flashlamp-pumped pulsed dye lasers and, 493
Epidermis in erbium skin remodeling, 147
Epinephrine, 421–422
  beta-blockers, 453
  blepharoplasty, 727
  Cook Weekend Alternative to the Facelift, 644
  hair transplantation, 815
  infralash blepharoplasty, 759
  transconjunctival lower-lid blepharoplasty, 760
  tumescent lidocaine, 452–454
  tumescent liposuction, 547
EPTFE, 289, 324
  chemical structure, 290
  facial implants, 929
    complications, 935
  infection, 928
Equipment, 14–15
  actinic cheilitis, 864
  dermabrasion, 856
  earlobe repair, 859–860
  erbium skin remodeling, 142–144
  fat transplantation, 244
  flaps and grafts, 388, 393
  laser resurfacing, 857
  scars surgical excision, 849
  suction-assisted lipectomy, 578

[Equipment]
superficial chemical peels, 31
ultrasonic-assisted lipectomy, 578
Weekend Alternative to the Facelift, 644–645
Erbium laser machine, 142–143
Erbium skin remodeling, 123–162
acne scarring, 135–137, 150
birth marks, 140
with carbon dioxide laser resurfacing, 151
complications, 154–158
consultation, 127–135
drapes, 144
ear muffs, 144
EMLA cream, 145
equipment, 142–144
erbium laser machine, 142–143
exophytic skin lesions, 140, 151
eye protection, 144
face masks, 144
general anesthesia, 145
histology, 125–126
history, 123–124
immediate postsurgical care, 151–153
indications, 125–141
laser parameters, 146, 147
late postsurgical care, 153–154
local anesthetic infiltration, 145
neck lesions, 140
nerve blocks, 145
paperwork, 142
pigmentation, 137, 150–151
presurgical instructions, 141
presurgical skin care, 142
presurgical treatment, 141–144
scan pattern, 146
sedation, 144
smoke evacuation systems, 144
surgery room, 144
technique, 145–149
tumescent infiltration, 145
visual end points, 146–148
wrinkles, 127, 149–150
Erbium:YAG lasers, 164–165
vs. carbon dioxide lasers, 123–124
physical properties, 124
risks, 167
solar lentignes, 502–503
Erythema
erbium skin remodeling, 154–155
laser hair removal, 891
Ester anesthetics, 413–415
Etidocaine, 417
Excessive fat removal in blepharoplasty, 744
Excessive scarring in hair transplantation, 825
Exfoliative cheilitis, 863
Exophytic skin lesions, erbium skin remodeling and, 140, 151
Expanded polytetrafluoroethylene (ePTFE), 289, 324
chemical structure, 290
facial implants, 929
complications, 935
infection, 928
Expectations, unrealistic, 128, 132–133, 913
Extracting cannulas, 246
Extrafacial wrinkles, erbium skin remodeling and, 150
Extraocular muscle injury, blepharoplasty and, 765
Extrusion, soft-tissue augmentation and, 309
Eyebrows
aging, 679–681, 774
BTX-A, 343
configuration, 681
Spock, 341–342
Eyelids
blepharoplasty
lower. *See* Lower eyelids
upper. *See* Upper eyelid blepharoplasty
ectropion, 84
laser resurfacing, 170–171
lift, patient instructions for, 352
lower
elasticity, 752
hyperpigmentation, Q-switched ruby lasers and, 496
malposition, 764, 765
skin, 47
wrinkles, erbium skin remodeling and, 149
Eyes
patients', and laser safety, 166
protection in erbium skin remodeling, 144

Face
aging. *See* Aging face
assessment, 941
liposuction, 581–584
surgical anatomy
lower, 684–685
upper, 679–681

[Face]
tumescent liposuction, 555
Weekend Alternative to the Facelift, 646–647
Facelift, 699–701, 931
alloplastic chin and molar implants, 704
ancillary techniques, 701–707
anesthesia, 440
autologous fat injections, 703–704
camouflage cosmetics, 708
complications, 708–710
dermal strip grafts, 705–707
evaluation, 688–689
historical perspective, 685–686
informed consent, 690, 715, 717
laser resurfacing, 705
medical history, 716
microliposuction, 701–703
multivector analysis, 688–689
postsurgical care, 707–708
pregnancy test waiver, 718
presurgical instructions, 689–690
skin care, 708
twilight sedation, 691–692
video imaging, 686–688
weekend alternative, 555
Face masks, in erbium skin remodeling, 144
Facial aesthetics, 925–927
facial profile relationships, 926–927
transverse proportions, 926–927
vertical proportions, 926
Facial growth deformities, genioplasty and, 953
Facial hemiatrophy, fat transplantation and, 256, 257–258
Facial implants, 925–936
chin augmentation, 931–932
complications, 934–935
glabellar creases, 933–934
GORE, 929
historical development, 927
informed consent, 928
malar augmentation, 930–931
marionette lines, 933–934
nasolabial folds, 933–934
postsurgical instructions, 934
presurgical considerations, 933–934
presurgical planning, 927–928
types, 929
Facial nerve, frontal branch, 772
Facial rejuvenation, options, 296
Facial restructuring, examination, 940
Facial resurfacing, anesthesia in, 439
Facials, 877–888
Facial skeleton, evaluation, 940
Facial surgery
and body liposuction, 788–790
BTX-A, 348
Facial telangiectasias
argon lasers, 459
argon-pumped tunable dye lasers, 459
vs. PDLs, 466
cause, 462
copper lasers, 461
vs. PDLs, 466–467
KTP laser, 461
laser therapy, 462–467
PDLs, 463
photoderm VL, 462
Factitious cheilitis, 863
Familial multiple lipomatosis, 367
Famvir, erbium skin remodeling and, 152
Fascian, 322–323
Fat embolisms, 622
Fat removal in blepharoplasty
excessive, 744
incomplete, 744
Fat transfer adaptor, 249
Fat transfer, informed consent for, 240
Fat transplantation, 241–261
adipocyte processing, 250
collected fat treatment, 247–249
complications, 256–258
equipment, 244
historical development, 241–242, 319
indications, 251–256
informed consent, 263–264
lipoextraction, 244–245
patient instructions, 264–265
postsurgical care, 251
presurgical considerations, 242–243
presurgical instructions, 243
reimplantation, 249–251
technique, 244–251
Feathered hairline, diagram, 820
FeatherTouch laser system, 107
Fee schedule for sclerotherapy, 541, 543
Female breast liposuction, 587–590
Female pattern androgenetic alopecia (FPAA), 821–822
Fentanyl, 59
dermabrasion, 184–185
Fibrel, 323
Field block, 429

Filling substances
  future, 328–329
  human-derived, 269
  perfect, 316–318
Film, in photography, 903
Filtered flashlamp, hair removal and, 888
Filtration masks, laser safety, 166
Fire, laser safety and, 166
Fisher, Giorgio, 545
Fitzpatrick's classification of skin types, 38–42
Fitzpatrick Sun-Reactive Skin Type, 20–23
Flanks
  liposuction, 613–614
  tumescent liposuction, 559
Flaps
  postsurgical care, patient instructions for, 409
  random-pattern movements, 383
Flaps and grafts, 379–407
  anesthesia, 391–394
  disadvantages, 382
  equipment, 388, 393
  indications, 382
  informed consent, 387–388
  patient history, 379–380
  presurgical consultation, 380
  presurgical instruction, 380–386
  presurgical treatment, 380–386
  techniques, 394–404
    complications, 405–407
    full thickness skin graft, 394–397
    porcine xenografts, 401
    postsurgical care, 404–405
    split-thickness skin graft, 397–404
Flashlamp-pumped pulsed dye lasers, 462–464
  adverse effects, 463
  hypopigmentation, 533–534
  pigmented lesions, 483, 490–491
  varicose veins, 533–534
5-fluorouracil, dermabrasion in, 181
Focal mucinosis, 363–365
Folliculitis, hair transplantation and, 826
Foot drop, 622
Forehead
  aging, 679–681
  BTX-A, 339, 341
  rejuvenation algorithm, 783
  vascular supply, 681
  wrinkles, erbium skin remodeling and, 149–150
Fournier, Pierre, 242, 545
FPAA, 821–822
Frechet Scalp Extension, 826
Free flaps, 383
Freer elevator, 364
Frequency doubled Nd:YAG lasers and varicose veins, 531–532
Freud, Sigmund, 411
Frey's syndrome, 348
Frontal forelock design, 804
Frontalis muscle, 680, 772
  aging, 681
  BTX-A, 343
Front office, 9
Frosting, skin, 48–49
Frozen fat augmentation in structural lipoaugmentation, 235–237
FTSG, 394–397
Full thickness skin graft (FTSG), 394–397
Fungal infection
  scarring, 157

Galvanic electrolysis, 874
Gardner's syndrome, 367
General anesthesia
  erbium skin remodeling, 145
  liposuction, 573–635
Genioplasty for facial growth deformities, 953
Genital warts, copper vapor lasers and, 476
Gigli saw, 941
Glabella
  BTX-A, 335–336, 338–339, 343
  lines
    collagen implantation, 201
    facial implants, 933–934
    fat transplantation, 251, 260
Glandular cheilitis, 862–863
Globe perforation in blepharoplasty, 743
Glogau photoaging classification, 18–23, 39
Gloves, 13–14
Glycolic acid, 28
  protocols, 33
Glycolic acid peel
  nevi accentuation, 35
  proinflammatory hyperpigmentation, 35
Glycopyrolate, facelift surgery and, 691
Goggles, 13
GORE facial implants, 929
Gortex, 289–310, 323–352
  advantages, 289–291
  disadvantages, 289–291

[Gortex]
histopathology, 290
historical development, 289
new, 292
old, 291
patient instructions, 311
Grafts. *See also* Flaps and grafts
hair transplantation, 806–812
postsurgical care, patient instructions for, 409
terminology, 806
Granulomatous cheilitis, 863
Greater saphenous vein (GSV), 514
Green light lasers, for pigmented lesions, 491–494
Green light nonpulsed (quasicontinuous wave) lasers, for pigmented lesions, 494
Green tattoos, Q-switched Nd:YAG lasers and, 504
GSV, 514
Gustatory sweating, 348
Gynecomastia
liposuction, 584–587
tumescent liposuction, 557

Hair
anatomy, 881–883
growth, medications causing, 889
physiology, 881–883
removal, laser. *See* Laser hair removal
Hair bulb, 881
Hair follicles
growth phases, 881–883
units, 881
Hairline
design, in hair transplantation, 799–806
feathered, diagram, 820
zone, 819
Hair loss, facelift and, 710
Hair transplantation, 795–826
anesthesia, 815–817
bandages, 823–824
and blepharoplasty, 792
complications, 825–826
donor area excision, 817–819
donor strip, 801
grafts, 806–812
graftting, 823
hairline design, 799–806
hairs transplanted, 814
informed consent, 846
and neck liposuction, 792
[Hair transplantation]
photograph consent, 845–846
postsurgical care, 823–826
postsurgical instructions, 839–845
presurgical consultation, 796–812
presurgical instructions, 812–815, 836–838
recipient area, 819–823
scalp expansion, 828–830
and soft-tissue augmentation, 792
surgical technique, 817–823
Hands
fat transplantation, 256
senile lipoatrophy, 259
solar keratoses, 141
total body peel, 69–78
Hand washing, 13
Headache, BTX-A and, 341
Hemangiomas, PDLs and, 463
Hematoma, 677
AP, 529
in blepharoplasty, 743, 763
cyst removal, 360–361
facelift, 709
flaps and grafts, 406
Hemorrhage, 677
AP, 529
flaps and grafts, 382
hair transplantation, 825
laser resurfacing, 857
retrobulbar blepharoplasty, 762–764
Herpes infection, 135
scarring, 157
Herpes labialis, 102
Herpes simplex, 40, 65, 88, 168, 268
Hidrocystoma, 363
High-intensity pulsed light lasers for varicose veins, 534–537
Histrionic personality, in dissatisfied patient, 915
HIV, dermabrasion and, 180–181
Hour-Glass procedure, 559–560
Human collagen structure, 194
Human-derived filling substances, 269
Human placental collagen, 326
Hyaluronidase, facial resurfacing and, 439
Hydrocolloid masks, 877
Hydrocortisone, 87–88
Hydroquinones, 72
laser resurfacing, 173
Hylaform gel, 325
Hylan B gel, 325

Hyperhidrosis, BTX-A and, 348, 350
Hyperkeratotic warts, PDLs and, 476–477
Hyperpigmentation, 80–81
  carbon dioxide laser resurfacing, 112
  laser hair removal, 891
  PDLs, 464
Hyperthyroidism, epinephrine and, 454
Hypertrophic scars
  argon lasers, 459
  facelift, 709
  laser therapy, 470–473
  PDLs, 463, 472–473
  treatment, 86
  type V collagen, 472
Hypopigmentation, 80–82
  erbium skin remodeling, 155–156
  flashlamp-pumped pulsed dye lasers, 533–534
  laser hair removal, 891
  laser resurfacing, 173
Hypotension, clonidine and, 454–455

Ice, in blepharoplasty, 762
Ideal patient, 912
Illouz, Yves G., 545
Immune-mediated symptoms, 425
Implant removal, soft-tissue augmentation, 309
Incisor teeth, assessment, 940–941
Inclusion cysts, hair transplantation and, 825
Incompetent saphenous veins, 526
Incomplete fat removal in blepharoplasty, 744
Infection, 87–88
  bacterial, 157
  in blepharoplasty, 744
  carbon dioxide laser resurfacing, 112–113
  ePTFE, 928
  facelift, 708
  fungal, 157
  hair transplantation, 825
  herpes, 135, 157
  laser resurfacing, 167, 857
  peel complications, 87, 89
  scarring, 156, 157
  soft-tissue augmentation, 309
  staphylococcus, facelift and, 708
  wound, flaps and grafts and, 406–407
Inferior tarsal muscle, 722
Informed consent, 79
  AlloDerm, 288
  body peel, 77
[Informed consent]
  carbon dioxide laser resurfacing, 119
  chemical peel, 97
  cosmetic blepharoplasty, 756
  cosmetic laser blepharoplasty, 353, 767, 769
  facelift, 690, 715, 717
  facial implants, 928
  fat transplantation, 263–264
  flaps and grafts, 387–388
  hair transplantation, 846
  isolagen, 287
  laser hair removal, 894
  laser resurfacing, 177
  lipoaugmentation, 240
  orthognathic surgery, 958–960
  photography, 907, 910
  sclerotherapy, 543
  soft-tissue augmentation, 271–272
  structural lipoaugmentation, 234–235
  TCA, 77
  varicose veins, 542
  Weekend Alternative to the Facelift, 653–656
Infralash blepharoplasty, 758–760
  anesthesia, 759
  incision, 759–760
  skin redraping, 760
  Webster suture, 760
Infraorbital nerves
  midpupillary line, 433
  nerve block, 435, 436, 438
  sensory changes, 950
Infrared light lasers, for pigmented lesions, 491
Infundibulum, 881
Injectable anesthetics, 412
Instruments, in blepharoplasty, 725–727
Internal ultrasonic liposuction, tumescent, 552
Intravenous sedation in erbium skin remodeling, 145
Iodine, 13
Iontophoresis, 420–421
Island pedicle flaps, 383, 386
Isolagen, 269, 272–276, 319–320
  informed consent, 287
Isthmus, 881

Jaw, underdeveloped, 944
Jawline, aging, surgical anatomy, 684–685
Jessner's solution, 29, 43

Jessner's-TCA peel procedure, 48–49
Job descriptions, 6
Johnnie-Lok device, 248
Jowls
  surgical anatomy, aging and, 684–685
  tumescent liposuction, 553–555
  Weekend Alternative to the Facelift, 646–647

Kaposi's sarcoma, argon lasers and, 459
Keith needle, 300–302
Keloids
  argon lasers, 459
  laser resurfacing, 169
  laser therapy, 470–473
  PDLs, 463, 472–473
Keratoconjunctivitis sicca, blepharoplasty and, 743, 762
Kick buckets, 15
Klein, Jeffrey A., 545
Klein infiltrating cannula, 245
Kligman formula, in erbium skin remodeling, 154
Koken Atelocollagen, 208, 320
Krypton lasers, 457, 461, 467–469
Krypton triphosphate (KTP) lasers, 461, 467–469
  blepharoplasty, 740–741
  varicose veins, 531–532

Labial incompetence, facial characteristics, 954
Labile affect, in dissatisfied patient, 915
Labiomental crease, 685
Laboratory, 11
Lacrimal gland, 722
Lancet point needle, 250
Laryngeal edema, in deep peel, 92
Laser blepharoplasty, 739–741
  carbon dioxide laser, 739–740
  complications, 741
  KTP laser, 740–741
  ND:YAG laser, 740–741
  patient instructions, 352, 768
  safety, 742
Laser hair removal, 498–499, 881–892
  complications, 890–891
  informed consent, 894
  lasers and light sources, 882, 884–888
  patient history, 889
  patient instructions, 895
  physical examination, 889
[Laser hair removal]
  physics, 883–884
  postsurgical care, 890–891
  presurgical considerations, 889–890
  timing, 884
  treatment guidelines, 890
Laser protocol, in carbon dioxide laser resurfacing, 105–108
Laser resurfacing, 163–174, 856–859
  anesthesia, 169
  BTX-A, 347–348
  vs. chemical peeling, 163–164
  clinical endpoints, 170
  complications, 857–859
  vs. dermabrasion, 163–164
  equipment, 857
  eyelids, 170–171
  facelift, 705
  future, 173–174
  indications, 166–168
  informed consent, 177
  laser safety, 166
  postsurgical care, 171–173, 857
  presurgical considerations, 856–857
  presurgical instructions, 857
  presurgical patient evaluation, 168–169
  risks, 166–168
  skin interaction, 164–166
  techniques, 169–171, 857
  troubleshooting, 171–173
Lasers
  safety, 166
  Weekend Alternative to the Facelift, 645
Lateral canthal tendons, 722
Lateral subdermic venous system (LSVS), 514
Leg telangiectasias, laser therapy for, 530, 533
Lemperle, Gottfried, 321
Lens, 899
Lesser saphenous vein (LSV), 514
Levator apneurosis, Asian eye and, 728–729
Levator labii, BTX-A and, 346
Levator labii superioris, 681
Levator labii superioris alaque nasi, 681
Liability in photography, 907
Lidocaine, 415
  AP, 527
  cosmetic blepharoplasty, 757
  hair transplantation, 815
  infralash blepharoplasty, 759
  laser resurfacing, 169

[Lidocaine]
toxicity, 422
transconjunctival lower-lid blepharoplasty, 760
tumescent. *See* Tumescent lidocaine
tumescent liposuction, 547
Weekend Alternative to the Facelift, 644
Lighting, 10
Lip, upper, wrinkles in, 345
Lip augmentation
AlloDerm, 283
bovine collagen, 205–207
Dermalogen, 281–282
Lipoaugmentation, informed consent for, 240
Lipoextraction, in fat transplantation, 244–245
Lipomas, 366
diagnosis, 368
histopathology, 368
surgery, 368–371
distant incision technique, 369–370
excision, 370
incision technique, 369
liposuction, 370–371
presurgical evaluation, 368–369
tumescent liposuction, 565
types, 366
Liposuction, 370–371
abdomen, 600–604
contouring, 669
evaluation, 600
marking, 601–602
surgery, 601–604
arm, 590–600
evaluation, 590–592
marking, 593
surgery, 593–600
blood loss, 579
body, and facial surgery, 788–790
cannulas, 577–578, 580
face and neck, 581–584
evaluation, 581
marking, 581
surgery, 581–584
female breast, 587–590
evaluation, 587
marking, 587–588
surgery, 587–590
flanks and back, 613–614
general anesthesia, 573–635
gynecomastia, 584–587
evaluation, 584–585
[Liposuction]
marking, 584–585
surgery, 584–587
historical development, 573–574
internal ultrasonic tumescent liposuction, 552
lower extremity, 615–621
evaluation, 615–616
marking, 616–617
surgery, 616–621
male breast, 584–587
marking, 576
multiple procedures, 609–612
neck, in hair transplantation, 792
patient evaluation, 574–577
patient positioning, 577
photography, 576
postsurgical care, 579–580
presurgical counseling, 575
presurgical planning, 576
surgical preparation, 576
surgical technique, 577–579
tumescent. *See* Tumescent liposuction
tumescent solution, 577
waistline cincture, 605–608
Lips
fat transplantation, 251
SoftForm, 298
Local anesthesia
delivery methods, 428–429
historical development, 411
Local anesthetics
additives, 421–422
adjuncts, 427–428
allergic constituents, alternatives to, 427
allergy, skin testing, 426
classification, 411–412
contraindications, 422–423
drug interactions, 424
esters, 413–415
infiltration, in erbium skin remodeling, 145
injectable, 412
mechanism of action, 412–413
metabolism, 413
pharmacology, 411–412
presurgical considerations, 422–427
toxicity, 425, 427
Local flaps, 383
Loller, Carl, 411

Long Face Syndrome, 947–950
facial characteristics, 951–952
Long-pulse alexandrite laser, for hair removal, 886
Long-pulse infrared alexandrite laser, for varicose veins, 534
Long-pulse ruby laser, for hair removal, 884–886
Lower extremity liposuction, 615–621
Lower eyelid blepharoplasty, transconjunctival. *See* transconjunctival lower eyelid blepharoplasty
Lower eyelids
blepharoplasty, 730–739
complications, 734, 738
fat repositioning, 736–739
malposition, 764, 765
patient selection, 732
technique, 758–762
elasticity, 752
hyperpigmentation, Q-switched ruby lasers and, 496
orbicularis hypertrophy, BTX-A and, 345
Lower face, aging, surgical anatomy, 684–685
Lower facelift, 699–701
Luer Lok extraction cannula, 226
Lupus profundus, fat transplantation and, 253, 255–256
Lymphatic drainage, cellulite, 872–873

Madelung's disease, 366
Maintenance and repair, 11
Makeup, 132
Malar augmentation
botox, 349
presurgical considerations, 930–931
surgical procedure, 931
Male breast liposuction, 584–587
Male pattern baldness (MPB), 795–800
Norwood classification, 797–798
Mandibular asymmetry, 944–946
correction, 946
Mandibular body, excessive growth, 943
Mandibular dental arch, 941
Mandibular prognathism
facial characteristics, 942
subcondylar osteotomy, 941–943
Mandibular rami
external approach, 944
vertical oblique osteotomy, 943
Mandibular retrognathia, facial characteristics, 945
Manual dermabrasion, 788
Marionette lines
facial implants, 933–934
Gortex, 324
Marzola Lateral Lift, 829
Masks, 13
Maxillary retrognathia, 947
facial characteristics, 948
Mayo stands, 14, 31
Medazolam, dermabrasion, 184–185
Medial canthal tendon, 722
Median nerve compression, acute, 622
Medical history
blepharoplasty, 723
cosmetic blepharoplasty, 750
facelift, 716
Weekend Alternative to the Facelift, 656–659
Medical photography specialists, 908
Medication errors, tumescent lidocaine and, 451–452
Medications causing hair growth, 889
Medium chemical peels, 42–53, 786
agents, 42–53
indications, 38–42
patient selection, 38–42
postsurgical care, 51
presurgical care, 43
sedation, 43
TCA, 43–44
Melanosomes, Q-switched ruby lasers and, 489–490
Melasma, Q-switched ruby lasers and, 496, 498
Melolabial furrow, fat transplantation and, 251, 260
Mentalis, BTX-A and, 346
Mental nerves
midpupillary line, 433
nerve block, 437, 438–439
Meperidine, in alopecia reduction, 831
Meperidine, dermabrasion and, 184–185
Mepivacaine, 415
Methylxanthine, cellulite and, 872
Micrografting, 807
Microlipoinjection, 242
Microliposuction in facelift, 701–703
Midazolam, 59
facelift surgery, 691
tumescent liposuction, 547

Midface
augmentation, complications, 934
lift, 696–699
aging, surgical anatomy, 681–684
Midline ellipse, 827
Midpapillary dermis, in erbium skin remodeling, 148
Milia, 89, 362
in blepharoplasty, 745
carbon dioxide laser resurfacing, 112
laser resurfacing, 173
Mini-browlift, 693–696
Minoxidil and female pattern androgenetic alopecia, 821
Mirror II imaging software, 686
Mission statement, 5
Moderate photoaging skin, in medicum chemical peel, 51, 55
Modified Bitemporal Flap, 829
Modified crescent abdominal tuck, in abdominal contouring, 669–670
Modified Klein solution in tumescent anesthesia, 225
Moisturizers
erbium skin remodeling, 153
postsurgical skin care, 878–879
Moist wound healing, in laser resurfacing, 171
Molar implants, in facelift, 704
Monitors, 15
tumescent liposuction, 550–551
Monoamine oxidase inhibitors, epinephrine, 454
Mood disorder, in dissatisfied patient, 915
Morphea, in fat transplantation, 253, 255–256
Mouth wrinkles, erbium skin remodeling of, 150
MPB (Male pattern baldness), 795–800
Norwood classification, 797–798
Mucoceles, 365–366
Mucoid cysts, 363–365
Mucous cysts, 363–366
Mucus retention cysts, 365–366
Muller, Robert, 525
Muller hook, 526
Muller's muscle, stimulation of, 339
Multiple lipomas, 366, 367
Multivector face/neck/brow lift
multidirectional forces of pull, 692
surgical technique, 692–701
topographical markings, 693
Musculature changes in the aging face, 24
Myxoid cysts, and carbon dioxide laser vaporization, 364–365
Myxomatous cysts, 363–365

Narcissism, in dissatisfied patient, 914
Nasalis, BTX-A and, 345
Nasion, aging, 679–681
Nasolabial lines
BTX-A, 345
collagen implantation, 202–203, 274–275, 278
expanded polytetrafluorethylene, 324
facial implants, 933–934
fat transplantation, 251
Gortex, 297
Nasolabial transposition flaps, 390–391
Nd:YAG lasers, 173–174, 470
blepharoplasty, 740–741
frequency doubled, varicose veins and, 531–532
Q-switched, 499–509
varicose veins, 531
Neck
aging, surgical anatomy, 684–685
lesions, erbium skin remodeling and, 140
lift, 699–701
liposuction, 581–584
and hair transplantation, 792
total body peel, 69–78
tumescent liposuction, 553–555
Weekend Alternative to the Facelift, 646–647
Necrosis, flaps and grafts, 406
Necrotizing fasciitis, 622
Neo-synephrine, 339
Nerve blocks, 429–435
erbium skin remodeling, 145
Nerves
ear, 432
nose, 431
palsy, in facelift, 709–710
scalp, 430
Neurotic, as dissatisfied patient, 915
Nevi, Q-switched alexandrite lasers vs. Q-switched Nd:YAG lasers, 497–498
Nevus of Ito, Q-switched ruby lasers and, 495
Nevus of Ota
Q-switched Nd:YAG lasers, 501–502
Q-switched Nd:YAG lasers, 501
Q-switched ruby lasers, 495–497

New Botox, 335
Nikon cameras, sources, 908
Nikon N70 camera, 898
Nitrous oxide, 428
Nongenital warts, carbon dioxide lasers and, 476
Nordstrom suture, 826
Norwood classification, male pattern baldness, 797–798
Nose, nerves, 431

Obsessive-compulsive disorder, in dissatisfied patient, 915
Obwegesser bilateral sagittal osteotomy, 944
Oculinum, 335
Oesch's hook, 526
Office setup, 10
Office surgical facilities, surgical suite design, 2
Open brow rejuvenation, 777–778
Operating tables, 14
Opsite, in erbium skin remodeling, 152
Oral and maxillofacial surgery
- postdischarge instructions, 956
- postsurgical pain, 956

Oral antibiotics, in erbium skin remodeling, 152
Oral antiviral medications, in erbium skin remodeling, 152
Oral comissures, fat transplantation and, 251
Oral painkillers, in erbium skin remodeling, 153
Oral retinoids, scarring, 156
Oral rhytides, 47, 50
Oral steroids, in erbium skin remodeling, 153
Orbital hemorrhage in blepharoplasty, 742
Orbital septum in blepharoplasty, 733, 737
Orentriech, Norman, 328
Orthognathic surgery, informed consent for, 958–960
Outdoors, 132

Painkillers, in erbium skin remodeling, 153
Palmar/plantar hyperhidrosis, BTX-A and, 350
Palmar warts, PDLs and, 477
Paperwork, in erbium skin remodeling, 142
Papillary dermis, erbium skin remodeling and, 147
Papillary-reticular dermal junction, erbium skin remodeling and, 148
Paraffin, 315
Paralysis, BTX-A and, 354
Parotid cyst, facelift and, 710
Patient. *See also* Dissatisfied patient
- carbon dioxide laser resurfacing, 120
- oral and maxillofacial surgery, 956

Patient flow, 9
Patient history, laser hair removal, 889
Patient instructions
- actinic cheilitis, 864
- blepharoplasty, 770
- carbon dioxide laser resurfacing, 102–104, 120
- chemical peels, 97
- cosmetic blepharoplasty, 755–756
- dermabrasion, 96, 856
- earlobe repair, 859
- erbium skin remodeling, 141
- facelift, 689–690
- facial implants, 934
- fat transplantation, 243, 264–265
- flap postsurgical care, 409
- flaps and grafts, 380–386
- gortex, 311
- graft postsurgical care, 409
- hair transplantation, 812–815, 839–845
- laser blepharoplasty, 352, 768
- laser hair removal, 895
- laser resurfacing, 857
- oral and maxillofacial surgery, 956
- post-skin chemical peels, 97–98
- scars surgical excision, 849
- sclerotherapy, 544
- soft-tissue augmentation, 296, 299
- structural lipoaugmentation, 222–224
- superficial chemical peels, 30, 31
- TCA, 78
- Total Body Peel, 70
- Weekend Alternative to the Facelift, 643–644
- zyderm collagen, 211–219
- zyplast collagen, 211–219

PDLs. *See* Pulsed dye lasers
Peel, Total Body, 69–78
- complications, 72
- history, 70
- materials, 71
- postsurgical considerations, 72
- presurgical care, 70
- presurgical instructions, 70
- procedure, 71–72

Peripheral nerve block, flaps and grafts, 391–392
Periungual warts
carbon dioxide lasers, 476
PDLs, 476–477
Perleche, 862
Permacol, 326
Persistent erythema
deep chemical peels, 64–66
peel complications, 87–88
Personnel manual, 6
Phenol concentration limitation, 54
Phenothiazines, epinephrine, 454
Photoaging of aging face, 18–20
Photoderm VL, 457, 462, 534–536
Photograph consent in hair transplantation, 845–846
Photographic equipment, sources, 908–909
Photographic suite setup, 902
Photography, 897–910
archiving, 904
background, 903–904
cameras, 897–899, 905
setting, 900
cosmetic blepharoplasty, 753
digital, 906–907
exposure, 899–901
film, 903
informed consent, 907, 910
lens, 899
liability, 907
lighting, 901–902
record keeping, 904
view standardization, 903
Photophobia, 344
Photothermolysis, 457
selective, 883
Phototyping index, 41
Physical examination
blepharoplasty, 724
cosmetic blepharoplasty, 751–753
laser hair removal, 889
Picture quality information exchange (PQIE), 905
Pigmentary changes, 80–83
Pigmentary dyschromias, medicum chemical peel and, 51, 56
Pigmentary system, aging face and, 20–22
Pigmentation, erbium skin remodeling and, 137, 150–151, 155
Pigmented lesions
flashlamp-pumped pulsed dye lasers, 490–491
laser treatment, 489–500
Pigment gel forte, in erbium skin remodeling, 154, 155
Pilar cysts, 361
Placental collagen, human, 326
Plantar warts
carbon dioxide lasers, 476
PDLs, 476–477
Plasma cell cheilitis, 863
Platysma, BTX-A and, 347
Platysma muscle, 684
Pleomorphic lipomas, 368
Plethysmography of varicose veins, 514, 516
Poikiloderma of Civatte
argon-pumped tunable dye lasers, 459
PDLs, 469–470
Polaroid camera, 897–899
Policanol, 522–523
Polyethylene facial implants, 929
complications, 935
Polytetrafluoroethylene. *See* Expanded polytetrafluoroethylene (ePTFE)
Porcine xenografts, 401
Port wine stains
argon lasers, 459
argon-pumped tunable dye lasers, 459–460
PDLs, 463, 464
photoderm VL, 462
Postdischarge instructions for oral and maxillofacial surgery, 956
Posterior gluteal fold asymmetry, 635
Postoperative instruction sheet for carbon dioxide laser resurfacing, 120
Postsclerosis pigmentation, 530
Post-skin chemical peels, patient instructions, 97–98
Postsurgical care
abdominal contouring, 674–677
actinic cheilitis, 866–867
blepharoplasty, 742–743, 762
brow rejuvenation, 781
dermabrasion, 856
earlobe repair, 861–862
erbium skin remodeling, 151–153
facelift, 707–708
fat transplantation, 251
flaps, patient instructions, 409
grafts, patient instructions, 409

[Postsurgical care]
  hair transplantation, 823–826
  laser hair removal, 890–891
  laser resurfacing, 171–173, 857
  liposuction, 579–580
  medium chemical peels, 51
  structural lipoaugmentation, 233–234
  superficial chemical peels, 33–34
  tumescent liposuction, 566
Postsurgical instructions
  facial implants, 934
  hair transplantation, 839–845
Potassium titanyl phosphate (KTP) lasers, 457
PQIE, 905
Pregnancy test waiver, in facelift, 718
Preoperative checklist for carbon dioxide laser resurfacing, 121
Preoperative instructions for structural lipoaugmentation, 222–224
Preoperative skin preparation for carbon dioxide laser resurfacing, 104–105
Preparatory solutions, 12–13
Presurgical care
  medium chemical peels, 43
  superficial chemical peels, 29–31
  Total Body Peel, 70
Presurgical instructions
  actinic cheilitis, 864
  dermabrasion, 856
  earlobe repair, 859
  erbium skin remodeling, 141
  facelift surgery, 689–690
  fat transplantation, 243
  flaps and grafts, 380–386
  hair transplantation, 812–815, 836–839
  laser resurfacing, 857
  scars surgical excision, 849
  soft-tissue augmentation, 296, 299
  superficial chemical peels, 30, 31
  Total Body Peel, 70
  Weekend Alternative to the Facelift, 643–644
Presurgical skin care in erbium skin remodeling, 142
Presurgical treatment
  erbium skin remodeling, 141–144
  flaps and grafts, 380–386
Prilocaine, 415
Primum non nocere, 793
Problem patient, 912–914
Procaine, 413
Procerus muscle, 680, 772
Profil, 326
Prognathic mandible, 941
Proliferating trichilemmal tumor, 361
Promethazine in tumescent liposuction, 547
Prominent mandible, surgical correction of, 941
Proparacaine
  infralash blepharoplasty, 759
  transconjunctival lower-lid blepharoplasty, 760
Propofol
  cosmetic blepharoplasty, 756–757
  facelift surgery, 691
Protective eyewear, laser safety, 166
Pruritus, as peel complications, 87–88
Pseudogynecomastia, tumescent liposuction of, 557
Psychotic, as dissatisfied patient, 915
PTFE. *See* Expanded polytetrafluoroethylene (ePTFE)
Ptosis, 694
  in blepharoplasty, 743–744
  BTX-A, 339
Pulmonary edema, 622
Pulsed dye lasers (PDLs), 470
  actinic poikiloderma, 471
  vs. argon-pumped tunable dye lasers, facial telangiectasias, 466
  cherry angiomas, 469
  copper vasor lasers, facial telangiectasias and, 466–467
  flashlamp-pumped. *See* Flashlamp-pumped pulsed dye lasers
  scars, 471–472
  striae, 475
  tattoos, 504–505
  vascular lesions, 174
  warts, 476–478
Pulsed lasers vs. continuous wave lasers, pigmented lesions, 491
Pyogenic granulomas
  argon lasers, 459, 569
  copper lasers, 461, 469
  PDLs, 463, 469

Q-switched alexandrite lasers
  vs. Q-switched Nd:YAG lasers for nevi, 497–498
  solar lentignes, 500
  tattoos, 503, 506

Q-switched Nd:YAG lasers, 499–500
  nevus of Ota, 501–502
  vs. Q-switched alexandrite lasers for nevi, 497–498
  vs. Q-switched ruby lasers for tattoos, 505
  solar lentignes, 492–494
  tattoos, 503–509
Q-switched ruby lasers
  congenital nevus, 499
  melanosomes, 489–490
  pigmented lesions, 494–498
  vs. Q-switched Nd:YAG lasers for tattoos, 505
  tattoos, 500–501, 503, 505
Quality improvement, 8–9
Quasicontinuous wave lasers, 457
Questionnaire, for patient selection, 103

Ramelet's hook, 526
Reassurance, of dissatisfied patient, 917
Recombinant human collagen, 326
Recovery time, 129
Rectus plication, abdominal contouring, 669
Red light lasers for pigmented lesions, 491, 494
Red tattoos, Q-switched Nd:YAG lasers and, 504, 508
Re-epithelialization, in deep chemical peels, 64
Relaxed skin tension lines (RSTL), 380, 847
Resoplast, 208, 321, 326
Restrooms, 11
Restylane, 326–327
Resurfacing
  and blepharoplasty, 788
  carbon dioxide laser. *See* Carbon dioxide laser resurfacing
  facial anesthesia, 439
  laser. *See* Laser resurfacing
  and rhytidectomy, 788
  techniques, combining, 785–788
Reticular veins, diagnosis of, 513–522
Retinoic acid, 72
Retinoids, scarring, 156
Retrobulbar hemorrhage, blepharoplasty and, 762–764
Retrogenia, facial characteristics, 954
Rhinophyme, dermabrasion, 187
Rhytidectomy and resurfacing, 788
Rhytides
  carbon dioxide laser resurfacing, 111
  carbon dioxide *vs.* erbium:YAG laser, 167, 170
[Rhytides]
  dynamic, Botox and, 314–315
  expanded polytetrafluorethylene, 324
  fat transplantation, 251
  Gortex, 324
  oral, 47, 50
Ring block, 429
Risk management, 8–9
  dissatisfied patient, 920
Ropivocaine, 145
Rosacea, 40
  argon-pumped tunable dye lasers, 459, 467
  copper vasor lasers, 467
  KTP lasers, 467
  PDLs, 463
Rotation flaps, 383–384, 388–389
Rothmund-Thomson syndrome, 470
Relaxed skin tension lines, 380, 847
Ruby lasers, 498–499

Sacral scar, presurgical photograph, 852–853
Salary, 7
Salivary glands, mucous cysts and, 365–366
SAM, 323. *See also* Gortex
  histopathology, 291
  multistranded implants, 296
  single stranded implants, 295
Saphenopopliteal junctions, 526
Scalp
  expansion, hair transplantation and, 828–830
  extender, 827
  nerves, 430
  reduction patterns, 828
Scars, 83–87
  argon lasers, 459
  bacterial infection, 157
  carbon dioxide lasers, 470
  contact dermatitis, 157–158
  cyst removal, 360
  ectropion, 158
  electrolysis, 876
  erbium skin remodeling, 156–157
  excessive, hair transplantation and, 825
  facelift, 709
  fungal infection, 157
  laser therapy, 470–473
  PDL, 471–472
  peel complications, 83–87
  revision, 847–849
    historical development, 848
    presurgical considerations, 849

[Scars]
risk factors, 86
surgical excision, 849–856
anesthesia, 850
equipment, 849
paperwork, 849
postsurgical care, 853–856
presurgical instructions, 849
technique, 850–853
Schizophrenia, in dissatisfied patient, 915
Sclerodex, Dextrose, 522–523
Sclerolaser, 464
Sclerolaser Plus, 464
Sclerosing solutions, 522–523
Sclerotherapy
fee schedule, 541, 543
informed consent, 543
patient instructions, 544
telangiectasias, 522–524
varicose veins, 519–522
Sebaceous cysts, 361
Sebaceum, dermabrasion and, 183
Second opinion, for dissatisfied patient, 920
Sedation. *See also* Anesthesia
AP, 527
deep chemical peels, 52–53
erbium skin remodeling, 144
intravenous, in erbium skin remodeling, 145
twilight, in facelift surgery, 691–692
Selective photothermolysis, 883
Senile lipoatrophy
cheeks, 252
hands, 259
Sensory zones, 433
Seromas, 567, 631, 677
cyst removal, 360–361
Short Face Syndrome, 953
Signed written orders for tumescent lidocaine, 451
Silicone, 327–328
facial implants, 929
complications, 934–935
SilkTouch, 107, 165
Single lens reflex camera, 897
Skeletal malocclusions, 939, 946
Skin, frosting, 48–49
Skin care
facelift, 708
postsurgical, 878–879
superficial chemical peels, 30
Skin interaction in laser resurfacing, 164–166
Skin kneading, cellulite and, 872–873
Skin lightening gel, in erbium skin remodeling, 154
Skin testing, allergy and local anesthetics, 426
Slave flash system, sources, 908
Slit grafting, 807
SMAS, 380, 680–681
Smoke evacuation systems, in erbium skin remodeling, 144
Smoker's lines. *See* Rhytides
Smoking, 132
Snap test, 752
Sodium tetradecyl sulfate, 522–523
SoftForm, 292, 294, 295, 320
implantation, 304–305
device, 305
SoftLight system of hair removal, 888
Soft-tissue augmentation, 267–284, 790
anesthesia, 299
complications, 309
consultation, 295–299
and hair transplantation, 792
histopathology, 293
historical development of, 315–316
indications, 270, 293–294
informed consent, 271–272
injection techniques, 270
patient selection, 270
postsurgical period, 305–309
preoperative consultation, 271
presurgical considerations, 268–271
presurgical instructions, 296, 299
procedure, 299–305
Solar keratoses on the hand, 141
Solar lentignes
carbon dioxide lasers, 500
Er:YAG lasers, 502–503
Q-switched alexandrite lasers, 500
Q-switched Nd:YAG laser, 492–494
Q-switched ruby lasers, 495, 497
Solitary lipomas, 366
Space planning, surgical suite design, 9–10
Spasm of frontalis, BTX-A and, 341
Spider angiomas
copper bromide/copper vapor lasers, 467–469
copper lasers, 461
krypton lasers, 467–469
KTP lasers, 467–469

Spindle cell lipomas, 368
Split-thickness skin graft (STSG), 397–404
Spock eyebrow, 341–342
Staphylococcus infection, in facelift, 708
Static wrinkles, 314
Steatocystoma multiplex, 363
Sterilization, 12
Steroids, in erbium skin remodeling, 153
Storage, 11
Stretch marks, laser therapy for, 474–475
Striae distensae, laser therapy and, 474–475
Structural lipoaugmentation, 221–237
 cheek infiltration, 231
 complications, 234–235
 extraction technique, 224–226
 fat preparation, 227–228
 forehead infiltration, 232–233
 frozen fat augmentation, 235–237
 indications, 222
 informed consent, 234–235
 longevity, 235
 mandibular infiltration, 230–231
 patient selection, 222
 perioral infiltration, 229
 periorbital infiltration, 231–232
 postsurgical care, 233–234
 preoperative instructions, 222–224
 recipient site
 anesthesia, 226–227
 preparation, 226
 transplantation technique, 228–229
STSG, 397–404
Subcision, 320
Subcondylar osteotomy and mandibular prognathism, 941–942
Subcutaneous augmentation material (SAM), 323. *See also* Gortex
 histopathology, 291
 multistranded implants, 296
 single stranded implants, 295
Subcutaneous fat loss in the aging face, 22–24
Submalor augmentation, 931
Submental scar, presurgical photograph, 851–852
Suction-assisted lipectomy (SAL), 575. *See also* Liposuction
 complications, 622–635
 equipment, 578
Suction lipectomy, 574
Sufentanyl, in cosmetic blepharoplasty, 756–757
Sunscreens
 erbium skin remodeling, 153
 postsurgical skin care, 879
Superficial chemical peels, 27–35, 786
 complications, 34–35
 consultation, 29–31
 depth
  classification, 28
  determination, 28
 equipment, 31
 postsurgical care, 33–34
 presurgical care, 29–31
 presurgical instructions, 30, 31
 resurfacing agents, 29
 skin care regimen, 30
 technique, 31–33
Superficial mimetic muscles, 681
Superficial musculoaponeurotic system (SMAS), 380, 680–681
Superficial resurfacing agents, 29
Supraorbital nerve block, 434, 435, 437
Supraorbital nerves
 midpupillary line, 433
 nerve block, 434
Supraorbital sensory nerves, 772
Supratrochlear nerve block, 434
Supratrochlear sensory nerves, 772
Surgery room for erbium skin remodeling, 144
Surgical addict, as dissatisfied patient, 914
Surgical attire, 13
Surgical instrumentation for abdominal contouring, 667
Surgical lift, 685
Surgical scars, dermabrasion and, 181, 183
Surgical scrub, 13
Surgical scrub suites, 13
Surgical site preparation, 12
Surgical suites, 1–15
 AAAHC accreditation, 2–5
 administration and staffing, 5–9
 ambulatory surgery centers, 1–2
 design, 9–15
  equipment, 14–15
  space planning, 9–10
  surgical practices, 12–14
 office surgical facilities, 2
 size, 10
SurgiPulse, 165
Synechiae, scarring and, 158
Synovial cysts, 363–365
Syringomas, dermabrasion and, 183

TAC, 419
Tattoos
  dermabrasion, 181, 186
  green, 504
  laser therapy, 500–502
  Q-switched ruby lasers vs. Q-switched Nd:YAG lasers, 505
  Q-switched Nd:YAG lasers, 504, 508
  red, 504, 508
  yellow, 504
TCA, 28
  after-care instructions, 78
  deep chemical peels, 52–53
  informed consent, 77
  medium chemical peels, 43–44
Tegaderm, erbium skin remodeling and, 152
Telangiectasias
  ankle, laser therapy for, 532
  facial. *See* Facial telangiectasias
  leg, laser therapy for, 530
  sclerotherapy, 522–524
  varicose veins, 516
Telangiectatic matting, 530
Temporal lift, 696
Tetracaine, 413, 415
  blepharoplasty, 727
Tetracaine-adrenaline-cocaine (TAC), 419
Thighs, tumescent liposuction of, 562–565
Topical anesthetics, 417–419
Topical therapy, in erbium skin remodeling, 152
Topical Vitamin C, in erbium skin remodeling, 154
Torn earlobe, presurgical photograph, 860–861
Total strip collection, 816
Touch laser system, 107
Toxic shock syndrome, 622
Transconjunctival blepharoplasty, 731–736
  and carbon dioxide resurfacing, 792–793
  presurgical, 722
Transconjunctival lower eyelid blepharoplasty, 760–762
  anesthesia, 760
  incision, 760–762
  marking, 760
Transcutaneous blepharoplasty, 730
Transillumination of varicose veins, 519–521
Transposition flaps, 384–385
Tretinoin, dermabrasion and, 188
Tretinoin, laser resurfacing and, 173
Triamcinolone acetonide, tumescent liposuction and, 547
Trichilemmal cysts, 361
Trichloroacetic acid (TCA), 28
  after-care instructions, 78
  deep chemical peels, 52–53
  informed consent, 77
  medium chemical peels, 43–44
Trichoepitheliomas, dermabrasion and, 184–185
Tricyclic antidepressants, epinephrine, 454
Triple Flap Procedure, 826
TruPulse laser, 107–108
Tumescent anesthesia, 244–245, 547–549
  historical development, 662
  modified Klein solution, 225
Tumescent infiltration, in erbium skin remodeling, 145
Tumescent lidocaine
  absorption, 445–446
    delay, 445
  bioavailability, 447–448
  bulk spread, 444
  clonidine, 455
  diffusion, 445
  dilution, 446
    definitions, 450
  elimination, 447
  epinephrine, 452–454
  formulation, 449–450
  irrational dosage limits, 444
  medication errors, 451–452
  peak concentration, 446
  pharmacokinetics, 443–452
  postsurgical sedatives, 452
  safe dosage, 448
  safety, 443
  sentinel cases, 448–449
  signed written orders, 451
  slow-release, 445
  toxicity, 446
  vascularity, 446
  vasoconstriction, 447
Tumescent liposculpture, Weekend Alternative to the Facelift, 644–645
  lower face, jowls, neck, 646–647
Tumescent liposuction, 545–567
  abdomen, 559–561
  anesthesia, 547–549
  ankles, 565
  arms, 556
  banana roll, 562

[Tumescent liposuction]
bra fat, 557
buffalo hump, 558
calves, 565
complications, 567
face, 555
fat collection, 565
flanks, 559
follow-up care, 566
gynecomastia, 557
internal ultrasonic liposuction, 552
lipomas, 565
neck and jowls, 553–555
pharmacology, 443–455
postsurgical care, 566
postsurgical procedure, 565–567
presurgical consultation, 545–546
presurgical procedure, 546–547
pseudogynecomastia, 557
surgical procedure, 547–553
thighs, 562–565
violin deformity, 561–562
Tumescent solution
hair transplantation, 815
Weekend Alternative to the Facelift, 644
"Turkey neck," 642
Twilight sedation, for facelift surgery, 691–692
Tylenol, in erbium skin remodeling, 153
Type IV delayed hypersensitivity, 425
Type V collagen for hypertrophic scars, 472

UAL, 578
complications, 622–635
equipment, 578
Ultrapulse, 106–107, 165
Ultrasonic-assisted lipectomy (UAL), 578
complications, 622–635
equipment, 578
Ultrasonic machine for tumescent liposuction, 550
Ultrasound, Weekend Alternative to the Facelift, 645
Underdeveloped jaw, 944
Unger Prolonged Acute Tissue Expansion, 826
Unger's safe donor zone, 818
Unilateral condylar hyperplasia, 946
Unna, 848
Unrealistic expectations, 128, 132–133, 913
Upper eyelid blepharoplasty, 727–730
complications, 735
surgical technique, 729–730, 757
Upper face, surgical anatomy, 679–681
Upper lip wrinkles, BTX-A and, 345

Valtrax
erbium skin remodeling, 152
laser resurfacing, 171
Varicose veins
AP, 525–529
diagnosis, 513–522
diode lasers, 534
flashlamp-pumped pulsed dye lasers, 533–534
frequency doubled Nd:YAG lasers, 531–532
high-intensity pulsed light lasers, 534–537
informed consent, 542
KTP lasers, 531–532
laser therapy, 529–536
long-pulse infrared alexandrite, 534
Nd:YAG lasers, 531
sclerotherapy, 519–522
transillumination, 519–521
Vascular lesions
laser removal, 457–479
pulsed dye laser, 174
Venous lakes
argon lasers, 459
PDLs, 463, 469
Ventilation, 11
Verapulse, 461–462, 533
Versed used in blepharoplasty, 756–757
Vertical maxillary excess
facial characteristics, 949
surgical correction, 947
Vertical oblique osteotomy, mandibular rami, 943
Video imaging of facelift surgery, 686–688
Vigilon, in erbium skin remodeling, 152
Vinyl-based masks, 877
Violin deformity, tumescent liposuction and, 561–562
Virus transmission, AlloDerm implants and, 928
Vision loss, Zyderm Collagen and, 205
Vitamin A and scarring, 156
Vitamin C, in erbium skin remodeling, 154
V to Y flap, 855

Wacon tablet, 686
Waistline cincture, liposuction and, 605–608
Warp tool, 686
Warts, laser therapy for, 475–478
Waste receptacles, 14–15
Wax-based masks, 877
Webster suture in infralash blepharoplasty, 760
Weekend Alternative to the Facelift, 555, 641–652
  anesthesia, 644, 646
  chin augmentation, 645, 648
  clinical evaluation, 643
  complications, 649
  dermis resurfacing, 648
  equipment, 644–645
  fat vaporization, 648
  historical overview, 642
  indications, 642–643
  informed consent, 653–656
  laser surgery, 645
  lower face, jowls, neck, 646–647
  marking, 645–646
  medical history form, 656–659
  neck septae transection, 647
  patient preparation, 645
  platysma plication, 648–649
  platysma resurfacing, 648
  platysma separation, 647
  postsurgical considerations, 649–651
  presurgical considerations, 642–644
  presurgical evaluation, 642–643
  presurgical instructions, 643–644
  presurgical work-up, 643
  submental skin resection, 647
  subplatysmal fat pad, tumescent liposculpture of, 647
  surgical procedure, 646–649
  tumescent liposculpture, 644–645
  ultrasound, 645
Wen, 361
Wire brush dermabrasion, 788
Wound care
  blepharoplasty, 762
  flaps and grafts, 404
Wound dehiscence, 677
  in blepharoplasty, 745
  flaps and grafts, 407
  laser resurfacing, 857
Wound healing
  deep chemical peels, 64–66
  delayed, 84–85
  facelift, 709
  moist, in laser resurfacing, 171
Wound infection, flaps and grafts, 406–407
Wound necrosis, laser resurfacing, 857
W-plasty, 855
Wrinkles. *See also* Botox, CO_2 resurfacing, Collagen, *and* Chemical peels
  cheek, erbium skin remodeling, 150
  dermabrasion, 181
  dynamic, 314
  erbium skin remodeling, 127, 149–150
  static, 314
  upper lip, BTX-A and, 345
Written orders, signed, for tumescent lidocaine, 451

Yellow tattoos, Q-switched Nd:YAG lasers, 504

Zithromax, in erbium skin remodeling, 152
ZP, 199–200
Z-plasty, 855
Zyderm Collagen Implant
  consultation record, 220
  historical development of, 315
  implantation techniques, 197–198
  patient handout, 211–219
  vision loss, 205
Zyderm Collagen Implant-I, 199
Zyderm Collagen Implant-II, 199
Zyderm/zyplast collagen
  composition, 196–197
  historical development, 194–196, 320–321
Zygomaticus ligament, 683
Zygomaticus major, 681
Zygomaticus minor, 681
Zyplast collagen, 280
  consultation record, 220
  patient handout, 211–219
Zyplast (ZP), 199–200

About the Editor

Rhoda S. Narins is the Director of the Dermatology Surgery and Laser Center of Manhattan and White Plains, New York, and is Clinical Professor of Dermatology and Chief of the Liposuction Surgery Unit at the New York University Medical Center, New York, New York. The author of numerous books, journal articles, and book chapters, she is a Fellow of the American Academy of Dermatology and the American Society of Dermatologic Surgery, where she has been on the Board of Directors, as well as a member of the American Society of Liposuction Surgery, the American Society for Laser Medicine and Surgery, the American Academy of Cosmetic Surgery, and the International Society for Dermatologic Surgery, where she also served on the Board of Directors. Selected by her peers as one of only 12 dermatologists in the United States listed in "Best Doctors in America" under Aesthetic Surgery and named by *New York* magazine as one of the "Best Doctors in New York" (June, 2000), Dr. Narins received her M.D. degree (1965) from the New York University School of Medicine, New York, and is board certified by the American Board of Dermatology. Dr. Narins is on the liposuction council of both the American Academy of Dermatology and the American Academy of Dermatologic Surgery.